Handbook of Experimental Pharmacology

Continuation of Handbuch der experimentellen Pharmakologie

Vol. 70/I

Pharmacology of Intestinal Permeation I

Contributors

W. McD. Armstrong · J. A. Barrowman · V. Capraro · K. E. Carr
T. Z. Csáky · G. Esposito · L. R. Forte · E. C. Foulkes · A. Gangl
J. F. Garcia-Diaz · B. Hildmann · H. Huebers · H. Murer
D. S. Parsons · W. Rummel · A. E. Spaeth · W. D. Stein · P. G. Toner
K. Turnheim · H. G. Windmueller

Editor

T. Z. Csáky

Springer-Verlag
Berlin Heidelberg New York Tokyo 1984

Tihamér Z. Csáky, M.D.
Professor of Pharmacology
Department of Pharmacology
University of Missouri-Columbia
School of Medicine
Columbia, MO 65212
USA

With 164 Figures

ISBN-13: 978-3-642-69507-0 e-ISBN-13: 978-3-642-69505-6
DOI: 10.1007/978-3-642-69505-6

Library of Congress Cataloging in Publication Data. Main entry under title: Pharmacology of intestinal permeation. (Handbook of experimental pharmacology; vol. 70/I–II) Includes bibliographical references and index. 1. Intestinal absorption. 2. Gastrointestinal agents – Physiological effect. I. Armstrong, W. McDermott (William McDermott) II. Csáky, T.Z. III. Series: Handbook of experimental pharmacology; v. 70/I–II. [DNLM: 1. Intestinal Absorption. 2. Intestines – metabolism. 3. Cell Membrane Permeability – drug effects. 4. Drugs – metabolism. W1 HA51L v. 70 pt. 1–2/WI 402 P536] QP905.H3 vol. 70/I–II 615′.1 s 84-5558 [QP156] [612′.33]

2122/3130-543210

List of Contributors

W. McD. ARMSTRONG, Department of Physiology, Indiana University, School of Medicine, 635 Barnhill Drive, Indianapolis, IN 46223, USA

J. A. BARROWMAN, Faculty of Medicine, Health Sciences Centre, Memorial University of Newfoundland, St. John's, Newfoundland, Canada A1 B 3V6

V. CAPRARO, Dip. di Fisiologia Generali e Biologica Chimica, Università di Milano, Via Celoria, 26, 20133 Milano, Italy

K. E. CARR, Department of Anatomy, University of Glasgow, Glasgow, G12 8QQ, Scotland

T. Z. CSÁKY, Department of Pharmacology, University of Missouri-Columbia, School of Medicine, Columbia, MO 65212, USA

G. ESPOSITO, Istituto di Fisiologia Generale e Chimica Biologica, Facultà di Farmacia, Università di Milano, Via Saldini, 50, 20133 Milano, Italy

L. R. FORTE, Department of Pharmacology, School of Medicine, University of Missouri-Columbia, M-523, Medical Sciences Building and Harry S. Truman Memorial Veterans Hospital, Columbia, MO 65212, USA

E. C. FOULKES, Department of Environmental Health, University of Cincinnati, College of Medicine, Cincinnati, OH 45267-0056, USA

A. GANGL, Allgemeines Krankenhaus der Stadt Wien, I. Universitätsklinik für Gastroenterologie und Hepatologie, Lazarettgasse 14, 1090 Wien, Austria

J. F. GARCIA-DIAZ, Department of Physiology, Indiana University School of Medicine, 635 Barnhill Drive, Indianapolis, IN 46223, USA (present address: Department of Physiology, Boston University, School of Medicine, 80 E. Concord Street, Boston, MA 02118, USA)

B. HILDMANN, Medizinische Klinik, Universitätsklinikum der Gesamthochschule Essen, Hufelandstr. 55, 4300 Essen 1, FRG

H. HUEBERS, Hematology Research Laboratory of the University of Washington, School of Medicine, 500 17th Ave., C-34008, Seattle, WA 98124, USA

H. MURER, Physiologisches Institut der Universität Zürich, Rämistraße 69, 8028 Zürich, Switzerland

D. S. Parsons, Department of Biochemistry, University of Oxford, South Parks Road, Oxford OX1 3QU, Great Britain

W. Rummel, Institut für Pharmakologie und Toxikologie der Universität des Saarlandes, 6650 Homburg/Saar, FRG

A. E. Spaeth, Laboratory of Cellular and Development Biology, National Institute of Arthritis, Diabetes and Digestive and Kidney Diseases, Bldg. 10, Room 5N-102, National Institutes of Health, Bethesda, MD 20205, USA

W. D. Stein, Department of Biological Chemistry, The Hebrew University of Jerusalem, Institute of Life Sciences, Jerusalem, 91904, Israel

P. G. Toner, University Department of Pathology, Glasgow Royal Infirmary, University of Glasgow, Glasgow G4 OSF, Scotland. Present Address: Department of Pathology, The Queen's University of Belfast, Royal Victoria Hospital, Grosvenor Road, Belfast BT12 6BN, Ireland

K. Turnheim, Pharmakologisches Institut der Universität Wien, Währingerstraße 13a, 1090 Wien IX, Austria

H. G. Windmueller, Laboratory of Cellular and Developmental Biology, National Institute of Arthritis, Diabetes and Digestive and Kidney Diseases, Building 10, Room 5N-102, National Institutes of Health, Bethesda, MD 20205, USA

Preface

The intestine, particularly the small bowel, represents a large surface (in the adult human approximately $200\,m^2$) through which the body is exposed to its environment. A vigorous substrate exchange takes place across this large surface: nutrients and xenobiotics are absorbed from the lumen into the bloodstream or the lymph, and simultaneously, the same types of substrate pass back into the lumen. The luminal surface of the intestine is lined with a "leaky" epithelium, thus the passage of the substrates, in either direction, proceeds via both transcellular and intercellular routes. Simple and carrier-mediated diffusion, active transport, pinocytosis, phagocytosis and persorption are all involved in this passage across the intestinal wall.

The term "intestinal permeation" refers to the process of passage of various substances across the gut wall, either from the lumen into the blood or lymph, or in the opposite direction. "Permeability" is the condition of the gut which governs the rate of this complex two-way passage.

The pharmacologist's interest in the problem of intestinal permeation is twofold: on the one hand, this process determines the bioavailability of drugs and contributes significantly to the pharmacokinetics and toxicokinetics of xenobiotics; on the other hand, the pharmacodynamic effects of many drugs are manifested in a significant alteration of the physiological process of intestinal permeation.

The material in these volumes was collected in order to present some of the fundamental aspects of the permeability and the permeation of the intestine. An attempt has been made to include morphological, physicochemical, physiologic, biophysical, biochemical, pharmacologic and toxicologic aspects. Clearly, intestinal permeation cannot be properly studied from the perspective of one or a few displines; the subject cuts across a wide spectrum of disciplines. Consequently, it is hoped that the information provided in these volumes will be useful to scientists working in a variety of specialties.

I would like to express my thanks to those colleagues who accepted my invitation and contributed to this publication. It is somewhat unfortunate that the collection of the material required a considerable amount of time, but in a publication of this size, with a large number of contributors, some delay is inevitable. One prospective contributor was prevented from completing his task by a fatal heart attack, while others had to be excused because they failed to find enough time for the work. Furtunately, outstanding replacements were secured, but not without some holdup. Our knowledge of fundamental principles seldom changes in a revolutionary fashion, thus, despite the spread in time, it is hoped that these volumes will provide the reader with the information necessary to form a correct contemporary image of the complex process of intestinal permeation and the conditions of permeability.

Finally, I would like to thank my wife for lending me a helping hand, amidst her own professional duties, in various aspects of the editorial work.

T. Z. Csáky

Contents

CHAPTER 1

Morphology of the Intestinal Mucosa. K. E. CARR and P. G. TONER
With 35 Figures

CHAPTER 2

Intestinal Permeation and Permeability: an Overview. T. Z. Csáky
With 4 Figures

CHAPTER 3

Permeability and Related Phenomena: Basic Concepts. V. Capraro
With 15 Figures

CHAPTER 6

The Use of Isolated Membrane Vesicles in the Study of Intestinal Permeation
H. MURER and B. HILDMANN
With 13 Figures

CHAPTER 7

The Transport Carrier Principle. W. D. STEIN
With 21 Figures

CHAPTER 8

Energetics of Intestinal Absorption. D. S. PARSONS
With 5 Figures

CHAPTER 9

Polarity of Intestinal Epithelial Cells: Permeability of the Brush Border and Basolateral Membranes. G. ESPOSITO

CHAPTER 10

Electrical Phenomena and Ion Transport in the Small Intestine
W. McD. ARMSTRONG and J. F. GARCIA-DIAZ. With 6 Figures

CHAPTER 11

Intestinal Permeation of Water. K. TURNHEIM
With 4 Figures

CHAPTER 12

Intestinal Permeability to Calcium and Phosphate. L. R. FORTE
With 1 Figure

CHAPTER 13

Protein-Mediated Epithelial Iron Transfer. H. HUEBERS and W. RUMMEL
With 6 Figures

CHAPTER 16

Pharmacologic Aspects of Intestinal Permeability to Lipids (Except Steroids and Fat-Soluble Vitamins). A. GANGL. With 1 Figure

CHAPTER 17

Intestinal Absorption of the Fat-Soluble Vitamins: Physiology and Pharmacology. J. A. BARROWMAN. With 8 Figures

Contents of Companion Volume 70, Part II

CHAPTER 1

Morphology of the Intestinal Mucosa

K. E. CARR and P. G. TONER

A. Introduction

I. General Considerations

The three anatomic divisions of the small intestine are the duodenum, the jejunum, and the ileum. These total about 6 m in length in the human. The intestine receives the gastric chyme, which mixes with the secretions of Brunner's glands, the crypts of Lieberkühn, the liver, and the pancreas. It provides the environment for digestion and absorption, while its muscular layers propel the dietary residue to the large bowel. Here water is reabsorbed, leading progressively to the formation of the feces.

The outermost layer of this muscular tube is the serosal or adventitial layer, depending on the peritoneal relations of the part in question. A serosal layer consists of a covering of flattened mesothelial cells with underlying loose connective tissue. The adventitial coat of the retroperitoneal parts of the gut lacks the smooth-surfaced mesothelial layer associated with the mobility of the intraperitoneal parts.

The main thickness of the gut is made up of smooth muscle. The lamina muscularis externa has an outer longitudinal layer and an inner circular layer, between which lie the ganglion cell bodies and nerve trunks of Auerbach's plexus. A second autonomic plexus, Meissner's plexus, lies in the submucosal layer of the gut. The autonomic nerve supply to the intestines consists of the usual antagonistic components of the sympathetic and parasympathetic nerves, the parasympathetic being, in general, motor to the gut tube and inhibitory to the sphincters.

Internal to the muscularis externa lies the lamina submucosa. This consists of a rather dense connective tissue with plentiful elastic fibers and occasional clusters of fat cells, along with blood vessels of various sizes, lymphatic channels, and unmyelinated nerves. The submucosa is demarcated from the mucosa by the lamina muscularis mucosae. This, as its name implies, is the deepest layer of the mucosa, consisting of a thin layer of smooth muscle which forms a mobile underlay to the intestinal mucosa. From here, occasional individual smooth muscle cells extend up towards the mucosal surface.

The final innermost layer of the intestine is termed the mucosa (Fig. 1). It is this layer that holds the key to most of the digestive and absorptive functions of the gut. The mucosa has a lining of epithelium, specialized according to site and function. This is supported by a delicate vascular connective tissue stroma, the lamina propria mucosae, which in turn lies upon the muscularis mucosae. The

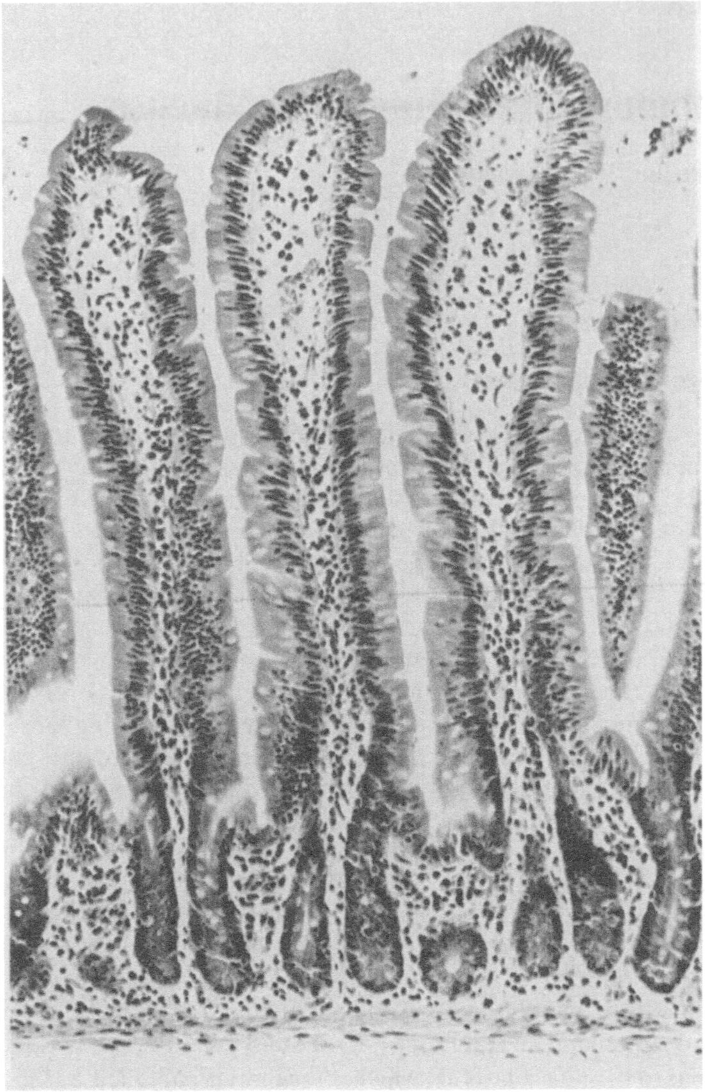

Fig. 1. Light micrograph of normal human jejunal mucosa obtained by capsule biopsy. The entire mucosa is shown here, including the intestinal villi and crypts, the lamina propria and the underlying muscularis mucosae. The ratio of the length of the villi to the length of the crypts is around 3:1, which is within normal limits. Notice the inflammatory cell infiltrate of the lamina propria, a normal part of mucosal anatomy. Courtesy of Dr. F. D. Lee, × 180

lamina propria is an important site for those cells of the lymphoreticular system which are associated with the gut. These lymphoid components play an important part in the state of balanced antagonism between the internal environment of the host and the potentially lethal microbial contents and other antigens present in the lumen of the bowel.

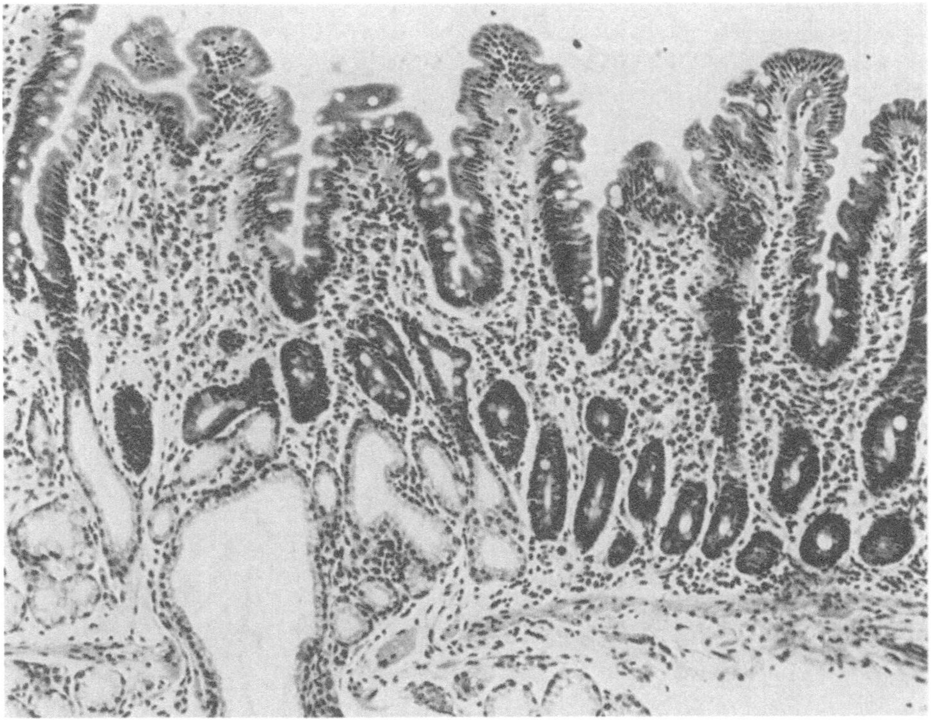

Fig. 2. Light micrograph of normal human duodenal mucosa obtained by biopsy. The villi are markedly shorter and the crypts longer than in normal jejunum. The submucosal glands of Brunner are seen opening into the foot of several crypts. These features lie within the range of normality at this site, despite the differences from the normal jejunal pattern. Courtesy of Dr. F. D. LEE, × 150

This basic pattern of serosa, muscularis externa, submucosa, muscularis mucosae, and mucosa is repeated throughout the gut, although there are regional variations such as the mucosal folds, or Kerckring's valves, seen in the small bowel, or the discontinuity of the external longitudinal muscle coat which gives rise to the teniae coli in the large bowel. The protective mucus-secreting submucosal Brunner's glands are found only in the most proximal part of the small bowel, in direct contact with the gastric acid (Fig. 2). The lymphoid tissue of the mucosa becomes especially prominent in the ileum, forming the aggregated lymphoid masses known as Peyer's patches. Finally, of course, the small intestine is distinguished from the large by its elaborate villous pattern, contrasting with the almost flat colonic mucosal surface. It is with these mucosal specializations, and in particular with their epithelial components, that this chapter will largely be concerned.

II. Heterogeneity of Intestinal Epithelium

The anatomic complexity of the gut hinted at in the previous section is only part of the reality. The intestinal epithelium itself is not a homogeneous structural en-

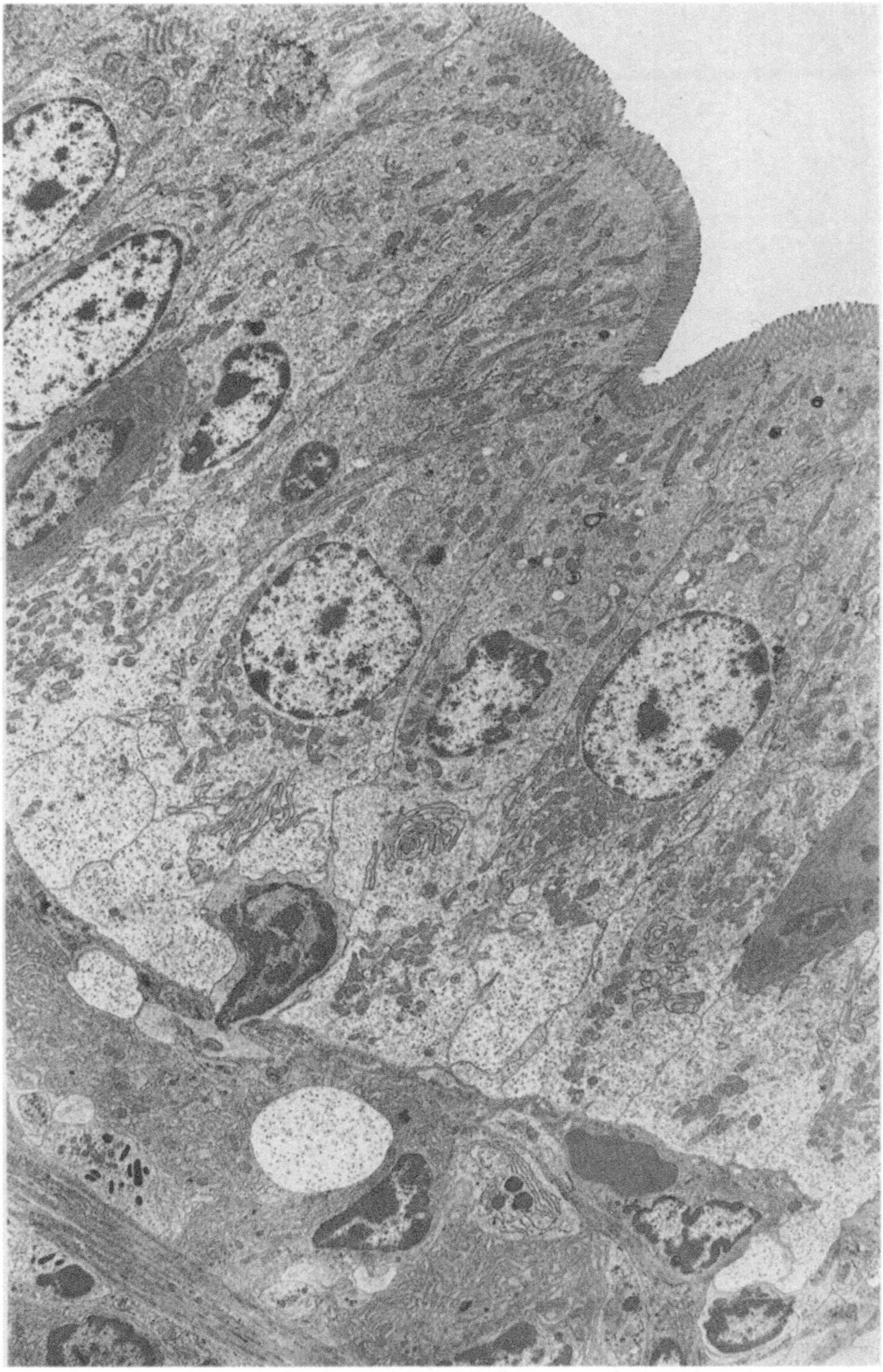

tity, composed simply of absorptive cells, but contains cells of widely differing identity and function. The individual cell types will be examined in greater detail in Sect. E, but their enumeration at this stage may help those who are unfamiliar with this subject.

The principal cells of the intestinal villus, often known as columnar absorptive cells or enterocytes, are indeed the most numerous (Fig. 3). They are distinguished by the presence of an apical striated border which forms the absorbing surface in contact with the luminal contents. The striated border consists of many closely packed microvilli. The second most obvious epithelial cell type is the goblet cell, a unicellular mucus-secreting gland, the carbohydrate-rich secretions of which can be stained by special histologic techniques. A third cell type, present in quite small numbers, is the intestinal endocrine cell. It is not often realized that the intestinal mucosa contains, in these cells, a total mass of endocrine tissue larger than many of the more anatomically localized endocrine glands. Specialized columnar cells known as tuft cells and M cells are present in small numbers in certain sites. Finally, nonepithelial components are present within the epithelial layer. The most common of these are the wandering lymphoid cells. They may amount to as much as 20% of the total of nucleated cells in the epithelium.

The intestinal crypt of Lieberkühn is a simple test-tube-shaped gland. It contains the precursor cell populations, dividing to supply the mucosal surface with a continuous stream of new recruits to maintain mucosal integrity and function. The life span of an individual cell is only a matter of days, since the daughter cells of this precursor population migrate from the crypt to the villus and are finally sloughed off at the extrusion zone, located at the tip of the villus. Nothing in the mucosa is stable; the epithelium of the villus is moving like an escalator, each cell, on average, moving up one position closer to the villus tip every hour.

The precursor cells are termed enteroblasts. They are distinct from the cells of the villus in various respects, maturing to their final form as they emerge from the crypt. The other cell types mentioned previously are also seen in the crypt, the endocrine cells being more numerous than on the villi. Finally, the distinctive Paneth cells, containing large eosinophilic apical secretion granules, are found only at the foot of the crypt, where their turnover is very slow.

The colonic mucosa consists, essentially, of cells similar to those of the small bowel (Fig. 4). Goblet cells are more numerous in large bowel mucosa, while Paneth cells are normally absent. Endocrine and tuft cells are found and migratory lymphoid cells are plentiful. In ultrastructural essentials, the chief cells match those of the small bowel, with only minor differences that will be mentioned in Sect. D.VII.

Fig. 3. Transmission electron micrograph of small intestinal epithelium from villous surface. The micrograph shows the lumen in the top right-hand corner, with the adjacent microvillous border. The columnar epithelial cells display their typical well-organized pattern. Parts of two goblet cells are distinguished by their denser cytoplasm, rich in granular endoplasmic reticulum. A basally situated lymphocyte can be observed, partly within, partly outside the epithelium. The lamina propria is densely packed with the processes of inflammatory cells, mostly plasma cells. A red blood cell can be seen lying within a subepithelial capillary vessel. × 3,400

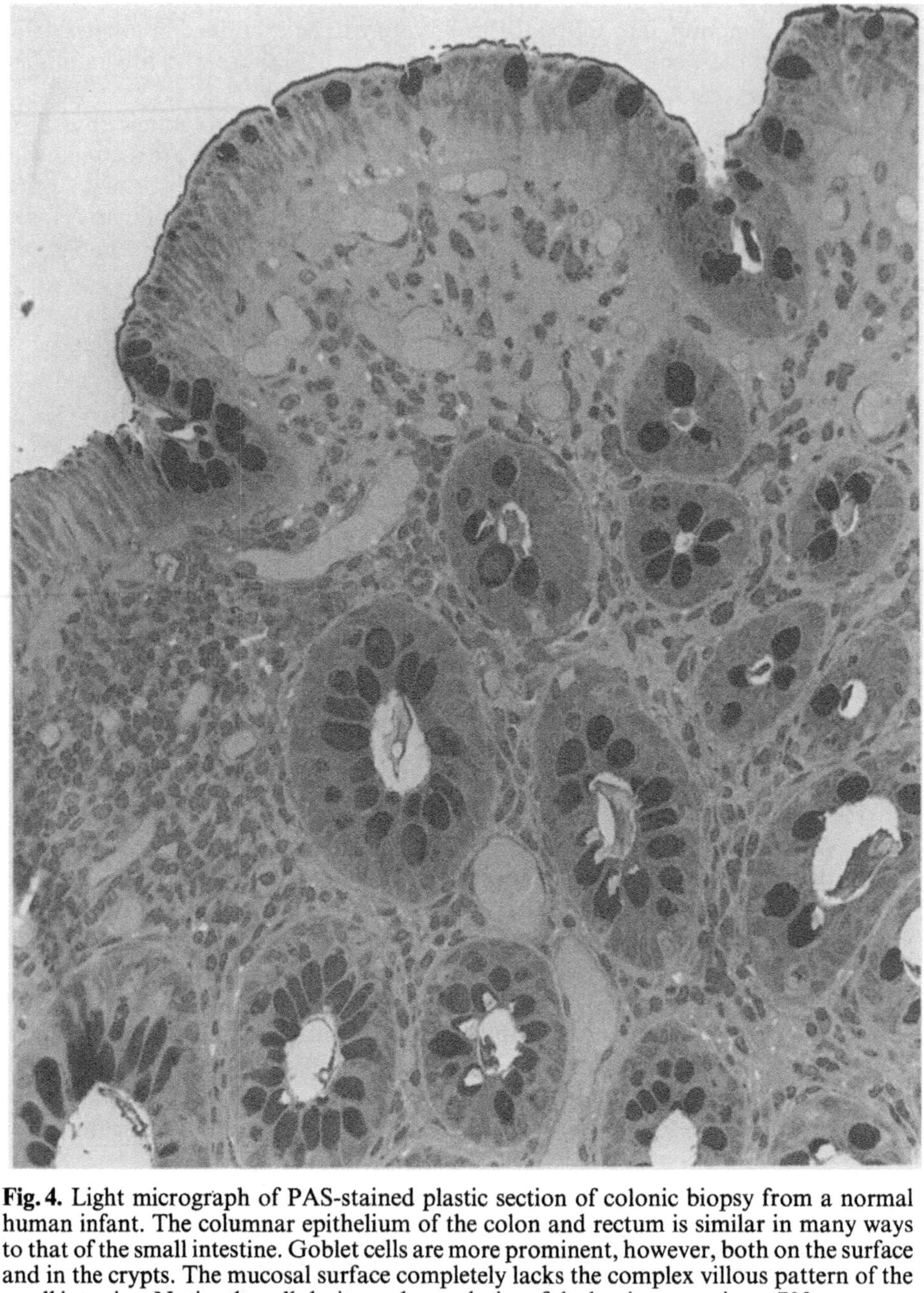

Fig. 4. Light micrograph of PAS-stained plastic section of colonic biopsy from a normal human infant. The columnar epithelium of the colon and rectum is similar in many ways to that of the small intestine. Goblet cells are more prominent, however, both on the surface and in the crypts. The mucosal surface completely lacks the complex villous pattern of the small intestine. Notice the cellularity and vascularity of the lamina propria. × 700

In conclusion, therefore, the intestinal mucosa is a complicated interface, made up of various cells of widely differing structure and function. This heterogeneity must always be considered in experimental situations, where interest often tends to focus on just one of these cell types, the mature enterocyte.

B. Morphological Techniques

Histologic technique is the basis of our present knowledge of gut structure, but over the last 30 years, this has been supplemented increasingly by information gained from conventional transmission electron microscopy (CTEM) (TONER et al. 1971). In both cases, the specimen takes the form of a section of suitably prepared tissue. For light microscopy (LM), the tissue is fixed in formaldehyde, dehydrated, embedded in paraffin wax, sectioned at 5 µm thickness, mounted on glass slides, and stained by colored dyestuffs. For CTEM, glutaraldehyde fixation gives better preservation; resin embedding gives more support, allowing <0.1-µm sections; "stains" are chosen for their electron scattering power rather than their color.

Cross-fertilization between the technology of the histologist and that of the electron microscopist has given rise to valuable hybrid techniques. The light microscopist is now making increasing use of glutaraldehyde-fixed, resin-embedded tissue, sectioned at 1 µm, and stained by modifications of conventional histologic techniques. The superior image quality of such preparations provides the ideal bridge between the upper range of the light microscope and the lower register of the electron microscope.

Special techniques based on LM remain invaluable for the experimental and diagnostic morphologist. Histochemistry uses specific markers for tissue components, such as the fat-soluble Sudan dyes for localizing lipids, or the Schiff reagent which binds to oxidized carbohydrates. Nuclear DNA can be identified by the Feulgen procedure, utilizing a process of mild hydrolysis. Tissue enzymes can be localized by the recognition of microscopically visible precipitates of insoluble reaction products. Other useful techniques for LM include the immunofluorescence and immunoperoxidase methods for the identification of tissue antigens, and those of autoradiography, which introduce a functional and a time dimension into the studies of tissues. Nuclear labeling with tritiated thymidine allows the migration of cells to be studied, opening up the field of cell renewal kinetics.

Each of these special techniques now has its ultrastructural equivalent. Differential stains and enzyme histochemical tests rely on heavy metal precipitates for electron microscopic identification. Ultrastructural immunoperoxidase procedures allow the subcellular localization of specific antigens. The use of appropriate radioactive labels and fine grain emulsions leads to the recognition of specific sites for particular subcellular metabolic functions.

All of these techniques, whether for LM or for CTEM, utilize sectioned tissues. There are, however, other aspects of biologic specimens which can best be studied "in the round". The contours of the mucosal surfaces of the gut have long been studied by the dissecting light microscope, an instrument still often used by the pathologist to make a rapid first assessment of the health of a mucosal biopsy of the small intestine (LEE and TONER 1980). The information available, however, is limited both in terms of resolution and of depth of field.

The ultrastructural homolog of the dissecting microscope is the scanning electron microscope (SEM), operated in the secondary emissive mode. The SEM produces surface scanning images of much greater clarity and detail than those available from the dissecting light microscope. In conceptual terms, however, the images are essentially the same, conveying topographic details of the contours of the specimen surface.

The surface of the intestinal mucosa is particularly suitable for study with the SEM. For this reason, some emphasis will be placed on the use of scanning micrographs in this chapter. In general, however, much of the information on which current concepts of intestinal structure and function are based is derived from more conventional LM and CTEM investigations.

Various techniques have been developed to assist in the experimental study of the intestine, some of which may be of interest to the experimental pharmacologist. Most important among these are attempts to develop an organ culture system in which intestinal mucosal specimens, whether from biopsies, or from adult, fetal or neonatal animals, can be maintained in a defined environment without serious prejudice to the essential structure and function of the mucosa. Various approaches in different species have met with differing degrees of success, as reviewed by TRIER (1976) and by SHIELDS et al. (1979).

At a different level of resolution, the isolated enterocyte is a valuable experimental preparation. TOWLER et al. (1978), have outlined a satisfactory isolation procedure, yielding cells which meet appropriate biochemical criteria of functional integrity. These authors call for a greater concentration of effort on the study of the metabolic role of the enterocyte, which they believe has a wider significance than its normally defined role in digestion and absorption. Cell culture of the intestinal mucosa has met with some success (LICHTENBERGER et al. 1979). The cell population retained some epithelial characteristics for 2 weeks, including rudimentary brush borders. After 2 weeks, however, a fibroblast-like growth of cells predominated. Rudimentary crypt-like structures survived until 10 days. Finally, FREIBURGHAUS et al. (1978) have presented a micromethod for the study of the intestinal mucosal enzymes. This method, using less than 15 mg wet weight of tissue, leaves ample material for the histopathologist while achieving an assessment of the digestive capacity of the tissues.

C. The Mucosal Interface

I. Surface Morphology of Small Intestine

The digestive and absorptive functions of the small bowel rely upon the availability of a large mucosal surface, specialized in several ways to maximize efficiency. Kerckring's valves, or plicae circulares, provide fixed folding of the mucosal surface, while the numerous villi increase the available area by a factor of eight. The villi are clothed with epithelial cells of different types which are produced in the numerous test-tube-shaped intestinal crypts of Lieberkühn, from which they

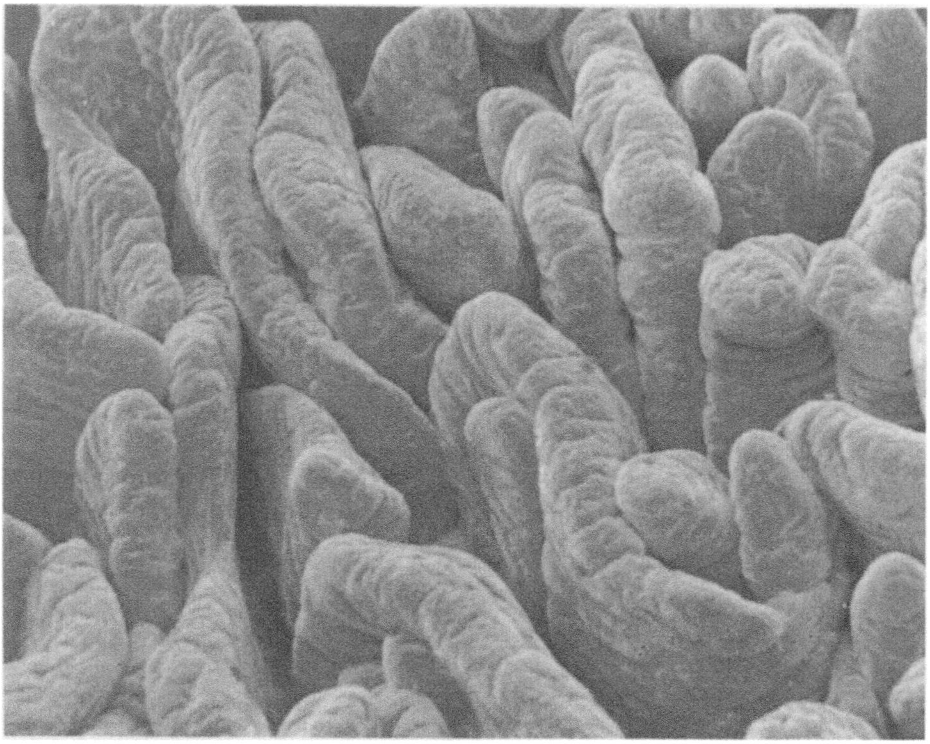

Fig. 5. Scanning electron micrograph of human jejunal biopsy. The villi are of various shapes and configurations. × 140

emerge to migrate across the villous surface, being shed finally at the tip. The villi have characteristic shapes and patterns in different species, being, for example, finger-shaped in the mouse, tongue-shaped in the rat (CARR and TONER 1968), and adopting a zigzag ridged configuration in the hen.

The human small intestinal mucosa consists ideally of finger-shaped villi, although there are wide individual variations (Fig. 5). In suitable specimens, the crypt orifices (Fig. 6) may be seen by SEM in the intervillous basin (TONER and CARR 1969; MARSH and SWIFT 1969). Duodenal villi are often shorter and broader than jejunal, and may be quite atypical in pattern. Diet and environment can materially affect mucosal morphology, as seen in studies of intestinal biopsies from groups of healthy individuals from tropical countries (BANWELL et al. 1964).

The surface features of the individual villus are also clearly seen by SEM (TONER and CARR 1979). A crisscross pattern of shallow creases is apparent (Fig. 7), while at higher magnification the outlines of the individual epithelial cells are shown by the presence of polygonal contours marking their margins (Fig. 8). Goblet cell mouths, sometimes discharging mucus, may be seen as pockmarks on the villous surface (Fig. 9). At higher resolution still, the pattern of individual enterocyte microvilli can often be recognized (Fig. 10). At the tip of the villus, the orderly smooth surface of the epithelium is usually broken by an irregular linear

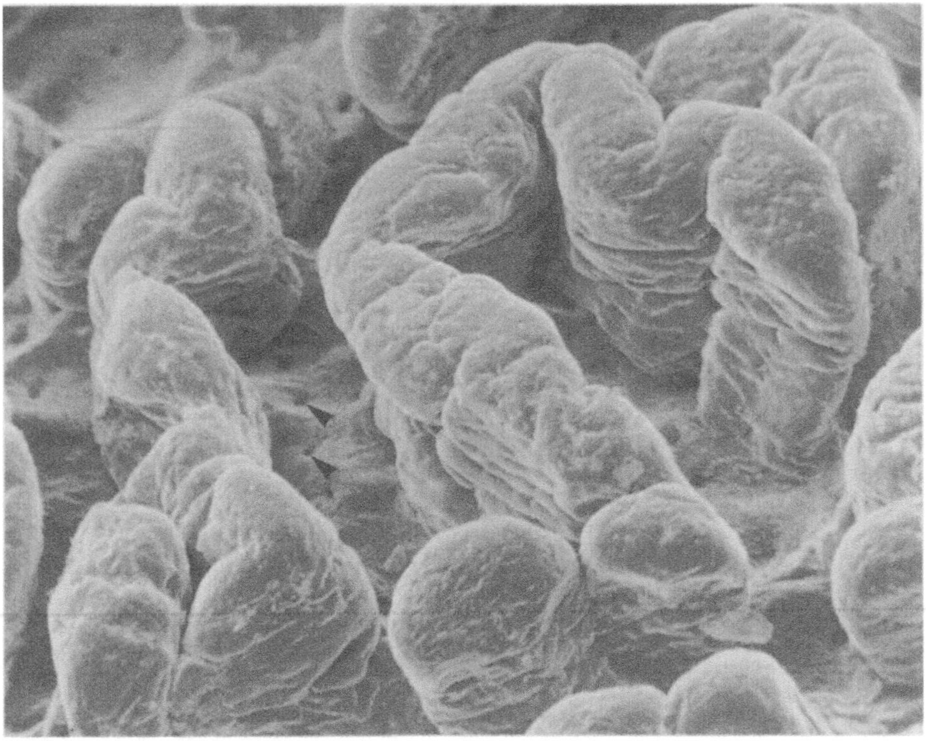

Fig. 6. Scanning electron micrograph of human duodenal mucosa. The villous pattern is atypical. The orifices of intestinal crypts can be seen opening between the bases of the intestinal villi (*arrows*). × 200

indentation corresponding to the extrusion zone at which the majority of cells are intermittently shed from the villus at the end of their useful life (POTTEN and ALLEN 1977). Cell extrusion, which may also occur focally elsewhere on the villous surface, is as essential a part of the orderly process of epithelial turnover as the continuous mitotic division of the enteroblasts, or intestinal precursor cells, within the crypts of Lieberkühn.

Fig. 7. Scanning electron micrograph of intestinal villus, showing the pattern of circumferential creases or indentations in the mucosal surface. × 400

Fig. 8. Scanning electron micrograph of the apical surfaces of intestinal absorptive cells, showing the polygonal outlines which mark the boundaries between individual cell territories. Faint details of the underlying microvillous pattern can just be made out. × 3,400

Fig. 9 a, b. Low (**a**) and high (**b**) magnification scanning electron micrographs from the same area of colonic surface. The goblet cell within the box in **a** is shown at higher magnification in **b**, its apical dome of mucus bulging into the lumen. In the colon this elevated bulging appearance is more typical than the pockmark pattern more often seen in the small intestine. × 680 and × 6,800

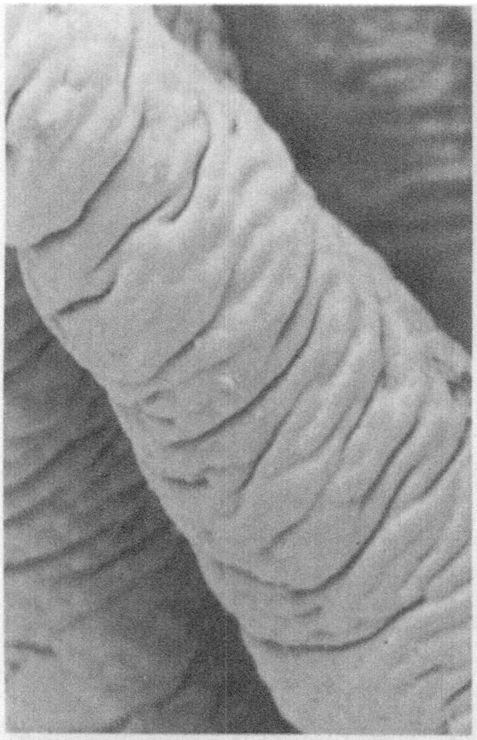

7

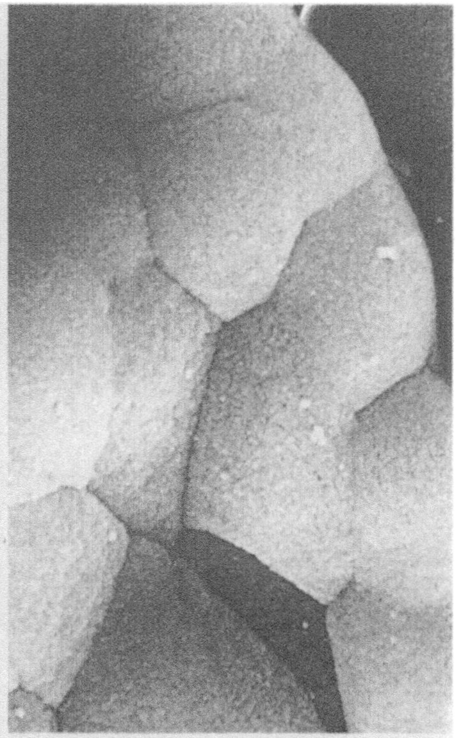

8

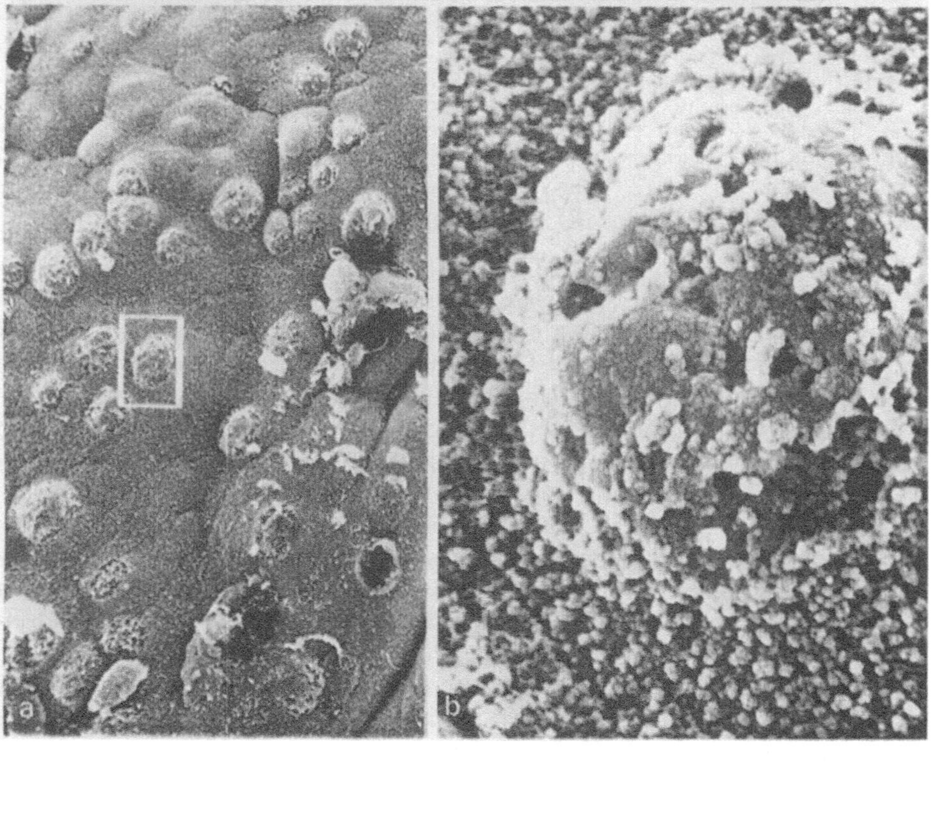

9

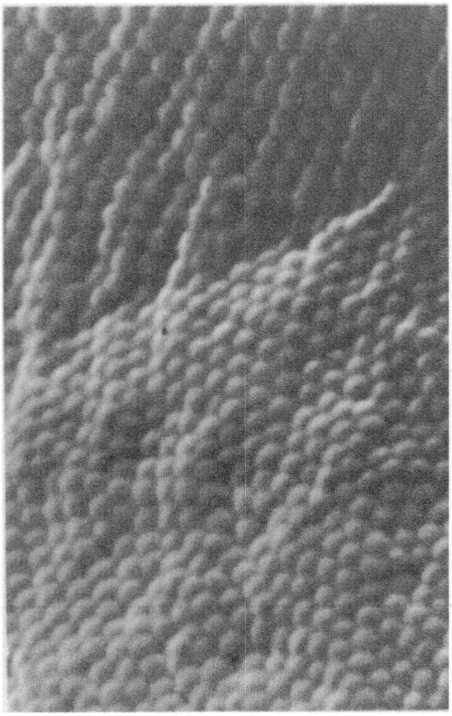
10

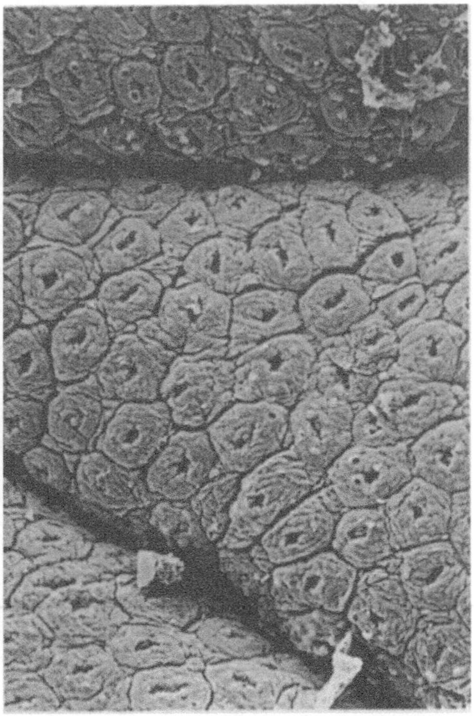
11

Fig. 10. Scanning electron micrograph of the tips of microvilli on the surface of an intestinal absorptive cell. The close packing and regularity of the processes are well demonstrated. ×27,200

Fig. 11. Scanning electron micrograph of the surface of human colon. Two deep creases divide the mucosa up into patches. Individual crypt orifices can be clearly made out, each surrounded by a collar of cells and each demarcated by a circular groove marking the territories of the individual crypt units. ×200

II. Surface Morphology of Large Intestine

Although devoid of villi (Fig. 11), the mucosal surface of the colon and rectum is far from "flat" and there are wide variations seen in normal individuals (RIDDELL and LEVIN 1977). The mouths of the crypts of Lieberkühn are often observed opening on to the mucosal surface. Furrows of two types are often present. The first outlines a low cuff of epithelium around the mouth of the crypt. Each polygonal area so outlined is termed a crypt unit. The second pattern of furrowing consists of long creases into which open the mouths of the crypts. The mucosal surface in the normal human colon may show either pattern, or a mixture of both.

At higher magnification, the crypt orifices are often slit-shaped, while the polygonal outlines of the surrounding cells sometimes tend to be exaggerated by dome-shaped cell apices. Individual microvilli may again be observed, although they are sometimes joined by a fine latticework of mucus (KAYE et al. 1979). Goblet cells are randomly distributed in the epithelium, their appearance varying from the pockmarks of discharged cells, as described in the small bowel, to the smooth convex projections of cells distended by mucus. Microvilli are present on some goblet cells, but when seen are sparser than enterocyte microvilli.

D. The Enterocyte

I. The Striated Border

The apical microvillus border of the enterocyte is its most distinctive specialization (Fig. 12). The apical membrane of the cell is itself specialized, being noticeably thicker (Fig. 13), at 10.5 nm, than the 7.5 nm unspecialized cell surface at its lateral and basal aspects. This membrane is highly contoured, forming numerous closely packed microvilli which project into the lumen. Each process measures rougly 0.1 μm in width and 1 μm in length. MARSH and SWIFT (1969) have calculated that a single enterocyte bears 3,700 microvilli, although there are wide variations in the literature, depending on the basis of calculation used. Their spatial concentration is species dependent, ranging from 65 per μm^2 in rats to 34 per μm^2 in dogs, (TAYLOR and ANDERSON 1972), although the effective absorbing surface per unit area is kept relatively constant, at around 25 μm^2 per μm^2 villous surface, through variations in their absolute size. The microvillous border, in other words, increases the surface area available for absorption by a factor of 25.

It is in matters such as these that an appreciation of the dynamic aspects of the intestinal mucosa is essential. As already mentioned, the enterocytes of the villus closest to the crypt mouth are those which have just undergone maturation from the crypt cell pattern to that of the villous enterocyte. These cells are still relatively immature in functional terms, their full capacity, as measured by enzymic activity, being gained as they climb up towards the tip of the villus (PADYKULA et al. 1961; PEARSE and RIECKEN 1967). These variations in functional capacity are paralleled by ultrastructural variations in the microvilli. BROWN (1962) and IANCU and ELIAN (1976) identified these variations and showed that the cells closest to the tip of the villus were those with the longest microvilli. Others, however, (MERRILL et al. 1967; BRUNSER et al. 1976; PHILLIPS et al. 1979) have identified the cells of the midregion of the villus as those best adapted for digestion and absorption, at least as judged by their villous morphology. There is a possibility that the situation differs in children and in adults (PHILLIPS et al. 1979). Whatever the truth of this matter may be, the existence of well-marked functional and structural variations from point to point on a single villus highlights the importance of standardized sampling procedures in any experimental or clinical investigations of enterocyte morphology.

A further interesting feature of the villous surface, as seen both by SEM and CTEM, is the presence of linear grooves or creases, recognized as a constant feature of mucosal organization in different parts of the gut (PFEIFFER 1971). These correspond to "microcrypts", or surface indentations seen in CTEM and familiar even from conventional histology as "kinks" indenting the contours of the sectioned villus. These correspond to linear arrangements of short cells, which are not otherwise specialized. How these creases arise is still unclear, but their reality and their gutter-like configuration is emphasized by occasional chance observations of epithelial damage, showing splitting along the line of the indentation. It remains unknown whether these contours may contribute in some special way to certain aspects of absorption by virtue of their sheltered and presumably relatively stagnant microenvironment.

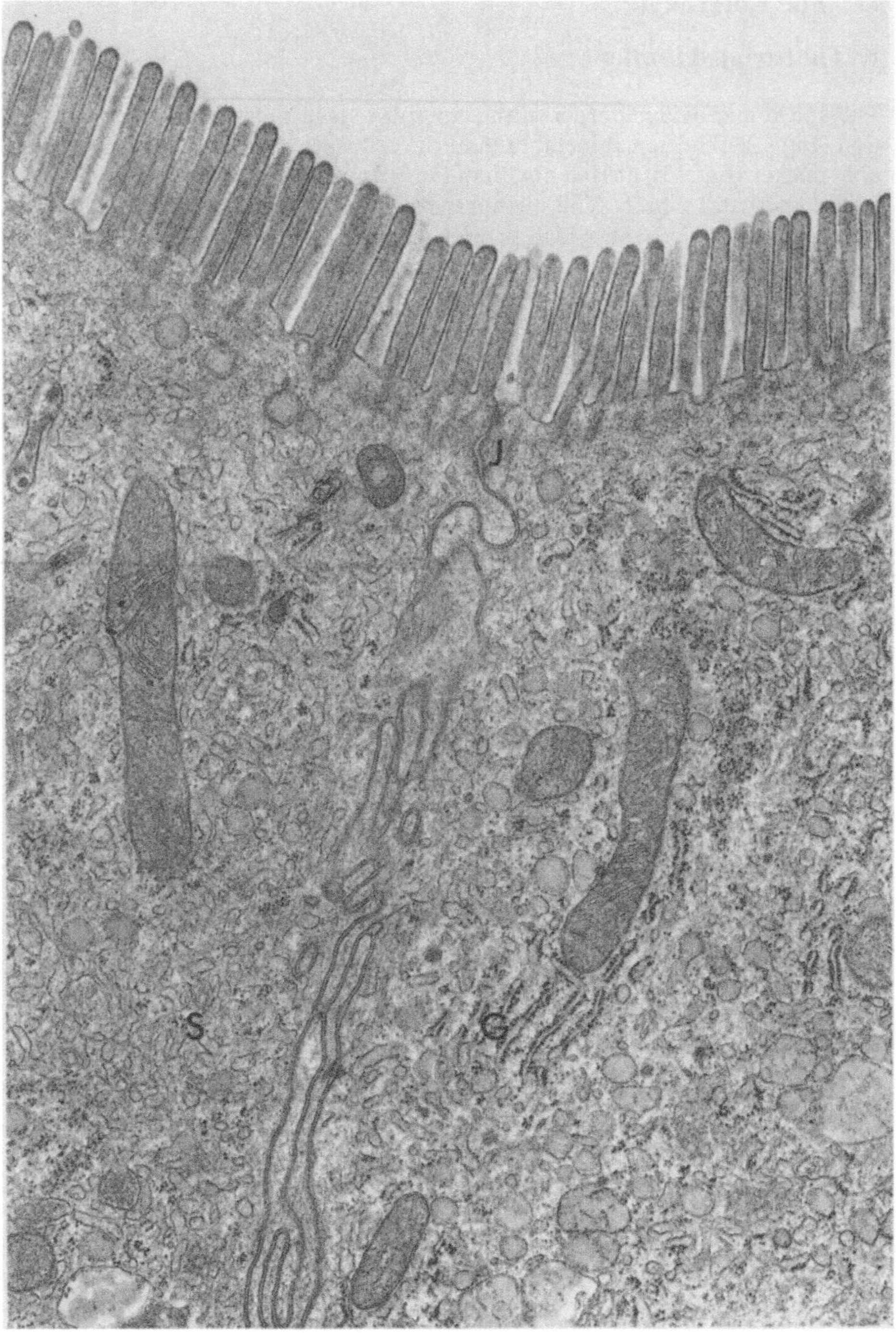
J
S
G

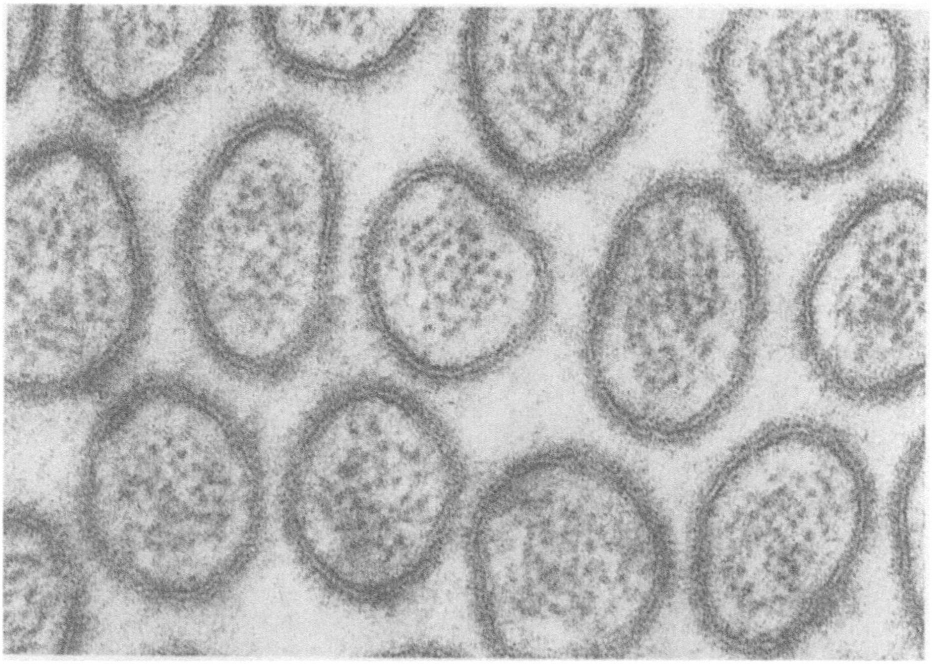

Fig. 13. Transmission electron micrograph of transverse section through intestinal microvilli, showing the trilaminar structure of the cell membrane. The space between the microvilli is filled by fine filamentous cell coat material originating from the outer surfaces of the cell membrane. The cores of the microvilli display cross-sectioned filaments similar in their dimensions to actin filaments. ×222,000

II. The Apical Cell Coat and Cell Membrane

The striated border is notably periodic acid – Schiff (PAS) positive, indicating the presence of a carbohydrate-rich glycoprotein cell coat, or glycocalyx. An external layer exists at all cell surfaces, but is quite elaborate in the gut, forming a "fuzzy coat" of fine filaments (Fig. 14) extending from the outer aspect of the membrane to a distance of around 0.1 μm from the tips of the microvilli, and filling the intermicrovillous space (Ito 1974). The cell coat material has been studied by autoradiographic techniques, which have shown its carbohydrate component to be synthesized by the Golgi apparatus on a continuous renewal basis. It may change in thickness from one cell to the next and it varies in ultrastructural prominence from species to species. Heterogeneity from cell to cell was shown also by a procedure for labeling anionic sites using polycationic ferritin (Jersild and Crawford 1978). The role of the glycocalyx is obscure, but many of the surface en-

Fig. 12. Transmission electron micrograph of apical cytoplasm of two adjacent columnar absorptive cells. The microvillous border is clearly seen in association with the underlying filamentous area of the terminal web. The boundary between the two cells is indicated by the complex interwoven contours of the lateral cell surfaces with the apical junctional complex (*J*). The cells are engaged in fat absorption, as indicated by the presence of numerous pale lipid droplets within the cytoplasm. Amongst the organelles to be seen are mitochondria, smooth endoplasmic reticulum (*S*), and granular endoplasmic reticulum (*G*). ×24,000

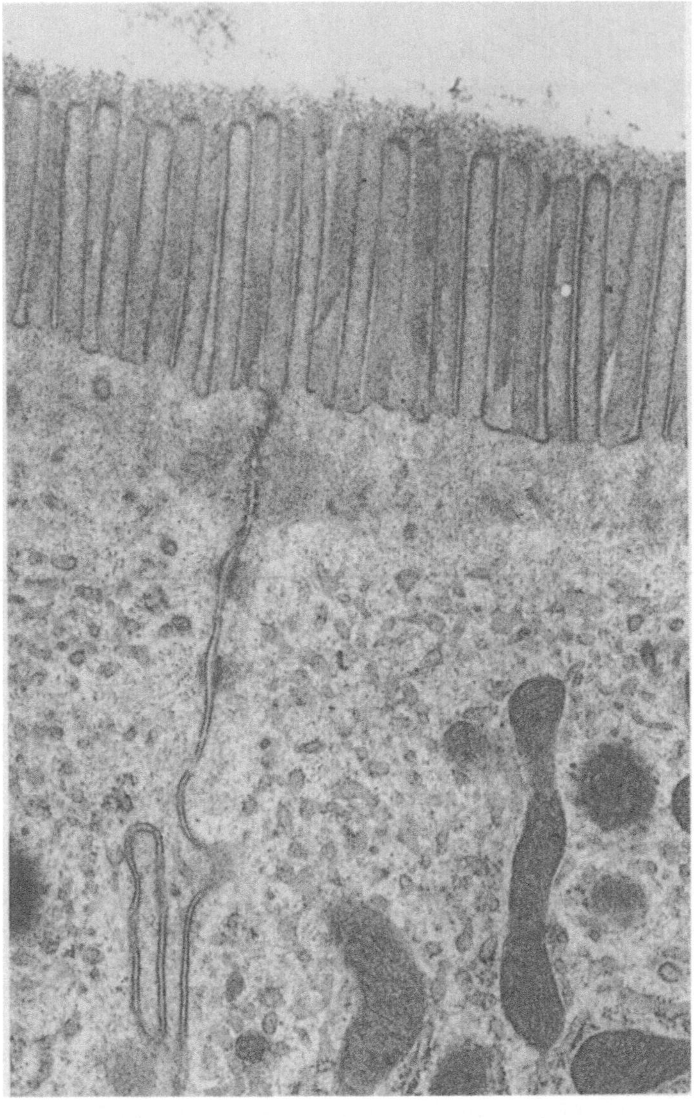

Fig. 14. Transmission electron micrograph of intestinal epithelial cells, showing close packing of microvilli, with processes overlain by a dense feltwork corresponding to the glycocalyx. This fuzzy coat is more prominent in some cells than in others and in some species than in others. × 35,000

zymes of the enterocyte involved in the digestive process are located at this region. It might also have some selective physicochemical role in relation to access of luminal contents to the actual membrane surface.

The membrane itself has a trilaminar structure when viewed in sections of fixed tissue, as with biologic membranes elsewhere. The early "unit membrane" concept proposed a basic common molecular pattern, although the simple bilamellar phospholipid–protein sandwich models of the past have now given way to more sophisticated concepts such as the fluid mosaic model of SINGER and NICHOLSON (1972). The continuous lipid bilayer remains in such models, accommodating the cholesterol and polar phospholipids which make up half of the membrane substance. The protein component is integrated into this lipid matrix, some molecules protruding from one surface only, while others occupy the entire thickness of the membrane. This allows an explanation of the different properties of the inner and outer aspects of the cell membrane, the outer being rich in random antigenic sites, the inner in proteins concerned with the regulation of cellular metabolism and control. The transmembrane proteins may represent the pores and carrier mechanisms involved in selective permeability and in the transport of electrolytes, amino acids, and glucose in and out of the cell.

Through the techniques of rapid freezing, followed by fracturing of the frozen tissue and etching of the exposed surface, valuable new data have emerged on membrane structure in the unfixed cell. Such techniques show that frozen membranes have a natural tendency to cleave along their median plane. Some transmembrane proteins are revealed as structural units by these methods, which allow their distribution to be studied in detail. Specific protein subunits, for example, have been shown to be involved in intercellular links at areas of specialized cell contact (MCNUTT 1977).

Recent studies of the striated border of colonic enterocytes have shown the presence of functionally unexplained linear arrays of intramembranous particles, (NEUTRA 1979), mostly located on the inner P face of the fractured membrane structure, with corresponding grooves on the outer E face. This suggests that such particles are not likely to be related to the glycocalyx, but are integral membrane proteins or protein complexes, perhaps with some specific functional connotation with regard to absorption.

There is now wide recognition of the fact that the apical surface of the enterocyte forms a complex digestive–absorptive specialization into which numerous metabolic functions are built through the incorporation of enzymes into the membrane structure (UGOLEV and DELAEY 1973). Although it was once thought that terminal digestion was essentially an intraluminal process, achieved by the release of digestive enzymes in the intestinal secretions, it was later recognized that the intraluminal concentration of free enzymes was inadequate to explain the rate of such processes. In fact, most of the supposedly free enzymes were only present in shed cells. It was finally recognized that many of the digestive enzymes carry out their physiologic function at the absorptive surface of the cell, rather than at large within the lumen. Many of the enzymes concerned with terminal digestion and absorption have now been shown to be present in high concentration in the apical membrane and cell coat regions (EICHHOLZ 1969; EICHHOLZ and CRANE 1974). Some, strictly speaking, are external to the membrane, such as aminopeptidase and sucrase, although anchored to the membrane by small hydrophobic extensions (LOUVARD et al. 1976). Structural subunits of the brush border membrane measuring 6 nm diameter have been associated with disaccharidase activity (JOHNSON 1969). Others are totally integrated within the membrane structure, or function at the cytoplasmic surface of the membrane, as is also the case with certain transport proteins.

Micropinocytosis occurs to a limited extent at the enterocyte surface, but is not a quantitatively significant process, except in the neonate (CLARKE 1959). Small vesicles or caveolae occasionally seen at the bases of microvilli in adult intestine were formerly thought to provide a pathway for the direct particulate absorption of lipid. This would, however, conflict with what is already known of the physiology of fat absorption, which proceeds largely through intraluminal hydrolysis, with molecular micelle formation and absorption. There is subsequent resynthesis of triglyceride from absorbed components within the cell apex (PORTER 1969; FRIEDMAN and CARDELL 1977).

The uptake of unaltered material from the lumen does not, therefore, occur to any major nutritional extent in the adult, although antigen uptake from the lumen may be a function of the specialized M cells described in Sect. E.V. In neonatal suckling mammals, however, widespread apical endocytosis occurs in the ileal enterocytes, enabling the infant to acquire substantial passive immunity through large-scale uptake of maternal antibodies from the colostrum (CLARKE 1959). The channels through which this takes place are visualized at the ultrastructural level by the presence, in freeze-fractured specimens, of arrays of uniform 7.5-nm intramembrane particles arranged in rows, closely packed together to form two-dimensional lattices. These membrane arrays are seen only in the tubular micropinocytic invaginations of the cell surface and are not found on the surfaces of the adjacent microvilli (KNUTTON et al. 1974). They are consistently associated with the E face of the fractured membrane, its external component, with small complementary grooves on the P face, its cytoplasmic component. These particles correspond to lattices which can be demonstrated by other techniques at the surface of the apical endocytic complex of the ileal epithelial cell (PORTER et al. 1967; WISSIG and GRANEY 1968). Further characterization of this specialized membrane has shown an association with the presence of *n*-acetylglucosaminidase, an enzyme involved in the hydrolysis of milk disaccharides (JAKOI et al. 1976), and a connecting protein.

III. The Cores of Microvilli and the Terminal Web

The cores of the intestinal microvilli consist of bundles of up to 50 parallel filaments, which have the dimensions and appearance of actin; this has been confirmed by immunologic labeling, opening up a new perspective of microvillous functional morphology (MOOSEKER and TILNEY 1975). The subsequent identification of myosin in the terminal web (MOOSEKER et al. 1978) has led to an inevitable, if somewhat surprising analogy being drawn with the sarcomere of striated muscle. The actin filaments are anchored to the cell membrane at the tip of the microvillus at an area of increased density in which the Z-line protein α-actinin has been shown to reside. The actin filament core of the microvillus thus corresponds to the I-band of striated muscle, while the region of interdigitation between the core and the terminal web would correspond to the A-band. The microvilli, formerly thought of as fixed and immobile, may therefore have a contractile capacity. Presumably, this might operate a pumping mechanism, just as the intestinal villi themselves shorten in a pumping action through contraction of the longitudinal smooth muscle strands in their cores. If this is so, the microvilli may have a hitherto unsuspected mechanical role in speeding the diffusion of absorbed metabolites from the apical region of the cell.

The terminal web of the intestinal epithelial cell is the horizontal feltwork of filaments which extends across the apical cytoplasm just beneath the microvilli (see Fig. 12). It appears to be structurally linked not only to the microvilli, as already described, but also to the apical junctional complex adhesion specializations. It contains not only actin and myosin components, but also filaments of 10 nm diameter, the so-called intermediate filaments (LAZARIDES 1980).

A stratification of the terminal web was described by HULL and STAEHELIN (1979), resulting from the association of different sets of filaments with the three structural components of the junctional complex (FARQUHAR and PALADE 1963). The apical zone of the terminal web contained filaments associated with the tight junction seals, the cores of the microvilli, and the apical membrane between microvilli. The adherens zone of the web contained individual actin-like filaments distinct from those of the microvillous cores, associated with the zonula adherens of the junctional complex. Here also were seen 10 nm intermediate filaments, or tonofilaments, presumed to stabilize the orientation of the actin-like filaments. The basal zone of the terminal web contained closely woven tonofilament bundles anchored to and linking up the spot desmosomes of the junctional complex. Transmembrane linkages between cells were observed at the region of these spot desmosomes, their function, presumably, being mechanical coupling, related to the need for stability at the cell apex in the face of trauma to the epithelial surface.

The intestinal striated border, thanks to the presence of this resilient and structurally coherent terminal web, can survive cell homogenization procedures intact (ANDERSEN et al. 1975). SEM shows the structural integrity of these preparations with particular clarity. Separated from their mutual interconnections and from their integrated cytoskeletal connections, these isolated brush borders curl up like hedgehogs through contraction of the filament meshwork.

IV. Other Enterocyte Surfaces

Concentration upon the apical striated border tends to distract attention from the other surfaces of the enterocyte. As a cell in an orderly polarized columnar epithelial sheet, the enterocyte has lateral surfaces in contact with its epithelial neighbors and a basal surface applied to the underlying basal lamina. The basal surface is usually flat and is separated from the homogeneous basal lamina of the epithelium by a narrow electron-lucent interspace of uniform width, the lamina rara interna. The cells may be detached from this underlay, exposing it to view by SEM (Fig. 15). This may be done by controlled autolysis of the cellular component of the gut (CREAMER and LEPPARD 1965), leaving the residual connective tissue framework of the mucosa, which retains the original mucosal contours (FERGUSON et al. 1969). Alternatively, the epithelial sheet can be shaken free of the basal lamina by trauma during preparation (Fig. 16), or by ultrasonic disintegration.

Circular discontinuities seen by SEM in the basal lamina have been attributed to lymphocytes migrating across this boundary (TONER et al. 1970). Occasionally, thin sections show the basal portion of an intestinal epithelial cell projecting through a gap in the basal lamina, to come into contact with cells in the lamina

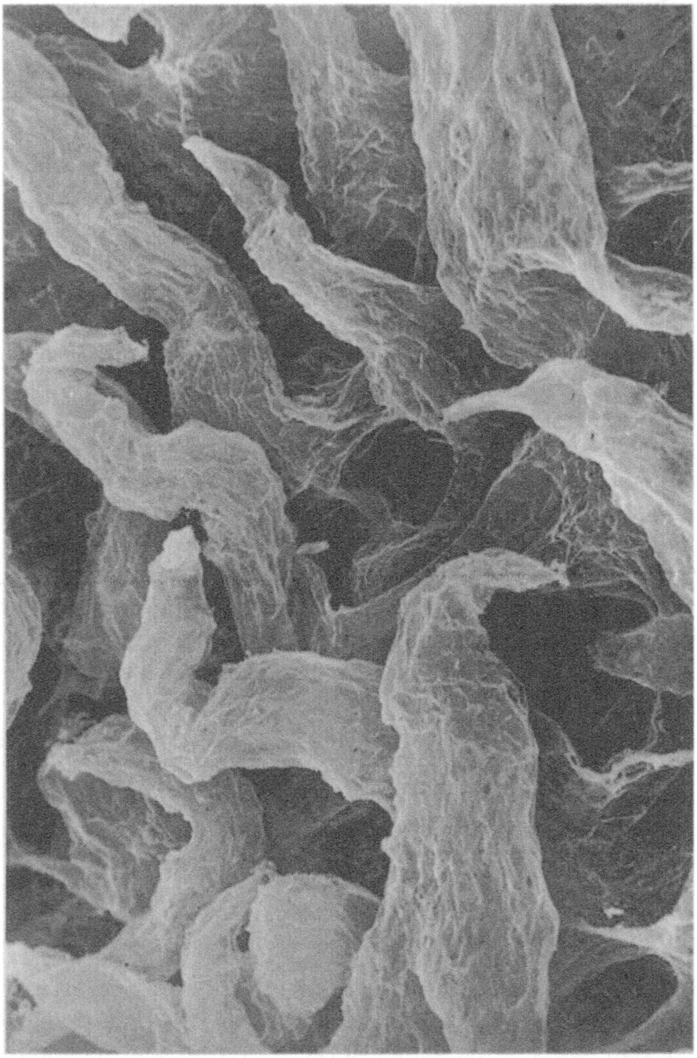

Fig. 15. Scanning electron micrograph of intestinal mucosa following autolysis to permit the disintegration of the cellular component of the mucosa. The remaining skeletons of the intestinal villi and crypts convey information on the mucosal surface pattern irrespective of the lack of an epithelial covering. The crypt orifices are wider than in the epithelialized specimen, for obvious reasons. × 500

propria. Such epithelial "herniations" may also be produced by the mechanical forces exerted by migrating lymphocytes (TONER and FERGUSON 1971). The basal aspect of the enterocyte has no contact specializations. It should be noted that preparations which display the surface of the connective tissue core show no sign of the distinctive patterns of surface creases already described as a feature of the epithelial sheet and attributed to linear arrays of short cells. If, as is often claimed,

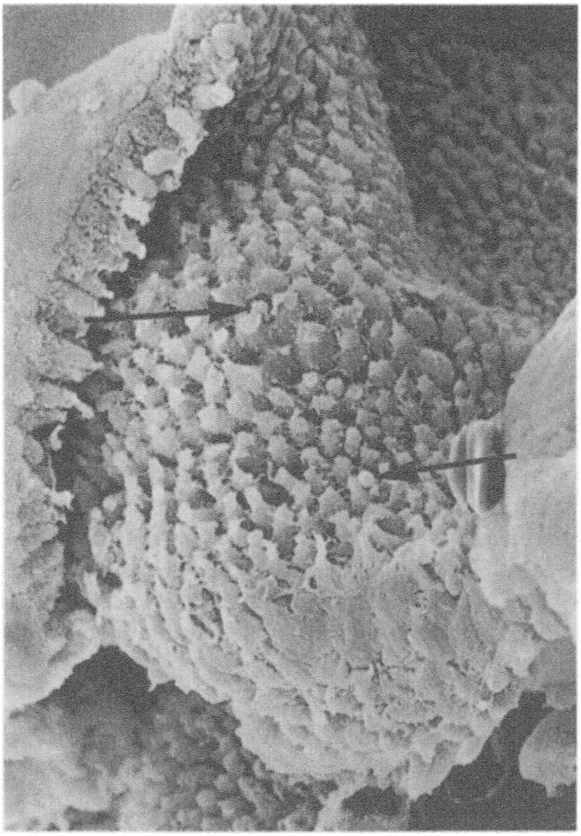

Fig. 16. Scanning electron micrograph of a portion of the epithelial surface artifactually detached from the villus. Over most of the specimen illustrated it is the basal aspect of the epithelial cells which is available for view. The basal intercellular spaces are clearly visualized in this case. This demonstrates the cohesion of the epithelial sheet of the intestinal mucosa. Several round cells just seen between the bases of the epithelial cells probably correspond to intraepithelial lymphocytes (*arrows*). ×800

these indentations were simply due to contraction of the smooth muscle in the core of the villus, the surface of "stripped" villi should reproduce the distinctive crisscross pattern of grooves. Such a pattern, however, is not seen on the connective tissue surface.

The lateral faces of the enterocytes lie in mutual contact. Their relationships vary from close contact with interdigitating processes, to wide separation, especially at their bases, with only fragmentary contact retained. Basal intercellular spaces, the Greunhagen-Mazzanini spaces, are more pronounced towards the villus tip, where absorption is most efficient, and are believed (MELLIGOTT et al. 1975), as in the gallbladder (TORMEY and DIAMOND 1967), to be associated with physiologic transport of fluid (HOLMAN et al. 1979). These lateral intercellular spaces may be occupied by masses of chylomicrons, or lipid droplets, during active fat absorption. The wandering lymphocytes, described in detail in Sect. E.VI also occupy these intercellular spaces.

As in other columnar epithelia, each cell is firmly attached to its neighbors by adhesion specializations, the most prominent of which is the apical junctional complex (FARQUHAR and PALADE 1963). This is a band around the apex of the cell (see Fig. 12), consisting of zones of special forms of close cellular contact. As described previously, filaments of the terminal web are associated with the components of the junctional complex (HULL and STAEHELIN 1979).

Most apically situated is the zonula occludens or tight junction, where the outer leaflets of the opposed cell membranes fuse together, eliminating the intercellular "space" at this point. Proximal to this is the zonula adherens, or intermediate junction, where the intercellular space is increased to 20 nm. Desmosomes form the third identified component of the junctional complex. Here there is a localized disc-shaped contact specialization, rather than a girdle or zonula surrounding the cell apex. Several interconnected small desmosomes or spot desmosomes often occur together at this site. The intercellular space at the desmosome is increased to 25 nm and there is a dense linear midline condensation of extracellular substance. Tonofilaments, cytoplasmic filaments of the 10 nm diameter intermediate class, are inserted into the cytoplasmic dense plates of desmosomes. Multiple desmosomes occur at different points along the intercellular contact surfaces of the intestinal epithelial cells.

The occludens specialization is thought to provide a "seal" at the epithelial surface, limiting passive intercellular diffusion and thus compelling the epithelial cells to control interchange between lumen and circulation. The adherens and desmosome specializations, with their associated structural filaments, probably contribute to the mechanical stability of the epithelium and to its resistance to traumatic disruption from contact with luminal contents.

The technique of freeze-fracture, followed by replication of the fractured surface, has already been mentioned in relation to intramembrane particles at the cell apex. This technique has greatly increased our knowledge of the morphology of cell junctions (STAEHELIN 1974). Particular interest has centered on the tight junctions (HULL and STAEHELIN 1976; KNUTTON et al. 1978) which form the most apical portion of the epithelial junctional complex and which are generally regarded as being of functional significance in sealing off the intercellular space from the gut lumen. In freeze-fractured preparations these junctions display anastomosing linear arrays of intramembrane particles, forming continuous networks around the cell apex (FRIEND and GILULA 1972). It has now been shown (TICE et al. 1979) that such junctional specializations may be more labile than one might expect and that their detailed morphology, at least in crypt epithelial cells, can be modified by mitotic activity. Quite extensive areas of crypt cell contact surface were observed to lack entirely the particle arrays which characterize these junctions. This finding leads to new questions about the biologic significance of the permanent "seal" that the apical tight junction is supposed to provide for the epithelium. If this "seal" is regularly absent for periods of time over large areas of the crypt cell surface in relation to mitosis, its functional meaning here and elsewhere may require reinterpretation.

V. The Enterocyte Cytoplasm

The columnar absorptive cell, as measured by morphometric techniques (PLATTNER and KLIMA 1969) has a volume of 253.7 μm^3, of which the nucleus accounts for 14.3%. Within the enterocyte, three cytoplasmic compartments are recognized, forming, respectively, the supranuclear, paranuclear, and infranuclear regions of the cell. The major membrane systems are found above the nucleus. These include the elaborate Golgi apparatus, the granular or rough endoplasmic reticulum, and the agranular or smooth reticulum, the relative proportions of which have been estimated by morphometric techniques (PLATTNER and KLIMA 1969). The Golgi system, 1.4% of the cytoplasmic volume, consists of parallel membrane lamellae, forming closed sacs, partly collapsed and partly dilated to form vacuoles. Around these membranes lie numerous small Golgi vesicles. With the exception of small pale fragments of lipoprotein material, the cavities of the Golgi membrane system are electron lucent, except when active fat absorption is in progress, in which case lipid droplets distend the system. The carbohydrate component of the glycocalyx or fuzzy coat of the intestine is synthesized within the Golgi system and then discharged at the cell surface (ITO 1974).

The granular endoplasmic reticulum of the enterocyte is not particularly prominent, amounting to 2.5% of cytoplasmic volume. Elongated single strands are sometimes present both above and below the level of the nucleus and cisternae are sometimes seen draped around mitochondria. Attached and free ribosomes are found in moderate numbers. The agranular endoplasmic reticulum, of variable extent, is usually best seen in the supranuclear cytoplasm. It takes the form of small, closely knit groups of membrane profiles without attached ribosomes, the individual cisternae in any plane of section being short or even vesicular in cross-section. Granular and agranular segments may be in continuity. The endoplasmic reticulum is presumed to form a functionally interconnecting system, linked also to the nuclear envelope, as shown by the occurrence, at times, of droplets of absorbed lipid at any point within these various cavities.

These membrane systems of the enterocyte are as important for absorption as the microvillous border itself, since it is here that most of the cellular control of absorption is exercised through cytoplasmic metabolism. The involvement of these various systems in fat absorption has already been referred to; the enthusiasm of electron microscopists for this subject is, of course, accounted for by the structurally identifiable nature of lipids in electron micrographs. The lipid micelles absorbed at the molecular level through the apical membrane of the cell provide the substrate for the resynthesis of triglyceride within the agranular endoplasmic reticulum. The cisternae within which the fat gathers provide a transport system capable of carrying lipid throughout the cytoplasm. The Golgi system (Fig. 17), appears to act as a staging post, from which lipid is passed to the lateral surfaces of the cell, where it is discharged as chylomicrons into the lateral intercellular spaces from where it passes to the intestinal lacteal (DOBBINS 1971). The normal synthesis of the apoprotein component of β-lipoprotein by the enterocyte is an essential step in the orderly discharge of absorbed fat. In abetalipoproteinemia, lipid is absorbed but not correctly discharged, leading to a buildup within the cell (DOBBINS 1966).

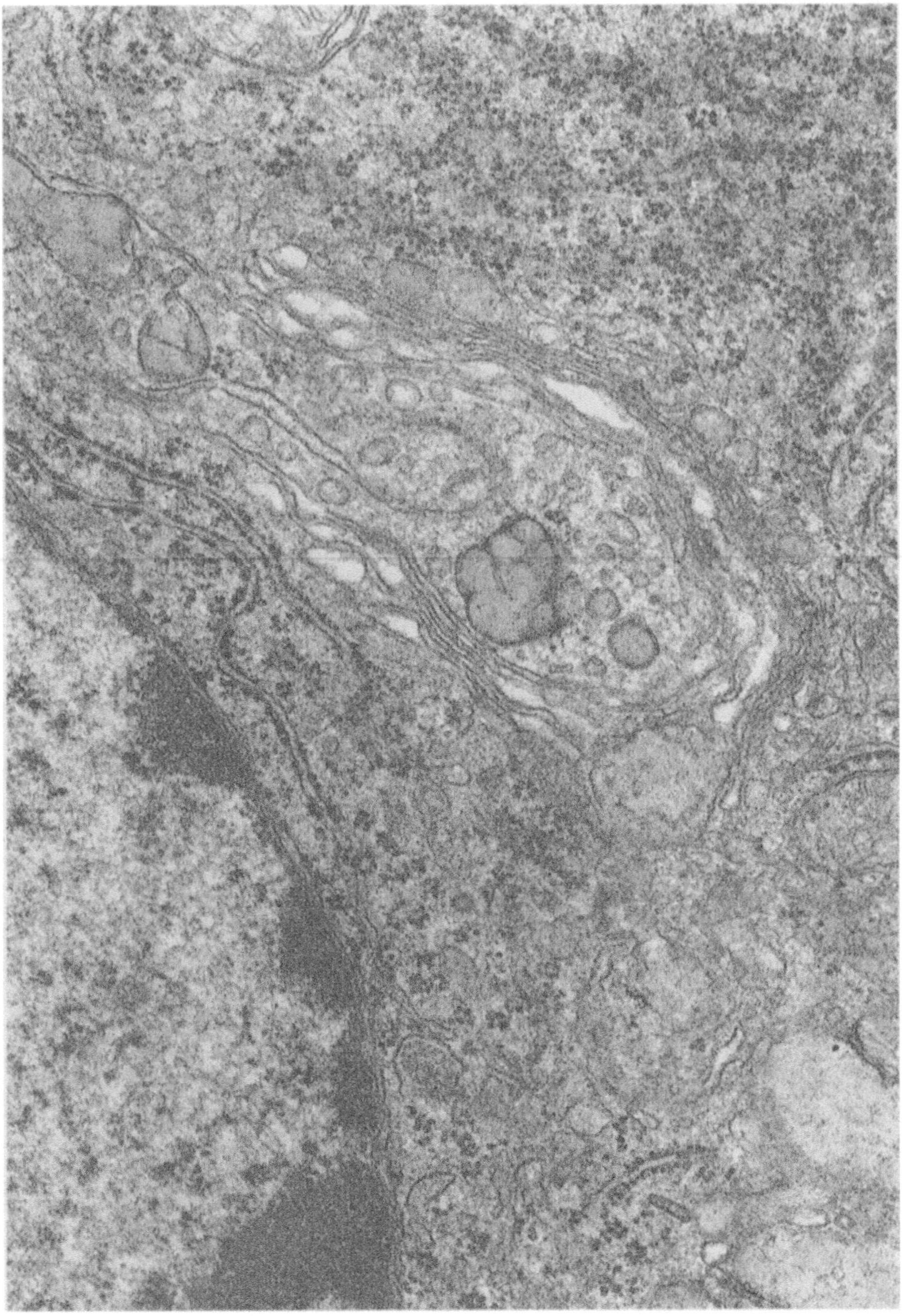

Fig. 17. Transmission electron micrograph of supranuclear portion of intestinal epithelium cell during fat absorption. The Golgi apparatus is well seen, with contained fat droplets. Several strands of granular endoplasmic reticulum lie nearby. ×83,700

The other organelles common to most cell types are also found in the enterocyte. Mitochondria measure up to 3 μm in length and are around 0.3 μm in diameter. Each cell, on average, has around 150 mitochondria. Above the nucleus the mitochondria often align themselves parallel to the long axis of the cell, but below it they are more randomly arranged. The cristae are not arranged in any particularly distinctive pattern and the mitochondrial matrix is unremarkable. Lysosomes are present, as dense bodies, usually in the apical part of the cell. They are scanty in normal cells, but more numerous in abnormal states, such as celiac disease. Multivesicular bodies, generally classified with lysosomes, are occasionally seen. Centrioles are rarely encountered in the mature enterocyte, although they are often found in the apex of crypt cells. Microtubules are present in small numbers in the cytoplasmic substance, along with cytoplasmic filaments, the two presumably combining to form a cytoskeleton of potential structural significance (BRUNSER and LUFT 1970). To what extent these structural units might also define selective diffusion pathways remains to be seen.

VI. The Precursor Cells of the Crypt and Epithelial Dynamics

The intestinal crypts house the precursor cell population of the gut, as well as several fully differentiated epithelial cell types. The enterocytes of the villus can be compared, in population terms, to the mature erythrocytes of the circulating blood. The enteroblasts of the crypt, from which the enterocytes arise by mitotic division and maturation (WATSON and WRIGHT 1974), correspond to the hemopoietic precursor cells of the marrow. Although at first sight this analogy may seem rather strained, it has helped to illuminate various features of the population dynamics of the gut in health and disease.

The daughter cells of mitosis either remain in the crypt to divide again, or migrate from crypt to villus, undergoing maturation in structural and functional terms as they emerge from the crypt orifice. This progressive migration continues, the cells travelling slowly towards the tip of the villus where 50 million cells each day are finally shed, mostly at the so-called extrusion zones. The enterocyte life span is around 3 days, depending on species. This escalator of cells is not driven by "pressure" of mitosis, since migration and extrusion continue when mitosis is halted by irradiation.

Epithelial shedding is itself a cyclic process, as has been demonstrated by crypt cell mitotic activity, which also displays a circadian rhythm. POTTEN and ALLEN (1977) have illustrated the morphology of cell shedding by SEM, correlating the appearances with the presence of cellular degeneration by CTEM. GEYER (1979), has observed two patterns of cell extrusion. Degenerate cells may become vacuolated and swollen, squeezing themselves out of the epithelium, detaching, rounding off, and floating free before disintegrating in the lumen. Alternatively, the cells may disintegrate in situ, leading to the piecemeal shedding of cellular debris rather than the loss of whole cells.

In either case, the process of cell shedding is apparently associated with the presence of transient gaps in the intestinal epithelial covering of the villi. Although these gaps will slowly close, they represent an important exception to the general rule that the epithelial sheet is sealed against uncontrolled macromolecu-

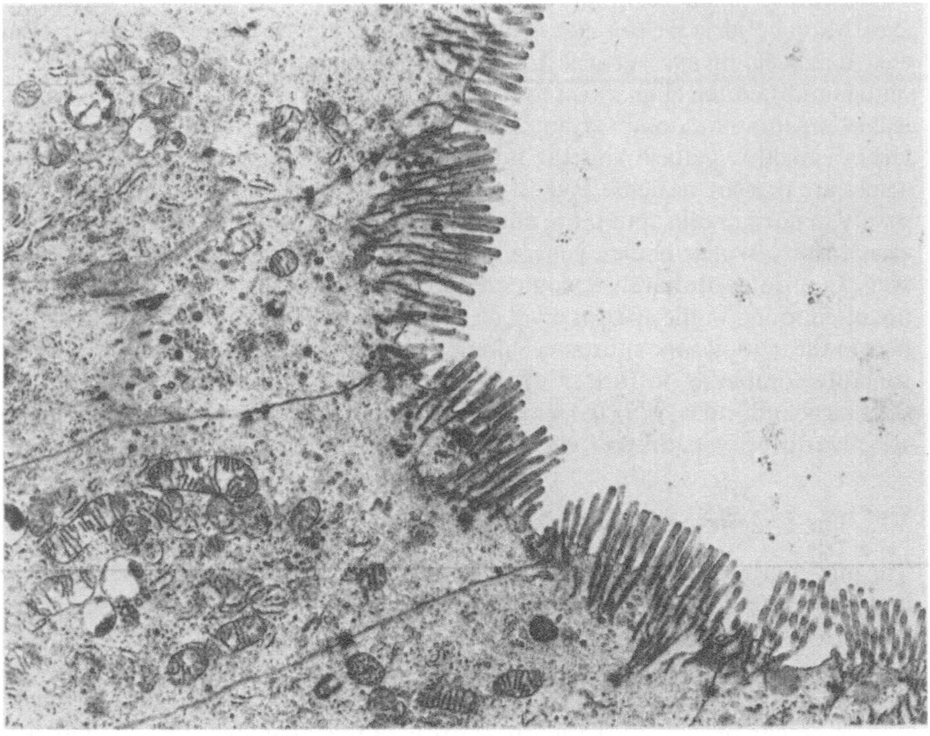

Fig. 18. Transmission electron micrograph, showing the apical region of the crypt cells of small intestine. The microvilli tend to lie at various angles and are less regimented than on the villus surface. The relatively undifferentiated nature of the cells is made clear by comparison with the mature enterocytes shown in Fig. 12. × 7,400

lar diffusion in either direction. These gaps, present as part of the system of normal dynamic renewal of the epithelium, must allow the focal ingress of antigenic and other substances and the focal loss of macromolecules from the intestinal mucosal tissue fluids. The normal gut is slightly "leaky" with respect to plasma proteins such as albumin and with respect also to access for particles of substantial size, such as starch and pollen grains (BAZIN 1976). It is tempting to associate this phenomenon with the gaps in epithelial continuity provided by physiologic cell extrusion. In the same way, the increased cell shedding which characterizes many intestinal diseases might also explain the often associated protein-losing enteropathy and the increased incidence of secondary food allergies. In this case, the gaps caused by cell shedding may not be the whole story, in view of the observations of TICE et al. (1979), on modifications to crypt cell tight junctions related to mitotic activity. The clinical immunologic implications of this remain uncertain (FERGUSON 1976), although it is well known that dietary proteins can produce immunologic sensitization by the oral route, even in the case of the normal gut.

The normal mucosal pattern of villi is dependent upon the orderly maintenance of cell renewal and cell loss. It is apparent that the mucosal surface pattern is sensitive to changes in cellular dynamics, responding to any relative shortfall of supply by remolding to a pattern more easily covered by a reduced population of mature cells. In the extreme case of severe celiac disease, there is a continued imbalance of cell loss through injury by gluten, and cell renewal, despite compensatory changes in the dynamics of the system (WATSON and WRIGHT 1974). Despite elongation of the crypts, which increases the precursor population, and an increased mitotic rate, which enhances the output of new cells, the supply can only be made to fit the demand by regression of the intestinal mucosa to the "flat" pattern which characterizes this disease and which explains the severity of the malabsorption from which such patients suffer. Morphology and cell renewal kinetics are inextricably interconnected in the gut.

When one examines the individual precursor cells, one finds the ultrastructural features which are typical of a rapidly dividing population. Their microvilli are rather scanty and are not organized into a regular array like those of the mature cell of the villus (Fig. 18). The membrane systems and other organelles are scanty, while free ribosomes are abundant, contributing to the basophilia of the crypt cell on LM. Centrioles are commonly seen towards the cell apex. Some crypt cells contain small apical secretion granules, indicating a contribution towards the intraluminal environment (TRIER 1963, 1964). These crypt cell features are lost as the cells cross the threshold of the crypt mouth, simultaneously with the acquisition of the enzyme apparatus characteristic of the mature enterocyte (PADYKULA et al. 1961).

VII. Special Features of Large Bowel Enterocytes

The colonic enterocyte has much in common with that of the small bowel, at least in structural terms. The microvilli of the striated border are often longer in the colon, with a rather less orderly arrangement. The glycocalyx (SWIFT and MUKHERJEE 1976) is less compact than in the small intestine, consisting of loosely arranged radial filaments extending perpendicular to the surface membrane, rather than the dense feltwork more typical of the small bowel (Fig. 19). The microvilli are often distinguished by the presence of streamers of small vesicles lying parallel to their long axes and close to their surfaces. These are formed of typical trilaminar membrane material, but their origin is debatable. They have been attributed variously to degeneration of the microvilli and discharge of multivesicular bodies, as well as being erroneously identified as virus particles.

The colonic enterocyte has cytoplasmic features which again are similar to those of the small intestinal counterpart. The large multivesicular bodies of colon are distinctive (BIEMPICA et al. 1976), apparently lacking the acid phosphatase activity seen in other sites. Their contained vesicles are often rod-shaped rather than spherical, whence the term "R-body" coined to identify them. Such bodies are numerous in colonic crypt cells and progressively more scanty towards the surface, matching the progressive increase in frequency of the microvillous vesicles already described, termed coccoidal or "C-bodies". STONE et al. (1977) propose that R-bodies give rise to C-bodies by progressive discharge, but the functional significance of this hypothetical relationship remains obscure.

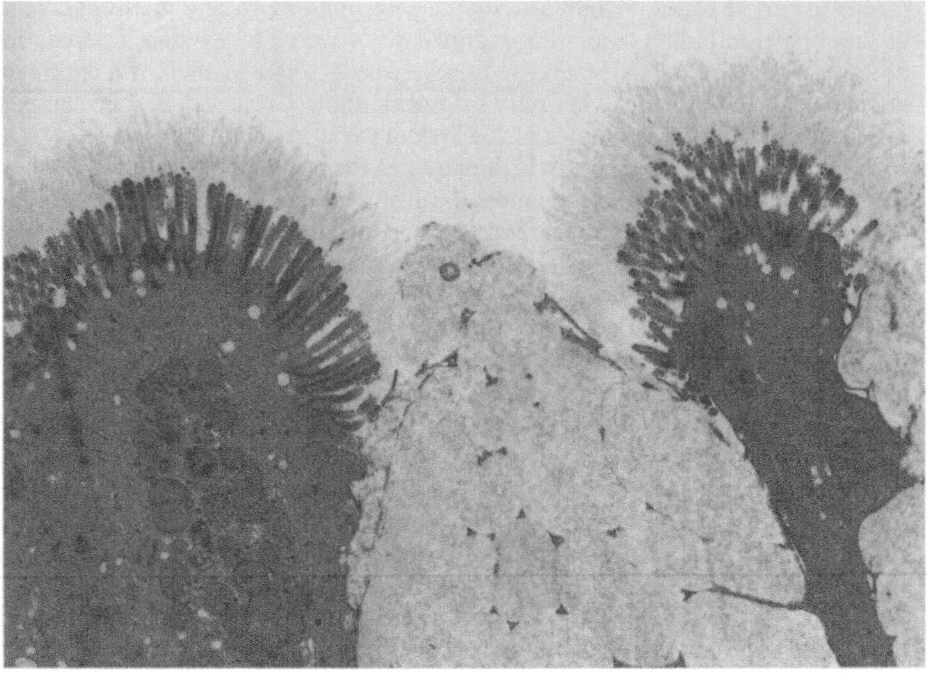

Fig. 19. Transmission electron micrograph of colonic surface epithelium, showing a goblet cell between two enterocytes. These have been purposely rather overprinted to bring up the detail in the elaborate but loosely knit glycocalyx extending out from the microvilli. Note also the streamers of small vesicles between the microvilli. × 6,700

The colonic crypts (LORENZSONN and TRIER 1968) contain a precursor cell population, as do small intestinal crypts. These are pyramidal cells with scanty microvilli, indented nuclei, free ribosomes, and a small Golgi system. Such cells correspond to precursor cells elsewhere in their general lack of ultrastructural markers of specific differentiation patterns. The precursor cell population appears to differentiate towards the enterocyte or goblet cell pattern through different intermediate stages (Fig. 20) as described by KAYE et al. (1973).

E. Other Cell Types of Intestinal Mucosa

I. Goblet Cells

Goblet cells are found in the crypts, where they mature from stem cell precursors, and migrate to the villus surface. They occur singly, their typical shape being determined by the pressure of surrounding enterocytes, balanced by the accumulation of secretion within the cell apex. The goblet cell is a unicellular gland, secreting mucus into the lumen for lubrication and protection.

The nucleus is basal, with a compressed, dense appearance, associated with a high proportion of heterochromatin. There is an extensive granular endoplas-

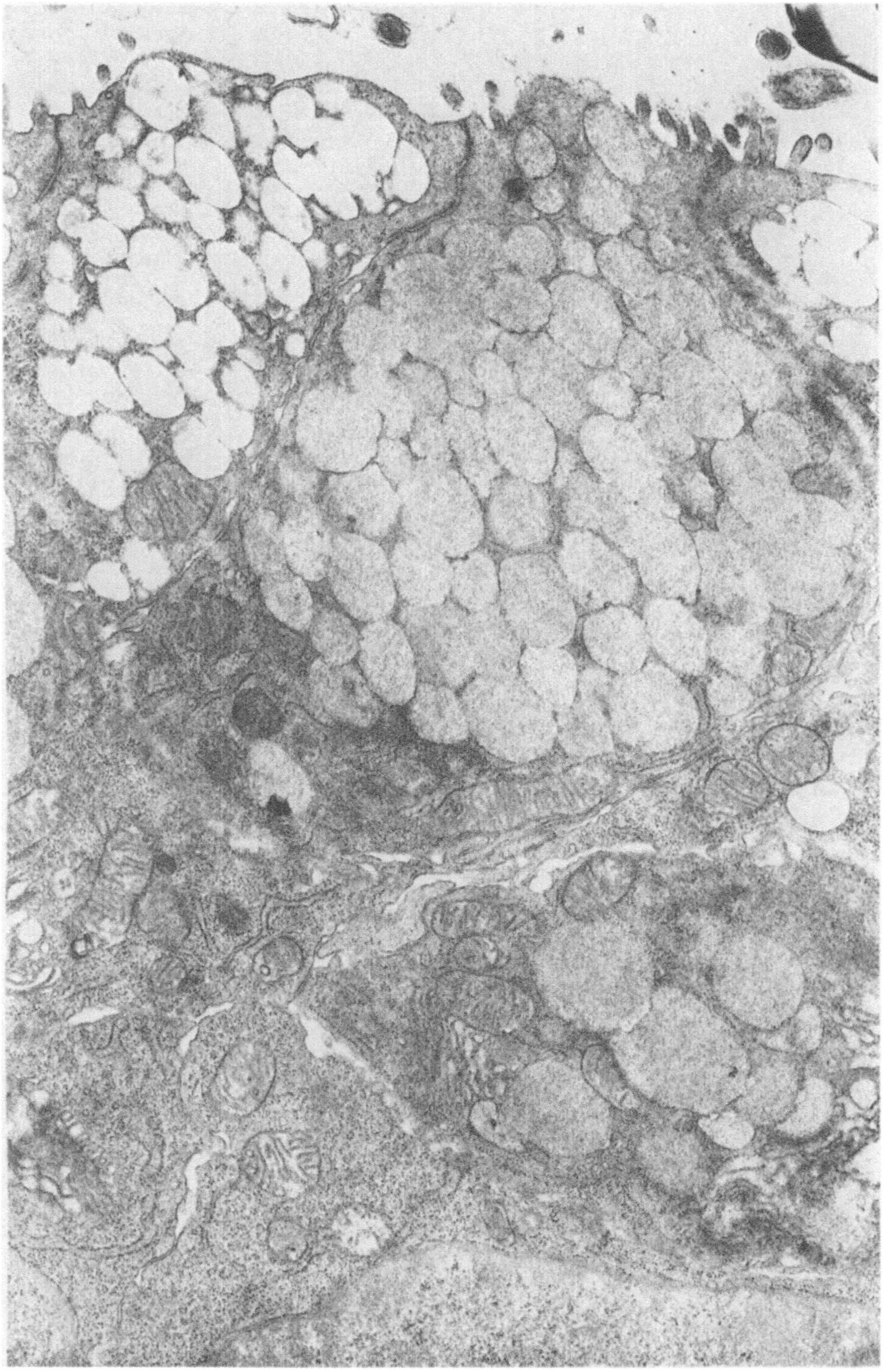

Fig. 20. Transmission electron micrograph of epithelial cells from colonic crypt, showing accumulating mucus granules of a goblet cell, with adjacent cells showing apical vacuoles of paler content. × 16,750

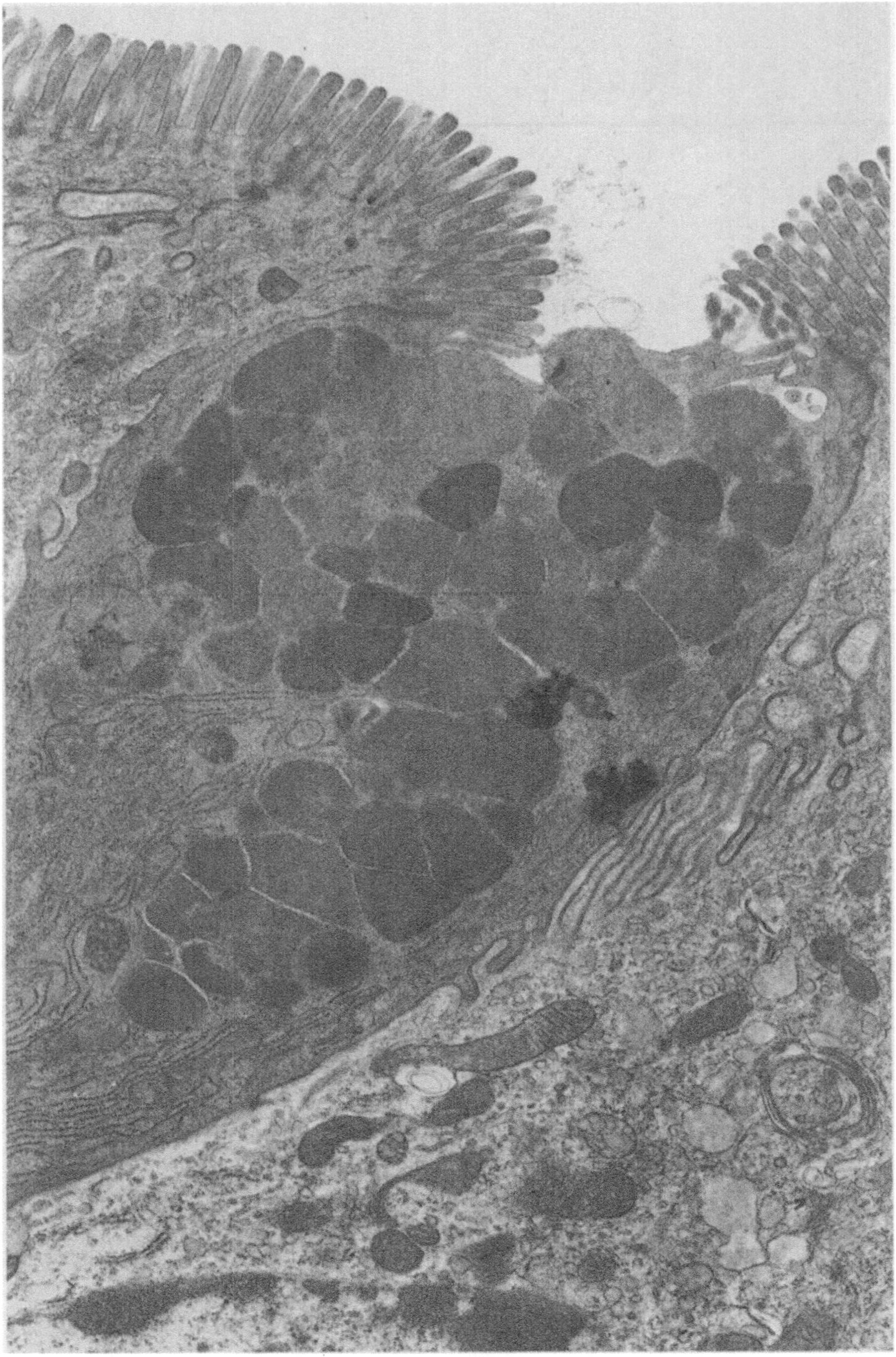

Fig. 21. Transmission electron micrograph of intestinal epithelium, showing goblet cell opening between adjacent columnar epithelial absorptive cells. The pit-like indentation of the epithelial surface produced in this case is well seen. The apical secretion granules are of variable density and are closely packed. Abundant granular endoplasmic reticulum is well seen in the subapical region. × 16,750

mic reticulum, consisting of parallel, well-organized cisternae, often containing dense flocculent material. The Golgi system is extremely elaborate, forming a collar above or around the apical pole of the nucleus. Mucus granules, pale and flocculent, form here as condensing vacuoles, become detached, and join the apical mass (Fig. 21). It has been estimated that one granule is released every 2–4 min from the Golgi apparatus under normal conditions (NEUTRA and LEBLOND 1966). The granules are stored until required for discharge in the merocrine mode, one or two granules at a time. The explosive discharge of goblet cells following exposure to irritant substances cannot be taken as the normal physiologic condition. The maturing goblet cell has microvilli like those of the surrounding crypt cells, although these become less and less apparent as the apical mucus mass swells and distends the cell. The granules contain abundant carbohydrate and a sulfated component, both of which are added to the initial protein component as it is processed through the Golgi system (BERLIN 1967). These chemical characteristics determine the distinctive staining reactions of the goblet cell by LM. The histochemistry of the intestinal mucosubstances is dealt with in detail by FILIPE and BRANFOOT (1976), who lay particular emphasis on the possible clinical significance of variations in the proportions of the sulfomucins, normally dominant, and the sialomucins, which increase in situations of cellular atypia.

II. Intestinal Endocrine Cells

These are distinctive epithelial cells, which have the features of endocrine gland cells, scattered throughout the mucosa of the gut. These cells were first identified by LM silver stains. The argentaffin and argyrophil reactions were the two main categories of the early classification of these cells, the former group being distinguished also by the chromaffin reaction, from which the term "enterochromaffin cell" arose. The old histologic terminology is now redundant, since a common endocrine identity now justifies the general term "intestinal endocrine cells". PEARSE has proposed that these cells have a common biochemical identity and lineage, characterized by the uptake and decarboxylation of amines and amine precursors. These "APUD" cells are seen as part of a general system of neuroendocrine cells, distributed widely throughout the body. They contain and secrete the various polypeptide local hormones of the gastrointestinal tract (PEARSE et al. 1977), along with a variety of biologically active amines such as 5-hydroxytryptamine, the physiologic role of which has not yet been adequately explained.

Although this group of endocrine cells is now known to have widely diverse functions, they share certain common structural features. They may be identified in histologic sections either as "clear" cells (Fig. 22), located towards the basement membrane, or as basal granulated cells with fine eosinophilic granules. By CTEM, both clear cells and basal granulated cells contain small endocrine secretion granules (Fig. 23). In the crypts, the apical parts of these endocrine cells may reach the lumen, reflecting their differentiation from common columnar crypt precursor cells (Fig. 24). As they migrate, they lose their apical extension, becoming pyramidal in shape and basal in location.

The typical endocrine secretion granules are membrane limited and vary in shape, size, and appearance, from large discoid or elliptical forms to uniform

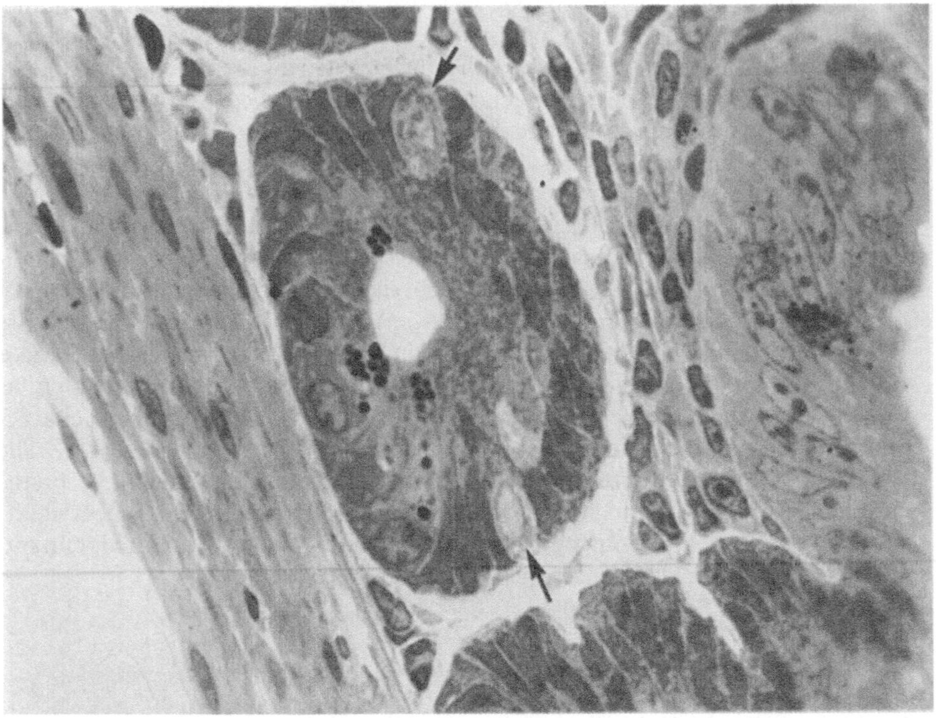

22

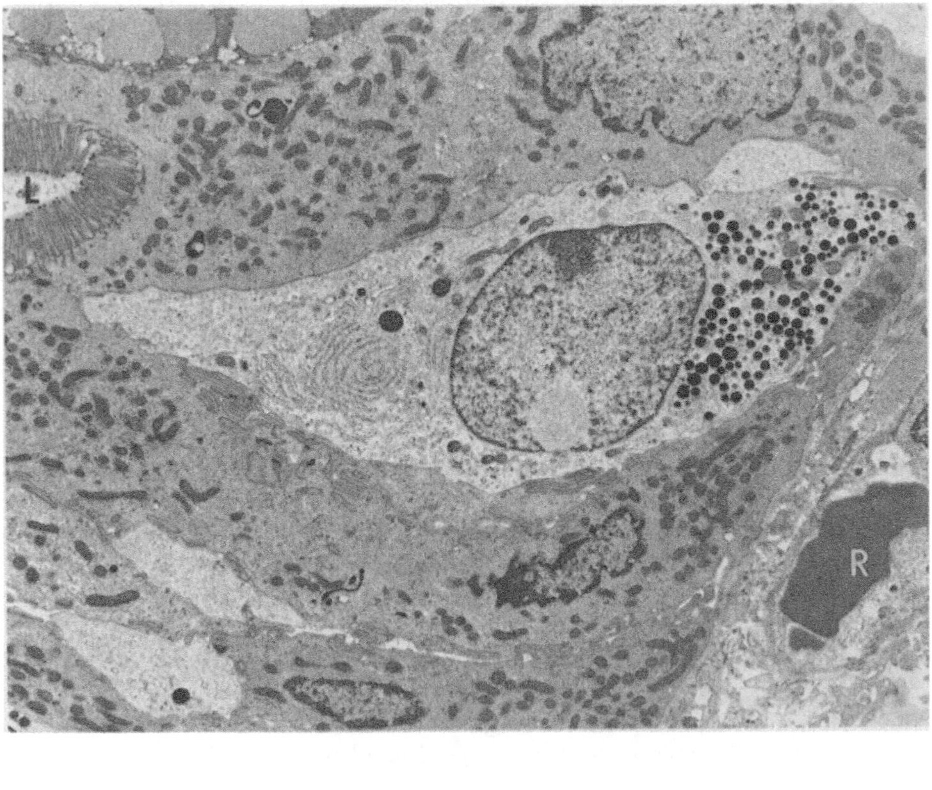

23

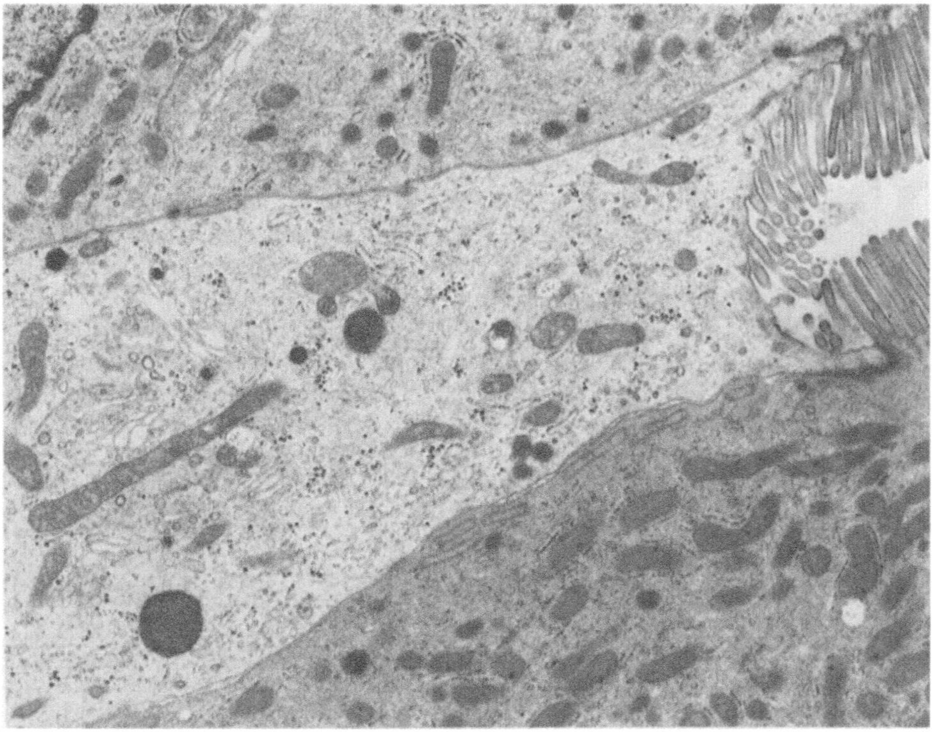

Fig. 24. Transmission electron micrograph of apical portion of an intestinal endocrine cell, showing the apical extension occasionally seen in this cell type. The endocrine cell is connected by apical junctional complexes to the adjacent enterocytes. The endocrine cell has surface microvilli, although these are rather less well organized than those of the adjacent absorptive cells. Only a few granules of the endocrine cell are seen in this portion of the cytoplasm, since the bulk of the secretion accumulates below the nucleus, preparatory to its discharge into the connective tissue. × 11,550

Fig. 22. Light micrograph of 1 µm azure B-stained thick section from plastic-embedded intestinal mucosa. This micrograph shows the foot of an intestinal crypt, in which two pale or clear cells (*arrows*) can be seen, identifiable as intestinal endocrine cells. The basal situation of these clear cells is typical of this cell type. Several Paneth cells can be seen nearby. × 1,400

Fig. 23. Transmission electron micrograph showing an intestinal endocrine cell with typical basal granules. A red blood cell (*R*) lies in an underlying capillary in the lamina propria. The apex of the cell extends close to, but does not reach, the lumen on the left-hand side (*L*). × 4,000

small round granules. The granules are always predominantly basal in location, being discharged eventually through the basal membrane of the cell and dispersing in the tissue fluid to reach the circulation. They are formed in the Golgi system, usually in a supranuclear position. The cell contains a moderately well-organized granular endoplasmic reticulum, consistent with a polypeptide secretory role.

The various cell types now recognized in this category can be identified by a combination of ultrastructural features and histochemical stains, and in particular by the immunohistochemical demonstration of specific polypeptide hormone products. Elaborate systems of classification exist, indicating a diversity the functional meaning of which remains to be fully explained. However, the intestinal endocrine cells, taken together, constitute one of the biggest endocrine glands in the body, their composite bulk being concealed by their anatomic dispersion. In functional terms, this endocrine system must be seen as one of the most important of the controlling mechanisms of the gut, although the details and clinical significance of this control still remain, for the most part, to be explained (BLOOM and POLAK 1979).

III. Paneth Cells

These are found only at the foot of the small intestinal crypts (Fig. 25), where they form a stable population arising from the common crypt cell precursors. They do not move from the crypts, unlike the enterocytes and goblet cells. When they die, they are phagocytosed in situ by neighboring crypt cells. The Paneth cell is pyramidal in shape and contains many apical eosinophilic refractile exocrine secretion granules. The cell apex, where the granules are released, bears a few microvilli (Fig. 26). The membrane systems are typical of a protein-secreting cell, with abundant granular endoplasmic reticulum and a large Golgi system. The presence of many complex lysosomes in addition to the Paneth cell granules distinguishes these cells from zymogenic cells, along with which they have often been classified in the past.

Morphometric analyses of the Paneth cell has produced the following figures (LOPEZ-LEWELLYN and ERLANDSEN 1979). The nucleus occupies 11.8% of the cellular volume. The cytosol, including granular endoplasmic reticulum, accounts for 55.7% of the total cytoplasmic volume; secretory granules take up 26.8%, Golgi areas 8.8%, and mitochondria 4.4%, respectively. Structures associated with the lysosome system occupy 4.3% of cytoplasmic volume. The average Paneth cell has a volume of 1,327 μm^3. The Paneth cells in the rat have been estimated to account for 5% of the cells of the small intestinal epithelium, while in the human a population of 2×10^8 Paneth cells has been calculated (CREAMER 1967).

The assumption of a zymogenic role for the Paneth cell was not proved by the identification of any specific digestive enzyme, but the identification of lysozyme in Paneth cell granules (PEETERS and VAN TRAPPEN 1975) along with the presence of immunoglobulins as shown by RODNING et al. (1976), suggests some possible antibacterial role; in support of this, Paneth cells have been shown to be able to ingest and destroy certain intestinal microorganisms (ERLANDSEN and CHASE

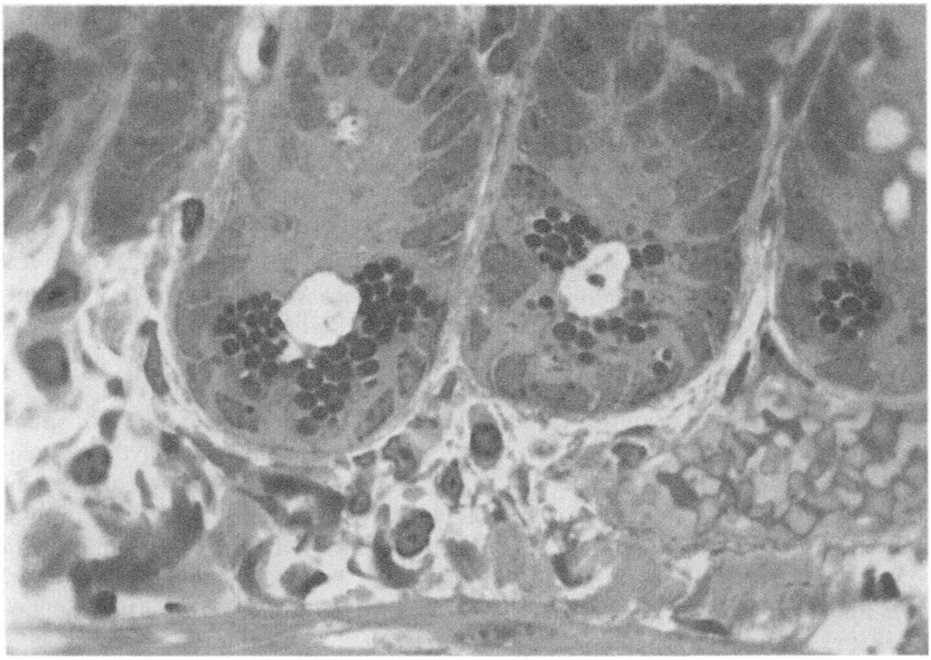

Fig. 25. Light micrograph of 1-μm section from plastic-embedded intestinal mucosa. The section shows the foot of several crypts with adjacent lamina propria. The Paneth cells are particularly prominent, distinguished by their dense apical secretion granules. × 1,150

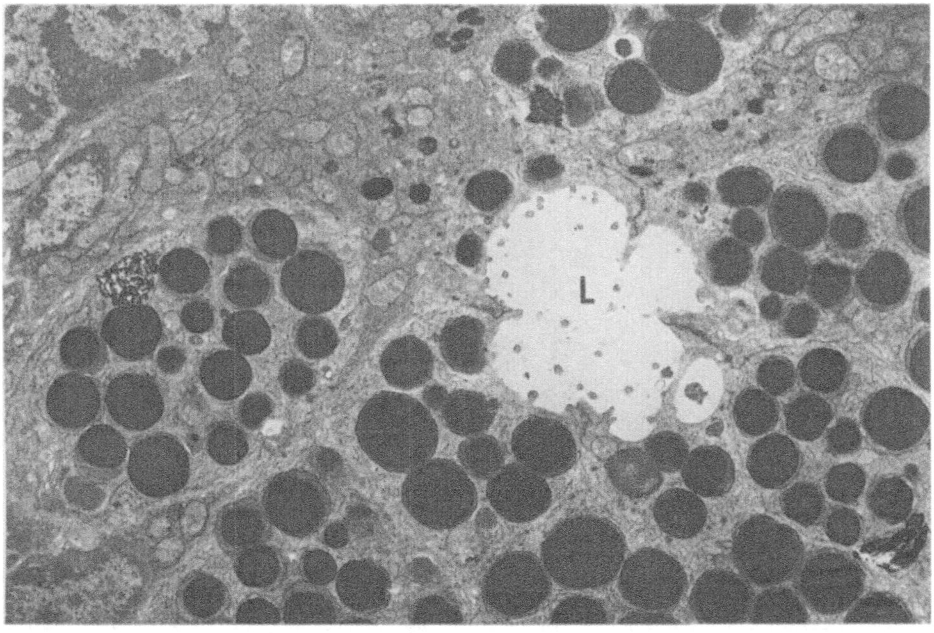

Fig. 26. Transmission electron micrograph of intestinal crypt showing numerous Paneth cells, distinguished by their apical dense granules grouped around the crypt lumen (*L*). × 5,600

1972). Perhaps, therefore, this unusual cell exerts some control over the microbial flora in the intestinal crypt.

IV. Tuft Cells

These have been described under a variety of names, including "multivesicular cells", "caveolated cells", "fibrillovesicular cells", "brush cells", and so on (ISOMAKI 1973; NABEYAMA and LEBLOND 1974). They are not confined to the gut, since similar cells have been seen in the respiratory, biliary, and urinary tracts, as well as stomach, duodenum, and colon. These cells take their name from a pronounced tuft of microvilli, taller and thicker than those of the enterocytes (Figs. 27, 28). Each cell has about 90 of these microvilli, the filamentous cores of which extend well down into the supranuclear cytoplasm. Deep micropinocytotic invaginations of the apical membrane are seen in association with the apical filament bundles. Lysosomes, mitochondria, Golgi profiles, and some glycogen are found, but endoplasmic reticulum is scanty. The function of the tuft cells remains obscure. They might be specialized absorptive cells, but their widespread distribution and their unusual ultrastructural features suggest other possibilities, such as a sensory role in relation to luminal contents.

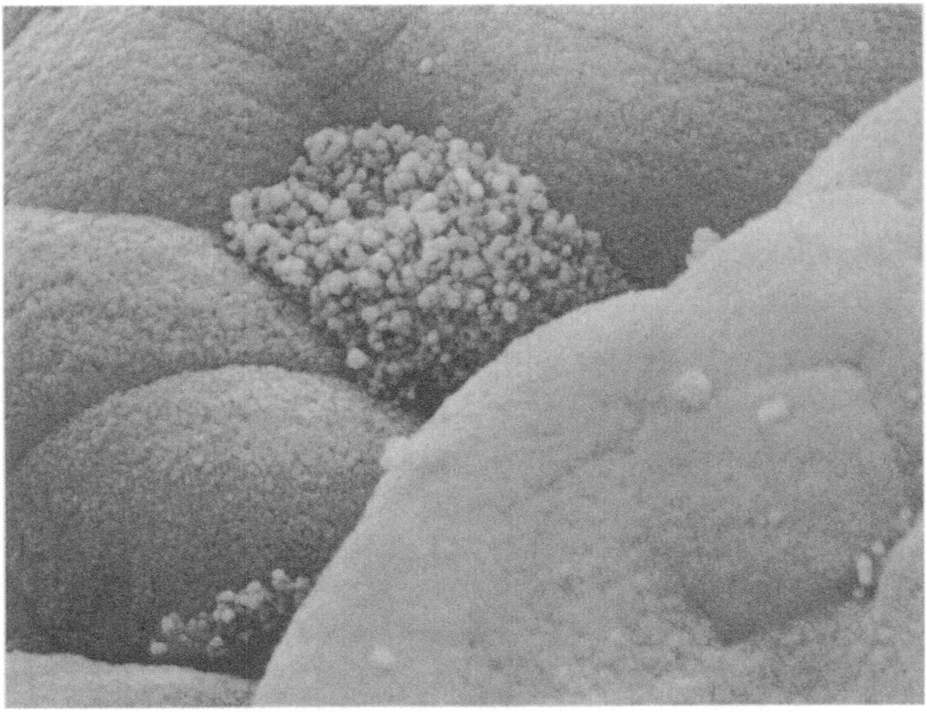

Fig. 27. Scanning electron micrograph of epithelial surface of small intestine, showing the apical portions of several columnar enterocytes surrounding a cell with more prominent thicker microvilli extending above the general surface of the mucosa. The appearances correspond to those of the tuft cell. × 5,900

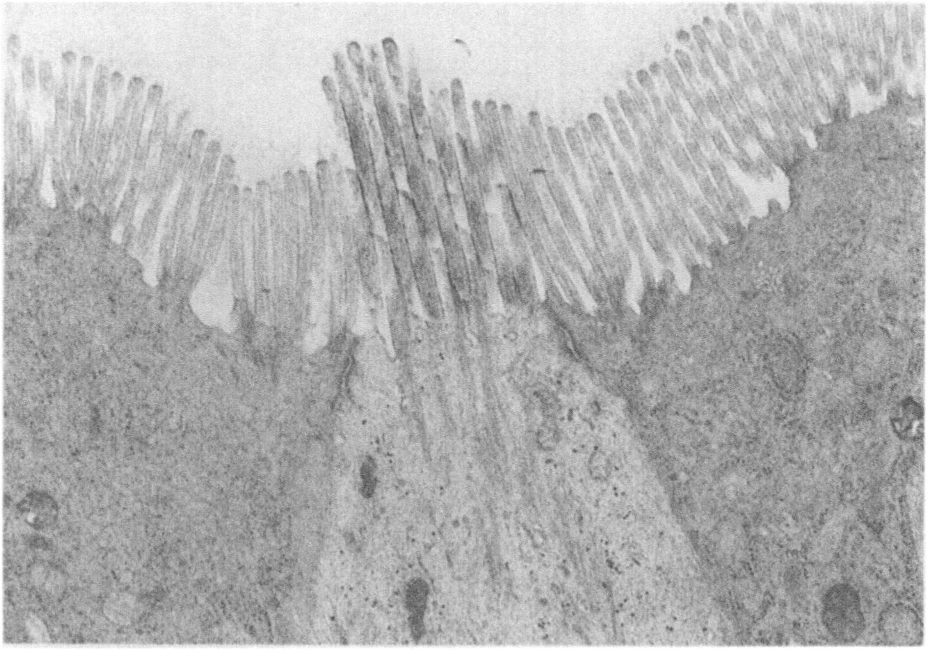

Fig. 28. Transmission electron micrograph, showing tuft cell with typical elongated microvilli extending above the general surface of the surrounding enterocytes. Apical junctional complexes connect the tuft cell to the surrounding epithelial cells. The fibrillar cores of the microvilli can be seen extending deep into the apical cytoplasm. × 18,500

V. M Cells

These originally took their name from their apical surface contours, consisting of anastomosing microfolds or convolutions (Fig. 29), rather than microvilli (Owen and Jones 1974). These cells are found overlying the intestinal lymphoid aggregates. They have a special relationship to the intraepithelial lymphoid cells which gather in clusters surrounded by the M cell and separated from the lumen by only a narrow apical shell of M cell cytoplasm. These cells have been shown to be able to take up antigens from the gut lumen and pass them to the underlying lymphocytes. It has been proposed that they act as part of the afferent limb of the intestinal immune responses (Owen 1977).

VI. Intraepithelial Lymphocytes

Up to 20% of the total cell population of the intestinal epithelium consists of nonepithelial cells. These are the intestinal lymphocytes, or theliolymphocytes, the possible biologic significance of which has only recently been recognized, with the growth of interest in the gut-associated lymphoid tissues (Otto 1973; Marsh 1975; Parrott 1976).

The intraepithelial lymphocytes are similar to lymphocytes in other locations, with pale cytoplasm, few formed organelles, and a relatively high nucleocytoplas-

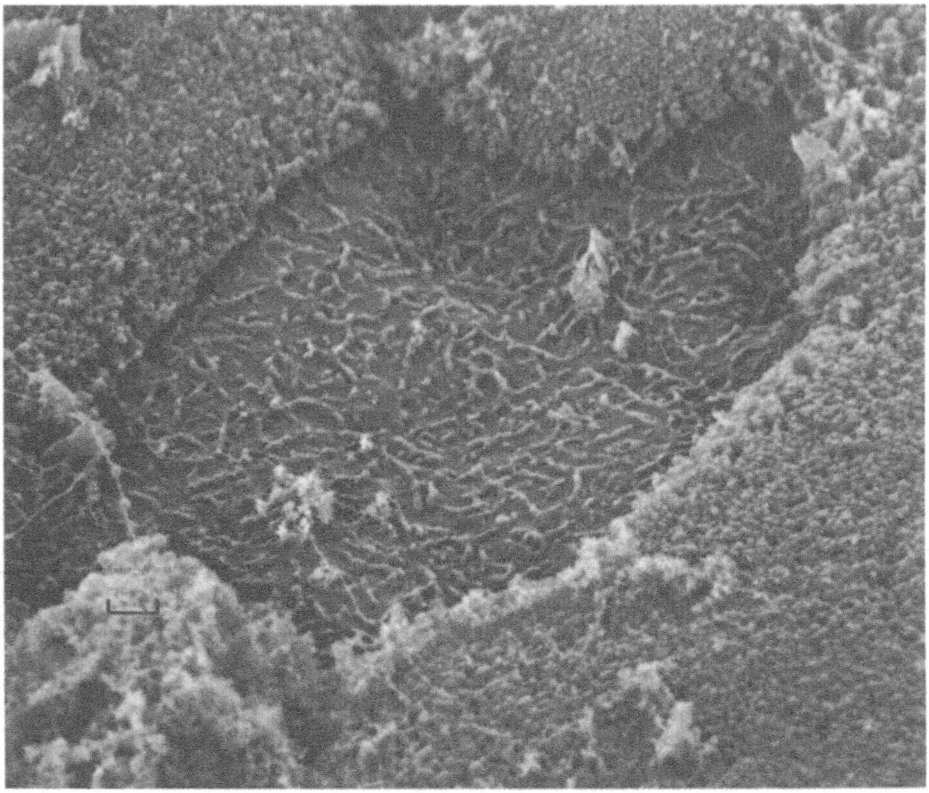

Fig. 29. Scanning electron micrograph of the surface of an intestinal M cell, showing the contrast between its low convoluted ridges and the microvilli of the surrounding enterocytes. Courtesy of Dr. R. L. OWEN, × 6,500

mic ratio. Some larger lymphoid cells have features suggestive of blast cells, with paler nuclei, large nucleoli, more abundant cytoplasm, and increased numbers of polyribosomes. None of these cells ever displays adhesion specializations (TONER and FERGUSON 1971), unlike the columnar cell populations, which adhere to one another by means of desmosomes and junctional complexes. These lymphoid cells

Fig. 30. Light micrograph of 1-μm section from plastic-embedded intestinal mucosa. The illustration shows a cross section of a single villus. The regular columnar cells are distinguished by the well-formed striated border. A basally situated intraepithelial lymphocyte is observed in the process of crossing the basement membrane of the epithelium (*arrow*). The pale cytoplasm of this cell distinguishes it from the surrounding enterocytes. × 1,000

Fig. 31. Transmission electron micrograph of the base of the intestinal epithelium, showing a migrating lymphocyte similar to that shown in the preceding figure. The pale cytoplasm contains no recognizable formed organelles in this plane of section. The amoeboid outlines of the cytoplasm suggest active migration. While the bulk of the cell lies within the epithelium, a portion of the cytoplasm lies in the lamina propria. The direction of migration cannot be confidently identified from such a micrograph. × 9,200

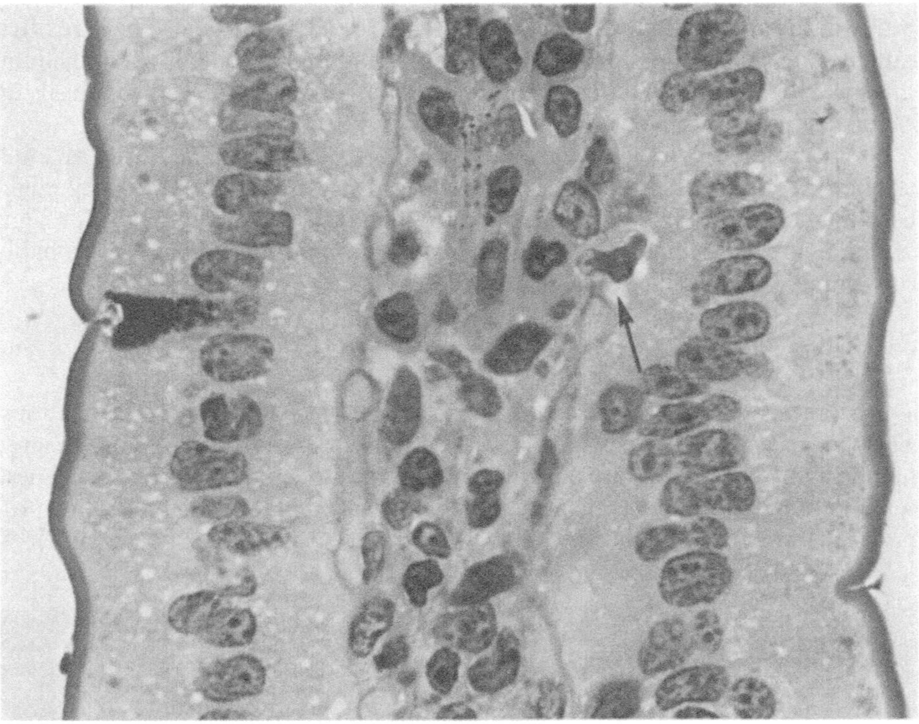

30

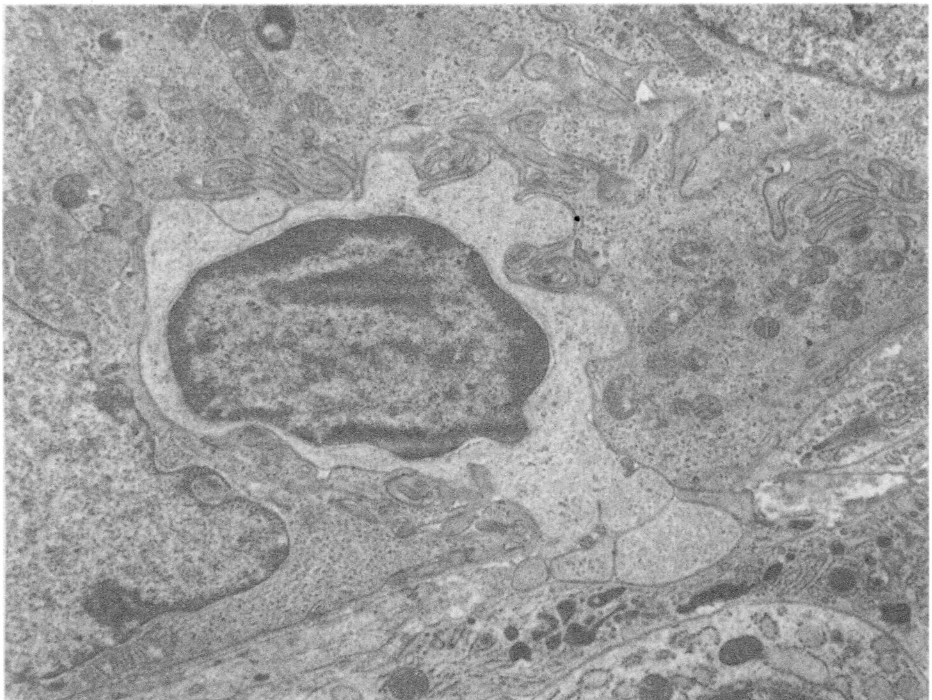

31

are clearly not fixed in position to their neighbors, and give every indication of being on the move, varying in their shape from round to ameboid. They are often caught in the act of crossing the basal lamina, half in, half out of the epithelium, causing a breach in the continuity of the basal lamina which presumably heals up again quickly once the cell passes through (Figs. 30, 31).

It is presumed that these migratory lymphoid cells, which are mostly of T cell origin, are of importance in the immunologic responses of the gut. They might be thought of as being on patrol, sampling the antigenic environment for signs of immunologic incursions. Their significance in relation to disease is probably considerable, although not yet fully understood.

VII. Globule Leukocytes

These are also transient intraepithelial cells, lacking adhesion specializations. They occur as part of the response to parasitic infestation, being found in large numbers during the self-cure of experimental nematode infections in mice. These cells are found not only in the intraepithelial situation, but also in the lamina propria. They are now thought to be derived from mast cells (MURRAY et al. 1968).

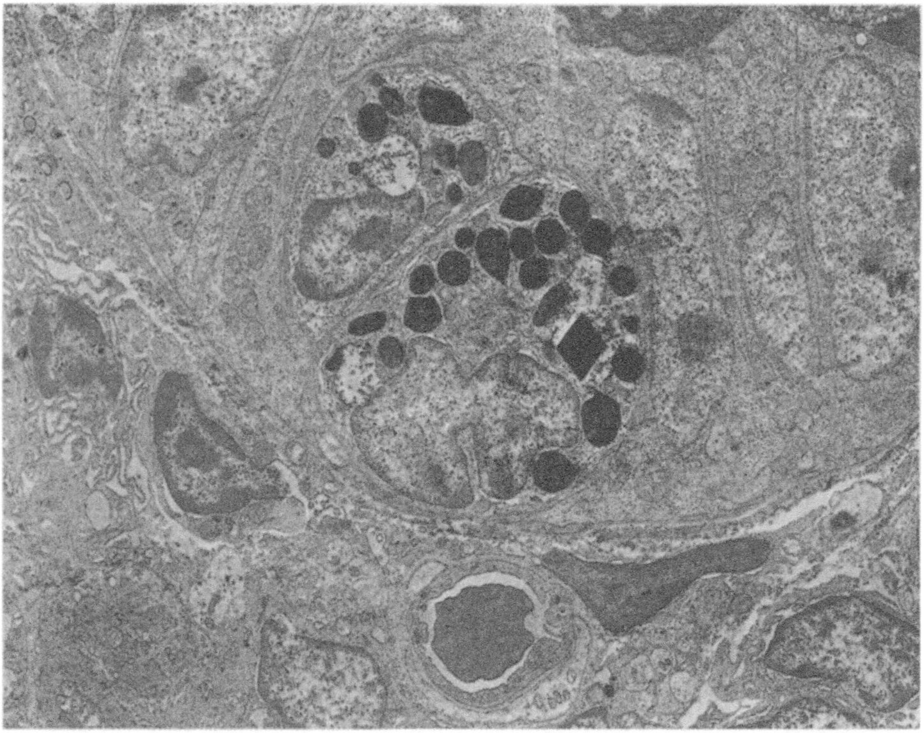

Fig. 32. Transmission electron micrograph, showing two globule leukocytes in the intestinal epithelium of the mouse. The cytoplasmic inclusions are distinguished by the presence of several crystalline structures. A red blood cell is seen within an underlying capillary vessel. ×2,900

The characteristic feature of the globule leukocyte is the presence of large cytoplasmic inclusions, or globules, which often contain complex crystalline or fibrous material (Fig. 32), variable according to species (CARR 1967; CARR and WHUR 1968). In other respects these cells are not particularly distinctive, but they are clearly different from intraepithelial eosinophil leukocytes, with which they have been confused in the past.

F. Deeper Layers of the Intestine

I. Lamina Propria

The intestinal lamina propria mucosae is the layer of loose vascular connective tissue immediately adjacent to the epithelium (Fig. 33), filling in the spaces between the crypts of Lieberkühn and forming the cores of the villi. It consists of a loose network of fibrocytes or fibroblasts, connective tissue fibers, and ground substance, with the addition of a large number of transient interstitial "inflammatory" cells, such as lymphocytes, plasma cells, polymorphs, macrophages, and occasional mast cells.

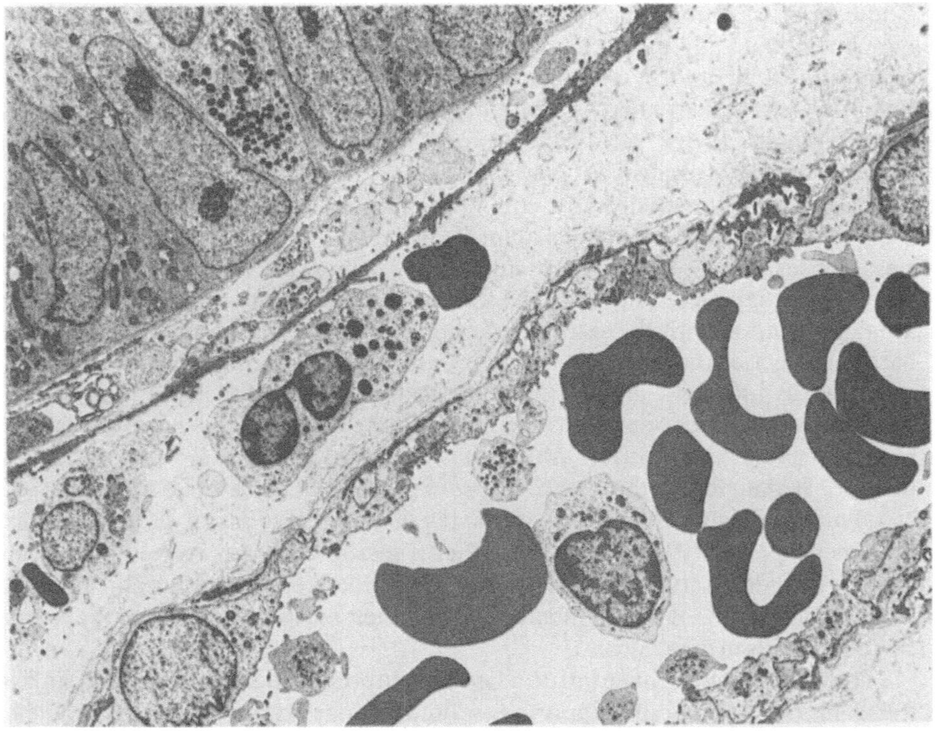

Fig. 33. Transmission electron micrograph, showing the lamina propria of the small intestine, immediately beneath the epithelium. A venule contains red and white blood cells and platelets. An eosinophil leukocyte lies between this vessel and the epithelium. An intestinal endocrine cell base can be observed within the epithelium. × 3,350

The fibrocyte or fibroblast is responsible for the maintenance of the connective tissue matrix which forms the framework of the mucosa. Such cells are present throughout the stroma, but a particular population has been recognized by its location and special behavior. This is the pericryptal fibroblast sheath, a single layer of fibroblasts that lie just below the basal lamina of the crypts. Labeling studies (MARSH and TRIER 1974) have shown that the cells of this sheath proliferate and migrate in parallel with the movement of epithelial cells. Presumably, this is an important factor in mucosal morphogenesis and response to injury and disease.

The "inflammatory" cells present in the lamina propria are a part of the normal anatomy of the gut. They represent the healthy state of balanced antagonism between the normal defense mechanisms and the various types of environmental challenge, such as food antigens and microorganisms, both commensal and pathogenic. Indeed, the presence of the normal flora of the gut influences intestinal morphology in more ways than this; the intestines of animals raised in a germ-free environment show marked variations from conventional structure, accompanied by differences in patterns of epithelial cell renewal (ABRAMS et al. 1963; GORDON 1968).

The germ-free small bowel appears thin walled and well filled, while the cecum is markedly distended by semi fluid contents. Inflammatory cells are few: this includes both the lamina propria infiltrate and the population of intraepithelial lymphocytes already mentioned. These changes are accompanied by shortening of intestinal villi, and by a markedly reduced rate of cell turnover in the epithelium, the average life span of the enterocyte doubling by comparison with conventional animals. In the germ-free cecum (GUSTAFSSON and MAUNSBACH 1971), there are equally striking histologic changes.

The inflammatory cells most commonly found in the normal lamina propria are lymphocytes and plasma cells, most of the latter being of the IgA-secreting class. This is the secretory form of immunoglobulin, which is taken up by the adjacent epithelial cells, transported to the cell apex, and discharged into the lumen after conjugation with the secretory component which makes this process possible. The effect of the secretion of IgA by the mucosal surfaces has been likened to a coat of "antiseptic paint" on the epithelium, but the full significance of this transport of antibody remains to be worked out. The lymphocytes of the lamina propria include both diffusely infiltrating cells and aggregated lymphoid nodules, the most striking being those of the Peyer's patches of the ileum. This gut-associated lymphoid tissue is now seen as playing an important part in gastrointestinal immune responses (PARROTT 1976). Other transient cell types seen in the lamina propria include macrophages, mast cells, globule leukocytes, eosinophil and neutrophil polymorphs. Their numbers vary, but their individual morphology is typical of such cells in other sites.

The vascular component of the lamina propria is an important final link in the chain of intestinal absorption. A submucosal arterial plexus gives branches of two types, the first ending in a deep capillary network above the muscularis mucosae and surrounding the crypts, the second specifically servicing the cores of the villi. Each villus has one or more such branches, leading to a subepithelial capillary network which can be visualized by injection replica techniques or even by the simple expedient of ultrasonic disintegration of the overlying epithelium. Small veins run from the villous capillary network to meet the venous plexus which surrounds the crypts, draining finally into the submucosal venous plexus. The capillary vessels are lined by fenestrated endothelial cells with numerous micropinocytotic vesicles, around which an external or basal lamina is situated. Arterioles have a surrounding smooth muscle layer; venules lack this, but have a wider diameter and an irregular contour on cross section.

Lymphatic vessels are important for absorption, particularly of fat. Each villus contains a terminal branch of the lymphatic plexus, known as a lacteal (DOBBINS 1971; DOBBINS and ROLLINS 1970). This is a thin-walled vessel, lined by endothelial cells, without a basal lamina. Smooth muscle cells run parallel to the lacteal, emptying its contents by their contraction.

Nerve fibers are abundant in the lamina propria, virtually all being of unmyelinated type. It has been shown that a single colonic gland can have up to 150 axons lying nearby in the connective tissue of the lamina propria. There is, however, little if any evidence for neuroepithelial synapses or intraepithelial nerve endings. The identity and location of receptor structures for afferent impulses remains obscure.

II. Muscle Layers and Their Autonomic Innervation

There are two distinct muscle coats in the intestine, the lamina muscularis mucosae and the lamina muscularis externa. Both consist of smooth muscle, with associated autonomic nerve components (GABELLA 1979). The muscularis mucosae is the deepest layer of the mucosa, the boundary with the submucosa. It consists of two thin layers of smooth muscle cells, the inner component circular, the outer longitudinal with respect to the gut. Individual smooth muscle cells run from here up into the core of the villus. An elastic and reticular fiber network surrounds the smooth muscle of this layer. The associated autonomic nerve system is Meissner's plexus, located in the submucosa. The muscularis externa is also composed of two layers, an inner circular and an outer longitudinal, although both adopt, strictly speaking, a spiral configuration of short and long pitch respectively. The myenteric autonomic nerve plexus of Auerbach lies between these two layers. The innermost part of the circular muscle coat, at the boundary of the submucosa, is distinctive, being composed of muscle cells which are smaller, darker, and more richly innervated than those of the main part of the muscularis externa.

The features of the smooth muscle of the gut are similar to those seen in other sites (Fig. 34). Individual fusiform cells are surrounded by an external lamina, with the exception of those points at which close cellular contact occurs, the so-called nexus specializations, permitting ionic movement between cells. Micropinocytotic caveolae are numerous at the cell surface. The cytoplasm of smooth muscle has abundant filaments, with associated cytoplasmic and subsurface dense attachment zones. The cigar-shaped dense bodies which are present throughout the cell are also associated with the cellular filaments concerned with the process of contraction. Actin and myosin filaments make possible a sliding mechanism, different in detail from that of skeletal muscle, but the same in principle.

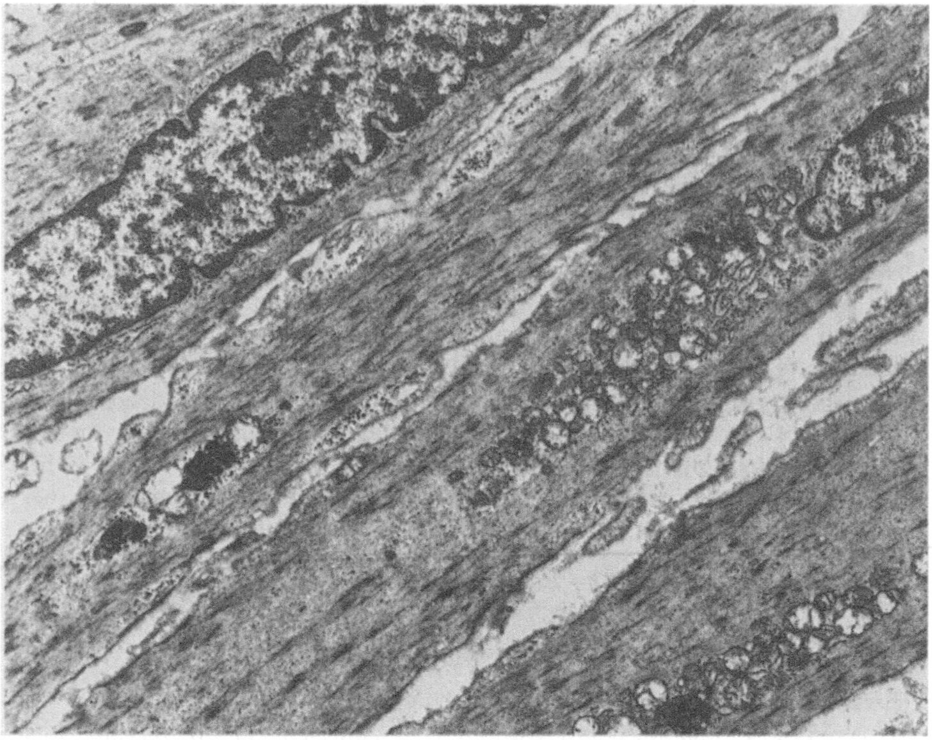

Fig. 34. Transmission electron micrograph of intestinal smooth muscle cells, showing the typical fusiform cell shape, with elongated nuclei. The cytoplasm is largely filled by longitudinally oriented filaments. Courtesy of Dr. A. A. M. Gibson, $\times$ 6,600

In functional terms, the nexus specializations are probably of major importance, allowing as they do for spreading excitation between cells in a muscle sheet. Freeze-fracture studies show that these junctions are distinguished by the presence of closely packed intramembranous particles, 9 nm in diameter, which appear to provide the pathway for ionic movement between cells. The circular muscle of the gut has been shown to be rich in nexuses in the species studied, whereas the longitudinal muscle layer is variable in this respect in different species. Nexuses may be few, or may be totally absent from the teniae coli.

The morphology of the autonomic nerve plexuses of the gut has been reviewed in detail by Gabella (1979), although there remain many unexplained features. The neural components are tightly packed together, without intervening collagen fibers or other connective tissue components, an appearance that has more in common with the central nervous system than with peripheral nerve. There is a basal lamina surrounding the associated nerve cell bodies and processes. The non-neuronal cells outnumber neural cells in the plexuses.

Attempts have been made to classify the various nerve endings seen within the myenteric plexus. Up to eight different morphologic types have been recognized, although such classifications can only be regarded as provisional, pending the

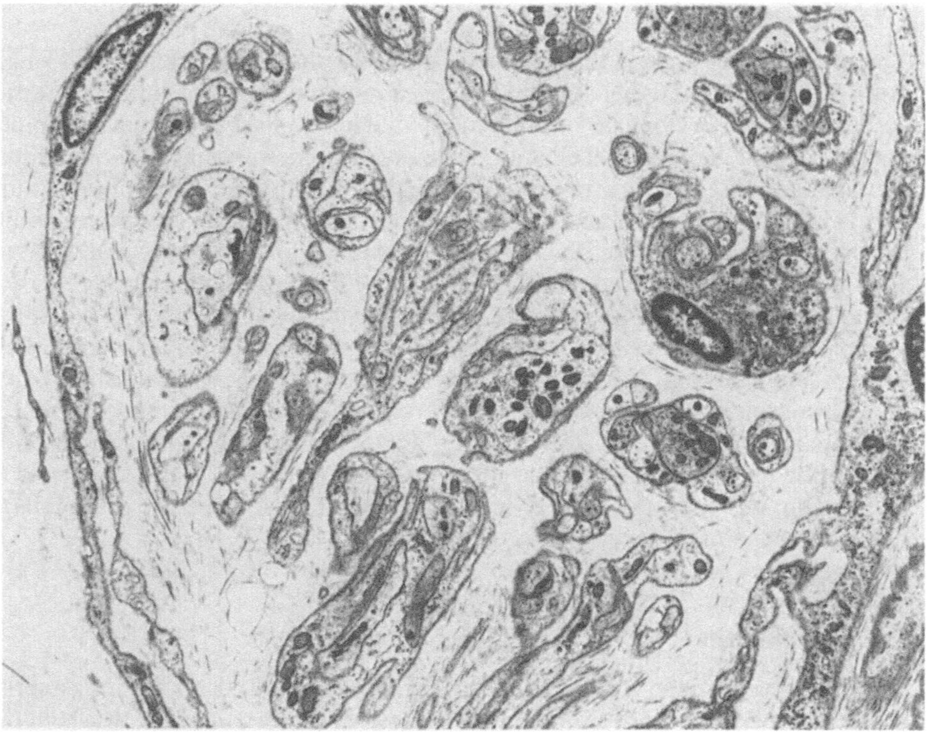

Fig. 35. Transmission electron micrograph of cross-sectioned nerve bundle in the intestinal wall. Groups of axons are ensheathed within common Schwann cell cytoplasmic tubes. Courtesy of Dr. A. A. M. GIBSON, × 4,600

availability of more functional data. Specializations are seen in the synaptic membranes and aggregates of vesicles of different pattern are found. Three broad types of transmitter vesicle have been tentatively identified, the small empty type, presumably cholinergic, the small dense-cored type, presumably adrenergic, and the large pleomorphic type, possibly polypeptide in nature.

The peripheral innervation (Fig. 35) of the intestinal smooth muscle cells remains largely unexplained. In general, nerve bundles containing up to several dozen axons within a single Schwann cell sheath run between muscle cells. The axons have expansions or varicosities along their length, containing synaptic vesicles in aggregates. The average distance from such presumptive functional nerve endings to the adjacent smooth muscle cells is over 80 nm, a distance substantially greater than the corresponding figure in other varieties of smooth muscle. Some axons, however, reach to within 15 nm of a muscle cell surface. In general, the patterns of nerve endings within the muscle are similar to the patterns seen in the myenteric plexus itself. There remain many questions in this area, such as the exact role of the puzzling autonomic interstitial cells. Are they merely fibroblasts, or could they play some part in the coordination of muscle activity? Much work remains to be done on this area of the gut wall.

III. The Serosa

The intestinal serosa is a thin external connective tissue layer lined by a single layer of flattened mesothelial cells. There is an underlying basal lamina. The mesothelial cells carry elongated surface microvilli, have apical and basal micropinocytotic caveolae and are attached to one another by desmosomes and junctional complexes. Solitary cilia often project from the cell surface. The concentration and length of the serosal microvilli vary according to the site: the more mobile the organ, the more elaborate the surface specialization (ANDREWS and PORTER 1973). External to the cell surface lies a mucopolysaccharide-rich glycocalyx, which takes the form of fine strands radiating from the microvilli. The combination of microvilli and cell coat is thought to provide the slippery surface typical of serosa, a functional specialization little regarded until the mechanical problem of adhesions points out its absence. The serosal layer has itself a marked absorptive capacity, as shown by the rapid uptake of intraperitoneally administered medication and by the therapeutic effectiveness of peritoneal dialysis in nephrology. Again, however, the biology of this important part of the gut wall remains only poorly explored.

G. Conclusion

The intestines provide for digestion and absorption, but also have an essential protective role, in view of the potential hazards of the environment to which the intestinal mucosa is exposed. The complex interconnected systems of absorption, defense, mechanical propulsion, neural and endocrine contral are as yet only partly understood in structural and functional terms. This chapter has tried to place the histologic and ultrastructural data in a functional perspective, indicating various points of current interest and identifying several unsolved problems. It has tried to show that the pharmacology of absorption and permeability can only be properly understood against a background of detailed ultrastructural knowledge. The application of modern microscopic techniques now allows a much clearer appreciation of the cellular aspects of intestinal function.

Acknowledgements. We are grateful to Professor R. J. SCOTHORNE and R. B. GOUDIE for the use of departmental facilities, and to Mrs. C. WATT and Mr. J. ANDERSON, FIMLS, for their enthusiastic help. We would also like to thank Miss M. HUGHES, Mr. O. REID, Miss J. MUNRO and Mr. W. RITCHIE for their assistance and advice. We are indebted to Mrs. M. THOMSON for her painstaking work in typing the manuscript. Many of the transmission electron micrographs were provided by Mr. H. S. JOHNSTON and we are glad to acknowledge his contribution to the chapter.

References

Abrams GD, Bauer H, Sprinz H (1963) Influence of the normal flora on mucosal morphology and cellular renewal in the ileum. A comparison of germ free and conventional mice. Lab Invest 12:355

Andersen KJ, Von der Lippe G, Morkrid L, Schjonsby H (1975) Purification and characterization of guinea pig intestinal brush borders. Biochem J 152:157–159

Andrews PM, Porter KR (1973) The ultrastructural morphology and possible functional significance of mesothelial microvilli. Anat Rec 177:409
Banwell JG, Hutt MSR, Tunnicliffe R (1964) Observations of jejunal biopsy in Ugandan Africans. East Afr Med J 41:46–54
Bazin H (1976) The secretory antibody system. In: Ferguson A, MacSween RNM (eds) Immunological aspects of the liver and gastrointestinal tract. MTP Press, Lancaster
Berlin JD (1967) The localization of acid mucopolysaccharides within Golgi complex of intestinal goblet cells. J Cell Biol 32:760
Biempica L, Sternlieb I, Sohn HB, Ali M (1976) R-bodies of human rectal epithelial cells. Arch Pathol Lab Med 100:78–80
Bloom SR, Polack JM (1979) Alimentary endocrine system. In: Sircus W, Smith AN (eds) Scientific foundations of gastroenterology. Heinemann, London, pp 101–122
Brown AJ (1962) Microvilli of the human jejunal epithelial cell. J Cell Biol 12:623–627
Brunser O, Luft JH (1970) Fine structure of the apex of absorptive cells from rat small intestine. J Ultrastruct Res 31:291
Brunser D, Castillo C, Araya M (1976) Fine structure of the small intestinal mucosa in infantile marasmic malnutrition. Gastroenterology 70:495–507
Carr KE (1967) Fine structure of crystalline inclusions in the globule leukocyte of the mouse intestine. J Anat 101:793
Carr KE, Toner PG (1968) Scanning electron microscopy of rat intestinal villi. Lancet 2:570
Carr KE, Whur P (1968) Ultrastructure of globule leukocyte inclusions in the rat and mouse. Z Zellforsch mikrosk Anat 86:153
Clarke SL (1959) The ingestion of proteins and colloidal materials by columnar absorptive cells of the small intestine in suckling rats and mice. J Biophys Biochem Cytol 5:41
Creamer B (1967) Paneth-Cell Function. Lancet 1:314
Creamer B, Leppard P (1965) Post mortem examination of a small intestine in celiac syndrome. Gut 6:466–471
Dobbins WO (1966) Abetalipoproteinemia. Gastroenterology 50:195–210
Dobbins WO (1971) Intestinal mucosal lacteal in transport of macromolecules and chylomicrons. Am J Clin Nutr 24:77–90
Dobbins WO, Rollins EL (1970) Intestinal mucosal lymphatic permeability: An electron microscopic study of endothelial vesicles and cell junctions. U Ultrastruct Res 33:29
Eichholz A (1969) Fractions of the brush border. Fed Proc 28:30–34
Eichholz A, Crane RK (1974) Isolation of plasma membranes from intestinal brush borders. In: Fleischer A, Packer L (eds) Methods Enzymol 31, part A:123–134
Erlandsen SL, Chase DG (1972) Paneth cell function. Phagocytosis and intracellular digestion of intestinal microorganisms. 1. Hexamita muris. J Ultrastruct Res 41:296–318
Farquhar MG, Palade GE (1963) Junctional complexes in various epithelia. J Cell Biol 17:375
Ferguson A (1976) Celiac disease and gastrointestinal food allergy. In: Ferguson A, MacSween RNM (eds) Immunological aspects of the liver and gastrointestinal tract. MTP Press, Lancaster
Ferguson A, Maxwell JD, Carr KE (1969) Progressive changes in the small intestinal villous pattern with increasing length of gestation. J Pathol 99:87–91
Filipe MI, Branfoot AC (1976) Mucin histochemistry of the colon. In: Morson BC (ed) Pathology of the gastrointestinal tract. Curr Top Pathol 63:143–178
Freiburghaus AU, Hauri HP, Green J, Hadorn B (1978) Micromethod for separation and identification of digestive enzymes in brush border membrane fragments of single human intestinal biopsies. Clin Chim Acta 86:227–234
Friedman HI, Cardell RR (1977) Alterations in the endoplasmic reticulum and Golgi complex of intestinal epithelial cells during fat absorption and after termination of this process. A morphological and morphometric study. Anat Rec 188:77–102
Friend DS, Gilula NB (1972) Variations in tight and gap junctions in mammalian tissues. J Cell Biol 53:738–776
Gabella G (1979) Innervation of the gastrointestinal tract. Int Rev Cytol 59:129–193
Geyer G (1979) Decay of murine intestinal epithelial cells under extrusion. Acta Histochem (Jena) 64:213–225

Gordon HA (1968) Is the germ-free animal normal? A review of its anomalies in young and old age. In: Coates ME (ed) The germ-free animal in research. Academic, London, pp 127–150
Gustafsson BE, Maunsbach AB (1971) Ultrastructure of the enlarged cecum in germ-free rats. Z Zellforsch Mikrosk Anat 120:555–578
Holman GD, Naftalin RJ, Simmons NL, Walker M (1979) Electrophysiological and electron-microscopical correlations with fluid and electrolyte secretion in rabbit ileum. J Physiol (Lond) 290:367–386
Hull B, Staehelin LA (1976) Functional significance of the variations in the geometrical organization of tigh junction networks. J Cell Biol 68:688–704
Hull BE, Staehelin LA (1979) The terminal web. A re-evaluation of its structure and function. J Cell Biol 81:67–82
Iancu T, Elian E (1976) The intestinal microvillus – ultrastructural variability in coeliac disease and cow's milk intolerance. Acta Paediatr Scand 65:65–73
Isomaki AM (1973) A new cell type (tuft cell) in the gastrointestinal mucosa of the rat. Acta Pathol Microbiol Scand [A] Suppl 240
Ito S (1974) Form and function of the glycocalyx on free cell surfaces. Philos Trans R Soc Lond [Biol] 268:55–66
Jakoi ER, Zampighi G, Robertson JD (1976) Regular structures in membranes. II. Morphological and biochemical characterization of two water-soluble proteins isolated from suckling rat ileum. J Cell Biol 70:97–111
Jersild RA, Crawford RW (1978) The distribution and mobility of anionic sites on the brush order of intestinal absorptive cells. Am J Anat 152:287–305
Johnson CF (1969) Hamster intestinal brush border surface particles and their function. Fed Proc 28:26
Kaye GI, Fenoglio CM, Pascal RR, Lane N (1973) Comparative electron microscopic features of normal, hyperplastic and adenomatous human colonic epithelium. Gastroenterology 64:926–945
Kaye MD, Brody AR, Whorwell PJ, Beeken WL (1979) Scanning electron microscopy of rectal mucosa in Crohn's disease. Dig Dis Sci 24:369–375
Knutton S, Limbrick AR, Robertson JD (1974) Regular structures in membranes. I. Membranes of the endocytic complex of ileal epithelial cells. J Cell Biol 62:679–694
Knutton S, Limbrick AR, Robertson JD (1978) Structure of occluding junctions in ileal epithelial cells in suckling rats. Cell Tissue Res 191:449–462
Lazarides E (1980) Intermediate filaments as mechanical integrators of cellular space. Nature 283:249–256
Lee FD, Toner PG (1980) Biopsy pathology of the small intestine: Chapman and Hall, London
Lichtenberger LM, Lechago J, Miller TA (1979) Cell culture of human intestinal mucosa. Gastroenterology 77:1291–1300
Lopez-Lewellyn J, Erlandsen SL (1979) Morphometric analysis of a polarized cell. The intestinal Paneth cell. J Histochem Cytochem 27:1554–1556
Lorenzsonn V, Trier JS (1968) The fine structure of human rectal mucosa. The epithelial lining of the base of the crypt. Gastroenterology 55:88–101
Louvard D, Semeriva M, Maroux S (1976) The brush border intestinal aminopeptidase, a transmembrane protein as probed by macromolecular photolabeling. J Mol Biol 106:1023–1035
Marsh MN (1975) Studies of intestinal lymphoid tissue. I. Electron microscopic evidence of "blast transformation" in epithelial lymphocytes of mouse small intestinal mucosa. Gut 16:665–674
Marsh MN, Swift JA (1969) A study of small intestinal mucosa using the scanning electron microscope. Gut 10:940–949
Marsh MN, Trier JS (1974) Morphology and cell proliferation of subepithelial fibroblasts in adult mouse jejunum. I. Structural features. Gastroenterology 67:622
McNutt NS (1977) Freeze fracture techniques and applications to the structural analysis of the mammalian plasma membrane. In: Poste G, Nicolson GL (eds) Dynamic aspects of cell surface organization. Elsevier-North Holland Biomedical, Amsterdam, pp 75–126

Melligott TF, Beck IT, Dinda PK, Thompson S (1975) Correlation of structural changes at different levels of the jejunal villus with positive net water transport in vivo and in vitro. Can J Physiol Pharmacol 53:439–450
Merrill TG, Sprinz H, Tousimis AJ (1967) Changes of intestinal absorptive cells during maturation. An electron microscopic study of prenatal, postnatal and adult guinea-pig ileum. J Ultrastruct Res 19:304–326
Mooseker MK, Tilney LG (1975) Organization of an actin filament-membrane complex. Filament polarity and membrane attachment in the microvilli of intestinal epithelial cells. J Cell Biol 67:725–743
Mooseker MK, Pollard TD, Fujiwara K (1978) Characterization and localization of myosin in the brush border of intestinal epithelial cells. J Cell Biol 79:444–453
Murray M, Miller HRP, Jarrett WFH (1968) The globule leukocyte and its derivation from the subepithelial mast cell. Lab Invest 19:222
Nabeyama A, Leblond CP (1974) Caveolated cell characterised by deep surface invaginations and abundant filaments in mouse gastro-intestinal epithelial. Am J Anat 140:147–166
Neutra MR (1979) Linear arrays of intramembrane particles on microvilli in primate large intestine. Anat Rec 193:367–382
Neutra M, Leblond CP (1966) Synthesis of the carbohydrate of mucus in the Golgi complex as shown by electron microscope autoradiography of goblet cells from rats injected with glucose-H^3. J Cell Biol 30:119
Otto HF (1973) The interepithelial lymphocytes of the intestinum. Morphological observations and immunological aspects of intestinal enteropathy. Curr Top Path 57:81–122
Owen RL (1977) Sequential uptake of horseradish peroxidase by lymphoid follicle epithelium of Peyer's patches in the normal unobstructed mouse intestine: an ultrastructural study. Gastroenterology 72:440–451
Owen RL, Jones AL (1974) Epithelial cell specialization within human Peyer's patches: an ultrastructural study of intestinal lymphoid follicles. Gastroenterology 66:189–203
Padykula HA (1962) Recent functional interpretations of intestinal morphology. Fed Proc 21:873–879
Padykula HA, Strauss EW, Ladman AJ, Gardner FH (1961) A morphologic and histochemical analysis of the human jejunal epithelium in non-tropical sprue. Gastroenterology 40:735
Parrott DMV (1976) The gut-associated lymphoid tissue and gastrointestinal immunity. In: Ferguson A, MacSween RNM (eds) Immunological aspects of the liver and gastrointestinal tract. MTP Press Lancaster, pp 1–32
Pearse AGE, Riecken EO (1967) Histology and cytochemistry of the cells of the small intestine, in relation to absorption. Br Med Bull 23:217
Pearse AGE, Polack JM, Bloom SR (1977) The newer gut hormones. Cellular sources, physiology, pathology and clinical aspects. Gastroenterology 72:746–761
Peeters T, Van Trappen G (1975) The Paneth cell; a source of intestinal lysozyme. Gut 16:553
Pfeiffer CJ (1971) Mucosal surface convolutions. Cellular aggregates observed on the enteric surface of various species. Biol Gastroenterol (Paris) 3 (Suppl 3):225–229
Phillips AD, France NE, Walker-Smith JA (1979) The structure of the enterocyte in relation to its position on the villus in childhood: an electron microscopical study. Histopathology 3:117–130
Plattner H, Klima J (1969) In: Shmerling DH, Berger H, Prader A (eds) Intestinal absorption and malabsorption. S. Karger, New York, p 18
Porter KR (1969) Independence of fat absorption and pinocytosis. Fed Proc 28:35–40
Porter KR, Kenyon K, Badenhausen S (1967) Specializations of the unit membrane. Protoplasma 63:262–274
Potten CS, Allen TD (1977) Ultrastructure of cell loss in the intestinal mucosa. J Ultrastruct Res 60:272–277
Riddell RH, Levin B (1977) Ultrastructure of the "transitional" mucosa adjacent to large bowel carcinoma. Cancer 40:2509–2522

Rodning CB, Wilson ID, Erlandsen SL (1976) Immunoglobulins within human small intestinal Paneth cells. Lancet 1:984–987
Shields HM, Yedling ST, Blair FA, Goodwin CL, Alpers DH (1979) Successful maintenance of suckling rat ileum in organ culture. J Anat 155:375–389
Singer SJ, Nicolson GL (1972) The fluid mosaic model of the structure of cell membranes. Science 175:720–731
Staehelin LA (1974) Structure and function of intercellular junctions. Int Rev Cytol 39:191–283
Stone J, Mukherjee TM, Hecker R (1977) C-bodies and R-bodies in the epithelial cells of normal and diseased human rectum. Arch Pathol 101:437–441
Swift JA, Mukherjee TM (1976) Demonstration of the fuzzy surface coat of rat intestinal microvilli by freeze etching. J Cell Biol 69:491–495
Taylor AB, Anderson JH (1972) Scanning electron microscopic observations of mammalian intestinal villi, intervillus floor and crypt tubules. Micron 3:430–453
Tice LW, Carter RL, Cahil MB (1979) Changes in tight junctions of rat intestinal crypt cells associated with changes in their mitotic activity. Tissue Cell 11:293–316
Toner PG, Carr KE (1969) The use of scanning electron microscopy in the study of the intestinal villi. J Pathol 97:611
Toner PG, Carr KE (1979) The digestive system. In: Hodges GM, Hallowes RC (eds) Biomedical research applications of scanning electron microscopy. Academic, London, pp 203–272
Toner PG, Ferguson A (1971) Intraepithelial cells in the human intestinal mucosa. J Ultrastruct Res 34:329–344
Toner PG, Carr KE, Ferguson A, MacKay C (1970) Scanning and transmission electron microscopic studies of human intestinal mucosa. Gut 11:471–481
Toner PG, Carr KE, Wyburn GM (1971) The digestive system. An ultrastructural atlas and review. Butterworths, London
Tormey JM, Diamond JM (1967) The ultrastructural route of fluid transport in rabbit gallbladder. J Gen Physiol 50:2031–2060
Towler CM, Pugh-Humphreys GP, Porteous JW (1978) Characterization of columnar absorptive epithelial cells isolated from rat jejunum. J Cell Sci 29:53–75
Trier JS (1963) Studies of small intestinal crypt epithelium. I. The fine structure of the crypt epithelium of the proximal small intestine of fasting humans. J Cell Biol 18:599–620
Trier JS (1964) Studies of small intestinal crypt epithelium. II. Evidence for and mechanisms of secretory activity by undifferentiated crypt cells of the human small intestine. Gastroenterology 47:480–495
Trier JS (1976) Organ culture methods in the study of gastrointestinal mucosal function and development. N Engl J Med 295:150–155
Ugolev AM, Delaey (1973) Membrane digestion. A concept of enzymatic hydrolysis on cell membranes. Biochim Biophys Acta 300:105–128
Watson AJ, Wright NA (1974) Morphology and cell kinetics of the jejunal mucosa in untreated patients. In: Cooke WT, Asquith P (eds) Celiac disease. Clin Gastroenterol 3(1):20
Wissig SL, Graney DO (1968) Membrane modifications in the apical endocytic complex of ileal cells. J Cell Biol 39:564–579

CHAPTER 2

Intestinal Permeation and Permeability: an Overview

T. Z. CSÁKY

A. Introduction

The objective of this chapter is to provide a broad, bird's-eye view of the problems of intestinal permeation and permeability. The aim of the subsequent chapters is to discuss these problems in more detail. Two parts of the intestinal tract can be clearly distinguished both morphologically and functionally in the human, in other mammals, in birds, and in some amphibians: the small intestine and the large intestine. The small intestine begins at the pylorus as duodenum, continues as jejunum into the aboral part called ileum. The large intestine, or colon, originates at the ileocecal junction and, in humans, has three parts: the ascending, transverse, and descending colon; the latter continues into the rectum. The cecum is a blind sac at the beginning of the colon; in humans this part of the gut apparently is of minor functional significance.

B. Diffusion Processes

Intestinal permeability refers to the intestinal wall's property which modifies the permeation, i.e., the flow of substances into or across the organ. The modification consists mostly of a degree of resistance to the free diffusional flow. The resistance depends on the structure of the intestine as a biologic membrane as well as on the physicochemical nature of the permeant.

Diffusion is the unrestricted flow of substances from one compartment to the other. It is caused by thermal agitation of the molecules. The rate of diffusion is quantitatively expresed by Fick's law (FICK 1855).

$$\frac{\mathrm{d}n}{\mathrm{d}t} = DA\frac{\mathrm{d}c}{\mathrm{d}x},$$

where $\mathrm{d}n$ is the number of molecules (ions) crossing an area A in time $\mathrm{d}t$ in proportion to the concentration difference $\mathrm{d}c$ over a distance of $\mathrm{d}x$. D is the diffusion coefficient and is expressed by the amount of substance diffusing across unit area per unit time where $\mathrm{d}c/\mathrm{d}x = 1$.

If the free diffusion is restricted by interposing a membrane between the two compartments having different concentrations, the rate of movement will depend not only upon the concentration gradient, but upon the resistance presented by the membrane. If the membrane is very loosely structured so that it does not offer any resistance, the flow process will be essentially diffusion. By knowing the diameter of the membrane, however, the term $\mathrm{d}x$ is included in a new coefficient which is now called the permeability coefficient P and has the dimensions of a velocity. P includes not only the thickness, but other physical properties of the membrane which are responsible for its resistance to transport. Fick's law in terms of the permeability constant P is thus modified

$$\frac{dn}{dt} = PA\,dc\,.$$

Permeation is essentially a two-way process; thus, in the intestine the flow of substances from the lumen into the bloodstream (absorption) and the flow from the bloodstream into the lumen (exorption) occur simultaneously. The primary physiologic function of the intestine is absorption; the organ is differentiated both anatomically and physiologically to fulfill this function. This differentiation results in a preferential directional flow for most substances, i.e., the net result of permeation is usually absorption. Nonetheless, exorption cannot be completely neglected (see Sect. D.III).

The small intestine is the principal site of the absorption of most nutrients, the large intestine is mainly involved in the absorption of electrolytes and water. Consequently, the small intestine is endowed with a more elaborate system which determines its permeability. This is the reason why considerably more research effort has been directed toward elucidating the permeability of the small intestine than that of the large bowel. As a result the monographs dealing with intestinal absorption (VERZÁR and MCDOUGALL 1936; WILSON 1962; WISEMAN 1964; CODE 1968) and secretion (BINDER 1979) concentrate on the small intestine. The small intestine is also the principal site of drug absorption and, because of its complex physiologic function, is the target of drug actions. Consequently, when discussing the pharmacology of intestinal permeation, a good deal of emphasis is placed on the small intestine although some drugs, particularly those which produce catharsis by increasing the bulk, act in the colon (see Chap. 28).

C. The Intestine

The small intestine represents a large surface. Taking the infoldings of Kerckring, the macrovilli, and microvilli into consideration, the surface of the small intestine in the adult human is estimated to be 200 m^2 (WILSON 1962). Through this very large surface the body is exposed to the environment. It should be emphasized that at least two significant functions are connected with the permeability of the small intestine (CSÁKY 1981): one relates to the nutrition of the body, the other to the maintenance of the body's homeostasis. The first function is involved in the intestinal absorption of nutrients and other substances foreign to the body (xenobiotics) which are present in the intestinal lumen. Since permeability is a two-way process, valuable nutrients (sugars, amino acids, electrolytes, etc.) are continuously oozing from the blood into the intestine. Because of the large intestinal surface, this continuous leak could lead to the loss of substantial quantities of nutrients, upsetting the body's homeostasis. Owing to the vigorous active transport ability of the intestine (see Sect. D.II.1.c), the nutrient molecules are continuously reabsorbed from the lumen into the bloodstream, thus the homeostasis is preserved.

The rate of permeation across any biologic membrane depends on the structure of the membrane as well as upon the physicochemical properties of the permeant. In general, biologic membranes display the property of a porous lipid membrane through which water and a few small polar particles can easily pass, but the passage of the vast majority of hydrophilic molecules is markedly restricted. The intestine is no exception to this rule. Yet, many essential polar nutrients pass across the intestinal barrier. Such passage requires a specific transport mechanism. This mechanism can be either carrier mediation or pinocytosis. Under special conditions very large particles can be taken up from the lumen and released into the circulation through phagocytosis by migrating leukocytes or can enter the intestinal villi across the gap created by the sloughing off of enterocytes at the tip of the villi (persorption).

D. Passage of Substances Across Biologic Membranes

This section summarizes the various ways substances can pass biologic membranes, including the intestine.

I. Simple Diffusion

Simple diffusion is caused by the thermal agitation of the solvent and solute particles. The rate of net transfer is described by Fick's law (see Sect. B). Lipids or lipid-soluble substances, including the majority of drugs and other xenobiotics, are transported by simple diffusion.

II. Specific Transport Mechanisms

There is ample evidence that highly polar substrates pass across the lipid intestinal membranes occasionally, even against a higher concentration or electrochemical gradient. In these cases the involvment of a specific transport mechanism is assumed.

1. Carrier Mediation

A detailed discussion of the carrier concept is given in Chap. 8. The basic function of the carrier could be visualized as a mechanism enabling the polar substrate to break its hydrogen bonding with the water and enter the lipid phase of the membrane. Although several theories have been proposed in this regard, the exact mechanism of this function remains to be clarified.

Although transport carriers have not yet been chemically isolated, purified, and structurally clarified, a good deal is known about them from kinetics and affinity studies. Because of the distinct selectivity and apparent structural versatility, it is assumed that the carriers are of proteinaceous nature, perhaps glycoproteins as are some of the receptors of which the structure is known (BLECHER and BAR 1981; COHEN and CHANGEUX 1975). Because of the limited density of carrier sites on the surface of the membrane, the kinetics of a carrier-mediated transport

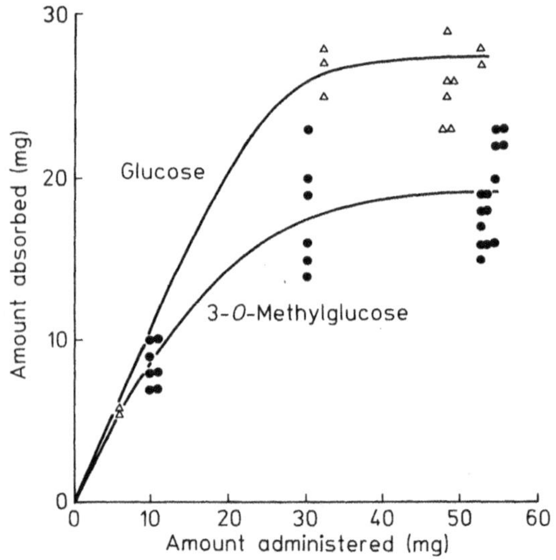

Fig. 1. Absorption of glucose and 3-*O*-methylglucose from the small intestine of the frog, *Rana pipiens*. Saturation absorption kinetics. When increasing the initial luminal concentration the rate of absorption increases only to the level at which the system is saturated. CSÁKY and FERNALD (1960)

is usually a saturation kinetics (Fig. 1). Another significant phenomenon connected with carrier-mediated transport is the mutual inhibition of transport by substrates of similar structure which can be assumed to share the same carrier.

One interesting analogy for the functioning of the carrier can be drawn from studies concerning the effect of dimethylsulfoxide (DMSO) upon the intestinal transport of sugars. DMSO, a solvent with both hydrophylic and hydrophobic properties, acts as a "carrier" for the transport of glucose the kinetics of which is changed from a saturation to a straight diffusion kinetics in the presence of the solvent (Fig. 2). It is theorized that DMSO may form a loose complex with the glucose molecule thereby "masking" its hydrophilic hydroxyl groups (CSÁKY and HO 1966).

a) Facilitated Diffusion

As its basic function the carrier simply facilitates the permeation of the polar substrate across the lipid membrane. Consequently, as long as the carrier sites are not saturated, the kinetics of the transport is a diffusion kinetics, i.e., the net transport ceases when equilibrium is reached on both sides of the barrier. The term "facilitated diffusion" (DANIELLI 1954) was coined for such euqilibrating transport involving the carrier.

b) Exchange Diffusion (Countertransport)

The carrier may combine with the substrate on one side of the membrane and deliver it to the other side where it may combine with another substrate of similar structure, facilitating its transport in the opposite direction. This process is called exchange diffusion or countertransport.

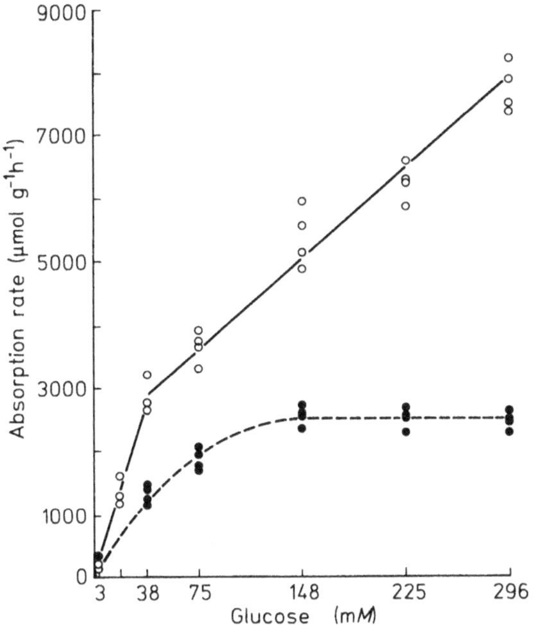

Fig. 2. *Broken line:* saturation absorption kinetics of glucose from the small intestine of the rat. *Full line:* in the presence of 4% DMSO the kinetics is converted into a straight diffusion kinetics. CSÁKY and HO (1966)

c) Active Transport

In certain cases the carrier-mediated transport of a substrate proceeds against a higher concentration or electrochemical gradient. Clearly, in this case the free energy of the substrate increases, consequently the process requires the expenditure of metabolic energy. Such a process is called active transport which thus could be accurately defined as an energy-requiring process whereby a substance permeates across a membrane barrier from a lower to a higher concentration (or electrochemical) gradient, yet the substance is neither bound on either side of the membrane nor produced or consumed during the transport. The energy for the active transport is usually derived from the hydrolysis of high energy phosphate bounds contained in such compounds as adenosine triphosphate (ATP), creatinine phosphate, or arginine phosphate.

2. Pinocytosis

This is a process in which the cell membrane produces a deep infolding which is eventually detached as a intracellular vesicle (LEWIS 1931). Subsequently, the membrane of this vesicle is dissolved and its content is emptied into the cytosol. Alternately the pinocytotic vesicle attaches itself to the opposite membrane of the cell, fuses with it, and "defecates" its content into the opposite extracellular space. The first step in the process of pinocytosis is a specific binding of an inducing molecule to the outer surface of the membran (BENNET 1956; BRANDT 1958; SHUMAKER 1958; HOLTER 1959; MARSHALL et al. 1959; MERCER 1959). The kinetics of the binding process indicates the present of distinguishing receptors at the outer surface of the membrane (Brandt and Pappas 1960). The possible involvement of factors present in the nutrient in the process of intestinal absorption by pinocytosis has not yet been explored despite some observations which may point in that direction. It has been found that certain metabolic inhibitors were more effective if offered to kidney-tubular epithelial cells dissolved in an albumin solution; it was assumed that the inhibitor enters the cells combined with the protein by pinocytosis (György and Kinne 1971). Also botulinus toxin A, which is a high molecular weight toxin, is better absorbed from the intestine if given to a well-fed than to a starved animal (May and Whaler 1958).

Pinocytosis can produce an uphill transport against a higher concentration. The energy in this case is needed for the movements of the membrane. It has even been proposed that pinocytosis may play a significant role in the active transport of electrolytes and water (Bennet 1956). However, such a proposal does not seem feasible on the basis of calculations by Parsons (1963). According to these calculations, for the human intestine to absorb daily about 7 l water, which is the average load offered to the human gut, each cell has to produce one thousand vesicles per second, which is practically impossible.

III. Persorption

This is a special permeation across the intestinal wall in which the cell membranes are not involved. The intestinal epithelium turns over very rapidly. New cells are continuously produced in the crypts of Lieberkühn. These cells migrate toward

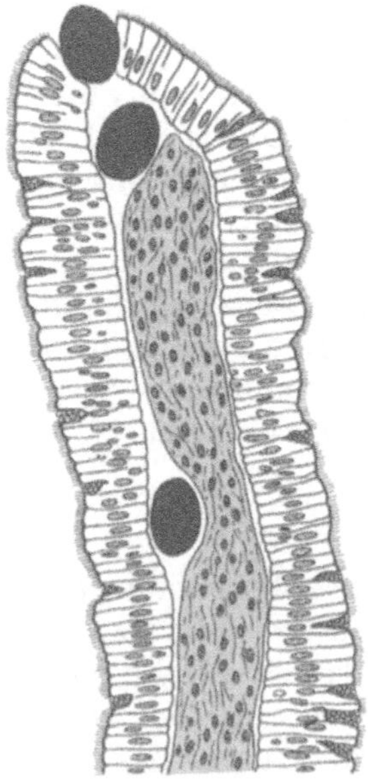

Fig. 3. Persorption of starch particles. The particles are taken up at the tip of the villus where the epithelial cells are sloughed off. The particles travel along the submucosal space and end up in the lymph. Courtesy of Professor G. Volkheimer, Berlin

the tip of the villi where they are sloughed off, leaving temporarily a hiatus in the cell layer. Apparently, rather large particles can slip int the circulation (Fig. 3; VOLKHEIMER 1972). At this moment the physiologic significance, if any, of persorption is unclear. A pharmacotoxicologic significance is obvious as potentially harmful particles, e.g., asbestos fiber, can be absorbed from the intestine into the circulation. It is important to remember that there is a basic difference between pinocytosis and persorption: the former is a transcellular, the latter an intercellular transport process.

E. Intestinal Permeation

Let us now examine the involvement of these transport mechanisms in the complex process of intestinal permeation. Figure 4 illustrates schematically the intestinal permeation barriers and the mechanisms of passing across them. Because of intestinal motility it is assumed that the bulk phase within the lumen is well mixed. However, there is a layer in the watery content immediately adjacent to the intestinal wall which consists of a series of poorly mixed stationary lamellae. The average thickness of this layer is estimated to be approximately 300 nm and is referred to as the unstirred water layer, UWL. (For a detailed discussion of the significance of UWL in the intestinal permeability see Chap. 22.) Substances pass through this layer by diffusion.

Another thin layer (not more than 20 nm) lies immediately adjacent to the brush border. This layer provides an acidic microclimate which in turn influences the passage of weak acids and bases into the membrane. (A more detailed discussion of the significance of this layer is found in Chap. 21.)

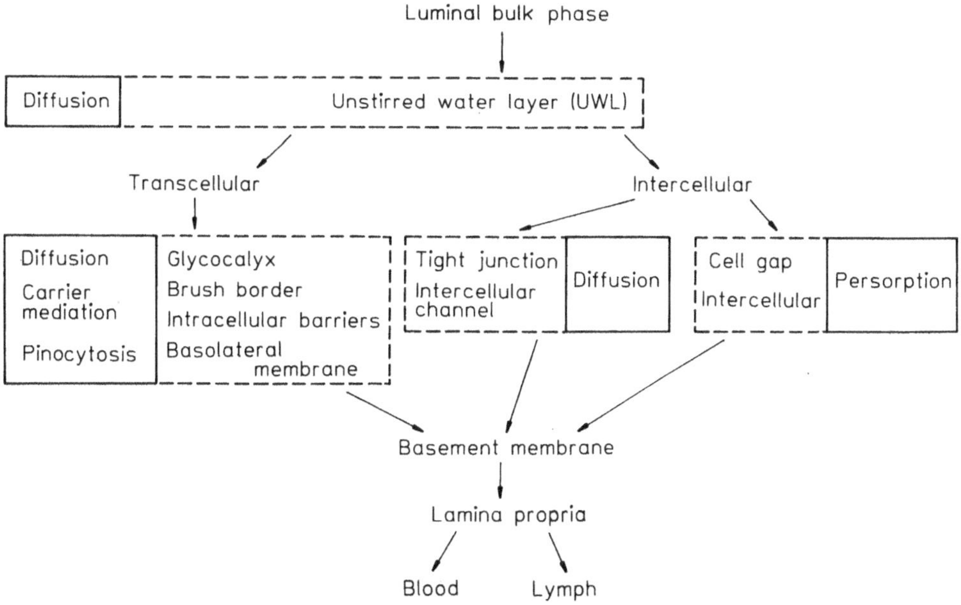

Fig. 4. The principle routes of substrate flux from the lumen of the gut into the bloodstream or lymph. *Full lines,* transport mechanism; *broken lines,* barrier sites

Two routes of permeation exist below these barriers: a transcellular and an intercellular. In the transcellular passage, the substance has to be translocated first through the brush border. This membrane behaves essentially as a lipid barrier. The passage may proceed by simple diffusion, by carrier mediation, or by pinocytosis. The basolateral membrane is, both morphologically and in its permeability properties, not unlike plasma membranes of other bodily cells, e.g., erythrocytes. The passage again proceeds by diffusion, carrier mediation, or pinocytosis. The thin structure dividing the enterocyte and the intercellular space from the lamina propria is called the basement membrane. As far as is known today, the basement membrane does not offer a permeability barrier. From the cells the permeant passes across the basement membrane into the subepithelial space, called the lamina propria, or into the intercellular space and from there into the lamina propria.

The intercellular passage commences with the tight junction which morphologically appears to fuse the brush border membranes of adjacent enterocytes into a continuum. Functionally, however, the tight junction is not tight, but allows the passing of both water and solutes. In fact, a major portion of the intestinal salt and water absorption is channeled through the tight junction and intercellular channels (FRÖMTER and DIAMOND 1972). Calcium chelation enhances the permeability of the tight junction to nonelectrolytes, but not to sodium (CSÁKY and AUTENRIETH 1975). There is no evidence for a specific transport mechanism across the tight junction and intercellular channels. Substances which pass through this route eventually cross the basement membrane and end up in the lamina propria just like the permeants across cells. The lamina propria is richly endowed with capillaries in which permeants can rapidly be taken up. Substrates which cannot readily pass the capillary wall, end up in the lymph and are carried through the mesenteric lymph vessels into the thoracic duct which empties into the bloodstream (DEAK 1977).

So far, the mechanism of intestinal absorption has been outlined. When considering intestinal permeation by definition one refers to a two-way process: absorption and exorption, i.e., secretion or excretion. While a good deal of knowledge has been accumulated concerning intestinal absorption, knowledge about the mechanisms of exorption is rather limited. There is continuous leak of both electrolytes and nonelectrolytes from the bloodstream into the lumen of the gut. Manipulations which increase the permeability of the tight junction, enhance the exorption. This indicates that, at least in part, the intercellular route is involved in the process of exorption.

The intestine actively transports sugars, amino acids, purines, pyrimidines, and other essential nutrients along with sodium, chloride, and other ions from the lumen into the bloodstream against a higher concentration. This active transport mechanism assures the steady reabsorption of the essential nutrients as soon as they are leaked into the UWL. Thus, active transport provides an important and essential mechanism for the maintenance of the body's homeostasis. Recent observations concerning an active uphill secretion of certain drugs clearly indicate the involvement of carrier in the exorption process. It has even been suggested that the same carrier may be involved in both absorption and exorption (TURNHEIM and LAUTERBACH 1981).

References

Bennet HS (1956) The concept of membrane flow and membrane vesiculation as mechanisms for active transport and ion pumping. J Biophys Biochem Cytol [Suppl]2:99

Binder HJ (ed) (1979) Mechanism of intestinal secretion. Alan R. Liss, New York

Blecher M, Bar RS (1981) Receptors and human disease. Williams and Wilkins, Baltimore, pp 2–23

Brandt PW (1958) A study of the mechanism of pinocytosis. Exp Cell Res 15:300

Brandt PW, Pappas GJ (1960) An electronmicroscopic study of pinocytosis in amoeba. J Biophys Biochem Cytol 8:675

Code CF (ed) (1968) Intestinal absorption. American Physiological Society, Washington DC (Handbook of physiology, vol 3)

Cohen JB, Changeux JP (1975) The cholinergic receptor protein in its membrane environment. Ann Rev Pharmacol 15:83–103

Csáky TZ (1981) Factors involved in the integrated mechanism of intestinal absorption. In: Advances in physiological sciences. Proceedings of the 28th international congress of physiological sciences, Budapest, 1980, Pergamon, Oxford, vol 12, p 411

Csáky TZ, Autenrieth B (1975) Transcellular and intercellular intestinal transport. In: Csáky TZ (ed) Intestinal absorption and malabsorption. Raven, New York, pp 177–185

Csáky TZ, Fernald (1960) Absorption of 3-methylglucose from the intestine of the frog, Rana pipiens. Am J Physiol 198:445–448

Csáky TZ, HO PM (1966) The effect of dimethylsulfoxide on the intestinal sugar transport. Proc Soc Exp Biol Med 122:860–865

Danielli JF (1954) The present position in the field of facilitated diffusion and selective active transport. Proc Symp Colston Res Soc 7:1–4

Deak ST (1977) Factors regulating the intestinal lymphatic absorption of nutrients and drugs. Dissertation, University of Kentucky

Fick A (1855) Über Diffusion. Ann Physik U Chem 94:59–86

Frömter E, Diamond JM (1972) Route of passive ion permeation in epithelia. Nature 235:9–13

György AZ, Kinne R (1971) Energy source for transepithelial sodium transport in rat renal protineal tubules. Pflugers Arch 327:234–260

Holter H (1979) Problems of pinocytosis with special regard to amoebae. Ann NY Acad Sci 78:524–537

Lewis WR (1931) Pinocytosis. Bull Johns Hopkins Hosp 49:17–27

Marshall DA, Shumaker VN, Brandt PW (1959) Pinocytosis in amoebae. Ann NY Acad Sci 78:515–523

May AJ, Whaler BC (1958) The absorption of clostridium botulinum type A toxin from the alimentary canal. Br J Exp Pathol 39:307–317

Mercer EH (1959) An electron microscopic study of amoeba proteus. Proc R Soc Lond B 150:216

Parsons DS (1963) Quantitative aspects of pinocytosis in relation to intestinal absorption. Nature 199:1192–1193

Shumaker VN (1958) Uptake of protein from solutions by amoeba proteus. Exp Cell Res 15:314

Turnheim K, Lauterbach F (1980) Interaction between intestinal absorption and secretion of monoquaternary ammonium compounds in guinea pigs. A concept of the absorption kinetics of organic cations. J Pharmacol Exp Ther 212:418–424

Verzár F, McDougall EJ (1936) Absorption from the intestine. Longmans, London

Volkheimer G (1972) Persorption. Thieme, Stuttgart

Wilson TH (1962) Intestinal absorption. Saunders, Philadelphia

Wiseman G (1964) Absorption from the intestine. Academic London

CHAPTER 3

Permeability and Related Phenomena: Basic Concepts

V. CAPRARO

A. Introduction

The overall permeability of the intestinal wall is a complex phenomenon in which simple diffusion, across the cellular layer and the intercellular space, and carrier-facilitated transport are involved. The carrier mediation results in facilitated diffusion or in an energy-requiring transport (active transport). Furthermore, the intestinal permeability of water is clearly distinguishable from the permeability to solutes.

The original model of membrane carriers (diffusing carriers) has been recently subjected to a deep revision (see for instance KLINKENBERG 1981); however, the mechanism of the experimental phenomena is formally well described also by theoretical considerations based on diffusing carriers.

B. Passive Transport of Nonelectrolytes in Solution

The driving force for passive transport always originates in a nonequilibrium and vanishes as the equilibrium is reached. The driving force for active transport causes a state of nonequilibrium and the nonequilibrium is permanent because the living organism is continuously supplying energy of metabolic origin which maintains this driving force.

I. Nonequilibria Determining a Passive Net Flux

The existence of a concentration difference in a solute between two aqueous solutions separated by a permeable membrane determines a net flux of the solute as long as the concentration difference remains. However such a nonequilibrium tends to disappear with the passage of the solute and when the concentration difference vanishes, the net passage disappears too. The existence of a pressure difference between two aqueous phases separated by a membrane permeable to water is the cause of a pressure nonequilibrium. This nonequilibrium determines the filtration of water as long as the nonequilibrium remains. As a consequence of the passage of water the pressure difference tends to equilibrate and when this difference is zero filtration ceases.

The existence of a solubility difference of a substance between two immiscible phases (water/oil) causes a partition nonequilibrium; as long as the concentration ratio between the two phases is different from the partition coefficient a net flux of the solute takes place from the lower to the higher affinity phase. This flux tends to

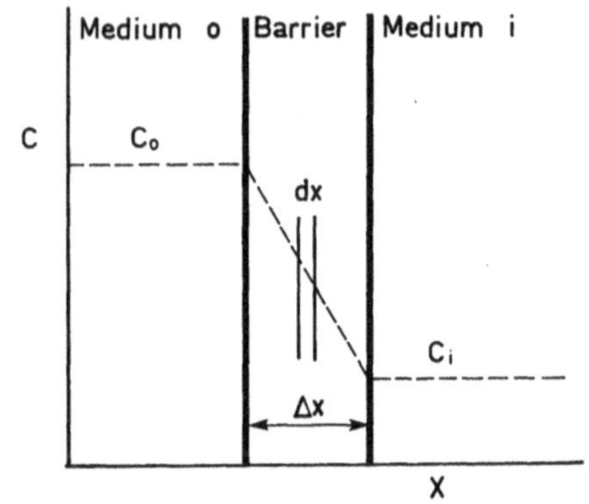

Fig. 1. Schematic representation of a biological barrier dividing two media o and i. The thickness of the barrier is Δx. The aqueous concentrations of the diffusing substance are c_0 and c_i, respectively. The concentration gradient dc/dx is assumed to be constant throughout the barrier

draw the system nearer to a partition equilibrium; when this equilibrium is reached, the net flux disappears.

In spite of a concentration equilibrium between two solutions separated by a membrane permeable to the solute, when a nondiffusible reactant is added to one of the two phases, a new nonequilibrium sets in because the reactant reacts with the solute and takes the solute away from the solution. A net flux of the solute from one of the solutions to the reaction medium begins. The chemical reaction spontaneously tends towards a chemical equilibrium and, when this equilibrium is reached together with the concentration equilibrium between the two solutions, the solute net flux ceases.

II. Kinetics of Polar Solute Passage Driven by a Concentration Difference

If a porous membrane separates two aqueous solutions at different molar concentrations of a diffusible substance c_0 and c_i, respectively, and we assume that: (a) the pores crossing the membrane are regularly cylindrical and all have the same dimensions; (b) there is no fluid movement through the membrane; (c) the diffusing substance does not interact with the pores, we can calculate the driving force on 1 mol solute as follows (BAYLISS 1959).

The work which can be done by 1 mol solute diffusing isothermally and reversibly through a plane within the membrane and diluting itself by an infinitesimal quantity, is

$$RT \, d\ln a \,,$$

where R is the gas constant, T is the absolute temperature and $d\ln a$ is the logarithmic decrement of the chemical activity a of the solute along the distance dx perpendicular to the plane (Fig. 1).

If we divide this equation by dx we obtain a force

$$RT \, d\ln a/dx$$

and if we divide the force acting on 1 mol by N (Avogadro's number), we obtain the force which acts on a single molecule of the solute. Furthermore, by dividing the force acting on a single molecule by the resistence encountered in its movement in water, the molecular friction coefficient f, we obtain $\bar{v}$, the mean velocity of the molecules through the plane

$$\bar{v} = (RT/Nf)(\mathrm{d}\ln a/\mathrm{d}x)\,.$$

Assuming that

$$\mathrm{d}\ln c/\mathrm{d}\ln a = 1$$

we get

$$\bar{v}(RT/Nf)(\mathrm{d}\ln c/\mathrm{d}x) = (RT/Nfc)(\mathrm{d}c/\mathrm{d}x)\,.$$

The net flux of the substance $\dot{n}$ (mol/s) through the plane is proportional to the mean velocity, to the local concentration c and to the total surface of the pores A_p

$$-\dot{n} = A_p c\bar{v} = A_p(RT/Nf)(\mathrm{d}c/\mathrm{d}x) = A_p D(\mathrm{d}c/\mathrm{d}x)\,.$$

By integrating this equation between c_o and c_i and between 0 and Δx, the total thickness of the membrane, and assuming that c_o and c_i are equal to the concentrations at the external and internal borders of the membrane, we can write

$$\dot{n} = A_p D(c_o - c_i)/\Delta x\,.$$

The area of the pores A_p and the membrane thickness Δx, in many cases, may be assumed constant, but unknown, and the formula becomes

$$\dot{n} = AP(c_o - c_i)\,.$$

Where A is the apparent surface of the membrane, D is the diffusion coefficient of the solute considered, and P is the permeability coefficient of the same solute through the membrane.

If the physical quantities are expressed in mol, s, cm, cm^2, cm^3, the physical dimensions of D are cm^2/s and those of P are cm/s.

Graphical examples of thermal diffusion following these kinetics are reported in Fig. 2. As a matter of fact, the linearity of the relationship between net fluxes and concentration differences over a wide range of concentration difference strongly suggests a passive diffusion (see Sect. D). The diffusion coefficient D and the permeability coefficient P which is linearly proportional to D, decrease as the molecular weight of the solute M increases, following the equation

$$\log D = \alpha - \beta \log M\,.$$

The value of β is not constant and depends on the molecular weight of the diffusing substance (STEIN 1967). For diffusion in water, a molecular weight of 250 appears to be a transition point between two values of β; above this value the following equation seems to be valid

$$M^{1/3}D = \text{constant}$$

i.e., β, has a value of $\frac{1}{3}$; below 250 another equation seems to be valid

$$M^{1/2}D = \text{constant}\,.$$

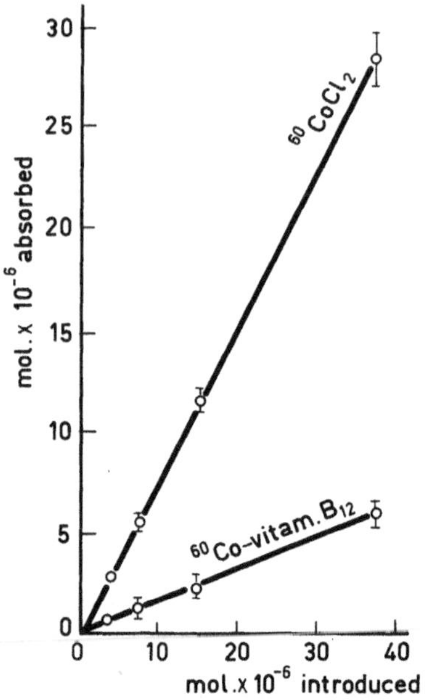

Fig. 2. Intestinal absorption, by apparently thermal diffusion kinetics, of Vitamin B_{12} ^{60}Co and of $^{60}CoCl_2$. Rat small intestine was separated by ligatures from the upper and lower sections of the gut, yet retaining its vascular and nervous connections with the body. The intrinsic factor is absent so that the facilitated absorption process does not appear under these experimental conditions. CAPRARO and CRESSERI (1964)

In this case the value of β is $\frac{1}{2}$.

The diffusion coefficient D is lower than the theoretical value when the wall offers an appreciable resistance to the diffusing substance, i.e. when the pore radius r_p is less than ten times the molecular radius r_m. In this case, we have a reduced diffusion coefficient D'. The quotient D'/D is (RENKIN 1955)

$$D'/D = (1 - r_m/r_p)^2[1 - 2.10(r_m/r_p) + 2.09(r_m/r_p)^3 + 0.95(r_m/r_p)^5]\,.$$

III. Kinetics of Nonpolar Solute Passage Driven by a Concentration Difference

The lipidic nature of most biological membranes has already been extensively illustrated. OVERTON (1899) made the fundamental observation that lipophilic substances overcome the cellular plasma membrane easier than water-soluble ones. Therefore the kinetics of such a transport is of great biological interest. Let us imagine a lipidic film with a thickness Δx, dividing two aqueous media o and i (Fig. 3).

If we assume that the passage of the lipophilic substance from the aqueous to the lipidic phase, and vice versa, are processes which are quicker than the transport within the lipidic film, the kinetics of such a transport is describable by the following equation

$$\dot{n} = ADq(c_o - c_i)/\Delta x\,,$$

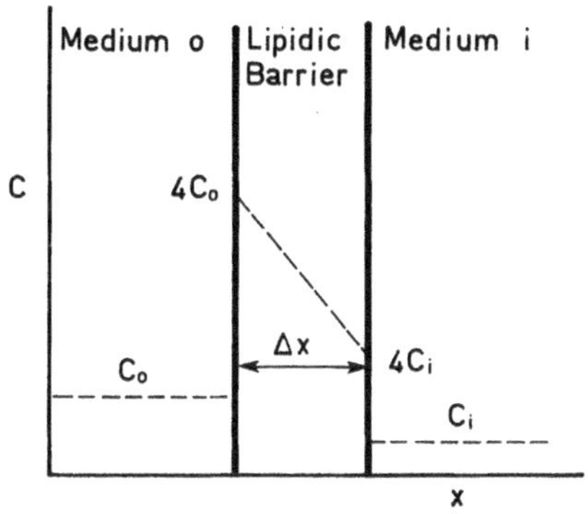

Fig. 3. Schematic representation of a lipidic barrier dividing two aqueous media o and i. The aqueous concentrations of the diffusing lipophilic substance are c_0 and c_i, respectively. In this example the partition coefficient oil/water is 4

where q is the partition coefficient between fat and water (the value of q is 4 in Fig. 3) and D is the diffusion coefficient of the lipophilic substance within the lipidic material. The thickness of the lipidic film Δx in many cases may be assumed constant, but unknown and therefore the equation can be written as follows

$$\dot{n} = AP(c_o - c_i),$$

where P also includes the value of q together with Δx. This equation has been supported by several experimental data. In fact if we take into account the reported relationship between D or P (including q) and M values for a series of lipophilic substances crossing a biological barrier, we obtain

$$PM^{1/2}/q = \text{const}.$$

IV. Calculation of the Relative Values of the Permeability Coefficients of a Substance Across Two Membranes in Series

If two media are separated by two membranes in series, as for example the plasma mucosal membrane and the basolateral membrane of an epithelial layer, the relative values of P for the two membranes can easily be calculated, under conditions of steady state passive transport, with a given water-soluble substance. The intracellular concentration c_c as well as the concentration in the external medium c_o and the concentration in the internal medium c_i must be experimentally determined in order to calculate the P values (P_m and P_s respectively). The kinetics of the two transmembrane transport processes are defined by the following equations

$$\dot{n}_{oc} = AP_m(c_o - c_c),$$

$$\dot{n}_{ci} = AP_s(c_c - c_i).$$

Under conditions of steady state net transport the two molar transport rates are equal ($\dot{n}_{oc} = \dot{n}_{ci}$), and therefore we have

$$AP_m(c_o - c_c) = AP_s(c_c - c_i)$$

and if the two apparent surface areas are considered equal

$$P_m/P_s = (c_c - c_i)/(c_o - c_c).$$

Obviously, if the two apparent membrane areas are not equal, a surface factor must be included, in the term P_m/P_s.

C. Passive Transport of Univalent Electrolytes

I. Kinetics of the Passive Net Transport of Univalent Electrolytes Across a Porous Membrane

Two forces are responsible for passive movement of electrolytes across a porous membrane, the force originating from a concentration gradient dc/dx and the force originating from an electrical potential gradient dE/dx. The kinetics of the net passage through an infinitely small layer dx of the membrane and an aqueous pore area A_p is defined by the following equation

$$-\dot{n} = A_p Dc\{(d\ln c/dx) \pm (F/RT)dE/dx)\},$$

where F is the quantity of electricity transported by an ion equivalent (Faraday). In fact the two forces acting on one equivalent of the charged univalent ion are respectively

$$RT\,d\ln c/dx \quad \text{and} \quad \pm F\,dE/dx.$$

If we introduce the concept of the mobility of the ion u ($D = uRT$), expressed in the physical dimensions $cm^2\,mol/s^{-1}J^{-1}$, the equation becomes

$$-\dot{n} = A_p uc\{RT(d\ln c/dx) \pm F\,dE/dx\}.$$

The current i transported by the net movement of one kind of ion becomes

$$\pm i = \dot{n}F.$$

If we consider a unit area and we assume that the friction coefficient f is independent of the concentration and that the electrical field inside the membrane is constant ($dE/dx = \Delta E/\Delta x$), these flux or current equations can be integrated with respect to x between the limits of zero and Δx and between the concentrations c_o and c_i of the ion at the borders of the membrane (BAYLISS 1959).

Integration for the net flux of a univalent ion gives the following result

$$\dot{n} = \pm\{c_o Fu(\Delta E/\Delta x)/[1 - \exp(\mp F\Delta E/RT)]\}\exp(\mp F\Delta E/RT)$$
$$\mp\{c_i Fu(\Delta E/\Delta x)/[1 - \exp(\mp F\Delta E/RT)]\}.$$

The two terms in this equation are the inward and outward ion fluxes, respectively.

II. Transmembrane Potentials

From the equations giving all single passive ion currents which cross the membrane and assuming that the algebraic sum of these currents is zero we can derive the equation for the transmembrane potential ΔE as a function of the ion concentrations in the two media (o and i respectively) and of the permeability coefficients of the same ions through the membrane. In the case of the plasma cell membrane the i and o media are the cellular and the external medium of the cell, respectively. Assuming that Na, K and Cl are the only ions crossing the cell membrane, this equation becomes the GOLDMAN equation

$$\Delta E=(RT/F)\ln\{(P_{\mathrm{Na}}[\mathrm{Na}]_i+P_{\mathrm{K}}[\mathrm{K}]_i+P_{\mathrm{Cl}}[\mathrm{Cl}]_o)/(P_{\mathrm{Na}}[\mathrm{Na}]_o+P_{\mathrm{K}}[\mathrm{K}]_o+P_{\mathrm{Cl}}[\mathrm{Cl}]_i)\}$$

In many cases, this formula fits the experimental data much better than the NERNST formula

$$\Delta E=(RT/F)\ln(c_i/c_o),$$

where c is the concentration of a single diffusible ion in the media o and i, respectively; the more highly concentrated medium is the numerator of the concentration ratio. This equation was derived from the assumption that the membrane is passively permeable to one or more ions, but not all ions, and that the intracellular composition is, therefore, in a state of true equilibrium. However, in many cases the cell composition is in a condition of steady nonequilibrium, and changes throughout the course of the in vitro experiment.

Other types of electrical potential originate in the movement of ions in the biological structures. Let us suppose that a solution of a permeable electrolyte such as NaCl in the medium o is in contact, through a porous membrane with a solution of the same electrolyte at a lower concentration in the medium i. If the mobilities of the two ions of the salt are different, a potential difference appears, called the diffusion potential.

The mean velocity of the sodium ion $\bar{v}_{\mathrm{Na}}$ must become equal to the mean velocity of the chloride ion $\bar{v}_{\mathrm{Cl}}$ and both velocities depend on the forces acting on ions (driving forces and resistance of the medium). If we consider a unit pore area and if the mobility of sodium ion u^+ is higher than the mobility of chloride ion u^-, the velocities are respectively

$$\bar{v}_{\mathrm{Na}}=(u^+/F)(RT\,\mathrm{d}\ln c/\mathrm{d}x-F\mathrm{d}E/\mathrm{d}x),$$

$$\bar{v}_{\mathrm{Cl}}=(u^-/F)(RT\,\mathrm{d}\ln c/\mathrm{d}x+F\mathrm{d}E/\mathrm{d}x).$$

From these equations we obtain

$$\mathrm{d}E/\mathrm{d}x=\{(u^+-u^-)/(u^++u^-)\}(RT/F)\,\mathrm{d}\ln c/\mathrm{d}x$$

and by integration with respect to x between the limits of 0 and Δx (the thickness of the membrane), between c_o and c_i and between E_o and E_i, we obtain

$$\Delta E=\{(u^+-u^-)/(u^++u^-)\}(RT/F)\ln(c_o/c_i).$$

The diffusion potential, at room temperature, increases by a factor inferior to 0.058 V for a tenfold increase of c_o/c_i; in fact, this factor is

$$\{2.3(u^+-u^-)/(u^++u^-)\}RT/F.$$

An example of diffusion potential is illustrated in Fig. 4.

Let us suppose that two equally concentrated solutions of NaCl are separated by a porous membrane permeable to the salt. A transmembrane potential may

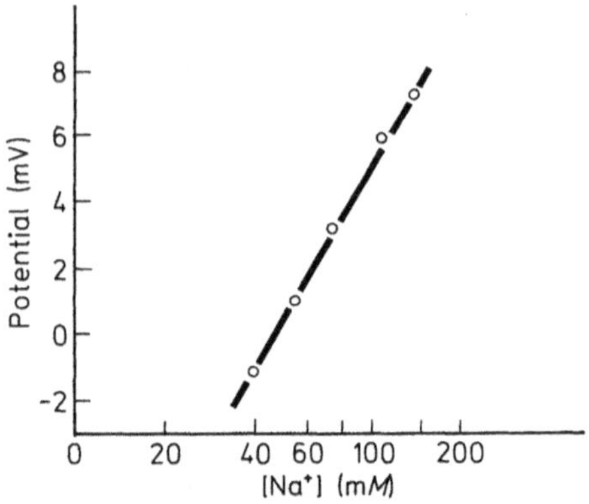

Fig. 4. Rabbit gallbladder mucosa perfused in vitro and poisoned with amphotericin B 40 μg/ml. Under normal conditions the transepithelial potential difference is negligible. After the addition of amphotericin, a positive potential appears on the serosal side and the net flow of water ceases. The figure shows that when the NaCl of the bathing fluids is gradually replaced by isotonic mannitol, the potential decreases linearly with the logarithm of the NaCl concentration. The slope of this function is 15.5 mV for a tenfold change of the NaCl concentration. Therefore, this potential seems to be due to the diffusional entry of NaCl through the brush border of the epithelial cell. The entry is noticeably increased as a consequence of the permeability induced by amphotericin B. HENIN and CREMASCH (1975)

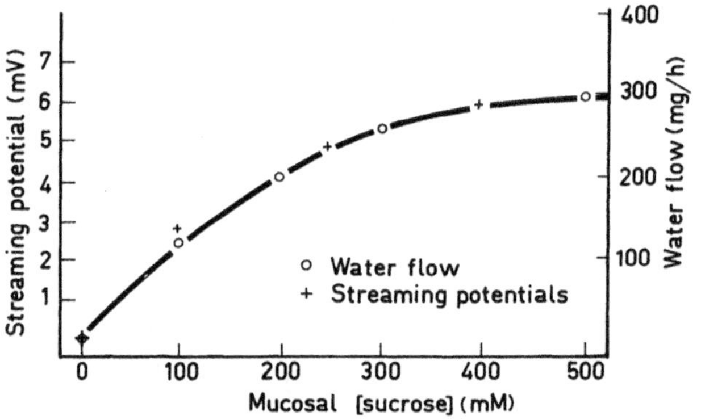

Fig. 5. Streaming potentials (*crosses*) and gravimetrically measured water flows (*circles*) in the gallbladder epithelium in vitro. The bathing solutions are Na_2SO_4 Ringer's solutions; the mucosal solution is made hypertonic by the addition of sucrose at the concentrations indicated. A positive water flow means flow from serosa to mucosa; a positive streaming potential means that the mucosa is electrically positive. DIAMOND (1966)

arise, even in this case, if there is a net water flow through the membrane due for instance to an osmotic gradient. This potential (streaming potential) is caused by the fact that the resistance to one of the two ions during the passage through the membrane is higher than the resistance to the other; for instance, the fixed charges of the pore walls attract one of the two ions and repulse the other. The streaming potential is proportional to the volumetric flow; for rabbit gallbladder in vitro the average value of the proportionality coefficient is, in this case, 1 mV for 0.002 $cm^3 cm^{-2} h^{-1}$ of volumetric flow (Fig 5; DIAMOND 1966).

III. Transepithelial Potentials

The intestinal epithelial cell, from an electrophysiological point of view, may be represented by an electrical model (Fig. 6). At least two sources of electrical potential are present in the cell, one linked to the mucosal membrane and the other linked to the basolateral one (ΔE_m and ΔE_s, respectively). The transepithelial potential is not the algebraic sum of these potentials because an electrical current circulates through the resistances R_m and R_s in the cell and R_{sh} in the paracellular channels. As a matter of fact, the epithelial battery is short-circuited through these channels.

Keeping in mind this model the short-circuiting current i is equal to

$$i=(\Delta E_m+\Delta E_s)/(R_{sh}+R_m+R_s)$$

and the measured transmembrane electrical potentials (this measurement is possible by the impaling of the cell with microelectrodes) which are named V_m and V_s, respectively, are equal to

$$V_m=\Delta E_m-iR_m=\Delta E_m-(\Delta E_m+\Delta E_s)\{R_m/(R_{sh}+R_m+R_s)\},$$

$$V_s=\Delta E_s-iR_s=\Delta E_s-(\Delta E_m+\Delta E_s)\{R_s/(R_{sh}+R_m+R_s)\}.$$

In the intestinal epithelium as in other low resistance epithelia, V_m and V_s have opposite electrical signs, so that the transepithelial potential V_{ms} is equal to the difference between V_m and V_s, and is usually positive in the serosal medium. V_m and V_s have values somewhere around 40–60 mV (HENIN and CREMASCHI 1975) and V_{ms} has a value of about 5–10 mV. The electrical profile through a single cell is represented in Fig. 7.

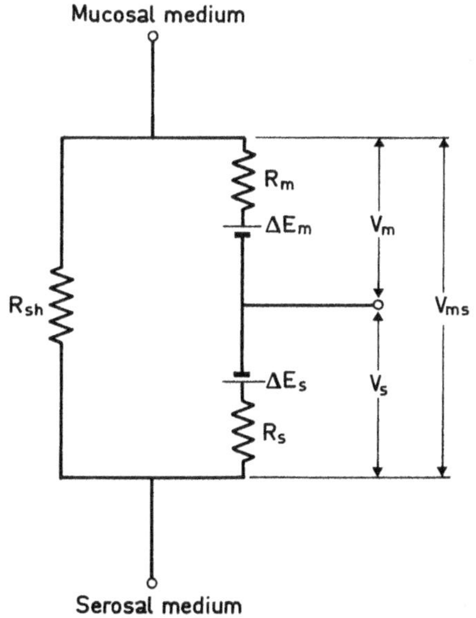

Fig. 6. Electrical equivalent circuit of the intestinal epithelial cell. The shunt resistance of the paracellular channels R_{sh} is low, i.e., this epithelium is a low resistance epithelium

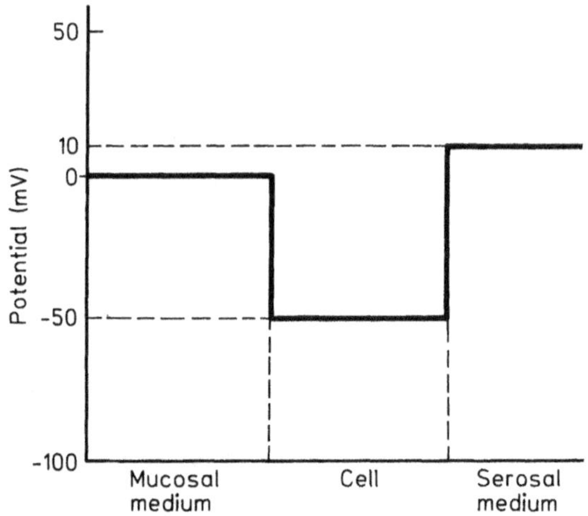

Fig. 7. Electrical profile through the intestinal epithelial cell. The potential values are plotted on the ordinate against the tissue compartments on the abscissa

D. Transport Across Biological Membranes

I. Passive Transport of Polar Nonelectrolytes Through Biological Membranes

Even if pores are present in biological membranes, they presumably are not regular and their resistance to diffusion is not uniformly distributed within the membrane. Therefore Fick's equation

$$-\dot{n} = A_p D \mathrm{d}c/\mathrm{d}x$$

cannot be integrated between 0 and Δx, because A_p is an unknown function of x.

However, a different conclusion may be drawn if we wish to determine only the ratio between the two unidirectional fluxes of the same substance through the same membrane and in the same time. These fluxes are termed ϕ_{oi} and ϕ_{io}, respectively. In order to determine these fluxes we must use two tracers for the same substance (for instance thiourea ^{36}S and thiourea ^{14}C) by adding each tracer to one medium only (tracer o in medium o and tracer i in medium i) and by measuring the corresponding radioactivity emerging on the other side.

The flux quotient is

$$\phi_{oi}/\phi_{io} = A_p D_o (\mathrm{d}c_o/\mathrm{d}x)/A_p D_i (\mathrm{d}c_i/\mathrm{d}x)\,.$$

Since at a given value of x the area of the pores are equal and the diffusion coefficients of the two tracers D_o and D_i are equal too, we can say

$$\phi_{oi}/\phi_{io} = (\mathrm{d}c_o/\mathrm{d}x)/(\mathrm{d}c_i/\mathrm{d}x)\,.$$

This equation can be integrated with respect to x between the limits of 0 and Δx (the thickness of the membrane) and between c_o and 0 for tracer o and between c_i and 0 for tracer i

$$\phi_{oi}/\phi_{io} = c_o/c_i\,.$$

This flux equation is physically valid for every concentration profile within the membrane. However, three exceptions must be considered:

a. When the unidirectional fluxes are "single-file fluxes" (BAYLISS 1959). In this case the pores are so narrow that only a single molecule at a time can enter the pore and the molecules are placed in single file in the pore. The flux quotient is

$$\phi_{oi}/\phi_{io}=(c_o/c_i)^n,$$

where n depends on the number of sites in the file. Obviously if $c_o/c_i=1$, n is irrelevant and $\phi_{oi}/\phi_{io}=1$.

b. When the fluxes obey the law of exchange diffusion (see Sect. E). In this case, even if c_o is different from c_i the flux quotient remains close to 1.

c. When the fluxes are modified by a simultaneous volumetric flow (see Sect. F). In order to avoid such an error we can try to prevent the net passage of water.

II. Passive Transport of Polar Electrolytes Through Biological Membranes

The kinetics of the passage of an electrolyte cannot be described by the equation given in Sect. C because the mechanical and electrical forces are not uniformly distributed within the membrane. The equation can be written as follows

$$-\dot{n}=(A_p c/Nf)(RT\,\mathrm{d}\ln c/\mathrm{d}x \pm F\mathrm{d}E/\mathrm{d}x).$$

Now let us consider the unidirectional fluxes of the sodium ion through a membrane with thickness Δx from a medium o to a medium i (with tracer o), or vice versa (with tracer i) in the case in which the concentration of sodium ion in medium o is lower than that in medium i, and a transmembrane potential which is positive in medium i is present. The unidirectional fluxes, at a given value of x, can be expressed by the following equations

$$-\phi_{oi}=(A_p c_o/Nf)(RT\,\mathrm{d}\ln c_o/\mathrm{d}x - F\mathrm{d}E/\mathrm{d}x),$$

$$-\phi_{io}=(A_p c_i/Nf)(RT\,\mathrm{d}\ln c_i/\mathrm{d}x + F\mathrm{d}E/\mathrm{d}x).$$

Now we introduce an auxiliary variable c', which is defined as follows

$$RT\,\mathrm{d}\ln c' = RT\ln c + FE,$$

where c and E are the concentration and the potential at a given value of x. We can also derive the following equations

$$c'=c\exp(FE/RT),$$

$$c=c'\exp(-FE/RT),$$

$$RT\,\mathrm{d}\ln c'/\mathrm{d}x = RT\,\mathrm{d}\ln c/\mathrm{d}x \pm F\mathrm{d}E/\mathrm{d}x.$$

By introducing these expressions in the equations for the unidirectional fluxes, we obtain

$$-\phi_{oi} = (A_p/Nf)c'_o \exp(-FE/RT)RT\,\mathrm{d}\ln c'_o/\mathrm{d}x$$
$$= (A_p/Nf)\exp(-FE/RT)RT\,\mathrm{d}c'_o/\mathrm{d}x$$
$$\phi_{io} = (A_p/Nf)c'_i \exp(-FE/RT)RT\,\mathrm{d}\ln c'_i/\mathrm{d}x = (A_p/Nf)\exp(-FE/RT)\mathrm{d}c'_i/\mathrm{d}x\,.$$

Now, by dividing the two expressions we obtain

$$\phi_{oi}/\phi_{io} = (\mathrm{d}c'_o/\mathrm{d}x)/(\mathrm{d}c'_i/\mathrm{d}x)\,.$$

By integrating this equation with respect to x between the limits of 0 and Δx, we have

$$\phi_{oi}/\phi_{io} = c'_o/c'_i,$$

where c'_o and c'_i are the values of c' for tracers o and i in media o and i, respectively.

Therefore

$$\phi_{oi}/\phi_{io} = c_o\exp(FE/RT)/(c_i\exp-(F(E+\Delta E)) = (c_o/c_i)\exp(-F\Delta E/RT),$$

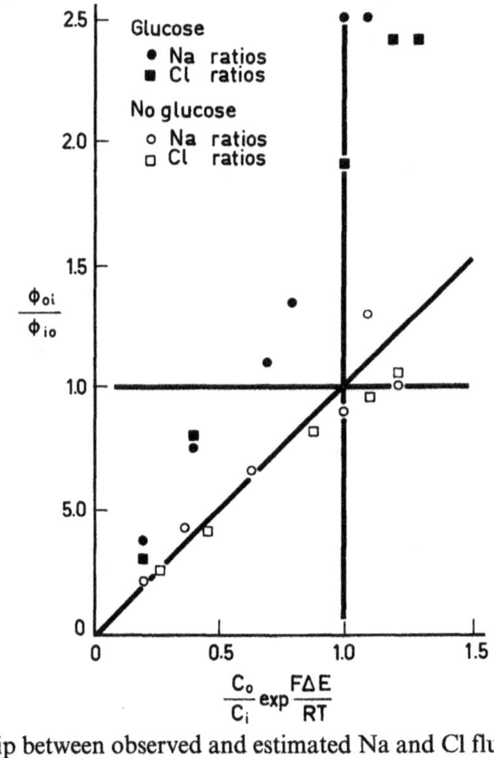

Fig. 8. Relationship between observed and estimated Na and Cl flux quotients in rat ileum in vitro. The line fits the expected values. ϕ_{oi}/ϕ_{io} values reported on the ordinate are the values of the quotient of mucosal to serosal medium flux divided by serosal to mucosal medium flux; c_o/c_i values reported on the abscissa are the values of the mucosal concentration of the ion considered divided by the serosal concentration of the same ion. In the presence of glucose, the observed values do not fit the expected line because there is an active transport of Na as well as Cl. In the absence of glucose no active transport is possible, since metabolism is decreased and the observed values fit the expected line. CURRAN (1960)

where c_o and c_i are the concentrations of tracers o and i in media o and i, respectively.

The flux equation of a univalent electrolyte (USSING 1949) like the flux equation of a nonelectrolyte, is physically valid for every concentration and potential profile within the membrane, with the exceptions already mentioned, and may be used in order to check the passive nature of an ion transport process (Fig. 8; see Sect. G).

E. Passive Transport by Carrier Facilitation[1]

I. Kinetics of Carrier-facilitated Transport

Most biological transport phenomena do not have the kinetics of thermal diffusion. In fact there are many water-soluble substances which, in spite of their high molecular weights (monosaccharides, amino acids etc.), are readily able to cross plasma membranes. Furthermore, substances of equal molecular weight and similar structure (D-glucose and D-mannose) differ substantially in their capacity to cross certain biological barriers (intestinal mucosa).

A chemical combination between these specifically facilitated substances and a carrier present in the membrane has been supposed to occur (WILBRANDT and ROSENBERG 1961). Only the complex of transported substance and the carrier CS crosses the membrane, owing to the affinity between the carrier and the membrane (more precisely, the affinity between the carrier and the lipids of the membrane).

Let us assume that on each side of the membrane (medium o and medium i) the equilibrium of the chemical reaction between the substance S and the carrier C is reached instantaneously

$$S_o + C \rightleftharpoons CS_o,$$

$$S_i + C \rightleftharpoons CS_i.$$

When the equilibria are reached, we have

$$([C]_t - [CS_o])[S_o]/[CS_o] = K_m,$$

$$([C]_t - [CS_i])[S_i]/[CS_i] = K_m.$$

From these equations we reach the following expressions for the concentration of CS at the two limits of the membrane

$$[CS]_o = [C]_t[S_o]/(K_m + [S_o]),$$

$$[CS]_i = [C]_t[S_i]/(K_m + [S_i]),$$

where $[C]_t$ is the sum of free and combined [C] and K_m is the apparent affinity constant.

If we now apply Fick's equation to the diffusion of CS through the membrane we have an equation which describes the kinetics of the chemically facilitated transport

$$\dot{n} = AD_{CS}([C]_t/\Delta x)\{([S_o]/(K_m + [S_o]) - [S_i]/(K_m + [S_i])\},$$

where D_{CS} is the diffusion coefficient of CS inside the membrane itself.

1 This topic is also discussed in Vol. 70/II, Chap. 21

II. Calculation of the Apparent Affinity Constant

If equilibration of a chemically facilitated transport process is considered at the beginning of the reaction, the second term in brackets in the final equation of Sect. E.I is close to zero, so that we may say

$$\dot{n} = AD_{CS}([C]_t/\Delta x)([S_o]/(K_m + [S_o])\,.$$

If $[S_o]$ is high enough, the flux becomes maximal ($\dot{n}_{max}$)

$$\dot{n} = AD_{CS}([C]_t/\Delta x) = \dot{n}_{max}$$

so that the expression may be written as follows

$$\dot{n} = \dot{n}_{max}[S_o]/(K_m + [S_o])\,.$$

This equation is similar to the Michaelis-Menten equation for enzymatic processes. In our case K_m is not the equilibrium constant of the reaction between the substrate and the specific enzyme, but the equilibrium constant of the reaction between the transported substance and the specific carrier. Following the Lineweaver-Burk method, the Michaelis-Menten equation can be modified to the reciprocal equation

$$1/\dot{n} = 1/\dot{n}_{max} + (K_m/\dot{n}_{max})1/[S_o]\,.$$

In this equation, the reciprocal of the molar net flux is a linear function of the reciprocal of the outside concentration (Fig. 9; DIEDRICH 1966).

The intercept on the ordinate ($1/[S_o] = 0$) gives the reciprocal of the maximal flux. The intercept on the abscissa ($1/\dot{n} = 0$)

$$1/K_m = -1/[S_o]$$

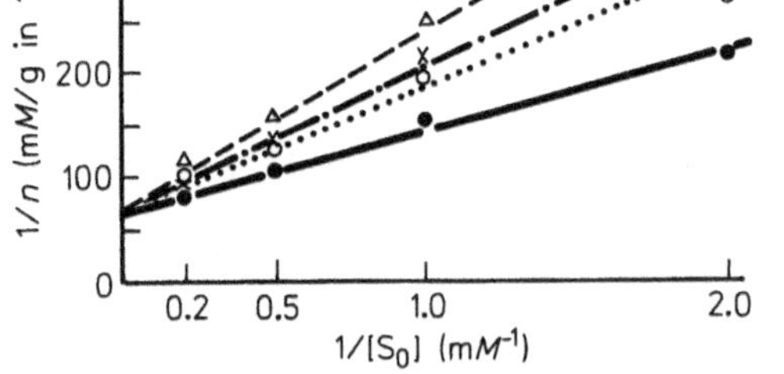

Fig. 9. Lineweaver-Burk plot of the reciprocal of D-glucose concentration in medium o on the abscissa against the reciprocal of D-glucose entry into the tissue on the ordinate. Small intestine of a golden hamster incubated in vitro. *Full circles* control experiments; other symbols indicate intestine treated with increasing concentrations of phlorizin: *open circles* 4 μM; crosses 5 μM; *triangles* 8 μM. DIEDRICH (1966)

i.e., the reciprocal of K_m, is equal to the reciprocal of the outside concentration $[S_o]$. Therefore, by means of the Lineweaver–Burk plot it is easy to determine the maximal net flux as well as the formal affinity constant of a chemically facilitated transport process. However, this method, like other similar ones, under a variety of experimental conditions, is liable to overestimate the mucosal concentration $[S_o]$ because of inadequate stirring of the outside medium; for this reason the bulk concentration of S is higher than the concentration of S in the aqueous layer facing the mucosal surface because of the continuous removal of S for transport. A correction must be introduced in order to have acceptable values of K_m (see Chap. 21).

III. Saturation Kinetics

If we consider the kinetics of a chemically facilitated transport process, we first of all observe that when $[S_o]$ and $[S_i]$ are low these kinetics can not be distinguished from simple diffusion kinetics, i.e., the net transport is linearly proportional to the concentration difference of the transported substance between medium o and medium i. But by increasing these concentrations, the flux rate loses its linearity and tends towards a limiting value. This behaviour can also be derived mathematically from the general equation if we suppose that concentrations of S are close to carrier saturation. In fact, under these conditions, the equilibrium equations are approximately

$$([C]_t-[CS_o])[S_o]/[C]_t=K_m\,,$$

$$([C]_t-[CS_i])[S_i]/[C]_t=K_m$$

and the CS concentrations at the two limits of the membrane are

$$[CS]_o=[C]_t\{1-K_m/[S_o]\}\,,$$

$$[CS]_i=[C]_t\{1-K_m/[S_i]\}\,.$$

Therefore, the general equation of the facilitated transport process becomes

$$\dot{n}=AD_{CS}([C]_t/\Delta x)K_m\{1/[S_i]-1/[S_o]\}\,.$$

Now, if we suppose that while $[S_i]$ remains constant, $[S_o]$ progressively increases, the second term in brackets tends to vanish and $\dot{n}$ becomes constant, in spite of the fact that the concentration difference increases. This may be the case for intestinal absorption of some nutrients in vivo, when the luminal concentration of the transported substance increases and the concentration of the same substance in the blood remains almost constant (Table 1, first condition). On the other hand, if we suppose that while $[S_o]$ remains constant $[S_i]$ progressively decreases, $\dot{n}$ increases many times more than the concentration difference (Table 1, second condition). This may be the case of facilitated transport from the extracellular space, $[S_o]$, to the intracellular space, $[S_i]$. The intracellular concentration decreases owing to higher utilization. Chemically facilitated transport may permit a much more efficient adaptation to the needs of the cell than simple diffusion.

Finally, if we suppose that the outside and inside concentrations grow together in spite of the fact that the concentration difference remains constant, the net flux

Table 1. Values of $[S_o]-[S_i]$ and of $1/[S_i]-1/[S_o]$ calculated from hypothetical values of $[S_o]$ and $[S_i]$ under three different conditions (see text)

Experimental condition	$[S_o]$	$[S_i]$	$[S_o]-[S_i]$	$1/[S_i]-1/[S_o]$
First	10	5	5	0.1
condition	50	5	45	0.18
	100	5	95	0.19
Second	10	5	5	0.1
condition	10	2	8	0.4
	10	1	9	0.9
Third	10	5	5	0.1
condition	50	45	5	0.002
	100	95	5	0.000

tends to vanish and the unidirectional influx becomes equal to the unidirectional outflux (Table 1, third condition); each molecule migrating in one sense is counterbalanced by the migration of another molecule in the opposite sense (exchange diffusion).

IV. Substrate Competition

Owing to their stereochemical similarity, two or more transported substances (for instance D-glucose and D-galactose) may compete for the same carrier. In this case the addition of one of these substances to the medium o inhibits the transport of the other. This case is illustrated in Fig. 9. Phlorhizin and derivatives inhibit the intestinal absorption of D-glucose, presumably because they are competing with the same carrier. Obviously the existence of competition phenomena is another argument in favour of the existence of carrier-transported substances.

V. Countertransport

The concentration equilibrium between medium o and medium i of a chemically facilitated transport process is reached when $[S_o]$ is equal to $[S_i]$. If, at equilibrium, we add to the medium i a substance S′ in competition with S for the same carrier, for example D-glucose to a system in which D-xylose has reached its concentration equilibrium, a transient state appears in which S moves against its concentration gradient from the medium o to the medium i. The uphill movement is possible because of the simultaneous downhill movement of S′ from medium i to medium o (Fig. 10; SALOMON et al. 1961). The countertransport phenomenon is very clearly seen if we apply the chemical concepts already mentioned.

Let us suppose that at each side of the membrane there are two substances, S and S′, competing for the same carrier. The chemical equilibria at each side are respectively

$$([C]_t-[CS]_o-[CS'_o])[S_o]/[CS]_o=K_m,$$

$$([C]_t-[CS]_i-[CS'_i])[S_i]/[CS]_i=K_m.$$

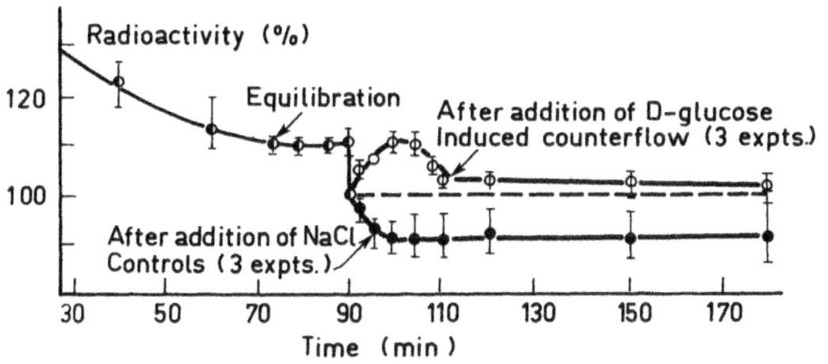

Fig. 10. The entire empty everted small intestine of guinea-pig incubated under air bubbling though an initial volume of 6.5 ml containing 1.95 mg D-xylose and 1 μCi D-xylose-1-^{14}C until equilibration between medium o and tissue is considered complete. Following periodic removal of samples of the incubation fluid, 0.5 ml cold 2*M* glucose or 1 *M* NaCl was added to the remaining 4.5 ml. Periodic fluid aliquots are counted as Ba $^{14}CO_3$. Incubation temperature 37 °C from 0 to 75 min and 0 °C thereafter. Relative levels of radioactivity after the addition of 2*M* glucose and 1 *M* NaCl are given. SALOMON et al. (1961)

Since

$$[CS]_o/[CS]'_o = [S_o]/[S'_o],$$
$$[CS]_i/[CS]'_i = [S_i]/[S'_i]$$

so we can derive the following CS concentrations

$$[CS_o] = [C]_t[S_o]/(K_m + [S_o] + [S'_o]),$$
$$[CS_i] = [C]_t[S_i]/(K_m + [S_i] + [S'_i])$$

and obtain the following kinetic equation

$$\dot{n} = AD_{CS}([C]_t/\Delta x)\{[S_o]/(K_m + [S_o] + [S'_o]) - [S_i]/(K_m + [S_i] + [S'_i])\}.$$

From this formula the conclusion can be drawn that as long as S'_i is higher than S'_o the system remains in a state in which S_i is also higher than S_o, because the two terms in brackets tend to become equal

$$[S_o]/[S_i] = (K_m + [S'_o])/(K_m + [S'_i]).$$

F. Passive Transport of Water

I. Driving Forces

The driving forces which determine the net passage of water across a porous membrane are caused by osmotic and/or pressure nonequilibria and there are two theoretically predictable kinetics: the kinetics arising from a diffusion process for water (molecular flow) and those arising from a water filtration process (bulk flow).

Let us imagine a porous membrane separating two media, o and i, at different osmotic pressure. The thickness of the membrane is Δx and the pores are regularly cylindrical. The net water flow is expressed in ml/s ($\dot{V}$) instead of mol/s ($\dot{n}$)

$$\dot{n} = \dot{V}/\bar{V}_{H_2O}.$$

Where $\bar{V}_{H_2O}$ is the molar volume of water.

If water transport is a simple diffusion process, we have the following expression

$$\dot{V} = A_p D_{H_2O} \bar{V}_{H_2O} \Delta c_{H_2O} / \Delta x .$$

Where D_{H_2O} is the diffusion coefficient of water in water. For sufficiently diluted solutions, two equations may be used to define the osmotic pressure difference $\Delta\pi$

$$\Delta\pi = \Delta c RT \quad \text{(van't Hoff's law)},$$

$$\Delta\pi = \Delta c_{H_2O} RT .$$

This latter equation is obtained by assuming that the driving force for the movement of water is caused by the diffusion of water from the medium in which we have a dilute solution to the medium in which a more concentrated solution is present, taking into account the fact that, in pure water

$$\bar{V}_{H_2O} c_{H_2O} = 1 .$$

From these expressions

$$\Delta c_{H_2O} = \Delta c = \Delta\pi / RT .$$

Therefore, the kinetics of net water transport, following the hypothesis of a molecular diffusion process, can be modified

$$\dot{V} = (A_p D_{H_2O} \bar{V}_{H_2O} / RT) \Delta\pi / \Delta x$$

or

$$\dot{V} = A P_{H_2O} \Delta\pi .$$

On the other hand, if we consider the kinetics to depend on a filtration process under a pressure difference ΔP (bulk flow), we have

$$\dot{V} = (N_p \pi r_p^4 / 8\eta) \Delta P / \Delta x .$$

This is the Poiseuille equation, where N_p is the number of the cylindrical pores crossing the area A, r_p is the pore radius and η is the viscosity coefficient of the fluid moving through the channels.

$$N_p = A_p / r_p^2 \pi .$$

Introducing this value of N_p in the Poiseuille equation, we obtain

$$\dot{V} = (A_p r_p^2 / 8\eta) \Delta P / \Delta x .$$

The behaviour of the transport of water through some biological membranes (frog skin, kidney tubules, frog urinary bladder) under the action of vasopressin suggests that an osmotic gradient also provokes a bulk flow of water as does a hydrostatic pressure gradient, so that the kinetics of water flow seems to be described in all cases by the Poiseuille equation in which ΔP can be substituted by $\Delta\pi$. As a matter of fact, if we determine, by using labelled water (D_2O, T_2O) added to one of the media, the unidirectional flux of water (ϕ_{oi} or ϕ_{io}) across one of the biological membranes mentioned (for instance frog skin, KOEFOED-JOHNSEN and USSING 1952; CAPRARO and BERNINI 1952) in the absence of an osmotic gradient, we

Table 2. Effect of vasopressin on the unidirectional flux ϕ_{oi} and the flux of water $\dot{V}$ before and after the addition of the hormone. Serosal solution Ringer's mucosal solution 1/10 Ringer's for amphibia. Each experimental period lasts 1 h. KOEFOED-JOHNSEN and USSING (1952)

Experiment	Experimental parameters (($\mu l\, cm^{-2}\, h^{-1}$)	Control periods		Periods after hormone	addition
1	ϕ_{oi}	441	460	532	551
	$\dot{V}$	12	13	30	36
2	ϕ_{oi}	305	319	292	310
	$\dot{V}$	6.7	5	10.8	7.7
3	ϕ_{oi}	343	370	334	404
	$\dot{V}$	9.7	7.4	16	17
4	ϕ_{oi}	326	287	344	369
	$\dot{V}$	11.7	8	21	25

observe that such a flux undergoes slight changes when vasopressin is added to the serosal side of the skin; thus vasopressin does not modify the pore area A_p. Nevertheless, water net flux across the same membrane in the presence of an osmotic gradient, significantly increases when vasopressin is added to the serosal medium (Table 2). The variable which is modified by vasopressin under these conditions seems to be the pore radius r_p and pore radius appears explicitly only in the bulk flow kinetics of Poiseuille, not in the diffusion kinetics of Fick.

II. The Hydrophilic Pores and Their Radius

By using the equation giving the unidirectional flux of water (diffusion equation) and the equation giving the bulk flow of water (the Poiseuille equation) it is possible to solve the system of equations for r_p (MALHOTRA and VAN HARREVELD 1968). From the diffusion equation we have

$$A_p/\Delta x = \phi/D_{H_2O}\,.$$

By introducing the term $A_p/\Delta x$ in the Poiseuille equation we obtain

$$r_p^2 = \dot{V} D_{H_2O} 8\eta/\phi\Delta P\,.$$

Such a calculation implies that: (a) the biological membrane has regularly cylindrical pores; (b) the Poiseuille equation actually describes the kinetics of net water transfer under the driving force originating from an osmotic gradient.

III. The Reflection Coefficient of Staverman

The Poiseuille equation applied to water net flow under an osmotic gradient contains the term $\Delta\pi$, the difference in osmotic pressure between the two media separated by the membrane

$$\dot{V} = (A_p r_p^2/8\eta)\Delta\pi/\Delta x\,,$$

where A_p, Δx and r_p are unknown but constant for a given biological membrane. Therefore, we can say, in the case of filtration, as well as in the case of osmotic net flow

$$\dot{V} = AL_p\Delta\pi \quad \text{or} \quad \dot{V} = AL_p\Delta P\,,$$

where L_p is known as the coefficient of hydraulic permeability and has the physical dimensions ml s^{-1} cm^{-2} atm^{-1}.

These equations are valid only in the case of a semipermeable membrane. On the other hand, when the solute too crosses the membrane, the difference $\Delta\pi$ must be corrected by a coefficient $\leqslant 1$, the reflection coefficient of Staverman (STAVERMAN 1951). This coefficient is zero when the membrane does not distinguish between water and solute and the filtrate has the same composition as the solution before the filtration.

Many methods have been proposed for the determination of the reflection coefficient. All methods are based on the comparison between the volumetric flux when the solute is present in one medium only, and the volumetric flux when an impermeable substance is present in the same medium and in the same osmolar concentration as that used for the tested solute.

In these two cases we have

$$\dot{V}_1 = AL_p\sigma\Delta\pi\,,$$
$$\dot{V}_2 = AL_p\Delta\pi\,,$$

where σ is the reflection coefficient and from these equations we obtain

$$\sigma = \dot{V}_1/\dot{V}_2\,.$$

WRIGHT and DIAMOND (1969) determined the streaming potential (see Sect. C) rather than the volumetric flow, in order to calculate the reflection coefficient. In fact the streaming potential is linearly proportional to the volumetric flux (Fig. 11).

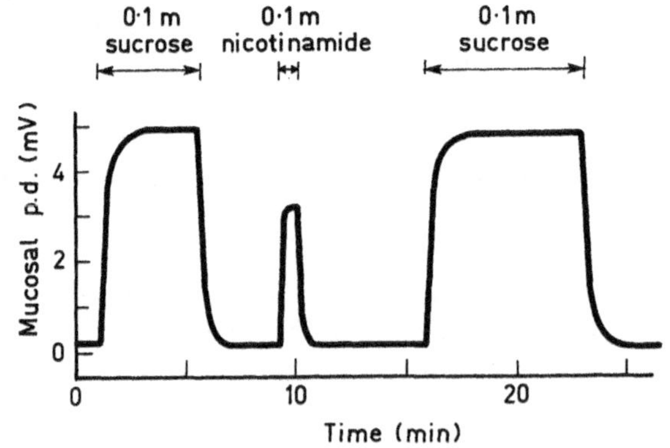

Fig. 11. Behaviour of the streaming potential in the isolated and everted rabbit gallbladder. The electrical potential (positive in the mucosal bathing solution) is plotted against the time of incubation. The serosal solution is Ringer's; the mucosal solution is Ringer's except during the periods indicated by the *arrows*; during these periods, Ringer's solution is made hypertonic by the addition of 0.1 *M* sucrose or nicotinamide. The nicotinamide reflection coefficient is obtained by dividing the nicotinamide potential by the sucrose potential. WRIGHT and DIAMOND (1969)

IV. Solvent Drag

Under most biological conditions, a diffusion process of a solute takes place with a simultaneous volumetric flux through the same pores in the same or the opposite direction. The water net flux causes a drag effect on the solute and this supplementary flux of the solute must be added to, or subtracted from the diffusional flux. The kinetic equation taking into account such a phenomenon following (KEDEM and KATCHALSKY 1958) is a

$$\dot{n} = A\omega RT(c_o - c_i) \pm (1-\sigma)\bar{c}\dot{V},$$

where ω is a mobility coefficient and $\bar{c}$ is a mean concentration. This mean concentration may be calculated as an arithmetic mean, when $(c_o - c_i)/c_i$ is less than 1; otherwise $\bar{c}$ is obtained from the following equation

$$\bar{c} = (c_o - c_i)/\ln(c_o/c_i).$$

G. Active Transport

I. Identification

The passage of a solute through a biological barrier is assumed to be an active one when the kinetics of the passage does not obey the flux equation (Sect. D) or does not follow the consequences of this equation, i.e., when a net transport against a chemical or an electrochemical gradient is present (see also Chap. 8).

II. Dependence of Water Transport on Metabolism

The passage of water is assumed to be dependent on metabolism when it takes place between two isotonic media or against an osmotic gradient; obviously the water movement considered here is a net one. This net passage of water, notwithstanding its dependence on metabolism, is not directly involved in metabolism itself, but is secondary to the active passage of solutes.

The hydration layer of the actively transported solute molecules seems not to be implicated in the coupling mechanism of this transport, because the transport rate of water by far exceeds the amount of water linked to the hydrated molecules or ions. The mechanism mainly taken into account in order to explain the net passage of water between two isotonic media divided by a biological barrier is the Curran model (CURRAN and MACINTOSH 1962). This model assumes the presence of an intermediate hyperosmotic space inside the separating barrier. This space (Fig. 12) is bordered on one side by a nearly semipermeable membrane and on the other by a nonselective membrane. The first membrane, in the intestinal epithelium, is the plasma cell membrane facing the paracellular space and the other membrane is formed by the subepithelial layers (DIAMOND and TORMEY 1966; KAYE et al. 1966). The paracellular space becomes hyperosmotic because of the active transport of sodium salts across the first membrane.

Water moves in the same direction, driven by the osmotic pressure difference and enlarges the paracellular space. During this process, water comes predomi-

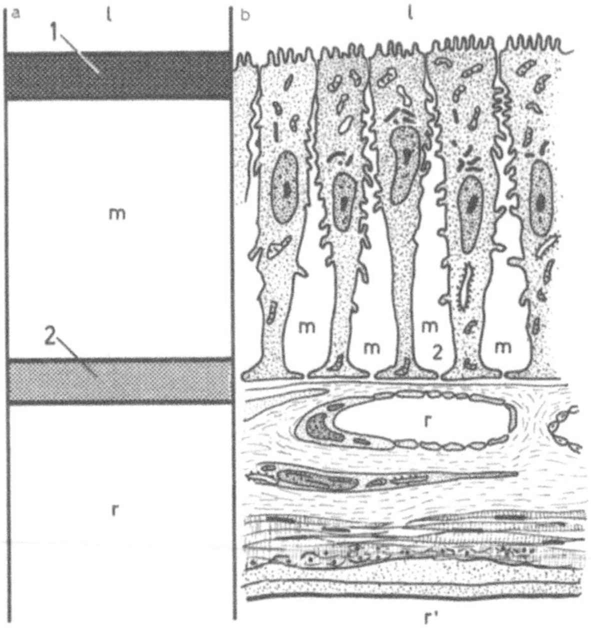

Fig. 12a, b. Schematic representation of the serial membrane model (**a**) and the epithelium of the rabbit gallbladder (**b**). Membrane 1 is a semipermeable membrane separating the lumen of the bladder (medium 1) and the paracellular space (medium m). Membrane 2 is a non-selective membrane separating the paracellular space and the serosal compartment (medium r). KAYE et al. (1966)

nantly through the cells and the tight junctions from the mucosal space and also to a lesser degree, through the subepithelial layers from the serosal space. In fact, the osmotic pressure difference in the last case is corrected by a reflection coefficient which is nearly zero.

Because of the resistance of the tissue, the enlargement of the paracellular space gives rise to a hydrostatic pressure inside the paracellular space. This pressure causes a bulk flow of water (and solutes), predominantly through the nonselective membrane. In fact, the hydraulic coefficient of permeability of this membrane is higher than that of the semipermeable membrane. Therefore a net flow of almost isotonic fluid crosses the entire barrier. This mechanism was first demonstrated in the gallbladder epithelium of the rabbit (Fig. 12).

III. Countercurrent Exchange

In some cases, the capillary arrangement in the blood circulation of organs (kidney medulla, intestinal villi, etc.) may be taken into account in order to evaluate the solute concentration in the subepithelial space in vivo. Let us consider the straight blood capillary loops which run parallel to the length of the intestinal villi. When the arterial blood enters the villus core it is invaded by solutes coming from the absorbing cells, but when the blood leaves the top of the villus, counterflow oc-

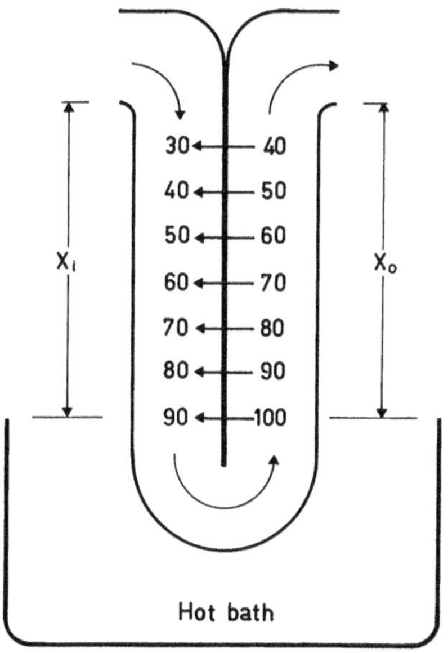

Fig. 13. Schematic representation of an example of countercurrent exchange. A stream of water passes through a hot bath by means of a tube loop; the heat taken up by the exit tube is partially returned to the entrance tube. Therefore, the heat drained by the stream of water is reduced

curs between entering and leaving capillaries and part of the solutes may be lost. In other words, there is a local recirculation of the solutes in a system of counterflowing blood which may decrease the drainage capacity of blood circulation. Therefore, this phenomenon is responsible for a possible stagnation in the villi of solutes which are permeable through the capillary walls (Fig. 13). A similar situation may occur for oxygen; the partial pressure of oxygen may be lower at the top than at the base of the villi.

IV. Thermodynamic Efficiency

1. Thermodynamics of Active Transport

Active transport requires a continuous energy supply because physical work must be carried out in order to overcome a chemical or an electrochemical gradient and, in the absence of a gradient, in order to overcome the internal resistance (see also Chap. 8). Let us imagine an actively transporting barrier dividing two media, o and i, where the o concentration of the uncharged transported substance is lower than the i concentration. In this transporting system the flux quotient must be higher than the concentration quotient

$$\phi_{oi}/\phi_{io} > c_o/c_i$$

and

$$RT\ln(\phi_{oi}/\phi_{io}) > RT\ln(c_o/c_i).$$

Since the two terms of this inequality have the dimensions of physical work, the difference must also be a work term, i.e., the minimal work L performed in order to transport 1 mol substance from medium o to medium i

$$L = RT\ln(\phi_{oi}/\phi_{io}) + RT\ln(c_i/c_o).$$

In this equation we have a term for the external osmotic work and one for the internal resistance to the movement: $RT\ln(\phi_{oi}/\phi_{io})$.

If the actively transported substance is a positively charged ion (for instance the Na ion), and in addition to a concentration difference there is also an electrical potential difference ΔE in opposition to the movement, the flux quotient must be higher than the expression for passive transport

$$\phi_{oi}/\phi_{io} > (c_o/c_i)\exp(-F\Delta E/RT)$$

and

$$RT\ln(\phi_{oi}/\phi_{io}) > \mathrm{RT}\ \ln(c_o/c_i) - F\Delta E.$$

Here, too, the two terms of this inequality have the dimensions of work and the difference must also be a work term

$$L = RT\ln(\phi_{oi}/\phi_{io}) + RT\ln(c_i/c_o) + F\Delta E.$$

L is the sum of the work done by the system per equivalent of transported ion to overcome the concentration difference, i.e., the external osmotic work, the work done in order to overcome the potential gradient (the external electrical work), plus the work necessary to overcome the resistance to movement inside the barrier. The total work needed for the functioning of this ion pump has been measured together with the energy expenditure in several epithelia.

In the case of frog skin (ZERAHN 1956), the oxygen consumed in the absence of sodium was determined first; the oxygen consumption while the sodium pump was functioning was then determined. The difference between the two consumptions is called the suprabasal oxygen consumption and is assumed to be the oxygen consumed by the sodium pump. The unidirectional fluxes (with the aid of two sodium tracers, ^{22}Na and ^{24}Na) and the net flux of sodium were determined simultaneously. Now it is possible to calculate the values of the three terms in the equation. For this purpose we must remember that

$$R = 1.9865\,\text{cal equiv.}^{-1}\ \text{V}^{-1}.$$

$$F = 23000\,\text{cal equiv.}^{-1}\ \text{V}^{-1}.$$

The quotient: transported sodium equivalents/oxygen moles consumed has a constant and very high value, 16–18. The efficiency of the process, i.e., the quotient: total thermodynamic work/total energy consumed may reach the value of 0.5, an astonishingly high value. Similar values have been obtained in other sodium pumping systems. In the epithelium of the small intestine of vertebrates a value of only 11 has been obtained (ESPOSITO et al. 1966); this may be due to the fact that the net sodium transport determined in the whole epithelium is the difference between the net sodium absorbed by the villi and the net sodium excreted by the crypts.

2. Energy Requirement for Active Transport

a) Cotransport

Active transport is always, directly or indirectly, dependent on chemical energy. A specific carrier is always involved, but the kinetics of this transport is not an equilibrating one as in the case of passive chemical facilitation. The affinity of the carrier for the actively transported substance may be different on one side ($K_{m(o)}$) from the other ($K_{m(i)}$) of the biological membrane

$$\dot{n} = AD_{CS}([C]_t/\Delta x)\{[S_o]/([S_o]+K_{m(o)}) - ([S_i]/([S_i]+K_{m(i)})\}$$

so that a steady nonequilibrium is reached only when

$$[S_o]/[S_i] = K_{m(o)}/K_{m(i)}\,.$$

A well-known example of an active transport process based on the difference between $K_{m(o)}$ and $K_{m(i)}$ is that offered by the intracellular accumulation of sugars and other nutrients in the absorbing enterocytes (CRANE's 1965 cotransport hypothesis). In this case it is assumed that sodium combining with the carrier allosterically influences the carrier's affinity to the transported substance. Since there is a difference in the sodium concentration between the plasma of the enterocyte and the luminal fluid, the affinity of the carrier for the transported substance is different, both outside and inside the brush border, and this difference allows for the accumulation of the transported substance inside the cell (Fig. 14). We have a simultaneous entry of sodium and transported substance into the cell by means of a ternary compound (sodium ions plus carrier plus transported substance) and the energy needed for the accumulation process is supplied by the downhill movement of the sodium ion. Sodium ion is maintained at a low concentration inside the cell because of the active extrusion process of sodium

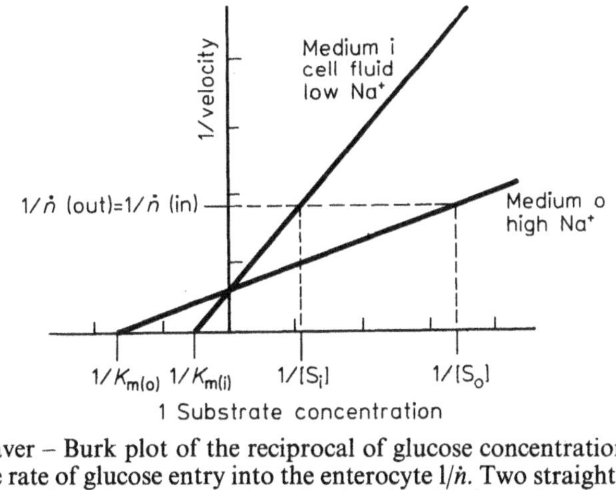

Fig. 14. Lineweaver – Burk plot of the reciprocal of glucose concentration 1/S against the reciprocal of the rate of glucose entry into the enterocyte $1/\dot{n}$. Two straight lines are reported, one in a high Na^+ medium o, and the other in a low Na^+ medium, i. When the inflow (straight line in medium o) and the outflow (straight line in medium i) of sugar are equal ($1/\dot{n}$ (out) $= 1/\dot{n}$(in) the sugar concentration in the cell (medium i) is higher than that in the outside medium, o. CRANE (1965)

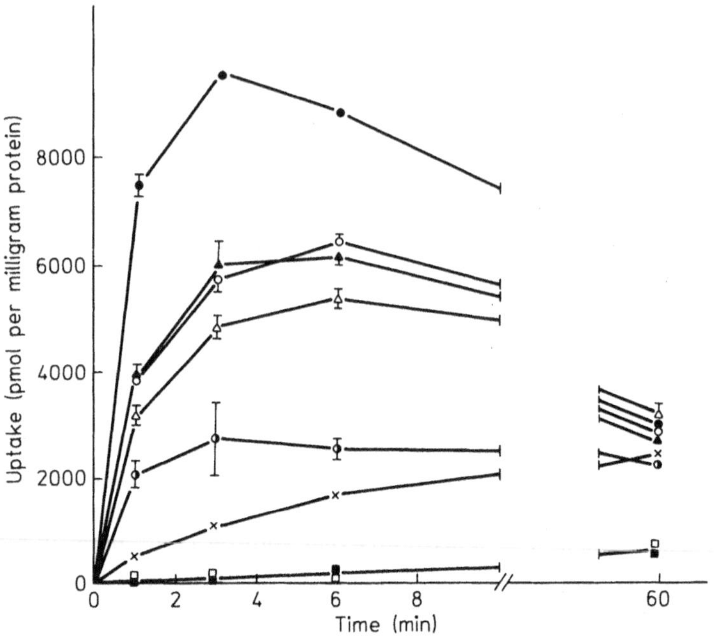

Fig. 15. Uptake of L-phenylalanine and D-glucose by membrane vesicles from *Philosamia cynthia* midgut. L-phenylalanine (1 m*M*) uptake in the presence of an initial gradient (100 m*M* outside and 0 inside) of: KSCN (*full circles*); NaSCN (*open circles*); KCl (*full triangles*); NaCl (*open triangles*). L-phenylalanine (1 m*M*) uptake in the absence of any salt gradient, with (*half-filled circles*) or without (*asterisks*) KCl (100 m*M*) outside and inside). D-glucose (1 m*M*) uptake in the presence of an initial gradient (100 m*M* outside and 0 inside) of KSCN (*full squares*) or NaSCN (*open squares*). The buffer in all cases was 10 m*M* HEPES-Tris pH 7.5. The results are the mean ± standard error of a typical experiment carried out in triplicate. When not given, standard error is smaller than the symbols used. Hanozet et al. (1979)

through the basolateral membrane into the serosal fluid. In other words, the accumulation of the transported substance is a secondary, useful, effect of the sodium pump.

This hypothesis has been strongly supported by accumulation experiments performed on isolated brush border membrane vesicles (Schmitz et al. 1973; Kessler et al. 1978). In fact, by breaking the brush border microvilli it is possible to prepare spherical vesicles surrounded by the brush border membrane and containing a fluid whose composition is known. These vesicles are then suspended in different media with the desired composition.

If the chemical or electrochemical activity of Na is higher outside than inside the vesicles, and if labelled D-glucose or a labelled neutral L-amino acid is added to the outside medium, a transient accumulation of the substance whose transport is Na dependent, takes place in the vesicle fluid. This accumulation is possible only so long as a Na concentration difference is present, and is proportional to the value of this concentration difference.

The cotransport process seems not always specific for sodium. In fact the mid gut of lepidopteran larvae (*Philosamia cynthia*) does not absorb sugar by a mechanism of cotransport and the brush border vesicles of such species are not capable of accumulating D-glucose. On the other hand, the vesicles themselves are able to accumulate L-phenylalanine in the presence of a Na gradient as well as in the presence of a K gradient (Fig. 15; HANOZET et al. 1979).

b) Direct Metabolic Involvement

Other mechanisms for active transport are possible in which the chemical metabolism is directly involved. The carrier may be inactivated on one side by one chemical reaction and reactivated on the other side of the membrane by another reaction

$$C_o + a_o \rightleftharpoons z_o + b_o ,$$

$$C_i + a_i \rightleftharpoons z_i + b_i \cdot$$

where z_o and z_i are the inactivated carrier on sides o and i, respectively.

Assuming that the concentrations of a and b are constant on the same side of the membrane, we can derive the following expressions from the chemical equilibria.

$$[z_o] = K_o[C_o] ,$$

$$[z_i] = K_i[C_i] .$$

The concentrations of the free carrier $[C_o]$ and $[C_i]$ on each side of the membrane are respectively

$$[C_o] = [C]_t - [CS]_o - K_o[C_o] ,$$

$$[C_i] = [C]_t - [CS]_i - K_i[C_i] .$$

From these expressions we obtain

$$[C_o] = ([C]_t - [CS]_o)/(1 + K_o) ,$$

$$[C_i] = ([C]_t - [CS]_i)/(1 + K_i) .$$

Now these expressions can be introduced into the equilibrium equations of the reaction between the free carrier with the actively transported substance on the two sides of the membrane o and i respectively

$$([C]_t - [CS_o])[S_o]/[CS]_o(1 + K_o) = K_m ,$$

$$([C]_t - [CS_i])[S_i]/[CS]_i(1 + K_i) = K_m \cdot$$

The expressions for $[CS]_o$ and $[CS]_i$ may be derived from these equations and, therefore, the transport kinetics is

$$\dot{n} = (AD_{CS}[C]_t/\Delta x)\{[S_o]/([S_o] + K_m(1 + K_o)) - [S_i]/([S_i] + K_m(1 + K_i))\} .$$

From this kinetic equation it appears that the net flux through the membrane stops only when the two terms in brackets are equal or when

$$[S_o]/[S_i] = (1 + K_o)/(1 + K_i) .$$

If K_i is higher than K_o, $[S_i]$ must also be higher than $[S_o]$ and an active accumulation of the transported substance in medium i takes place.

The source of chemical energy in these cases may be the high energy phosphate bond of ATP. The enzyme which hydrolyses ATP (ATPase) is involved in active transport of this kind. SKOU (1957) discovered in the nerves of crabs a specific ATPase associated with the membrane and dependent on Mg as well as on Na and K. The reaction of the enzyme with ATP giving the phosphorylated enzyme is Na dependent and the reaction of hydrolysis of the phosphorylated enzyme seems to be K dependent. Many authors (e.g., CHARNOCK and OPIT 1968) have put forward the hypothesis that ATPase itself is the specific carrier for the sodium pump (which in many cases is a cationic pump) located in the membrane of the cells, and, where the intestinal epithelium is concerned, in the basolateral membrane of the enterocyte. Congruent with this hypothesis is the fact that ouabain and other cardiac glycosides (see Chap. 9) inhibit the Na^+, K^+-ATPase in vitro as well as the cationic pump in vivo. This inhibition only appears when ouabain is added to the serosal perfusing of the intestinal epithelial cells, a medium which faces the basolateral membrane where the cationic pump seems to be located.

References

Bayliss LE (1959) Principles of general physiology, vol I. Longmans, London, pp 105–108, 138–142, 443–449, 453–460

Capraro V, Bernini G (1952) Mechanism of action of extracts of the posthypophysis on water transport through the skin of the frog (Rana Esculenta). Nature 169:454–455

Capraro V, Cresseri A (1964) Absorption, distribution and excretion of vitamin B_{12}. In: Santamaria L (ed) Research progress in organic, biological, and medicinal chemistry, vol I. Soc Ed. Farmaceutica, Milano, p 109

Charnock JS, Opit LJ (1968) Membrane metabolism and ion transport. In: Bittar EE, Bittar N (eds) The biological basis of medicine, vol I. Academic, London, pp 69–103

Crane RT (1965) Na^+-dependent transport in the intestine and other animal tissues. Fed Proc 24:1000–1006

Curran PF (1960) Na, Cl and water transport by rat ileum "in vitro". J Gen Physiol 43:1137–148

Curran PF, MacIntosh JR (1962) A model system for biological water transport. Nature 193:347–348

Diamond JM (1966) Non linear osmosis. J Physiol (Lond) 183:58–100

Diamond JM, Tormey J McD (1966) Role of long extracellular channels in fluid transport across epithelia. Nature 210:817–820

Diedrich DF (1966) Competitive inhibition of intestinal glucose transport by phlorizin analogs. Arch Biochem Biophys 117:248–256

Esposito G, Faelli A, Capraro V (1966) Metabolism and sodium transport in the isolated rat intestine. Nature 210:307–308

Hanozet G, Giordana B, Sacchi V (1979) Metabolite transport by membrane vesicles isolated from the midgut of Philosamia cynthia larvae. Rend Fisici Acc Naz Lincei fasc 5:455–460

Henin S, Cremaschi D (1975) Transcellular ion route in rabbit gallbladder. Pflugers Arch 355:125–139

Kaye GJ, Wheeler HO, Whitlock RT, Lane N (1966) Fluid transport in the rabbit gallbladder. J Cell Biol 30:237–268

Kedem O, Katchalsky A (1968) Thermodynamic analysis of the permeability of biological membranes to non-electrolytes. BBA 27:229–245

Kessler M, Acuto O, Storelli C, Murer H, Müller M, Semenza G (1978) A modified procedure for the rapid preparation of efficiently transporting vesicles from small intestinal brush border membranes. BBA 506:136–154

Klinkenberg M (1981) Membrane protein oligomeric structure and transport function. Nature 290:449–454
Koefoed-Johnsen V, Ussing HH (1952) The contribution of diffusion and flow to the passage of D_2O through living membranes. Acta Physiol Scand 28:60–76
Malhotra SK, Van Harreveld A (1968) Molecular organisation of the membranes of cells and cellular organelles. In: Bittar EE, Bittar N (eds) The biological basis of medicine, vol I. Academic, London, pp 3–68
Overton E (1899) Über die allgemeinen osmotischen Eigenschaften der Zelle, ihre vermutlichen Ursachen und ihre Bedeutung für die Physiologie. Vierteljahresschr Naturforsch Ges 44:88
Renkin EM (1955) Filtration, diffusion and molecular sieving through porous cellulose membranes. J Gen Physiol 38:225–243
Salomon LL, Allums JA, Smith DE (1961) Possible carrier mechanism for the intestinal transport of D-xylose. Biochem Biophys Res Commun 4:123–126
Schmitz J, Preiser H, Maestracci D, Ghosh BK, Cerda JJ, Crane RK (1973) Purification of the human intestinal brush border membranes. BBA 323:98–112
Skou JC (1957) The influence of some cations on an adenosintriphosphatase from peripheral nerves. BBA 23:394–401
Staverman AJ (1951) The theory of measurement of osmotic pressure. Recl Trav Chim Pays-Bas 70:344–352
Stein WD (1967) The movement of molecules across cell membranes. Academic, New York, pp 66–69
Ussing HH (1949) The distinction by means of tracers between active transport and diffusion. Acta Physiol Scand 19:43–56
Wilbrandt W, Rosenberg TH (1961) The concept of carrier transport and its corollaries in pharmacology. Pharmacol Rev 13:109–183
Wright EM, Diamond JM (1969) An electrical method of measuring non-electrolyte permeability. Proc R Soc Lond [Biol] 172:203–225
Zerahn K (1956) Oxygen consumption and active sodium transport in the isolated and short circuited frog skin. Acta Physiol Scand 36:300–318

CHAPTER 4

Methods for Investigation of Intestinal Permeability

T. Z. CSÁKY

A. Introduction

The definition of permeability refers to a specific property of a biologic membrane which modifies the passage of a given substrate, the permeant. Clearly, the distinction between free diffusion and permeation resides in the particular limitation presented to the freedom of diffusion by the membrane. The degree of limitation is determined both by the structure of the membrane and by the physicochemical nature of the permeant.

To a first approximation, the intestine may be considered as a complex biologic membrane. Thus, the overall permeability of the intestine is a composite of the permeability properties of the unstirred water layer, the epithelial cells, and the intercellular crevices. Furthermore, the permeability of the epithelial cell is a composite of the permeabilities of the glycocalyx, the brush order, the various intercellular barriers, and the basolateral membrane.

Basically permeation is a two-way process, thus, in the intestine the flux from the lumen into the bloodstream (absorption) and the flux from the bloodstream into the lumen (exorption) can occur simultaneously. The anatomic and physiologic differential of the intestinal wall favors a net absorption for most substances, nonetheless the intestinal exorption cannot be neglected, particularly in the case of some drugs or other xenobiotics.

Intestinal permeability can be examined at different levels of integration: in the whole animals with the intestine in situ, in the isolated intestinal loop, in isolated sheets composed of primarily epithelial cells with some connective and muscle tissues, in isolated enterocytes, or in their isolated membranes. This chapter attempts to summarize briefly the various techniques which can be employed in the study of intestinal permeation primarily in experimental animals. The specific methods used in the study of intestinal permeability in humans are summarized in Chap. 31, vol. 70/II.

B. In Vivo Techniques

I. In Conscious Animals

1. The Thiry–Vella Fistula

The classical method of the study of intestinal permeation which is most frequently used was originally described in 1864 by THIRY and modified in 1880 by VELLA. The Thiry–Vella fistula is prepared in larger animals, usually dogs. Under ether

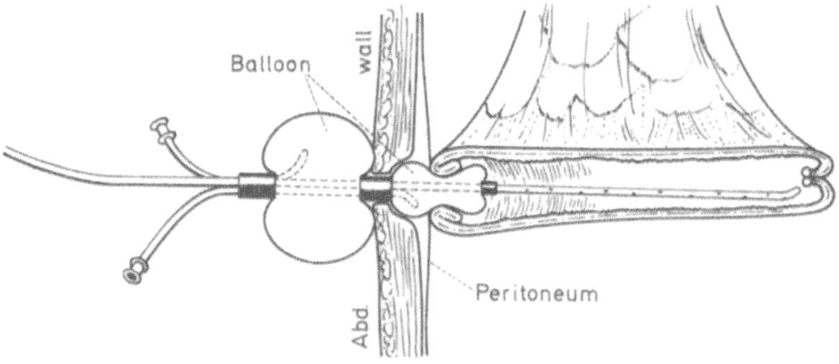

Fig. 1. Practical application of the Thiry–Vella principle. A loop is isolated from the intestinal ract; one end is closed, the other is open and sutured to the abdominal wall. The loop is kept fixed in position by two inflatable rubber balloons. Inside the loop is a 14F soft rubber catheter, freely perforated, through this the loop can be filled, emptied, and washed out. Johnston (1932)

anesthesia, a segment of the intestine, with its blood supply and lymphatic connection intact, is isolated from the intestinal tract and one or both ends are brought out to the skin surface. The rest of the intestine is restored to its continuity by an end-to-end anastomosis. Several modifications have bee made to the original Thiry–Vella fistula. One practical modification of this method, described by Johnston (1932) is depicted in Fig. 1. The solution of the substrate, the absorption of which is to be examined is introduced into the loop; after a given time the loop is emptied and the amount of substrate left in the lumen is analyzed. The disappearance is assumed to be a quantitative measure of absorption.

2. Blood Level After Placing the Substrate into the Intestinal Lumen

Another approach to the study of the intestinal transport in conscious animals is the placing of the substrate into the gut lumen with the help of a duodenal tube and monitoring of its appearance in the blood. A somewhat more realistic picture can be obtained if the blood is withdrawan from the portal vein which collects the venous outflow from the entire small bowel and a great part of the large bowel. London (1935) described a rather complicated method which allows the sampling of the portal venous blood in conscious animals. This method was simplified by Dent and Schilling (1949). Figure 2 depicts the simplified technique.

3. The Method of Cori

Cori (1925) introduced a simple technique for the quantitative examination of gastrointestinal absorption in rats. A measured volume of a solution of the substrate at known concentration is introduced into the stomach by a tube. After a given time the animal is killed, the entire gastrointestinal tract removed, thoroughly washed out, and the washing analyzed. Absorption is quantitated by the disappearance of the substrate and is expressed per 100 g body weight per hour.

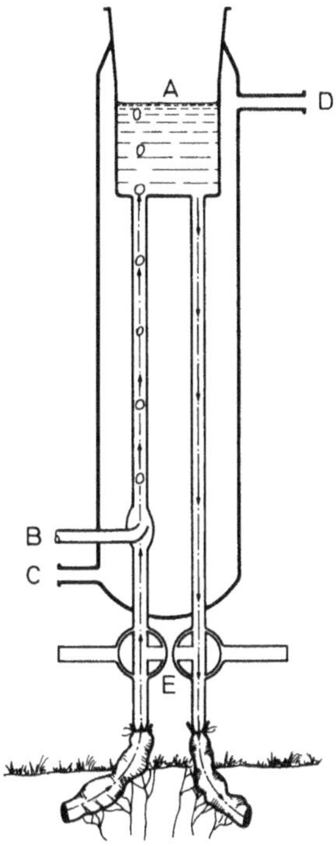

Fig. 3. Apparatus for luminal perfusion of an intestinal segment in vivo. *A*, reservoir; *B*, gas lift; *C*, inlet; *D*, outlet to water jacket maintained at 38 °C. Rapid rinsing of the segment is facilitated through a two-way tap E. Sheff and Smyth (1955)

(Verzár 1936) in their classical studies of intestinal absorption. The principal drawback of the closed loop system is the almost complete lack of mixing within the intestinal lumen, which enlarges considerably the unstirred layer effect and may lead to erroneous results and conclusions (see Chap. 22, vol. 70/II).

2. Open System (Luminal Perfusion)

The in situ intestinal loop preparations can be improved by perfusing the lumen of the gut with an appropriate solution containing the substrate under examination. Sols and Ponz (1947) described a method in which both ends of an in situ intestinal loop were cannulated, the upper cannula was connected to a funnel, while the caudal end was directed into a collecting flask. They poured the solution into the funnel, let it go through the gut, and collected it at the other end. This preparation could be used for repeated experiments. A modification of this technique was introduced by Horváth and Wix (1951). After cannulation, the intestinal loop was replaced into the abdomen, and the animal was allowed to recover from the anesthesia before the perfusion started.

A more elaborate method was developed independently by Scheff and Smyth (1955) and Fullerton and Parsons (1956). Figure 3 illustrates the method of Scheff and Smyth. In essence it allows the recirculation of the same fluid which is kept at body temperature. Jervis et al. (1956) and Jacobs and Luper (1957)

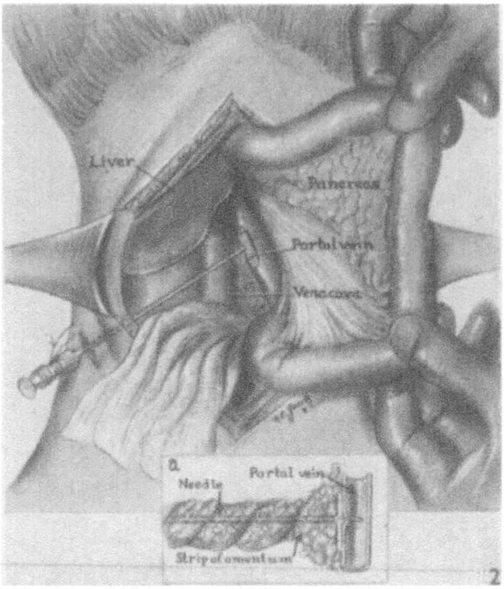

Fig. 2. The London cannula as modified by DENT and SCHILLINGS (1949). A strip of omentum is wrapped round the cannula, as shown in the *inset*, before the abdomen is finally closed. To withdraw portal blood the trocar is removed and a long needle inserted through the cannula until the wall of the vein is pierced

Cori called this value the absorption coefficient. According to Cori's measurements the absorption coefficient for glucose in the rat was 200. The value for galactose was somewhat higher (220), and lower for other sugars; fructose 86; mannose 38; xylose 30; and arabinose 18. The principal complicating factor in Cori's method is related to the fact that the substance the absorption of which is to be examined is administered into the stromach. Gastric emptying may drastically influence the rate of absorption; this is not taken into account in Cori's method.

II. In Anesthetized Animals

1. Closed System (Tied Loops)

The simplest approach is the following. The abdomen is opened, a loop of the intestine is ligated (some workers rinse the intestine with a lukewarm saline solution before ligation), and a known volume of the solution of the substrate is introduced into the closed loop. The intestine is replaced and the abdomen is closed. After a given time the animal is killed, the abdomen reopened, the ligated intestinal loop carefully isolated, opened, rinsed, and its contents analyzed. The remaining amount of substrate is substracted from the amount placed into the loop and is expressed as the amount absorbed per unit length of gut per unit time. Since the length of the intestinal loop may vary with the contraction, thus making it difficult to determine exactly, many investigators expressed the absorption not by unit length but by unit dry weight of the gut. This method was extensively used by HÖBER and co-workers (HÖBER and HÖBER 1937) and VERZÁR and co-workers

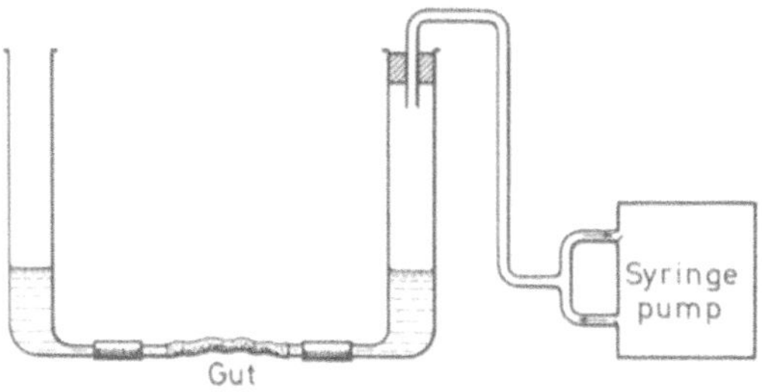

Fig. 4. Apparatus for agitating the contents of an intestinal segment in vivo. The segment is connected to two small containers in which the fluid is agitated with the help of a syringe pump or small-animal respirator. CSÁKY and HO (1965)

used a similar method, while CSÁKY and HO (1965) used a fingerpump to recirculate the fluid. CSÁKY and HO (1965) also described a method in which the intestinal fluid was not recirculated, but kept mixed by swishing back and forth. Figure 4 describes the method, the advantage of which is that it accommodates small volumes (6–12 ml) when using rats as experimental animals.

In all the in situ experiments it is important to keep the rate of the luminal fluid recirculation relatively high. It should be kept in mind that the absorption in vivo is essentially a translocation from the luminal into the blood compartment. If the rate of blood flow is higher than the rate of luminal perfusion, it may result in the measurement of luminal clearance rather than intestinal transport. Such measurements may yield disturbing results, such as those described by RIDER et al. (1967) who concluded that in vivo glucose is absorbed from the intestine of the rat by a straight diffusion rather than by saturation kinetics.

In situ perfusion techniques can be utilized exorption, i.e., blood–lumen flux. By perfusing the lumen with the calcium chelator EDTA or with a solution with pH > 9.0 (which did not cause irreversible damage to the mucosa) CSÁKY and AUTENRIETH (1975) could show a marked increase of the blood–lumen flux of glucose, of intravenously injected inulin, and of polyethylene glycol. The in situ luminal perfusion techniques can be applied combined with a limited interference with the blood or lymph supply. MATTHEWS and SMYTH (1954) drained the blood from the mesenteric vein from the loop in which the absorption was examined, the blood was replaced by transfusion from another animal. DEAK (1977) combined this method with cannulation of the lymph vessel coming from the same loop; this way the distribution of the absorbed substrate between the blood and lymph can be quantitated. The blood flow can be artifically regulated either mechanically or pharmacologically. Preparations involving simultaneous vascular and luminal perfusion are well suited for studies of two-way fluxes. They are described in detail in Chap. 5.

C. In Vitro Techniques

I. Isolated Loops

The oxygen demand of the small intestine is relatively large. Consequently, without proper oxygenation the isolated tissue will rapidly exhibit dysfunction and eventually die. For this reason the most important factor in any method involving isolated intestine, is proper oxygenation.

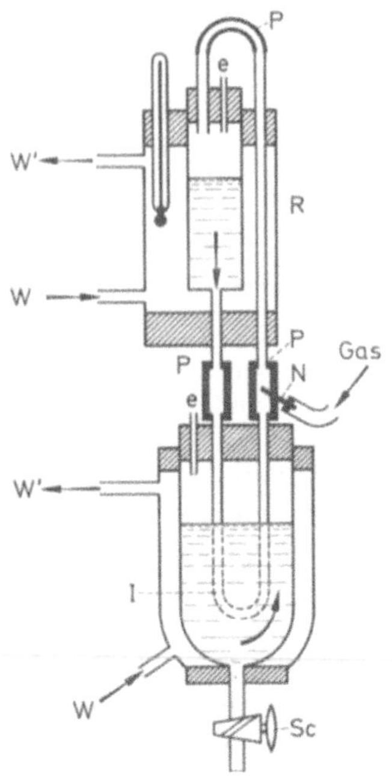

Fig. 5. Simplified version of the circulation unit described by FISHER and PARSONS (1949) for investigation of transport in an isolated intestinal loop in vitro. N hypodermic needle thrust through one of the rubber tubes P to function as a gas lift. The intestine I is in a container kept at constant temperature in a water jacket (W inlet; W'outlet). Only the fluid in contact with the mucosal surface is recirculated; *arrows* indicate direction of flow of fluid in mucosal circuit. Sc drain for lower reservoir. PARSONS and WINGATE (1961)

1. Unеverted Loops

Studies on excised gut segments were performed more than a century ago (ROBINSON 1857). About the turn of the century REID (1900) performed a number of elegant experiments in the isolated intestine of the rabbit. Later in the same preparation, it was clearly demonstrated that glucose is more rapidly transferred than xylose (AUCHINACHIE et al. 1930). The first viably in vitro preparation suitable for quantitative flux studies was described by FISHER and PARSONS (1949). The intestinal loop was mounted on two cannulae immersed in the warm, oxygenated serosal fluid and perfused with a warm, oxygenated mucosal medium. The medium was a Krebs–Ringer bicarbonate solution. With proper dimensions a circulation rate of 35–45 ml/min was achieved. The method was modified by FISHER (1960) and by PARSONS and WINGATE (1961) (Fig. 5). WISEMAN (1953) described a perfusion apparatus by which several intestinal loops could be simultaneously employed (Fig. 6). DARLINGTON and QUASTEL (1953) designed a simple apparatus which they used to study the absorption of sugars from the isolated small intestine of the guinea pig (Fig. 7). This apparatus was further simplified by PASENCHYCH (1961).

The intestine of poikylotherms is less sensitive to oxygenation than that of homoiotherms. CSÁKY and THALE (1960) described a simple apparatus in which

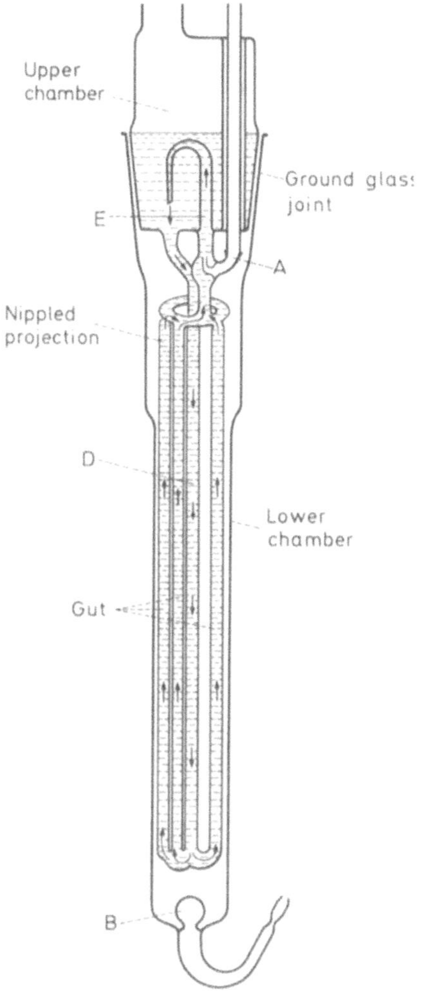

Fig. 6. Apparatus accommodating three isolated segments of intestine maintained in vitro. Gas enters through A, carrying mucosal fluid up the tube E into the upper chamber from which it flows down the glass tube D. The lower end of D is connected to the intestinal segments. *Arrows* indicate the direction of flow in the mucosal compartment. Gas also enters through B to mix the serosal fluid. WISEMAN (1953)

only the mucosal bathing solution is oxygenated (Fig. 8). The method has been applied to the intestine of the toad, the green frog, and the bullfrog. The preparation was found to be viable for at least 5 h as witnessed by the steady active transport of 3-*O*-methylglucose (Fig. 9; CSÁKY and HARA 1965).

2. Everted Loops

The introduction of the everted intestinal loop as a research tool was a significant development (WILSON and WISEMAN 1954). In this method the intestine, mostly of rodents, is excised and everted over a glass or stainless steel rod, 1.5 mm in di-

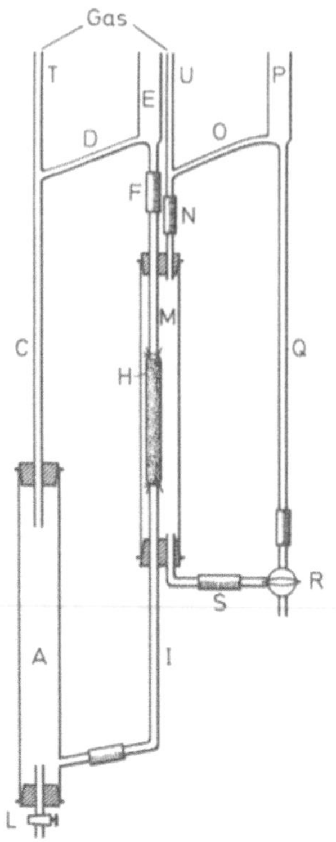

Fig. 7. Apparatus for the study of transport in the intestine in vitro by DARLINGTON and QUASTEL (1953). Fluid in contact with mucosal surface passes from *A* along *C* and *D* to reservoir *E* which is open. From *E* the fluid passes down *F* through the lumen of the segment *H* to return, via *I* to *A*. Circulation of the fluid is maintained by gas entering at *T* and bubbling along *D* to escape from *E*. The fluid *M* bathing the serosal surface of the segment circulates from the reservoir *P* down through *Q* and *S* and is returned along *N* and *O*, where it mingles with gas injected at *U*, *L*, and *R*: stopcocks through which samples may be removed during the experiment

ameter. The principle advantage of the technique is that it exposes the mucosal cells to a relatively large volume of well-oxygenated and mixed nutrient medium. Initially the method was a closed one. A sac 2–3 cm long was tied off at both ends, and the inside (which is the serosal side) is filled with a nutrient solution. The sac is placed in an Erlenmeyer flask containing the mucosal medium, oxygenated, and incubated at 38 °C. Despite some reservations (PARSON 1968; LEVINE et al. 1970) the everted intestinal preparation is widely used in studies of intestinal permeation, particularly in the form of modified open loop technique.

The first open loop everted gut method was described by CRANE and WILSON (1958). In this method, the gut is mounted on a glass cannula, 0.5 cm outside diameter. The lower end is tied, the loop is filled with a nutrient solution, and after filling, it is placed in a plastic centrifuge tube containing a well-gassed nutrient solution. Through the cannula, sampels can be taken repeatedly from the serosal compartment. A modified version of this technique was described by JORGENSEN et al. (1961). This modification allows the mixing or complete withdrawal and replacement of the serosal medium (Fig. 10).

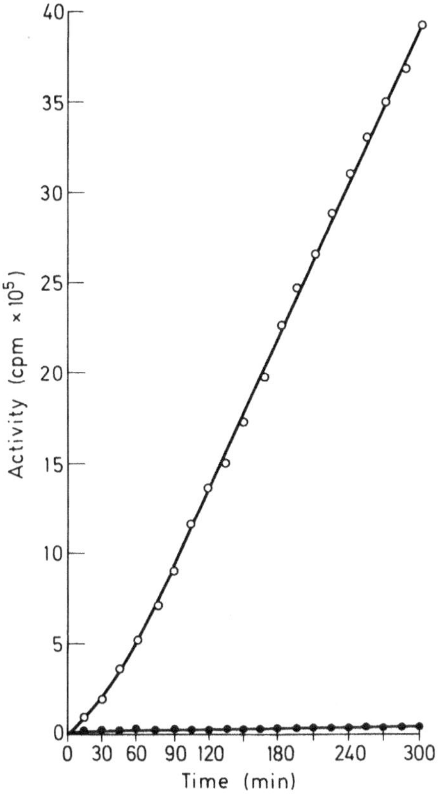

Fig. 9. Mucosal–serosal (*crosses*) and serosal–mucosal (*circles*) flux of labeled 3-*O*-methyl-glucose in the isolated small intestine of the bullfrog mounted in the apparatus depicted in Fig. 8. The steady flux asymmetry indicates that active transport was maintained over the entire period of 300 min. CSÁKY and HARA (1965)

both equilibrating and concentrating, can be measured. AGAR et al. (1954) studied the uptake of histidine by rings prepared from rat intestine. CRANE and MANDELSTAM (1960) used everted hamster intestinal rings for the examination of sugar transport, while BOARS and WILSON (1963) studied the uptake of vitamin B_{12}. The interpretation of the data obtained by the use of intestinal rings is limited by the fact that in these preparations the polarity of the epithelial cells is disregarded. Thus, this method does not allow the quantitative measure of translocation across the intestinal wall. On the other hand, under in vitro condition, the substrates which are taken up by accumulative transport are extruded into the subepithelial tissues. This way, an overall concentrative uptake of the substrate by the tissue is produced. Thus, the ring method is useful for demonstrating concentrative uptake of a given substrate by the intestine. Another advantage is that a large number of rings can be incubated simultaneously.

5. Intestinal Sheets

To a first approximation, the intestinal wall can be considered as a biologic membrane. By analogy the techniques designed for other biologic membranes can thus

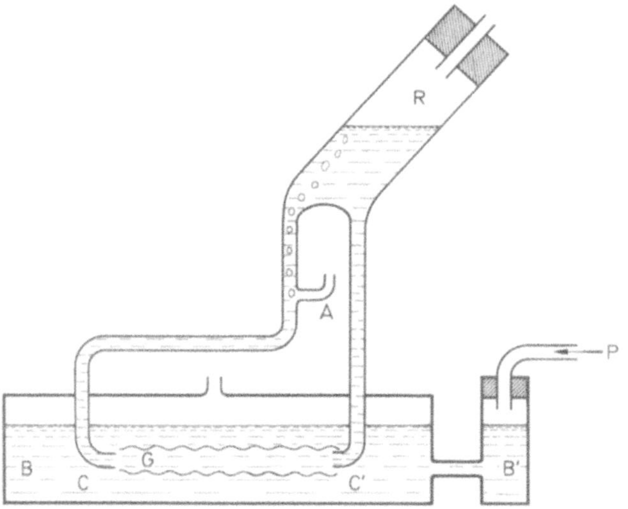

Fig. 8. Apparatus used for the study of transport in surviving intestine of frog or toad. The gut *G* is mounted on cannulae *C* and *C'* through which the mucosal surface is perfused from reservoir *R*. Air bubbles through opening *A* keep the contents in steady circulation. The serosal surface is in contact with the liquid in the bath *B*, the contens of which are gently agitated with a small respiratory pump *P* connected through container *B'*. CSÁKY and THALE (1960)

CLARKSON and ROTHSTEIN (1960) described a simple method which can be carried out with the least sophisticated equipment. In this technique, an everted intestinal sac is tied over the muzzle of the barrel of a 2-ml glass syringe which is floating attached to a cork sheet upon an oxygenated solution in a large beaker. ESPOSITO and CSÁKY (1974) described a simple apparatus in which an everted loop of intestine can be suspended in an oxygenated medium and the serosal compartment can be mixed manually (Fig. 11).

3. Loops Consisting Mainly of Mucosa

One of the disadvantages of both everted and uneverted isolated intestinal preparations is that they allow measurements only of the flux across the entire intestinal wall and not across the mucosal layer. However, with in situ preparations with intact blood circulation, the blood vessels reach into the lamina propria immediately under the layer of mucosal epitelial cells. The in vitro preparation could be improved if the mucosal layer could be separated from the bulky subepothelial tissues. PARSONS and PATERSON (1965) described a preparation of rat colon from which the subepithelial layer could be peeled off, leaving the mucosa with the muscularis mucosae which was everted and mounted on the apparatus depicted on Fig. 12. With proper oxygenation the preparation was viable for several hours. Attempts to make a similar preparation from the small intestine of the rat have not met with success.

4. Intestinal Rings

Small (1–5 mm) rings can be cut from everted or uneverted isolated intestine, suspended in oxygenated medium containing a given substrate. The rate of uptake,

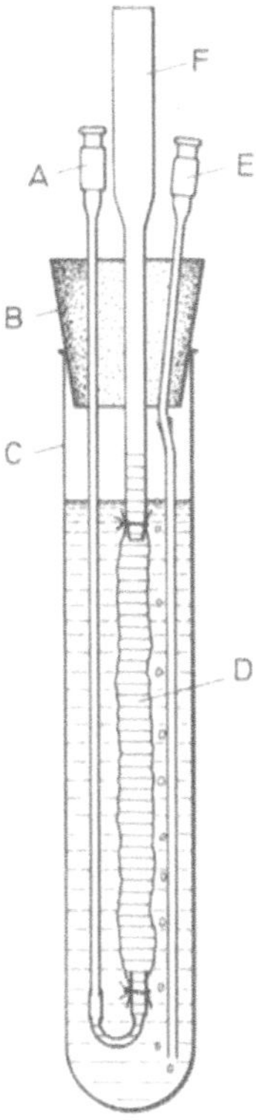

Fig. 10. Apparatus for measuring transport in the everted small intestine. *A* 13-cm no. 19 spinal needle (with stylette). This is attached to a polyethylene tube to which the lower end of the intestine *D* is tied. *E*, gas inlet; *F*, glass cannula to hold the intestine; *C*, test tube 150 × 20 mm; *B*, rubber stopper. The serosal solution can be withdrawn completely and replaced after removing the stylette from *A*. JORGENSEN et al. (1961)

be employed for the study of the permeability of the intestine. A biologic membrane that has been studied extensively is frog skin. This preparation was used by USSING and his co-workers in the examination of the relationship between the generation of electric potential and active ion transport. For such studies the Ussing chamber (USSING and ZERAHN 1951) was extensively used. This chamber, depicted in Fig. 13, allows the measurement of transport of various substrate across the sheet of isolated frog skin under short-circuit conditions. The chamber can be employed in the study of intestinal permeation. In this case the gut is excised, opened, and mounted as a sheet between the two sides of the chamber. If vigorous stirring is desired, small electrically driven stirrer blades can be arranged in each compartment. The Ussing chamber for intestinal permeation studies has been repeatedly modified. One practical modification automatically keeps the system short-circuited and registers continuously the short-circuit current (ROTHE et al. 1969).

For the study of rapid uptake of substrates at either the mucosal or serosal surface, SEMENZA (1969) designed a simple method: the everted gut is cut into 1.2–

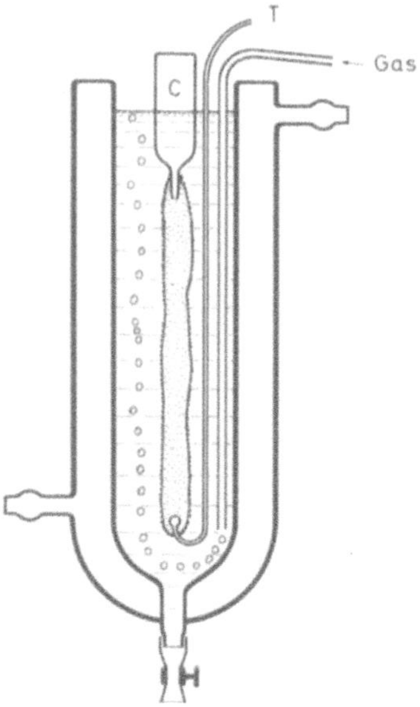

Fig. 11. Apparatus for incubation of isolated intestinal loop consisting of a water-jacketed container with an inlet tube for gassing. One end of the everted gut is mounted on cannula *C*; the other is mounted on a semirigid polyethylene tube with closed end *T*; by lifting and lowering the latter the contents of the serosal compartment can be mixed. EXPOSITO and CSÁKY (1974)

1.5-cm long pieces. These are then "sandwiched" between two plexiglass discs kept apart by a rubber ring of 1.4 mm diameter; this creates a space between the two discs. One of the discs has a circular opening through which one side of the tissue is exposed to the bath. This can be either the mucosal or the serosal side. The discs are clamped together and shaken in the medium containing the substrate. At the end of the incubation a circular piece is cut from the mounted gut and analyzed. With some animal species it is possible to strip away part of the subepithelial tissues, leaving essentially the mucosa, some submucosal connecting tissue, and muscularis mucosae intact. This "mucosal sheet" can then be mounted in the Ussing chamber (FIELD et al. 1971).

LAUTERBACH (1977) developed a technique in which the mucosa of the guinea pig small intestine is carefully lifted off the submucosal tissue with a razor blade. The epithelial sheet is them mounted on a sheet of nylon mesh and placed as a membrane between two small (0.2-ml) chambers. This preparation was successfully used in studies of both intestinal absorption and secretion (LAUTERBACH 1977; TURNHEIM and LAUTERBACH 1980).

6. Isolated Villi

In animals with finger-like intestinal villi, these can be cut off carefully with a sharp scalpel or ophthalmic scissors. CRANE and MANDELSTAM (1960) prepared villi from hamster small intestine by forcing the intestinal mucosa through syringe

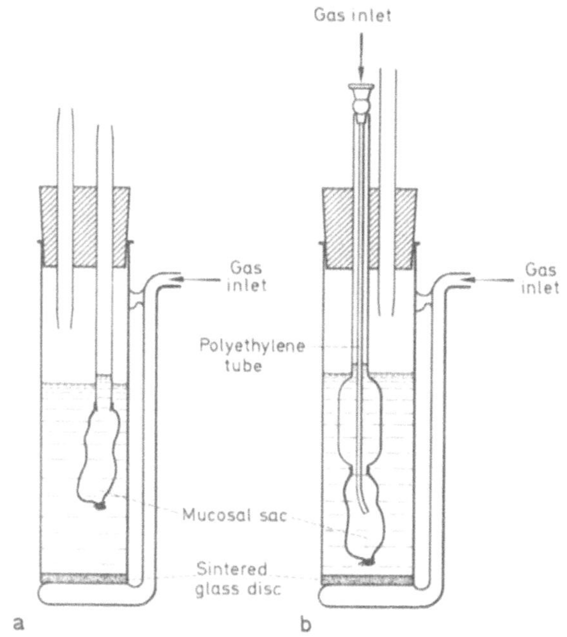

Fig. 12 a, b. Apparatus for incubation of everted sacs of colonic mucosa. **a** small sac attached to a plain glass cannula, initial volume of transmucosal fluid 0.5–1.0 ml; this fluid is unstirred; **b** larger sac attached to a cannula with bulb, initial volume of transmucosal fluid 5.0 ml, stirred by gas bubbles. The volume of mucosal fluid in both instances is 50 ml. The apparatus is immersed in a constant temperature bath. PARSONS and PATERSON (1965)

needles of decreasing diameter. The resulting suspension accumulated sugars. WRIGHT and LINE (1976) cut 5-mm rings from everted hamster jejunum. These rings were frozen in a Krebs–Ringer bicarbonate medium and lyophilized. The dry tissue was placed in a vial and by gentle tapping the powdery surface consisting of the salts of the medium, removed. Under a low power dissecting microscope, the dry villi were brushed off with a microspatula and analyzed. This method has been applied successfully to the intestine of small (30-day-old, but not older) rats (FONDACARO et al. 1974).

7. Isolated Enterocytes

One of the drawbacks of isolated mucosal preparations is the unfavorable ratio of epithelial cells to inert connective and muscle tissues. Even if part of this inert layer is stripped away, the preparation is not freed of subepithelial connective tissue and muscularis mucosae. Isolated intestinal mucosal cells would have the distinct advantage of freeing the cells which are primarily involved in intestinal transport from the other functionally inert living material.

Early attempts to prepare isolated cells by scraping the mucosa with a microscope slide and suspending the scrapings in an appropriate nutrient solution (DICKENS and WILE-MALHERBE 1941), did not yield viable preparations, as judged

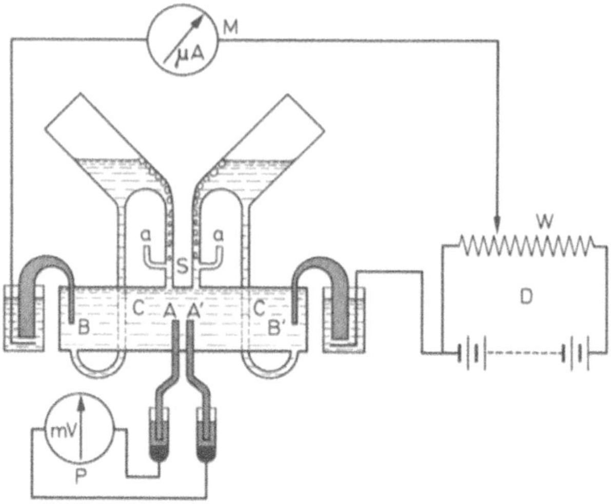

Fig. 13. The Ussing chamber for the determination of fluxes and short-circuit current through an isolated membrane. The membrane *S* separates the two chambers *C*. Two agar–Ringer bridges, *A* and *A'*, connect the bathing solutions with calomel electrodes. The potential difference across the membrane is measured by the valve potentiometer *P*. By means of the battery *D* and the potential divider *W* a variable current can be passed through the membrane via the agar bridges *B* and *B'*. The current passing in the circuit is read on the microammeter *M*. The bathing solutions are aerated and mixed by air from the inlets a. USSING and ZERAHN (1951)

by the rapid decline of the glycolytic rate accompanied by a considerable loss of weight. This indicated that perhaps proteolytic enzymes were released from the damaged cells, causing autolysis. Subsequently, methods were developed for freeing intestinal epithelial cells with less physical damage and at the same time freeing them from the mucus which caused clumping of the cells. SJOSTRAND (1968) everted the gut over a glass rod which was then mounted on a stirring motor and rotated in a medium at various speeds to remove the mucus; subsequently the mucosa was scraped off by applying gentle pressure on the rotation.

HARRISON and WEBSTER (1969) everted the intestine over a steel rod which was then attached to a Vibra-Mix motor and mechanically vibrated first for 5 min to remove the mucus and more loosely attached older cells, then for 30 min to free the rest of the cells. Judging by the degree of swelling of the isolated cells, the rate of lactic acid production and phosphorus : oxygen ratio of mitochondria isolated from these cells, the vibration method yielded preparations superior to those obtained by the rotation technique (IEMHOFF et al. 1970).

Several techniques have been developed in which the intestinal tissue was treated with chelating agents or enzymes to release the epithelial cells. STERN and REILLY (1965) used trypsin–pancreatin, but after the damaging effect of trypsin was demonstrated (HARRER et al. 1964) they employed a calcium chelation technique using citrate (STERN and JENSEN 1966; STERN 1966). These preparations exhibited glycolysis and accumulated glucose. REISER and CHRISTIANSEN (1971) combined the citrate chelation method with exposure to the enzyme hyaluroni-

Table 1. Characteristics of intestinal epithelial cells isolated by various techniques. Adapted from KIMMICH (1975)

Procedure	O_2 consumption (µl/h per milligram protein)	Lactate production (µmol/h per milligram protein)	CO_2 production (µmol/h per milligram protein)	Transport capability		Reference
				Sugars	Amino acids	
Trypsin–pancreatin + mechanical pressure	5–10	0.3–0.35	N.D.	Variable	N.D.	STERN (1966)
Lysozyme treatment of minced intestine	3.3	N.D.	2.1	4-fold gradients for 3-*O*-methyl-glucose	4-fold gradients for tyrosine	HUANG (1965)
Hyaluronidase treatment of everted sacs	21.6	N.D.	N.D.	+	N.D.	PERRIS (1966)
EDTA treatment with mechanical agitation	12.5	N.D.	N.D.	No active accumulation	< 2-fold gradients	SOGNEN (1967)
Mechanical pressure applied to surface of rotating intestine	N.D.	0.12	N.D.	N.D.	N.D.	IEMHOFF et al. (1970)
Vibration of everted sac in media containing EDTA	N.D.	0.6	0.19	N.D.	N.D.	REISER and CHRISTIANSEN (1971)
Citrate + hyaluronidase treatment + mechanical pressure	N.D.	N.D.	N.D.	N.D.	< 2.5-fold gradients	KIMMICH (1970)
Hyaluronidase treatment + mechanical agitation	1.35	0.3–0.5	0.5	4–8-fold gradients	4–8-fold gradients	

N.D. = not determined

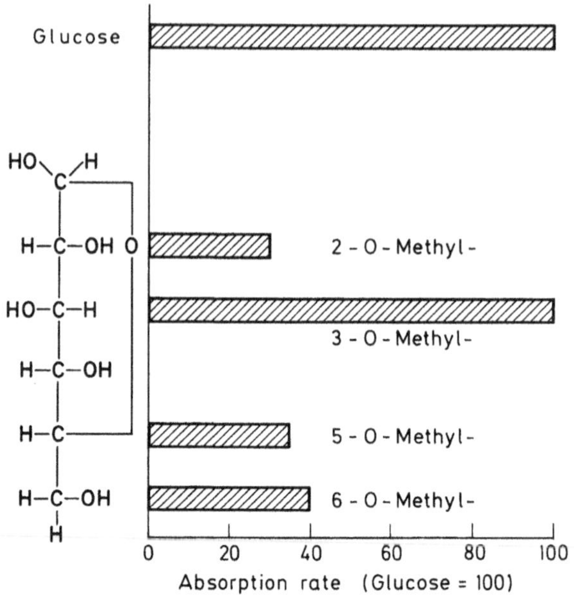

Fig. 14. The rate of absorption of glucose and its monomethyl ethers from the small intestine of the rat. The rate of absorption of glucose is arbitrarily set at 100. 3-*O*-Methylglucose is absorbed almost as fast as glucose while the absorption of 2-, 5-, and 6-*O*-methylethers is significantly slower. CSÁKY (1942) redrawn by WILSON (1962)

dase to prepare a cell suspension from the rat small intestine. They could demonstrate accumulation of amino acids in these preparations. PERRIS (1966) described a technique in which hyaluronidase was utilized to free the cells. Another method employing calcium chelation with EDTA was described by SOGNEN (1967). In this preparation an accumulation of glycine was observed, but not of 3-*O*-methylglucose.

HUANG (1965) used lysozyme for the isolation of the intestinal epithelial cells. In this technique, the intestine is exposed to lysozyme from both the venous and luminal sides. This is followed then by vigorous stirring, filtering through gauze, and centrifuging. The pellet which probably consisted of tissue fragments and isolated cells accumulated for a short period 3-*O*-methylglucose and 1-tyrosine.

KIMMICH (1970, 1975) developed a technique in which rings are prepared from the isolated small intestine of 6- to 8-week-old chickens. These rings are incubated with hyaluronidase in a Krebs–Ringer medium containing serum albumin. After a period of gentle stirring, the mixture is poured through a nylon mesh filter and the cells are isolated by gentle centrifugation (100 *g* for 1–2 min). The preparation accumulates sugars and amino acids. The accumulation is sodium dependent. Apparently the method is successfully applicable only for the intestine of the chicken. Table 1, slightly modified from the original compilation of KIMMICH (1975), summarizes the main features of the isolated intestinal cells obtained by various techniques.

Isolated cells have the advantage of a preparation consisting primarily of the cells involved in the intestinal transport, reasonably free of such inert tissues as muscle or connective tissue. With adequate methodology, viable preparations can be obtained, as judged by the oxidative (O_2 consumption and CO_2 production) and fermentative (lactic acid production) functions, and concentrative ability. The obvious limitation of the isolated cell preparation lies in the fact that it does not allow the study of one significant feature of the intestinal permeability, namely directional flux. The directional transport can be best studied by letting the intestine divide two compartments as a membrane and examining the fluxes between the two compartments. This approach is lost once the cells are isolated. Furthermore, in the isolated form both membranes of the cells are simultaneously exposed to the medium. This renders it difficult to assign the quantitative participation of either of the two membranes in the uptake or concentration of a given substrate. In some instances, this difficulty can be overcome by the use of different inhibitors which more or less specifically inhibit the transport of a given substrate in one membrane, but not in the other. Simultaneously in some cases it is known that a given substrate is transported readily across one of the membranes, but barely across the other. Examples for the specific inhibitors are phlorhizin which is a competitive inhibitor of aldose transport at the brush border, while its aglucone, phloretine, inhibits specifically the sugar transport across the basolateral membrane. For the specificity of substrate transport, α-methylglucoside can be mentioned which is almost selectively transported by the brush order, but not by the basolateral membrane, while 2-deoxyglucose is a specific substrate for the transport across the basolateral membrane (BOYD and PARSONS 1979).

8. Isolated Epithelial Membranes

This will be discussed in Chap. 7.

D. Modifications of the Permeant

The study of the permeation of a natural substrate is frequently complicated by the fact that it is metabolized in the intestinal tissue during transport. This difficulty can be overcome by the use of nonmetabolized analogs of the natural products, provided that the analogs are transported by the same mechanism as the parent substrate.

I. Artificial Sugar Compounds

In the study of the intestinal transport of sugars, the first attempt was made by CSÁKY (1936, 1942) who synthesized a number of glucose monomethyl ethers, injected them into a ligated loop of small intestine kept in situ in anesthetized rats, and examined the rate of disappearance from the gut lumen. Figure 14 illustrates that the rate of transport from the lumen of the 3-*O*-methyl compound was almost as fast as that of glucose, while the absorption of the 2-, 5-, and 6-methylethers was significantly slower. Subsequently it was shown that 3-*O*-methylglucose is actively transported in the intestine, sharing the same carrier with glucose. Moreover, the 3-*O*-methyl ether of glucose is not metabolized by the animal tissues (Csáky and Glenn 1957; Csáky and Wilson 1956). Interestingly, the 3-*O*-ethyl, -propyl, and -butyl ethers of glucose are not actively transported in the small intestine (Wilson and Landau 1960).

Subsequently, a large number of other artificial glucose derivatives were tested; several of these were found to be actively transported: 1-deoxyglucose, glucoheptulose, α- and β-methyl, -ethyl, -phenyl glucosides, β-isopropyl-, butyl-, phenyl-, *p*-chlorophenyl-, hydroxyquinone glucosides, and α- and β-methylgalactosides are all actively transported in the gut (Landau et al. 1962).

II. Artificial Amino Acid Analogs

In the study of intestinal amino acid transport, α-aminoisobutyric acid, isovaline, and cycloleucine (1-aminocyclopentane-1-carboxylic acid) were found to be typical artificial nonmetabolized analogs transported by one of the amino acid transport systems (Christensen 1962).

III. Radioisotopes

The study of intestinal permeability was greatly aided by the introduction of radiolabeled substrates. A discussion of the methodology involved in the use of radioisotopes is beyond the scope of this chapter. The method has been extensively studied and described (Andrews et al. 1966; Cohen 1971; Coursaget 1958; Roth 1965; Ussing 1948, 1952, 1978; Waser 1969). There is only one caveat which should be reemphasized here. The analysis of a labeled compound is based on the measurement of the radiation emitted by the radioactive atom within the labeled molecule. If the molecule undergoes metabolic change during its transport, the label will be present in one or more metabolites and is assayed as radiation energy. Consequently, the measuring of radiation alone will not indicate the permeation of the original substrate. Such measurement is reliable only if it is certain that the label is in the original substrate during permeation and nowhere else. The radiolabeled substrate can be visualized in the gut wall with the aid of autoradiography. This method has been described in detail (Rogers 1979) and explored in the study of intestinal absorption (Kinter and Wilson 1965; Stirling 1967).

References

Agar WG, Hird FJR, Sidhu GS (1954) The uptake of amino acids by the intestine. Biochim Biophys Acta 14:80–84

Andrews GA, Kniseley RM, Wagner HN (eds) (1966) Radioactive pharmaceuticals. US Atomic Energy Commission, Washington DC

Auchinachie DW, McCleod JJR, Magee HE (1930) Studies on diffusion through surviving isolated intestine. J Physiol (Lond) 69:185–209

Boars A, Wilson TH (1962) Development of mechanisms for intestinal absorption of vitamin B_{12} in the growing rat. Fed Proc 21:469

Boyd CAR, Parsons DS (1979) Movements of monosaccharides between blood and tissues of vascularly perfused small intestine. J Physiol (Lond) 278:371–391
Christensen HN (1962) Intestinal absorption with special reference to amino acids. Fed Proc 21:37–42
Clarkson TW, Rothstein A (1960) Transport of monovalent cations by the isolated small intestine of the rat. Am J Physiol 199:898–906
Cohen Y (1971) Radionuclides in pharmacology I and II. Pergamon, Oxford
Cori CF (1925) The fate of sugar in the animal body. 1. The rate of absorption of hexoses and pentoses from the intestinal tract. J Biol Chem 66:691–715
Coursaget J (ed) (1958) The method of isotopic tracers applied to the study of active ion transport. Pergamon, New York
Crane RK, Mandelstam P (1960) The active transport of sugars by various preparations of hamster intestine. Biochim Biophys Acta 45:460–476
Crane RK, Wilson TH (1958) In vitro method for the study of the rate of intestinal absorption of sugars. J Appl Physiol 12:145–146
Csáky TZ (1936) Einfluß der Methylierung und der Lage der Methylgruppen auf die Glukose-Resorption aus dem Dünndarm. Ber Gesamte Physiol Exp Pharmacol 94:662
Csáky TZ (1942) Über die Rolle der Struktur des Glukosemoleküls bei der Resorption aus dem Dünndarm. Hoppe-Seyler's Zeitschr Physiol Chem 277:47–57
Csáky TZ, Autenrieth B (1975) Transcellular and intercellular intestinal transport. In: Csáky TZ (ed) Intestinal absorption and malabsorption. Raven, New York pp 177–185
Csáky TZ, Glenn JE (1957) Urinary recovery of 3-methylglucose administered to rats. Am J Physiol 188:159–162
Csáky TZ, Hara Y (1965) Inhibition of active intestinal sugar transport by digitalis. Am J Physiol 209:467–472
Csáky TZ, Ho PM (1965) Intestinal transport of D-xylose. Proc Soc Exp Biol Med 120:403–408
Csáky TZ, Thale M (1960) Effect of ionic environment on intestinal sugar transport. J Physiol (Lond) 151:59–65
Csáky TZ, Wilson JE (1956) The fate of 3-O-$^{14}CH_3$-glucose in the rat. Biochim Biophys Acta 22:185–186
Darlington WA, Quastel JH (1953) Absorption of sugars from isolated surviving intestine. Arch Biochem Biophys 43:194–207
Deak ST (1977) Factors the intestinal lymphatic absorption of nutrients and drugs. Dissertation, University of Kentucky
Dent CE, Schilling JA (1949) Studies on the absorption of proteins: the amino-acid pattern in the portal blood. Biochem J 44:318:332
Dickens F, Weil-Malherbe H (1941) Metabolism of normal and tumor tissues. 19. The metabolism of intestinal mucus membrane. Biochem J 35:7–15
Esposito G, Csáky TZ (1974) Extracellular space in the epithelium of rat's small intestine. Am J Physiol 226:50–55
Field M, Fromm D, McColl I (1971) Rabbit ileum consisting of epithelium, lamina propria and muscularis mucosae. Am J Physiol 220:1388–1396
Fisher FB (1960) Quoted from J. H. Quastel (1961): Techniques for studies of intestinal absorption in vitro. Methods Med Res 9:273–286
Fisher RB, Parsons DS (1949) A preparation of surviving rat small intestine for the study of absorption. J Physiol (Lond) 110:36–46
Fondacaro JD, Nathan P, Wright WE (1974) Methionine accumulation in villi isolated from maturing rat intestine. J Physiol (Lond) 241:751–760
Fullerton PM, Parsons DS (1956) Absorption of sugars and water from the rat intestine in vivo. Q J Exp Physiol 41:387
Harrer DS, Stern BK, Reilly RW (1964) Removal and dissociation of epithelial cells from the rodent gastrointestinal tract. Nature 203:319–320
Höber R, Höber J (1937) Experiments on the absorption of organic solutes in the small intestine of rats. J Cell Physiol 10:401–419
Horváth I, Wix G (1951) Hormonal influences on glucose resorption from the intestine. Acta Physiol Acad Sci Hung 2:435–443

Huang KC (1965) Uptake of L-tyrosine and 3-O-methylglucose by isolated intestinal epithelial cells. Life Sci 4:1201–1206

Iemhoff WGJ, Van den Berg JWO, De Pijper AM, Hulsmann WC (1970) Metabolic aspects of isolated cells from rat small intestinal epithelium. Biochim Biophys Acta 215:229–241

Jacobs FA, Luper M (1957) Intestinal absorption by perfusion in situ. J Appl Physiol 11:136–138

Jervis EL, Johnson FR, Sheff MF, Smyth DH (1956) Effect of phlorizin on intestinal absorption and intestinal phosphatase. J Physiol (Lond) 134:675–688

Johnston CG (1932) A method for making quantitative intestinal studies. Proc Soc Exp Biol Med 30:193–196

Jorgensen CR, Landau BR, Wilson TH (1961) A common pathway for sugar transport in hamster intestine. Am J Physiol 200:111–116

Kimmich GA (1970) Preparation and properties of mucosal epithelial cells isolated from small intestine of the chicken. Biochemistry 9:3659–3668

Kimmich GA (1975) Preparation and characterization of isolated intestinal epithelial cells and their use in studying intestinal transport. Methods Membrane Biol 5:57–115

Kinter WB, Wilson TH (1965) Autoradiographic study of sugar and amino acid absorption by everted sacs of hamster intestine. J Cell Biol 25:19–39

Landau BR, Bernstein L, Wilson TH (1962) Hexose transport by hamster intestine in vitro. Am J Physiol 203:237–240

Lauterbach F (1977) Passive permeabilities of luminal and basolateral membranes in the isolated mucosal epithelium of guinea pig small intestine. Naunyn-Schmiedeberg's Arch Pharmacol 297:201–212

Levine RR, McNary WF, Korrguth PJ, Leblanc R (1970) Histological reevaluation of everted gut technique for studying intestinalabsorption Eur J Eur J Pharmacol 9:211–219

London ES (1935) Angiostomie und Organestoffwechsel. All-Union Institute for Experimental Medicine, Moscow

Matthews DM, Smyth DH (1954) Intestinal absorption of amino acid enantiomorphs. J Physiol (Lond) 126:96–100

Pasenchych (1961) Addendum in J. H. Quastel: Technics for studies of intestinal absorption in vitro. Methods Med Res 9:283–84

Parson DS (1968) Intestinal absorption. In: Code CF (ed) Alimentary canal. American Physiological Society, Washington DC, p 1199 (Handbook of physiology, sect 6, vol 3)

Parsons G, Paterson CR (1965) Fluid and solute transport across rat colonic mucosa. Q J Exp Physiol 50:220–231

Parsons DS, Wingate DL (1961) The effect of osmotic gradients on fluid transfer across rat intestine in vitro. Biochim Biophys Acta 46:170–183

Perris AD (1966) Isolation of the epithelial cells of the rat small intestine. Can J Biochem 44:687–693

Reid EW (1900) On intestinal absorption, especially on the absorption of serum, peptone and glucose. Philos Trans R Soc Lond [Biol] 102:211–297

Reiser S, Christiansen P (1971) The properties of the preferential uptake of L-leucine by isolated intestinal epithelial cells. Biochim Biophys Acta 225:123–139

Rider AK, Schedl HP, Nokes G, Shining S (1967) Small intestinal glucose transport. Proximal-distal kinetic gradients. J Gen Physiol 50:1173–1182

Robinson G (1857) Contributions to the physiology and pathology of the circulation of the blood. Longmans London

Rogers AW (1979) Techniques of autoradiography, 3rd edn. Elsevier, Amsterdam

Roth LJ (ed) (1965) Isotopes in experimental pharmacology. The University of Chicago Press, Chicago

Rothe CF, Quay JF, Armstrong W McD (1969) Measurement of epithelial electrical characteristics with an automatic voltage clamp devise with compensation for solution resistance. IEEE Trans Bio Eng 16:160–164

Semenza G (1969) Studies on intestinal sucrose and sugar transport. VII. A method for measuring intestinal uptake, the absorption of the anomeric forms of some monosaccharides. Biochim Biophys Acta 173:104–112

Sheff MF, Smyth DH (1955) Apparatus for study of in vivo intestinal absorption in the rat. J Physiol (Lond) 128:67P
Sjostrand FS (1968) A simple and rapid method to prepare dispersions of columnar epithelial cells from the rat intestine. J Ultrastruct Res 22:424–442
Sognen E (1967) A method for the preparation of suspensions of intestinal epithelial cells by means of calcium chelation. Acta Vet Scand 8:76–82
Sols A, Ponz F (1947) New method for the study of intestinal absorption. Rev Esp Fisiol 3:207–211
Stern BK (1966) Some biochemical properties of suspensions of intestinal epithelial cells. Gastroenterology 51:855–864
Stern DK, Jensen WE (1966) Active transport of glucose by suspensions of isolated rat intestinal epithelial cells. Nature 209:789–790
Stern BK, Reilly RW (1965) Some characteristics of the respiratory metabolism of suspensions of rat intestinal epithelial cells. Nature 205:563–565
Stirling CE (1967) High-resolution radioautography of phlorizin-^{3}H in rings of hamster intestine. J Cell Biol 35:605–618
Thiry L (1864) Über eine neue Methode den Dünndarm zu isolieren, Sitzungsber Akad Wiss Wien Kl. I 50:77–906
Turnheim K, Lauterbach F (1980) Interaction between intestinal absorption and secretion of monoquaternary ammonium compounds in guinea pigs. A concept of the absorption kinetics of organic cations. J Pharmacol Exp Ther 212:418–424
Ussing HH (1948) The use of tracers in the study of active ion transport across animal membranes. Cold Spring Harbor Symp Quant Biol 13:193–200
Ussing HH (1952) Some aspects of the application of tracers in permeability studies. Adv Enzymol 13:21–65
Ussing HH (1978) Interpretation of tracer fluxes. In: Tosteson DC (ed) Membrane transport in biology, vol 1, concepts and models. Springer, Berlin, pp 115–140
Ussing HH, Zerahn K (1951) Active transport of sodium as the source of electric current in the short-circuited isolated frog skin. Acta Physiol Scand 23:110–127
Vella L (1880) Nuovo methodo per avere il succo enterico puro e stabilirne le proprieta fisiologiche. Mem Acad Sci Inst Bologna Ser 4 2:515–535
Verzár F, McDougall EJ (1936) Absorption from the intestine. Longman, London
Waser PG, Glasson B (eds) (1969) International conference on radioactive isotopes in pharmacology. Wiley-Interscience, London
Wilson TH (1962) Intestinal absorption. Saunders, Philadelphia
Wilson TH, Landau BR (1960) Specificity of sugar transport by the intestine of the hamster. Am J Physiol 198:99–102
Wilson TH, Wiseman G (1954) The use of sacs of inverted small intestine for the study of the transference of substances from the mucosal to serosal surface. J Physiol (Lond) 123:116–125
Wiseman G (1953) Absorption of amino-acids using an in vitro technique. J Physiol (Lond) 120:63–72
Wright WE, Line VD (1976) Preparation of isolated intestinal villi useful for studying hydrolysis rates of penicillin and cephalosporin esters. Antimicrob Agents Chemother 10:861–863

CHAPTER 5

Vascular Perfusion of Rat Small Intestine for Permeation and Metabolism Studies

H. G. WINDMUELLER and A. E. SPAETH

A. Introduction

Vascular perfusion is a technique which permits the study of a living, intact organ while it is partially or totally isolated from other organs and in which the delivery of metabolic substrates and removal of metabolic products is through the normal vascular channels. The technique has particular relevance for the study of the small intestine, an organ with highly polarized muscosal epithelial absorptive cells engaged in transport from the lumen to the blood and the lymph, while at the same time taking up certain compounds from the blood. Thus, the arterial vasculature and the lumen serve as dual sources of substances entering these cells; and the venous vasculature, the lymphatics, and the lumen serve as departure routes for substances leaving the cells. Perfusion methods permit separate access to each of these channels, making it possible to study a wide variety of intestinal functions under relatively normal physiologic conditions.

Two vascular perfusion methods developed in our laboratory for rat small intestine will be described. The rat serves well as the experimental animal for a number of reasons. Rats are readily available, are easy to maintain, and are relatively inexpensive, which is particularly important during the developmental stages of a procedure. Their small size makes them convenient subjects for study in the average laboratory. The availability of highly inbred rat strains improves the uniformity of the experimental material and the reproducibility of results. And finally, the long history of the rat as a research animal in most areas of mammalian biology and biochemistry makes available a vast and invaluable reference literature. Although surgical procedures with the rat frequently require the use of a dissecting microscope or other means of magnification, the small amounts of tissue perfused and the relatively small perfusate volumes seldom pose analytic problems with the advent of newer enzymatic, immunologic, and chromatographic methods of high sensitivity and specificity.

The first procedure to be described involves vascular perfusion of the entire small intestine, isolated and removed from the animal. The cecum and part of the colon are generally included. The preparation also allows for lymph collection. The second preparation is an autoperfused segment of small intestine in vivo. Here, the arterial, neural, and lymphatic connections to the segment remain intact while the venous outflow from the segment is totally collected. This preparation is relatively easy to set up, is highly versatile, and has, in our opinion, received too little attention as an experimental tool. We will present a description of each preparation and the steps involved in setting it up and conducting a typical experiment, and will follow with some examples of its application. We have tried to be rather comprehensive in describing equipment and technique. Methodological details, mostly missing from the usual journal articles, are important for the convenience and often the very success of a perfusion procedure and are typically the product of much trial and error. The comparative advantages and disadvantages of the two preparations will become evident from the separate discussions and will be summarized in a concluding section.

Table 1. Vascular perfusion of isolated rat small intestine

Reference	Perfusing medium [a]	Comments
ÖHNELL (1939); ÖHNELL and HÖBER (1939)	Saline plus bovine erythrocytes and gum acacia	Studied sugar absorption; observed spastic motility, rapid functional deterioration, and edema
HESTRIN-LERNER and SHAPIRO (1954)	Dialyzed bovine serum plus bovine erythrocytes	Studied glucose absorption; few details given
JACOBS et al. (1966)	Buffer plus dextran and insulin	Studied iron absorption
GERBER and REMY-DEFRAIGNE (1966)	Heparinized rat blood plus Ringer's solution	Studied incorporation and metabolism of thymidine
KAVIN et al. (1967)	Modified Ringer's solution plus bovine erythrocytes and dextran	Viability for 1 h indicated by oxygen uptake (low), glucose transport and utilization, and histology; edema observed
FORTH (1968)	Electrolyte solution plus bovine serum albumin, polyvinylpyrrolidone, human erythrocytes, heparin, papaverine, and promethazin; pH 7.0 (single pass)	Measured iron and cobalt absorption
LEE and DUNCAN (1968)	Heparinized rat blood plus pentobarbital	Measured water absorption into blood and lymph
DUBOIS et al. (1968); DUBOIS and ROY (1969); ROY et al. (1970)	Buffer plus bovine erythrocytes, albumin, dextran, and polyol surfactant (single pass)	Measured oxygen uptake (low), glucose utilization, and hexose transport
JOHNSON et al. (1969)	Rat blood pumped directly from donor rat	Very few details or results given
OLSON and DELUCA (1969)	Krebs–Ringer buffer plus rat serum and dextran	Studied calcium transport; very few details given
WINDMUELLER et al. (1970, 1973); WINDMUELLER and SPAETH (1972, 1974)	Heparinized rat blood plus dexamethasone, norepinephrine, penicillin, and streptomycin	See accompanying text for details

Table 1 (continued)

Reference	Perfusing medium[a]	Comments
HÜLSMANN (1971)	Krebs–Henseleit buffer plus human erythrocytes, albumin, polyvinylpyrrolidone, papaverine, promethazin, and heparin	Measured uptake of oxidative substrates at 33 °C for 1 h
LAMERS and HÜLSMANN (1972)	Krebs–Henseleit buffer plus varying additions, including a fluorocarbon	Measured glucose utilization, lactate production, and tissue nucleotide levels
KATZ and O'BRIEN (1979)	Krebs–Ringer buffer plus dextran, glucose, heparin, dexamethasone, and propranolol	Studied vitamin B_{12} absorption; edema developed after 45 min.
OCHSENFAHRT (1979)	Rat blood pumped directly from donor rat	Studied absorption of antipyrene, salicylic acid, and urea
MATSUTAKA et al. (1973)	Rat blood plus saline	Metabolic studies indicate short-term viability (10 min)
HANSON and PARSONS (1976, 1977, 1978)	Krebs–Ringer buffer plus bovine erythrocytes, albumin, penicillin, and streptomycin	Used distension pressure of 15 cm saline in lumen to reduce excessive motility; measurements of oxygen, glucose, and glutamine utilization and lactate release indicate viability for 1 h; used for metabolic studies
ELOY et al. (1977)	Heparinized rat blood (single pass)	Used low arterial blood pressure and flow rate; appearance of mucosal enzymes in lumen indicates tissue damage
SMITH et al. (1978)	Krebs–Ringer buffer plus rat serum, dextran, dexamethasone, and norepinephrine	Studied zinc absorption
HENDERSON and GROSS (1979a, b)	Modified Krebs–Ringer buffer plus albumin, dexamethasone, and norepinephrine	Studied transport and metabolism of niacin and niacinamide
LEVIN et al. (1979)	Krebs–Ringer buffer plus bovine albumin and dextran (single pass)	Preparation includes stomach and spleen; sloughing of epithelial cells evident within 1 h; active glucose transport not demonstrable
BRONK and INGHAM (1979)	Ringer's bicarbonate buffer plus bovine serum albumin and human erythrocytes (single pass)	Studied hexose transport

[a] Not including the additions of metabolic substrates

B. Isolated Intestine with Lymph Collection

I. Historical Aspects

The idea of using an isolated, vascularly perfused intestinal preparation for studying intestinal function is by no means new, but dates back at least to the work of SALVIOLI (1880). Over the intervening years, numerous laboratories have attempted to establish such a preparation for mammalian intestine. The early history is discussed by ROESE (1930). PARSONS and PRICHARD (1968), after reviewing the literature accounts published between 1880 and 1966 from more than 30 different laboratories, noted the "singular ill-success" of the procedure throughout its history and concluded that "few of these attempts have produced a viable preparation suitable for studies of intestinal absorption." ÖHNELL (1939) was apparently the first to use small intestine from the rat, and subsequently rat preparations have been described from at least 20 laboratories (Table 1). Few of these preparations have been described in any detail. Most were designed to meet very limited experimental objectives and have not reappeared in the literature. From a consideration of the described methodology, in the light of our own experience with perfused intestine, it seems justifiable to question the prolonged viability of most of these preparations. However, some appear to have been used successfully for short-term metabolic and transport experiments of 1 h or less, despite evidence of abnormalities such as spasmodic bowel contractions (HANSON and PARSONS 1976). Other troublesome problems common to many earlier perfusion attempts include tissue edema, detachment of the mucosa, high vascular resistance, and progressive cellular necrosis. Procedural differences in the various methods, other than perfusate composition, include the anesthetic agent used, the surgical technique employed, the duration of the anoxic interval preceding the beginning of perfusion, the length of intestine being perfused, and the pharmacologic agents used to control the adverse effects.

It is not the purpose of this chapter to compare critically the various preparations that have been published; too few performance data are provided in most instances to justify this. A critical evaluation of several methods has been made by ROSS (1972). Instead, we will describe our own preparation in some detail – its development, the procedure as presently used, and its applications to date.

II. Development of Procedure

1. Problems Encountered and Remedies Tested

The development of an isolated intestinal preparation was undertaken in our case to study the biosynthesis of the protein moieties of chylomicrons and other lipoproteins by the small intestine (WINDMUELLER et al. 1970). Prolonged lymph collection from a vascularly perfused intestine had not been previously described, but was essential since intestinal chylomicrons reach the blood by way of the lymphatics. Two other shortcomings of many earlier preparations, deficiencies that contributed to the general lack of success, were the use of unphysiologic perfusing media and the often prolonged interval during surgery when the tissue was not being perfused at all and was obviously anoxic. At the outset, therefore, we used as the perfusate whole heparinized rat blood, freshly drawn from ether-anesthetized donors, and developed a surgical procedure that minimized traumatic handling of the intestine and insured an uninterrupted flow of oxygenated blood through the tissue. (Details of the updated technique appear in Sect. B. III.) Briefly, the entire small intestine, the cecum, and part of the colon were isolated en bloc with a series of ligatures, leaving the superior mesenteric artery, which supplies this portion of the gut, and the superior mesenteric vein uninterrupted. An arterial cannula, primed with blood pumped from a rotating spherical flask (oxygenator–reservoir) gassed with 95% O_2/5% CO_2, was inserted into the superior mesenteric artery and pumping of perfusate begun immediately. The superior mesenteric vein was similarly cannulated and venous blood recycled back to the oxygenator–reservoir. The rat was killed and both cannulae secured with ligatures. Arterial and venous pressure, temperature, and the blood glucose concentration were all maintained in the normal range.

Within minutes after perfusion was begun, however, several clear indications of bowel abnormality became evident.

a. Hypersecretion: the small intestinal lumen became progressively distended owing to the accumulation of a slightly alkaline, nearly clear, pale yellow fluid having an ionic composition resembling the duodenal secretion in dogs stimulated with cholera exotoxin (CARPENTER and GREENOUGH 1968).

b. Hypermotility: by 2 min, intense spasmodic contractions appeared, first in the proximal colon and cecum but, within 15 min, in all regions of the intestine. The contractions continued for more than 1 h, until the bowel was severely distended with fluid.

c. Hyperemia: within 15–30 min the bowel developed an inflamed, red appearance.

d. Low vascular resistance: the perfusate flow rate needed to maintain a normal arterial blood pressure was approximately twice the intestinal blood flow rate measured in vivo.

Vasoconstriction sufficient to prevent even normal blood flow, apparently seen by others who routinely added papaverine to the perfusate, (FORTH 1968; HÜLSMANN 1971) was observed only when the start of perfusion was delayed and the tissue became anoxic. As further evidence of inadequate conditions, histologic examination of the tissue after several hours of perfusion revealed edema and epithelial necrosis.

Various procedural modifications were tested, without success, to prevent the rapidly appearing hypersecretion and hypermotility.

a. The perfusate was changed to one of the following: heparinized rat blood diluted with Krebs–Ringer buffer containing 5% bovine albumin; washed rat or bovine erythrocytes in Krebs–Ringer buffer plus 5% or 9% bovine albumin; Krebs–Ringer buffer plus 5% albumin perfused only once and not recycled through the tissue; minimum essential tissue culture medium (EAGLE 1959) plus hemoglobin; washed erythrocytes in Krebs–Ringer buffer plus dextran (molecular weight 25,600); defibrinated rat blood; and albumin-containing buffer previously recycled through a perfused rat liver.

b. The rotating flask oxygenator was eliminated by recycling the heparinized blood perfusate through isolated rat lungs ventilated with air by means of a respirator.

c. An antihistamine (2-diphenylmethoxy-*N*,*N*-dimethylethylaminediphenhydramine) was added to the perfusate.

More encouraging results were obtained in additional experiments where the perfusion circuitry was designed so that the intestine could be perfused alternately with: (a) heparinized blood pumped directly from the aorta of a second rat; and (b) heparinized rat blood equilibrated with O_2/CO_2 in the oxygenator. Hypermotility and hypersecretion subsided immediately whenever aortic blood was perfused directly, and they resumed immediately when the perfused blood had been exposed to the oxygenator. After several erroneous interpretations of this result, it was established that the subdued motility and secretion were due to the ether present in the blood pumped directly from the ether-anesthetized blood donor rat. Once the blood passed to the oxygenator, the ether was rapidly lost.

2. Effects of Drugs and Hormones

The foregoing explanation for the observations emerged from further experiments in which various drugs and hormones were added to heparinized rat blood recycled through the intestine and the oxygenator. The results of these experiments are summarized in Table 2. When added alone, dexamethasone (9-α-fluoro-16α-methylprednisolone), a potent synthetic glucocorticoid, reduced the hyperemia, but failed to prevent the other deleterious responses to perfusion. However, further supplementation with pentobarbital, ethyl ether, or propranolol(1-isopropylamino-3-(1-naphthyloxy)-2-propanol), a β-adrenergic blocking agent that at high concentrations exhibits strong local anesthetic activity (ARIENS 1967), prevented the hypersecretion and hypermotility as well. The low vascular resistance remained, and, following 5 h of perfusion, evidence of epithelial necrosis remained. Similar results were obtained with atropine sulfate. The most successful results were achieved by adding dexamethasone to the perfusate and continuously infusing a regulated dose of norepinephrine (0.06–0.21 μg/min) into the arterial cannula. The infusion rate of this hormone, which increases vascular resistance in the intestine, was regulated to maintain normal arterial blood pressure, with the blood flow rate being held constant at a normal rate. While addition of dexamethasone alone had improved the perfusion only slightly, its presence in the perfusate was essential for the prolonged salutary effects of norepinephrine. Without dexamethasone, the responsiveness of the preparation to norepinephrine began to decline after 5–30 min. Progressively higher infusion rates of norepinephrine, up to ten times the initial rate, were then needed to maintain normal arterial pressure. The bowel also developed a marked hyperemia. When, after 60 min of perfusion in the absence of dexamethasone, the steroid was added to the perfusate (6×10^{-7} *M*), there was a gradual but dramatic return in norepinephrine responsiveness – the blood pressure could be maintained with progressively lower rates of norepinephrine infusion, and within 30 min the gross

Table 2. Response of isolated intestine to drugs and hormones. WINDMUELLER et al. (1970)

Additions to perfusate	Perfusate concentration (M)	Response by intestine[a]				
		Hyper-secretion	Hyper-motility	Hyper-emia	Low vascular resistance	Epithelial necrosis[b]
None		+	+	+	+	N.E.
Dexamethasone[c] (DEX)	6×10^{-7}	+	+	−	+	N.E.
Propranolol + DEX[d]	1×10^{-5}	−	−	−	+	+
Pentobarbital[e] + DEX	2×10^{-4}	−	−	−	+	+
Ethyl ether[f] + DEX	Anesthetic	−	−	−	+	+
Atropine[g] + DEX	9×10^{-5}	−	−	−	+	+
Norepinephrine[h] + DEX	$4–8\times10^{-8}$	−	−	−	−	−

[a] + Positive response; − negative response; N.E. not examined because perfusion was terminated after 2–3 h
[b] Determined from histologic examination after 5 h perfusion
[c] 25 μg/100 ml perfusate; added to the reservoir
[d] A 3.2 mg/ml solution of propranolol hydrochloride was continuously infused into the arterial inflow cannula at 10 μl/min; + DEX indicates that the perfusate also contained 6×10^{-7} M dexamethasone
[e] Sodium pentobarbital, 5 mg/100 ml perfusate; added to the reservoir
[f] Ether was added to the oxygenator O_2/CO_2 gassing mixture in the same ratio used for ether: O_2 in anesthesia (see Fig. 5)
[g] Atropine sulfate, 6.25 mg/100 ml perfusate; added to the reservoir
[h] L-Arterenol-D-bitartrate-H_2O; a 0.153 mg/ml solution was continuously infused into the inflow cannula at 1.0–2.2 μl/min

appearance of the tissue had returned to normal. On the basis of these studies, the use of dexamethasone and norepinephrine have become standard in our preparation. Other glucocorticoids and catecholamines have not been tested.

Evidence from several sources (see WINDMUELLER et al. 1970) indicates that loss of sympathetic innervation is the cause of the abnormal behavior of the intestine following isolation and is compensated for in our procedure by the continuous infusion of norepinephrine. Anatomic (NORBERG 1964), physiologic (DRESEL and WALLENTIN 1966; KEWENTER 1965), and pharmacologic (PATON and VIZI 1969) studies indicate that the adrenergic innervation of the intestine has at least two functions: vasomotor regulation of vascular smooth muscle and modulation of acetylcholine release within the tissue, by way of fibers terminating near parasympathetic ganglion cells of the intramural enteric plexus. Severing the adrenergic nerves disrupts vasomotor regulation, producing lowered vascular resistance, redistribution of blood flow through the tissue (FOLKOW 1967), and consequently cellular destruction. Denervation also leads to an increased release of acetylcholine, responsible for the hypermotility and hypersecretion. Atropine and also the anesthetic agents block these actions of acetylcholine, but are unable to correct the loss of vasomotor control.

The dexamethasone requirement, while it cannot as yet be satisfactorily explained on a molecular level, is related to other observations that have led to the concept of a permissive effect of glucocorticoids on catecholamine action (FRITZ and LEVINE 1951; RAMEY and GOLDSTEIN 1957). For example, hypermia and venous engorgement are observed in the mesenteric blood vessels of adrenalectomized rats. Furthermore, norepinephrine administered to such animals produces vasomotor exhaustion, vascular stasis, and loss of vasomotion, all reversible within 30 min by the local administration of glucocorticoids to the mesentery. The striking requirement for added glucocorticoid in our isolated intestinal preparation may be related to the stress and elevated circulating catecholamine concentrations associated with the method.

III. Description of Procedure

1. Equipment and Surgical Tools

The perfusion technique (WINDMUELLER et al. 1970; WINDMUELLER and SPAETH 1972) has undergone continuing development, and the most recent refinements in procedure and apparatus will be described. A schematic diagram of the perfusion circuit is shown in Fig. 1. The perfusate used is whole rat blood. The membrane lung has been described in detail (KOLOBOW et al. 1968). This model, formerly manufactured by Dow Corning Corporation, Midland, Michigan, is not now commercially available. A simpler membrane oxygenator constructed from thin-walled silicone rubber tubing, such as the one described by HAMILTON et al. (1974), would probably serve as well. The perfusate reservoir is an envelope fabricated from two sheets of silicone rubber (see Fig. 2). (The edges and joints of the reservoir, as well as those of all other items fabricated from silicone rubber, are cemented with silicone glue.) The reservoir holds up to 250 ml blood and can be cleared of air, providing, together with the membrane lung, a perfusion circuit devoid of any direct blood–air interface. This may be important when working with plasma lipoproteins and other blood proteins that are readily denatured. The reservoir is laid on the platform of a mechanical rocker (see B in Fig. 12), tilted down slightly toward the reservoir outlet. The rocker oscillates at approximately 30 cycles/min, achieving gentle mixing. Pumps A and B (Model RL-175 Holter pump, Extracorporeal Medical Specialties, King of Prussia, Pennsylvania) each have dual silicone rubber pumping chambers. Only one chamber of pump B is used. One chamber of pump A supplies the arterial circuit. The other chamber of pump A and also pump B, which is set to pump at a slow and constant rate of about 3 ml/min, operate the venous circuit and also the bypass loop. The filter contains 1.7 g glass wool compressed between stainless steel screens (see Fig. 2). The pressure-regulating valve in the venous circuit (see Fig. 2) is made of two 1-mm thick silicone rubber sheets glued together at their edges, with an inflow tube going to a space across the top and a polytetrafluoroethylene (PTFE) outflow tube passing snugly through an opening in the bottom. The valve functions as follows. The pumps and reservoir are at a lower level than the intestine, and, with blood in the system, negative pressure draws the walls of the valve together, tending to form a seal just above the end of the PTFE tube and blocking further transmission of the siphoning effect. The blood entering the valve from the intestine creates a thin channel through the "seal"; the venous line upstream from the valve remains under a positive pressure determined by the height of the valve above the preparation. The end of the PTFE tube within the valve is adjusted low enough to permit the "sealing" effect, but not lower, otherwise there will be intermittent filling and outflow. By use of the valve, venous pressure, monitored with a water manometer, is easily regulated and relatively stable, requiring only minor adjustments for changes in blood flow rate.

To permit periodic monitoring of the oxygen saturation of arterial and venous blood, a specially fabricated flow cell (Fig. 2) is interposed in the venous circuit and a similar one in the bypass loop, which contains fully oxygenated blood from the reservoir. These flow cells, lined with silicone rubber, are mounted with the glass windows facing down on a reflection oximeter (catalog No. 10841, American Optical Company, Buffalo, New York) modified so that the two cells can be alternately positioned over the instrument's light source. The blood volume of the cells is 0.3 ml. All tubing shown in Fig. 1 is of transparent silicone rubber. A cabinet thermoregulated at 37 °C contains all the components shown

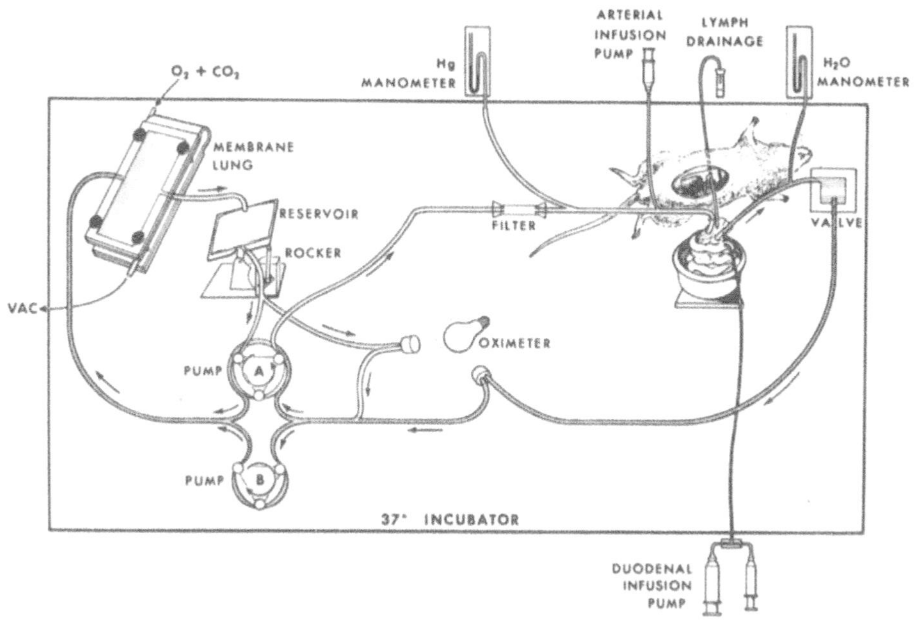

Fig. 1. Schematic diagram of apparatus for perfusing isolated rat intestine. In the perfusion circuit, *stippling* indicates venous blood from the intestine and *no stippling* indicates fully oxygenated blood. WINDMUELLER and SPAETH (1977)

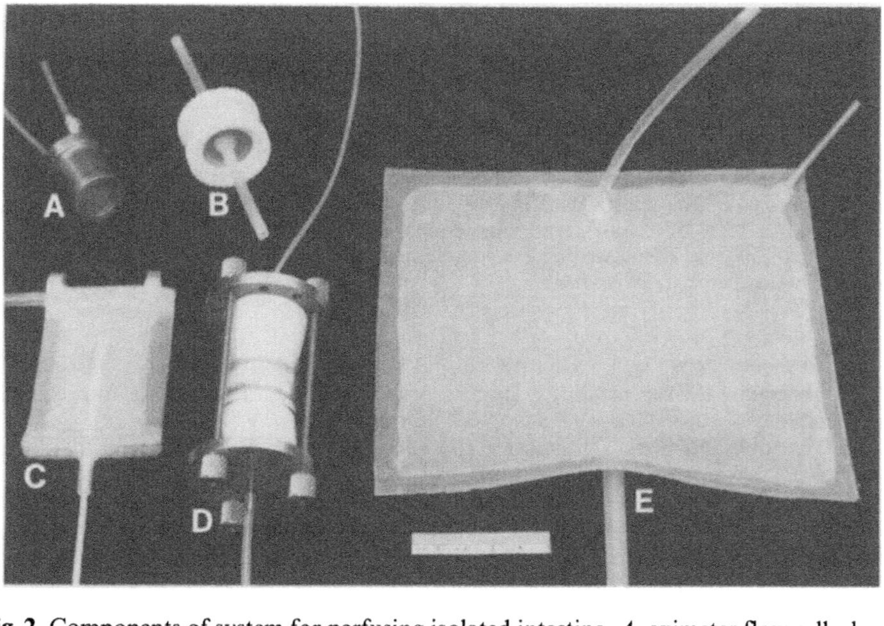

Fig. 2. Components of system for perfusing isolated intestine. *A*, oximeter flow cell, showing transparent glass window in its base; *B*, blood prefilter; *C*, valve for regulating venous pressure; *D*, glass wool blood filter; *E*, blood reservoir. Scale shown is 5 cm

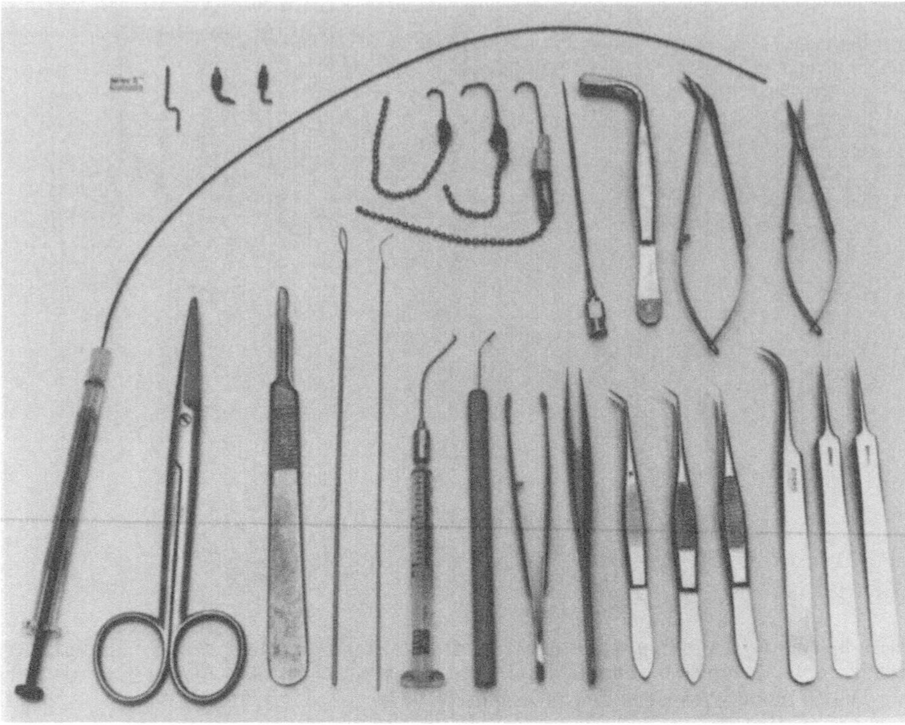

Fig. 3. Cannulae needles and surgical tools for perfusing isolated rat intestine. Upper row, left to right: 12-mm scale; duodenal infusion cannula; needle for superior mesenteric vein cannula; needle for superior mesenteric artery cannula; three retractors; trocar for positioning lymph cannula; forceps for grasping the rectangular brass blocks on the arterial and venous cannula needles during cannulation; two microdissecting scissors, extra-fine and fine. *Lower, row, left to right*: syringe and polyethylene lymph cannula (darkened for photographic contrast); general surgical scissors; scalpel; two of several stainless steel thread holders, one with double thread; tool for puncturing lymph vessel; aorta probe, used during cannulation of superior mesenteric artery; forceps with silicone rubber-covered tips, for handling intestine; fine microdissecting forceps, Swiss-style, modified for grasping lymph cannula; three pairs of extra-fine angular dissecting forceps, modified to achieve varying degrees of additional fineness; fine microdissecting forceps, curved, Swiss-style; two fine microdissecting forceps, Swiss-style

within the rectangle in Fig. 1 except the rat, gut bath, and surgical platform. These are on a table adjacent to the cabinet during surgery, after which they are brought within the thermoregulated space by means of a transparent canopy.

The cannulae and most of the surgical tools are shown in Fig. 3. Several deserve special mention. The venous cannula needle is constructed from thin-walled 16-gauge stainless steel tubing. It has a shallow bevel, about 25°, a sharpened point, and a shallow circumferential groove just behind the bevel. The arterial cannula needle is of thin-walled 20-gauge stainless steel tubing. It has a steep bevel, approximately 45°, a smooth, rounded point, and also has a shallow groove behind the bevel. To minimize crimping and increased flow resistance, the angles in the tubing are made by inserting a tight-fitting wire or bundle of wires, bending the tubing over a rounded support, then removing the wires. The shafts of both cannula needles are fitted with rectangular brass blocks, which can be firmly grasped with forceps during cannulation. The lymph cannula is polyethylene, 0.58 mm inside diameter and 0.97 mm outside diameter. The end inserted into the rat is cut to a steep bevel, approximately 45°, and immediately behind the bevel there is a very slight bulge, produced by directing a stream of hot air at that point while the tubing is rotating. The thread holders are 15 cm lengths of stainless steel tubing, 18- or 21-gauge. The threads, 4-0 and 6-0 surgical silk, are readily inserted by applying a vacuum to one end of the holders.

2. Preparing for Perfusion

Suitable rats, various infusion solutions, and the equipment must all be prepared and in readiness on the day of an experiment. Blood donor rats are typically 450–700 g males, usually Osborne-Mendel or Sprague-Dawley strain ex-breeders fed a stock ration. Intestine donors are 240–290 g Osborne-Mendel males, generally fasted overnight. In our experience, rats of this strain typically have a single, well-defined mesenteric lymph channel that is more readily cannulated than in Sprague-Dawley rats.

Before assembling the perfusion circuit, all tubing and components that contact the perfusate are soaked for several hours in a solution of crude trypsin, to digest any adhering residual protein. They are then rinsed thoroughly with distilled water, sterilized by autoclaving, and allowed to dry.

The following infusion solutions (room temperature) are loaded bubble-free into pump-driven syringes for delivery: (1) 0.5 *M* $NaHCO_3$; (2) 0.5 *M* glucose; (3) 0.04 *M* glutamine in 0.15 *M* NaCl; and (4) 0.4 m*M* norepinephrine, as L-arterenol-D-bitartrate-H_2O (Mann Research Laboratories, New York), in 0.15 *M* NaCl. Gas-tight glass syringes with PTFE plungers (Hamilton Company, Reno, Nevada) are particularly well suited for infusion because they resist leaking and also jamming, without the need for lubrication. Pumps having continuously variable speed (for example Model 906, Harvard Instrument Company, Millis, Massachusetts) are required for delivery of $NaHCO_3$ and norepinephrine. All infusion pumps are placed outside the 37 °C cabinet, and the solutions delivered through small holes in the cabinet by way of small-bore polyethylene tubing. The gut bath solution is prepared by making the following additions to Earle's balanced salt solution (EARLE 1943) (per 100 ml): glucose, 1.1 mmol; glutamine, 65 µmol; penicillin G, 10,000 USP units; streptomycin sulfate, 6.7 mg. The solution is warmed to 37 °C and the flask continuosly flushed with 95% O_2/5% CO_2, to maintain the pH at 7.4 and to prevent the precipitation of calcium salts. Earle's solution was chosen because it is similar in composition to peritoneal fluid (BOEN 1961).

The perfusate is prepared immediately before surgery. Blood is drawn from the abdominal aorta of ether-anesthetized rats with syringes containing sufficient sodium heparin solution (10 mg/ml in 0.15 *M* NaCl) to give a final blood concentration of approximately 30 USP units per milliliter blood. The blood is delivered through a prefilter (see Fig. 2) into the blood reservoir (see Fig. 2), which is submerged in an ice slurry. The prefilter was fabricated from a Millipore filter holder and silicone rubber and has a stainless steel screen for removing any clots. Approximately ten donor rats are required to obtain the 150 ml blood usually used. The following additions to the blood are then made (per 100 ml): dexamethasone, 25 µg; glucose, 0.3 mmol; penicillin G, 10,000 USP units; and streptomycin sulfate, 6.7 mg. The additions are made as isotonic solutions with a total volume of about 3 ml. Any air in the reservoir is removed. The reservoir and perfusate are then warmed to 37 °C in a water bath and transferred onto the rocker in the 37 °C cabinet. The perfusate is recycled slowly through the membrane lung until perfusion of the intestine is begun.

3. Surgical Procedure

The intestine donor rat, anesthetized with ether, is placed in a supine position on an adjustable, sloping surgical platform (see Fig. 4). The rat's head is inserted into a rectangular box through the tight-fitting circular opening in the rubber diaphragm (cut from a surgical glove) covering one end (Fig. 4; the bi-level steel platform and cannulae are initially not present). During surgery, the rat can conveniently be kept well oxygenated and lightly anesthetized by continuously flushing the box with a regulated mixture of oxygen and ether,

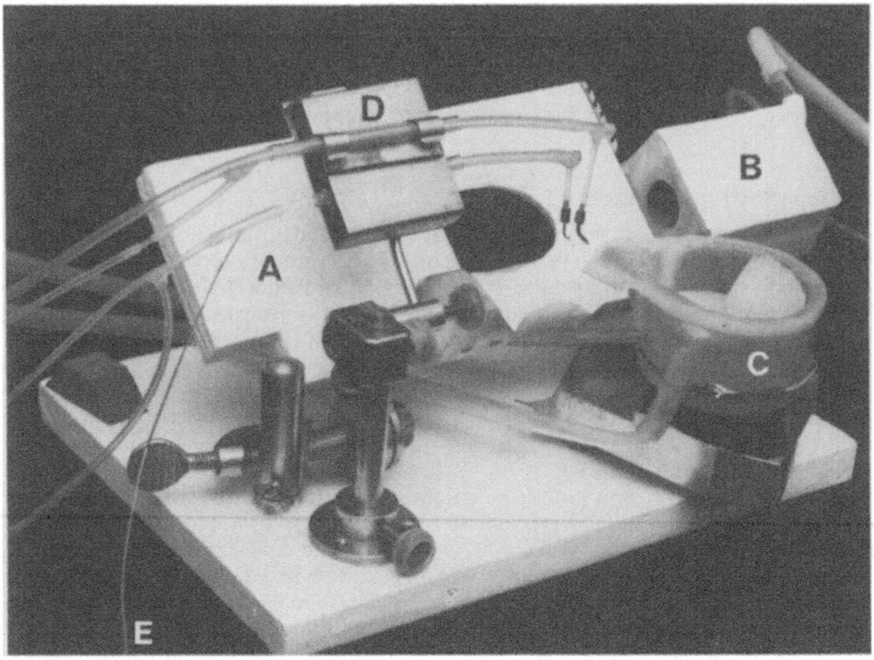

Fig. 4. Surgical platform and gut bath for perfusing isolated rat small intestine. *A*, surgical platform with hole for lymph cannula; *B*, box for rat's head, for delivery of oxygen and ether; *C*, jacketed gut bath, thermoregulated with 37 °C water; *D*, bi-level steel platform supporting the arterial and venous cannulae, each with T-connections for manometers; *E*, tubing for norepinephrine infusion into the arterial cannula

as shown in Fig. 5. The flow of oxygen is set at 1 l/min. The composition of ether–oxygen mixture delivered to the rat is regulated with a needle valve that controls the proportion of the oxygen flow passing through the flask of ether and the proportion going through the bypass. With an ether volume of 50–100 ml, light anesthesia can be maintained for long periods with a flow through the flask of about 0.25 l/min. Temporarily clamping the bypass will quickly deepen anesthesia if the rat starts to awaken. Body temperature, monitored rectally (telethermometer, Model 43TA, Yellow Springs Instrument Company, Yellow Springs, Ohio), is maintained at 37 °C with a heat lamp and transformer.

The hair on the abdomen is clipped and a midline incision made from the xiphoid cartilage to the pubis. The entire intestine from duodenum to midcolon is exteriorized, wrapped with a gauze pad moistened with warmed gut bath solution, and gently laid up on the rat's right side. The thermoregulated gut bath (see Fig. 4) is then positioned with its lip protruding into the abdominal cavity, nearly reaching to the vena cava. The contact surface between the front of the gut bath and the shaved abdomen is coated liberally with petrolatum, to prevent loss of the bath fluid by siphoning. The uncovered intestine is now allowed to slide into the bath, which is then filled with about 20 ml gut bath solution. The solution volume required to cover the tissue is minimized by use of a spacer (see Fig. 4), adjustable in size to accommodate the widely different cecal volumes of germ-free rats and conventional rats fed different types of diet. The bath is covered with a transparent plastic lid.

The mesenteric lymph channel and the superior mesenteric artery and vein are brought into view (Fig. 6) by gently retracting the liver and the cut edge of the abdominal opening. The ligament between the duodenum and colon is cut, and the overlying mesentery adja-

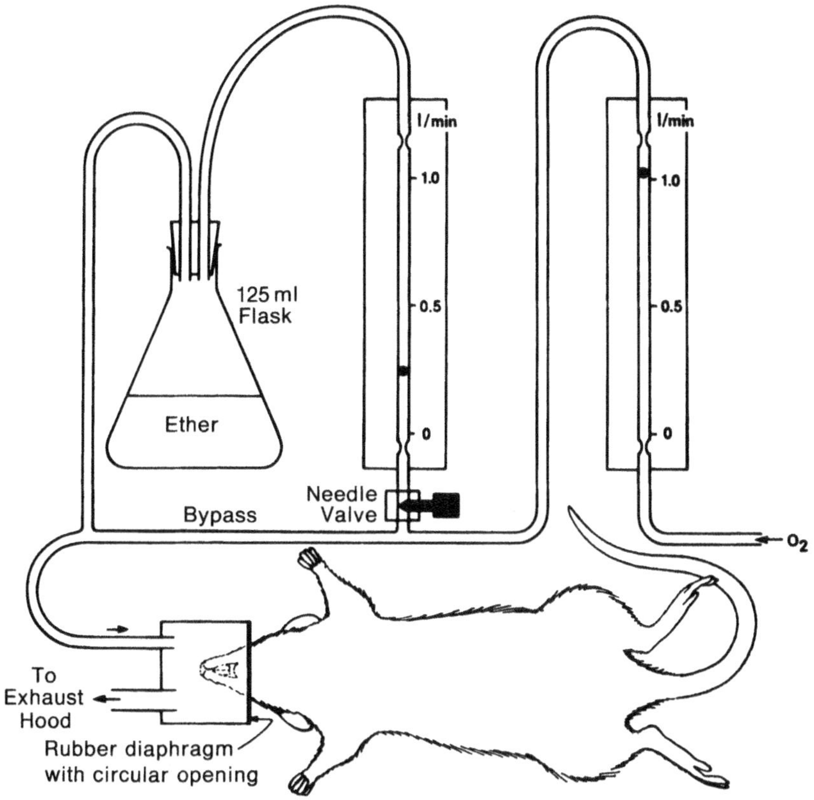

Fig. 5. Schematic diagram of apparatus for maintaining ether anesthesia. Total oxygen flow is 1 l/min. The ether content of the gas flow to the rat is regulated with the needle valve

cent to the vena cava is carefully removed with microscissors to expose the vessels fully. This and subsequent surgery are accomplished with the aid of a dissecting microscope that provides ×4–16 magnification and is illuminated with a fiber-optic light, to minimize drying of the tissue. The lymph cannula is positioned for insertion by the aid of a trocar, which is tunneled under the vena cava and out through the opposite abdominal wall and the hole in the surgical platform. The distal end of the cannula is attached to a syringe and filled with a 4% solution of sodium ethylenediaminetetraacetate, pH 7. The lymph channel is punctured with the point of a tool made from a 21-gauge disposable needle (see Fig. 3). The point is temporarily left in the channel to serve as a guide for insertion of the tip of the cannula beneath it. The syringe is detached and lymph begins to flow immediately. The cannulated lymph channel is then carefully separated from the superior mesenteric artery with extra fine angular forceps, and a 6-0 ligature is placed around each vessel with the aid of thread holders (see Fig. 3). The ligature around the lymph cannula is tied just behind the slight bulge near the cannula tip. The ligature around the artery remains loose.

A series of four additional contiguous ligatures is then placed as shown in Fig. 6, around the colon, duodenum, superior mesenteric vein, and the base of the mesenteric pedicle. All are tied except the one surrounding the vein. The duodenal tie also includes the bile duct and secures the duodenal infusion cannula. The bi-level steel platform for supporting the arterial and venous cannulae is now put into place, and, with the aid of magnetic holders, both cannulae are carefully positioned for insertion (see Fig. 4). The upper level of the platform is hinged in the rear. This allows the venous cannula to be temporarily

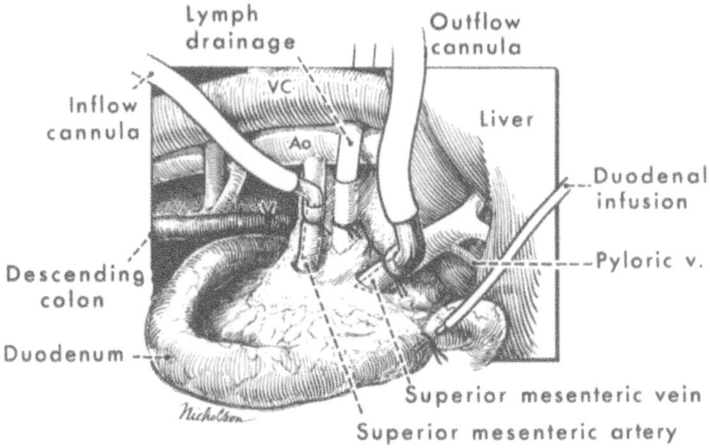

Fig. 6. Location of ligatures and cannulae for perfusing isolated rat intestine. View is through the midline abdominal incision, with the rat's head to the right and the remainder of the intestine in the foreground. *VC*, vena cava; *Ao*, aorta. WINDMUELLER et al. (1970)

tilted back and out of the way during arterial cannulation, then rapidly repositioned for venous cannulation. Immediately prior to cannulation, the venous circuit, from the pumps up to the T-connection for the water manometer, is primed with perfusate; the manometer is temporarily disconnected. The entire arterial circuit is also primed, out to the very tip of the arterial cannula, to avoid pumping any air into the tissue. Cannulation can now proceed.

Two procedures have been used for arterial cannulation: (a) the artery is punctured directly with a sharpened cannula while an opposing force is applied with a probe (see Fig. 3) by pushing against the aorta adjacent to the origin of the artery; or (b) an additional ligature is secured around the base of the artery, at its junction with the aorta; the artery is then nicked with microscissors and a cannula with a rounded bevel is inserted. In either case, the flow of perfusate is begun immediately, at 8–10 ml/min, and then the ligature around the cannula is tied in the groove behind the bevel. The 10–15-s interval when the tissue is not being perfused in the second method does not appear to damage the intestine, and this method is now generally preferred. Once the arterial cannula is secured, the rat is killed by cutting the left jugular vein and carotid artery. Then the venous cannula is swung into position, the vein cannulated by direct puncture, and the ligature around this cannula likewise tied. Once venous blood from the preparation has filled the tubing out to the T-connection for the water manometer, the manometer is reconnected and the recycling of venous blood begun.

At the same time, the infusion of norepinephrine is begun at 0.4 nmol/min into the arterial circuit at a point about 15 cm upstream from the arterial cannula needle (see Fig. 4). Also, the height of the venous valve is adjusted to achieve a pressure of 15 cm H_2O in the superior mesenteric vein. Next, the intestine is totally excised by cutting across the duodenum, the colon, and the mesenteric pedicle just outside the arc formed by the six contiguous ligatures. The surgical platform can then be rotated some 15°–20° around its supporting post and away from the gut bath, to separate the gut bath from the body of the rat. This allows the cannulae and supporting bi-level platform to be lowered, totally submerging the perfused intestine in the gut bath. As described, the preparation will include the proximal half of the colon, the cecum, the entire small intestine (except the proximal 1.5 cm) and the associated mesentery, a total of about 10–12 g tissue, including intestinal contents. The dry weight of the perfused tissue, minus contents, averages 2.8 g.

4. Routine Procedures During an Experiment

Once the recycling of perfusate is under way, attention is directed toward maintaining constancy, as far as possible, in the physiologic and biochemical parameters of the system: arterial and venous pressure, blood flow rate, perfusate pH, and the supply of oxidative substrates for the tissue.

Venous pressure is controlled by use of the venous valve. Arterial pressure can be controlled by adjustments in the perfusion rate and also the norepinephrine infusion rate. In practice, we establish a constant rate of perfusion such that the extraction of perfusate oxygen by the preparation is about 18% of the total, as determined from oximeter readings of hemoglobin oxygen saturation in the arterial and venous circuits. Since blood in the arterial circuit is always 96%–98% saturated with oxygen, the flow rate is adjusted to achieve oxygen saturation in the venous circuit of 78%–80%. This is usually attained at a flow rate of near 12 ml/min. With the flow rate constant, arterial pressure is then adjusted to 95–110 mm Hg by regulating the infusion rate of norepinephrine, typically between 0.4 and 1.2 nmol/min. The manometer reading must always be corrected to reflect the flow-rate-dependent resistance (previously determined) in the arterial circuit between the manometer and the artery.

The perfusate pH, if not adjusted, will gradually decrease, mainly owing to an accumulation of lactic acid produced by the blood cells. Under our perfusion conditions, the rate of lactic acid production was found to be 0.29 mmol/h per 100 milliliter perfusate (hematocrit 40%). Perfusate pH can therefore be conveniently maintained at pH 7.4 by a continuous infusion of 0.5 *M* $NaHCO_3$ at an equimolar rate. The pH is determined every 30 min and adjustments made in the $NaHCO_3$ infusion rate if necessary. The pH can be conveniently measured with a microelectrode unit (Type E5021a, Radiometer, Copenhagen, Denmark). This unit requires only a small capillary tube full of perfusate, less than 100 µl, which can be delivered directly into the capillary from a T-connection in the arterial circuit. As an alternative to the use of $NaHCO_3$, pH can be controlled by gradually reducing the CO_2 content of the 95% O_2/5% CO_2 gassing mixture drawn through the membrane lung. Perfusate pH has been satisfactorily controlled throughout a 5-h experiment by reducing the proportion of CO_2 stepwise to zero. This is easily accomplished with two flowmeters, by mixing different proportions of 95% O_2/5% CO_2 and 100% O_2 in the intake port of the membrane lung.

Supplying the preparation with energy-yielding substrates seems advisable, although endogenous substrates alone will support a surprisingly high rate of respiration when small intestine is incubated in vitro (see, e.g., LESTER and GRIM 1975). Lactate produced by the blood cells will serve as a respiratory fuel, particularly after higher than normal concentrations accumulate in the perfusate (WINDMUELLER and SPAETH 1978). However, glutamine is a preferred substrate and glucose is also utilized to some extent (WINDMUELLER and SPAETH 1974, 1977). We therefore continuously infuse both 0.04 *M* glutamine and 0.5 *M* glucose into the perfusate. The glutamine utilization rate is about 75 µmol/h. The glucose utilization rate is approximately 130 µmol/h for the tissue plus 290 µmol/h for each 100 ml perfusate, to supply the blood cells. Oxygen consumption by the preparation averages 18% higher when glucose and glutamine are supplied than with glucose alone. Glutamine, glucose, and $NaHCO_3$ are infused separately into the venous circuit tubing between the pumps and membrane lung. The glucose may also be infused into the duodenum, from where it is absorbed into the perfusate without undergoing appreciable metabolism (WINDMUELLER and SPAETH 1972). Recent studies have identified acetoacetate and 3-hydroxybutyrate as additional respiratory fuels for small intestine (WINDMUELLER and SPAETH 1978; HANSON and PARSONS 1978). The have not been tested with our isolated intestine, but, from available data, infusing each of these ketone bodies at a rate equimolar to that of glutamine would be appropriate. Compounds infused luminally are dissolved in Earle's balanced salt solution. Typically, luminal infusion is begun at 0.15 ml/min for 10 min (priming dose) and continued at 2.5 ml/h.

Clots appearing in the lymph cannula during surgery can be removed with a 0.13-mm diameter metal stylus having a slight hook at one end. It is convenient to have this stylus already in place within the cannula at the time of lymph cannulation and then to withdraw it, and also any clots, once perfusion is begun. No additional clots will form owing to the presence of heparin.

For the purpose of monitoring the metabolic and permeation activity of the preparation, perfusate may be sampled periodically from the reservoir, to determine cumulative changes, or samples can be taken simultaneously from the arterial and venous circuits, to determine concentration changes in a single pass through the preparation. When ^{14}C-labeled compounds are administered, $^{14}CO_2$ production can be measured by bubbling the effluent gas mixture from the membrane lung through 4 *M* NaOH. Frothing of the NaOH solution can be controlled by adding several drops of octyl alcohol. The loss of CO_2 by diffusion across the walls of the silicone rubber tubing in the perfusion circuit will be small.

For postperfusion histologic examination, it is practical and frequently desirable to fix the tissue in situ by administering the fixative vascularly through the existing arterial cannula. This was found to be the preferred method of fixation with 1% glutaraldehyde in Tyrode's solution in preparation for electron microscopy (WINDMUELLER et al. 1970).

5. Departures from Basic Procedure

During development of the method and later for particular applications, various modifications in apparatus and technique were used. The rats used as intestine donors for the preparation may be germ free, to eliminate the possible influence of the intestinal microflora on the results (WINDMUELLER and SPAETH 1974). The spacer in the gut bath must be adjusted to accommodate the greatly enlarged cecal volume in germ-free rats. With conventional or germ-free animals, the cecum and colon can be excluded from the preparation, leaving only the small intestine. This is accomplished during surgery by excision after first ligating the cecal branch of the ileocolic artery and the middle and right colic arteries and their accompanying veins.

We have compared pulse-free perfusion, obtained with the pumps described in Sect. B. III. 1, with pulsatile perfusion at 300 cycles/min and a pulse height of 40 mm Hg, approximating conditions in the rat aorta (WINDMUELLER and SPAETH 1972). The results of pulsatile and nonpulsatile perfusion were not clearly different–similar to findings in vivo (SHOOR et al. 1979).

Heparin can be omitted from the perfusate, if necessary, by using defibrinated rat blood. An initial mild vasoconstriction occurs when defibrinated blood is first perfused. This diminishes gradually and within 10–15 min hemodynamic parameters of the system are similar to those observed with heparinized blood. We have had little experience using dexamethasone and norepinephrine in perfusates other than whole blood. Preliminary results with a medium containing 40% washed rat erythrocytes in an artificial plasma were encouraging, but further evaluation is needed. The plasma contained 5% crystalline bovine serum albumin and antibiotics in Eagle's minimum essential tissue culture medium (EAGLE 1959). In several recent reports (SMITH et al. 1978; HENDERSON and GROSS 1979a, b), dexamethasone and norepinephrine were used with cell-free perfusion media composed of a buffered salts solution plus dextran or albumin. The oxygen solubility in such media is about 0.023 v/v (DEAN 1973), and utilization of oxygen by the isolated intestinal preparation perfused with blood is about 0.38 ml/min. Therefore, to meet the oxygen demand, the flow rate of cell-free media would have to be at least 16.5 ml/min, or 1.4 times the usual blood flow rate, assuming that complete oxygen extraction by the tissue were possible.

The use of norepinephrine and dexamethasone was introduced in 1970, and thereafter at least seven research groups have used isolated, perfused rat gut preparations in which neither hormones nor any other agent was used to counteract the deleterious effects of intestinal denervation (see Table 1). Pentobarbital was the anesthetic agent used in each case. It seems possible that the perfused tissue retained sufficient anesthetic to suppress excessive motility or secretion, although not completely (HANSON and PARSONS 1976; LEVIN et al. 1979). Additional mitigating factors could have been the generally low arterial pressure and perfusate flow rates used and the relatively short duration of the experiments, 60 min or less. While preparations such as these may be adequate for very short-term studies, they are likely to deteriorate quite rapidly.

IV. Evidence for Sustained Viability

From morphological and functional indications, the preparation, as described, remains alive for at least 5 h. Longer experiments have not been done. There is little change in the gross appearance; the surface of the bowel retains a pink, moist, glistening appearance. Infrequently there is a small loss of blood into the lumen. Continuous peristaltic activity is evident throughout the small intestine, somewhat more vigorous than in vivo in anesthetized rats, but free of spasmodic contractions. Morphology remains essentially normal (Figs. 7 and 8). By electron microscopy, the intestinal epithelium also retains well-preserved ultrastructure (Fig. 9).

Lymph flow is continuous at 0.6–1.2 ml/h and the lymph protein concentration remains constant. There is no evidence for accumulation of any luminal fluid when a total of 14 ml isotonic solution is infused intraduodenally over a 5-h period, indicating that fluid absorption from the lumen is continuous. The rates of utilization of oxygen, glucose, and glutamine remain essentially unchanged. When sodium taurocholate plus soybean oil and lecithin totalling 225 μmol fatty acid are infused into the duodenum, more than 50% of the fatty acid is recovered in the lymph, 90% of this in triacylglycerols of which 75% appears in chylomicrons with average diameters estimated to be 100–200 nm (WINDMUELLER and SPAETH 1972). This indicates that the isolated intestine can perform all the required steps in the mucosal as well as luminal phase of the lipid transport pro-

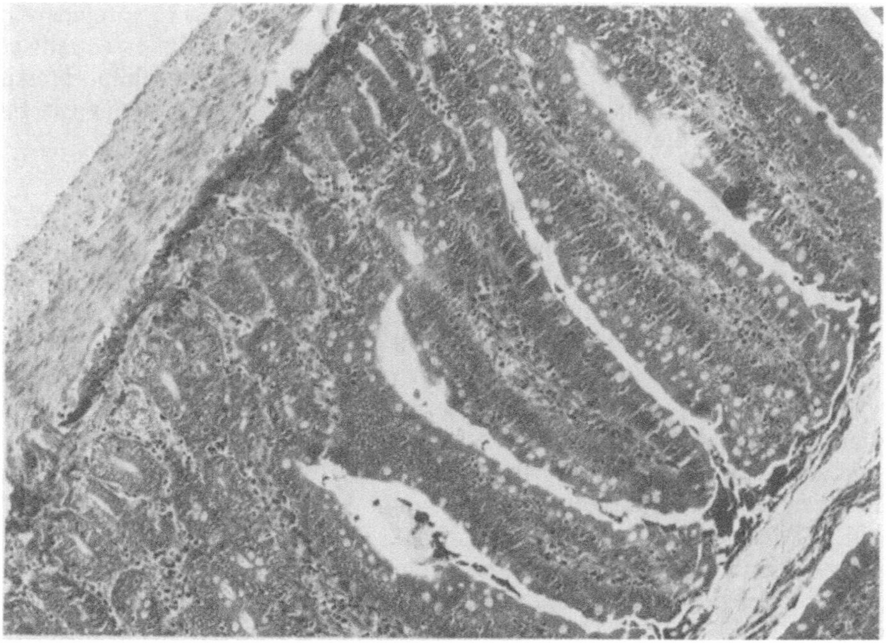

Fig. 7. Cross section of jejunal wall after 5 h of perfusion with heparinized rat blood plus norepinephrine and dexamethasone. Hematoxylin–eosin. WINDMUELLER et al. (1970), × 125

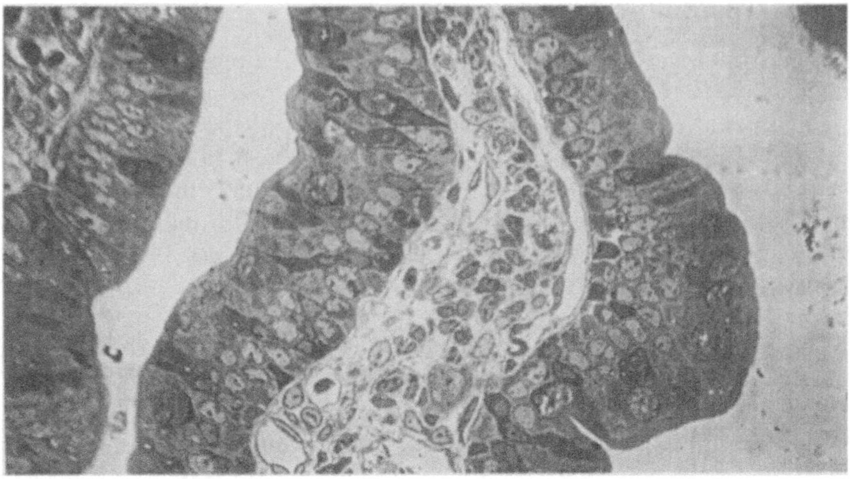

Fig. 8. Cross section of jejunal villus after 5 h of perfusion as in Fig. 7. Tissue was fixed by vascular perfusion with 1% glutaraldehyde in a modified Tyrode's solution (WINDMUELLER et al. 1970). Toluidine blue, ~ × 480

cess, including partial hydrolysis of luminal triacylglycerols and phospholipids, absorption of the products into the mucosal cells, reesterification, biosynthesis of chylomicron proteins, assembly of lipid and protein components, and discharge of the lipoprotein complexes into the lymph.

Finally, the preparation retains its vascular responsiveness to norepinephrine – the necessary infusion rate to maintain blood pressure remains essentially constant. Interrupting the infusion at any time results in a prompt fall in pressure. Uptake and metabolism of norepinephrine by the perfused tissue (VANE 1969; LANDSBERG 1976) prevent its accumulation in the perfusate.

V. Perfusate Composition During Recirculation

The composition of the perfusing medium will tend to be altered by the metabolic activity of the cells in the perfusate and in the tissue. The production of hydrogen ions and lactate and the utilization of glucose and glutamine have been mentioned (Sect. B. III. 4). Glutamine metabolism will lead to an increase in the perfusate concentration of alanine, citrulline, and proline (WINDMUELLER and SPAETH 1974). The presence of endogenous or exogenous protein in the lumen may lead to increases in the concentration of other amino acids. On the other hand, if there is no source of luminal amino acids, the levels of essential amino acids will decrease, the result of uptake and incorporation into proteins by the tissue (WEBER et al. 1979; WINDMUELLER and SPAETH 1980). The concentration of ammonia will increase, partly from the action of microbial urease in the lumen and partly from glutamine deamidation by the tissue. Ammonia levels during glutamine infusion will reach 3 mM, 30 times the normal arterial blood level. No deleterious effects due to the ammonia have been identified. Perfusate concentrations of long-chain fatty acids will increase roughly twofold in 5 h, the combined result of small amounts of lipoprotein lipase in the perfusate (WINDMUELLER and SPAETH 1972)

ditions, simulating as closely as possible conditions in vivo, or after the system has been perturbed, for instance by adding a specific metabolic inhibitor or by altering the normal perfusate metabolite concentrations.

Experiments revealing the physiologic significance of glutamine metabolism by intestine serve as examples (WINDMUELLER and SPAETH 1974). In each pass of perfusate through the tissue, intestine was found to extract about 25% of the total plasma glutamine, but no other plasma amino acid. The resulting rate of utilization is sufficient to account for a turnover of the animal's total plasma glutamine in vivo every 4.6 min, particularly significant since glutamine is the most abundant amino acid in rat plasma. From arteriovenous concentration difference measurements across the preparation, the net rate of glutamine uptake was found to be a function of the perfusate glutamine concentration. In 1 h the glutamine concentration in the recycling perfusate fell from 0.6 m*M*, the normal blood level, to 0.2 m*M*; it fell no further unless 4 m*M* L-methionine sulfoximine, an inhibitor of glutamine synthetase, was added to the perfusate, in which case the glutamine concentration fell to near zero. These findings reveal a capacity by at least some of the cells in the preparation to synthesize glutamine and indicate that the net uptake observed is a balance between a low production rate and a much larger utilization rate.

In single-pass perfusion experiments with the perfusate glutamine uniformly labeled with ^{14}C, the radioactivity taken up was partly incorporated into the tissue (14%) and the remainder reappeared with little delay in the venous blood in CO_2 (57%), citrulline (6%), proline (5%), and organic acids (18%), mostly lactate and citrate. Single-pass experiments have the advantage that the identified metabolites are clearly primary products, not secondary or tertiary products resulting from the uptake of recirculated metabolites. Perfusate glutamine was the source for 32% of the total CO_2 produced by the preparation, indicating the quantitative importance of this amino acid as an intestinal energy source. Glutamine nitrogen taken up could be accounted for by the quantities of ammonia, citrulline, alanine, and proline that were discharged into the perfusate. Identification of these products has provided new insight into metabolic pathways important for the intestine. Also revealed was a wider metabolic role for this organ – processing circulating glutamine, a major nitrogenous end product from muscle, into other nitrogenous compounds that serve as precursors for urea biosynthesis in the liver and, in the case of citrulline, as precursors for endogenous arginine synthesis in the kidneys.

By using simpler, plasma-free perfusion media, access by the intestine can be limited to individual or selected groups of potential metabolic substrates (HÜLSMANN 1971; LAMERS and HÜLSMANN 1972; HANSON and PARSONS 1976, 1977, 1978). When compared with the use of whole blood, however, the resulting increase in control over experimental conditions must be weighed against the further departure from physiologic normalcy.

2. Permeation and Metabolism of Luminal Compounds

The accessibility of the lumen, the blood, and the lymph makes a wide variety of permeation studies obviously possible. Prepared solutions can be easily infused into the duodenum or into more distal portions of the intestine. However, pro-

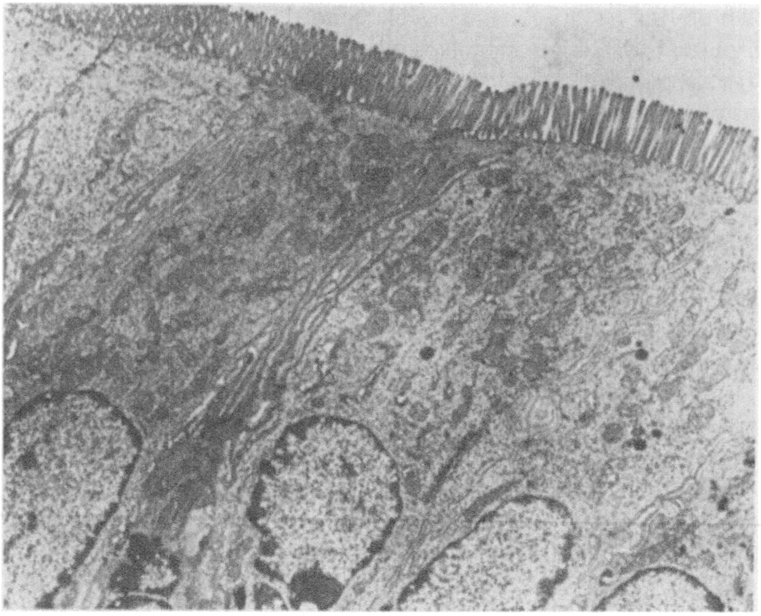

Fig. 9. Low magnification electron micrograph of absorptive cells (enterocytes) from jejunum of isolated intestine after 5 h of perfusion. Conditions for perfusion and tissue fixation were as in Fig. 8. Postfixation was in osmium tetroxide and staining was with uranyl acetate and lead citrate (WINDMUELLER et al. 1970). Ultrastructural appearance of nuclei and cytoplasm is similar to nonperfused controls, except perhaps for slight swelling of mitochondria. ~ × 4800

and of poor utilization of fatty acids as oxidative substrates by intestine (WINDMUELLER and SPAETH 1978). In 5 h, the radioimmunoassayable plasma insulin concentration increases nearly fourfold, from 130 to 480 μU/ml, the product of pancreatic tissue associated with the duodenal mesentery. As a result of slight hemolysis, the free hemoglobin concentration also increases, from 0.6 to 1.4 mg/ml in 5 h (WINDMUELLER and SPAETH 1972). The plasma concentrations of sodium and potassium ions remain relatively unchanged. No doubt there are marked changes, still unidentified, in the levels of other constituents, some quite possibly crucial to the long-term survival of the organ.

VI. Applications

1. Metabolism of Vascular Compounds

Several types of information can be obtained with regard to the uptake and utilization of compounds from the blood. First, the overall utilization rate of a substance by the entire intestine can be determined from its rate of disappearance from the recirculating perfusate. Second, if the compound can be labeled with radioactivity, information about the pathway of metabolism in intestine can be derived from an analysis of the labeled products discharged into the perfusate or retained in the perfused tissue. Such studies can be carried out under normal con-

longed control over the concentration of luminal constituents is difficult. This would require continuous luminal perfusion, not practical for the entire intestine, but possible if the intestine is divided into segments (KAVIN et al. 1967). The isolated intestine is capable of absorbing fatty acids, assembling chylomicrons and other lipoproteins, and discharging them into the lymph. It could therefore be used to study the permeation of other water-insoluble substances, for instance vitamins A, D, E, and K and water-insoluble drugs. Metabolic transformation of substances during permeation can be investigated from an analysis of the metabolic products appearing in the perfusate or lymph, as has, for example, been done with niacin and niacinamide (HENDERSON and GROSS 1979b).

3. Biosynthesis of Specific Proteins, Peptides, and Lipids

The capacity of intestine to synthesize the various protein moieties of chylomicrons and high density lipoproteins of lymph and plasma was first demonstrated unequivocally with the isolated, vascularly perfused gut preparation (WINDMUELLER et al. 1973). Lysine ^3H was added to the perfusate, and after 5 h the labeled apolipoproteins from the lymph and from the perfusate were recovered by ultracentrifugation, delipidation, and polyacrylamide gel electrophoresis. The relative rates of synthesis of the various proteins were determined from the relative amounts of label incorporated. These studies revealed that rat intestine can synthesize B apolipoprotein, one or more of the A apolipoproteins, but little or none of any of the low molecular weight C apolipoproteins. These C apolipoproteins, which can be synthesized by liver, constitute, however, a significant portion of the mass of lymph chylomicron protein. It thus became apparent that chylomicrons, discharged from intestine virtually devoid of C apolipoproteins, acquire these proteins in the lymph, into which they have filtered from the blood. Furthermore, these studies showed that all the B apolipoprotein of intestinal origin reaches the blood by way of mesenteric lymph. On the other hand, only part of the intestinally made A apolipoproteins follow this route; the remainder bypass the lymph by direct transfer into the blood. Similar radioactive labeling techniques and also immunochemical and biologic assay methods should be applicable for measuring the biosynthesis of other proteins of intestinal origin, for example immunoglobulins and peptide hormones.

In other unpublished studies, using a technique previously applied in isolated perfused rat liver (WINDMUELLER and SPAETH 1966), we measured the capicity of intestine to synthesize longchain fatty acids. At the start of perfusion, a 25 mCi dose of ^3H_2O was divided between the perfusate and the gut bath solution. Within minutes all the water in the system, including tissue water, reaches a uniform and constant specific radioactivity. Fatty acids were isolated from the total lipids extracted from the tissue, the lymph, and the perfusate following 4 h of perfusion. Only newly synthesized fatty acid molecules incorporate tritium. The rate of fatty acid biosynthesis was calculated from the specific radioactivity of the water and the tritium content of the fatty acids. Preliminary results show that under our experimental conditions the rate of fatty acid synthesis is not large, about 10 µmol/h, and takes place largely in the mesenteric adipose tissue (60%) and in the mucosa of the small intestine (20%). The use of tritiated water should also permit quantification of intestinal cholesterol biosynthesis (WINDMUELLER and SPAETH 1966).

4. Other Applications

This isolated preparation is not under the influence of an anesthetic agent and may therefore be particularly well suited for studying the physiologic and biochemical responses to drugs and hormones. In a preliminary study, for example, we have infused prostaglandin E_1 (PGE_1) into the arterial circuit at a rate of 0.6 µg/min (perfusate concentration, 0.05 µg/ml). Within 1 min, vascular resistance and intestinal motility were dramatically reduced and hyperemia developed. The advantage of such studies with the isolated organ is, of course, that only the intestine would be exposed to the agent, eliminating secondary or tertiary effects involving other tissues.

C. Autoperfused Intestinal Segment In Vivo

As an alternative to the isolated, pump-perfused intestinal preparation, a segment of rat small intestine can be very effectively studied in situ by preserving the arterial, lymphatic, and neural connections of the segment, but collecting its entire venous drainage. With appropriate adaptations, this technique allows for virtually the entire range of experimentation possible with the isolated preparation.

I. Description of Basic Procedure

The basic procedure is illustrated schematically in Fig. 10. In principle, a portion of the small intestine is exteriorized into a 37 °C gut bath and a 2–5-cm segment drained by a single vein is selected for study. The ends of the segment are ligated, and the single vein draining the segment is cannulated. Replacement blood is infused from a reservoir into a saphenous vein. Another cannula lying in the aorta serves to monitor arterial blood pressure and to permit sampling of arterial blood. Body temperature is maintained by a heating pad and anesthesia by a continuous infusion of pentobarbital.

1. Apparatus and Surgical Tools

The surgical platform and associated equipment are shown in Fig. 11. The platform has a metal surface that accepts magnets, useful for positioning and securing the various cannulae. The rat lies in as supine position on a 5 × 15 cm silicone rubber heating pad (No. BSS-26, Briscoe Manufacturing Company, Columbus, Ohio) thermoregulated by way of a proportional temperature controller (Versatherm, No. 2156, Cole-Parmer Instrument Company, Chicago, Illinois) and a rectal thermistor to maintain body temperature at 37 °C (monitored with a rectal telethermometer). The voltage applied to the heating pad is further reduced with a rheostat to prevent overshoot of the rat's body temperature. The rat's head is inserted into a plastic box through the circular opening in the rubber diaphragm covering one end. The box is continuously flushed with oxygen at 1 l/min, to insure that the rat is well oxygenated. The gut bath is fabricated from the cut-down base of a plastic bottle which supports a molded top and sides made of stainless steel wire mesh covered with silicone rubber sheeting. Water at 37 °C is circulated through the body of the bath to warm the bottom and sides of the shallow intestinal compartment. The heat exchanger for warming the replacement blood contains a coil of silicone rubber tubing and is also thermoregulated with 37 °C water. The blood collection ice bath has a two-way valve, made by cementing short

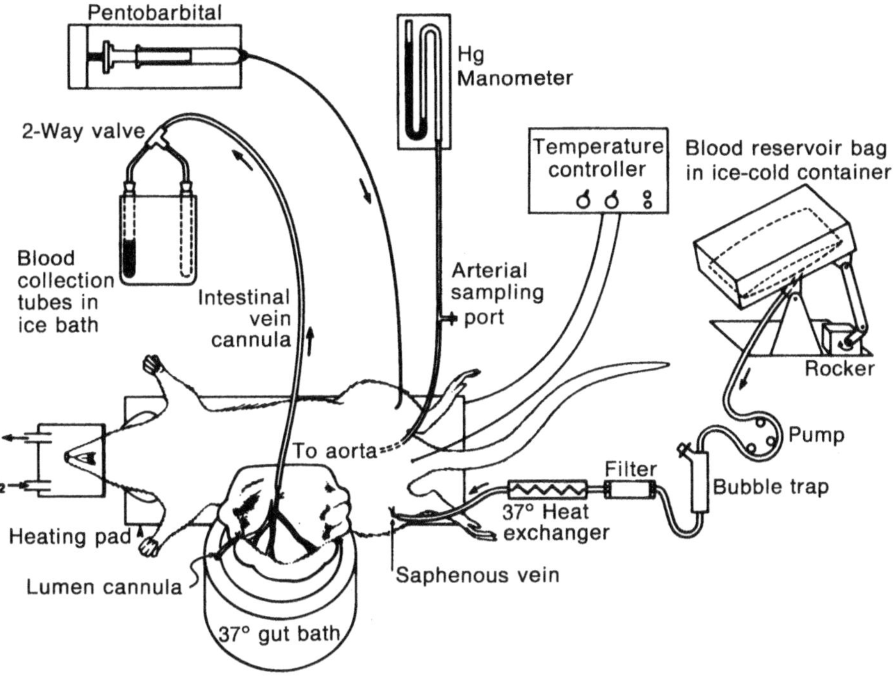

Fig. 10. Schematic diagram of apparatus for autoperfused intestinal segment in vivo

lengths of 19-gauge stainless steel tubing into the orifices of a plastic Luer three-way stopcock. This bath is filled with an ice slurry and has an outlet near the bottom connected to a length of rubber tubing (not visible in Fig. 11); the open end of the tubing is positioned over a sink at a height such that the bath remains filled, but excess water drains automatically whenever more ice is added.

The apparatus for perfusing replacement blood is pictured in Fig. 12. An envelope made of silicone rubber (see Fig. 2) serves as the blood reservoir. It lies within a flat metal box surrounded in turn by an expanded polystyrene box. Ice water is circulated by pump through the space between the two boxes to maintain the blood temperature near 0 °C. To mix the blood gently and to prevent the cells from settling out, the unit is rocked mechanically at 30 cycles/min. The pump and glass wool filter are the same as used for the isolated intestinal preparation (see Sect. B. III. 1). The surgical tools and retractors are shown in Fig. 13. Thread holders made of metal tubing, as shown in Fig. 3, are also helpful. The various cannulae used are made from silicone rubber tubing terminating in a short length of sharpened stainless steel needle tubing. The intestinal vein cannula is pictured in Fig. 14. It is critical that the bore diameter of the needle and silicone rubber tubing used for this cannula be sufficiently large to prevent excessive resistance to blood flow. Use of the intestinal artery cannula, also pictured in Fig. 14, will be discussed later (Sect. C. II. 3). For pentobarbital infusion, 27-gauge needle tubing is used and for the aorta, 23- or 25-gauge.

2. Preparing for Experiment

The rats, solutions, apparatus, and blood require preparation in advance. We have used male rats of the Sprague-Dawley or Osborne-Mendel strains. Blood donors weigh 450–700 g and are typically fed a stock diet. Intestine donors weigh 350–400 g. They may be fasted or fed any diet consistent with the purposes of the experiment.

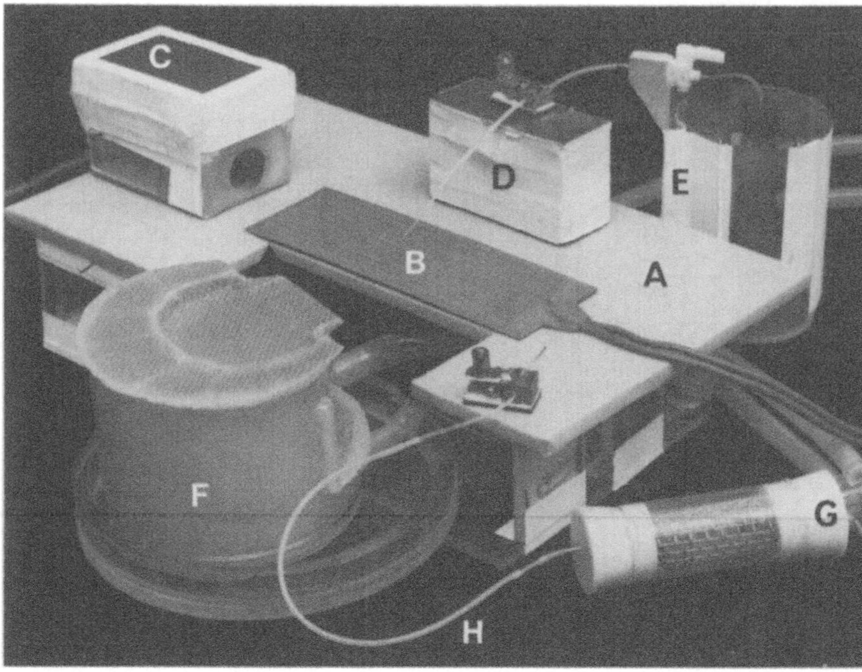

Fig. 11. Surgical platform and associated apparatus for autoperfused intestinal segment. *A*, acrylic plastic surgical platform with surface covered by a thin metal sheet; *B*, heating pad; *C*, box for rat's head; *D*, block supporting intestinal vein cannula – the top surface of the block is metal, the bottom surface is a magnet, and the cannula is held in a modified chromatography clip lined with silicone rubber sponge tape (Connecticut Hard Rubber Company, New Haven, Connecticut) and also attached to a magnet; *E*, ice bath with two blood collection tubes and two-way valve; *F*, gut bath thermoregulated with 37 °C water; *G*, 37 °C heat exchanger, containing a coiled length of silicone rubber tubing; *H*, blood infusion cannula held in a clip attached to a magnet and positioned approximately for saphenous vein cannulation

The gut bath solution is Earle's balanced salt solution (EARLE 1943) with the addition of 0.56 mmol glucose and 0.06 mmol glutamine per 100 milliliters. A 250 ml supply is warmed to 37 °C and the flask flushed continuously with 95% O_2/5% CO_2. An aqueous solution of sodium pentobarbital, 50 mg/ml, is freshly prepared. A 4-ml portion for continuous infusion is loaded into a gas-tight syringe (Hamilton Company, Reno, Nevada) mounted on an infusion pump with continuously variable speed (e.g., model 906, Harvard Apparatus Company, Millis, Massachusetts). Sodium heparin is prepared as a 10 mg/ml solution in 0.15 *M* NaCl. Any compounds to be luminally administered are prepared in Earle's balanced salt solution. A series of venous blood collection tubes, usually 6–12 ml capacity, are numbered and the tare weights recorded. All needle cannulae are inspected (× 40 magnification) and resharpened if necessary. It is important that needles be extremely sharp and free of visible burrs.

To prepare the replacement blood, donor rats are anesthetized with an intraperitoneal injection of sodium pentobarbital, 5 mg per 100 gram body weight. Blood is drawn from the abdominal aorta into syringes containing sodium heparin solution to give a blood concentration of about 30 USP units/ml. The blood is injected through the metal screen prefilter (see Fig. 2) into the silicone rubber blood reservoir, which is submerged in an ice slurry. The length of the experiment will determine the blood volume required (see Sect. C. III).

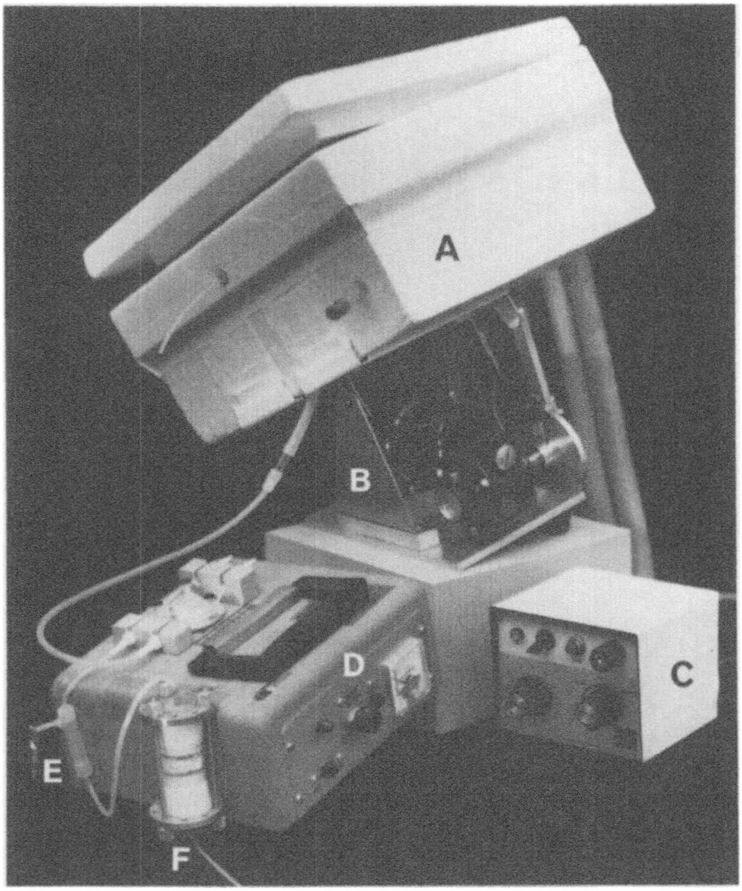

Fig. 12. Blood infusion apparatus for autoperfused intestinal segment. *A*, expanded polystyrene box surrounding a metal box containing the silicone rubber blood reservoir bag – ice water circulates through the space between the two boxes; *B*, motor-driven rocker; *C*, controls for rocker; *D*, peristaltic pump; *E*, bubble trap; *F*, blood filter

After removing the air, the reservoir is transferred to the cooled box atop the rocker and mixing is begun.

The aorta cannula is attached to the manometer and the tubing filled with 0.15 *M* NaCl. The blood infusion cannula, including a 15-cm length of silicone rubber tubing, is filled with heparin solution, and the pentobarbital infusion cannula is primed. Finally, the gut bath and heat exchanger are warmed to 37 °C.

3. Surgical Procedure

The intestine donor rat is anesthetized with an intraperitoneal injection of sodium pentobarbital (5 mg per 100 gram body weight); care is taken to avoid damaging the intestine. Alternatively, ethyl ether anesthesia can be used, in which case anesthesia is maintained throughout the experiment with the apparatus described in Fig. 5, and ether in lieu of pentobarbital is used to anesthetize the blood donor rats. We prefer pentobarbital to ether for metabolic experiments because blood glucose and lactate concentrations remain normal (WINDMUELLER and SPAETH 1978). The rat is laid on the heating pad in a supine position,

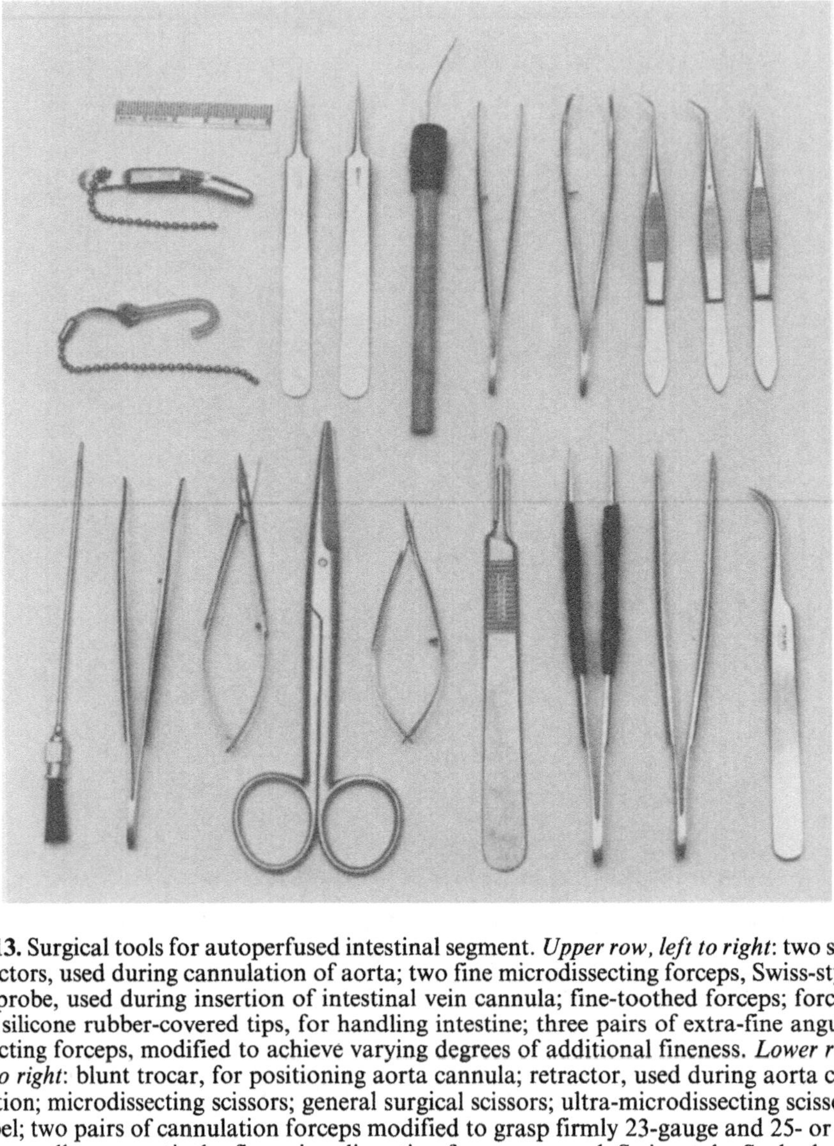

Fig. 13. Surgical tools for autoperfused intestinal segment. *Upper row, left to right*: two skin retractors, used during cannulation of aorta; two fine microdissecting forceps, Swiss-style; fine probe, used during insertion of intestinal vein cannula; fine-toothed forceps; forceps with silicone rubber-covered tips, for handling intestine; three pairs of extra-fine angular dissecting forceps, modified to achieve varying degrees of additional fineness. *Lower row, left to right*: blunt trocar, for positioning aorta cannula; retractor, used during aorta cannulation; microdissecting scissors; general surgical scissors; ultra-microdissecting scissors; scalpel; two pairs of cannulation forceps modified to grasp firmly 23-gauge and 25- or 27-gauge needles, respectively; fine microdissecting forceps, curved, Swiss-style. Scale shown is 5 cm

with feet taped to the surgical platform (see Figs. 10 and 11). The hair is clipped from the abdomen, from both thighs, and from around the base of the tail. Through a midline incision, made from the xiphoid to the pubis, the small intestine and cecum are gently exteriorized, wrapped in gauze moistened with warm gut bath solution, and laid up on the left side of the rat's abdomen. The gut bath is now positioned up against the rat with its lip extending into the abdominal cavity. The bath is held in place with an elastic strap. The contact surface between the front of the bath and the abdomen is coated liberally with petrolatum, to prevent loss of bath fluid by siphoning. The intestine is placed into the bath, which is then filled with 10 ml warmed gut bath solution. Using moistened swabs to handle the in-

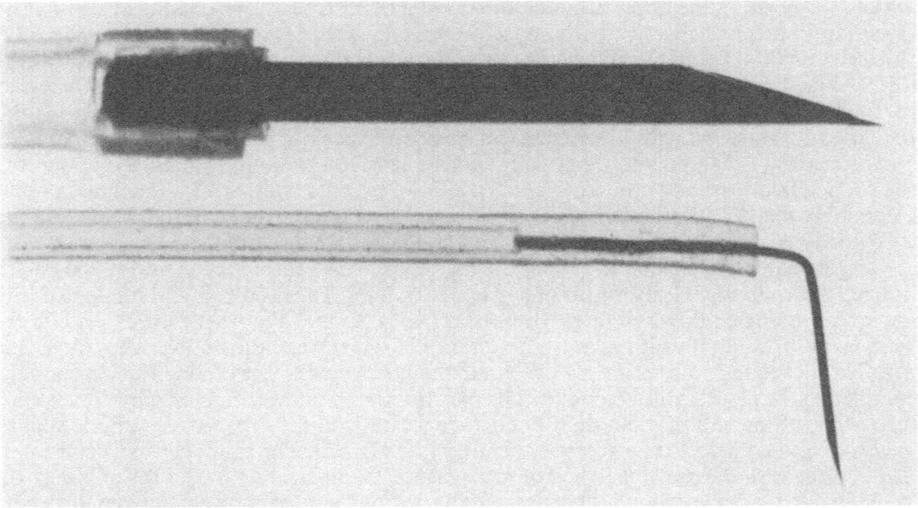

Fig. 14. Needles of cannulae for autoperfused intestinal segment. *Upper*: 23-gauge thin-walled intestinal vein cannula, attached by a polyethylene collar to a 3-cm length of silicone rubber tubing, inner diameter 0.64 mm, which is attached to a 10-cm length of silicone rubber tubing, inner diameter 1.02 mm; an identical needle is used for the blood infusion cannula. *Lower*: 36-gauge needle of intestinal artery cannula. × 12.4

testine, an experimental segment drained by a single vein is selected and positioned as shown in Fig. 10. A triangular 5-mm thick gauze pad is used to elevate and support the segment. Suitable segments are generally available in the distal two-thirds of the jejunum and in the ileum. The cecum and remaining intestine are returned to the abdomen, and the bath is covered with a thin, transparent plastic sheet.

The left saphenous vein is exposed, by making a skin incision and separating overlying fascia with forceps, and the vein is cannulated by direct puncture for infusion of pentobarbital. A dissecting microscope with × 4–8 magnification and a fiber-optic light are used for this and subsequent surgery. The cannula tubing is secured to the surgical platform with tape, and a continuous pentobarbital infusion is begun. A suitable level of anesthesia is generally maintained with an infusion rate of 3.3 mg/h. Next, working through an opened flap in the plastic cover, the selected intestinal vein is fully exposed near its junction with the larger superior mesenteric vein by carefully removing the overlying mesentery with the finest microforceps and ultra-microscissors. A 6–0 silk ligature is passed under the intestinal vein, being careful not to go deep or wide enough to include the lymphatic drainage from the segment. These steps in the surgery are completed early to allow time for any constriction of the intestinal vein caused by the surgical trauma to disappear before cannulation. Uncovered areas of tissue are kept moistened with gut bath fluid at all times, using swabs.

The right saphenous vein is then also exposed and a 6–0 ligature passed under the vein and, for sake of ease, also under the adjoining artery and nerve. The blood infusion cannula, primed with heparin solution and positioned with the aid of a magnetic clip (see Fig. 11), is inserted into the vein by direct puncture and the ligature securely tied around the needle. At this time the 15-cm cannula remains attached to a 0.5-ml syringe filled with heparin solution.

Next, 4–0 ligatures are secured around each end of the selected segment, forming a closed sac with an infusion cannula (a bent piece of 20-gauge needle tubing with a silicone rubber-coated tip) inserted into the proximal end (see Figs. 10 and 15, E). The cecum and remainder of the small intestine are temporarily returned to the bath, and the edges of the abdominal incision are retracted to expose the aorta near the iliac bifurcation. A 10–15-mm section of aorta is cleared by wiping with dry swabs. Care is taken to avoid tearing blood vessels. To position the aorta cannula, the tip of a blunt trocar is inserted near the iliac bifurcation and tunneled toward the base of the tail, where it is pushed out of the body through a small skin incision. The aorta cannula, attached to the manometer and filled with 0.15 *M* NaCl, is positioned with its needle lying over the cleared portion of aorta. A retractor made from a pair of forceps (see Fig. 13) serves to keep the aorta fully exposed. At this time the rat is injected with 0.3 ml heparin solution by way of the blood infusion cannula. Now the aorta is cannulated by direct puncture, and the cannula secured by taping it to the surgical platform near the rat's tail. The blood pressure will be 135–150 mmHg (100–110 mmHg if ether anesthesia is used). All retractors are removed, and the cecum and unused portions of small intestine are replaced into the abdomen.

The intestinal vein cannula is then precisely positioned for insertion and blood collection, as shown in Fig. 11, by means of a magnetic holder. The needle should be aligned with the vein and angled down slightly with respect to it, so that the needle bevel, once in the vein, is not pressing upward against the interior surface. Also, the bubble trap, filter, and 37 °C heat exchanger are primed with blood and connected to the blood infusion cannula, completing the blood infusion circuit. The intestinal vein is now cannulated by direct puncture, while lifting and pushing slightly on its junction with the superior mesenteric vein by means of a fine probe with a specially bent tip (see Fig. 13). The cannula needle is securely tied in place with the previously positioned ligature. Coincident with the flow of blood, the infusion of replacement blood is begun, initially at 1.5–2.0 ml/min, depending on the length of the segment. The venous blood is collected through the two-way valve into tared tubes in the ice bath (Fig. 11).

4. Routine Procedures During an Experiment

The rate of blood infusion is adjusted to equal the rate of blood collection, determined gravimetrically on samples collected over 4–8-min intervals, plus an additional amount to compensate for a slow but continuous surgical loss, typically 0.3 ml/min. Blood collections are timed with the aid of an electric interval timer. When the experiment involves taking arterial samples, the volume of these will, of course, also be replaced. Normal arterial blood pressure serves to indicate an adequate infusion rate. An excessive infusion rate will eventually be reflected in engorgement of the liver, one lobe of which is usually visible. Thus, adjustments in the infusion rate are made to parallel changes in the collection rate and also as needed to maintain arterial blood pressure and the normal appearance of the liver. A relatively shallow level of anesthesia is maintained by making small adjustments in the pentobarbital infusion rate if necessary. We aim to preserve a strong costal respiration (respiration becomes less costal and more diaphragmatic as anesthesia deepens) and to retain a tail-pinch response.

To determine the weight of perfused tissue at the end of an experiment, the segment and associated mesentery are grossly excised and transferred to ice-cold 0.15 *M* NaCl. There, under magnification, the tissue drained by the cannulated vein is precisely excised, the mesenteric and intestinal portions separated with microscissors, and the intestine opened longitudinally and rinsed free of mucus and diet residue. Intestine and mesentery are thoroughly blotted, weighed separately (wet weight), dried for 18 h at 110 °C, and reweighed (dry weight).

5. Some Physiologic Parameters

Experimental segments are 2–5 cm in length. The wet weight averages 0.40 g for intestine and 0.15 g for associated mesentery. The mean dry: wet weight ratio for intestine is 0.20:1 and for mesentery it is 0.68:1, reflecting its high lipid content. The mean blood flow rate for jejunal segments from rats fasted for 18 h is 1.2 ml/min, equivalent to 3.0 ml/min, per gram intestine. For nonfasted rats it is 4.0 ml/min per gram intestine. The pale pink color and overall gross appearance of the segments remains normal. If the needle and tubing used to cannulate the intestinal vein are not sufficiently large, excessive resistance to flow will produce engorgement and tortuosity of the mesenteric veins, and a darkening in color of the tissue. Peristaltic activity is weak, owing to anesthesia. The rat's body temperature remains constant at 37 °C and a normal blood pressure of 135–150 mmHg can be maintained for at least 3 h, the longest experiments done to date.

II. Specialized Techniques and Adaptations

1. Luminal Infusion or Perfusion

To study the permeation or metabolism of luminally administered substances, a single dose can be given, in which case the segment is prepared as a closed sac with a lumen infusion cannula, or the lumen can be perfused. For a single administration, a volume of 0.3 ml or less is used, to prevent distension. A 0.5-cm segment of silicone rubber tubing on the exterior end of the infusion cannula is clamped with a small serrefine clamp to prevent leakage. The arrangement used for luminal perfusion is shown in Fig. 15. The dual system permits rapid switching from one solution to another. The solutions are delivered with peristaltic pumps or from syringes driven by infusion pumps. The lumen is initially cleared of diet residue by perfusing Earle's balanced salt solution at 2 ml/min for 5–10 min. Subsequent continuous perfusion is customarily at 0.1–0.2 ml/min. The large bore of the outflow cannula (3 mm inside diameter) normally prevents clogging by mucus or diet. However, pinching the tube is necessary on occasion to relieve an obstruction and prevent luminal distension.

2. Arteriovenous Concentration Difference Measurements

Arteriovenous difference measurements are useful to determine net uptake or release of blood metabolites and also to determine the net permeation rate from the lumen into the venous blood. Arterial blood samples are obtained from the aorta cannula, by opening the

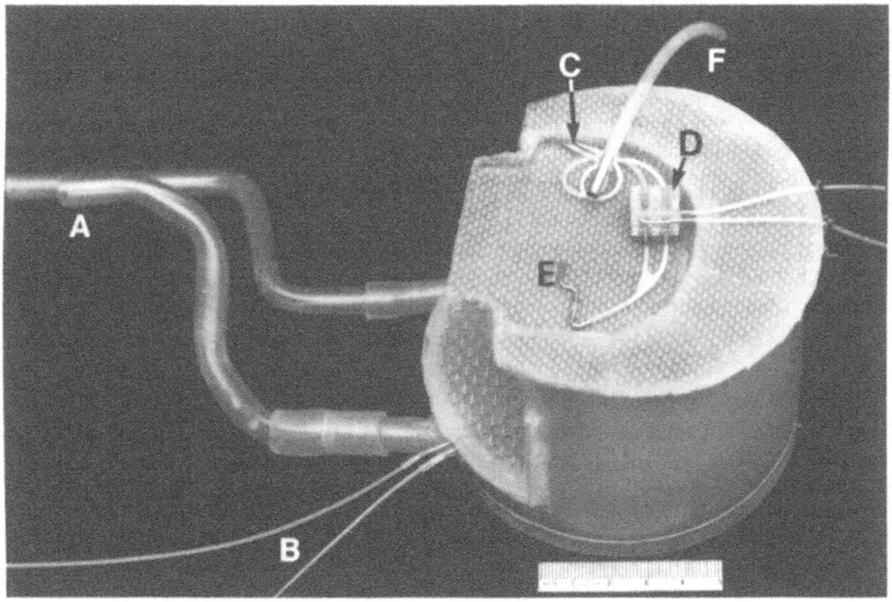

Fig. 15. Adaptation of gut bath for perfusing lumen of autoperfused intestinal segment. The arrangement shown allows two different solutions to be perfused alternately. *A*, inflow and outflow tubes for 37 °C water; *B*, dual vinyl or polyethylene tubes for delivery of luminal perfusates – tubing connects with dual stainless steel tubes that extend through the water compartment and exit above, at *C*, in the intestinal compartment; *D*, dual-chambered bubble trap, with all silicone rubber tubing connections; *E*, lumen inflow cannula, made from 20-gauge needle tubing and having a silicone rubber-covered tip; *F*, lumen outflow cannula. Scale shown is 5 cm

sampling port after temporarily clamping the tubing between the port and the manometer (see Fig. 10). The first ten drops of blood flush the cannula and are discarded. Arterial and venous samples should ideally be collected simultaneously. This can be approximated by sampling arterial blood manually midway through collection of the corresponding venous sample. For completely simultaneous sampling, important when arteriovenous concentration differences are small and the arterial concentration is fluctuating (e. g., for CO_2), blood from the intestinal vein cannula and from the aorta cannula can be withdrawn at identical rates into paired syringes mounted in parallel on a withdrawal pump. For analyses of blood oxygen and CO_2, in addition, the silicone rubber cannulae, which are permeable to these gasses, are replaced with vinyl tubing; also, all dead space in the withdrawal tubing and syringes is filled with mercury, to prevent any contact of the blood with air.

3. Arterial Infusion

To achieve single-pass vascular exposure, a substance can be either injected or continuously infused into the single artery that supplies the segment. Figure 10 illustrates the characteristic parallel arrangement of arterial and venous branches in the mesentery. The artery is cleared by microdissection adjacent to the site selected for intestinal vein cannulation and near the artery's junction with the superior mesenteric artery, which courses beneath the superior mesenteric vein. Trauma should be minimized to prevent the intestinal artery from constricting. Arterial cannulation immediately precedes intestinal vein cannulation in the surgical routine. The artery is entered with a 36-gauge needle, bent and sharpened as shown in Fig. 14. The needle is grasped in a groove filed across one tip of a pair of Swiss-style microdissecting forceps (see Fig. 13). Once in place, the heel of the needle, at the bend, rests against the superior mesenteric vein, which prevents the needle from being gradually expelled by the arterial pressure. The needle and silicone rubber tubing (0.25 mm inside diameter) are previously primed with 0.15 *M* NaCl from a pump-driven syringe (free of bubbles). Infusion is continuous at 0.01 ml/min, initially with isotonic saline and later with an isotonic solution of the experimental compound or compounds. The small size of the needle prevents any interference with normal blood flow through the artery.

A few words about the fabrication and care of this very delicate cannula seem warranted. The bore of the silicone rubber tubing is larger than the shaft of the 36-gauge needle (see Fig. 14). To make the connection, the end of the tubing is first sealed with a plug of silicone glue. After it hardens, the plug is pierced with a sharpened metal stylus, 0.08 mm diameter, forming a channel for the needle shaft. The needle, like all the others, is sharpened under $\times 40$ magnification with hard Arkansas stones (rotating wheel and hand held). All solutions infused through this cannula should be filtered to remove particles. Sonication has been very successful in opening the needle when it gets clogged.

4. Stabilizing Collected Blood Samples

Stabilization may be necessary to protect compounds that are chemically labile or subject to enzymatic conversion in plasma or to metabolism by blood cells. The routine procedure of collecting venous blood in ice will gradually lower the blood temperature to 0 °C over 5–10 min. Almost immediate rapid chilling can be achieved by inserting a simple heat exchanger, such as shown in Fig. 16, into the intestinal vein cannula between the preparation and the collection tubes. A single pump circulates ice water through the exchanger and the blood reservoir container. Blood will be cooled from 37° to 0 °C at flow rates through this exchanger of up to 2.5 ml/min. A similar exchanger can be used to cool arterial blood collected from the aorta cannula.

Chemical stabilizers may also be employed, either by adding them to the collection tubes, or, for more immediate effect, by continuously infusing them directly into the collection cannula, as shown for the intestinal vein cannula in Fig. 16. As examples, in metabolic studies with arginine, it was necessary to infuse sodium borate to inhibit blood arginase (WINDMUELLER and SPAETH 1976), and in studies with glucose, sodium fluoride was infused to inhibit glycolysis by the blood cells (WINDMUELLER and SPAETH 1978).

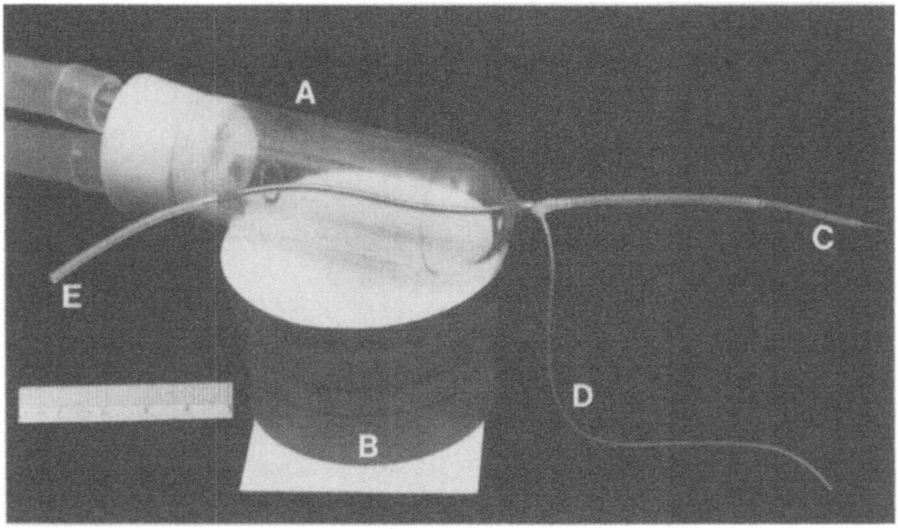

Fig. 16. Heat exchanger (0 °C) for cooling blood collected from autoperfused intestinal segment. *A*, heat exchanger, made by cementing a length of 15-gauge thin-walled stainless steel tubing within, and through the walls of, a 28.4 × 78 mm polycarbonate centrifuge tube – ice-cold water is continuously circulated through the centrifuge tube, shown without insulaton; *B*, heat exchanger support, fastened below to a magnet; *C*, intestinal vein cannula; *D*, optional side arm, for infusing compounds to stabilize blood constituents; *E*, to collection tubes in ice bath. Scale shown is 5 cm

5. Collection of Mesenteric Lymph

The small size and inaccessibility of the lymph vessels makes lymph collection from an individual intestinal segment difficult. As a useful compromise, however, one may collect the rat's entire mesenteric lymph output after administering labeled precursor compounds either arterially or luminally to the segment. Since no venous blood from the segment returns to the systemic circulation, only the segment will be exposed to the label, and any labeled products appearing in the mesenteric lymph will be uneqivocally derived from that segment (Wu and Windmueller 1978). Animals with a cannula in the main mesenteric lymph channel are prepared, essentially as described by Warshaw (1972), 18–24 h before the study, to allow for recovery and to insure a stable flow of lymph. During recovery, a 0.15 *M* NaCl solution, sometimes containing glucose or other nutrients, is continuously infused intraduodenally at 2.4 ml/h. When subsequently setting up the intestinal segment preparation, the distal end of the lymph cannula is taped to the front edge of the surgical platform, near the rat's right front paw, where the lymph is collected in tubes in ice. To maintain lymph flow at about 1.5 ml/h, a 0.15 *M* NaCl solution is infused continuosly through a T-connection into the blood infusion cannula at 2 ml/h throughout the experiment.

III. Applications

1. Net Uptake, Metabolism, and Release of Vascular Compounds

Arteriovenous difference measurements coupled with the technique of arterial infusion open the way for studying the uptake and metabolism of normal as well as abnormal blood constituents. This dual experimental approach can yield detailed, quantitative results, as illustrated by the data in Table 3, an analysis of the

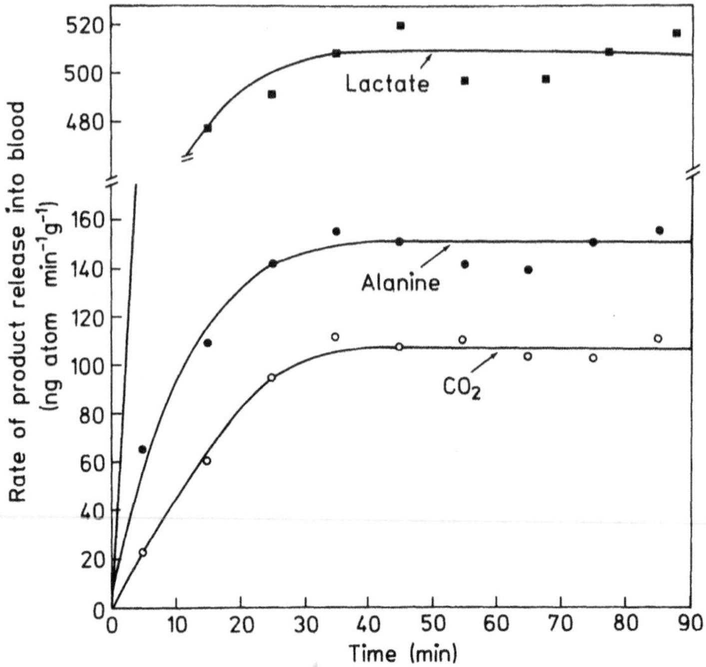

Fig. 17. Metabolism of arterial glucose to venous products by autoperfused jejunal segment. Starting at zero time, a tracer dose of D-glucose ^{14}C(ul) was infused continuously at 0.01 ml/min into the blood of the single artery supplying a 0.31-g jejunal segment. Venous blood from the segment was collected in a series of nine samples over the next 85 min. A 1.5-ml blood sample was taken from the aorta every 10 min to monitor the arterial plasma glucose concentration and thereby to calculate the specific radioactivity of glucose carbon perfusing the segment. The total radioactivity in CO_2, alanine, and lactate was determined in each venous sample. Results were calculated as ng atom glucose carbon in product per minute per gram intestine. WINDMUELLER and SPAETH (1978)

circulating respiratory fuels utilized by the intestine. Quantitatively important substrates were first identified from arteriovenous difference measurements of the major oxidative substrates present in blood. A substantial net uptake was found for glucose, glutamine, and ketone bodies. The metabolic fate of these substrates in intestine was then determined in separate experiments by continuously infusing a tracer dose of each, uniformly labeled with ^{14}C, into the artery supplying the segment and then quantifying the release rates of labeled metabolic products into the venous blood. Thus, product formation was measured while the segments were being perfused with normal blood having one constituent radioactively labeled. The release rates of ^{14}C-labeled products reach a steady state under these conditions in about 30 min, as illustrated for the main glucose products in Fig. 17. The conversion rate of substrate carbon into each product was calculated from the steady state rate of appearance of labeled product in venous blood and the specific radioactivity of the substrate carbon atoms in the arterial blood. This, in turn, was calculated from the arterial substrate concentration, determined on blood sampled periodically from the aorta, and the known infusion rate of radioactivity. Routine examination of aortic blood samples for radioactivity

Table 3. Utilization of arterial substrates by jejunum of postabsorptive rats [a]

Arterial substrate	Concentration in arterial blood (m*M*)	Net uptake rate [b] (nmol/min per gram intestine)	Metabolism of substrate [c]			
			Flux metabolized (%)	Metabolic products released into venous blood		Contribution to total CO_2 produced by jejunum (%)
				Product	Substrate carbon (%)	
Acetoacetate + 3-hydroxybutyrate	0.8	333	12	CO_2	68	50
				Lactate	11	
				Glucose	7	
				Other	14	
Glutamine	0.6	191	31	CO_2	64	35
				Lactate	10	
				Proline	6	
				Citrulline	5	
				Glucose	5	
				Other	10	
Glucose	7.5	220	2	CO_2	15	7
				Lactate	58	
				Alanine	17	
				Other	10	
Lactate	0.5	– 170	10	CO_2	24	5
				Alanine	66	
				Other	10	
Unesterified fatty acids	0.7		1	CO_2	65	3
				Other	35	
(Total)						(100)

[a] From studies with autoperfused jejunal segments in vivo using rats fed a stock diet and fasted for 18 h (Windmueller and Spaeth 1978)
[b] Calculated from the flow rate through the segments multiplied by the arteriovenous concentration difference in simultaneously collected arterial and venous blood samples
[c] Calculated from results obtained during the continuous infusion of the substrates, uniformly labeled with ^{14}C, into the arterial blood supplying the segment

never revealed more than traces of ^{14}C, showing the absence of significant anastomoses between blood vessels of the experimental segment and the remainder of the systemic circulation. The traces of ^{14}C could have reached the systemic blood via mesenteric lymph. As seen from Table 3, the important ^{14}C-labeled metabolic products from the various substrates were CO_2, lactate, alanine, and, in the case of glutamine, also proline, citrulline, and glucose. Although there was a net release of lactate, some arterial lactate was also metabolized, largely to alanine. For each substrate, one can calculate the amount metabolized as a proportion of the total amount flowing through the tissue (flux). The proportion metabolized varied from 1% for unesterified long-chain fatty acids to 31% for glutamine (Table 3).

Also revealing is a comparison of metabolic rate values determined, on the one hand, from arteriovenous difference measurements and, on the other hand, from the single-pass perfusions with ^{14}C-labeled substrates (Table 4). The gener-

Table 4. Comparison of results from arteriovenous measurements and from single-pass perfusions with ^{14}C-labeled substrates [a]

Parameter	From arteriovenous concentration difference (nmol/min per gram intestine)	From vascular perfusion with ^{14}C-labeled substrates (nmol/min per gram intestine)
Glutamine uptake	191	215
Glucose uptake	220	179
CO_2 production	1,650	1,704
Lactate production	290 [b]	232
Alanine production	138	148

[a] From studies in vivo with autoperfused jejunal segments from postabsorptive rats (WINDMUELLER and SPAETH 1978). The results are from the experiments described in Table 3

[b] Net release into blood (170 nmol/min per gram intestine) plus the rate of lactate metabolism, based on single-pass perfusions with L-lactate ^{14}C(ul) (120 nmol/min per gram intestine)

ally good agreement indicates that the sum of the reaction pathways measured radiochemically approximately accounts for all the net uptake or release measured chemically. For example, a total CO_2 yield of 1704 nmol/min per gram intestine was obtained by summing the calculated steady state yields from the individual substrates. This value is in good agreement with the actual net rate of CO_2 release, determined from arteriovenous difference measurements by the Van Slyke manometric method (Table 4). Since metabolism of the substrates listed in Table 3 fully accounts for all the CO_2 produced, the results show that no additional oxidative substrates of any quantitative significance remain to be identified. The results also showed that 85% of the CO_2 produced by jejunal segments in fasted rats is derived from the oxidation of circulating ketone bodies and glutamine.

The largely unanswered question of the relative importance of arterial blood and luminal contents as nutrient sources for small intestine can also be approached with this preparation. One type of experiment is illustrated in Fig. 18. With glucose as the only oxidative substrate present in the lumen, the steady state rate of CO_2 production from arterial glutamine was 480 nmol/min per gram intestine. The addition of 6 m*M* glutamine or 30 m*M* glutamate to the luminal perfusate reduced this value about 25%–40%, indicating a sparing effect of the luminal substrate on its utilization from the blood. We could also determine the total rate of glutamine metabolism from both sources, by combining arteriovenous difference measurements (chemical) and radiochemical measurements on segments being luminally perfused with glutamine ^{14}C (WINDMUELLER and SPAETH 1975).

2. Permeation and Metabolism of Luminal Compounds

Having access to the total venous outflow for 1 h or more and optically also to the lymph makes the preparation ideally suited for permeation and metabolism studies with compounds administered luminally, either as a single dose into closed

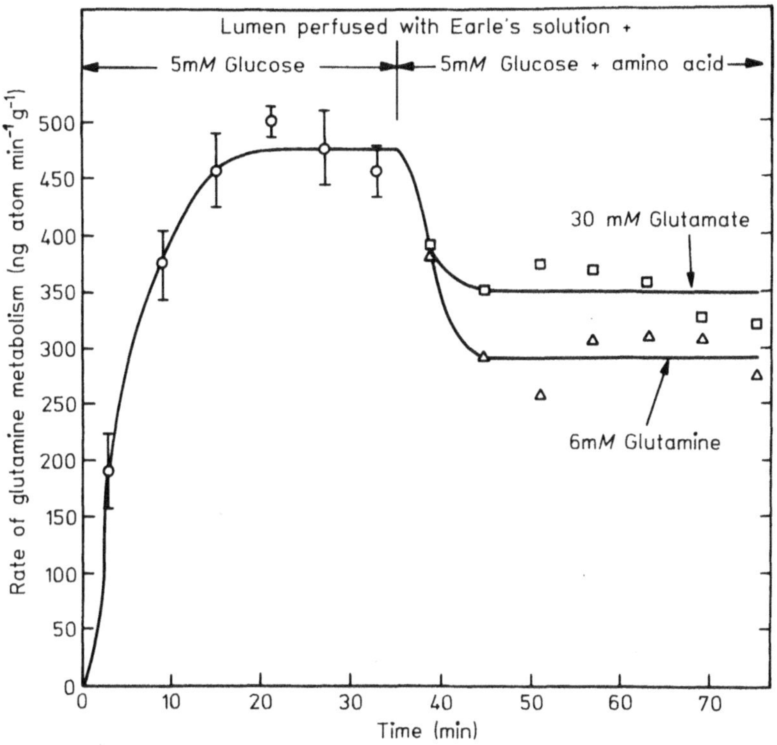

Fig. 18. Effect of luminal glutamine and glutamate on the rate of metabolism of arterial glutamine to CO_2. The lumen of autoperfused jejunal segments was perfused with 5 m*M* glucose in Earle's balanced salt solution, with the addition of glutamine or glutamate as indicated. Starting at zero time, a solution of L-glutamine ^{14}C (ul) was infused continuously at 0.01 ml/min into the blood of the artery supplying the segment. Venous blood was collected at 5–6-min intervals and the $^{14}CO_2$ content determined; 1 ml aortic blood was sampled every 10 min to monitor the arterial glutamine concentration. The results are plotted as ng atom arterial glutamine carbon metabolized to CO_2 per minute per gram tissue WINDMUELLER and SPAETH (1975)

segments or perfused continuously. Our own interest has been in amino acids and glucose. Figure 19 shows the cumulative appearance of ^{14}C in the venous blood following the luminal administration of a single dose of uniformly labeled amino acid. Except for glutamate, absorption was virtually complete within 30 min, as indicated by the nearly 100% recovery of ^{14}C in the blood. The unrecovered ^{14}C was largely incorporated into the tissue (Table 5). Rates of permeation were probably reduced by the decrease in intestinal motility produced by the anesthesia. WINNE et al. (1979) have shown in a similar autoperfused rat intestinal preparation (WINNE 1966; OCHSENFAHRT and WINNE 1969) that the permeation rate of L- and D-phenylalanine was increased when the intraluminal solution was more efficiently mixed by the simultaneous luminal perfusion of air. This is due apparently to a reduction in thickness of the effective unstirred layer, and possibly limits the usefulness of the preparation for estimating maximal permeation rates. Nevertheless, relative rates should be valid. Thus, we were surprised to find a

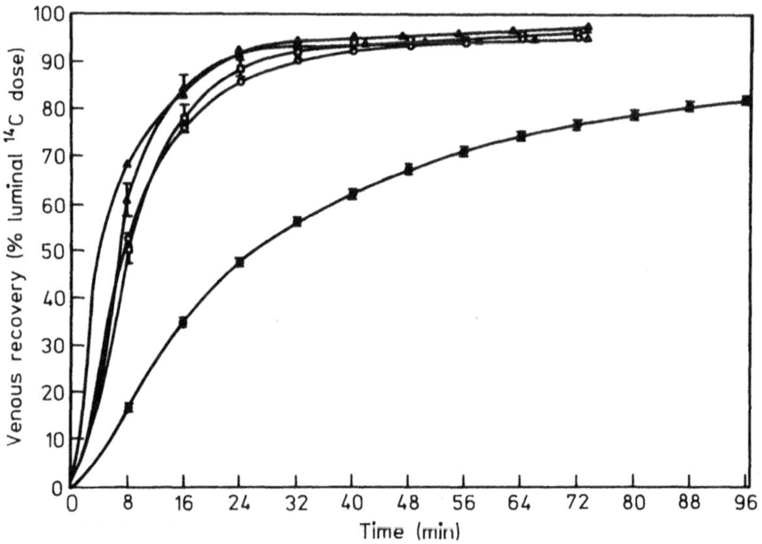

Fig. 19. Time course for appearance of radioactivity in intestinal venous blood following the luminal administration of L-amino acids ^{14}C(ul) into autoperfused jejunal segments. For each compound, 0.3 ml 6 *mM* solution in Earle's balanced salt solution, pH 7.4, was administered into closed segments. Results show cumulative recovery of ^{14}C in the administered amino acid plus metabolic products. *Open circles* glutamine; *open triangles* asparagine; *squares* aspartate; *full triangles* arginine; *full circles* glutamate. WINDMUELLER and SPAETH (1976)

large difference, previously unreported, in the uptake rates for aspartate and glutamate.

The extent to which these amino acids and also glucose are metabolized during their movement across the intestinal wall is shown in Table 5. Less than 3% of the glutamate or aspartate escaped metabolism, effectively ruling out any significant permeation by a paracellular pathway, for example by way of the tight junctions between cells (SCHULTZ and FRIZZELL 1975). Glutamine and arginine were also partially metabolized, while asparagine was transported unchanged. This is explained by the specificity of the phosphate-dependent glutaminase, which catalyzes the first step in the intestinal metabolism of glutamine, but which will not hydrolyze asparagine (PINKUS and WINDMUELLER 1977). The results with arginine were the same whether the rat was conventional or germ free, showing unambiguously that the arginase activity, evident from the stoichiometric appearance of labeled urea, was of tissue rather than microbial origin. Studies like those in Table 5 with L-lysine, L-leucine, L-phenylalanine, and L-proline revealed no measurable metabolism during their transit across the intestine.

The separate metabolic fates of a compound taken up both from the blood and from the lumen can be determined and compared. Such a comparison can be made for glutamine from the results in Tables 3 and 5. The product distribution of glutamine carbon was similar for both routes of entry, consistent with the presence of a single metabolic pool for amino acid entering mucosal cells through the brush border and through the basolateral membrane.

Table 5. Fate of nutrients absorbed from the lumen of autoperfused jejunal segments

Fate of administered radioactivity	^{14}C-labeled compound administered into the lumen (Percentage of absorbed ^{14}C)					
	Glutamate [a]	Glutamine [a]	Aspartate [b]	Arginine [a]	Asparagine [a]	Glucose [c]
Recovered in jejunal venous blood in:						
Unchanged compound	2.8	35.3	0.4	62.9	95.4	97.1
CO_2	60.5	34.6	53.6	5.0		0.8
Lactate	15.1	9.6	20.3	1.0		1.1
Citrate	1.3	1.1	1.5	0.3		0.1
Glucose	2.5	1.6	7.4	0.1		
Proline	3.9	3.5	1.4	3.8		0.0
Citrulline	3.0	2.7	1.0	5.8		0.1
Ornithine	0.9	1.3	0.4	10.7		0.0
Alanine	3.1	2.4	6.9	0.4		0.6
Urea				5.7		
Other products	4.4	4.4	4.4	0.7	0.6	0.1
Incorporated into jejunal tissue:	2.5	3.5	2.7	3.6	4.0	0.1
Total	100	100	100	100	100	100

[a] 0.3 ml Earle's balanced salt solution, pH 7.4, containing 6 m*M* L-amino acid ^{14}C (ul), was administered into closed jejunal segments. Venous blood collected from the segments for 60–100 min was analyzed (WINDMUELLER and SPAETH 1975, 1976)

[b] Experimental protocol as in [a]. Similar results were obtained when 6 m*M* L-aspartate ^{14}C (ul) was administered together with 67 m*M* glucose + 18 other L-amino acids, 0.7–5.3 m*M* each, all unlabeled (WINDMUELLER and SPAETH 1976).

[c] A solution containing 70 m*M* D-glucose ^{14}C(ul) plus 20 unlabeled L-amino acids, 0.5–6.5 m*M* each, was perfused continuously through the lumen and the steady state rate of ^{14}C appearance in venous blood was determined (WINDMUELLER and SPAETH 1980)

A glucose permeation rate of 3370 nmol/min per gram intestine was determined from the steady state rate of release of ^{14}C to venous blood during the continuous luminal perfusion with 70 m*M* D-glucose ^{14}C(ul). Only 3% was metabolized, less than observed in earlier experiments with similar autoperfused intestinal preparations, but where the blood flow rate through the tissue was artificially low (KIYASU et al. 1956; ATKINSON et al. 1957). These results emphasize the importance of maintaining the normally high flow rate.

The physiologic significance for the intestine of metabolizing nutrients taken up from the lumen can also be evaluated. Thus, the large capacity of intestine to metabolize aspartate, glutamate, and glutamine suggested that, following a meal, these three amino acids, as oxidative substrates, may contribute importantly to the tissue's energy requirement, particularly since together they constitute approximately 30% of the total weight of the usual dietary proteins. To test this hypothesis, jejunal segments were luminally perfused with a glucose–amino acid mixture, to simulate a meal (Fig. 20). Production of CO_2 from the three luminal

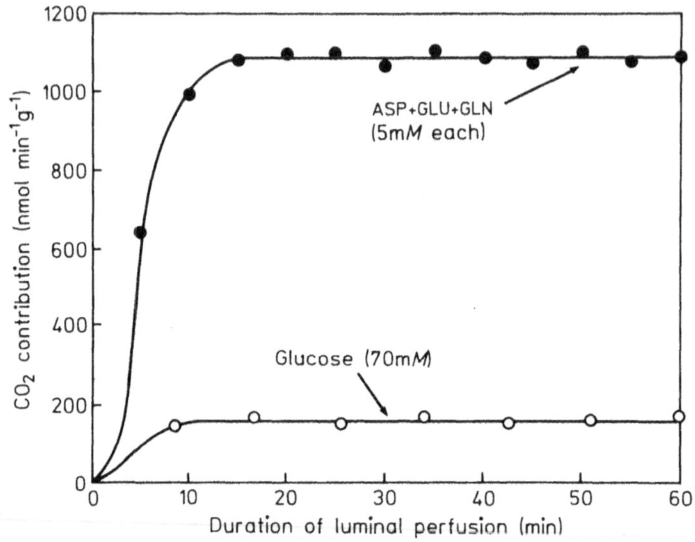

Fig. 20. Contribution of luminal substrates to respiratory CO_2 in autoperfused jejunal segments. The lumen was perfused continuously with Earle's balanced salt solution containing 70 m*M* glucose plus 20 L-amino acids, 0.5–6.5 m*M* each, to simulate a meal. *Full circles*: aspartate, glutamate, and glutamine in the perfusate were uniformly labeled with ^{14}C; the specific radioactivity of carbon atoms in all three compounds was the same. *Open circles*: perfusate glucose was uniformly labeled with ^{14}C. The CO_2 yield was calculated in all experiments from the specific radioactivity of the substrate carbon in the luminal perfusate and the rate of appearance of $^{14}CO_2$ in the venous blood. WINDMUELLER and SPAETH (1980)

amino acids totalled about 1100 nmol/min per gram intestine and from luminal glucose it was about 160 nmol/min per gram intestine as calculated from radiochemical measurements. Total CO_2 output, determined by arteriovenous difference measurements, was about 2800 nmol/min per gram intestine. Under these conditions, therefore, 39% of all the CO_2 produced was derived from luminal aspartate, glutamate, and glutamine, and 5.7% from glucose. Since the metabolism of glutamine from the blood also continues following a meal, the overall importance of amino acids as energy sources for small intestine becomes evident.

Permeation and metabolism of drugs, xenobiotics, and metabolic intermediates, as well as the normal nutrients, can, of course, be studied. BARR and RIEGELMAN (1970 a, b) have examined the permeation of salicylamide and its conjugation with glucuronic acid in autoperfused rabbit intestine. The rat preparation has been extensively used by WINNE and co-workers to study the permeation and metabolic transformation of a number of drugs (OCHSENFAHRT and WINNE 1969; WINNE and REMISCHOVSKY 1971; BOCK and WINNE 1975; JOSTING et al, 1976; BREYER and WINNE, 1977) and by WEBER et al. (1979) to measure the transamination of keto analogs of amino acids to the corresponding amino acids. Access to the lymph makes the preparation suitable as well for studying the fate of fat-soluble compounds absorbed from the lumen.

3. Biosynthesis of Lymph and Plasma Proteins

The ability of an intestinal segment to synthesize a specific protein can be determined by administering a labeled precursor, e.g., an amino acid, and subsequently isolating the protein and examining it for radioactivity. In this way we have further identified the circulating apolipoproteins synthesized by small intestine (WU and WINDMUELLER 1978). A dose of leucine ^3H was administered into the lumen of jejunal segments from fat-fed rats cannulated for mesenteric lymph drainage. Apolipoproteins were then isolated from 3-h collections of the lymph and venous blood. Any apolipoprotein containing tritium was unequivocally synthesized by the experimental segment, the only tissue exposed to the leucine ^3H. Approximately 4% of the dose was incorporated into tissue proteins and 0.5% into lymph and plasma proteins, mostly lymph, of which about half was in lipoproteins. Lymph and plasma lipoprotein analyses confirmed the earlier findings with the isolated, vascularly perfused intestine (Sect. B. VI. 3), and, with the recent advent of improved methods of apolipoprotein separation and identification, provided additional details regarding synthesis of specific proteins. Since the leucine ^3H was administered luminally, only mucosal cells had access to the label, thus further localizing the site of intestinal apolipoprotein production. The relative synthetic rates of the various proteins, determined from the relative amounts of label they incorporated, established the intestinal pattern of apolipoprotein synthesis. The pattern was found to be very different from that for liver, the other source of plasma lipoproteins. Further use was made of the jejunal segment preparation, in conjunction with related experiments in isolated, perfused rat livers and in intact rats, to determine the relative contribution of intestine and liver to each of the major apolipoproteins in the circulation. The results showed that in fat-fed rats, more than 50% of two of the major proteins of plasma high-density lipoproteins – apolipoproteins A-I and A-IV – are produced by the small intestine (WU and WINDMUELLER 1979).

4. Localized Exposure to Drugs, Hormones, and Radioactive Labels

The leucine ^3H experiments described in the preceding section illustrate a potentially useful principle, i.e., that only mucosal cells become exposed to soluble compounds administered luminally while all cells in the preparation become exposed if the compound is administered into the arterial blood supply to the segment. An example of this differential exposure is provided by experiments with two analogs of glutamine, each of which can completely and irreversible inhibit the glutamine-hydrolyzing enzyme, glutaminase (PINKUS and WINDMUELLER 1977). L-2-amino-4-oxo-5-chloropentanoic acid administered luminally into autoperfused jejunal segments resulted in 50% inhibition of whole tissue glutaminase activity, but completely inhibited the hydrolysis of glutamine subsequently absorbed from the lumen. The hydrolysis of glutamine taken up from arterial blood was little affected. In contrast, 6-diazo-5-oxo-L-norleucine administered arterially resulted in nearly 100% inhibition of whole-tissue glutaminase and inhibited the hydrolysis of glutamine taken up from the arterial blood as well as the lumen. Such use of the two alternate routes of delivery may be advantageous in studies with other drugs, hormones, or labeled compounds to localize their target cells or to identify the site for a particular biochemical activity in the intestine.

D. Concluding Remarks

I. Advantages of the Isolated Intestinal Preparation

A comparison of the two perfusion methods can be made in terms of the relative advantages of each. An advantage listed for one method can be considered as a corresponding disadvantage for the other. Advantages of the isolated preparation are as follows:

1. Since the perfusate can be repeatedly recycled through the tissue, small perfusate compositional changes reflecting the metabolic activity of the tissue will become amplified, aiding detection and quantification.
2. The composition of the perfusate can be more varied and more easily controlled, providing greater experimental flexibility.
3. The intestine is studied in the absence of an anesthetic agent, inasmuch as the ether used during surgery is rapidly lost from the tissue once isolated perfusion is started.
4. Perfusion with blood in the absence of heparin is possible by blood defibrination.
5. The entire lymph collection will be derived from the part of the intestine under study.
6. Since the tissue studied is nearly the whole of the small intestine and may also include the cecum and proximal colon, the results will directly reflect the metabolic impact on the animal of this entire portion of the gastrointestinal system.
7. The method affords an opportunity to study intestine for several hours in the absence of central neural control.

II. Advantages of the Autoperfused Intestinal Preparation

1. Establishing and maintaining the preparation are surgically and technically less demanding. Temperature regulation and blood pumping are simplified, no membrane lung is needed, and no pH control or nutrient infusions are necessary.
2. The composition of the perfusing blood remains both constant and physiologically normal, except for the presence of heparin and an anesthetic.
3. The innervation of the intestine remains intact, obviating the requirement for norepinephrine and steroid hormones.
4. Perfusing the lumen, to control the composition of the luminal contents, is facilitated.
5. Single-pass perfusion of both the vasculature and lumen for long periods offers wide experimental possibilities. Compounds arterially infused and metabolic products released cannot recycle through the tissue. With tissue weight and blood flow rate both known, absolute rates for permeation and metabolic conversion can be determined.
6. For comparative purposes, specific regions along the small intestine can be studied independently, or, with modifications in technique (GALLUSER et al. 1976), possibly even simultaneously.
7. By selecting the route of administration, one has the choice to permit all the cells of an intestinal segment to have access to a compound, or only the mucosal cells.

References

Ariens EJ (1967) The structure-activity relationships of *beta* adrenergic drugs and *beta* adrenergic blocking drugs. Ann NY Acad Sci 139:606–631

Atkinson RM, Parsons BJ, Smyth DH (1957) The intestinal absorption of glucose. J Physiol (Lond) 135:581–589

Barr WH, Riegelman S (1970 a) Intestinal drug absorption and metabolism. I: Comparison of methods and models to study physiological factors of in vitro and in vivo intestinal absorption. J Pharm Sci 59:154–163

Barr WH, Riegelman S (1970 b) Intestinal drug absorption and metabolism. II: Kinetic aspects of intestinal glucuronide conjugation. J Pharm Sci 59:164–168

Bock KW, Winne D (1975) Glucuronidation of l-naphthol in the rat intestinal loop. Biochem. Pharmacol 24:859–862

Boen ST (1961) Kinetics of peritoneal dialysis. Medicine 40:243–287

Breyer U, Winne D (1977) Absorption and metabolism of the phenothiazine drug perazine in the rat intestinal loop. Biochem Pharmacol 26:1275–1280

Bronk JR, Ingham PA (1979) Sugar transfer from the lumen of the rat small intestine to the vascular bed. J Physiol 289:99–113

Carpenter CCJ, Greenough WB III (1968) Response of the canine duodenum to intraluminal challenge with cholera exotoxin. J Clin Invest 47:2600–2607

Dean JA (ed) (1973) Lange's handbook of chemistry, 11th edn. McGraw-Hill Book Company, New York, p 10–7

Dresel P, Wallentin I (1966) Effects of sympathetic vasoconstrictor fibers, noradrenaline and vasopressin on the intestinal vascular resistance during constant blood flow or blood pressure. Acta Physiol Scand 66: 427–436

Dubois RS, Roy CC (1969) Insulin stimulated transport of 3–0-methyl glucose across the rat jejunum. Proc Soc Exp Biol Med 130:931–934

Dubois RS, Vaughan GD, Roy CC (1968) Isolated rat small intestine with intact circulation. In: Norman JC (ed) Organ perfusion and preservation. Appleton Century Crofts, New York, p 863

Eagle H (1959) Amino acid metabolism in mammalian cell cultures. Science 130:432–437

Earle WR (1943) Production of malignancy in vitro. IV. The mouse fibroblast cultures and changes seen in the living cells. J Nat Cancer Inst 4:165–212

Eloy R, Raul F, Pousse A, Mirham R, Anana A, Grenier JF (1977) Ex vivo vascular perfusion of the isolated rat small bowel: Importance of the intestinal brush border enzyme-release in basal conditions. Eur Surg Res 9:96–112

Folkow B (1967) Regional adjustments in intestinal blood flow. Gastroenterology 52:423–434

Forth W (1968) Eisen- und Kobalt-Resorption am perfundierten Dünndarmsegment. In: Staib W, Scholz R (eds) 3. Konferenz der Gesellschaft für Biologische Chemie. Springer, Berlin, Heidelberg, New York, p 242

Fritz I, Levine R (1951) Action of adrenal cortical steroids and norepinephrine on vascular responses of stress in adrenalectomized rats. Am J Physiol 165:456–465

Galluser M, Pousse A, Ferard G, Grenier JF (1976) Mise au point d'une technique d'étude de l'absorption intestinale des monosaccharides chez le rat, in vivo. Biomedicine 25:127–132

Gerber GB, Remy-Defraigne J (1966) DNA metabolism in perfused organs. II. Incorporation into DNA and catabolism of thymidine at different levels of substrate by normal and X-irradiated liver and intestine. Arch Int Physiol Biochim 74:785–806

Hamilton RL, Berry MN, Williams MC, Severinghaus EM (1974) A simple and inexpensive membrane "lung" for small organ perfusion. J Lipid Res 15:182–186

Hanson PJ, Parsons DS (1976) The utilization of glucose and production of lactate by in vitro preparations of rat small intestine: effects of vascular perfusion. J Physiol (Lond) 255:775–795

Hanson PJ, Parsons DS (1977) Metabolism and transport of glutamine and glucose in vascularly perfused rat small intestine. Biochem J 166:509–519

Hanson PJ, Parsons DS (1978) Factors affecting the utilization of ketone bodies and other substrates by rat jejunum: effects of fasting and of diabetes. J Physiol (Lond) 278:55–67
Henderson LM, Gross CJ (1979a) Transport of niacin and niacinamide in perfused rat intestine. J Nutr 109:646–653
Henderson LM, Gross CJ (1979b) Metabolism of niacin and niacinamide in perfused rat intestine. J Nutr 109:654–662
Hestrin-Lerner S, Shapiro B (1954) Absorption of glucose from the intestine. II. In vivo and perfusion studies. Biochim Biophys Acta 13: 54–60
Hülsmann WC (1971) Preferential oxidation of fatty acids by rat small intestine. FEBS Lett 17:35–38
Jacobs P, Bothwell TH, Charlton RW (1966) Intestinal iron transport: studies using a loop of gut with an artificial circulation. Am J Physiol 210:694–700
Johnson L, Nylander G, Svensson Å (1969) A new experimental device for in vitro study of the functions of the small intestine. Acta Chir Scand 135:241–247
Josting D, Winne D, Bock KW (1976) Glucuronidation of paracetamol, morphine and 1-naphthol in the rat intestinal loop. Biochem Pharmacol 25:613–616
Katz M, O'Brien R (1979) Vitamin B_{12} absorption studied by vascular perfusion of rat intestine. J Lab Clin Med 94:817–825
Kavin H, Levin NW, Stanley MM (1967) Isolated perfused rat small bowel – technic, studies of viability, glucose absorption. J Appl Physiol 22:604–611
Kewenter J (1965) The vagal control of the jejunal and ileal motility and blood flow. Acta Physiol Scand 65:1–68, Suppl 251
Kiyasu JY, Katz J, Chaikoff IL (1956) Nature of the ^{14}C compounds recovered in portal plasma after enteral administration of ^{14}C-glucose. Biochim Biophys Acta 21:286–290
Kolobow T, Zapol W, Marcus J (1968) Development of a disposable membrane lung for organ perfusion. In: Norman JC (ed) Organ perfusion and preservation. Appleton Century Crofts, New York, p 155
Lamers JMJ, Hülsmann WC (1972) Pasteur effect in the in vitro vascularly perfused rat small intestine. Biochem Biophys Acta 275:491–495
Landsberg L (1976) Extraneuronal uptake and metabolism of [^{3}H]L-norepinephrine by rat duodenal mucosa. Biochem Pharmacol 25:729–731
Lee JS, Duncan KM (1968) Lymphatic and venous transport of water from rat jejunum: a vascular perfusion study. Gastroenterology 54:559–567
Lester RG, Grim E (1975) Substrate utilization and oxygen consumption by canine jejunal mucosa in vitro. Am J Physiol 229:139–143
Levin SR, Pehlevanian MZ, Lavee AE, Adachi RI (1979) Secretion of an insulinotropic factor from isolated, perfused rat intestine. Am J Physiol 236:E710-E720
Matsutaka H, Aikawa T, Yamamoto H, Ishikawa E (1973) Gluconeogenesis and amino acid metabolism. III. Uptake of glutamine and output of alanine and ammonia by nonhepatic splanchnic organs of fasted rats and their metabolic significance. J Biochem (Tokyo) 74:1019–1029
Norberg KA (1964) Adrenergic innervation of the intestinal wall studied by fluorescence microscopy. Int J Neuropharmacol 3:379–382
Ochsenfahrt H (1979) The relevance of blood flow for the absorption of drugs in the vascularly perfused, isolated intestine of the rat. Naunyn Schmiedebergs Arch Pharmacol 306:105–112
Ochsenfahrt H, Winne D (1969) Der Einfluß der Durchblutung auf die Resorption von Arzneimitteln aus dem Jejunum der Ratte. Naunyn Schmiedebergs Arch Pharmacol 264:55–75
Öhnell R (1939) The artificially perfused mammalian intestine as a useful preparation for studying intestinal absorption. J Cell Comp Physiol 13:155–159
Öhnell R, Höber R (1939) The effect of various poisons on the absorption of sugars and some other non-electrolytes from the normal and the isolated artificially perfused intestine. J Cell Comp Physiol 13:161–174
Olson EB, DeLuca HF (1969) 25-Hydroxycholecalciferol: direct effect on calcium transport. Science 165:405–407

Parsons DS, Prichard JS (1968) A preparation of perfused small intestine for the study of absorption in amphibia. J Physiol (Lond) 198:405–434
Paton WDM, Vizi ES (1969) The inhibitory action of noradrenaline and adrenaline on acetylcholine output by guinea pig ileum longitudinal muscle strip. Br J Pharmacol 35:10–28
Pinkus LM, Windmueller HG (1977) Phosphate-dependent glutaminase of small intestine: localization and role in intestinal glutamine metabolism. Arch Biochem Biophys 182:506–517
Ramey ER, Goldstein MS (1957) The adrenal cortex and the sympathetic nervous system. Physiol Rev 37:155–195
Roese HF (1930) Methoden zum Studium der Physiologie und Pharmakologie des künstlich durchbluteten Säugetierdarmes. Pflügers Arch 226:171–183
Ross BD (1972) Perfusion techniques in biochemistry. Clarendon Oxford, pp 356–394
Roy CC, Dubois RS, Philippon F (1970) Inhibition by bile salts of the jejunal transport of 3-0-methyl glucose. Nature 225:1055–1056
Salvioli G (1880) Eine neue Methode für die Untersuchung der Funktionen des Dünndarms. Arch Anat Physiol (suppl):95–112
Schultz SG, Frizzell RA (1975) Amino acid transport by the small intestine. In: Czáky TZ (ed) Intestinal absorption and malabsorption. Raven, New York, p 77
Shoor PM, Griffith LD, Dilley RB, Bernstein EF (1979) Effect of pulseless perfusion on gastrointestinal blood flow and its distribution. Am J Physiol 236:E28-E32
Smith KT, Cousins RJ, Silbon BL, Failla ML (1978) Zinc absorption and metabolism by isolated, vascularly perfused rat intestine. J Nutr 108:1849–1857
Vane JR (1969) The release and fate of vaso-active hormones in the circulation. Br J Pharmacol 35:209–242
Warshaw AL (1972) A simplified method of cannulating the intestinal lymphatic of the rat. Gut 13:66–67
Weber FL Jr, Deak SB, Laine RA (1979) Absorption of keto-analogues of branched-chain amino acids from rat small intestine. Gastroenterology 76:62–70
Windmueller HG, Spaeth AE (1966) Perfusion *in situ* with tritium oxide to measure hepatic lipogenesis and lipid secretion. J Biol Chem 241:2891–2899
Windmueller HG, Spaeth AE (1972) Fat transport and lymph and plasma lipoprotein biosynthesis by isolated intestine. J Lipid Res 13:92–105
Windmueller HG, Spaeth AE (1974) Uptake and metabolism of plasma glutamine by small intestine. J Biol Chem 249:5070–5079
Windmueller HG, Spaeth AE (1975) Intestinal metabolism of glutamine and glutamate from the lumen as compared to glutamine from blood. Arch Biochem Biophys 171:662–672
Windmueller HG, Spaeth AE (1976) Metabolism of absorbed aspartate, asparagine, and arginine by rat small intestine in vivo. Arch Biochem Biophys 175:670–676
Windmueller HG, Spaeth AE (1977) Vascular perfusion of rat small intestine: metabolic studies with isolated and in situ preparations. Fed Proc 36:177–181
Windmueller HG, Spaeth AE (1978) Identification of ketone bodies and glutamine as the major respiratory fuels in vivo for postabsorptive rat small intestine. J Biol Chem 253:69–76
Windmueller HG, Spaeth AE (1980) Respiratory fuels and nitrogen metabolism in vivo in small intestine of fed rats: Quantitative importance of glutamine, glutamate, and aspartate. J Biol Chem 255:107–112
Windmueller HG, Spaeth AE, Ganote CE (1970) Vascular perfusion of isolated rat gut: norepinephrine and glucocorticoid requirement. Am J Physiol 218:197–204
Windmueller HG, Herbert PN, Levy RI (1973) Biosynthesis of lymph and plasma lipoprotein apoproteins by isolated perfused rat liver and intestine. J Lipid Res 14:215–223
Winne D (1966) Der Einfluß einiger Pharmaka auf die Darmdurchblutung und die Resorption tritiummarkierten Wassers aus dem Dünndarm der Ratte. Naunyn Schmiedebergs Arch Pharmacol Exp Pathol 254:199–224

Winne D, Remischovsky J (1971) Der Einfluß der Durchblutung auf die Resorption von Harnstoff, Methanol, und Äthanol aus dem Jejunum der Ratte. Naunyn Schmiedebergs Arch Pharmacol 268:392–416
Winne D, Kopf S, Ulmer ML (1979) Role of unstirred layer in intestinal absorption of phenylalanine in vivo. Biochim Biophys Acta 550: 120–130
Wu AL, Windmueller HG (1978) Identification of circulating apolipoproteins synthesized by rat small intestine in vivo. J Biol Chem 253:2525–2528
Wu AL, Windmueller HG (1979) Relative contributions by liver and intestine to individual plasma apolipoproteins in the rat. J Biol Chem 254:7316–7322

CHAPTER 6

The Use of Isolated Membrane Vesicles in the Study of Intestinal Permeation

H. MURER and B. HILDMANN

A. Introduction

Until about 1972–1973 most of the knowledge on small intestinal epithelial transport processes was derived from studies with the intact epithelium in vivo or in vitro. It has been demonstrated that these epithelia are able to perform active transport of a variety of solutes from the lumen to the serosal compartment with a well-defined specificity for several groups of compounds. Even though the epithelial cell had to be treated as a black box in these studies, the experimental evidence obtained strongly supported the hypothesis that the energy inherent in the sodium gradient across the brush border membrane was utilized by the cell to perform active transepithelial transport of a considerable number of organic and inorganic solutes (for review see SCHULTZ 1979; SCHULTZ and CURRAN 1970; CRANE 1977).

A more direct approach in studies with intact epithelial preparations allowing an opening of the black box epithelial cell and an assessment of permeability properties of the individual plasma membranes was achieved in electrophysiological studies by measuring the electrical potential differences and their changes as a consequence of solute transport across the intestinal wall, or even across either the brush border or basolateral plasma membranes (e.g. ROSE and SCHULTZ 1970, 1971). Also, unidirectional influx measurement, a technique mainly developed by SCHULTZ and CURRAN (1970) as well as unidirectional transepithelial flux measurements (e.g. FRIZZELL et al. 1979) permitted a separate analysis of the events at the individual cell surfaces. In this context studies with isolated epithelial cells should also be mentioned, which made significant contributions to the understanding of the energetics of transepithelial transport in the small intestine (KIMMICH 1977; KIMMICH and RANDLES 1980).

An alternative possibility to open the black box of the epithelial cell is a biochemical one. Since 1973 isolated plasma membrane vesicles have been used to study small intestinal transport processes (HOPFER et al. 1973; HOPFER 1977a; MURER and KINNE 1980, 1982). By isolating the luminal as well as the contraluminal plasma membranes it is possible to detect a polar distribution of transport systems in the cell envelope. The principal advantage of this approach is the possibility of presetting and knowing the exact environmental conditions of the membranes containing the transport systems, because of the separation of the membranes from the cytosol and their suspension in solutions of known composition.

In this chapter a short outline of work performed thus far with plasma membrane vesicles isolated from small intestine is presented. It is not intended to present a complete review of the field. A more complete review also covering experiments with membrane vesicles from nonintestinal epithelia has been completed recently (MURER and KINNE 1980).

B. Methods for Membrane Isolation

I. Brush Border Membranes

In their attempt to isolate brush border membranes from small intestinal epithelium MILLER and CRANE (1961 a, b) have used two criteria for the recognition of the brush border fragments: (a) their morphology and (b) their high content of disaccharidases and alkaline phosphatase. Further studies performed by EICHHOLZ and CRANE (1965), PORTEOUS and CLARK (1965) as well as by HÜBSCHER et al. (1965) have demonstrated that invertase and aminopeptidase M (leucine aminopeptidase) are reliable marker enzymes for the identification of the luminal border of the small intestinal epithelial cell, too. Finally, cell fractionation experiments performed after exclusive labelling of the luminal surface with *p*-diazosulfobenzoic acid ^{35}S in intact intestinal preparations showed that sucrase is exclusively located in the luminal cell surface (MIRCHEFF and WRIGHT 1976).

Using these well-defined marker enzymes, FORSTNER et al. (1968) developed a technique for the isolation of brush border fragments with the subsequent isolation of brush border membranes free from the electron-dense core material. In the intact cell the core is made up of microfilaments, probably mainly actin (TILNEY and MOOSECKER 1971). More recently, proteins such as villin and calmodulin have been identified as components of these microfilaments (GLENNEY et al. 1980). LOUVARD et al. (1973) as well as the group led by CRANE described methods which permitted isolation of brush border membranes without prior isolation of brush border fragments (LOUVARD et al. 1973; SCHMITZ et al. 1973). These "direct" methods were based on the different reactivity of the luminal membrane and the other cellular organelles with magnesium or calcium (see following discussion).

Transport studies with isolated brush border membrane vesicles require vesiculation of isolated membrane fragments. In the method of HOPFER et al. (1973) brush border fragments are isolated in 5 mmol/l Na_3EDTA buffer first. Then, homogenization of the brush border fragments in a buffered mannitol solution of low ionic strength leads to depolymerization of the actin filaments. After addition of 0.1 mmol/l $MgSO_4$ vesiculated brush border membranes can be isolated by two differential centrifugation steps. The calcium precipitation procedures for vesicle preparation, originally described by BOOTH and KENNY (1974) for renal membrane preparations, are very simple methods and are today most frequently used to isolate brush border membrane vesicles (e.g. KESSLER et al. 1978 a; HILDMANN et al. 1980 a; HAUSER et al. 1980; BIBER et al. 1981). After addition of 10–20 mmol/l $CaCl_2$ (or $MgCl_2$) to a hypotonic homogenate of mucosal scrapings, brush border membranes can be isolated by differential centrifugation steps. The addition of $CaCl_2$ or $MgCl_2$ in appropriate proportion to the amount of material homogenized leads to agglomeration of most of the membranous material. The brush border membrane does not enter into these calcium–membrane

Table 1. Flow scheme for the isolation of brush border membranes from rabbit small intestine by a calcium precipitation method. This procedure corresponds to that described by HILDMANN et al. (1980a)

Discarded	Fraction	Procedure
	Intestine	Kill rabbit by a blow on the neck and bleeding from the carotid artery, quickly remove intestine, immerse in ice-cold Ringer's solution
Outer layers of intestinal wall ←	↓	Rinse with Ringer's solution evert segments of intestine, remove residual faeces and mucus, scrape mucosa gently
	Scraped mucosa	
	↓	Suspend scrapings in 300 m*M* mannitol, 12 m*M* HEPES-Tris, pH 7.1 (60 ml per 10 gram mucosa), dilute 6 times with water, homogenize for 3 min at maximum speed in a blender in portions not exceeding 300 ml
	Homogenate	
Discard pellet P1 ←	↓	Add 1 ml 1 *M* $CaCl_2$ to 100 ml of homogenate, leave for 15 min, centrifuge at 7000 rpm, Sorvall GSA rotor, 15 min (corresponds to 8000 *g* at the bottom of the tubes)
	Supernatant S1	
Discard supernatant S2 ←	↓	Centrifuge at 11500 rpm, Sorvall GSA rotor, 30 min (21600 *g*)
	Pellet P2	
Discard pellet P3 ←	↓	Resuspend in buffer needed for the uptake measurement (40 ml per 10 gram mucosa), add 1 ml 1 *M* $CaCl_2$ to 100 ml suspension, leave for 15 min, centrifuge at 8000 rpm, Sorvall SS 34 rotor, 15 min (7800 *g*)
	Supernatant S3	
Discard supernatant S4 ←	↓	Centrifuge at 13000 rpm, Sorvall SS 34 rotor, 30 min (20400 *g*)
	Pellet P4	
Discard pellet P5 ←	↓	Resuspend in buffer needed for the uptake measurement (1 ml per 10 gram mucosa), put into Eppendorf tubes, centrifuge at 4000 rpm, Sorvall SS 34 rotor, 5 min
	Supernatant S5	
Discard supernatant S6 ←	↓	Centrifuge in an Eppendorf table centrifuge at maximum speed for 30 min
	Pellet P6	
	↓	Resuspend with a syringe in appropriate amount of buffer needed for the uptake experiment
	Brush border membranes	

agglomerates, mots probably protected by the glycocalyx (fuzzy coat) (BOOTH and KENNY 1974). Table 1 presents as an example a flow scheme for the isolation of brush border membranes from rabbit small intestine (HILDMANN et al. 1980a). For different species and different purposes different volumes and centrifugation conditions have been used.

With respect to membrane purification, the method of HOPFER et al. (1973) is superior to the methods based on a single calcium precipitation, as judged by the enrichment factors of brush border marker enzymes. However, membrane vesicles can be obtained more quickly and with higher yields by calcium precipitation methods. Furthermore, the latter membranes show less nonspecific leak permeabilities than those obtained by the method of HOPFER et al. (1973). A membrane purity similar to that obtained by the method of HOPFER et al. (1973) can be obtained by repeating the precipitation step, e.g. after two Mg^{2+} precipitations (HILDMANN et al. 1982b).

II. Basolateral Plasma Membranes

It is generally accepted that Na^+, K^+-ATPase can be considered as a reliable marker for the basolateral membrane of the small intestinal epithelial cell. This was documented by the microautoradiographic determination of bound labelled ouabain, a high affinity inhibitor of Na^+, K^+-ATPase (STIRLING 1972). Furthermore, membrane fractionation experiments with density gradient centrifugation and separation by free-flow electrophoresis separation consistently showed that marker enzymes for the brush border membrane and Na^+, K^+-ATPase migrate independently (e.g. QUIGLEY and GOTTERER 1969; FUJITA et al. 1972; MURER et al. 1974, 1976b; MIRCHEFF and WRIGHT 1976; MIRCHEFF et al. 1979; SCALERA et al. 1980). Finally, the study of LEWIS et al. (1975) revealed that, after iodination of epithelial cell sheets, Na^+, K^+-ATPase activity can be found associated only with iodinated membranous material, i.e. Na^+, K^+-ATPase is exclusively located in the surface membrane of the enterocytes. Summarizing all these observations one can be assured that Na^+, K^+-ATPase is located exclusively in the basolateral cell membranes. Cell fractionation studies of PARKINSON et al. (1972), MURER et al. (1976b) and WALLING et al. (1978) revealed that adenylate cyclase is also an excellent marker enzyme for enterocyte basolateral membranes.

Many different procedures have been developed over the past 10 years for the isolation of basolateral plasma membranes (e.g. WRIGHT et al. 1979; FUJITA et al. 1972; MURER et al. 1976). The main drawbacks of these methods for the isolation of basolateral membranes were their long duration, their low yields and the use of equipment not generally available in laboratories orientated more towards research in physiology or pharmacology. Therefore, recently a more simple procedure for the isolation of basolateral membranes based on Percoll density gradient centrifugation (Pharmacia, Uppsala, Sweden) was developed (SCALERA et al. 1980). This method allows isolation of basolateral plasma membranes with high speed centrifugation ($\leq 48\,000$ *g*) and requires only a short time (3–4 h). The enrichment of Na^+, K^+-ATPase is about 20, compared with its activity in the homogenate, and thus equals that of the other methods mentioned. The yield, however, of basolateral membranes, as estimated by the recovery of the Na^+, K^+-ATPase in the membrane fraction, is definitely higher (up to 10% of cell homoge-

Table 2. Flow scheme for the isolation of basolateral plasma membranes from rat small intestinal epithelial cells. The method corresponds to that published by SCALERA et al. (1980)

Isolated epithelial cells (3 rats, 180–200 g)

- 50 ml sucrose buffer (250 mM sucrose, 10 M triethanolamine HCl, pH 7.6, and 0.1 mM phenylmethylsulfonylfluoride
- homogenize for 3 min with blender
- dilute 1:1 with sucrose buffer

↓

Homogenate

- centrifuge at 4600 rpm, Sorvall SS 34 rotor, 15 min (2500 g)
- discard pellet

↓

Supernatant

- centrifuge at 13 000 rpm for 20 min (20 5000 g)
- discard supernatant and dark pellet

↓

Fluffy layer of pellet

- resuspend in 350 ml sucrose buffer
- homogenize in glass–polytetrafluoroethylene homogenizer (20 strokes at 1200 rpm)

↓

Crude plasma membranes

- 31.5 ml membrane suspension + 3.5 ml Percoll (final concentration = 10%)
- homogenize in glass–polytetrafluoroethylene homogenizer (3 strokes at 1200 rpm)
- centrifuge at 20 000 rpm, Sorvall SS 34 rotor, 60 min (48 000 g)

↓

Fractions of Percoll gradient

nate). The cross-contamination of the basolateral membrane fraction obtained by the Percoll centrifugation method by other cellular components is not higher than that of other methods. However, one has to consider that different isolation procedures might produce significant differences in the cross-contamination with respect to the nature of contaminating constituents. An example of a flow scheme of the Percoll centrifugation method is presented in Table 2. In the course of recent experiments we found it necessary to modify centrifugation conditions slightly with each new batch of Percoll used. The crude plasma membrane fraction was centrifuged with different concentrations of Percoll (10%–12% v/v) and for different times (30–60 min). In such preliminary experiments gradients were selected by eye for fractionation with the criterion that two bands were clearly separated: one in the upper third of the tube and one in the lower quarter of the tube, both of which may split into double bands depending on the amount of material centrifuged in the gradient. The gradients separated into 50–60 fractions were assayed for the distribution of protein, Na^+, K^+-ATPase, aminopeptidase M (see Fig. 1 a) and in addition for alkaline phosphatase, succinate: cytochrome *c*-oxi-

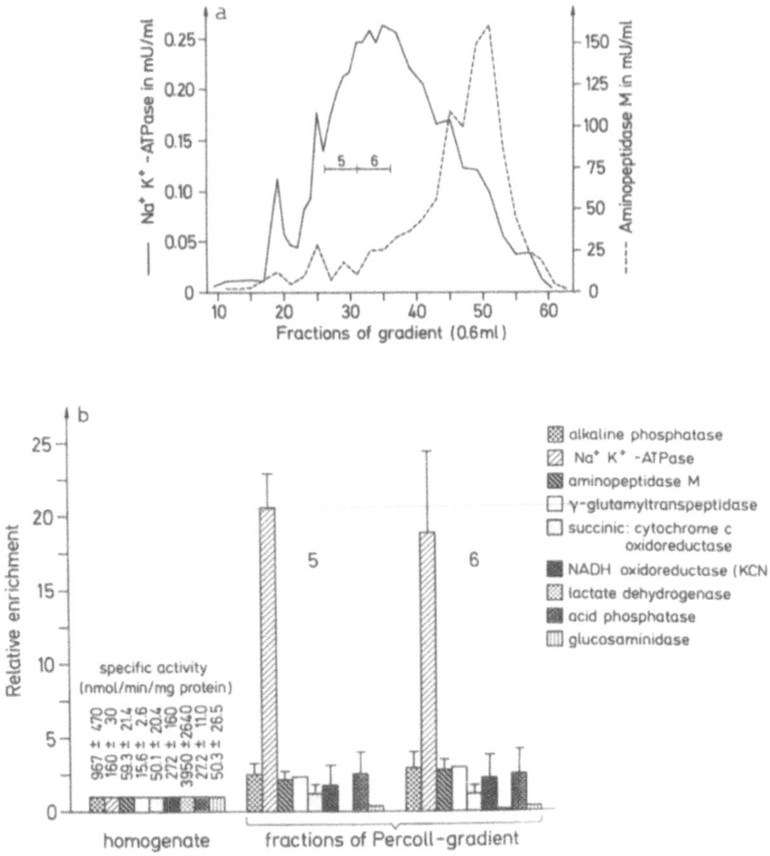

Fig. 1. a Isolation of basolateral membranes from rat small intestine. Distribution of Na^+, K^+-ATPase (marker enzyme for basolateral membranes) and aminopeptidase M (marker enzyme for the brush border membrane) in a Percoll gradient (10% v/v in 250 m*M* sucrose; 10 m*M* triethanolamine hydrochloride, pH 7.6) after centrifugation of a heavy microsomal fraction from rat enterocytes at 48,000 *g* for 1 h. **b** Relative enrichments of marker enzymes obtained in pooled fractions from the Percoll gradient ($N=5$; means ±S.D.). After SCALERA et al. (1980)

doreductase. NADH: (acceptor)-oxidoreductase (not shown in Fig. 1 a). The conditions leading to migration of Na^+, K^+-ATPase to the middle third of the gradient and clear separation of the upper and lower protein bands containing contaminating enzyme activities were chosen for preparative purposes. Thereby the basolateral membrane fraction was defined by the volumes which had to be pumped out of the tubes from above the band and containing the band. An example of enrichment factors obtained in a preparative scale isolation is given in Figure 1 b. It is hoped that the ease now achieved with the isolation of basolateral membranes from small intestinal epithelial cells will enable investigators to perform more extensive transport studies with these membranes to make up the deficiency in knowledge about their permeability characteristics.

Table 3. Asymmetric distribution of cell surface membrane bound enzymes in rat small intestinal epithelial cells (proximal duodenum). In this table it is assumed that Na^{+},K^{+}-ATPase and sucrase activity are restricted to the basolateral and brush border membrane, respectively (see text). The enzyme activity in each fraction is given as the percentage of that in the initial homogenate. These data are taken from WRIGHT et al. (1979)

	Basolateral membranes	Brush border membranes
	Percentage distribution	
Na^{+},K^{+}-ATPase	100	
Adenylate cyclase	100	
Sucrase		100
Aminopeptidase M		100
γ-Glutamyl transpeptidase		100
Ca^{2+}-ATPase	66	34
Acid phosphatase [a]	28	4
Mg^{2+}-ATPase [a]	20	6
Guanylate cyclase [a]	11	63
Alkaline phosphatase	35	65
HCO_3^--ATPase [a]		

[a] The sum is not 100% because the remaining enzyme activity is found to be associated with intracellular structures
Experiments suggest that anion-stimulated Mg^{2+}-ATPase is also a constituent of brush border membranes (HUMPHREYS et al. 1980; HUMPHREYS and CHOU 1979)

III. Enzyme and Polypeptide Content of Isolated Brush Border and Basolateral Membranes

Table 3 summarizes the distribution of marker enzymes of different enterocyte components. The results of this study by WRIGHT et al. (1979) suggest that Na^{+}, K^{+}-ATPase and adenylate cyclase can be considered as reliable marker enzymes for the basolateral plasma membrane, whereas sucrase, aminopeptidase M and γ-glutamyl transpeptidase are the best marker enzymes for the brush border membrane. According to these results, alkaline phosphatase is predominantly but not exclusively localized in the brush border membrane. Since comigration of alkaline phosphatase and Na^{+}, K^{+}-ATPase was also found after attempts to further separate by free-flow electrophoresis a rat intestinal basolateral membrane fraction isolated by sorbitol density gradient centrifugation, it has to be concluded that alkaline phosphatase can be a constituent of basolateral membranes and should not be taken as the only marker for the luminal membrane in separation experiments (MIRCHEFF and WRIGHT 1976; WRIGHT et al. 1979; WALLING et al. 1978; BIBER et al. 1981). According to the multiplicity of functions of the brush border as well as of the basolateral plasma membrane of small intestinal epithelial cells, it is not surprising that the protein pattern found in sodium dodecylsulphate polyacrylamide gel electrophoresis (SDS PAGE) is very complex (e.g. WRIGHT et al. 1979: SHLATZ et al. 1978; KIMBERG et al. 1979).

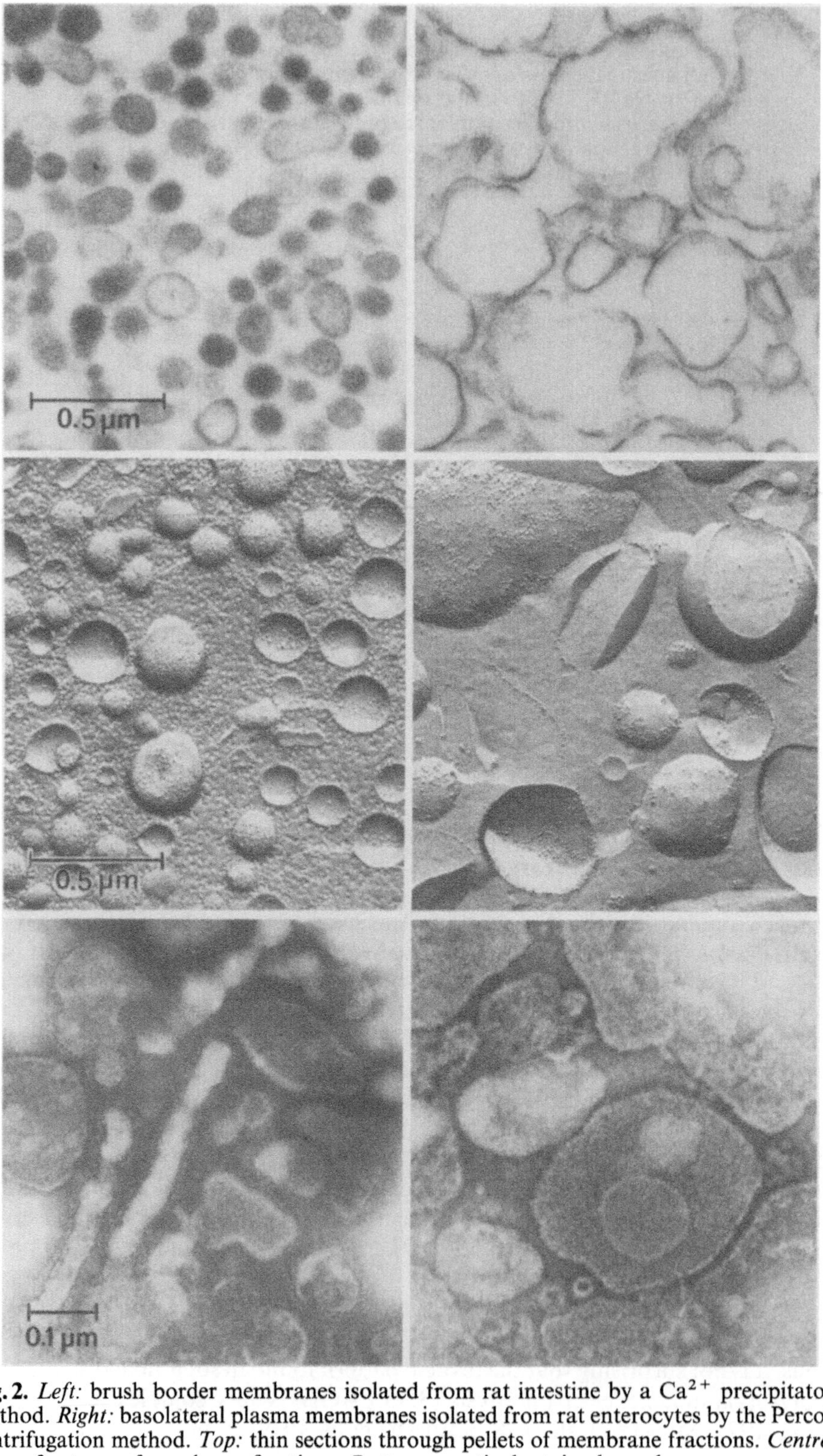

Fig. 2. *Left:* brush border membranes isolated from rat intestine by a Ca^{2+} precipitaton method. *Right:* basolateral plasma membranes isolated from rat enterocytes by the Percoll centrifugation method. *Top:* thin sections through pellets of membrane fractions. *Centre:* freeze-fractures of membrane fractions. *Bottom:* negatively stained membranes.

IV. Morphology and Orientation of Isolated Brush Border and Basolateral Membranes

As illustrated by the electron micrographs (Fig. 2), brush border membranes and isolated basolateral membranes can also be distinguished by their morphological appearance. The external surface of the brush border membrane as seen in thin sections is coated by a fuzzy structure, probably representing the glycocalyx, which can be clearly recognized in high magnification thin section pictures, especially after staining with ruthenium red. The inner and outer surfaces of basolateral membranes cannot be distinguished in thin sections stained with routine techniques. Brush border membranes isolated from rat or rabbit intestine by the calcium precipitation method often appear in thin section preparations as membrane vesicles filled with an electron-dense material. Interestingly the filling of the vesicles with the electron-dense material depends on the species of animal used for membrane isolation. Membrane vesicles isolated from rat intestine are almost all filled, whereas membranes isolated from guinea-pig intestine appear to be mostly empty (B. STIEGER and H. MURER 1981, unpublished work). This electron-dense material is not observed in membrane vesicles isolated from rat intestine by the method of HOPFER et al. (1973). In contrast to the method of HOPFER et al. (1973), the conditions used in the calcium precipitation method do not favour depolymerization of the core material. Indeed, the presence of high amounts of actin can be demonstrated by SDS PAGE (KLIP et al. 1979a, b).

Negative staining pictures of brush border membranes show knob-like structures on the external membrane surface. This surface structure is typical for the brush border membrane and is not seen on the basolateral cell surface or in isolated basolateral membrane fractions. It is generally believed that these knob-like structures on the surface of the brush border membrane are protein particles containing hydrolases such as aminopeptidase M or sucrase (MAESTRACCI 1976). Accordingly, it could be found that enzymes located in these protein particles are rapidly digested by proteases, whereas enzymes (e.g. alkaline phosphatase) located deeper in the membrane are more resistant to protease treatment (MAESTRACCI 1976; ROHN et al. 1983).

Differences are also visible in freeze-fracture electron micrographs of the two membrane populations. In brush border membrane preparations the convex leaflets have a higher intramembranous particle density than the concave ones, whereas the particle densities in basolateral membranes are randomly distributed between convex and concave leaflets. Thin section, negative staining as well as freeze fracture preparations, all demonstrate that isolated brush border membranes as well as isolated basolateral membranes are closed membrane vesicles and that basolateral membranes form vesicles with considerably higher diameters.

A statistical analysis of the distribution of the intramembranous particles in isolated brush border fragments led to the conclusion that the isolated brush border membranes are almost exclusively orientated right side out. This finding was also supported in an immunological study on the accessibility of aminopeptidase M – known to be located in the knob-like structures on the external membrane surface – to its specific antibody (HAASE et al. 1978). Unfortunately, the orientation of isolated intestinal basolateral membranes was thus far not clearly defined. In analogy to similar experiments with renal preparations (KINNE et al. 1978) we speculate that isolated basolateral membrane fractions are randomly orientated.

C. Methods for Analysing Transport Properties of Isolated Membrane Vesicles

Uptake of solutes into isolated membrane vesicles can be studied by filtration techniques. The membranes are incubated with labelled solutes and the uptake reaction is terminated by dilution of an aliquot of the reaction mixture in ice-cold buffer solution (stop solution) and immediate collection of the membranes by filtration. If a specific inhibitor for the transport of a substrate is available (e.g. phlorhizin for D-glucose transport) it can be added to the stop solution to minimize loss of substrate from the vesicles. Radioactivity nonspecifically retained by the filters is washed off by 3–15 ml buffer solution (isotonic or hypertonic ice-cold buffer similar to that used for membrane dilution prior to filtration). Alternatively, the reaction mixture can be pipetted directly onto the membrane filters (e.g. 0.6 μm pore size, cellulose acetate or cellulose nitrate, e.g. Sartorius or Millipore) with subsequent washing (HILDMANN et al. 1980a). This latter procedure is appropriate when leakage into the ice-cold stop solution does occur. It is also possible to perform double-label experiments using two different substrates both being transported if a possible interaction of the two transport mechanisms does not interfere with the scope of the experiment or if their interaction can be controlled. The rapid filtration technique allows the study of the time course of solute uptake (HOPFER et al. 1973; MURER and HOPFER 1974; HILDMANN et al. 1980a). In the manner described it is possible to obtain the first time point at 15 s of incubation. If the dilution prior to filtration is omitted – this should be restricted only to solutes with little tendency to bind to the filters used – it is possible to obtain a first time point after 5 s of incubation. KESSLER et al. (1978b) developed a simple semiautomatic apparatus which permits one to take time points after 1–2 s of incubation. The possibility of taking time points at initial incubation periods, i.e. at time points where the amount of solute taken up is a linear function of the incubation time, is important for a kinetic analysis of transport mechanisms. Ion exchange chromatography has also been used for terminating the uptake reaction and separating membrane vesicles from the incubation medium containing the labelled substrate or substrates (GASKO et al. 1976).

Uptake of a solute by an isolated membrane fraction can be composed of transport into an intravesicular compartment and/or binding to the outer or inner membrane surface. It is possible to distinguish between binding and transport by analysing the osmotic sensitivity of solute uptake. The uptake of a solute at equilibrium in the case of uptake into an intravesicular compartment should be in direct linear relation to the vesicular volume. The vesicular volume can be modified by altering the osmolarity of the incubation medium by adding to the incubation medium different concentrations of a substance which does not penetrate to a significant extent across the membrane within the experimental time. With intestinal membrane preparations, the disaccharide cellobiose fulfils this requirement (HOPFER et al. 1973). In the experiment presented in Fig. 3 brush border and baso-

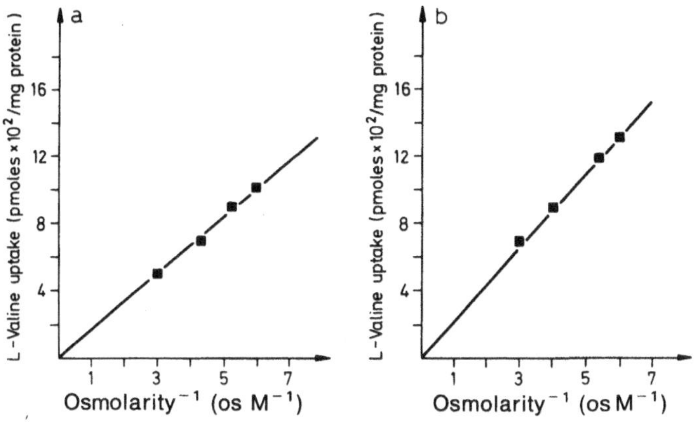

Fig. 3a, b. Effect of medium osmolarity on L-valine uptake. Brush border membranes (**a**) and basolateral membranes (**b**) were prepared by a sucrose density gradient technique (MURER et al. 1976) and suspended in 100 m*M* cellobiose. The incubation medium contained 25 m*M* NaSCN, 1 m*M* L-valine and sufficient cellobiose to give the osmolarity indicated. Incubation was carried out for 30 min at 25 °C. After HOPFER et al. (1976)

lateral plasma membranes were prepared in a cellobiose medium; cellobiose was also used to modify the osmolarity of the incubation medium. L-Valine uptake after 30 min (equilibrium uptake) was proportional to the inverse osmolarity of the incubation medium. Since no intercept can be found after extrapolating to infinite medium osmolarity values, it can be concluded that L-valine uptake under the conditions of analysis entirely represents transport into the intravesicular compartment. Furthermore, these results indicate that the membrane vesicles used for this particular experiment represent "perfect" osmometers in the range of differences of osmotic pressure applied in this experiment. Such ideal behaviour is not observed for all substrates, e.g. taurocholic acid shows a significant amount of binding (LÜCKE et al. 1978); neither is it observed for all membrane preparations. For example, we believe that shrinkage of brush border membrane vesicles isolated by the calcium precipitation method may be hindered, probably due to their presence in core material (HILDMANN et al. 1980a). Binding of substrate to the external membrane surface can be estimated by measuring rapid initial solute uptake by extrapolating the initial linear uptake component to a zero incubation period (e.g. STIEGER et al. 1983).

The existence of a transport system or a carrier in a biological membrane is usually inferred from observations such as different transport rates of structurally related compounds (stereospecificity), accumulation against a concentration gradient, saturation kinetics and the simulation of tracer flux by the same or related unlabelled compounds present on the transmembrane side (countertransport). Examples of these different types of experiments will be presented in the course of the discussion of the different solutes transported by the vesicles.

It is also feasible to study permeability characteristics of isolated membrane vesicles by spectroscopic techniques such as light scattering experiments, dual wavelength and fluorescence spectroscopy; also ion-selective electrodes might be used for an analysis of membrane permeability properties (DE GIER et al. 1978; MURER et al. 1977; MURER and KINNE 1980; YINGST and HOFFMANN 1978; BECK and SACKTOR 1978; BURCKHARDT et al. 1980). Recently, transmembrane proton or hydroxyl ion fluxes have been analysed by fluorescent, pH-sensitive dyes (e.g. WARNOCK et al. 1982; CASSANO et al., to be published).

D. Transport Studies

I. Systems Involved in Primary Active Transport

The transport of a solute is considered as primary active when direct coupling between an energy-providing chemical reaction and the transmembrane transport of a solute occurs. Examples for such mechanisms are the phosphoenolpyruvate-phosphotransferase system in bacterial membranes (KUNDIG 1976), ATP-driven Ca^{2+} transport in sarcoplasmic reticulum (MACLENNAN and HOLLAND 1976) and the Na^+, K^+-ATPase system in animal plasma membranes (ALBERS 1976). With respect to the different enzyme activities found to be associated with the luminal and the contraluminal membrane of intestinal epithelial cells (see Table 3) there are at least two candidates for primary active transport mechanisms: (1) Na^+, K^+-ATPase and (2) Ca^{2+}-ATPase.

1. Na^+, K^+-ATPase

Experiments to demonstrate transport of sodium and of potassium by isolated intestinal basolateral membranes have not yet been reported. However, using Na^+, K^+-ATPase preparations from other epithelial sources different laboratories have demonstrated that Na^+, K^+-ATPase mediates coupled exchange of Na^+ and K^+, e.g. for renal preparations (ANNER et al. 1977). It is also likely that the intestinal enzyme shows such ion exchange properties and is primarily involved in the extrusion of sodium from the cell and in the uptake of potassium into the cell. Studies with isolated basolateral membrane vesicles offer a chance to prove this assumption. Since the operation of Na^+, K^+-ATPase represents the metabolic energy-requiring reaction for transepithelial sodium and sodium-dependent solute transport, studies on the ion transport properties of this enzyme (stoichiometry between sodium and potassium flux, electrogenicity as well as stoichiometry between ion flux and ATP hydrolysis) are most important for an understanding of the energetics of the transcellular transport (KIMMICH 1977).

2. Ca^{2+}-ATPase

ATP-driven Ca^{2+} transport by basolateral membrane vesicles isolated from rat small intestinal epithelial cells by the Percoll centrifugation method (SCALERA et al. 1980) has been demonstrated by HILDMANN et al. (1979, 1982a). As shown in Fig. 4 the calcium uptake into basolateral plasma membrane vesicles is stimulated by ATP. In the presence of ATP calcium is transiently accumulated by the vesicles above the equilibrium uptake. The stimulation by ATP is not sensitive to addition of oligomycin, the inhibitor of the mitochondrial ATP-driven Ca^{2+} uptake (HILDMANN et al. 1979, 1982a). The finding that addition of the Ca^{2+} ionophore

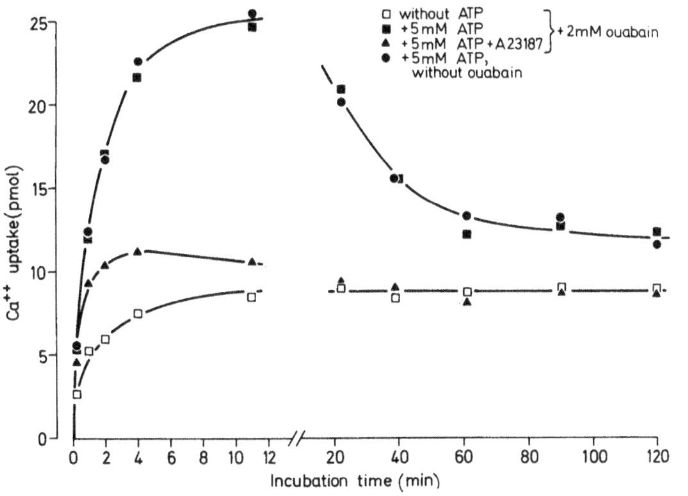

Fig. 4. ATP-driven accumulation of Ca^{2+} into rat intestinal basolateral membrane vesicles. Membranes were isolated by the Percoll centrifugation method (SCALERA et al. 1980). The incubation medium contained 100 m*M* KCl, 5 m*M* $MgCl_2$, 20 m*M* HEPES-Tris, pH 7.4, 2 m*M* ouabain and 0.05 m*M* $^{45}CaCl_2$ with or without ATP (5 m*M*). The uptake of Ca^{2+} was also measured in the presence of the ionophore A23187 (2 μg/ml) and without ouabain. The incubation was carried out at 25 °C

A23187 inhibits the ATP effect indicates that ATP increases the rate of calcium transfer across the membrane and does not cause binding of calcium to the membranes, e. g. provoked by an increase in surface negativity due to membrane phosphorylation. Since ATP is not considered to permeate plasma membranes and since the ATP site of the enzyme should be located on the cytoplasmic side of the membrane (VINCENZI and HINDS 1976), ATP-driven Ca^{2+} uptake by the isolated basolateral membrane preparation is most probably due to inside-out orientated membrane vesicles and represents a calcium extrusion mechanism in the intact cell.

II. Systems Involved in Secondary Active Transport

Transport of a solute is considered as secondary active, if it is transported against its chemical (in the case of uncharged particles) or its electrochemical gradient (in the case of charged particles) by virtue of the coupling of its transmembrane flux to the flux of another solute, whose transmembrane electrochemical potential difference is maintained by a transport process energized by a chemical energy-providing reaction, i. e. a solute which is transported primarily actively. This concept was proposed by the groups of CRANE and SCHULTZ in the so-called sodium gradient hypothesis for different sodium-dependently transported solutes (CRANE 1977; SCHULTZ 1979). To perform secondary active transepithelial transport the plasma membrane must have at least the following prerequisites: (1) a flux coupling (or cotransport) mechanism must be present; (2) the plasma membrane at the two cell poles must have different permeability properties (active or passive) for the solute concerned. In the following sections a few experiments will be pre-

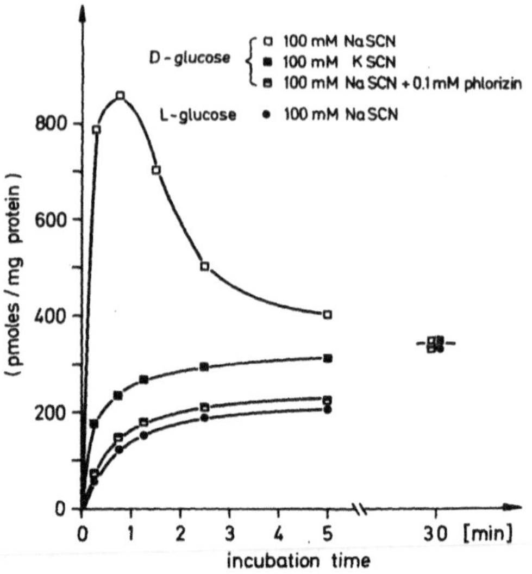

Fig. 5. Glucose transport by rat intestinal brush border membrane vesicles. Membranes were prepared by the method of HOPFER et al. (1973). The incubation medium contained 1 m*M* D-glucose ^{3}H or L-glucose ^{3}H, 100 m*M* mannitol, 1 m*M* HEPES-Tris, pH 7.5, and the indicated salts. Incubation temperature was 25 °C. KINNE and MURER (1976)

sented documenting the existence of cotransport mechanisms in the plasma membrane of the small intestinal epithelial cell. The transport of D-glucose will be discussed in more detail.

1. Transport of Glucose

a) Brush Border Membrane

When isolated rat small intestinal brush border membranes were incubated with the two stereoisomers of glucose D-glucose entry was more rapid than that of L-glucose (Fig. 5). The observation of stereospecificity of glucose uptake by the isolated membrane fraction is an indication of a "carrier mechanism". The difference between the two isomers was especially pronounced when sodium was present in the incubation medium. Phlorhizin inhibited the initial rate of D-glucose uptake, but had a negligible effect on the equilibrium value (Fig. 5). Thus, glucose transport across the isolated brush border membrane shows two properties also observed in transepithelial, concentrative glucose transport, namely sodium dependence and inhibition by phlorhizin. In studies with brush border membrane vesicles isolated from rat small intestine SIGRIST-NELSON and HOPFER (1974) found evidence for a distinct sodium-independent transport system for D-fructose.

b) Different Transport Properties of Brush Border and Basolateral Membranes

In brush border membranes the initial uptake of D-glucose was stimulated approximately fourfold in the presence of a sodium gradient, as compared with a potassium gradient of the same size (membranes isolated by sucrose gradient technique, HOPFER et al. 1976b). In contrast, glucose transport in the basolateral membranes was insensitive to sodium. Carrier mediated transport of D-glucose across the brush border as well as across the basolateral membrane was indicated by saturation and countertransport experiments (HOPFER et al. 1976b). Stereo-specificity in glucose uptake by isolated enterocyte basolateral membranes, D-glucose being transported faster than L-glucose, has also been shown (MIRCHEFF et al. 1980a).

According to CRANE (1968) and BARNETT et al. (1968, 1969) a free OH group on C-2 in the D-gluco configuration seems to be an essential requirement for active transepithelial hexose transport in the intestine. On this basis, specificity experiments were carried out using brush border and basolateral plasma membrane vesicles, in the hope of obtaining information on the polar organization of the epithelial cell, i.e. on the location of the "active" glucose transport site (Table 4; MURER et al. 1978). Since D-mannose and 2-deoxy-D-glucose inhibited D-glucose uptake only very slightly in the brush border vesicles, it could be concluded that these two glucose analogs did not share a common sodium-dependent transport system with D-glucose across this membrane (Table 4). In basolateral membranes, however, D-glucose transport was strongly inhibited by both D-mannose and 2-deoxy-D-glucose (Table 4). Similar properties have also been reported by WRIGHT et al. (1980). Thus, translocation of D-glucose across the isolated brush border membrane or at least interaction of the solute with the transport site also seems to require the OH group at C-2 of the glucose configuration, whereas for the transport across basolateral membranes this is not required. Different properties of the D-glucose transport system in the brush border and in the basolateral membranes could also be elicited by means of glucose transport inhibitors. Phloretine and cytochalasin-B, both inhibitors of facilitated glucose diffusion in erythrocytes (STEIN 1967; TAVERNA and LANGDON 1973), inhibited D-glucose transport in basolateral membranes much more strongly than in brush border membranes, whereas phlorhizin, an inhibitor of sodium-dependent glucose transport (CRANE 1968), had a much greater inhibitory effect in the brush border membranes (HOPFER et al. 1975, 1976b).

The results obtained on glucose transport into the vesicles thus far demonstrate that the two membrane fractions isolated from either cell pole contain glucose transport systems clearly different with respect to specificity, sodium sensitivity and susceptibility to specific inhibitors. Thus, the system which accomplishes uphill glucose uptake seems to be located in the brush border and to be stimulated by sodium. On the other hand, the characteristics of glucose transport in the basolateral membranes (i.e. low specificity, insensitivity to sodium and inhibition by phloretine and cytochalasin-B) suggest that they contain a transport system analogous to those demonstrated in erythrocytes and adipocytes, which catalyze "downhill" facilitated diffusion of glucose (STEIN 1967; LE FEVRE 1975). The energy for the exit of D-glucose from the cell would then be its own concentration gradient across the basolateral membrane. Recent experiments on intact rat small intestinal epithelia provided evidence for a glucose transport mechanism driving glucose out of the cell into the interstitium against its concentration gradient (ESPOSITO et al. 1981; see also Chap. 9).

Table 4. Effect of various sugars on D-glucose uptake into isolated plasma membrane vesicles. Incubation media contained 100 m*M* mannitol, 0,1 m*M* $MgSO_4$, 1 m*M* HEPES-Tris, pH 7.5, 100 m*M* NaSCN and 1 m*M* [^{14}C]-D-glucose. Plasma membranes were isolated by a sucrose density gradient technique (MURER et al. 1976) and suspended in a buffer containing 100 m*M* mannitol, 0.1 m*M* $MgSO_4$ and 1 m*M* HEPES-Tris at pH 7.5 (MURER et al. 1978)

Test inhibitor (40 m*M*	Brush border membranes	Basolateral plasma membranes
	D-Glucose uptake (pmol) (mg protein in 15 s)[a]	
D-Mannitol (control)	810 (0)	3,200 (0)
D-Glucose	250 (69)	1,590 (50)
D-Galactose	265 (67)	1,500 (53)
D-Mannose	730 (10)	1,710 (46)
2-Deoxy-D-glucose	765 (6)	1,935 (40)

[a] The percentage inhibition is given in parentheses

c) Glucose-Induced Sodium Flux

As seen from the experiments with the brush border membrane vesicles (Fig. 4), the application of a sodium gradient leads to a transient accumulation of D-glucose over the equilibrium value. The sodium gradient obviously provides an energy source for intravesicular glucose accumulation. These findings suggest cotransport of glucose with sodium. If sugars are cotransported with sodium, then a stimulation by sugars or amino acids of the sodium flux should also be demonstrable. An experiment indicating that this is really the case is presented in Fig. 6.

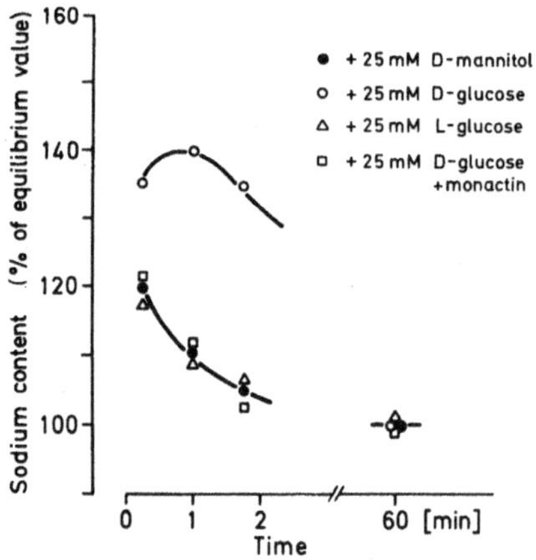

Fig. 6. Glucose-induced sodium accumulation by rat intestinal brush border membrane vesicles. Brush border membranes were isolated by a calcium precipitation method and incubated for 1 h at 25 °fC in a solution containing 100 m*M* mannitol, 5 m*M* HEPES-Tris, 95 m*M* KSCN, and 5 m*M* ^{22}NaSCN. At zero time, 30 µl containing 5 m*M* HEPES-Tris, 75 m*M* KSCN, and 150 m*M* nonelectrolyte (indicated in the figure) were added to 150 µl of membrane suspension. Values are expressed as percentages of new equilibrium reached after 60 min of incubation. MURER and KINNE (1977)

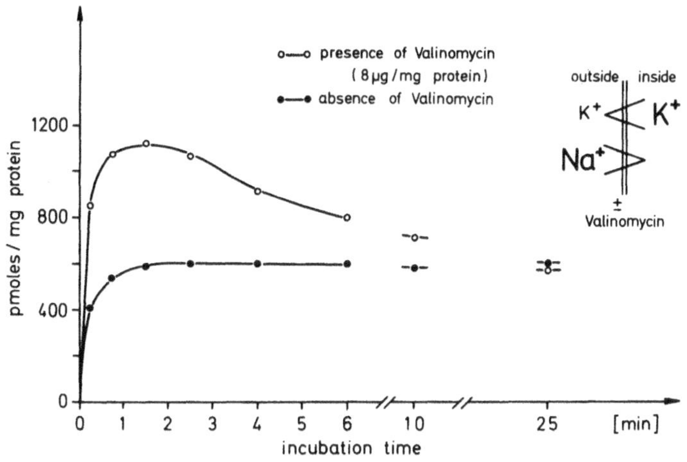

Fig. 7. Effect of potassium diffusion potential on D-glucose uptake by isolated brush border membrane vesicles. Brush border membranes were prepared according to HOPFER et al. (1973) and preloaded by an osmotic shock procedure with 100 m*M* mannitol, 50 m*M* K_2SO_4, 1 m*M* HEPES-Tris (pH 7.5) and 0.1 m*M* $MgSO_4$. D-Glucose uptake in the presence or absence of valinomycin was studied in an incubation medium with the following final composition: 100 m*M*/l D-mannitol, 50 m*M* Na_2SO_4, 1.0 m*M* [14C]-D-glucose, 5.6 m*M*/l K_2SO_4, and 1 m*M* HEPES-Tris, pH 7.5. MURER and KINNE (1979)

Brush border vesicles were preincubated for 1 h in a solution containing 95 mmol/l KSCN and 5 mmol/l ^{22}NaSCN. Concentrated solutions of D-glucose or mannitol were then added, and the changes in intravesicular Na^+ content were measured. Upon addition of mannitol a new equilibrium value, determined by dilution of the membrane suspension, was reached immediately. Upon addition of D-glucose $^{22}Na^+$ was transiently accumulated in the brush border membrane vesicles. This indicates that Na^+ entry can be driven by a gradient of D-glucose, i.e. that these transports are coupled. Elegant studies on glucose-induced sodium flux across isolated rabbit renal brush border vesicles were carried out by HILDEN and SACKTOR (1979) and for rabbit small intestinal brush border vesicles by KAUNITZ et al. (1982). These studies provided direct information on the stoichiometry of sodium and glucose flux.

d) Electrogenicity of Sodium-Dependent D-Glucose Transport

A cotransport of sodium with a nonelectrolyte is necessarily an "electrogenic", potential-sensitive process, unless it is coupled to a stoichiometric movement of an anion in the same direction or to a cation in the opposite direction. To verify a potential sensitivity of sodium-dependent nonelectrolyte transport experimentally, several approaches were developed to manipulate the membrane potential artificially. One of those experiments, in which valinomycin was used in the presence of a potassium gradient to induce a K^+ diffusion potential is shown in Fig. 7. The membranes were preloaded with potassium and then suspended in a potassium-free medium containing D-glucose and sodium. Addition of valinomycin which led to the development of a negative potential inside the membrane as compared with the control without valinomycin produced an overshoot in D-glucose uptake which was not observed in the absence of valinomycin. This and similar experiments strongly suggested that the sodium-dependent D-glucose uptake located in the brush border transport was indeed "electrogenic" (MURER and HOPFER 1974). In other words, it appears that the coupled translocation of Na^+ and D-glucose by a hypothetical ternary "Na^+-D-glucose-carrier" complex can occur with a net transport of an electrical charge. When this also occurs in vivo indicated by the electrophysiological observation made by ROSE and SCHULTZ (1970), the electrochemical potential difference of sodium across the brush border membrane would be the driving force for D-glucose transport.

Manipulations of the magnitude of the transmembrane electrical potential difference in studies with isolated vesicles can also be carried out by applying different anion gradients in the presence of the same cation gradient or by using protonophores (uncouplers) in the presence of transmembrane proton gradients (MURER and HOPFER 1974).

2. Transport of Amino Acids

As with the transport of D-glucose and its derivatives, it is generally accepted that "active" transepithelial transport of amino acids in the small intestine is sodium dependent (e.g. CRANE 1977; SCHULTZ 1978). In studies with isolated membrane vesicles only limited experiments have been carried out as far as the amount of different transport pathways and their specificity is concerned. Therefore, we will present only results obtained in studies with vesicles on the transport of neutral amino acids. However, from preliminary experiments with brush border membranes carried out in our laboratory as well as in SEMENZA's laboratory there is no doubt that the brush border membrane also contains distinct sodium-dependent transport pathways for acidic amino acids. Furthermore, a transport system for dipeptides has been described in brush border membrane vesicles isolated from rat small intestine (SIGRIST-NELSON 1975).

As with the transport of D-glucose, it was found that sodium stimulates uptake of L-valine in brush border membranes, but not in basolateral membranes (Fig. 8), indicating a polarity of the epithelial cell. Evidence for carrier mechanisms for L-valine in brush border membranes as well as in basolateral plasma membranes was obtained in saturation and countertransport experiments (HOPFER et al. 1976b).

Sodium-dependent transport of L-alanine in brush border membrane vesicles has been studied more extensively than sodium-dependent transport of L-valine. SIGRIST-NELSON et al. (1975) were able to demonstrate stereospecific uptake of L-alanine. Transport of D-alanine was also sodium dependent, but transported at a much slower rate than the L isomer. Furthermore, saturation and potential sensitivity of L-alanine transport was shown.

Recently, study on rabbit jejunal brush border membrane vesicles detected two major transport pathways for amino acids in these membranes: (1) Na-independent carriers and (2) Na-dependent carriers. Based on uptake kinetics and cross-inhibition profiles, at least two Na-independent and three Na-dependent carrer mediated pathways exist. One Na-independent pathway similar to the clas-

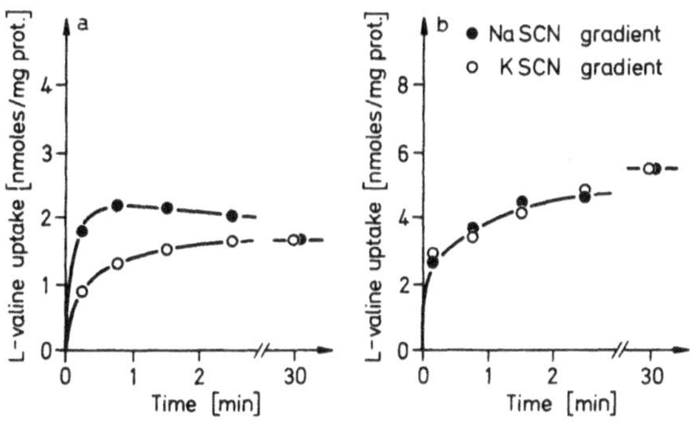

Fig. 8 a, b. Uptake of L-valine by isolated rat enterocyte membrane vesicles. Brush border (**a**) and basolateral membrane vesicles (**b**) were isolated by a sucrose density gradient technique (MURER et al. 1976). Incubation media contained 100 m*M* D-mannitol, 1 m*M* HEPES-Tris, pH 7.4, 1 m*M* L-valine and 100 m*M* salt as indicated in the figure. After HOPFER et al. (1976b)

sical L-system favours neutral amino acids, while an additional pathway accepts the dibasic amino acids. One Na-dependent pathway transports neutral L-amino acids. Another Na-dependent mechanism transports phenylalanine and methionine. The third pathway is selective for the imino acids. According to these findings, the intestinal mechanisms do not correspond to the classical A or ACS paradigms found in nonpolarized cells (LERNER 1978). Furthermore, the intestinal membrane in contrast to the renal membrane is lacking a transport mechanism for β-alanine and does not show interaction between proline and glycine transport (STEVENS et al. 1982; MIRCHEFF et al. 1982).

Experiments on the transport of L-alanine into basolateral plasma membrane were performed by MIRCHEFF et al. (1980a). These investigators concluded from their experiments that basolateral membranes of rat small intestinal epithelial cells contain sodium-independent as well as sodium-dependent transport mechanisms for L-alanine. Interestingly, for the sodium-independent alanine uptake only one pathway could be defined with properties similar to the classical L-system (CHRISTENSEN 1979), whereas for the sodium-dependent uptake three different pathways with different stereospecificities have been proposed. Thereby, the high capacity, low affinity sodium-independent transport system seems to represent the system involved in the transepithelial transport of neutral amino acids. On the other hand, the low capacity, high affinity sodium-dependent transport of L-alanine in the basolateral membranes could represent a transport system present in all plasma membranes and be responsible for the cellular uptake of amino acids needed in the protein and amino acid metabolism of the cell. The results of MIRCHEFF et al. (1980a) are not in contradiction to our results for sodium-independent L-valine uptake in basolateral membranes. The high concentrations of substrate used enabled us to see predominantly the sodium-independent mechanism.

3. Mutual Interaction Between Sugar and Amino Acid Transport

Studies with isolated small intestinal brush border vesicles have shown that the transport of L-amino acids as well as the transport of D-monosaccharides across

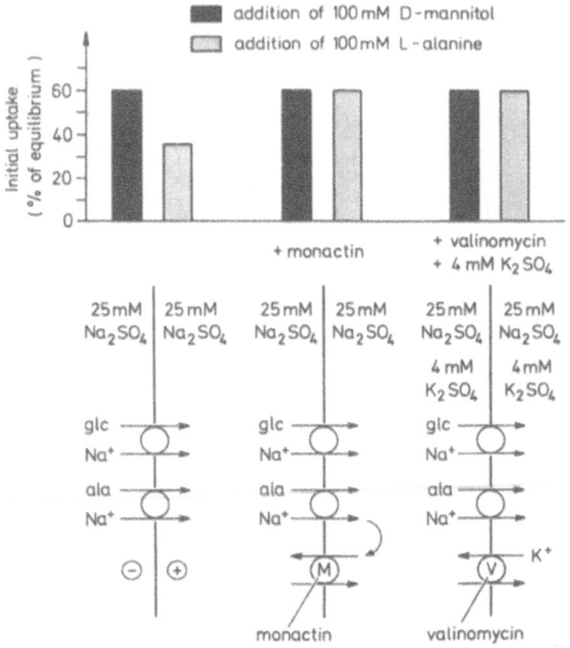

Fig. 9. Inhibition of D-glucose transport by alanine. Rat intestinal brush border membrane vesicles were isolated by a calcium precipitation method and were preincubated for 30 min at 25 °C with a buffer containing 100 mM D-mannitol, 1 mM HEPES-Tris (pH 7.4) and 25 mM Na_2SO_4. Uptake of D-glucose ^3H (1 mM) was initiated by addition of the glucose in the presence of 100 mM L-alanine or 100 mM mannitol. Other additions were as indicated: monactin 10 µg/per milligram protein, valinomycin 10 µg/per milligram protein, K_2SO_4 on both membrane sides 4 mM. Results from MURER et al. (1975); figure from MURER and KINNE (1977)

the brush border membrane is energized by the transmembrane electrochemical potential difference of sodium (see Sects. D. II. 1, 2). The presence of several sodium-dependent cotransport systems in one membrane implies interactions between sodium-dependent transport systems owing to the competition for the common driving force, the electrochemical potential difference of sodium across the membrane.

An experiment on this type of mutual interaction is presented in Fig. 9. Brush border membrane vesicles isolated from rat small intestine were equilibrated with sodium – this means the electrochemical potential difference of sodium was zero – and the uptake of D-glucose was measured. Addition of L-alanine inhibited D-glucose transport by the brush border vesicles. Control experiments performed under alanine-preequilibrated or nonpreequilibrated conditions, respectively, demonstrated that this inhibition only occurred when net transmembrane flux of L-alanine took place and could only be observed in the presence of sodium (MURER et al. 1975). Thus, this inhibition can be explained by an L-alanine-promoted influx of sodium ions, creating an electrochemical potential difference for sodium directed from the vesicle interior to the vesicle exterior, which inhibits net glucose influx. Consequently, L-alanine-dependent inhibition of D-glucose influx was not observed in experiments in which the sodium conductance of the membrane was artificially increased by the addition of ionophores such as monactin, which allow rapid equilibration of sodium (Fig. 9). Interestingly, the inhibition cannot be seen after "short-circuiting" the transmembrane electrical potential difference by the addition of valinomycin in the presence of equal potassium concentrations on both membrane sides. These findings led to the conclusion that mutual interaction can reflect an electrochemical coupling of two sodium-dependent potential-sensitive transport mechanisms and does not necessarily imply an interaction on the level of a common transport system for the two different solutes (MURER et al. 1975).

The experiments presented in Fig. 9 do not exclude the existence of a "polyfunctional" carrier (ALVARADO and ROBINSON 1979). However, since with vesicles several experimental parameters can be followed more closely than in the experiments with the intact epithelial tissue, it would be worthwhile to perform a few of the crucial experiments on the postulated "polyfunctional" carrier with the vesicles.

4. Transport of Anions

In this section evidence obtained from experiments with brush border vesicles will be presented which indicates that the energy inherent in the transmembrane electrochemical potential difference of sodium can be used to drive anion transport across the small intestinal brush border membrane by cotransport systems for some organic as well as inorganic anions (MURER and KINNE 1980 b).

Sodium stimulation of transmembrane anion flux needs more careful interpretation than sodium stimulation of the transmembrane flux of neutral compounds. Stimulation of anion flux for example by the sodium gradient does not necessarily imply that a sodium-anion cotransport system is present in the membrane as in the systems observed for D-glucose and other neutral sugars or amino acids, since indirect coupling, e.g. through generation of a positive diffusion potential within the vesicle in the presence of a sodium gradient could occur (MURER and KINNE 1977). Furthermore, through the action of the sodium-proton exchange system a transmembrane pH difference might develop and the entry of weak acids by nonionic diffusion might be favoured. Therefore, it is most important in experiments on sodium stimulation of anion flux to carry out appropriate control experiments in which diffusion potentials or transmembrane pH differences are imposed in the absence of a sodium gradient or in which the occurrence of such effects is excluded in the presence of a sodium gradient. A positive diffusion potential within the vesicle can be imposed by the addition of valinomycin to the membranes, when a potassium gradient (out > in) is present and its effect evaluated by comparison with a control in the absence of valinomycin. Transmembrane electrical potentials can be minimized by equilibrating potassium across the membrane and adding valinomycin to the membranes.

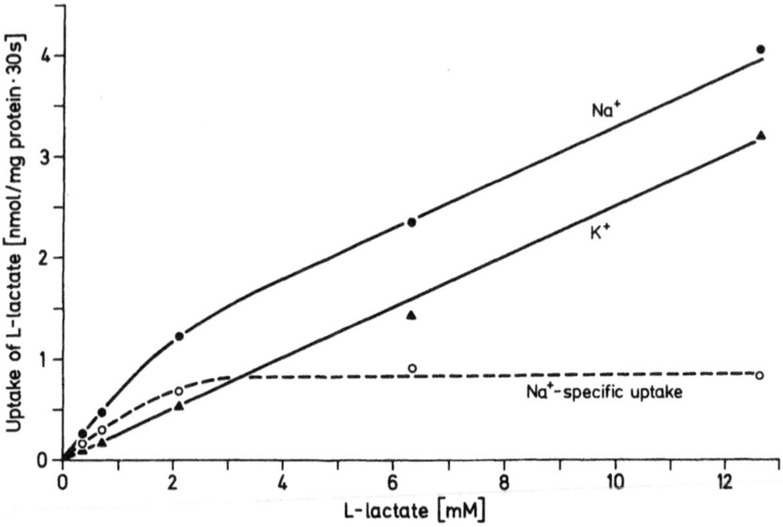

Fig. 10. Dependence of L-lactate uptake on substrate concentration. Brush border membranes from rabbit jejunum were isolated by a calcium precipitation method. 20 µl membrane suspension was added to 80 µl incubation medium containing 25 m*M* NaCl or 25 m*M* KCl and increasing concentrations of L-lactate. The sodium-specific uptake was calculated by subtracting the uptake with KCl from that with NaCl. HILDMANN et al. (1980)

a) Transport of Organic Anions

L-lactate transport into brush border membrane vesicles isolated from rabbit small intestine was studied by HILDMANN et al. (1980a). One of the experiments providing evidence for a sodium-L-lactate cotransport system is presented in Fig. 10. The initial uptake of L-lactate at a potassium or a sodium gradient was measured with different L-lactate concentrations in the incubation medium. In the presence of a potassium gradient the L-lactate uptake after 30 s is a linear function of the substrate concentration. With a Na^+ gradient a saturable component apparently adds to the unsaturable one. Saturation is expected for processes in which a limited number of distinct sites is involved. Thus, the fact that L-lactate uptake has a saturable component only in the presence of sodium is one piece of evidence that Na^+ activates a membrane component which is able to enhance L-lactate transport across the brush border membrane (HILDMANN et al. 1980a). Since a sodium concentration difference could be identified as the driving force for L-Lactate movement, sodium-L-lactate cotransport is suggested (HILDMANN et al. 1980a).

Several groups have studied intestinal transport of bile acids (LÜCKE et al. 1978a; WILSON and TREANOR 1979; BEESLEY and FAUST 1979; ROSE and LACK 1979). There is general agreement that a sodium gradient is able to stimulate predominantly bile acid uptake into brush border membrane vesicles isolated from ileal segments; in membrane vesicles isolated from duodenal or jejunal segments sodium stimulation of bile acid uptake is much smaller or nonexistent (e.g. LÜCKE et al. 1978a). This similarity in the segmental localization of sodium-dependent

Table 5. Effect of monactin on taurocholate transport into brush border membrane vesicles. The experiments were carried out in incubation media containing 100 m*M* mannitol, 20 m*M* HEPES-Tris at pH 7.4, 0.15 m*M* taurocholate ^{3}H- and 100 m*M* $NaNO_3$. Monactin concentration was 15 µg per milligram protein and was added as an ethanolic solution. Ethanol concentration in all incubation media was 1%. Incubation temperature was 37 °C. Samples were taken at 0.33 min, 1 min and 30 min (LÜCKE et al. 1978a)

Conditions in incubation medium	Taurocholate uptake (pmol per milligram protein)		
	0.33 min	1 min	30 min (equilibrium)
$NaNO_3$ gradient	440	447	333
$NaNO_3$ gradient plus monactin	112	163	272

bile acid transport between the findings obtained in vitro with the vesicles and the observation made on bile acid transport in the intact gut in vivo is a valuable control for the physiological significance of the specific action of sodium on transmembrane bile acid flux in ileal brush border membranes. Furthermore, a distinction between indirect coupling of transmembrane sodium flux and bile acid flux owing to generation of diffusion potentials and direct coupling of sodium flux and bile acid flux was carried out by artificially increasing the sodium conductance of the brush border membrane with ionophores. Addition of monactin, an electrogenic ionophore for monovalent cations (HENDERSON et al. 1969), prevents the intravesicular accumulation of taurocholate in the presence of an inwardly directed $NaNO_3$ gradient (Table 5). Since monactin increases the cation conductance of the membrane, an Na^+-gradient-dependent diffusion potential should be increased initially rather than decreased by the addition of the ionophore. Therefore, if Na^+-gradient-dependent movement of taurocholate is primarily the consequence of the increase in diffusion potential and not due to a direct coupling, an increased uptake rate of taurocholate in the presence of monactin should be observed. Its decreased uptake in the presence of monactin suggests a cotransport system for Na^+ and taurocholate in brush border membrane vesicles isolated from ileal segments (LÜCKE et al. 1978).

Unfortunately there is a disagreement in the reports on taurocholate uptake by isolated brush border membrane concerning the effect of the transmembrane electrical potential difference on sodium-dependent taurocholate transport. In the reports of LÜCKE et al. (1978a) as well as of WILSON and TREANOR (1979), it has been shown that an increased electrical negativity within the vesicle, as obtained after addition of valinomycin in the presence of an outwardly directed potassium gradient, leads to an increased transport rate for taurocholate in the presence of sodium. This would suggest that the negative charge of the taurocholate anion is overcompensated by the cotransported sodium ions during the transmembrane sodium-dependent movement of taurocholate across rat ileal brush border membranes. However, anion replacement experiments (another tool to modify the transmembrane electrical potential difference) did not show a stimulation of sodium-dependent taurocholate uptake by replacing relatively impermeable anions by more permeable anions, suggesting that sodium-dependent taurocholate uptake by brush border membrane vesicles isolated from the ileum of guinea-pig intestine is an electroneutral process (ROSE and LACK 1979). It is difficult to present an explanation for this apparent discrepancy. Possible reasons might be (a) a species difference; (b) a difference in the seasonal or another physiological status of the animals used; and (c) specific effects of the different anions used on the transport site itself (binding site for taurocholate on the carrier). The group led by SEMENZA reported that transport of L-ascorbic acid across isolated brush border membranes of guinea-pig intestine is also sodium dependent [SILIPRANDI et al. 1979).

Recently, the difference between transmembrane transport of L-lactate across brush border membranes and basolateral membranes isolated from rat small intestine has been studied (STORELLI et al. 1980). Sodium-L-lactate cotransport was identified in the brush border membranes, whereas L-lactate transport across the basolateral membrane was shown to be carrier mediated, but sodium independent. The transport of other organic anions across isolated basolateral membranes has not yet been reported.

b) Transport of Inorganic Anions

The best-studied examples of inorganic anion transport in the small intestine with isolated brush border membrane vesicles are phosphate transport and sulphate transport. Like rat kidney proximal tubule, the rat small intestinal brush border membrane contains a sodium phosphate cotransport system (BERNER et al. 1976; HOFFMANN et al. 1976). Sodium phosphate cotransport systems have also been described for brush border membrane preparations isolated from rabbit duodenum (HILDMANN et al. 1980b; 1982b) and from chicken intestine (FONTAINE et al. 1979). As will be shown in Sect. F, sodium phosphate cotransport is probably a site of regulation in transepithelial phosphate transport.

Recently, unidirectional fluxes of $^{35}SO_4^{2-}$ across and into rabbit ileal epithelium were measured under short-circuit conditions (SMITH et al. 1981). These experiments clearly suggest the existence of Na-coupled influx across the brush border membrane. Studies with brush border membrane vesicles isolated from rat ileum were in complete agreement with these observations. Transport of sulphate into the vesicles was stimulated specifically by sodium ions and was only saturable in the presence of sodium. Sodium sulphate cotransport was electroneutral (LÜCKE et al. 1981). Since the steady state of SO_4^{2-} in cell water appears to be, in the rabbit ileal epithelial cell, at a lower level than theoretically predicted (SMITH et al. 1981: LANGRIDGE-SMITH and FIELD 1981), there seems to be an uphill transport mechanism at the basolateral cell surface. A candidate for this mechanism would be an anion exchange. In favour of the anion exchange, efflux studies with basolateral membrane vesicles isolated from rat small intestine showed a strong inhibition by stilbene derivatives of transmembrane sulphate flux (GRINSTEIN et al. 1980). In exploring the substrate specificity of transmembrane transport systems, transstimulation experiments are useful tools. For sodium-dependent transport of inorganic sulphate across the rat ileal brush border membrane, it could be demonstrated that tracer sulphate uptake in the presence of Na^+ occurred fas-

Table 6. Transstimulation of Na^+-dependent sulphate uptake by SO_4^{2-}, $S_2O_3^{2-}$, MoO_4^{2-}. The amount of SO_4^{2-} taken up was measured at 1 min and at equilibrium after 60 min. Membrane vesicles loaded with 100 m*M* mannitol, 20 m*M* HEPES-Tris (pH 7.4) (control) and in addition with the listed unlabelled substances were incubated at 25 °C in a medium containing 100 m*M* mannitol, 20 m*M* HEPES-Tris (pH 7.4), 100 m*M* NaCl. Sulphate concentration in the incubation media was always 0.06 m*M*, as $Na_2\,{}^{35}SO_4$. The concentration in the incubation media of the different anions tested as substrates to induce transstimulation was 0.06 m*M* introduced by dilution of the membrane suspension or added before to the incubation media (individual controls). LÜCKE et al. (1980)

Conditions inside vesicles	Sulphate uptake (pmol per milligram protein)		
	0.33 min	1 min	60 min (equilibrium)
No further addition (control)	15	26	40
Plus unlabelled SO_4^{2-} (0.6 m*M*)	34	36	41
No further addition (control)	16	30	43
Plus unlabelled MoO_4^{2-} (0.6 m*M*)	25	32	41
No further addition (control)	16	30	46
Plus unlabelled $S_2O_3^{2-}$ (0.6 m*M*)	36	33	43

ter into membrane vesicles preloaded with unlabelled sulphate, thiosulphate or molybdate than into nonpreloaded controls (Table 6; LÜCKE et al. 1981).

For rabbit ileum it has been demonstrated that the luminal entry mechanism as well as the intracellular chloride concentration above equilibrium distribution are dependent on the presence of sodium in the luminal bathing fluid (for review see FRIZZELL et al. 1979). Thus, there is evidence for a NaCl cotransport mechanism in the luminal membrane. This mechanism is inhibited by furosemide and by mechanisms dependent on increased cellular levels of cAMP (for review see FRIZZEL et al. 1979). BIEBERDORF et al. (1972) proposed the existence of Na^+/H^+ and Cl^-/HCO_3^- exchanges in the luminal membrane of the enterocyte. Provided that apparent coupling of these two exchange mechanisms is possible via the proton/hydroxyl ion concentration in the microclimate of the transport systems, it is evident that the overall flux observed is an electroneutral sodium cloride cotransport. Recently, studies with isolated membrane vesicles were performed in order to analyse the transport mechanisms for chloride in brush border membranes from rat small intestine and rat proximal tubule. LIEDTKE and HOPFER (1982a), on the basis of kinetic arguments, denied the existence of a coupled NaCl cotransporter in experiments with brush border membrane vesicles isolated from rat small intestine. The Na^+/H^+ and Cl^-/OH^- exchange mechanisms were identified in studies with rat small intestinal brush border membrane vesicles by the use of pH meter techniques and tracer techniques (MURER et al. 1976a, 1980a; LIEDTKE and HOPFER 1977, 1982b). Thus, the two separate elements of an electroneutral coupled mechanism for sodium and chloride are present in isolated brush border membranes. The two exchange mechanisms are probably the components of transmembrane electroneutral chloride and sodium movement in the intestinal brush border membrane. The clinical observations of an impaired anion exchange mechanism (BIEBERDORF et al. 1972) and the experimental observation of inhibition of coupled NaCl absorption in the intact epithelia by azetazolamide are strong evidence that these mechanisms are indeed operating in the inact epithelial cell, too (NELLANS et al. 1975).

Little is known about the exit step at the contraluminal cell membrane. As intracellular chloride activities are above equilibrium, the movement of chloride follows its electrochemical potential difference and does not require metabolic energy. GRINSTEIN et al. (1980) found no significant effect of stilbene derivates on chloride efflux from basolateral membrane vesicles isolated from renal and small intestinal epithelium; as the stilbene derivates also had no effect on chloride efflux from brush border membranes, there might be some reason to doubt the results of this study. Stilbene sensitivity of transmembrane chloride flux has been unequivocally demonstrated in studies with brush border membranes (LIEDTKE and HOPFER 1982b).

5. Transport of Inorganic Cations

a) Transport of Sodium

A sodium/proton exchange system has been demonstrated in intestinal brush border membranes from rat, and flounder (MURER et al. 1977; EVELOFF et al. 1980; H. MURER 1980, unpublished work). This mechanism seems to be, at least in the vesicular system, the main mechanism for the transmembrane movement of sodium. Concerning the coupled transport of sodium and chloride across the small intestinal brush border membrane, one could think of a parallel coupled operation of two exchange mechanisms. Thus, a sodium/proton exchange system and a chloride/hydroxyl exchange system have been identified as possible elements for coupled electroneutral transport of sodium and chloride. However, the demonstration of their combined function has been very difficult or almost impossible (LIEDTKE and HOPFER 1980, 1982a, b) in studies with vesicles. Uncoupling of the two exchange processes might be explained by the absence of a pH microclimate in the vesicular system, which is required for coupling in the intact epithelium. It is also possible that other cellular factors are responsible for an obligatory combined operation of these two exchange mechanisms. Such coupling factors might be lost during membrane isolation.

b) Transport of Calcium

Considering the low intracellular calcium concentration it is certain that active steps in transepithelial calcium transport are located in the basolateral membranes. Thus, as described in Sect.D.I.2, a primary active, ATP-driven calcium pump was identified in basolateral membrane preparations (HILDMANN et al. 1979, 1982a).

From studies with basolateral membrane vesicles isolated from rat small intestine by the Percoll centrifugation method, evidence was obtained that sodium also plays an important role in the transport of Ca^{2+} across this membrane. It could be observed that replacing potassium by sodium inhibits ATP-driven Ca^{2+} uptake by basolateral membrane vesicles. This finding suggested that in the presence

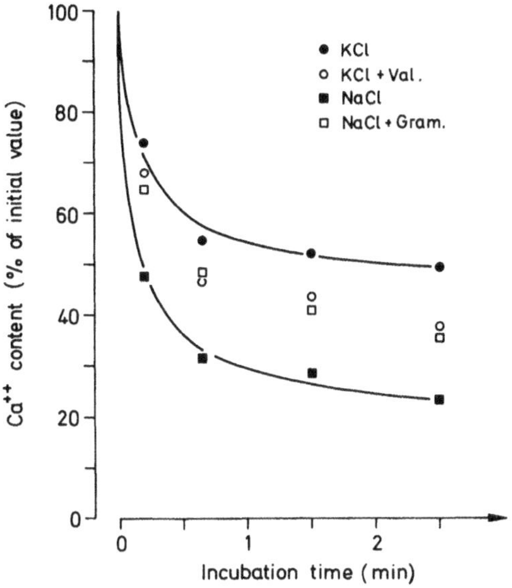

Fig. 11. Ca^{2+} efflux from basolateral membrane vesicles. Basolateral membrane vesicles were isolated by a Percoll centrifugation method (SCALERA et al. 1980) and incubated for 1 h at room temperature with 0.1 m*M* $^{45}CaCl_2$ in 300 m*M* HEPES-Tris, pH 7.4. 100 m*M* choline cyclamate, 5 m*M* $MgSO_4^{2-}$. Efflux of Ca^{2+} was initiated by addition of 10 μl 20 m*M* EGTA in 300 m*M* mannitol, 20 m*M* HEPES-Tris, pH 7.4, 5 m*M* $MgSO_4^{2-}$ and 1 m*M* NaCl or KCl, concentrations of valinomycin or gramicidin were 20 μg/per milligram protein. After HILDMANN et al. (1980b)

of sodium a "calcium leak" is opened in basolateral membrane vesicles counteracting ATP-driven Ca^{2+} accumulation. Furthermore, as shown in Fig. 11, an inwardly directed sodium gradient was able to accelerate calcium efflux from preloaded vesicles. Since increasing sodium conductance in isolated basolateral membranes by the addition of gramicidin D decreased the efflux rate in the presence of an inwardly directed sodium gradient, direct coupling of sodium influx with calcium efflux via a calcium/sodium exchange mechanism is suggested. Thus, besides the ATP-driven mechanism, an Na^+-gradient-dependent, secondary active extrusion mechanism seems to be located in the basolateral membrane of the epithelial cell (HILDMANN et al. 1979, 1982a).

These observations have been confirmed by other research groups (NELLANS and POPOVITCH 1981; GHIJSEN et al. 1982, 1983). It has also been shown that 1,25$(OH)_2$-vitamin D_3 regulates Ca^{2+}-ATPase activity and ATP-dependent Ca^{2+} uptake (GHIJSEN and VAN OS 1982).

Owing to the high amount of calcium bound to the membrane surface, studies with brush border membrane vesicles are difficult to carry out. Experimental evidence for the existence of a transport system mediating the passive entry of calcium across the brush border membrane was obtained by the group led by RASMUSSEN working with membrane vesicles isolated from chicken intestine (FONTAINE et al. 1979; RASMUSSEN et al. 1979). It was demonstrated that calcium entry into isolated brush border membranes is a saturable phenomenon and furthermore regulated by 1,25(OH)$_2$-vitamin D_3. Recently, it has also been shown with brush border membranes of rat or rabbit small intestine that the Ca^{2+} permeability is specifically altered by in vivo treatment with 1,25(OH)$_2$-vitamin D_3 (HILDMANN et al. 1980b; MILLER and BRONNER 1981).

E. Energetics and Kinetics

Studies with isolated brush border membrane vesicles have been used to study energetic and kinetic problems related to sodium-dependent transport. Experiments on the sodium dependence and electrical potential dependence contribute most important knowledge for energetic considerations of transmembrane transport on a qualitative level. Thus it can be decided if the sodium concentration difference or the electrochemical potential difference has to be considered as part of the driving force.

Attempts to evaluate the energetics of sodium-dependent D-glucose transport quantitatively have been reported (KESSLER and SEMENZA 1980). By estimating the Na^+-gradient-related driving force and comparing it with the experimentally observed D-glucose accumulation inside the vesicles, it has been concluded that: (1) the efficiency of energy conversion from an electrochemical potential difference for sodium to a chemical potential difference of D-glucose by the sodium-D-glucose cotransport system is very high; (2) the stoichiometry of sodium to glucose flux is one to one.

Kinetic properties of the transport systems have thus far been analysed in the vesicular system by two different methods. SEMENZA's group derives the kinetic parameters from initial, unidirectional (linear uptake rate) influx measurements under sodium gradient conditions (KESSLER et al. 1978b; SILIPRANDI et al. 1979) HOPFER's group determines kinetic parameters by tracer exchange procedures in the absence of chemical gradients for solute and sodium (HOPFER 1977b, 1981). Considering the arguments discussed by the authors (KESSLER et al. 1978b; SILIPRANDI et al. 1979; HOPFER 1977b, 1981) as well as the discussion by GECK and HEINZ (1976) it is not surprising that the numerical values obtained for K_m and V_{max} by the two different methods are clearly different.

Concluding this brief discussion, one has to realize that kinetic properties studied in the vesicular system strongly depend on the experimental conditions used. Therefore, it is difficult to correlate the numerical values obtained under different experimental conditions. However, saturation experiments with vesicles under similar incubation conditions seem to be most useful in comparative studies, e.g. comparing transport properties in vesicles isolated from different intestinal segments or comparing transport properties in vesicles isolated from animals with different physiological status (HILDMANN et al. 1980b, 1982b; HOPFER 1977a; HOPFER et al. 1976a; KESSLER et al. 1978b; RASMUSSEN et al. 1979).

F. Studies with Isolated Membrane Vesicles on the Physiological Regulation of Transepithelial Transport

It is known that transepithelial transport of solutes can be influenced by various physiological parameters, e.g. diet and hormones. Conceptually, regulation of

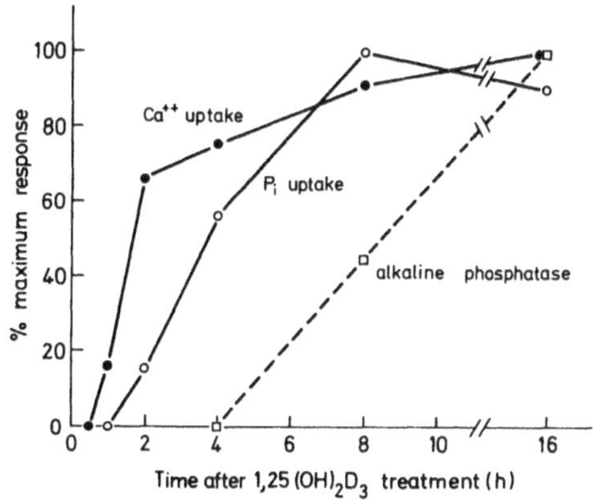

Fig. 12. Time course of the effect of in vivo treatment with 1,25(OH)$_2$-vitamin D$_3$ on chick intestinal brush border membrane vesicle calcium uptake, sodium-dependent phosphate uptake and alkaline phosphatase activity. FONTAINE et al. (1979)

transepithelial transport can occur at several distinct levels. Taking sodium-dependent transport as an example at least the following steps can be modified: (1) the sodium-dependent transport system itself; (2) the exit mechanism in the contraluminal membrane; (3) the driving force which corresponds to the electrochemical potential difference of sodium across the luminal membrane and can be altered, e.g. by a change in the pumping rate of Na^+, K^+-ATPase and/or by changes in the sodium permeability (or more general ion conductivity) of the plasma membrane, especially the brush border membrane. While it is difficult in the intact epithelium to distinguish between these possibilities, it is possible to detect changes of these transport properties in isolated membrane vesicles.

Thus, it was possible to attribute the differences among sodium-dependent solute transport in different intestinal segments observed in intact epithelial preparations to different transport properties of the brush border membrane for various solutes (HOPFER et al. 1976a; KESSLER et al. 1978b; LÜCKE et al. 1978a, b, 1980; MURER et al. 1980). Also, evidence was obtained that intracellular cAMP levels influence sodium-dependent transport in the intestinal brush border membrane, probably indirectly by altering the sodium conductivity of these membranes (MURER et al. 1980). With animals of different vitamin D status it has been shown that transport of calcium and phosphate across chicken and rabbit intestinal brush border membranes is, as in the intact epithelium, regulated by 1.25(OH)$_2$-vitamin D$_3$ (FONTAINE et al. 1979; RASMUSSEN et al. 1979; HILDMANN et al. 1980b, 1982b). The studies of the group led by RASMUSSEN are summarized in Fig. 12. Regarding the time course of the effect of 1,25(OH)$_2$-vitamin D$_3$ treatment of rachitic chicken on brush border membrane calcium uptake (after 30 min incubation), Na^+-dependent phosphate uptake (after 15 s incubation), and alkaline phosphatase activity, several interesting phenomena can be noticed: (1) all three activities, as studied with isolated brush border vesicles, increase after 1.25(OH)$_2$-vitamin D$_3$ administration to the animal before it is killed; (2) the time courses of these effects of the vitamin on the three different activities are dissociated, when referred to the maximum increase observed at 8–16 h. This finding

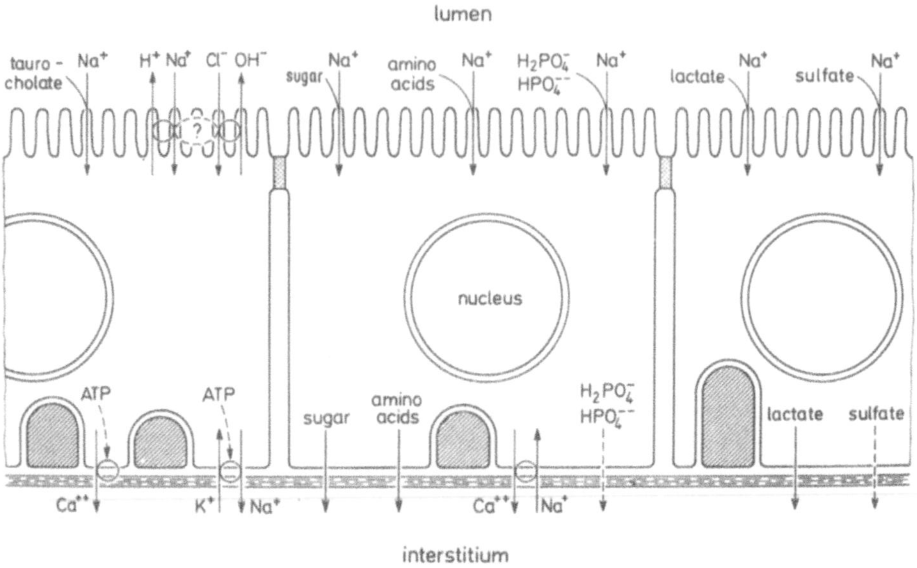

Fig. 13. Schematic representation of membrane-bound transport systems in the small intestinal enterocyte as identified in studies with isolated membrane vesicles

clearly indicates that these three activities represent separate properties of the brush border membrane. Furthermore, these studies demonstrate that physiological alterations observed in the intact epithelium may be retained on the level of brush border membranes. Recently, it has been shown that 1,25$(OH)_2$-vitamin D_3-dependent differences in the handling of inorganic phosphate in the rabbit duodenum can at least in part be attributed to an alteration of the sodium-dependent transport system (HILDMANN et al. 1980b, 1982b). From such studies it is evident that type and physiological status of animals used for performing membrane isolation and transport studies can considerably influence the transport properties observed. Finally, studies with isolated membranes now offer the possibility of analysing the biochemical basis for altered transmembrane transport (e.g. MAX et al. 1978; RASMUSSEN et al. 1979).

G. Conclusions

Studies with isolated intestinal membrane vesicles have by now been performed for several years. Although such studies can only be a piece of the puzzle of "transepithelial transport in the small intestine", the contribution to the understanding of membrane-bound phenomena involved in transepithelial transport obtained by this biochemical approach is significant. As summarized in the scheme (Fig. 13) studies with isolated membrane vesicles allowed investigators to define mechanisms involved in the intestinal transport of sugars, amino acids, organic and inorganic ions. If investigations with isolated membrane vesicles are carried out within the framework of our general knowledge of the physiology of epithelial transport and with the indispensable care which has to be taken in any approach making use of disintegrated systems in artificial media, relevant information improving our understanding of transepithelial transport can be expected in the future. Most promising seems to be the use of isolated membrane vesicles in the study of mechanisms involved in the physiological regulation of transepithelial transport.

Experiments with isolated membrane vesicles are now being performed to elucidate the biochemical nature of the transport systems. In several laboratories efforts are being made towards the isolation of carrier molecules. Such investigations will hopefully allow an insight into the molecular mechanisms involved in transmembrane movement of solute and epithelial transport (KLIP et al. 1979 a, b; FAIRCLOUGH et al. 1979; TOGGENBURGER et al. 1978; CRANE et al. 1979).

References

Albers RW (1976) The (sodium plus potassium)-transport ATPase. In: Martonosi A (ed) The enzymes of biological membranes, vol 3. Plenum, New York, p 283

Alvarado F, Robinson JWL (1979) A kinetic study of the interactions between amino acids and monosaccharides at the intestinal brush border membrane. J Physiol (Lond) 295:457–475

Anner BM, Pitts BJR, Crane LK, Schwartz A (1977) A reconstituted $Na^+ + K^+$ pump in liposomes containing purified $(Na^+ + K^+)$ ATPase from kidney medulla. Biochim Biophys Acta 467:340–345

Barnett JEG, Jarvis WTS, Munday KA (1968) Structural requirements for active intestinal sugar transport. The involvement of hydrogen bonds at C_1 and C_6 of the sugar. Biochem J 109:61–67

Barnett JEG, Ralph A, Munday KA (1969) Structural requirements for active intestinal transport. Biochem J 114:569–573

Beck JC, Sacktor B (1978) Membrane potential-sensitive fluorescence changes during Na^+-dependent D-glucose transport in renal brush border membrane vesicles. J Biol Chem 253:7158–7162

Beesley RC, Faust RG (1979) Sodium ion coupled uptake of taurocholate by intestinal brush border vesicles. Biochem J 178:299–303

Berner W, Kinne R, Murer H (1976) Phosphate transport into brush border membrane vesicles isolated from rat small intestine. Biochem J 160:467–474

Biber J, Stieger B, Haase W, Murer H (1981) A high yield preparation for rat kidney brush border membranes. Different behaviour of lysosomal markers. Biochim Biophys Acta 647:169–176

Bieberdorf FA, Gorden P, Fordtran JS (1972) Pathogenesis of congenital alkalosis with diarrhea. Implications for the physiology of normal ileal electrolyte absorption and secretion. J Clin Invest 51:1958–1968

Booth AG, Kenney AJ (1974) A rapid method for the preparation of microvilli from rabbit kidney. Biochem J 142:575–581

Burckhardt G, Stieger B, Murer H (1980) Optical monitoring of membrane potential changes as a tool to study sodium dependent substrate transport in brush border vesicles from rat kidney proximal tubules. Meeting Abstract, Experientia 36:C 719

Cassano G, Stieger B, Murer H (1983) Na^+/H^+ and Cl^-/OH^- exchange in rat jejunal brush border membrane vesicles. Pfluegers Arch (to be published)

Christensen HN (1979) Exploiting amino acid structure to learn about membrane transport. Adv Enzymol 49:41

Crane RK (1968) Absorption of sugars. In: Code CF (ed) Handbook of physiology, sect 6, vol III. American Physiological Society, Washington DC, p 1323

Crane RK (1977) The gradient hypothesis and other models of carrier mediated active transport. Rev Physiol Biochem Pharmacol 78:101–159

Crane RK, Malathi H, Preiser H, Fairclough P (1979) Some characteristics of kidney Na^+-dependent glucose carrier reconstituted into liposomes. Am J Physiol 284:E1–E5

De Gier J, Blok MC, Van Dijck PWM, Mombers C, Verkley AJ, Van der Neut-Kok ECM, Van Deenen LLM (1978) Relations between liposomes and biomembranes. Ann NY Acad Sci 308:85–100

Eichholz A, Crane RK (1965) Studies on the organization of the brush border in intestinal epithelial cells. I. Tris disruption of isolated hamster brush borders and density gradient separation of fractions. J Cell Biol 26:687–692

Esposito G, Faelli A, Tosco M, Carpraro V (1981) Hyperglycemia and net transintestinal glucose and sodium transport in the rat. Pfluegers Arch 390:202–206

Eveloff J, Field M, Kinne R, Murer H (1980) Sodium cotransport systems in intestine and kidney of the winter flounder. J Comp Physiol 135:175–182

Fairclough P, Malathi P, Preiser H, Crane RK (1979) Reconstitution into liposomes of glucose active transport from the rabbit renal proximal tubule. Biochim Biophys Acta 553:295–306

Fontaine O, Matsumoto T, Simionescu M, Goodman DBP, Rasmussen H (1979) Fundamental actions of 1,25$(OH)_2$ cholecalciferol in intestinal ion transport do not involve gene activation. In: Norman AW, Schaefer K, Coburn JW, DeLuca HF, Fraser D, Grigoleit HG, Henath DV (eds) Vitamin D. Biochemical, chemical and clinical aspects related to calcium metabolism. Walter de Gruyter, Berlin, p 693

Forstner GG, Sabesin SM, Isselbacher KJ (1968) Rat intestinal membranes. Purification and biochemical characterisation. Biochem J 106:381–390

Frizzell RA, Field M, Schultz SG (1979) Sodium coupled chloride transport by epithelial tissues. Am J Physiol 236:F1–F8

Fujita M, Ohta H, Kawai K, Matsui H (1972) Differential isolation of microvillus and basolateral membranes from intestinal mucosa. Biochim Biophys Acta 274:336–347

Gasko OD, Knowles AF, Shertzer HG, Suolinna EM, Racker E (1976) The use of ion-exchange resins for studying ion transport in biological system. Anal Biochem 72:57–65

Geck P, Heinz E (1976) Coupling in secondary transport, effect of electrical potentials on the kinetics of ion linked cotransport. Biochim Biophys Acta 443:49–63

Ghijsen WEJM, De Jong MD, Van Os CH (1982) ATP-dependent calcium transport and its correlation with Ca^{2+}-ATPase activity in basolateral plasmamembranes of rat duodenum. Biochim Biophys Acta 689:327–336

Ghijsen WEJM, De Jong MD, Van Os CH (1983) Kinetic properties of Na^+/Ca^{2+} exchange in basolateral plasma membranes of rat small intestine. Biochim. Biophys. Acta 730:85–94

Ghijsen WEJM, Van Os CH (1982) 1α,25-dihydroxy-vitamin D-3 regulates ATP-dependent calcium transport in basolateral plasma membranes of rat enterocytes. Biochim Biophys Acta 689:170–172

Glenny JR, Bretscher A, Weber K (1980) Calcium control of the intestinal microvillus cytoskeleton: Its implications for the regulation of the microfilament organizations. Proc Natl Acad Sci USA 77:6458–6462

Grinstein S, Turner RJ, Silverman M, Rothstein A (1980) Inorganic anion transport in kidney and intestinal brush border and basolateral membranes. Am J Physiol 238:F452–F460

Haase W, Schäfer A, Murer H, Kinne R (1978) Studies on the orientation of brush border membrane vesicles. Biochem J 172:57–62

Hauser H, Howell K, Dawson RMC, Boyer DE (1980) Rabbit small intestinal brush border membrane preparation and lipid composition. Biochim Biophys Acta 602:567–577

Henderson PJF, McGivan JD, Chapell JB (1969) The action of certain antibiotics on mitochondrial, erythrocyte and artificial phospholipid membranes. Biochem J 111:521–529

Hilden SA, Sacktor B (1979) D-glucose dependent sodium transport in renal brush border membrane vesicles. J Biol Chem 254:7090–7096

Hildmann B, Schmidt A, Murer H (1979) Ca^{++} transport in basal-lateral plasma membranes isolated from rat small intestinal epithelial cells. Pfluegers Arch 382:R23

Hildmann B, Storelli C, Haase W, Barac-Nieto M, Murer H (1980a) Sodium ion-L-lactate cotransport in rabbit small intestinal brush border membrane vesicles. Biochem J 186:169–176

Hildmann B, Storelli C, Schmidt A, Murer H (1980b) Mechanisms involved in small intestinal transport of calcium and phosphate ions: Studies with isolated membrane vesicles. In: Gáti T, Szollár G, Ungváry G (eds) Nutrition, digestion, metabolism. Advances in Physiological Science, vol 12. Pergamon, New York, pp 459–464

Hildmann B, Schmidt A, Murer H (1982a) Ca^{++} transport across basal-lateral plasma membranes from rat small intestinal epithelial cells. J Membrane Biol 65:55–62

Hildmann B, Storelli C, Danisi G, Bonjour P, Murer H (1982b) Regulation of Na-Pi cotransport by 1,25-dihydroxyvitamin D_3 in rabbit duodenal brush border membranes. Am J Physiol 242:G533–G539

Hoffmann N, Thees M, Kinne R (1976) Phosphate transport by isolated renal brush border vesicles. Pfluegers Arch 362:147–156

Hopfer U (1977a) Isolated membrane vesicles as tools for analysis of epithelial transport. Am J Physiol 236:F1–F8

Hopfer U (1977b) Kinetics of Na^+ dependent D-glucose transport. J Supramol Struct 7:1–13

Hopfer U (1981) Kinetic criteria for carrier mediated transport mechanisms in membrane vesicles. Fed Proc 40:2480–2485

Hopfer U, Nelson K, Perrotto I, Isselbacher KJ (1973) Glucose transport in isolated brush border membranes from rat small intestine. J Biol Chem 248:25–32

Hopfer U, Sigrist-Nelson K, Murer H (1975) Intestinal sugar transport: Studies with isolated plasma membranes. Ann NY Acad Sci 264:414–427

Hopfer U, Sigrist-Nelson K, Groseclose R (1976a) Jejunal and ileal D-glucose transport by isolated brush border membranes. Biochim Biophys Acta 426:349–353

Hopfer U, Sigrist-Nelson K, Ammann E, Murer H (1976b) Differences in neutral amino acid and glucose transport between brush border and basolateral membrane of intestinal epithelial cells. J Cell Physiol 89:805–810

Hübscher GG, West R, Bundley DN (1965) Studies on the fractionation of mucosal homogenates from the small intestine. Biochem J 97:629–642

Humphreys MH, Chou LYN (1979) Anion-stimulated ATPase activity of brush border from rat small intestine. Am J Physiol 236:E70–E76

Humphreys MH, Kaysen GA, Chou LY, Watson IB (1980) Anion-stimulated phosphohydrolase activity of intestinal alkaline phosphatase. Am J Physiol 238:G3–G9

Kaunitz JD, Gunther R, Wright EH (1982) Involvement of multiple sodium ions in intestinal D-glucose transport. Proc Natl Acad Sci USA 79:2315–2318

Kessler M, Semenza G (1979) On the efficiency of energy conversion in sodium driven D-glucose transport across small intestinal brush border membrane vesicles. An estimation. FEBS Lett 108:205–208

Kessler M, Acuto O, Storelli C, Murer H, Müller M, Semenza G (1978a) A modified procedure for the rapid preparation of efficiently transporting vesicles from small intestinal brush border membranes. Biochim Biophys Acta 506:136–154

Kessler M, Tannenbaum V, Tannenbaum C (1978b) A simple apparatus for performing short time (1–2 seconds) uptake measurements in small volumes; its application to D-glucose transport studies in brush border vesicles from rabbit jejunum and ileum. Biochim Biophys Acta 509:348–359

Kimberg VD, Shlatz LJ, Cattieu KA (1979) Cyclic nucleotide dependent protein kinase in membranes from rat small intestine. In: Binder H (ed) Mechanisms of intestinal secretion. Alan R Liss, New York, p 131

Kimmich GA (1977) Energetics of Na^+ dependent sugar transport by isolated intestinal cells: evidence for a major role for membrane potential. Am J Physiol 233:E357–E362

Kimmich GA, Randles J (1980) Evidence for an intestinal Na: sugar transport coupling stoichiometry of 2.0. Biochim Biophys Acta 596:439–444

Kinne R, Haase W, Gmaj P, Murer H (1978) ATP hydrolysis as driving force for transport processes in isolated renal plasma membrane vesicles. In: Guder WG, Schmidt U (eds) Biochem nephrology. Hans Huber, Bern, p 178

Klip A, Grinstein S, Semenza G (1979a) Transmembrane disposition of the phlorizin binding protein of intestinal brush border. FEBS Lett 99:91–96

Klip A, Grinstein S, Semenza G (1979b) Partial purification of the sugar carrier of intestinal brush border membranes. Enrichement of the phlorizin binding component by selective extractions. J Membrane Biol 51:47–53

Kundig W (1976) The bacterial phosphoenolpyruvate phosphotransferase system. In: Martonosi A (ed) The enzymes of biological membranes, vol 3. Plenum, New York, p 31

Langridge-Smith IL, Field M (1981) Sulfate transport in rabbit ileum: Characterization of the serosal border anion exchange process. J Membrane Biol 63:207–214

Le Fevre PG (1975) The present state of the carrier hypothesis. Curr Top Membr Transp 7:109–215

Lerner J (1978) A review of amino acid transport processes in animal cells and tissues, glossary of transport and associated terminology. University of Maine at Orano Press, Orano, pp 178–185

Lewis BA, Alkin A, Michell RH, Coleman R (1975) Basolateral plasma membranes of intestinal epithelial cells. Biochem J 152:71–84

Liedtke CM, Hopfer U (1977) Anion transport in brush border membranes isolated from rat small intestine. Biochem Biophys Res Commun 76:579–585

Liedtke CM, Hopfer U (1980) Chloride sodium symport versus chloride/hydroxide antiport across rat intestinal brush border membrane. Fed Proc 39:734

Liedtke CM, Hopfer U (1982a) Mechanism of Cl^- translocation across the small intestinal brush border membrane. I. Absence of NaCl cotransport. Am J Physiol 242:G263–G271

Liedtke CM, Hopfer U (1982b) Mechanism of Cl^- translocation across the small intestinal brush border membrane. II. Demonstration of Cl^-/OH^- exchange and Cl^- conductance. Am J Physiol 242:G272–G280

Louvard D, Maroux S, Baratti J, Desnuelle P, Mutaftschiev S (1973) On the preparation and some properties of closed membrane vesicles from hog duodenal and jejunal brush border. Biochim Biophys Acta 291:747–763

Lücke H, Stange G, Murer H (1978a) Taurocholate sodium cotransport by brush border membrane vesicles isolated from rat ileum. Biochem J 174:951–958

Lücke H, Stange G, Murer H (1978b) Sulphate sodium cotransport by brush border membrane vesicles isolated from rat ileum. Hoppe Seylers Z Physiol Chem 359:1115

Lücke H, Stange G, Murer H (1981) Sulfate sodium cotransport by brush border membrane vesicles isolated from rat ileum. Gastroenterology 80:22–30

MacLennan DH, Holland PC (1976) The calcium transport ATPase of sarcoplasmatic reticulum. In: Matonosi A (ed) The enzymes of biological membranes, vol 3. Plenum, New York, p 221

Maestracci D (1976) Enzymic solubilization of the human intestinal brush border membrane enzymes. Biochim Biophys Acta 433:469–481

Max EE, Goodman DBP, Rasmussen H (1978) Purification and characterization of chick intestine brush border membrane. Effects of 1α (OH)Vitamin D_3 treatment. Biochim Biophys Acta 511:224–239

Miller D, Crane RK (1961a) The digestive function of the epithelium of the small intestine. I. An intracellular locus of disaccharide and sugar phosphate ester hydrolysis. Biochim Biophys Acta 52:281–293

Miller D, Crane RK (1961b) The digestive function of the epithelium of the small intestine. II. Localization of disaccharidase hydrolysis in the isolated brush border portion of intestinal epithelial cells. Biochim Biophys Acta 52:293–298

Miller A, Bronner F (1981) Calcium uptake in isolated brush border vesicles from rat small intestine. Biochem J 196:391–401

Mircheff AK, Wright EM (1976) Analytical isolation of plasma membranes of intestinal epithelial cells. Identification of Na^+K^+-ATPase rich membranes and the distribution of enzyme activities. J Membrane Biol 28:309–333

Mircheff AK, Sachs G, Hanna SD, Labiner CS, Rabon E, Douglas AP, Walling MW, Wright EM (1979) Highly purified basal-lateral plasma membranes from rat duodenum. Physical criteria of purity. J membrane Biol 50:343–363

Mircheff AK, Van Os C, Wright EM (1980a) Pathways for L-alanine transport in intestinal basal-lateral membrane vesicles. J Membrane Biol 52:83–92
Mircheff AK, Harms V, Wright EM (1980b) Interaction of p-chloromercuriphenylsulfonate (PCMPS) with amino acid transport systems in intstinal basolateral membranes. Fed Proc 39:735
Mircheff AK, Klippen I, Hirayama B, Wright EM (1982) Delineation of sodium stimulated amino acid transport pathways in rabbit kidney brush border vesicles. J Membrane Biol 64:113–122
Murer H, Hopfer U (1974) Demonstration of electrogenic Na^+-dependent D-glucose transport in intestinal brush border membranes. Proc Natl Acad Sci USA 71:484–488
Murer H, Kinne R (1977) Sidedness and coupling of transport processes in small intestinal and renal epithelia. In: Semenza G, Carafoli E (eds) Biochemistry of membrane transport, FEBS-Symposium No 42. Springer, Berlin Heidelberg New York, p 292
Murer H, Kinne R (1980) The use of isolated membrane vesicles to study epithelial transport processes. J Membrane Biol 55:81–95
Murer H, Kinne R (1982) The role of sodium in anion transport across renal and intestinal cells. Studies with isolated plasma membrane vesicles. In: Zadunaiski JA (ed) Chloride transport in biological membranes. Acedemic, New York, pp 173–197
Murer H, Hopfer U, Kinne-Saffran E, Kinne R (1974) Glucose transport in isolated brush border and basal-lateral plasma membrane vesicles from intestinal epithelial cells. Biochim Biophys Acta 345:170–179
Murer H, Sigrist-Nelson K, Hopfer U (1975) On the mechanisms of sugar and amino acid interaction in intestinal transport. J Biol Chem 250:7392–7396
Murer H, Hopfer U, Kinne R (1976a) Sodium proton antiport in brush border membrane vesicles isolated from rat small intestine and kidney. Biochem J 154:597–604
Murer H, Ammann E, Biber J, Hopfer U (1976b) The surface membrane of the small intestinal epithelial cell. I. Localization of adenyl cyclase. Biochim Biophys Acta 433:509–519
Murer H, Hopfer U, Kinne R (1977) Sodium/proton antiport in brush border vesicles isolated from rat small intestine and kidney. Biochem J 154:597–604
Murer H, Hopfer U, Kinne R (1978) Molecular evidence for the sodium gradient hypothesis. In: Varro V, Balint G (eds) Current views in gastroenterology. Hungarian Society of Gastroenterology, Budapest, p 77
Murer H, Kinne-Saffran E, Beauwens R, Kinne R (1980a) Proton fluxes in isolated renal and intestinal brush border membranes. In: Schultz I, Sachs G, Forte IG, Ullrich KI (eds) Hydrogen ion transport in epithelia. Elsevier/North Holland Biomedical, pp 267–285
Murer H, Lücke H, Kinne R (1980b) Isolated brush border vesicles as a tool to study disturbances in intestinal solute transport. In: Field M, Fordtran JS, Schultz SG (eds) Secretory diarrhea American Physiological Society, Bethesda, pp 31–43
Nellans HW, Frizzell RA, Schultz SG (1975) Effect of a azetazolamide on sodium and chloride transport by in vitro rabbit ileum. Am J Physiol 228:1808–1814
Nellans HN, Popovitch JE (1981) Calmodulin-regulated, ATP-driven calcium transport by basolateral membranes of rat small intestine. J Biol Chem 256:9932–9936
Parkinson DK, Ebel H, Di Bona DR (1972) Localization of the action of choleratoxin on adenyl cyclase in mucosal epithelial cells of rabbit intestine. J Clin Invest 81:2292–2298
Porteous JW, Clark B (1965) The isolation and characterisation of subcellular components of the epithelial cells of rabbit small intestine. Biochem J 96:159–171
Quigley JD, Gotterer GS (1969) Distribution of Na^+-K^+ ATPase activity in rat intestinal mucosa. Biochim Biophys Acta 173:456–468
Rasmussen H, Fontaine O, Max EE, Goodman DBP (1979) The effect of 1α hydroxyvitamin D_3 administration on calcium transport in chick intestine brush border membrane vesicles. J Biol Chem 254:2993–2999
Rohn R, Biber J, Haase W, Murer H (1983) Effect of protease treatment on enzyme content and transport function of brush border membranes isolated from rat small intestine and kidney cortex. Mol Physiol 3:3–18

Rose L, Lack L (1979) Ion requirements for taurocholate transport by ileal brush border membrane vesicles. Life Sci 25:45–52
Rose RC, Schultz SG (1970) Alanine and glucose effect on the intracellular electrical potential of rabbit ileum. Biochim Biophys Acta 211:376–378
Rose RC, Schultz SG (1971) Studies on the electrical potential profile across rabbit ileum. J Gen Physiol 57:639–661
Scalera V, Storelli C, Storelli-Joss C, Haase W, Murer H (1980) A simple and fast method for the isolation of lateral basal membranes from rat small intestinal epithelial cells. Biochem J 186:177–181
Schmitz J, Preiser H, Maestracci D, Ghosh BK, Cerda JJ, Crane RK (1973) Purification of the human intestinal brush border membrane. Biochim Biophys Acta 323:98–112
Schultz SG (1979) Transport across small intestine. In: Giebisch G, Tosteson DC, Ussing HH (eds) Membrane transport in biology, vol IV B, chap 14. Springer, Berlin Heidelberg New York, p 749
Schultz SG, Curran PF (1970) Coupled transport of sodium and organic solutes. Physiol Rev 50:637–718
Shlatz LJ, Kimberg DV, Cattieu KA (1978) Cyclic nucleotide dependent phosphorylation of rat intestinal microvillous and basal-lateral membrane proteins by endogenous protein kinase. Gastroenterology 75:838–846
Sigrist-Nelson K (1975) Depeptide transport in isolated intestinal brush border membrane. Biochim Biophys Acta 394:220–226
Sigrist-Nelson K, Hopfer U (1974) A distinct D-fructose system in isolated brush border membranes. Biochim Biophys Acta 367:247–254
Sigrist-Nelson K, Murer H, Hopfer U (1975) Active alanine transport in isolated brush border membranes. J Biol Chem 250:5674–5680
Siliprandi L, Vanni P, Kessler M, Semenza G (1979) Na^+ dependent, electroneutral L-ascorbate transport across brush border membrane vesicles from guinea pig small intestine. Biochim Biophys Acta 552:129–142
Smith PL, Orellana SA, Field M (1981) Active sulfate absorption in rabbit ileum: Dependence on sodium and chloride and effects of agents that alter chloride transport. J Membr Biol 63:199–206
Stein WD (ed) (1967) The movement of molecules across cell membranes. Academic, New York
Stevens BR, Ross HI, Wright EM (1982) Multiple amino acid transport pathways in rabbit jejunal brush border vesicles. J Membr Biol 66:213–225
Stieger B, Stange G, Biber J, Murer H (1983) Transport of L-cysteine by rat renal brush border membrane vesicles. J Membr Biol 73:25–37
Stirling CE (1972) Radiographic localization of sodium pump sites in rabbit intestine. J Cell Biol 53:704–714
Storelli C, Corcelli A, Hildmann B, Murer H, Lippe C (1980) L-lactate transport by brush border and basal-lateral membranes of rat small intestine. Pfluegers Arch 388:11–16
Taverna RD, Langdon RG (1973) Reversible association of cytochalasin B with the human erythrocyte membrane. Inhibition of glucose transport and the stoichiometry of cytochalasin binding. Biochim Biophys Acta 323:207–219
Tilney LG, Mooseker MS (1971) Actin in the brush border of epithelial cells of the chicken intestine. Proc Natl Acad Sci USA 68:2611–2615
Toggenburger G, Kessler M, Rothstein A, Semenza G, Tannenbaum C (1978) Similarity in effects of Na^+-gradient and membrane potentials on D-glucose transport by, and phlorizin binding to, vesicles derived from brush borders of rabbit intestinal cells. J Membrane Biol 40:269–290
Vicenci FF, Hinds TR (1976) Plasma membrane calcium transport and membrane-bound enzymes. In: Martonosi A (ed) The enzymes of biological membranes. Plenum, New York, pp 261–281
Walling MW, Mircheff AK, Van Os CH, Wright EM (1978) Subcellular distribution of nucleotide cyclases in rat intestinal epithelium. Am J Physiol 235:E539–E545
Warnock DG, Reenstra WW, Jee JL (1982) Na^+/H^+ antiporter of brush border vesicles: studies with acridine orange uptake. Am J Physiol 242:F733–F739

Wilson FA, Treanor LL (1979) Glycodeoxycholate transport in brush border membrane vesicles isolated from rat jejunum and ileum. Biochim Biophys Acta 554:430–440
Wright EM, Mircheff AK, Hanna SD, Harms V, Van Os CH, Walling MW, Sachs G (1979) The dark side of the intestinal epithelium: The isolation and characterization of basolateral membranes. In: Binder H (ed) Mechanisms of intestinal secretion. Alan R Liss, Inc, New York, p 117
Wright EM, Van Os CH, Mircheff AK (1980) Sugar uptake by intestinal basolateral membrane vesicles. Biochim Biophys Acta, 597:112–124
Yingst DR, Hoffmann JF (1978) Changes of intracellular Ca^{++} as measured by Arsenazo III in relation to the K^{+} permeability of human erythrocyte ghosts. Biophys J 23:463–471

CHAPTER 7

The Transport Carrier Principle

W. D. STEIN

A. The Carrier Concept in Relation to Intestinal Transport

The transport of metabolites across the intestinal epithelium has been a subject of absorbing interest to physiologists and pharmacologists for over a century. This present chapter deals with the carrier concept as applied to intestinal absorption, especially of sugars and amino acids. In this first section we shall consider the historical aspects of the development of the carrier concept and its elaboration for the understanding of intestinal absorption processes; Sect. B deals with the kinetics of carrier transport, while Sect. C is concerned with the efficiency and, hence, the energetics of carrier transport in absorbing systems.

I. Early Development of the Carrier Concept

The Permeability of Natural Membranes, by H. DAVSON and J. F. DANIELLI (1943), gives a good picture of the state of understanding of biologic transport in the early 1940s. Their book shows how much of the transport data of that period could be comfortably encompassed in the membrane model of a lipid bilayer, distinguishing between solutes by virtue of their solublity in lipids. But the movement of some metabolites such as sugars, glycerol, and certain ions, could be understood only if "active patches" on the membrane were in some way specifically concerned in transport of these metabolites. HÖBER's treatise *Physical Chemistry of Cells and Tissues* (1945) gives a rather fuller treatment of the intestinal and kidney physiology of that period. HÖBER attempted to distinguish between a "physical" or "physicochemical permeability" of tissues (by which he meant the fundamental permeability of the cell membranes, which DAVSON and DANIELLI's treatment was beginning to make understandable), and a "physiological" permeability which required the direct intervention of the more complex cellular machinery of metabolism. It seemed to HÖBER that movement of a substance in a direction opposite to its electrochemical gradient could certainly not be accounted for by a purely physical permeability, and would require the intervention of some metabolic input for its operation.

Two types of experiment in particular, largely using intestinal preparations, were very influential in directing the attention of physiologists towards models more complex than the simple diffusion that DAVSON and DANIELLI were explaining so well. In the first class of such experiments, the rate of absorption of a substance from the lumen of the intestinal preparations was measured as a function of the concentration of the absorbed substance. For many substances, the rate of absorption was linearly dependent on the absorbate concentration, while for other substances the rate reached a limiting plateau value as the absorbate concentration was increased. Some experiments, for instance, on the absorption of malonamide or of asparagine, from loops of rat intestine, showed that for the former, but not for the latter substance, quadrupling the absorbate concentration quadrupled the rate of absorption (HÖBER and HÖBER 1937). For asparagine, the parallel increase in rate was only a doubling. Many such studies were performed with sugars and amino acids and in many, but not all, cases such "saturation behavior" was found.

In the second class of experiments, absorption was studied as a function of some additive suspected of being able to inhibit absorption. Many of these additives were drugs or poisons, such as the well-known case of phlorhizin acting on sugar absorption. In many cases, such additives indeed inhibited absorption and often did so specifically in that doses of additives could be found where the absorption of certain substances only, say sugars, was affected. "Such results suggested the belief that the selective absorption of [certain substances] is due to some kind of carrier system, which is seated in the intestinal wall and which is unable to shift more than the maximum load of these sugars at one time," as HÖBER put it in 1945. But what were these carriers? HÖBER felt that "the carrier may be looked upon as an adsorbent, or as a solvent, or as a chemical substrate undergoing a stoichiometric reaction with the transport substance," whereas "the energy required by the system would be utilized... for the loading process, for shifting the carrier across the cell, for setting free the substance from its attachment and for its elimination from the cell." Finally, "the unidirectional shift seems to be predetermined... by structural components of the protoplasm, like the filamentous mitochondria, providing through their arrangement, intracellular channels parallel to the long axis of the cell." A significant advance in our conceptual understanding of such specific membrane transport events came when physiologists turned away for a time from intestine and kidney to the simpler single-cell preparations. LEFEVRE's studies (1948) on sugar and glycerol movement across human red cells provided convincing kinetic data for the existence of specific but nonconcentrating transport systems in these cells, while his inhibitor studies strongly suggested a parallelism between the behavior of these specific membrane systems and specific enzymes. LEFEVRE still used the term "active transfer" or "active transport" to describe these specific, nonconcentrating systems, and it was left to DANIELLI (1954) to clear up the terminological problem by introducing the phrase "mediated transfer" to describe collectively all types of specific systems, the phrase "facilitated transfer" for that subclass where no concentration of the substrate could be observed, and leaving "active transport" to refer to transport against a prevailing electrochemical gradient of substrate. ROSENBERG's (1954) incisive theoretical arguments were very influential in supporting this distinction. The mathematicoanalytic treatment of the carrier model was established by WIDDAS, who worked first on placental transfer of sugar (1952), and then later applied his treatment to data on red cell sugar movements (1954). WIDDAS enunciated the carrier hypothesis in a very clear fashion, his analysis being sharpened by his succinct mathematical formulation. For WIDDAS, and for carrier kineticists since, the carrier was an entity which existed in two different states, facing the two sides of the membrane and able to combine with or discharge its substrate at each membrane face in turn. The interaction of carrier and substrate followed the simple law of mass action for the combination of ligand with a receptor, and the complex then flowed across the membrane by some process (perhaps diffusion) governed by a rate constant, to be broken down to free substrate and carrier at the opposite membrane face. WIDDAS's equations could be successfully applied to an analysis of the early data on red cell sugar transport. Over the years the kinetic treatment of transport across red cells has become increasingly sophisticated and successful (LIEB 1982).

With the carrier model established for the simpler nonconcentrating system of the red blood cell, it became possible to return to the analysis of the concentrating systems in intestine and kidney. A prevailing view was that phosphorylation of sugars was in some way concerned in their transmembrane movement and/or their accumulation by intestinal cells. This hypothesis was influenced by prevailing ideas on cellular metabolism, where phosphorylations were beginning to be revealed as the bases of many cellular metabolic activities, and was supported by evidence that inhibitors of phosphorylation, phlorhizin and iodoacetate (WILBRANDT and LASZT 1933), also inhibited sugar absorption. Many studies (reviewed by CRANE 1960) were generated by this hypothesis, but it was eventually abandoned as it was found that the inhibitor concentrations required to block sugar absorption were considerably smaller than those required to block phosphorylation. In addition, the sugar specificity of the absorption process was quite different from that of the phosphorylation of sugars. Other proposals included one in which a specific enzyme "mutarotase" catalyzed the interconversion between two isomeric forms of the sugars, trapping sugar within the cell. But could the carrier concept as such be invoked in the understanding of the concentrating systems? WIDDAS had already (1954) seen that the simple carrier could be capable of producing a concentration of a substrate, at the expense of an existing gradient of a second substrate that shared the same carrier. PARK et al. (1956) and ROSENBERG and WILBRANDT (1957) had clearly demonstrated such carrier-linked concentration by what was termed "countertransport." What was the "second substrate" in the case of sugar and amino acid concentration by the intestine?

That the concentrating ability of cells for amino acids could be linked to ion movements was shown by CHRISTENSEN et al. (1952), using duck erythrocytes. CHRISTENSEN and his colleagues saw clearly that the accumulation of amino acid within the cell could result from "the potential energy inherent in the asymmetric distribution" of an ion. Clear evidence for the obligatory requirement for sodium ions in intestinal sugar transport came from the important studies of CSÁKY and his colleagues (CSÁKY and THALE 1960; CSÁKY and ZOLLICOFFER 1960; CSÁKY et al. 1961). But CRANE could accurately write in his influential review on intestinal absorption of sugars (1960), that "no proposal advanced for a mechanism of active absorption of sugars ranks as more than speculation on the possible relationship to active absorption of ordinary metabolic events, structures and enzymes..." Indeed, his own speculation which concludes that review makes interesting reading when it is realized that just a year or so later CRANE would propose the now fully accepted model for such processes. In 1960, CRANE's model was still as follows. Microvilli in the intestine contained energy-driven sodium pumps. These established an osmotic gradient up which water would flow, carrying with it the contents of the lumen. Those substances for which specific carriers existed

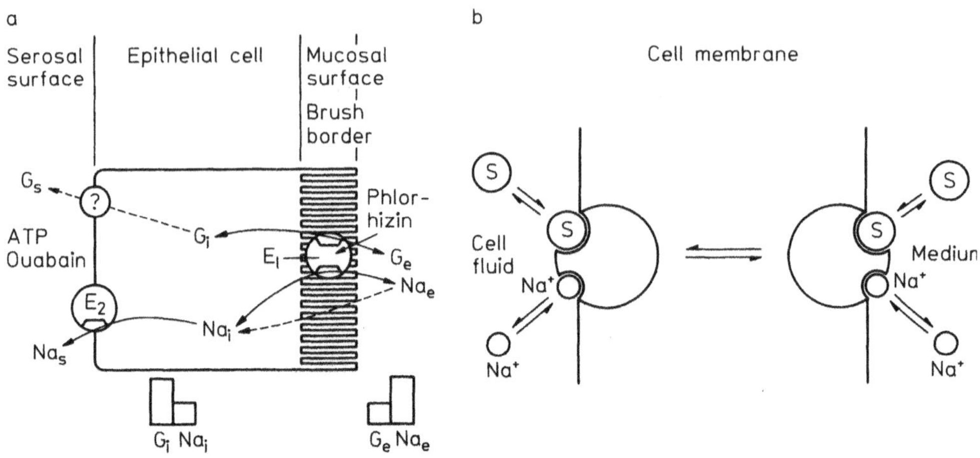

Fig. 1. a Schematic diagram of the model proposed by CRANE (1962) for the interrelations of sodium and glucose transport in intestine. E_1 is a cotransporting sodium- and glucose-requiring carrier system, sensitive to phlorhizin. E_2 is the sodium pump, sensitive to oubain and requiring ATP. The *question mark* represents a facilitated diffusion system, now considered to be sensitive to phloretine. The heights of the blocks at the foot of the figure represent the prevailing levens of glucose (G) and sodium (Na), in the lumen or cytoplasm. STEIN (1967). **b** Simple cotransport carrier model. CRANE et al. (1965)

would be able to flow into the lumen, carried along by the flow of water. Finally, "...sugar could be accumulated within the cell to the extent that Na^+ could be removed by the Na^+ pump. The maximal concentration to be expected if all the Na^+ were removed from the entering solution would be determined by the amount of an isotonic sugar solution which the cell could contain by swelling."

Perhaps the most critical experiment which led to our current view of the interrelations of sodium and sugar transport was that of BIHLER and CRANE (1962). These researchers studied the exchange of a nonmetabolized sugar across the cell membrane of cells of rat intestinal strips. The cells were allowed to take up sugar to equilibrium levels and then the uptake of labeled sugar into these cells was monitored as a function of the external sodium level. The uptake of sugar into the cell was directly proportional to external sodium, over a wide concentration rage of sodium. Clearly, sodium was directly needed for the entry of sugar and not for any trapping of sugar subsequent to its entry. CRANE (1962) made the final breakthrough into a full understanding of the link between sodium and sugar movements, and hence into the understanding of active transport by intestine (and many other tissues), with the model depicted in Fig. 1. The crucial idea in this scheme is that sugar and sodium ions together are needed for the movement of either across the membrane on the sugar carrier. The system is one of cotransport of sugar and ion. This explains the need for sodium ions, but if sodium is absolutely necessary for carrier-mediated transport of the sugar, then the low sodium ion concentration prevailing within cells, as a result of the action of the cell's sodium pump, would reduce the rate of exit of sugar from the cell. Thus, sugar would accumulate within the cell according to the prevailing sodium gradi-

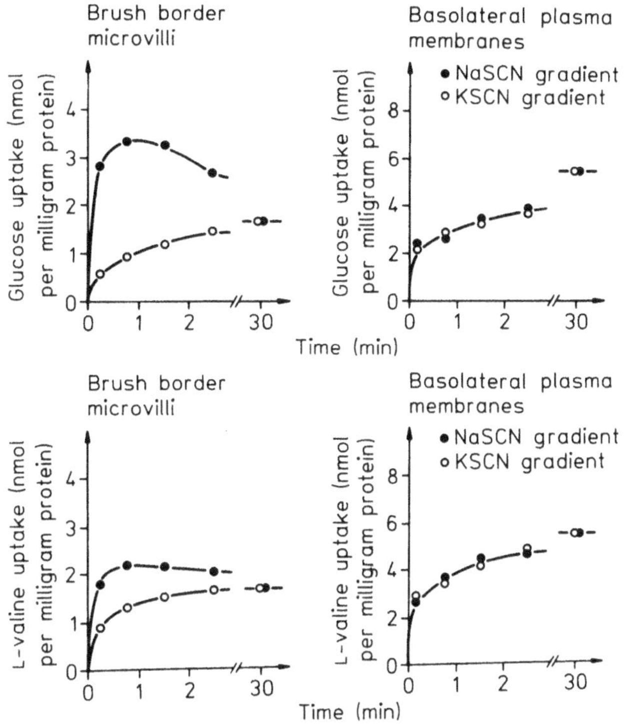

Fig. 2. Uptake of D-glucose and L-valine into membrane vesicles isolated from intestinal brush border and basolateral membranes, as indicated. Note the "overshoot" at early times, in the case of membranes isolated from brush border, but not from basolateral surfaces. After MURER and HOPFER (1977)

ent. Essential for the model is the aspect of the polarization of the cell membrane into that portion facing the intestinal lumen, and containing the sodium–sugar cotransport system and into that portion facing the serosal surface, where would be situated the sodium pump and some nonconcentrating system for the equilibration of cellular and serosal sugar concentrations. A similar polarization of epithelial cells into pumping and facilitated transporting regions was the basis of KOEFOED-JOHNSEN and USSING's famous (1958) model for transepithelial transfer of sodium ions by frog skin, a model which doubtless influenced CRANE's thinking on sugar transfer.

A great deal of work over the years following the enunciation of the CRANE cotransport model has fully confirmed the essential correctness of these insights. Thus, SCHULTZ and ZALUSKY (1964) soon showed that a flow of sodium across rabbit ileum accompanied the flow of sugar, according to the tenets of the cotransport model, and that the flow of sodium ions (measured as a short-circuit current) could be blocked by the addition of phlorhizin, the inhibitor of sugar transport. The final proof of the correctness of the model has come with the isolation, from the epithelium of the small intestine, of vesicles from the cell membranes facing the lumen and, separately, from the cell membranes facing the serosal surface of the epithelium (MURER et al. 1974).

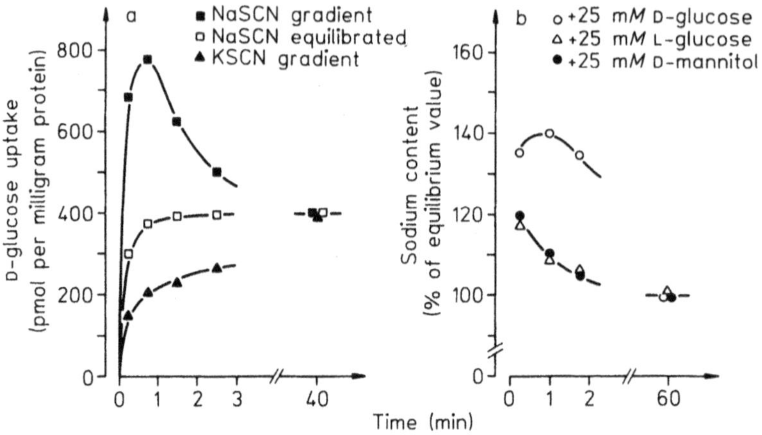

Fig. 3a, b. Uptake of D-glucose into membrane vesicles from brush borders (**a**), and uptake of sodium into these vesicles (**b**). Glucose uptake measured in the presence of a sodium gradient, sodium but no gradient, or a potassium gradient. Sodium uptake studied with a gradient of D-glucose, L-glucose, or mannitol. After Murer and Hopfer (1977)

In what has now become a routine procedure, these workers succeeded in isolating, identifying, and purifying membrane vesicles from brush border faces of the epithelium and from the basolateral surfaces of these cells. The left-hand side of Fig. 2 shows the time course of the uptake of glucose by a vesicle preparation from the brush borders, while the right-hand side shows such a time course for vesicles from the basolateral surface (Murer and Kinne 1977). The former, but not the latter preparation, demonstrates a sodium dependence for glucose accumulation. The former, but not the latter preparation, demonstrates the characteristic "overshoot" phenomenon at early time points when a sufficient gradient of sodium ions is still present across the vesicle so as to cause an accumulation of glucose above the level to be reached at equilibrium. Finally, the uptake curves in Fig. 3 show that a sodium gradient is required for the accumulation of glucose above the equilibrium level, that sodium enters the vesicles, once again is accumulated transiently above its equilibrium level, and that this accumulation depends on the presence of glucose, and D-glucose, at that. The basolateral preparation of the right-hand side of Fig. 2 contains a facilitated diffusion system for sugar movement which is independent of sodium, although it is these membranes which contain the sodium pump, as direct determination shows. The lower half of Fig. 2 shows very similar data on the sodium-dependent active accumulation of the amino acid valine by brush border membranes, but not by membranes from basolateral surfaces.

The significance of the carrier model for intestinal transport and for membranes in general has been very greatly extended by Mitchell's (1966, 1967, 1977) propounding of the chemiosmotic hypothesis on which cotransport and countertransport link, through membrane carriers, the movement of transportable substrates such as cations and especially protons, to the chemical reactions involved in ATP synthesis and in electron transfer during oxidative phosphorylation. It is the transition between two states of a membrane carrier, inward-facing and outward-facing, which appears to link these energy-storing chemical reactions with the flow of transportable substrates. While such reactions are, of course, found in most cells, and not confined to the intestine, they are essential to intestinal function and will also be discussed in the subsequent sections of this chapter. We shall now proceed to a kinetic analysis of the carrier model, so as to explore the consequences of the model of Fig. 1.

B. The Kinetic Approach to Membrane Carriers

In this section we shall develop the kinetic treatment of membrane carriers, starting with the very simplest model and proceeding to quite complex cases. Each level of complexity introduces new transport concepts and predicts new transport behavior for the carrier model, and we shall emphasize these in their turn as we proceed.

I. The Simple Pore and Simple Carrier

Am membrane carrier system is generally first identified by one of two criteria. (1) It is often seen that the transport of the substrate in question is not a linear function of substrate concentration, but rather saturates as the substrate concentration reaches a high level. Transport is then said to display "saturation behavior" or "saturation kinetics." (2) It may well be the case that transport is blocked or inhibited by the addition of some agent, perhaps similar in chemical structure to the substrate or perhaps very different in structure. Transport is then said to display "inhibition behavior" or "inhibition kinetics." Both these types of kinetic behavior are found also for most of the common enzymes, and it is thus very natural to attempt to base the kinetic analysis of transport systems on the well-established kinetic analyses of enzymes. This has, indeed, been the main trend of carrier kinetic analysis over the last 30 years and increasingly sophisticated use has been made of the very important advances during that period in the analysis of enzyme kinetics. We shall proceed in this spirit.

1. The Elementary Kinetic Analysis

Transport is the movement of a substrate from one face of the membrane to the other. We shall term the substrate at face 1 of the membrane S_1, while that at face 2 of the membrane will be S_2. We shall postulate that a transport enzyme E exists within the membrane (Fig. 4). It can combine at face 1 of the membrane with substrate S_1 and at face 2 with S_2 to form complex ES. For the case of an enzyme system it would be the combination with E that allows the transformation of reactant S_1 into product S_2. For the transport system we shall initially postulate that such a combination of S_1 or S_2 with E is sufficient to allow their interconversion, which is here their transport or movement from one membrane face to the other. Thus,

$$S_1 + E \underset{b_1}{\overset{f_1[S_1]}{\rightleftharpoons}} ES \underset{f_2[S_2]}{\overset{b_2}{\rightleftharpoons}} S_2 + E. \qquad (1)$$

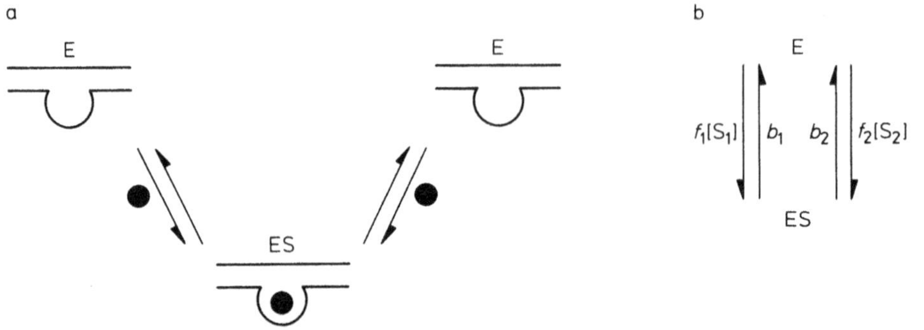

Fig. 4. a Schematic diagram of a simple pore, binding to substrate S to form complex ES. **b** Formal representation of this model in terms of the relevant rate constants

The rate constants in Eq. (1) are b_1 and b_2, which describe the rate of breakdown of the complex ES, and the constants f_1 and f_2, which describe the rate of formation of the complex at faces 1 and 2.

Equation (1) is then applicable both to enzyme systems and to transport systems. What features of transport systems does this very, very simple model account for? In order to compare this model and Eq. (1) with the experimental findings, we have to bring it into a form which describes how the rate of transport from face 1 to face 2 of the membrane depends on the concentrations of transported substrate at faces 1 and 2. The most general measure of rate is the *unidirectional flux* of substrate from one membrane face to the other. This we can measure by adding radioactively labeled substrate at one membrane face and measuring the rate at which label appears at the other membrane face. We shall, however, often find it convenient to measure the *net flow* of substrate from one membrane face to the other. This is measured by estimating the amount of substrate chemically or by its physicochemical effects, or else ensuring that the labeled substrate has the same specific activity at both faces of the membrane. Kinetically, the net flow is obtained by merely taking the (algebraic) difference between the unidirectional fluxes in the two directions across the membrane:

$$\mathrm{Net}_{1\to2} = \underset{v_{2\to1}}{\overset{v_{1\to2}}{\rightleftharpoons}}.$$

Both transport measures can be obtained, therefore, if we derive from Eq. (1) another equation which will describe how the rate of unidirectional flux is determined by S_1 and S_2.

To obtain the unidirectional flux from face 1 to face 2 of the membrane, we find out first the rate at which ES is formed from E and S_1. This is given by the product of the rate constant f_1 for ES formation, the concentration $[S_1]$ of substrate, and the concentration [E] of free enzyme, i.e. by $f_1[S_1]$ [E]. The rate at which ES now breaks down to yield S_2 is given by the fraction $b_2/(b_1+b_2)$, i.e., that part of the total breakdown of ES, (b_1+b_2), which occurs in the direction 1 to 2. Thus, the unidirectional flux of S from side 1 to side 2 is given by $v_{1\overset{3}{\to}2}$ in

$$v_{1\to2} = f_1[S_1][E]\frac{b_2}{(b_1+b_2)}. \tag{2}$$

To solve Eq. (2), we need to know the concentration of free enzyme [E]. We get this by applying the steady state assumption to Eq. (1). That is, we assume that at the steady state (and the steady state will always be reached in milliseconds after a transport reaction commences and hence far sooner than most transport determinations can be made), the rate of formation of ES is equal to its rate of breakdown, i.e., that

$$f_1[\mathrm{S}_1][\mathrm{E}]+f_2[\mathrm{S}_2][\mathrm{E}]=(b_1+b_2)[\mathrm{ES}] \tag{3}$$

while the total concentration of transport enzyme [Tot] is constant and given by

$$[\mathrm{Tot}]=[\mathrm{E}]+[\mathrm{ES}]. \tag{4}$$

Solving Eqs. (3) and (4) for the unknown [E] and [ES] yields

$$[\mathrm{E}]=\frac{(b_1+b_2)[\mathrm{Tot}]}{(b_1+b_2+f_1[\mathrm{S}_1]+f_2[\mathrm{S}_2]}. \tag{5}$$

and

$$[\mathrm{ES}]=\frac{(f_1[\mathrm{S}_1]+f_2[\mathrm{S}_2])[\mathrm{Tot}]}{(b_1+b_2+f_1[\mathrm{S}_1]+f_2[\mathrm{S}_2])} \tag{6}$$

and substituting, now from Eq. (5) into Eq. (2), gives

$$v_{1\to 2}=\frac{f_1 b_2[\mathrm{S}_1][\mathrm{Tot}]}{(b_1+b_2+f_1[\mathrm{S}_1]+f_2[\mathrm{S}_2])} \tag{7}$$

an equation which gives the unidirectional flux of substrate from face 1 of the membrane to face 2, in terms of the rate constants of the very simple model of Eq. (1), and in terms of the concentrations of the substrate at the two faces of the membrane and of total enzyme [Tot]. ([Tot] will be in units of moles of enzyme per unit volume of the reaction mixture for which $v_{1\to 2}$ is being measured, and will have to be brought into the more familiar units of amount of enzyme per unit area of the transporting membrane, by using appropriate conversion factors.) We can convert Eq. (7) into a form containing readily determinable experimental parameters, if we define a resistance term Q as

$$Q=\left(\frac{1}{f_1}+\frac{1}{f_2}\right)$$

and two coefficients of resistance terms as

$$R_{12}=\frac{1}{b_2[\mathrm{Tot}]}$$

and

$$R_{21}=\frac{1}{b_1[\mathrm{Tot}]}$$

when Eq. (7) becomes

$$v_{1\to2}=\frac{[S_1]}{Q+R_{12}[S_1]+R_{21}[S_2]}. \tag{8}$$

(To obtain Eq. (8) from Eq. (7), we divide top and bottom of the right-hand side of equation (7) by $f_1b_2=f_2b_1$. These products of rate constants are equal, since they represent the overall rate of conversion of 1 mol S_1 into S_2 or S_2 into S_1, respectively, at the same concentration, and these rates must be equal, since S is the same chemical substance on both sides of the membrane and must have the same chemical potential.)

Why are these "readily determinable experimental parameters"? Why are the R terms coefficients of resistance? Why is Q a resistance? We proceed to find answers to these questions.

2. Classification of Transport Experiments

The simplest transport experiment is known as the zero-trans procedure (Fig. 5a). Here the concentration of substrate at one face of the membrane (we will take this as face 2) is held at zero, while that at the other is varied and the flux, here a net flow as well as a unidirectional flux, is measured from the nonzero face into the solution containing no substrate. To obtain this condition from Eq. (8), we put $S_2=0$ and write

$$v^{zt}_{1\to2}=\frac{(1/R_{12})[S_1]}{(Q/R_{12})+[S_1]}. \tag{9}$$

Now Eq. (9) is of the familiar form of a Michaelis equation in enzyme kinetics. The maximum velocity of transport, $V^{zt}_{1\to2}$, is obtained by letting the concentration $[S_1]$ go to infinity in Eq. (9) and is readily seen to be given by $V^{zt}_{1\to2}=1/R_{12}$. The Michaelis parameter or half-saturation concentration, $K^{zt}_{1\to2}$, is given by setting $[S_1]=Q/R_{12}$, at which concentration the flux is $1/2R_{12}$ and is one-half of the maximal flux. The "maximum permeability" of the membrane for the substrate is to be determined at limitingly low concentrations of S_1, where the flux is linearly proportional to $[S_1]$, with the coefficient of proportionality being given by $1/Q$. The simple zero-trans experiment thus allows Q and R_{12} to be readily determined, while if the same experiment is performed in the reverse direction, with $[S_2]$ varying and $[S_1]$ held at zero, R_{21} can be found and a second estimate made of Q. This term Q is a "resistance" since it is the reciprocal of the effective permeability or conductance of the membrane for the substrate. The terms in R are coefficients of resistance, since in Eqs. (8) and (9), the term $[S_1]/v_{1\to2}$ gives the resistance to flow of substrate at concentration $[S_1]$, and the terms R_{12} and R_{21} are then the linear coefficients by which this resistance depends on concentration. These coefficients of resistance terms are the reciprocals of the maximum velocities that the membrane permits for the passage of the substrate in the two directions. A high coefficient of resistance will allow only a low maximum rate of transport, a low coefficient of resistance permits a high maximum rate of transport.

Another important experimental procedure is the equilibrium exchange experiment (Fig. 5b). Here the concentration of substrate is set equal at both faces

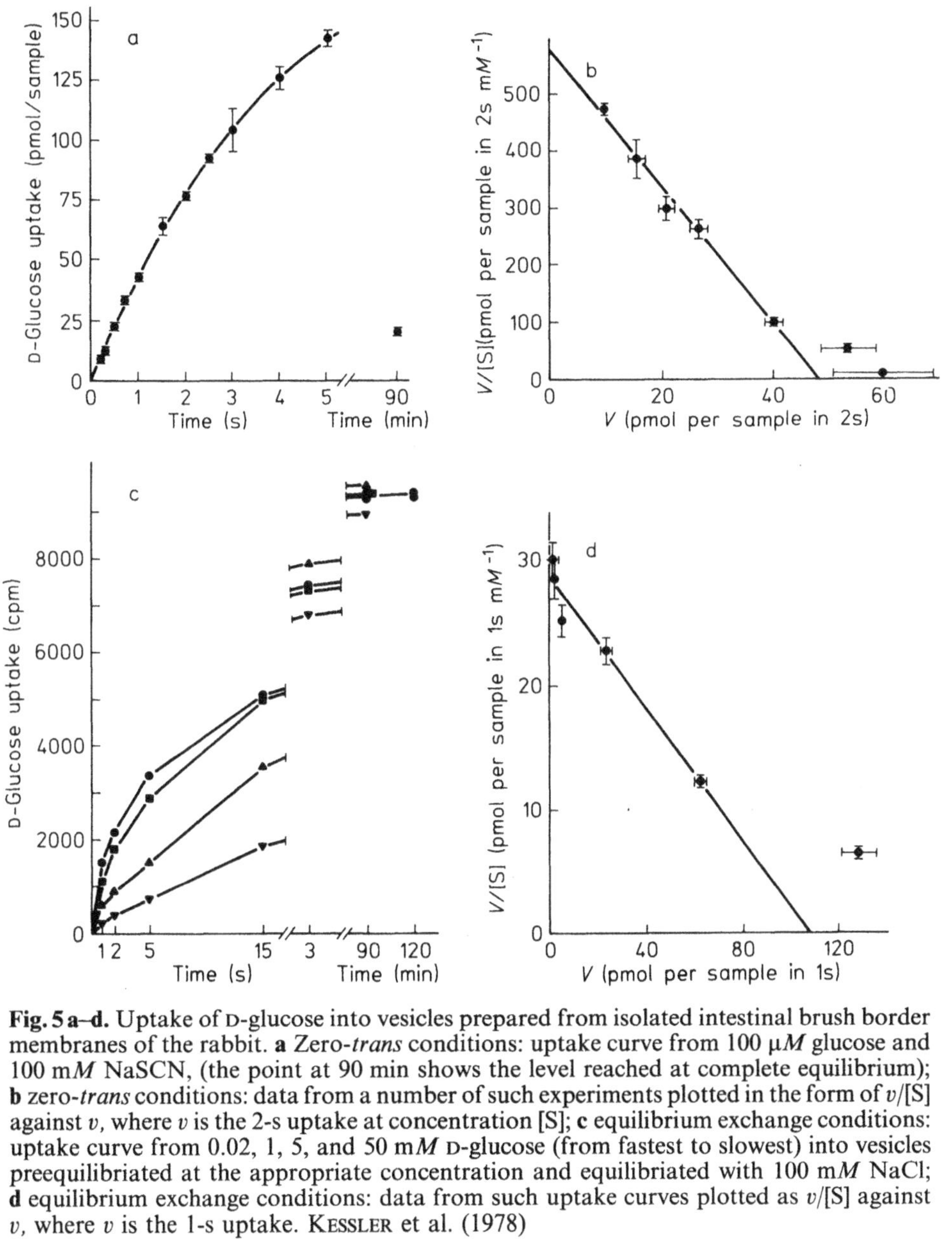

Fig. 5 a–d. Uptake of D-glucose into vesicles prepared from isolated intestinal brush border membranes of the rabbit. **a** Zero-*trans* conditions: uptake curve from 100 μ*M* glucose and 100 m*M* NaSCN, (the point at 90 min shows the level reached at complete equilibrium); **b** zero-*trans* conditions: data from a number of such experiments plotted in the form of $v/[S]$ against v, where v is the 2-s uptake at concentration [S]; **c** equilibrium exchange conditions: uptake curve from 0.02, 1, 5, and 50 m*M* D-glucose (from fastest to slowest) into vesicles preequilibriated at the appropriate concentration and equilibriated with 100 m*M* NaCl; **d** equilibrium exchange conditions: data from such uptake curves plotted as $v/[S]$ against v, where v is the 1-s uptake. KESSLER et al. (1978)

of the membrane, at $[S_1]=[S_2]=[S]$, while the unidirectional flux of labeled substrate is measured as a function of [S]. The flux in the two directions is necessarily the same. We obtain for the flux, putting $[S]=[S_1]=[S_2]$ in Eq. (8):

$$v_{1\to 2}^{ee}=v_{2\to 1}^{ee}=\frac{(1/R_{12}+1/R_{21})[S]}{(Q/R_{12}+Q/R_{21})+[S]}. \tag{10}$$

Here the maximum velocity, $V_{1\to2}^{ee} = V_{2\to1}^{ee} = 1/R_{12} + 1/R_{21}$, while the half-saturation concentration, $K_{1\to2}^{ee} = K_{2\to1}^{ee} = Q/R_{12} + Q/R_{21}$, and the "maximum permeability" is again given by $1/Q$. We see that the maximal velocity of exchange is exactly given as the sum of the maximal velocities of the two zero-trans experiments, the half-saturation parameter is given as the sum of the two values obtained for the two zero-trans experiments, while the resistance Q or its reciprocal, the maximum permeability $1/Q$, is identical for all three experiments. (The latter term must, of necessity, be identical in all three experiments since it is defined as the ratio of transport to substrate concentration in the limiting case of zero substrate concentration, when it cannot matter whether a zero-trans or an equilibrium exchange experiment is being performed – all concentrations are anyway zero!) If the maximal velocity and half-saturation concentrations are found experimentally not to be related as this simple treatment predicts (and such contradictory findings are very often observed), then it is apparent that the model of Eq. (1) does not apply.

A third type of procedure often performed on membrane systems is the infinite-trans experiment. In this procedure, the concentration of substrate at one face (here, say face 2) is held at a limitingly high value, defined as so high that a further increase in $[S_2]$ would make no difference to the rate of transport where this is measured as the unidirectional flux of labeled substrate from face 1 to face 2. If we now attempt to derive this procedure from Eq. (8) by setting $[S_2]$ infinitely high, we find the surprising result that the flux from face 1 to face 2 is zero at all concentrations of $[S_1]$ less than infinity! Yet this experiment is often performed for transport systems and gives perfectly reasonable values for the unidirectional flux. We shall give examples of such experimental findings in a later section. Clearly, any such experimental finding is inconsistent with the simple model of Eq. (1). Indeed, it is often found for transport systems that the unidirectional flux in an infinite-trans experiment is greater than that in a zero-trans experiment, at corresponding substrate concentrations at the cis face, yet the model of Eq. (1) fails to give this result. Equation (8) shows that for all values of $[S_2]$, the flux given by Eq. (8) is always less than the value for $[S_2]$ equal to zero, the zero-trans case.

The next two procedures that we should handle are conceptually less simple than the ones discussed up to now, but are experimentally often very tractable. One such procedure is the infinite-cis experiment. Here, substrate is held at limitingly high levels at one face of the membrane, say face 1, and the net flow of substrate from that cis face determined as a function of the substrate concentration at the trans face. Substituting into Eq. (8) gives:

$$\mathrm{Net}_{1\to2} = \frac{[S_1]-[S_2]}{Q+R_{12}[S_1]+R_{21}[S_2]} \tag{11}$$

which, when $[S_1]$ goes to infinity, yields a constant value of $1/R_{12}$ unaffected by altering $[S_2]$ at less than infinitely high levels. Yet when the infinite-cis experiment is performed, altering the concentration of substrate at face 2 does, in most cases, decrease the net flow of substrate, even when the concentration at face 1 is saturatingly high. Once again the model of Fig. 4 (and hence, Eq. (1)) fails to account for easily demonstrable experimental findings for a number of transport systems.

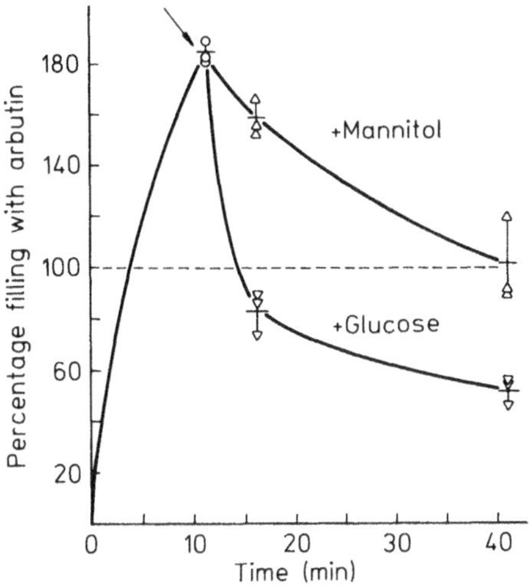

Fig. 6. Countertransport out of an intestinal preparation. Strips of hamster small intestine were loaded with arbitun, a phenylglucoside, nonmetabolizable but a substrate for the sugar-concentrating system. At the *arrow*, 2,4-dinitrophenol was added to prevent further accumulation together with arbutin at the original concentration and either mannitol or D-glucose. With D-glucose, a substrate for the system, arbutin moves out of the tissue to a level below that in the external medium. With mannitol, which is not a substrate for the system, arbutin flows out, but only to the level present externally. ALVARADO (1965)

The last transport procedure which we need to consider is that of the countertransport experiment. Here we start with the substrate present at equilibrium at both faces of the membrane, labeled to the same specific activity and at the same concentration. We then add, say to face 2 of the membrane, unlabeled substrate or a substrate analog and follow the time course of movement of label across the membrane in the 1 to 2 direction (Fig. 6). The high concentration of substrate at face 2 dilutes the effective concentration of label at that face and lowers the unidirectional flux of label in the 2 to 1 direction, while that in the 1 to 2 direction can remain unchanged. Thus, there can be a net flow of label in the 1 to 2 direction. The phrase "can be a net flow" is carefully chosen. Experimentally, there is often such a flow of label, but the model of Eq. (1), as we can demonstrate, does not predict this flow. To show this we proceed as follows. The flow of label in the 1 to 2 direction is given from Eq. (8) as $v_{1-2} = [S_1]/(Q + R_{12}[S_1] + R_{21}[S_2])$. The flow of material in the 2 to 1 direction is given by $[S_2]/(Q + R_{12}[S_1] + R_{21}[S_2])$ but the flow of *label* is only a fraction $[S_1]/[S_2]$ of this, since the label at face 2 is diluted to this extent by the addition of unlabeled substrate. Multiplying out, one sees that the expressions for the flow of label in the 1 to 2 and in the 2 to 1 directions are identical, so the net flow of label is zero. Yet in many experiments, as we have emphasized, a flow of label occurs. Such experiments demonstrate the inapplicability of the model of Fig. 4 and Eq. (1) to those systems for which countertransport can be demonstrated. Does this simplest model account, however, for the phenomenon of inhibition of transport, a phenomenon so important in the field of drug action? To test this point, we set up simple models for inhibition of the transport enzyme of Fig. 4.

3. Inhibition Kinetics of Transport Systems

An inhibitor will affect the rate of transport process by combining with the transport enzyme. Thus, for the model of Fig. 1, we might add to Eq. (1), which describes the combination of substrate with enzyme, an equation describing the combination of the inhibitor with the transport enzyme

$$I_1 + E \underset{d_1}{\overset{g_1[I_1]}{\rightleftharpoons}} EI \underset{g_2[I_2]}{\overset{d_2}{\rightleftharpoons}} I_2 + E . \tag{12}$$

For this type of inhibition, the substrate and inhibitor compete for the transport enzyme. Equations (1) and (12) can be solved simultaneously, and the unidirectional flux of S from side 1 to side 2 is then found to be given by

$$v_{1\to 2}^{S} = \frac{[S_1]}{Q^S(1+Q^I R_{12}^I[I_1]+Q^I R_{21}^I[I_2])+R_{12}^S[S_1]+R_{21}^S[S_2]} . \tag{13}$$

The terms in Q are the resistances for S and I, respectively, as labeled with the superscript S or I, while the terms in R are the coefficients of resistance for S and I, as labeled. With no inhibitor, Eq. (13) reduces to Eq. (8). At infinitely high [S], the same maximal velocity is found as in the absence of inhibitor, so the inhibition is competitive, the kinetic effect of the presence of the inhibitor being to increase the half-saturation concentration for S by a factor $(1+Q^I R_{12}^I[I_1]+Q^I R_{21}^I[I_2])$. A plot of $1/v_{1\to 2}$ against $1/[S_1]$, at different values of the inhibitor concentrations $[I_1]$ and $[I_2]$ gives a pencil of straight lines intersecting on the $1/v_{1\to 2}$ axis, at the value $R_{12}+R_{21}$ corresponding to the reciprocal of the maximal velocity of transport. This finding of a pencil of lines intersecting on the $1/v$ axis is the enzymologist's test for pure competitive inhibition.

According to Eq. (13), a high concentration of inhibitor at either face of the membrane will inhibit the unidirectional flux of S to the same extent when this is measured in the 1 to 2 or in the 2 to 1 direction. This is so since the denominator of Eq. (13) is unchanged when the subscripts 1 and 2 are interchanged. Thus, if a countertransport experiment is attempted with substrate originally at the same concentration at each membrane face, while a competitor is then added to one face only, then according to Fig. 4 flow of the substrate should not occur, although the inhibitor will be competing with substrate from one side of the membrane only. The finding of countertransport between two substrates (or substrate and competitive inhibitor) thus invalidates the simple model of Fig. 4.

Uncompetitive inhibition will result if the inhibitor is able to combine with the enzyme–substrate complex ES to form ESI. The appropriate kinetic scheme is

$$S_1 \text{ (or } S_2) + E \underset{b_1 \text{ (or } b_2)}{\overset{f_1[S_1] \text{ (or } f_2[S_2])}{\rightleftharpoons}} ES \underset{c_1 \text{ (or } c_2)}{\overset{h_1[I_1] \text{ (or } h_2[I_2])}{\rightleftharpoons}} ESI \tag{14}$$

which gives the unidirectional flux of S from 1 to 2 as

$$v_{1\to 2}^{S} = \frac{[S_1]}{Q^S+(R_{12}^S[S_1]+R_{21}^S[S_2])\{1+Q^I(R_{12}^I[I_1]+R_{21}^I[I_2])\}} \tag{15}$$

with the same meaning for the symbols in Q and R as in Eq. (13). For this case, the unidirectional flux of S does not reach the uninhibited maximal value as the concentration of S is raised, but rather a smaller value given by the factor $1/\{1+Q^{\mathrm{I}}(R^{\mathrm{I}}_{12}[\mathrm{I}_1]+R^{\mathrm{I}}_{21}[\mathrm{I}_1])\}$, which depends on the inhibitor concentration. Also, the half-saturation parameter is increased by this same factor. Thus, for the case where the inhibitor can combine with the transport enzyme–substrate complex, both the maximum velocity and the half-saturation concentration are increased by the same factor. The plot of $1/v_{1\to 2}$ against $1/[\mathrm{S}_1]$, at different values of the inhibitor concentrations $[\mathrm{I}_1]$ and $[\mathrm{I}_2]$, will give a set of parallel lines, the intercept on the $1/v_{1\to 2}$ axis and that on the $1/[\mathrm{S}_1]$ axis both being increased correspondingly by the presence of inhibitor. The slope of such lines gives the resistance, and this is not affected by the inhibitor. The finding of such a set of parallel lines is the enzymologist's test for purely uncompetitive inhibition.

It follows (and inspection of Eq. (15) will reveal) that, at limitingly low concentrations of substrate, no inhibition will be noticed, the conductance or permeability here being given simply by $1/Q$, unchanged from the value in the absence of inhibitor. This result is perhaps not surprising, since if the inhibitor has to combine with enzyme–substrate complex in order to inhibit, then at low substrate concentrations when little or no complex is present, there will be little or nothing to combine with it.

Finally, we might have the case that the ternary complex between transport enzyme, substrate, and inhibitor can form either through prior combination of E with S, or with I. The formal kinetic scheme is

$$\mathrm{E} \underset{b_1\ (\text{or } b_2)}{\overset{f_1[\mathrm{S}_1]\ (\text{or } f_2[\mathrm{S}_2])}{\rightleftharpoons}} \mathrm{ES} \underset{c_1\ (\text{or } c_2)}{\overset{h_1[\mathrm{I}_1]\ (\text{or } h_2[\mathrm{I}_2])}{\rightleftharpoons}}$$

$$\mathrm{EIS} \underset{e_1[\mathrm{S}_1]\ (\text{or } e_2[\mathrm{S}_2])}{\overset{a_1\ (\text{or } a_2)}{\rightleftharpoons}} \mathrm{EI} \underset{g_1[\mathrm{I}_1]\ (\text{or } g_2[\mathrm{I}_2])}{\overset{d_1\ (\text{or } d_2)}{\rightleftharpoons}} \mathrm{E}. \tag{16}$$

It is sufficient for our purposes to note that at sufficiently high concentrations of the inhibitor, all of the transport enzyme will be in the form of EI or EIS, and transport would then be occurring on the modified transport enzyme EI. In this situation the resistance of the system Q^{SI} is given by $(1/e_1+1/e_2)$, while the coefficients of resistance R^{SI}_{12} and R^{SI}_{21} are $1/a_1$ and $1/a_2$. If these values are greater than those for the unmodified transport enzyme, namely $1/b_1$ and $1/b_2$, we will see inhibition with a reduced maximal velocity of transport. If, however, $Q^{\mathrm{S}}/R^{\mathrm{S}}_{12}$ and $Q^{\mathrm{S}}/R^{\mathrm{S}}_{21}$ happen to be equal to the corresponding values in the absence of inhibitor, the half-saturation concentrations will not be affected by the inhibitor. A plot of $1/v_{1\to 2}$ against $1/[\mathrm{SI}]$ will here again give a pencil of lines, but this time the pencil intersects on the $1/[\mathrm{S}]$ axis. This result is often found for transport systems and their inhibitors.

On the whole, then, the fact of inhibition of transport and the types of inhibition found derive readily from the simple model of Fig. 4 and Eq. (1), although the phenomenon of countertransport of a competitor is not predicted by the simple model. In what way does one have to modify or expand the simple model in order to account for those properties of transport systems which are not consistent with Fig. 4?

Table 1. Steady state values for two forms of the simple pore (LIEB 1981)

$$v_{1\to 2}=\frac{[S_1]}{Q+R_{12}[S_1]+R_{21}[S_2]}$$

	One state for ES	Two states for ES
$nR_{12}=$	$\frac{1}{b_2}$	$\frac{1}{b_2}+\frac{1}{g_1}+\frac{g_2}{b_2 g_1}$
$nR_{21}=$	$\frac{1}{b_1}$	$\frac{1}{b_1}+\frac{1}{g_2}+\frac{g_1}{b_1 g_2}$
$nQ\ =$	$\frac{1}{f_1}+\frac{1}{f_2}$	$\frac{1}{f_1}+\frac{1}{f_2}+\frac{b_1}{f_1 g_1}$
Constraint:	$b_1 f_2=b_2 f_1$	$b_1 f_2 g_2=b_2 f_1 g_1$

These results are for the special case of an uncharged (neutral) permeant (LIEB and STEIN 1974a). $v_{1\to 2}$ is the unidirectional flux of permeant from solution 1 to solution 2; the reverse flux $v_{2\to 1}$ is obtained by simply interchanging subscripts 1 and 2 in the equation. In the absence of unstirred layers, $[S_1]$ and $[S_2]$ are the concentrations of permeant in solutions 1 and 2, while n is the total concentration of pores. Notice that the steady state equations for $v_{1\to 2}$ and $v_{2\to 1}$ are independent of the form used when expressed in terms of the observable transport parameters Q, R_{12}, and R_{21}

4. A First Attempt to Improve the Simple Transport Model

Those properties of transport systems which are not predicted by the model of Fig. 4 are all of them properties which concern interaction between transport substrates across the two faces of the membrane. We have, for instance, the phenomenon of infinite-trans flow of label, where the trans presence of a high substrate concentration should, in Fig. 4, interfere with flow of label; yet, if anything, it often speeds up this flow. Similarly, for countertransport, the flows of substrate in the two opposite directions do not interfere with each other, but rather aid one another. It would seem that a more correct model would be one in which the equilibria between transport enzyme and substrate at the two faces of the membrane are shielded from one another, in that substrate at the trans face cannot compete with substrate that is binding at the cis face of the membrane. Let us see to what extent it will help matters if we put into the model of Fig. 4 a step in which the complex between transport enzyme and substrate moves across the membrane, thereby, perhaps, isolating the substrate–enzyme equilibria at the two membrane faces. We introduce therefore a conformation change $ES_1 \rightleftharpoons ES_2$ into the equations of transport, getting

$$S_1+E \underset{b_1}{\overset{f_1[S_1]}{\rightleftharpoons}} ES_1 \underset{g_2}{\overset{g_1}{\rightleftharpoons}} ES_2 \underset{f_2[S_2]}{\overset{b_2}{\rightleftharpoons}} S_2+E \tag{17}$$

in place of Eq. (1). We find that if we solve Eq. (17) just as we solved Eq. (1), taking account of the flux of substrate and of the concentration of the various forms of the transport enzyme, now [E], $[ES_1]$, and $[ES_2]$, we obtain an equation for the unidirectional flux of substrate which is identical with that of Eq. (8). The meanings of the parameters Q, R_{12}, and R_{21}, in terms of rate constants are now different from those for the case of the simpler Eq. (1), (these results are recorded in Table 1), but the resulting equation and hence the *predictions of the model* are unchanged. The addition of an extra conformation change in the transport enzyme–substrate complex does not rescue the model and it fails again to predict easily made experimental observations. What other way do we have out of this impasse?

5. A Second Attempt at Rescuing the Model

Since introducing a conformation change of the transport enzyme–substrate complex has not helped us, would it help instead to introduce a conformational change of the free transport enzyme? We introduce a conformational change $E_1 \rightleftharpoons E_2$ into the equations of transport and get

$$S_1 + E_1 \underset{b_1}{\overset{f_1[S_1]}{\rightleftharpoons}} ES \underset{f_2[S_2]}{\overset{b_2}{\rightleftharpoons}} S_2 + E_2 , \tag{18}$$

$$E_1 \underset{k_2}{\overset{k_1}{\rightleftharpoons}} E_2 . \tag{19}$$

If we now solve Eqs. (18) and (19), just as we solved Eq. (1), we obtain this time, instead of Eq. (8), the equation

$$v_{1\to 2} = \frac{K[S_1] + [S_1][S_2]}{K^2 R_{oo} + KR_{12}[S_1] + KR_{21}[S_2] + R_{ee}[S_1][S_2]} , \tag{20}$$

where the meanings of the terms in K and R are as listed in Table 2. Now this equation is quite different from Eq. (8). Does it enable us to account for the properties of the transport systems? By putting $[S_2]=0$ in Eq. (20), we can derive the predictions of the zero-trans experiment. Inspection of Eq. (20) reveals that an equation of similar form to that of Eq. (9) is derived, with a maximum velocity, a maximum permeability, and a half-saturation concentration term given easily in terms of K and the R terms, as recorded in Table 3. Similarly, by putting $[S_1]=[S_2]=[S]$ in Eq. (20), we can derive the predictions of the equilibrium exchange experiment. Again, an acceptable form in terms of a maximum velocity of exchange and a half-saturation concentration is found, with the relevant parameters and their interpretation as recorded in Table 3. If, for the infinite-trans experiment, we now set $[S_2]$ equal to infinity in Eq. (20) and solve for the resulting unidirectional flux, we obtain

$$v_{1\to 2}^{it} = \frac{(1/R_{ee})[S_1]}{K\dfrac{R_{21}}{R_{ee}} + [S_1]} \tag{21a}$$

a form with a definite flux at any $[S_1]$, a maximum velocity, a maximum permeability, and half-saturation concentration (Table 3) perfectly able to account for the available experimental observations.

Table 2. Steady state values for two forms of the simple carrier (LIEB and STEIN 1974, 1976; LIEB 1982)

$$v_{1\to 2} = \frac{(K+[S_2])[S_1]}{K^2R_{oo}+KR_{12}[S_1]+KR_{21}[S_2]+R_{ee}[S_1][S_2]}$$

	One state for ES	Two states for ES
$nR_{12}=$	$\frac{1}{b_2}+\frac{1}{k_2}$	$\frac{1}{b_2}+\frac{1}{k_2}+\frac{1}{g_1}+\frac{g_2}{b_2g_1}$
$nR_{21}=$	$\frac{1}{b_1}+\frac{1}{k_1}$	$\frac{1}{b_1}+\frac{1}{k_1}+\frac{1}{g_2}+\frac{g_1}{b_1g_2}$
$nR_{ee}=$	$\frac{1}{b_1}+\frac{1}{b_2}$	$\frac{1}{b_1}+\frac{1}{b_2}+\frac{1}{g_1}+\frac{1}{g_2}+\frac{g_1}{b_1g_2}+\frac{g_2}{b_2g_1}$
$nR_{oo}=$	$\frac{1}{k_1}+\frac{1}{k_2}$	$\frac{1}{k_1}+\frac{1}{k_2}$
$K=$	$\frac{k_1}{f_1}+\frac{k_2}{f_2}$	$\frac{k_1}{f_1}+\frac{k_2}{f_2}+\frac{b_1k_1}{f_1g_1}$
Constraint:	$b_1f_2k_1=b_2f_1k_2$	$b_1f_2g_2k_1=b_2f_1g_1k_2$

These results are for the special case of an uncharged (neutral) permeant. Definitions as Table 1

At last, we have an equation for the unidirectional flux (Eq. (20)), which is able to account for the infinite-trans experiment! The equilibria of Eqs. (18) and (19) seem to be good candidates for the transport system model. The infinite-cis experiment is accounted for by taking Eq. (20) and deriving the net flux of substrate in the 1 to 2 direction, when the $[S_1]$ term goes to infinity. We obtain

$$\text{Net}^{ic}_{1\to 2} = \frac{K/R_{ee}}{K\frac{R_{12}}{R_{ee}}+[S_2]} \tag{21b}$$

an equation which adequately accounts for data for infinite-*cis* experiments. A measurable net flow $(=1/R_{12})$ is observed in the absence of substrate at face 2, and this flow is reduced by the addition of substrate at face 2, along a curve showing a typical half-saturation behavior (Table 3). Finally, for the countertransport experiment, Eq. (20) gives us the unidirectional flux in the 1 to 2 direction for substrate, while the flow of substrate in the opposite direction is given by the right-hand side of this equation with the subscripts 1 and 2 interchanged, and the flow of label in this direction being obtained by multiplying this expression by the dilution of label $[S_1]/[S_2]$. The numerator of the resulting expression is then $[S_1]([S_2]-[S_1])$ and will be positive whenever $[S_2]$ is greater than $[S_1]$. That is, a counterflow of S will occur if the label at the *trans* face is diluted by unlabeled substrate. The countertransport procedure (Fig. 6) is accounted for by Eqs. (18) and (19). We have then a model which accounts for the behavior of many systems. What is there special about Eqs. (18) and (19) which enables them to do such a good job of accounting for transport?

Table 3. Interpretation of experimental data in terms of the basic observable parameters for the simple pore and carrier. After LIEB (1982)

Procedure	v_{max}	K_m	Maximum permeability
	Simple pore		
Zero-trans	$v^{zt}_{1\to 2}=\frac{1}{R_{12}}$	$K^{zt}_{1\to 2}=\frac{Q}{R_{12}}$	$1/Q$
	$v^{zt}_{2\to 1}=\frac{1}{R_{21}}$	$K^{zt}_{2\to 1}=\frac{Q}{R_{21}}$	$1/Q$
Equilibrium exchange	$v^{ee}=\frac{1}{R_{ee}}$	$K^{ee}=\frac{Q}{R_{ee}}$	$1/Q$
Constraint:	$R_{ee}=R_{12}+R_{21}$		
	Simple carrier		
Procedure	v_{max}	K_m	Maximum permeability
Zero-trans	$v^{zt}_{1\to 2}=\frac{1}{R_{12}}$	$K^{zt}_{1\to 2}=K\frac{R_{oo}}{R_{12}}$	$1/KR_{oo}$
	$v^{zt}_{2\to 1}=\frac{1}{R_{21}}$	$K^{zt}_{2\to 1}=K\frac{R_{oo}}{R_{21}}$	$1/KR_{oo}$
Infinite-trans	$v^{it}=v^{it}_{1\to 2}$	$K^{it}_{1\to 2}=K\frac{R_{21}}{R_{ee}}$	$1/KR_{21}$
	$=v^{it}_{2\to 1}=\frac{1}{R_{ee}}$	$K^{it}_{2\to 1}=K\frac{R_{12}}{R_{ee}}$	$1/KR_{12}$
Infinite-cis	$v^{ic}_{1\to 2}=\frac{1}{R_{12}}$	$K^{ic}_{1\to 2}=K\frac{R_{12}}{R_{ee}}$	
	$v^{ic}_{2\to 1}=\frac{1}{R_{12}}$	$K^{ic}_{2\to 1}=K\frac{R_{21}}{R_{ee}}$	
Equilibrium exchange	$v^{ee}=\frac{1}{R_{ee}}$	$K^{ee}=K\frac{R_{oo}}{R_{ee}}$	$1/KR_{oo}$
Constraint:	$R_{ee}+R_{oo}=R_{12}+R_{21}$		

6. Transport on the Carrier Model

A pictorial representation of the model described by Eqs. (18) and (19) is seen in Fig. 7. This figure emphasizes the essential feature of all such models: the equilibrium at face 1 of the membrane between substrate and the transport enzyme is shielded from substrate at face 2. In contrast, in Fig. 4, substrate at both membrane faces was able simultaneously to interact with transport enzyme. The essential feature of Fig. 7 is that the enzyme undergoes a change of position, involving availability to substrate, as it transforms between the two forms E_1 and E_2. This

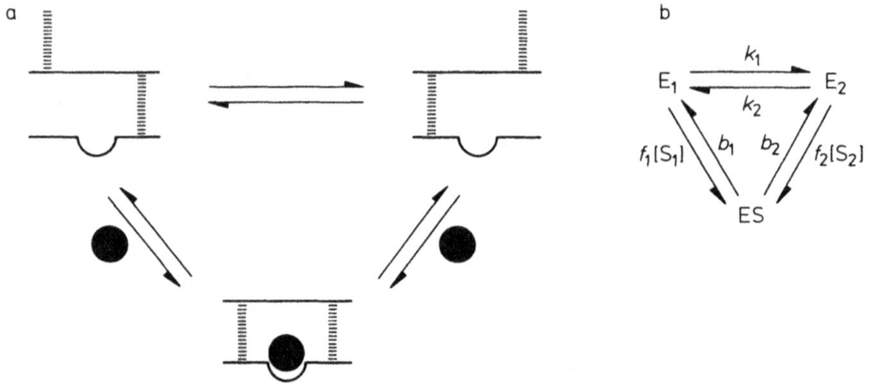

Fig. 7. a Schematic representation of the simple carrier, in its three-state form. The *spheres* represent a substrate molecule, while the *bars* represent "gates" which open or close with the conformation change of the carrier. **b** Formal representation of the model in terms of chemical reactions. LIEB and STEIN (1976)

transformation must involve a conformational change of the transport enzyme, a change which occurs as the free enzyme interconverts from E_1 to the E_2 form, in addition to that which occurs when the enzyme is bound to substrate. While the enzyme is bound to substrate and the conformational change occurs, the substrate itself is carried across the membrane. Thus, the transport enzyme which behaves as in Eqs. (18) and (19) is entitled to the designation of a carrier. We have called such a model the "simple carrier," while the model of Fig. 4 and Eq. (1), where there is no physical movement of the transport enzyme itself, we have termed a "simple pore" (LIEB and STEIN 1974a, b). Any transport experiment in which saturation behavior is demonstrated or in which inhibition is shown can be accounted for as well by a simple pore as by a simple carrier, but those experiments such as the infinite-*trans* or infinite-*cis* procedures or the phenomenon of countertransport need for their explanation the unique properties of the simple carrier. It is amusing to note that it is the conformational change of the free enzyme that is required for the kinetic treatment. If we allow for ES being in two states, as in Eq. (17) for the simple pore, i.e., if we replace Eq. (18) by

$$S_1 + E_1 \rightleftharpoons ES_1 \rightleftharpoons ES_2 \rightleftharpoons S_2 + E_2 \tag{22}$$

for the simple carrier, Eqs. (8) and (20) are derived. Table 2 records the interpretation of the K and R parameters of Eq. (20) in terms of the rate constants of Eq. (22).

It must be emphasized that the difference between pore and carrier is absolutely fundamental. From the fact of the conformational change that the carrier undergoes as it crosses the membrane, with or without substrate, follow the exceedingly important coupling properties which are the basis of the phenomena of bioenergetics. The active transport systems – bioenergetic machines – which we will go on later to describe, work only because their working substance is a transport enzyme which can exist in at least two different conformational forms, facing towards opposite sides of a biologic membrane.

We see, therefore, that the distinctive properties of membrane transport systems are well represented by the formalism of Eq. (20). It is worthwhile for us to enter a little more deeply into the meanings of the different terms of Eq. (20) for this will give us a broader picture of what behavior we might expect from a simple carrier. The terms in R are, again, coefficients of resistance. R_{12} determines the maximum velocity of the zero-*trans* flow in the 1 to 2 direction, R_{21} the same in the 2 to 1 direction and R_{ee} gives the maximum velocity of the equilibrium exchange experiment and also the infinite-*trans* experiment. It follows from the definition of these R terms (Table 2) that $R_{oo} = R_{12} + R_{21} - R_{ee}$. These R terms are themselves determined (see Table 2) by the rate constants for breakdown of the ES complex and the rate constants for transmembrane movement of the free carrier (or strictly speaking, the rate of the conformational change that transforms the E forms into one another). The parameter K is the sum of the dissociation constants for the breakdown of the ES complex into free carrier and substrate at side 1 and at side 2 of the membrane. It itself determines, together with combinations of the R terms, the half-saturation concentrations for substrate in the various experimental procedures (Table 3). Thus, for example, the half-saturation concentration for the zero-*trans* experiment in the 1 to 2 direction is given by $K\, R_{oo}/R_{12}$, while that for the reverse direction is the same expression with subscripts 1 and 2 interchanges. The "maximum permeability" of the membrane for the substrate, that is, the ratio of flow (or flux) to substrate concentration in the linear range of the flux versus concentration curve is given by $1/(K\, R_{oo})$, for all of the various experimental parameters. The following features of the carrier model can easily be understood from Eq. (20):

1. No net flow will occur against a concentration gradient of the substrate. The numerator of the expression for net flow in the 1 to 2 direction is $K([S_1] - [S_2])$ and has the same sign as the concentration gradient.
2. Flow or flux can show saturation behavior.
3. Transport behavior of the system can be markedly asymmetric; the maximum velocities of zero-*trans* flow are given by $1/R_{12}$ and $1/R_{21}$ and these can be quite different from each other, depending on the fine details of the reaction scheme and, hence, on the rate constants of Eqs. (18) and (19).
4. The "maximum permeability," however, being given by $K\, R_{oo}$, is the same in both directions.
5. Hence, it follows that, in spite of any possible asymmetry, the ratio of maximum velocity to half-saturation concentration in one direction must be equal to the same ratio in the other direction, both being given by the value of $K\, R_{oo}$.
6. The maximum velocity of the equilibrium exchange experiment or of the infinite-*trans* experiment can certainly be greater than that of the zero-*trans* experiment in either direction. That is, unlabeled substrate at the *trans* face will often speed up the unidirectional flux of substrate measured from the *cis* face. If the exchange experiment gives a faster maximum velocity than for a zero-*trans* procedure, it follows (Tables 2 and 3) that the fully loaded carrier breaks down to liberate substrate at a particular face more rapidly than the free carrier interconverts towards that face.
7. However, the exchange experiment may yield a lower maximum velocity than a zero-*trans* experiment, if the ES breakdown is slower than the relevant E_1

Table 4. Uridine transport across the human red blood cell membrane (LIEB 1982)

Experimental values (± standard error)

Procedure	Direction	v_{max} (mM/min)	K_m (mM)
Zero-trans	In→out	$v^{zt}_{1\to2}=1.98\ (\pm0.31)$	$K^{zt}_{1\to2}=0.40\ (\pm0.12)$
	Out→in	$v^{zt}_{2\to1}=0.53\ (\pm0.038)$	$K^{zt}_{2\to1}=0.073\ (\pm0.069)$
Infinite-cis	In→out	$v^{ic}_{1\to2}\equiv v^{zt}_{1\to2}$	$K^{ic}_{1\to2}=0.252\ (\pm0.096)$
	Out→in	$v^{ic}_{2\to1}\equiv v^{zt}_{2\to1}$	$K^{ic}_{2\to1}=0.937\ (\pm0.226)$
Equilibrium	Both	$v^{ee}=7.54\ (\pm0.45)$	$K^{ee}=1.29\ (\pm0.11)$

Simple carrier resistance parameters (± standard error)

R (min/mM)	nR (ms)
$R_{12}=(v^{zt}_{1\to2})^{-1}=0.505\ (\pm0.079)$;	$nR_{12}=10.1\ (\pm1.6)$
$R_{21}=(v^{zt}_{2\to1})^{-1}=1.887\ (\pm0.135)$;	$nR_{21}=37.7\ (\pm2.7)$
$R_{ee}=(v^{ee})^{-1}=0.133\ (\pm0.008)$;	$nR_{ee}=2.7\ (\pm0.16)$
$R_{oo}=R_{12}-R_{21}-R_{ee}=2.259\ (\pm0.157)$;	$nR_{oo}=45.1\ (\pm3.1)$

Independent estimates of simple carrier affinity parameter K (± standard error)

Estimated using:	Value (μM) (± standard error)
$K=K^{zt}_{1\to2}(R_{12}/R_{oo})$	89 (±31)
$K=K^{zt}_{2\to1}(R_{21}/R_{oo})$	61 (±58)
$K=K^{ic}_{1\to2}(R_{ee}/R_{12})$	66 (±28)
$K=K^{ic}_{2\to1}(R_{ee}/R_{21})$	66 (±17)
$K=K^{ee}(R_{ee}/R_{oo})$	76 (±10)
	Mean (± standard deviation) = 72 (±11) μM

Values calculated in terms of the simple carrier model, and the rate constants of Figs. 7 and 8

$27\ (\pm2)\,s^{-1}<k_1<29\ (\pm2)\,s^{-1}$

$99\ (\pm16)\,s^{-1}<k_2<135\ (\pm29)\,s^{-1}$

$b_1, b_2, g_1, g_2>370\ (\pm22)\,s^{-1}$

$f_1>3.7\ (\pm0.6)\times10^5\,M^{-1}s^{-1}$

$f_2>1.4\ (\pm0.3)\times10^6\,M^{-1}s^{-1}$

All inequalities involving b_1, b_2, f_1, f_2, k_1, and k_2 are valid for both the one-complex formulation and the two-complex formulation of the simple carrier. Solution 1 here refers to the cytoplasm. Values (± standard error) were calculated using the relationships given in Table 2 and the experimental values of K, nR_{12}, nR_{21}, nR_{ee}, and nR_{oo} listed. The experimental values are taken directly from CABANTCHIK and GINSBURG (1977), for uridine transport into and out of the human red blood cell at 25° C. The unit mM in both v_{max} and the resistance parameters is shorthand for mmol uridine per liter isotonic cell water. To obtain the values of nR in the table, LIEB used a value of $n=3.3\times10^{-4}$ mmol uridine transport systems per liter isotonic cell water. This value was obtained from the average number of nitrobenzylthioinosine high affinity binding sites (12500 sites per cell; CASS et al. 1974), assuming one site per transport system, and taking the average red cell volume to be 87 μm³ and the average water content to be 71.7% v/v

to E_2 (or E_2 to E_1) interconversion. Surprisingly, these situations are very infrequently found experimentally, transstimulation being almost invariably found, when a *trans* effect is noted.

We have seen that a number of different procedures can be used to derive the K and R parameters of the simple carrier. There are the equilibrium exchange experiment, the two zero-*trans* procedures (one in each direction), two infinite-*trans* and two infinite-*cis* procedures, and two countertransport experiments. The K and R terms themselves number just four independent variables (since the R terms are themselves interconnected) and, therefore, are heavily overdetermined experimentally. Consistent tests can thus be provided for the applicability of the carrier model to any transport systems. A full treatment, characterizing and testing the simple carrier model, has been applied to a number of transport systems (CABANTCHIK and GINSBURG 1977; LIEB 1982). The results of such testing for three well-studied systems in the human red blood cell are given by LIEB (1982). The most completely understood system is that for uridine transport in the human erythrocyte (Table 4). It behaves as a simple carrier, asymmetric and displaying transstimulation in both directions across the membrane. Yet it is, of course, a simple equilibrating (that is, not actively transporting) system, in spite of its clear asymmetry. Equation (20) applies exactly to this system.

A careful analysis of the relations between the various R terms allows bounds to be set to the ratio of the rate constants for the carrier model as described in Eqs. (18) and (19). These bounds are also listed in Table 4, for the case of the uridine carrier system. Certain of these bounds are sufficiently close together to provide quite good estimates of the values of certain rate constants, and here the absolute number of carrier molecules per cell has been estimated by labeling the transport system (CASS et al. 1974).

A particular case of the carrier model, important for the situations of the coupling of two flows that we will deal with later, is that where transport of the free carrier cannot occur. Only carrier bound to substrate can undergo a conformation change and thus all transport will be only the exchange of two substrates across the membrane, those two substrates sharing the same carrier. Equations (18) or (22) apply to this situation without the addition of Eq. (19), which describes the transformation of unloaded carrier. Solving the unidirectional flux equations for this model gives

$$v_{1\to 2}=\frac{[S_1][S_2](1/R_{ee})}{K_1[S_2]+K_2[S_1]+[S_1][S_2]}, \tag{23}$$

where the terms in K are the affinity parameters, defined for Eq. (18) as the *off* constants divided by the *on* constants (b/f), for the formation of ES complexes, while R_{ee} is a coefficient of resistance given by $(1/b_1+1/b_2)$. For Eq. (22) these terms are appropriately modified by g_1 and g_2.

$$K_1\frac{b_1}{f_1}\left(\frac{g_2}{g_1+g_2}\right)$$

K_2 is the same with subscripts 1 and 2 interchanged, while R_{ee} is as defined in Table 2 for the four-state model. For any value of the substrate concentration at the cis face $[S_1]$ the flux depends on the trans concentration $[S_2]$. Both the maximum velocity and the half-saturation concentration for $[S_1]$ are dependent on $[S_2]$, but the maximum permeability, at limitingly low $[S_1]$, is independent of $[S_2]$. The half-saturation parameter, K_m, when $[S_2]$ is limitingly large, is given by K_1.

7. Inhibition Kinetics of the Carrier

The existence of the interconversion between the two conformations of the carrier in the carrier model of Fig. 7 has some important implications for the kinetics of the inhibition of transport systems, and it is worthwhile for these findings to obtain a wider hearing among pharmacologists. Pioneering studies in the field of carrier inhibition kinetics have been made by BAKER and WIDDAS (1973), by DEVES and KRUPKA (1978, 1979), and by EDWARDS (1972, 1973 a, b, 1974), while the author, together with W. R. LIEB, has also published in this field (LIEB and STEIN 1976).

We must first distinguish between two major classes of inhibitors. In the first class are the irreversible inhibitors, whose effects are best understood as classic chemical reactions between the inhibitor or drug and the transport system. Washing away the inhibitor does not lead to the restoration of transport activity; hence, the action is irreversible. Like any chemical reaction, the process of inhibition takes a measurable, often quite considerable, time to develop, and with a high enough ratio of inhibitor to transport system, inhibition should eventually be total at any inhibitor concentration. In contrast, the reversible inhibitors will reach an equilibrium level of inhibition at any level of inhibitor concentration, and (hence) transport activity will be restored when the inhibitor concentration is reduced on washing the system in inhibitor-free medium. These reversible inhibitors can themselves be further subclassified into competitive and noncompetitive inhibitors, as we shall see.

a) Irreversible Inhibition Studies

The approach one can use to understand the effects of irreversible inhibitors on transport systems can be clarified by reference to Fig. 8. Here is depicted the conventional carrier model (two states of E and two states of ES), with reversible transport interconversions between the various conformations of this model given by the rate constants of the figure. Irreversible reactions with some inhibitor are described by the rate constant in q, each state of the model being able to react with the inhibitor at a different rate. If the irreversible inhibition does occur at a rate differing with the various states of the carrier, situations where the substrate is or is not present, or is present at different concentrations across the membrane, should cause a redistribution of the carrier and hence affect the rate of inhibition by the irreversible inhibitor. Only if all the rates, symbolized by the terms in q, are everywhere the same will a redistribution of the carrier in response to substrate gradient not affect the rate of inhibition. LIEB and STEIN (1976) have worked out the fully general treatment of the model of Fig. 8, of the model with only one form of ES (the case of Fig. 7), and a model with both the E and the ES forms existing as intermediate forms within the membrane. All these three models

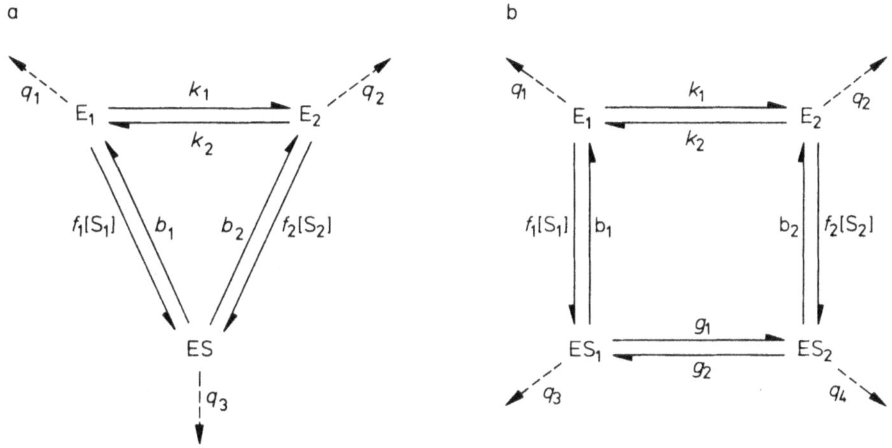

Fig. 8 a, b. Reactions leading to irreversible inhibition of the simple carrier. **a** three-state form; **b** four-state form. The terms in q are the rate constants for the irreversible interaction of inhibitor with corresponding forms of the carrier. LIEB and STEIN (1976)

give precisely the same mathematical form for the equation describing the effect of substrate concentrations on the rate of inhibition by an irreversible inhibitor. (Thus, such studies do not, once again, allow one to distinguish between the various types of models, within the framework of the carrier model, but do allow one further to test and characterize the carrier, in conjunction with transport studies.)

The relevant equation is

$$q=\frac{K^2Q_{oo}R_{oo}+KQ_{12}R_{12}[S_1]+KQ_{21}R_{21}[S_2]+Q_{ee}R_{ee}[S_1][S_2]}{K^2R_{oo}+KR_{12}[S_1]+KR_{21}[S_2]+R_{ee}[S_1][S_2]}, \tag{24}$$

where q is the rate of inactivation by the irreversible inhibitor, as a function of the substrate concentrations $[S_1]$ and $[S_2]$ at sides 1 and 2 of the membrane. The symbols in R and K are as defined in Table 2, for the carrier models, while the symbols in Q have the definitions listed in Table 5 and involve combinations of the rate constants for the irreversible inhibition step and for the transport steps. These parameters in Q are, once again, the experimentally derivable parameters, descriptive of the inactivation process in the various situations of transport experiments. Thus, considering Eq. (24), we find that:

1. For the situation in the absence of substrate, when $[S_1]=[S_2]=0$, the rate $q=Q_{oo}$.
2. For the zero-*trans* case (at infinite-*cis*), where $[S_1]\to\infty$, while $[S_2]=0$, $q=Q_{12}$.
3. For the corresponding case where $[S_1]=0$, while $[S_2]$ is limitingly high, $q=Q_{21}$.
4. Where both $[S_1]$ and $[S_2]$ are limitingly high (and equal), in the equilibrium exchange situation, $q=Q_{ee}$.

Thus, the terms in Q are analogous to the coefficients of resistance terms in R, are obtained in the same sorts of experimental situations and, for a system which behaves as a simple carrier, are related by $Q_{12}R_{12}+Q_{21}R_{21}=Q_{ee}R_{ee}+Q_{oo}-R_{oo}$. This relation is indeed a test for a simple carrier.

Table 5. Kinetic parameters for irreversible inhibition of the simple carrier

$$q=\frac{K^2Q_{oo}R_{oo}+KQ_{12}R_{12}[S_1]+KQ_{21}R_{21}[S_2]+Q_{ee}R_{ee}[S_1][S_2]}{K^2R_{oo}+KR_{12}[S_1]+KR_{21}[S_2]+R_{ee}[S_1][S_2]}$$

One state for ES	Two states for ES
$Q_{12}nR_{12}=\frac{q_2}{k_2}+\frac{q_3}{b_2}$	$\frac{q_2}{k_2}+\frac{q_4}{b_2}+\frac{q_3}{g_1}\left(\frac{b_2+g_2}{b_2}\right)$
$Q_{21}nR_{21}=\frac{q_1}{k_1}+\frac{q_3}{b_1}$	$\frac{q_1}{k_1}+\frac{q_3}{b_1}+\frac{q_4}{g_2}\left(\frac{b_1+g_1}{b_1}\right)$
$Q_{ee}nR_{ee}=q_3\left(\frac{1}{b_1}+\frac{1}{b_2}\right)$	$q_3\left[\frac{1}{b_1}+\frac{1}{g_1}\left(\frac{b_2+g_2}{b_2}\right)\right]+q_4\left[\frac{1}{b_2}+\frac{1}{g_2}\left(\frac{b_1+g_1}{b_1}\right)\right]$
$Q_{oo}nR_{oo}=\frac{q_1}{k_1}+\frac{q_2}{k_2}$	$\frac{q_1}{k_1}+\frac{q_2}{k_2}$
Constraint: $b_1f_2k_1=b_2f_1k_2$	$b_1f_2g_2k_1=b_2f_1g_1k_2$

Terms in [S], R, and K defined in Table 2. Rate constants defined in Fig. 9a for the one-state model of ES, Fig. 9b for the two-state model of ES

It is often convenient to look at the difference between the inactivation rate in the presence of substrate and the rate in the absence of substrate. We saw from Eq. (24) that the inactivation rate in the complete absence of substrate was Q_{oo}. Then, at any substrate concentration, we can define Δq as the effect of the substrate concentrations on the rate of inactivation; Δq is given by $q-Q_{oo}$, and we can rewrite Eq. (24) as

$$\Delta q=\frac{K(\Delta Q_{12})R_{12}[S_1]+K(\Delta Q_{21})R_{21}[S_2]+(\Delta Q_{ee})R_{ee}[S_1][S_2]}{K^2R_{oo}+KR_{12}[S_1]+KR_{21}[S_2]+R_{ee}[S_1][S_2]} \tag{25}$$

where $\Delta Q_{ee}=Q_{ee}-Q_{oo}$, $\Delta Q_{12}=Q_{12}-Q_{oo}$, and $\Delta Q_{21}=Q_{21}-Q_{oo}$. This equation now gives us the effect of the addition of substrate on the rate of the inactivation reaction. To take one example, we might consider the zero-trans situation where only the concentration $[S_1]$ is varied. Then, Eq. (25) reduces to the equation

$$\Delta q^{zt}_{1\to 2}=\frac{(\Delta Q_{12})[S_1]}{(KR_{oo}/R_{12})+[S_1]} \tag{26}$$

(for the zero-*trans* case in the 1 to 2 direction) which is a typical Michaelis form, analogous to that of enzyme kinetics. Thus, the effect of a zero-*trans* substrate on the rate of the inactivation reaction is describable in terms of a half-saturation concentration or Michaelis parameter (compare Table 3). This has exactly the same value as is found for the corresponding (zero-*trans*) transport experiment. An analogous result is found for the equilibrium exchange case. Thus, studies with irreversible inhibitors enable the Michaelis parameters of the transport model to be determined. These are useful in themselves, and the testing of their identity with the corresponding terms derived from pure transport experiments is in each case a validity test for the carrier model. The basis of this identity of results is clear. Both the rates of transport systems and the rates by which these are inhibited irreversibly depend on the distribution across the membrane of the various states of the carrier. Whether it is transport or inhibition that is being measured, the underlying carrier distribution will be identically determined by the substrate concentrations.

It is of interest also to see how the simple pore might be expected to behave in the presence of an irreversible inhibitor. The simple pore exists, of course, in only two kinetically distinguishable states, E and ES. If these react with the irreversible inhibitor at different rates, q_E and q_{ES}, respectively, then the rate of inactivation can readily be shown to be given by the equation

$$q = \frac{q_E Q + q_{ES}(R_{12}[S_1] + R_{21}[S_2])}{Q + R_{12}[S_1] + R_{21}[S_2]} \tag{26a}$$

where Q and the terms in R are as defined in Table 1. The rate of inactivation in the absence of any substrate is q_E, while the rate of inactivation when substrate is present at limitingly high concentrations at either side of the membrane, or at both sides, is the single value q_{ES}. Thus, in contrast to the simple carrier (where the rate of inactivation could be quite different for substrate at limitingly high concentrations at side 1, as opposed to side 2 of the membrane) for the pore no such difference exists. That the presence of substrate affects the rate of inactivation by an irreversible inhibitor is an indication merely of a conformational change when substrate binds to transport enzyme, and will be found both for the pore and for the carrier. However, a finding that the maximal effect of presence of substrate is different depending on whether substrate is on one side, on the other, or on both sides of the membrane, is a result that is inconsistent with a pore but perfectly consistent with a carrier, and is a result of the defining property of a carrier, that it exists free in two forms, interconversion between these forms being separated by an activation energy barrier. For both the glucose transport system of the human red cell (EDWARDS 1973; JUNG 1974) and the choline transport system of this cell (EDWARDS 1973a, b), different maximal values of inhibition were found (using the irreversible inhibitors *N*-ethyl-maleimide and 2,4-fluorodinitrobenzene) in experiments where the substrate was present on one side of the membrane, on the other, or on both sides. Thus, for these systems one must, once again, reject the simple pore as a model. The data for glucose are, apparently not consistent with the simple carrier model either (LIEB and STEIN 1976).

b) Reversible Inhibitor Studies, Nonpenetrating Inhibitors

We begin by considering reversible inhibitors that do not penetrate the membrane using the carrier system which they inhibit. This class comprises very many compounds of great pharmacologic interest, for instance, phlorhizin and phloretine as inhibitors of intestinal glucose transport, the drug cytochalasin-B as an inhibitor of red cell (and intestinal) transport of sugar, oubain as an inhibitor of the sodium pump in very many tissues, and so on. A general model for the action of such inhibitors on transport carriers is depicted in Figs. 9a and 9b, for the case of the simplified carrier (of Fig. 7) and for the conventional representation (of

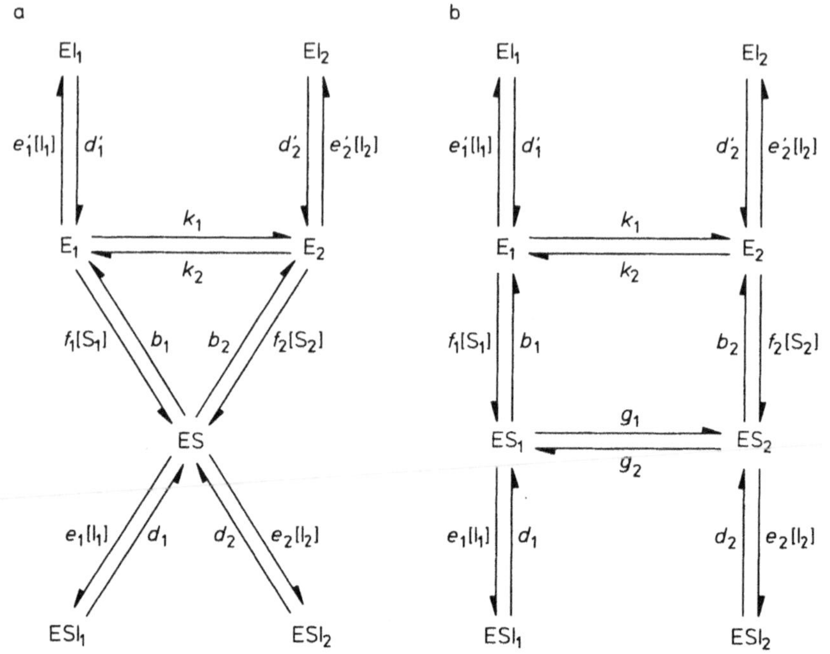

Fig. 9 a, b. Reactions leading to reversible inhibition of the simple carrier. **a** three-state form; **b** four-state form. I is the inhibitor

Fig. 8). We shall allow all forms of the carrier, E_1, E_2 and ES forms to bind reversibly to the inhibitor, with rate constants for these interactions as depicted in the figures. It can easily be shown that the kinetic analysis gives a very simple result: for Figs. 9a and 9b (and similar figures), it is sufficient merely to replace in the results collected in Table 2 any rate constant c leading *from* a form interacting with inhibitor, by the term $c/(1+e[\mathrm{I}]/d)$, where e is the on constant for the reaction leading to the formation of the inhibitor-form complex, while d is the off constant for this reaction, and [I] is the concentration of inhibitor. This result follows because the action of the inhibitor is to draw the equilibrium between unbound and bound form of any complex over into the bound form, reducing the effective concentration of the relevant unbound form, and hence reducing the reaction rates leading from that form. We can see immediately, therefore, by referring each time to Table 2, that if the inhibitor does not bind to either ES form but only to the free E forms, the b and g rate constants in Table 2 will be unaltered and, hence, R_{ee} will be unaffected by inhibitor. R_{ee} determines the maximum velocity of the equilibrium exchange reaction which is thus unaffected by such an inhibitor. On the other hand, if the inhibitor binds only to the ES form (or forms) and not to either E form, rate constants in k and f are unaffected by the presence of inhibitor, the term K is unaffected and likewise the term R_{oo}. Hence, the maximum permeability, i.e., the rate of transport at limitingly low concentrations of substrate, will be unaffected by inhibitor, although all maximum velocities will be so affected. Results worked out in this way for the various possible inhibition patterns are collected in a forthcoming monograph (Stein, manuscript in preparation).

We shall consider in greater detail two important cases. First, we consider the situation where the inhibitor binds only to the free carrier, so that it effectively competes with the transported substrate. Will this case always display the kinetics of competitive inhibition? Since only the E forms bind inhibitor, only rate constants in f and k will be affected. If we consider substrate to be present, now only at face 1 of the membrane, then in a zero-*trans* experiment in the 1 to 2 direction, the R_{12} term which determines the maximum velocity here, contains only terms in b_2 and k_2, and thus is unaffected by the inhibitor. The R_{oo} term is affected however, and the net result of adding inhibitor (see Table 3) is to increase K_m, leaving V_{max} unaffected. Such a result would be interpreted as pure competitive inhibition (correctly). However, for the zero-*trans* experiment in the 2 to 1 direction, the term R_{21} is affected by the inhibitor, as is R_{oo}. Thus, the maximum velocity would be reduced and K_m increased, although V/K would be unaffected. This would be interpreted (wrongly) as showing purely uncompetitive inhibition. Therefore, the same inhibitor, binding reversibly and competing with substrate at face 1 of the membrane would display competitive inhibition kinetics when transport in the 1 to 2 direction was measured, but would display uncompetitive kinetics when transport was measured in the 2 to 1 direction. Equilibrium exchange would display purely competitive kinetics. This result follows directly from the carrier model, and is indeed a test for the applicability of the carrier model (or rather, for the inapplicability of the simple pore model). The physical basis of the result is that the interaction between substrate or inhibitor and transport enzyme will be a real competition when these are present on the same side of the membrane, but when they are on opposite sides the activation energy barrier for the transition between the two forms E_1 and E_2 of the carrier prevents direct competition between the two ligands. This point has been clearly made by DEVES and KRUPKA (1978) in their penetrating analysis of the phenomenon of inhibition of glucose transport in human red cells by cytochalasin-B. This was shown by some workers to be a competitive, and by others an uncompetitive, inhibitor. DEVES and KRUPKA showed that these puzzling results could be reconciled by a full analysis of the kinetics of carrier inhibition, as we have already discussed.

The second case we shall consider is the use that can be made of nonpenetrating, noncompetitive inhibitors to enable a distinction to be made between the three-state model of Fig. 9a and the four-state model of Fig. b. The experimental approach which can be used is to study how the maximum velocities of the zero-*trans* procedures are differentially affected by the presence of nonpenetrating inhibitor on one or the other side of the membrane. To begin with, we consider the three-state model of Fig. 9a. From our theoretical considerations just discussed as well as from Tables 2 and 3, the slope of a plot of $1/V_{12}^{zt}$, the relevant maximum velocity, against the concentration of inhibitor when this is present at side 1 only, is given by $\{e_1/(d_1+d_2)\}/b_2$. Similarly, the slope of the plot of $1/V_{21}^{zt}$, for the experiment performed in the other direction, but with the inhibitor still present on side 1, is given by $\{e_1/(d_1+d_2)\}/b_1$. Thus, the *ratio* of these slopes, or the relative effectiveness of the inhibitor in inhibiting the two zero-*trans* flows is given by b_1/b_2. The rate constants for the inhibitor itself cancel out of the final expression. If this whole procedure is now repeated, with the nonpenetrating inhibitor present at side 2 of the membrane, the same considerations lead to precisely the same expression for the relative effectiveness of the inhibitor. It again inhibits these two flows in the term b_1/b_2, regardless of where the inhibitor itself is situated.

This result is not found for the case of the four-state model of Fig. 9b. If the entire analysis is performed for these experimental situations for the model in which the two states ES_1 and ES_2 are separated by an activation energy barrier, then the effectiveness of the inhibitor will depend upon which side of the membrane it is placed. Only if the rate constants g_1 and g_2 are very high in comparison with the rate constants b_1 and b_2, respectively, will the inhibitor show no sidedness of its effectivity. Indeed, if the inhibitor shows sidedness in its action, that is, if it affects the zero-*trans* flow much more strongly *from* the side at which it is present than *to* the side at which it is present, the simplified model of Fig. 9a can be ruled out in favor of the conventional model of Fig. 9b. The degree of sidedness of the inhibitor in inhibiting the two zero-*trans* flows gives a measure of the ratio of the rate constant for transmembrane movement of the loaded carrier to the rate constant for the dissociation of the carrier–substrate complex, the b and g terms in Fig. 9b. A comparison of a zero-*trans* flow and the equilibrium exchange flux can be interpreted in the same way, and again gives a means of deciding between the three-state and four-state models. As we have seen, inhibitor studies can be used to derive important information on the properties of transport systems, as well as being of importance in their own right as analyses of the mode of action of drugs and other pharmacologic agents.

c) Reversible Inhibitor Studies, Penetrating Inhibitors

Reversible inhibitors that penetrate the membrane, using the transport system which they inhibit, are nothing but substrate analogs. If *either* the substrate *or* its inhibitor (analog) can bind to the carrier, the two will interfere with each other when both are present at the same face of the membrane, but may well mutually speed up transport (in a countertransport) when present on opposite sides of the membrane. If both substrate and its analog bind simultaneously to the carrier, they are best considered as cosubstrates for each other. The properties of such counter- and cotransport systems will form the basis of most of the remainder of this chapter. At this stage we shall continue to consider the case of substrates that compete for binding to the carrier, and see what information such inhibition studies give as to the properties of the carrier.

The kinetic model for this case, for the simplified carrier, is given in Fig. 10a, while the conventional carrier is drawn in Fig. 10b. The two models cannot be distinguished by the use of penetrating competitive inhibitors. Analysis of the transport kinetics for the models of Fig. 10 gives the following equation describing the unidirectional flux of substrate S from side 1 to side 2 of the membrane with S present at $[S_1]$ and $[S_2]$, and the inhibitors P present at $[P_1]$ and $[P_2]$

$$\begin{aligned} v^{S}_{1\to 2} = {} & \{K^{P}[S_1]+[S_1][P_2]+(K^{P}[S_1])/(K^{S}[S_2])\}/ \\ & \cdot\{R_{oo}K^{S}K^{P}+K^{P}([S_1]R^{S}_{12}+[S_2]R^{S}_{21}) \\ & +K^{S}([P_1]R^{P}_{12}+[P_2]R^{P}_{21})+R^{SP}_{ee}[S_1][P_2]+R^{PS}_{ee}[S_2][P_1] \\ & +K^{P}(R^{S}_{ee}[S_1][S_2])/K^{S}+K^{S}(R^{P}_{ee}[P_1][P_2])/K^{P}\} \end{aligned} \tag{27}$$

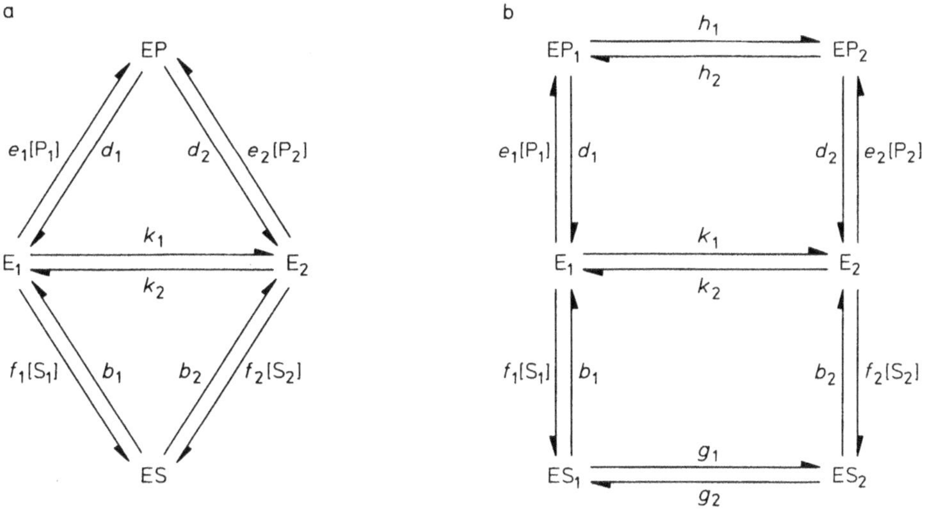

Fig. 10 a, b. Competitive inhibition on the simple carrier. **a** three-state form; **b** four-state form. S and P are two substrates of the common carrier E. The rate constants for each reaction are as indicated. The cross-resistance terms appearing in Eq. (27) are defined as

$$R_{ee}^{SP} = 1/b_2 + 1/d_1;$$
$$R_{ee}^{PS} = 1/b_1 + 1/d_2,$$

and are related to the straight resistances by

$$R_{ee}^{SP} + R_{ee}^{PS} = R_{ee}^{S} + R_{ee}^{P}$$

In addition to the symbols used in Eq. (20) for the case of pure S, here designated by the superscript S, Eq. (27) contains analogous symbols for the inhibitor (substrate) P, designated by superscript P. Furthermore, the equation contains symbols for those transport events in which both S and P take part. The relevant cross-terms are cross-resistances for the situation where S combines with carrier at one side of the membrane, while it is P that combines at the other side. These cross-resistances are defined in the legend to Fig. 10 and are related to the pure resistance terms as recorded in the legend. In all, seven parameters are required to define fully the behavior of a transport system that carries two different substrates. All terms are derivable by experiments on the individual substrates and the parameter R_{oo}, which describes the flow of carrier in the absence of any substrate, is clearly shared between all different substrates that share a common carrier. Indeed, the constancy of R_{oo} in such cases is a test of the validity of a single carrier as a model for all the substrates (competitors).

Equation (27) simplifies to a very easily handled form when the concentration of one substrate, say S, is set so low that it can be neglected in comparison with appropriate half-saturation parameters. Following DEVES and KRUPKA (1979), we shall study how the flux of S then varies as the concentration of the inhibitor P is varied at either side or at both sides of the membrane, using the equation

$$v_{1\to 2}^{S} = \frac{(K^P/K^S)(K^P + [P_2])[S_1]}{R_{oo}(K^P)^2 + K^P(R_{12}^P[P_1] + R_{21}^P[P_2]) + R_{ee}^P[P_1][P_2]} \tag{28}$$

for the case where $[S_2]$ and $[S_1]$ are limitingly low. The flux in the absence of inhibitor is found, of course, by putting $[P_1]=[P_2]=0$ in Eq. (28), so that the fractional inhibition of the transport of S becomes

$$\text{fractional inhibition} = \frac{R_{oo}K^P(K^P+[P_2])}{R_{oo}(K^P)^2+K^P(R_{12}^P[P_1]+R_{21}^P[P_2])+R_{ee}^P[P_1][P_2]} \tag{29}$$

an equation which is formally closely related to Eq. (20), our fundamental transport equation. Pursuing the analogy between Eqs. (20) and (29), we can specify three useful experimental conditions for studying competition:

a. In the zero-*trans* case, the concentration of the competitor [P] at side 2 of the membrane is zero. Equation (29) transforms to

$$\text{fractional inhibition (zero-trans)} = \frac{R_{oo}K^P}{R_{oo}K^P+R_{12}^P[P_1]}. \tag{30}$$

An inhibition of 50% will be found when the concentration of $[P_1]$ is equal to $R_{oo}K^P/R_{12}^P$. This is exactly the half-saturation concentration for the zero-trans experiment with pure P as substrate.

b. In the equilibrium exchange situation, the concentration of the competitor [P] at the two sides of the membrane is equal. Equation (29) yields

$$\text{fractional inhibition (equilibrium exchange)} = \frac{R_{oo}K^P}{R_{oo}K^P+R_{ee}^P[P]}. \tag{31}$$

An inhibition of 50% is found when $[P]=K^P(R_{oo}/R_{ee}^P)$, which is the very K_m for the equilibrium exchange experiment with pure P as substrate.

c. Similarly, an infinite-*trans* ($[P_2]=\infty$) procedure can be described, where the inhibitor is kept at a limitingly high concentration at face 2 of the membrane, while its concentration is varied at face 1. The flux of S in the direction 1 to 2, when $[P_2]$ is always limitingly high, will be reduced by adding P to side 1 and will be halved when $[P_1]$ is equal to $K^P R_{21}^P/R_{ee}^P$. This is exactly the same K_m as for the infinite-*trans* experiment using pure P as substrate.

In this way, half-saturation concentrations can be found for any substrate, even if no method is available for measuring the transport of that substrate (if it cannot readily be obtained labeled, for instance), when it is used to inhibit the transport of a readily measured permeant.

8. How the Kinetic Parameters of the Simple Carrier are Affected by an Applied Voltage

In many cases that have been studied, substrates of a transport system are electrically charged, e.g., the sodium ions or protons of many of the cotransport or countertransport systems we shall be discussing in the following sections of this chapter. It might also be the case that the free carrier is charged, while the carrier–substrate complex may be charged or not. To handle the case of the charged substrate, one has merely to replace any term referring to the concentration of substrate, in all of the many transport equations that we have already derived, by a term referring to the electrochemical potential of the substrate. Thus, if $\Delta\psi$ is the electrical potential difference across the membrane, in the 1 to 2 direction, we must replace terms $[S_1]$ and $[S_2]$ in our transport equations by $[S_1]\exp(zF\Delta\psi/2RT)$ and $[S_2]\exp(zF\Delta\psi/2RT)$, respectively, to obtain the appropriate transport equations.

The problem of the charged state of the carrier or of the carrier–substrate complex is more difficult, but more enlightening. We shall tackle here the formally simpler situation of the four-state carrier model of Fig. 8, the conventional carrier. The treatment of the three-state carrier of Fig. 7 can be found in STEIN (1977a). For the four-state carrier, we refer to Fig. 8. The rate constants that can be affected by an applied voltage across the membrane consist only of those which refer to processes occurring across the membrane. Thus, only the k and g terms can be affected by an applied voltage. If we now refer to Table 2, where the kinetic parameters in K and in R are defined in terms of the rate constants of the carrier model, we can see which of these parameters will be affected if either the k, the g, or both k and g terms are affected by the applied voltage. There are four cases to consider:

1. If the free carrier is uncharged, terms in k are not affected by the applied voltage, and R_{oo} is, therefore, not affected. If the substrate, but not the carrier, is charged, then the carrier complex is likewise charged, terms in g will be influenced by the applied voltage, and K and all the R terms, other than R_{oo}, will be affected.
2. If the free carrier is charged, while the substrate is uncharged, both the free carrier and the carrier–substrate complex bear the same charge and hence k and g terms are all affected by the applied voltage, those in the same direction being equally affected. K and all terms in R will be affected by voltage.
3. If the free carrier is charged, while the substrate is oppositely but equally charged, the complex ES will be uncharged. Terms in g will be unaffected by voltage, so that R_{ee} (giving the maximum velocity of the equilibrium exchange experiment) will be unaffected. The value of K will be affected as will all terms in R other than R_{ee}.
4. If the charge on the substrate does not neutralize that on the carrier, k and g terms will all be affected by voltage, each to a different extent. None of the parameters of the carrier need remain invariant with voltage. Thus, the finding that either R_{oo} or R_{ee} is invariant with applied voltage gives directly important information about the charged state of the different forms of the carrier.

These considerations apply whatever the detailed distribution of the electric field across the membrane. A more subtle analysis can be made of the voltage dependence of those parameters that do vary with the applied voltage (STEIN 1977 a). In certain cases it may be possible to identify the point, during the transmembrane movement of the carrier, at which the voltage drop is experienced.

II. Coupled Transport Systems

In all of our analyses so far, we have considered only cases where a single substrate molecule can bind to the carrier at any time, and for those situations where

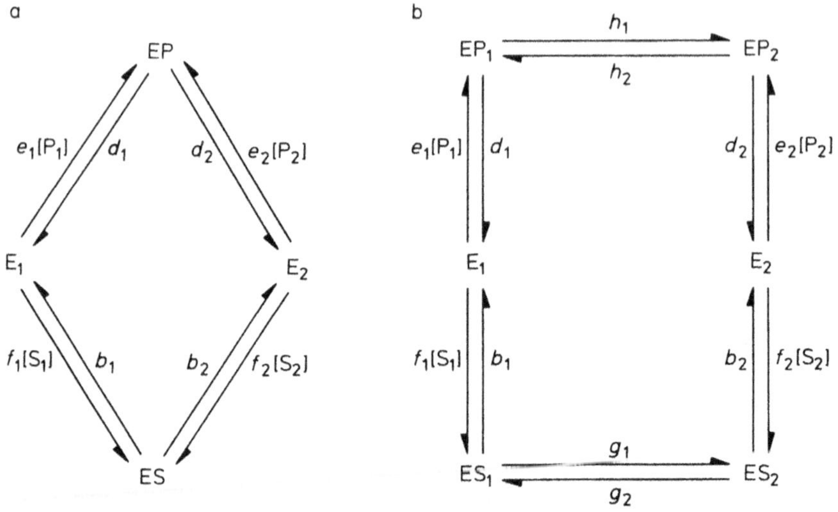

Fig. 11 a, b. Countertransport by the simple carrier. **a** model with only a single form of the carrier–substrate complex; **b** model with two interconverting forms of the complex. S and P are two alternate substrates of the carrier. Free carrier cannot interconvert between the two forms that face the different sides of the membrane

a substrate and its analog can bind in turn to the carrier, we have focused our attention on the role of the analog as an inhibitor of the flow of substrate. Important insights into physiology and, in particular, into the physiology and pharmacology of the intestine, arise when we relax these restrictions and consider the cases where two substrates must cooperate in the formation of an effective transporting complex with the carrier or where two substrates present at opposite faces of the membrane ride on the same carrier. In both these sets of phenomena we have a *coupling* between the substrate flows. The two substrates that combine simultaneously with the carrier move in the same direction across the membrane and their coupling is termed cotransport or symport. When the substrates bind alternatively to the carrier so that the coupling is of flows moving in opposite directions across the membrane, we have the phenomenon of countertransport or antiport. Much can be learned by a deeper analysis of the transport kinetics of these two phenomena.

1. The Analysis of Countertransport

The model we shall analyze is depicted as Fig. 11. We are now quite familiar with the view that the four-state model of Fig. 11 a is, of course, kinetically equivalent to the six-state model of Fig. 11 b, and we shall largely confine ourselves here to the further analysis of the four-state form. The unidirectional flux of substrate S in the presence of both S and P at both membrane faces is conveniently given by

$$v^{S}_{1\to 2} = \frac{([\bar{S}_1][\bar{S}_2]R^{P}_{ee}/R^{S}_{ee}) + [\bar{S}_1][\bar{P}_2]}{R^{P}_{ee}([\bar{S}_1]+[\bar{S}_2]+[\bar{S}_1][\bar{S}_2]) + R^{S}_{ee}([\bar{P}_1]+[\bar{P}_2]+[\bar{P}_1][\bar{P}_2]) + R^{PS}_{ee}[\bar{P}_1][\bar{S}_2] + R^{SP}_{ee}[\bar{P}_2][\bar{S}_1]} \tag{32}$$

The terms in R in this equation are resistances of the "equilibrium exchange" experiment for pure S and P or for experiments with only P at one side of the membrane and only S at the other. They are defined in terms of Fig. 11a in the legend to Fig. 10. The barred concentrations in Eq. (32) are "reduced concentrations", useful in the present context, and refer in every case to the concentration of substrate at any face divided by the relevant affinity parameter at that face (K_1^S, K_2^S, K_1^P, or K_2^P). The affinity parameter is defined in all cases as the off constant divided by the on constant for the reaction between the relevant substrate and the free carrier. Thus, for substrate S at side 1, its concentration is $[S_1]$, $K_1^S = b_1/f_1$, and the reduced concentration of S is $[\bar{S}_1] = [S_1]/(b_1/f_1)$.

The first point to establish with regard to Eq. (32) concerns the ratios of the substrate concentrations at equilibrium. Such an equilibrium will be reached when the net flow of substrate is zero and no further change occurs. We derive the net flow for S from Eq. (32) by subtracting the flux in the 1 to 2 direction from the flux in the 2 to 1 direction. On such a subtraction, the first term in the numerator of Eq. (32) drops out, leaving as numerator $([\bar{S}_1][\bar{P}_2] - [\bar{S}_2][\bar{P}_1])$. Whatever the denominator, the net flow is zero when the numerator is zero, that is, when $[\bar{S}_1][\bar{P}_2] = [\bar{S}_2][\bar{P}_1]$. We can rewrite this equation as

$$\frac{[S_1][P_2]}{[S_2][P_1]} = \frac{b_2 d_1 e_2 f_1}{b_1 d_2 e_1 f_2} \tag{33}$$

from the definitions of the barred terms. If P is at the same concentration [P] on both sides of the membrane, then S must be at some concentration [S], the same on both sides of the membrane, since there is no energy input into the system to keep S concentrated at one membrane face. Thus, the right hand side of Eq. [33] must be unity, and we have that $[S_1]/[S_2] = [P_1]/[P_2]$ at equilibrium. (We used the fact that this equation holds when $[P_1]/[P_2] = 1$, in order to derive it, but from Eq. (33) it is true for all values of $[P_1]/[P_2]$.) It follows that, whatever the details of the carrier model of Fig. 11, the equilibrium concentration of substrate S, which we may arbitrarily call the driven substrate, will be determined by the concentration of P, the driving substrate.

The two flows of S and of P are coupled and, if the concentration ratio of P can be held at some value other than unity (by the introduction of some metabolic energy link), the concentration ratio of S must be held at this same value if the model of Fig. 11 is adequate to describe the transmembrane movements of P and of S. Mechanistically, if P is at high concentration at face 1 of the membrane and low at face 2, it will compete effectively with S at face 1, preventing it from crossing the membrane in the 1 to 2 direction. At face 2, however, P will fail to compete effectively with S and thus S can flow from face 2 towards 1. The resultant flow of S is in the opposite direction (counter) to the flow of P, and will continue until, with the driven and driving substrates at the same concentration ratio, competition is mutual and no further net flow occurs. We note here that in the final relation for the equilibrium situation for S and P, any term connected with the affinities of the carrier for the substrates disappears. The significance of this result will be discussed in detail in Sect. C.II, where we shall deal with the design principles of carrier systems.

Next, we must discuss the kinetic consequences of Eq. (33) and, hence, of Fig. 11. It is clear, first, that the model does not allow for the net flow of either S or P when these are present alone. There is no transmembrane movement of free (unloaded) carrier. The only processes that can take place are the exchange of S with P or of labeled substrate with unlabeled substrate. If a net flow of substrate is found, for any experimental system with only a single substrate present, then the model of Fig. 10 is to be preferred, with an E_1 to E_2 transformation. Such a net flow rejects the simpler model of Fig. 11. Many systems appear to behave, however, in accordance with Fig. 11, and net flows are usually negligible in coupled countertransport systems. Second, the kinetic parameters of the model of Fig. 11 can be determined by the type of transport experiment with which we are now quite familiar. The terms in R are obtained from the maximum velocities of experiments with pure S or P, or with only S at one side of the membrane and only P at the other. A consistency test for the model is that the R terms so determined must be related by the expression $R^{S}_{ec} + R^{P}_{ee} = R^{SP}_{ee} + R^{PS}_{ee}$, if the model of Fig. 11 is to apply to the transport of S and P. The four half-saturation concentrations for the substrates S and P at each membrane face, in infinite-*trans* experiments with only S or P present, allow the determination of the affinity parameters in K. A consistency test for the countertransport carrier model is that $K^{S}_{1}K^{P}_{2} = K^{S}_{2}K^{P}_{1}$, a result which is equivalent to Eq. (33). If only P is present at side 2, while only S is present at side 1, and the flux of S in the 1 to 2 direction is followed, the maximum velocity is given by R^{SP}_{ee}, and the half-saturation concentration for this "hetero infinite-*trans*" experiment is given by the affinity parameter for S at face 1, modified by the appropriate resistance terms, i.e., as $K^{S}_{1} \times R^{P}_{ee}/R^{SP}_{ee}$. Corresponding results are found for the other three hetero infinite-*trans* experiments, and the interrelationships between the derived parameters provide many more consistency tests for the model of Fig. 11. If the model is well established, these experiments provide alternative routes for determining the parameters of the countertransport system. Finally, the half-saturation concentration for the equilibrium exchange experiment with pure S or P only is found to be the sum of the values determined in the two (homo) infinite-*trans* situations ($K^{ee} = K^{it}_{1\to 2} + K^{it}_{1\to 2}$), again a readily testable prediction. The energetics of countertransport will be discussed in Sect. C.II.

2. The Analysis of Cotransport

The model to be analyzed is drawn as Fig. 12; Fig. 12a gives the five-state form, while Fig. 12b shows the conventional six-state form, kinetically equivalent to Fig. 12a. the unidirectional flux of S in the presence of S and P at both membrane faces is given by (STEIN 1977b)

$$
\begin{aligned}
v^{S}_{1\to 2} = {} & \{D_2[\bar{P}_1][\bar{S}_1] + [\bar{P}_1][\bar{P}_2][\bar{S}_1][\bar{S}_2](1 + (1/[\bar{P}_1]) + (1/[\bar{P}_2]))/R_{SS}\}/ \\
& \cdot\{R_{SS}R_{PP}D_2D_1 + R_{SS}(D_2[\bar{P}_1] + D_1[\bar{P}_2]) \\
& + R_{PP}(D_2[\bar{S}_1] + D_1[\bar{S}_2]) + R^{*}_{12}D_2[\bar{P}_1][\bar{S}_1] + R^{*}_{21}D_1[\bar{P}_2][\bar{S}_2] \\
& + ([\bar{P}_1] + [\bar{P}_2] + [\bar{P}_1][\bar{P}_2])([\bar{S}_1] + [\bar{S}_2] + [\bar{S}_1][\bar{S}_2])\},
\end{aligned}
\tag{34}
$$

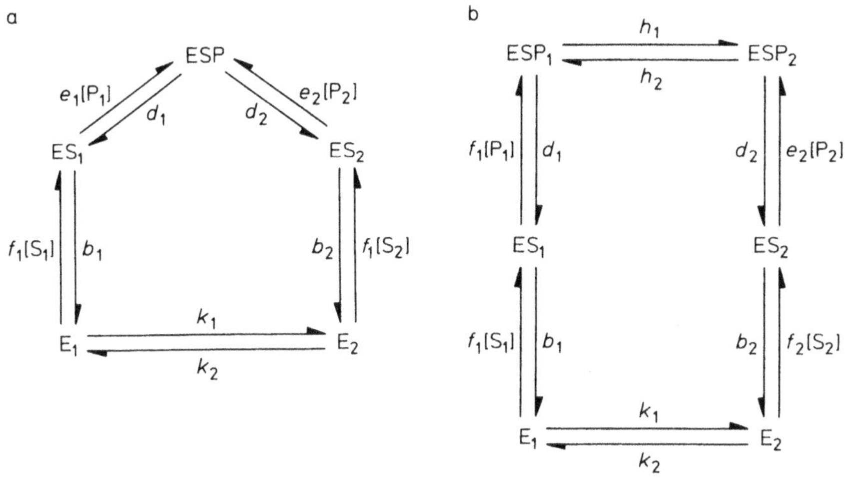

Fig. 12 a, b. Cotransport by the simple carrier. **a** model with only a single form of the terary ESP complex; **b** model with two interconverting forms of the ternary complex. The forms in ES cannot interconvert except after combination with P.

For **a**, we have

$$\begin{aligned} R_{ss} &= 1/b_1 + 1/b_2; \\ R_{PP} &= 1/k_1 + 1/k_2; \\ R^*_{12} &= 1/b_1 + 1/k_2; \\ R^*_{21} &= 1/b_2 + 1/k_1; \\ D_1 &= d_1; \\ D_2 &= d_2. \end{aligned}$$

For **b**, the terms containing b must be modified to take account of the transformations between the two forms of the ternary complex

where the terms in $[\bar{P}]$ and $[\bar{S}]$ are as defined following Eq. (32), while the terms in R and D are coefficients of resistance, defined in the legend to Fig. 12. (It should be pointed out that P and S are in each case the first and second substrate to be bound at each face, on this model. In practice it might well be the case that glucose, say, is bound first at side 1, but second at side 2. In this situation Eq. (34) will apply with P_1 being glucose at side 1, and S_2 being glucose at side 2.)

This formidable looking equation is for the simplest case of cotransport, that depicted in Fig. 12, where the order of addition of S and P to the carrier is specified, so that the formation of the ESP complex is an ordered reaction. In practice, the reaction might well be random. The solution of the unidirectional flux for such a random reaction system, where no prior assumptions are made as to whether carrier and substrates are or are not in equilibrium, is not yet available, although the distribution of the carrier between the various E, ES, EP, and ESP forms has been published for a related model where ESP isomerizes, but not E (BRITTEN 1977). The model of Fig. 12 is known in the enzyme kinetic literature as the "iso-Ordered BiBi model" (CLELAND 1963). Inasmuch as we shall show shortly how to decide whether the reaction between E, S, and P is or is not ordered, we might as well limit ourselves to this simpler case until solving the more difficult kinetic problem of the random model is demanded by experimental data. The model of Fig. 12 does not allow in addition the possibility of the transmembrane movement of S and of P uncoupled with movement of the second substrate. The consequences of such uncoupled movement will be discussed in a later section.

Let us first consider the ratio of substrate concentrations at equilibrium. Exactly as was shown for the countertransport model in the previous section, one can readily show that at zero net substrate flow, i.e., at equilibrium, the substrate concentrations across the membrane are related by the equation $[S_1]/[S_2]=[P_2]/[P_1]$, exactly the reverse of that found for countertransport. Since flow across the membrane demands, on the model, addition of both S and P to the carrier, a high concentration of the driving substrate, say P, will lead to transmembrane flow of the driven S. Thus, S will be low where P is maintained high. This relation between substrate concentrations at equilibrium will hold for all possible models in the general framework of Fig. 12, whatever the fine details of the reactions leading to formation of the ESP complex at either face of the membrane. The affinities of the carrier for the different substrates, defined as the quotient of the off divided by the on constants for the formation of the ES, EP, and ESP complexes, are related by the expression $(K_1^S K_1^P)/(K_2^S K_2^P)=k_2/k_1$, where k_2/k_1 is the equilibrium constant for the interconversion of the two forms of the free carrier and gives the value of $[E_1]/[E_2]$ in the steady state.

On the model of Fig. 12, there is no flow of S without flow of P. The two flows are fully coupled in the same direction and, hence, the system is termed one of cotransport. If the concentrations of one substrate across the membrane can be held (by linking to metabolism) at unequal values, a system behaving as in Fig. 12 will ensure the transmembrane concentration of the second, coupled substrate. In the absence of one of the substrates, there is no flux at all of the second substrate (every term in the numerator of Eq. (34) contains both an S_1 and a P_1). This is in complete contrast to the prediction of a countertransport situation of Fig. 11, where exchange of S with S, in the absence of P, would be expected. Again, the countertransport model demanded the presence of some substrate of the carrier, S or P, at the *trans* face of the membrane, for a flux to be measurable. In contrast, cotransport will take place readily with no *trans* S or P, since the model allows and indeed demands the ability of free carrier forms to interconvert across the membrane.

To explore the kinetic consequences of the cotransport model of Fig. 12, we take, to begin with, the zero-*trans* situation. Writing $[\bar{S}_2]=[\bar{P}_2]=0$ in Eq. (34), leads to

$$v_{1\to 2}^{S(zt)}=\frac{[P_1][S_1]}{K_1^P K_1^S R_{SS} R_{PP} D_1 + K_1^S R_{SS}[P_1] + K_1^P R_{PP}[S_1] + (R_{12}^* + 1/D_2)([P_1][S_1])} \qquad (35)$$

in terms of the affinity parameters K_1^P and K_2^S, rather than of reduced concentrations. Performing such zero-*trans* experiments in both directions across the membrane, with S and P in turn at each side at limitingly high concentrations, while the other is varied, leads to simple Michaelis forms, familiar to the enzyme kineticist. Maximum velocities and half-saturation concentrations derived from

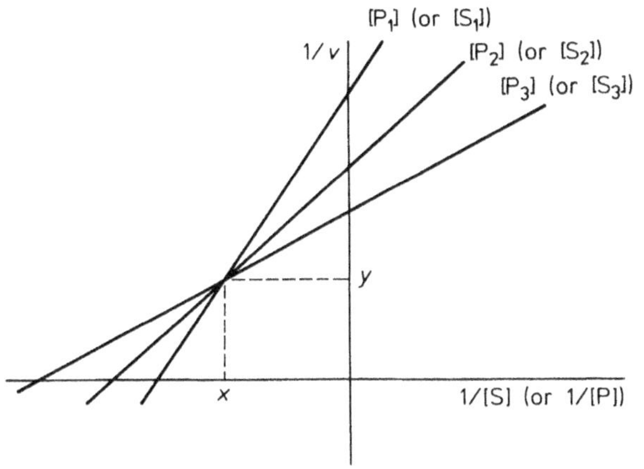

Fig. 13. Theoretical predictions for a cotransport system behaving according to Eq. (34) and Fig. 12. On the ordinate is plotted the reciprocal of the velocity of uptake of S (or P) as a function, on the abscissa, of the reciprocal of the concentration of S (or P). Each straight line represents data for a particular concentration of P (or S), the slope of the lines increasing with decreasing concentration of P. The point of intersection of the lines has coordinates of $-(1/b_1+1/b_2)K_1D_1$, $(R_{12}+1/D_2-1/D_1)$ when it is 1/[S] that is on the x-axis, and of $-(1/k_1+1/k_2)K_1D$, $(R_{12}+1/D_2-1/D_1)$ when it is 1/[P] that is on the x-axis

such experiments will yield the parameters D_1, D_2, R_{12}, R_{21} and to the products $K_1^S R_{SS}$, $K_1^P R_{PP}$, $K_2^S R_{SS}$, and $K_2^P R_{PP}$. One can, however, hold just S and then P at *less* than limitingly high concentrations, while P and S respectively are varied. One then obtains a series of plots. When these are drawn in the reciprocal form of 1/(unidirectional flux of P or S) against 1/(concentration of P or S), a series of straight lines will be obtained (Fig. 13). These lines intersect at a common point, having coordinates of $(R_{12}^*+1/D_2-1/D_1)$ on the $1/v$ axis and of $-(1/b_1+1/b_2)$ $K_1^S D_1$ (when $1/[S_1]$ is on the x-axis), and of $-(1/k_1+1/k_2)K_1^P D_1$ (when it is $1/[P_1]$ that is on the x-axis), with corresponding terms for the 2 to 1 fluxes. If, by coincidence, a relationship exists between rate constants such that $(R_{12}^*+1/D_2)=1/D_1$, the activating cosubstrate will appear to act by increasing only the maximum velocity of transport. Alternatively, the terms which determine the intercept on the x-axis may be very small (for instance, if rate constants d_1 and d_2 are very small in comparison with f_1 and f_2). In this case, the pencil of lines on the $1/v$ versus 1/[S] plot will almost intersect on the y-axis, and the activating cosubstrate will appear to act as a simple reducer of the half-saturation concentration, i.e., as if its whole effect was to increase the apparent affinity of the carrier for the activated substrate. Both of these two types of behavior have been found experimentally (CRANE et al. 1965; GOLDNER et al. 1969) and there has been much discussion of the possible significance of such so-called "V-Type" and "K-type" kinetics (SEMENZA 1967; HEINZ et al. 1972). It is becoming clear that such cases represent situations of no special significance and the general finding is rather that either slopes or intercepts, or both, of $1/v$ versus 1/[S] plots, can be altered depending on the details of the cotransport model in question. The model of Fig. 12 does, however, present some constraints to the possibility of V-type kinetics. From the condition already derived, V-type kinetics will be found for the flux from side 1, if $R_{12}+1/D_2=1/D_1$. This implies that $1/D_1$ is substantially bigger than $1/D_2$. If V-type kinetics are found also for the flux in the 2 to 1 direction, it would imply in addition that $1/D_2$ is bigger than $1/D_1$. Since both these conditions cannot hold for a particular system, the finding of V-type kinetics for fluxes in both directions across the membrane is sufficient to rule out the model of Fig. 12 for the system in question. I have no record of such a result being reported, but it would be of interest to test some system in this way.

We proceed to consider situations where the substrates can be present on both sides of the membrane. The simplest experiment is the equilibrium exchange flux with both substrates at limitingly high levels at both membrane faces. This maximum flux gives directly the reciprocal of R_{SS}, from Eq. (34). This, with the results already derived for the zero-*trans* experiments, allows all the steady state parameters of the model of Fig. 12 to be calculated. Any subsequent experiment is then a test of the consistency of the model chosen. There are many such experiments in which, for instance, one or other of the two substrates is at limitingly high levels at a *trans* face. (There are now four infinite-*trans* experiments.) Many of the possible experiments of this type were discussed in a previous paper (STEIN 1977b). We consider here only the main, more striking characteristics of the model.

We consider the flux from side 1 of either P or S, which in the particular model drawn in Fig. 12 will be the first or second substrate bound, respectively, in this ordered reaction for the formation of ESP. It will be helpful to refer continually to Fig. 12. We can draw several conclusions from a consideration of this:

1. When $[S_2]$ and $[P_2]$ are both limitingly high, there will be a definite flux of S from side 1 following a typical Michaelis form. This flux will occur in the complete absence of P at face 1. Thus, although the system is one of cotransport, when sufficient S and P are present at face 2, no P is needed at face 1 to ensure a flux of S in the 1 to 2 direction. Enough carrier can be returned to face 1 by the breakdown of ESP formed at face 2.

2. But when $[S_2]$ and $[P_2]$ are, in this way, limitingly high, there will be no flux of P from face 1 to face 2. The flux of S from face 1 may well be maximal, but that of P will be nonexistent. This arises because no free E will be present at side 1; all will shuttle between forms ESP and EP_1. This prediction forms a powerful test of the model of Fig. 12, and, indeed, enables the order of addition of substrates at either face of the membrane to be established by a simple experiment: ensure that substrates at the *trans* face are at limitingly high concentrations, then attempt to measure the flux of each substrate, in turn, from the *cis* face. If the flux of one substrate is high while that of the other is very low, the reaction of ESP is ordered and that substrate whose flux is low is the first to be bound at the *cis* face.

3. Indeed, as the concentration of substrate at the *trans* face is increased from zero, the flux from the *cis* face of one substrate (the second to be bound) may well increase, but the flux of the other (the first to be bound) will certainly decrease.

4. A final test of the model is the prediction for the case where P is present at limitingly high levels at side 2, while S is present there at some finite level. Then the flux of P from side 1 will be strictly dependent on the presence of S at *both* sides 1 and sides 2 of the membrane. These will be needed to form ESP at both faces. Yet, when at either face of the membrane the concentration of S is raised

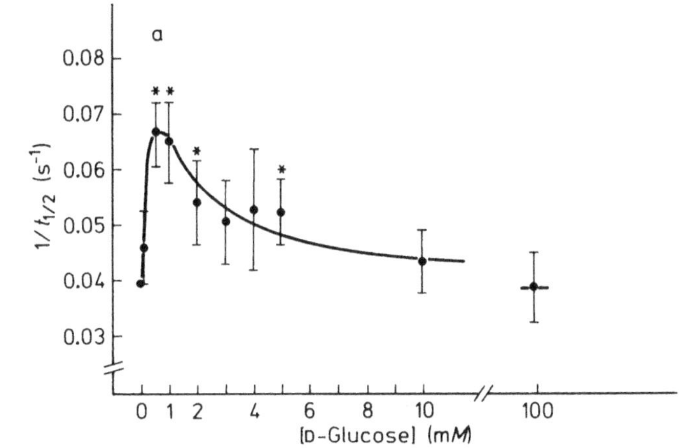

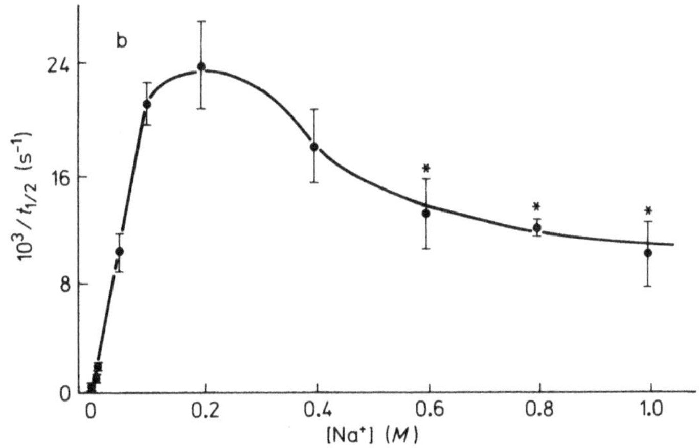

Fig. 14a, b. Uptake of D-glucose and sodium by membrane vesicles prepared from rabbit intestine brush borders. All experiments are performed under equilibrium exchange conditions. **a** rate of uptake of sugar shown as a function of the added sodium, the glucose being at 1 mM; **b** rate of uptake of sodium, the ion being present at tracer levels, shown as a function of the sugar concentration. HOPFER and GROSECLOSE (1080)

to limitingly high levels, the flux of P from side 1 will fall to zero. Its flux, therefore, goes through a maximum value as either $[S_1]$ or $[S_2]$ and is raised from zero to a limitingly high value.

Experiments along these lines have been performed on membrane vesicles isolated from rabbit intestine (HOPFER and GROSECLOSE 1980). These data are depicted in Fig. 14, where Fig. 14a shows how the rate of glucose uptake by these vesicles is first stimulated and then depressed as the sodium concentration is increased, while Fig. 14b shows similar data where glucose is the additive and sodium uptake is studied. These experiments were performed under equilibrium exchange conditions of both glucose and sodium, so that the two ligands are varied, always at both sides of the membrane. The reduction of substrate flow as the cosubstrate is varied is, as we have seen, indicative of an ordered reaction in which the varied substrate binds second to the carrier. How then can such a reduction be seen both for glucose and for sodium as the varying substrate? Can they both bind second to the carrier enzyme? An explanation could be that it is glucose that binds second to the carrier at one face of the membrane, but it is sodium that binds second at the other face. HOPFER and GROSECLOSE term this case the "first in, first out" case and propose such a model for the sodium/glucose cotransport system of intestine. Their experimental procedure, in which additives are varied simultaneously at both membrane faces, does not allow them to establish whether it is at the cytoplasmic face of the membrane or at the luminal face that glucose is the second substrate to bind. Data on the binding of the transport inhibitor phlorhizin to such membrane vesicles (which we shall discuss shortly) bears upon this point.

The last point we need to make about the kinetics of cotransport is this: when the first substrate to be bound to the carrier is at limitingly high concentrations at both sides of the membrane, the resulting system is a simple carrier for the second substrate. Thus, if the transport of S is studied (in the case of Fig. 12) at very high levels of $[P_1]$ and $[P_2]$, all of the predictions previously found for the simple carrier with S as substrate should hold. All of the inhibitor kinetics should apply without further analysis as well as all of the effects of an applied voltage. Studying a cotransport system in this way, with the situation simplified by having one substrate present in limitingly high concentrations, will lead to many insights into the behavior of the system.

3. An Inhibitor of a Cotransport System

In Sects. B.I.3 and B.I.7, we dealt with the kinetics of inhibition of simple pores and carriers. Much of the analysis of carrier inhibition applies, of course, directly to the inhibition of cotransport and countertransport systems in that these are carrier mediated. But there are some particular aspects of coupled transport systems which need further consideration. We shall describe these with reference to a study (ARONSON 1978) of the inhibition by phlorhizin of the sugar–sodium cotransport system (using data obtained on renal tissue, however, rather than on intestine – but the principles are no doubt the same; see TOGGENBURGER et al. 1978). Phlorhizin in this system is a competitive inhibitor of glucose binding. It is possible, therefore, that it binds at or near the site on the carrier to which the sugar binds. Binding of phlorhizin to membrane vesicles isolated from epithelial tissue can be directly measured and thus the influence of additives on this binding determined. Figure 15 shows ARONSON's data (1978) on the binding of phlorhizin to a membrane preparation from rabbit renal tissue. The upper curve shows data obtained in the presence of sodium ions, the lower in the absence of sodium. Binding of inhibitor, itself nontransported, is clearly dramatically affected by the ion in this cotransport system. Further studies showed that sodium ions increased the rate of binding of phlorhizin, that is, the rate of the on constant for the formation of the carrier–inhibitor complex, and decreased the off constant for phlorhizin already bound to membranes. Most interesting was the effect of altering the transmembrane potential on the rate of phlorhizin binding. Increasing the electro-

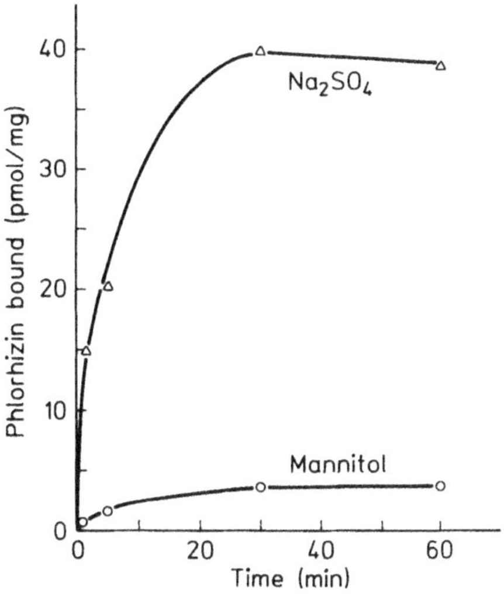

Fig. 15. Binding of the inhibitor phlorhizin to brush border membranes isolated from rabbit kidneys. The binding from 0.2 μ*M* phlorhizin was measured in the presence (*upper curve*) or the absence (*lower curve*) of 60 m*M* sodium sulfate. ARONSON (1978)

negativity *within* the vesicles increaes the binding of phlorhizin at the outer face of the membrane preparation, while increasing the electropositivity decreased the rate of binding of phlorhizin. Neither manipulation had an effect on the rate of release of already bound phlorhizin. These results are most readily interpreted on the hypothesis that the carrier itself is negatively charged in the free state, and is thus distributed across the membrane in accordance with the prevailing electrical potential, being driven outwards when the inside is negative. Finally, ARONSON found that sodium ions at the inner face of the vesicle membrane reduced the equilibrium binding of phlorhizin at the outer face, presumably by virtue of the fact that the sodium ions held the carrier within the vesicle, thereby reducing its availability to phlorhizin.

We can compare these data of ARONSON (1978) on binding of phlorhizin to kidney membrane vesicles with the data discussed previously of HOPFER and GROSECLOSE (1980), on the cotransport of glucose and sodium into intestinal vesicles. Phlorhizin is present, of course, at the outer face of such vesicles, and we have just seen that external sodium strongly increases binding of phlorhizin. If the binding sites for glucose and phlorhizin are identical, one can combine these two sets of data and attempt to establish the order of binding of sodium and sugar at the outer face of the membrane. If it is sodium that binds first at the outer face, the dependence of glucose (or phlorhizin) binding on the sodium concentration will be according to a simple hyperbola. If sodium binds second, binding of the cosubstrate is clearly independent of sodium concentrations over a wide concentration range (HOPFER and GROSECLOSE 1980). ARONSON's data support the first alternative, so that one can argue that the order of binding of sugar and sodium is: at the luminal face, sodium binds first, glucose second; at the cytoplasmic face, it is glucose that binds first and sodium that binds second. In the process of active glucose transport in the "physiologic" direction, i.e., from lumen to cytoplasm, sodium is the first substrate to bind to the carrier at the luminal face and the first to leave it at the cytoplasmic face. Such studies on inhibitor–carrier interactions at the level of isolated carrier systems are likely to be increasingly used in future analyses of drug–carrier interrelationships.

III. Chemiosmotic Coupling

It did not take many years after the original work of CHRISTENSEN, of CSÁKY, and of CRANE (referred to in Sect. A) before physiologists were able to grasp the "gradient hypothesis" and to cope with the concept that the flows of two substrates could be coupled if they used the same carrier, and that this coupling could lead to the net flow of one of the substrates against its concentration gradient. The corresponding concept of coupling between the flow of substrate and the progress of chemical reaction, propounded by MITCHELL over many years (MITCHELL 1966, 1967, 1977), took far longer to be accepted. But this proposal has had revolutionary effects on our understanding of bioenergetics and now dominates research in this field. MITCHELL's proposal of "chemiosmotic" coupling arises directly from the carrier concept, with its insistence on two states of a membrane carrier, interconverting only over an activation energy barrier.

It is easy for us to accept that substrate at side 1 of a membrane can interact with one form of the carrier, E_1, and yet be unable to reach and, hence, combine with E_2. It was MITCHELL's genius to generalize this concept to include also chemical reactions catalyzed by an enzyme. We shall suggest that the substrate A of a chemical reaction combines with one form of the enzyme, E_1, while the product, B, can combine only with E_2. Then, during the course of the enzyme-catalyzed chemical reaction $A \rightarrow B$, there is a conformation change of the enzyme $E_1 \rightarrow E_2$, the whole reaction being able to be written as

$$E_1 + A \rightleftharpoons E_B^A \rightleftharpoons E_2 + B \tag{36}$$

which is equivalent to our original Eq. (1). Now, if the enzyme E is here also a transport enzyme, all of our previous considerations apply to it. In particular, the cotransport scheme of Fig. 12 becomes a description of how the transport of a permeant S from side 1 to side 2 of a membrane can be coupled to the progress of a chemical reaction. This chemical reaction is the interconversion of two chemical substrances, P_1 and P_2, and the coupled processes are catalyzed by the *transport enzyme carrier* E_1, E_2. Similarly, the countertransport model of Fig. 11 is a description of a chemiosmotic coupling in which the interconversion of the two forms of the transport enzyme carrier is brought about *either* by the transfer of substrate S_1 to S_2 or by the progress of the chemical reaction of P_1 into P_2. The formal kinetics that we have developed in the present section apply both to osmotic-osmotic and to chemiosmotic coupling. The essential point of MITCHELL's theory is not, however, just that there is a formal analogy between the two processes, but that there is a mechanical identity. For both types of coupling the defining characteristic of a carrier, that it exists in two interconvertible forms, leads to the transformations of matter from one form to another, or of matter in one place into the same form of matter in another place.

There is one small point of detail by which our preceding treatment of carrier kinetics must be modified or, better, generalized in order to describe exactly the phenomena of chemiosmotic as well as osmotic-osmotic coupling. Consider first the transport of a permeant S. The flow of S will be at equilibrium, when this is not coupled to any other flow, when $[S_1]=[S_2]$. If we now consider the progress of a chemical reaction, the conversion of substance A into B, the flow of reaction uncoupled to any other flow, will cease when the concentrations of A and B are related by the equilibrium constant K_{eq} for the $A \rightarrow B$ reaction, i.e., at equilibrium $[A]/[B]=K_{eq}$. The equilibrium constant is determined by the molar free energy difference between A and B. Indeed, for permeants too, the concentration ratio at equilibrium is given by $[S_1]/[S_2]=K_{eq}$, but here $K_{eq}=1$, since there is no difference in free energy between S_1 and S_2, both at 1 *M*, these being the same chemical substance. Clearly, the equilibrium constant K_{eq} must appear somewhere in our equations describing coupled flows. It is easy to show (STEIN and HONIG 1977) that all that has to be altered, for countertransport, is our Eq. (33), in which the right-hand side of this equation becomes equal to K_{eq} instead of unity so that we have, at equilibrium

$$[S_1]/[S_2]=([P_1]/[P_2])\,K_{eq}\,, \tag{37}$$

where K_{eq} is the equilibrium constant for the chemical transformation of P_1 into P_2. For cotransport we must write for the equilibrium condition

$$[S_1]/[S_2]=([P_2]/[P_1])\,K_{eq}^{-1}\,. \tag{38}$$

These equations emphasize the fact that for a chemical reaction, the strength of the driving force is determined by the distance that the reactants and products of the reaction, P_1 and P_2, are from equilibrium, where $[P_2^{eq}]/[P_1^{eq}]=K_{eq}$. (The driving force for a permeant flow is likewise determined by the distance that S_1 and S_2 are from the equilibrium value, here unity.)

To take a concrete case, consider Fig. 16a, where we depict the pumping of sodium ions coupled to the hydrolysis of ATP (GLYNN and KARLISH 1975). Here E_1 and E_2 are two forms of the transport enzyme, which in the form E_1 can bind ATP to form a complex. When this complex now binds sodium ions, it splits off ADP, hydrolyzing the ATP, with the enzyme itself becoming phosphorylated to form the tertiary complex EPN_a. This can break down at side 2 of the membrane to release the sodium, leaving the enzyme in the form E_2P, phosphorylated still, but with its sodium binding site facing side 2 of the membrane. The enzyme now releases inorganic phosphate, forming E_2, which can interconvert to E_1, enabling the cycle to repeat itself. Flow of sodium and hydrolysis of ATP will continue until at equilibrium we have

$$[Na_1]/[Na_2]=([Pi\cdot ATP]/[ADP])/K_{eq}^{ATP/ADP\cdot Pi}$$

from Eq. (38). The forms E_1 and E_2 differ in that they have their binding sites for sodium facing sides 1 and 2 of the membrane, respectively, and can combine with ATP or with inorganic phosphate, respectively. Nothing so far written implies that the ATP binds and releases at side 1, while the inorganic phosphate does the same at face 2. On the contrary, everything that is known about such systems shows that the chemical reaction takes place entirely at one face of the membrane,

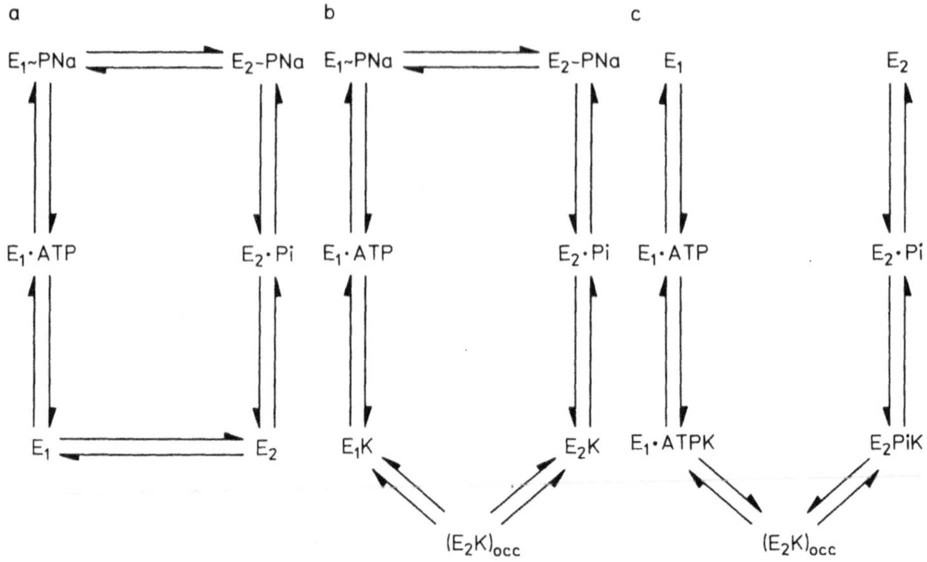

Fig. 16 a–c. Kinetic schemes for the mechanism of action of the sodium pump, seen as a chemiosmotic engine. **a** scheme for the case of sodium pumping, uncoupled to the movement of potassium ions; **b** scheme for the coupled Na, K pumping system; **c** scheme for potassium–potassium exchange. Pi symbolises PO_4, either covalently bound or complexed to the pump, while ATP may be complexed or else already split to ADPi, although still bound to the pump enzyme. "occ" is the occluded form of the pump enzyme

facing the cell interior (GLYNN and KARLISH 1975). It is the binding site for sodium ion that alters its accessibility across the membrane as the conformational change of the transport enzyme occurs.

The example of Fig. 16a describes the pumping of sodium ions coupled to the hydrolysis of ATP. The most commonly encountered mode of action of the sodium pump is that in which the flow of sodium and splitting of ATP are coupled also to the transmembrane flow of potassium ions, in a direction contrary to that of sodium flow. The model of Fig. 16b accounts for this phenomenon. The $E_2 \rightarrow E_1$ conversion of Fig. 16a is replaced in the sodium–potassium coupled pump, by a conversion involving the simultaneous translocation of potassium ions. The system can also catalyze the exchange of potassium ions, uncoupled to the movement of sodium ions. Figure 16c depicts this phenomenon. The form $(E_2K)_{occ}$ depicted in both of Figs. 16b and 16c is known as the "occluded" form, strong evidence existing (POST et al. 1972; BEAUGE and GLYNN 1979) that the potassium ions are here shielded in some way from access to bathing solution at side 1 or 2 of the membrane. Note that the flux of potassium in Fig. 16c needs the interaction with ATP or Pi only in order to bind to or become unbound from, the carrier. The flow of potassium is not coupled to any flow of ATP or Pi, nor any chemical interconversion of these ligands. Thus, potassium by itself can never be pumped by the system and its flux is never coupled, in the absence of sodium ions.

The sodium pump is, of course, essential to the operation of the intestine, since the sodium concentration gradient used by all the sodium cotransport systems is derived from it. The ATP of the cells of the intestine, like other body tissues, itself derives from the operation of proton–ATP countertransport chemiosmotic coupling (MITCHELL 1977). This proton gradient is itself formed by chemiosmotic coupling linked to the redox reactions of the oxidative phosphorylation pathways. Finally, the operation of calcium pumps linked chemiosmotically to ATP splitting, and osmotic-osmotically to sodium gradients, are essential for the activity of intestinal cells as well as so many other cells of the body.

C. The Thermodynamics and Energetics of Membrane Carrier Systems

If the carrier systems that we have been discussing existed quite on their own in the cell membrane, were able to cross the membrane only by the steps depicted in the models for the various systems, and were embedded in an otherwise perfectly impermeable membrane, the relationships between the concentrations of driven and driving permeants and of chemical reactants would be given precisely by the values listed in Eqs. (33), (37), and (38). The precise details of the molecular models would be quite irrelevant to their function. These conditions are never satisfied, however. All the cotransport and countertransport systems will display some measure of flow along paths which do not couple movements of driving and driven substrates. Thus, for the countertransport schemes, any movement of free carrier between conformations E_1 and E_2 provides a return path for the carrier, in a mode uncoupled to the substrate flows. This represents a leak of driving or driven substrate (or chemical reaction), leading to a loss of efficiency of the coupling. In cotransport systems, flow of carrier bound to a single substrate, rather than to both substrates, will be such a leak, breaking coupling between driving and driven substrates and leading to a loss of efficiency. We shall call all such flow by "forbidden" pathways of the carriers themselves "internal leaks." Any such internal leak will lead to a loss of efficiency in the coupling process and thus must be minimized for efficient working of a pumping system.

But there will also be, in general, pathways for leaks of driving and driven substrates by routes parallel to the carrier-linked movements. The driven substrate may flow down its built-up concentration gradient by simple diffusion through the membrane, or it may flow by a facilitated diffusion system in the membrane, parallel to the pumping system. The driving substrate may leak by simple diffusion or by riding on a parallel system, or if a chemical reaction is the driving force, the chemical reaction may take place along a path quite distinct from that of the coupling to flow of driven substrate. All such "external leaks" must be minimized in a cell by effective evolution of membrane properties, but such external leaks are not factors which evolution of the pumping system itself can affect. What can be effected by evolution of the pumping system is minimization of the relative importance of pump and leak pathways. This can be achieved by maximization of the rate of pumping. The efficiency of the pumping system, that is, the extent to which the theoretical relationship between the concentrations of driven and driving substrates of Eqs. (33), (37), and (38) are found to occur in practice, will depend directly on the relationship between pump and leak rates. An efficient pump will thus be one in which: (a) internal leaks are minimized by effective confining of carrier flows to those directly concerned in the coupling of driver and driven substrate; and (b) the pumping rate itself at (or near) equilibrium is maximized. The design principles of carrier systems (HONIG and STEIN 1978) operate on these functions and determine the precise details of carrier function, the thermodynamics and energetics of the pumping process itself.

I. Carrier Asymmetry

We shall want to consider, then, the rates of pumping systems and, in particular, to explore what molecular features of such systems lead to flow being favored in one direction, the direction of pumping, over flow in the opposite direction. It is not merely the rate of flow through the system that matters, but rather the net rate of flow in the direction of pumping. We shall need to look at the question of the asymmetry of pumping systems and, to make the phenomenon clear, we start by considering the asymmetry of the very simplest systems (WILBRANDT 1977) before going on to introduce the complexities of coupled flows.

We shall in all cases handle the problem of asymmetry by using an asymmetry parameter, A, defined as the flow of substrate at a particular concentration in the 1 to 2 direction divided by the flow in the 2 to 1 direction at the same concentration. It will often be helpful to define this value for net flows in zero-*trans* situations (i.e., where $[S_1]=[S]$, $[S_2]=0$ or $[S_1]=0$, $[S_2]=[S]$). Occasionally, we shall consider unidirectional flows or net flows of a particular substrate against infinitely high *trans* concentrations, i.e., in infinite-*trans* conditions. For the very simplest mediated transport system, the simple pore of Eq. (1) and Fig. 4, the asymmetry parameter A for zero-*trans* situations is given (using Eq. (9)) by

$$A=(R_{21}[S]+Q)/(R_{12}[S]+Q)\,. \tag{39}$$

At low values of the substrate concentrations, the asymmetry is unity, i.e., the system will behave symmetrically but, at high substrate concentrations, the system will be asymmetric, with a maximum asymmetry of $A=R_{21}/R_{12}$, the ratio of the maximum velocities. This result derived for the simple pore is generally true for carrier systems as well. At low substrate concentrations all systems will appear to behave symmetrically, whatever their underlying asymmetry. As the maximal flows are reached, however, asymmetry begins to be displayed and is maximal at saturation substrate concentrations. Even a simple pore can behave quite asymmetrically, and will act as a valve, permitting a high flow of substrate in one direction only. Such valve properties, therefore, are not carrier distinctive. Given a high enough substrate concentration, a simple pore will offer a different resistance to net flow of substrate in the two directions across the membrane. For the simple pore of Eq. (1), then, the maximal value of A is equal to the ratio of coefficients of resistance, which is also (Table 1) given by b_2/b_1 and f_2/f_1.

We can depict the energetics of this simple model in the diagram of Fig. 17. The horizontal lines in this and subsequent figures represent the values of the energy of the state considered, here the carrier E with substrate S_1, with substrate S_2, or the carrier–substrate complex. The humps represent activation energy barriers for the transitions depicted, transition states being denoted $ES_1^{\ddagger}$ and $ES_2^{\ddagger}$

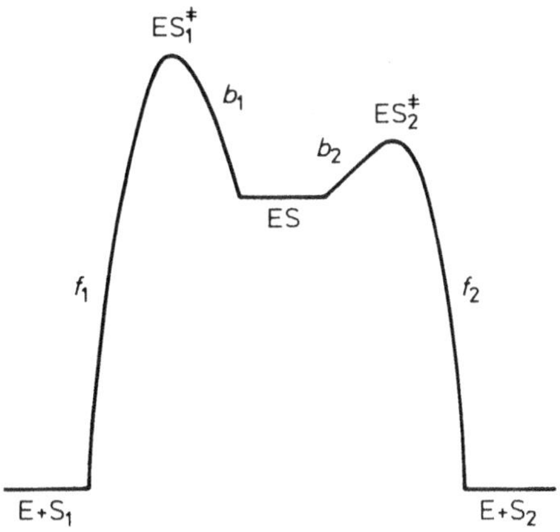

Fig. 17. Schematic representation of the energy levels for different states of the simple pore. In this and subsequent figures, the y-axis shows the energy levels of the different states, indicated by horizontal lines, lettered with reference to each state. The smooth curves represent transition paths between the different states, the hump representing the activation energy barrier for the transition. The concentration of transportable substrate is considered to be 1 *M* everywhere, i.e., the standard state. In this figure there is only one form of free E and one form of ES. The lowercase letters refer to rate constants for the steps shown

here, and correspondingly in later figures. The rate constants of Eq. (1) are represented on the figure as letters written next to the transition to which they refer. It is clear from the figure, and from the discussion in the previous paragraph, that the asymmetry of the pore system here results from the different heights of the energy barriers between the transition in the 1 to 2 and 2 to 1 directions. Since the state E is common to the transition in both directions, as is the state ES, altering the relative energies of E and ES will make no difference to the asymmetry of the system. Such changes will stabilize the ES complex or distabilize it, but will do so symmetrically towards the two membrane faces. But with the transition states $ES_1^\ddagger$ and $ES_2^\ddagger$ set at different energies, a markedly asymmetric valve-like system can be set up.

Consider now the exchange-only carrier system, described by Eqs. (18) or (22), for which the unidirectional flux is given as Eq. (23). We represent this in Fig. 18 a (one state of the carrier–substrate complex) and Fig. 18 b (two states of the ES complex). Such a system is, of course, the basic model for a countertransport situation). Then the asymmetry parameter here, defined for the infinite-*trans* situation (since there is no zero-*trans* flow) is given by

$$A = (K_2 + [S_2])/(K_1 + [S_1]) \tag{40}$$

In complete contrast to the situation for the simple pore, this system shows asymmetry at low values of the *cis* concentration, and the maximum value of A is given when both $[S_1]$ and $[S_2]$ are limitingly low in the separate infinite-*trans* experiments and is equal to K_2/K_1. At high values of $[S_1]$ and $[S_2]$, the asymmetry disappears. If we substitute for the rate constants in the expression for the maximum value of A, we obtain $A = b_2 f_1 / b_1 f_2$ for the single ES model and $A = b_2 f_1 g_1 / b_1 f_2 g_2$ for the two forms of ES model. If we now look at Fig. 18, we see that the

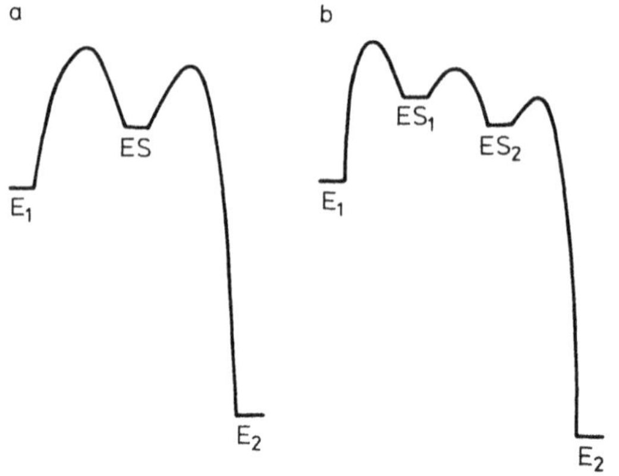

Fig. 18a, b. Schematic representation of the energy levels for the exchange-only carrier. **a** the model with one state of the complex; **b** the model with two states of the complex

implication of this result is that alterations in the heights of the activation energies for the transition states in this figure will make no difference to the asymmetry. Any such alteration always affects rate constants in pairs, and cancels out in the formulae for A. Similarly, any alteration in the relative energies of free carrier or bound forms has no effect, for the same reason. The only change which does affect the asymmetry is that made by altering the relative free energies of the unloaded carrier, E_1 and E_2. This affects, uniquely and unilaterally, the *on* constant f_1 or f_2, with direct effect on the asymmetry. A high rate of transport will occur from the side for which the free carrier has the highest free energy. This is the only factor which affects asymmetry for this model. The apparent affinity of carrier for substrate, given by the (reciprocal of) terms in K in Eq. (23), is highest at the side from which flow is greatest, i.e., at which the free carrier is of highest energetic state.

The models of Fig. 7 and 8 can be similarly treated. Figures 19a and b depict this model for the three-state and four-state situations, respectively. (Note, here, that we have the possibility of an interconversion of the free carrier transforming from E_1 to E_2. This is to be viewed as if in a different plane from the diagram for the interconversions of the bound carrier forms, since the latter diagram also includes energy contributions from the substrates.) For zero-*trans* situations and at high *cis* concentrations where the asymmetry is maximal, the asymmetry parameter is given by three-state model:

$$A=(1/b_1+1/k_1)/(1/b_2+1/k_2)\,, \tag{41 a}$$

four-state model:

$$A=(1/g_2+1/k_1)/(1/g_1+1/k_2) \tag{41 b}$$

for the case where g_1 and g_2 are far lower than b_1 and b_2.

Which energy state determines the asymmetry depends on whether it is the rate of movement of free or of loaded carrier that limits the overall transport event. If it is the unloaded carrier that moves slowly, a result often found, then in both models the terms in k dominate and the asymmetry is given by $A=k_2/k_1$, that is, by the free energy difference between the two forms of the free carrier.

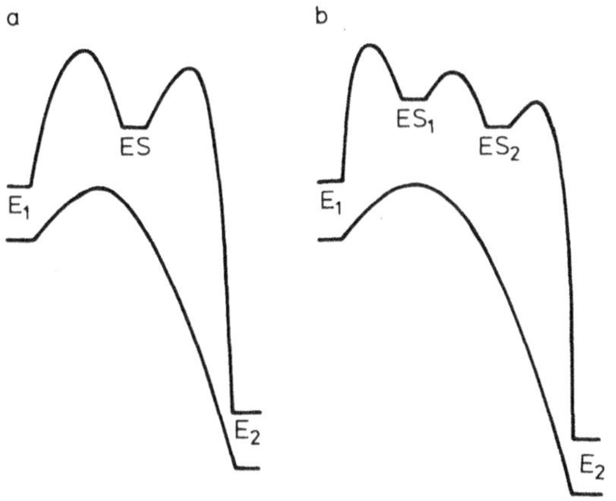

Fig. 19 a, b. Schematic representation of energy levels for the simple carrier. **a** one-state complex; **b** two-state complex. The energy levels of the free forms must be thought of as being on a different plane since they are drawn without addition of substrates S and P

That form of the free carrier which is most stable, i.e., which has lowest energy, is on the side *from* which net transport will be higher. Thus, if it is the unloaded carrier which moves slowly, none of the details of the energy states of the bound carrier forms will have the slightest effect on the asymmetry. This is precisely the same as the situation previously discussed for the exchange only system (where, of course, the free carrier movement is so slow as to be nonexistent). If, however, it is the movement of the loaded carrier that limits the overall rate of transport, the asymmetry parameter will be determined by the fine details of the energetics of the carrier substrate complex in its various forms. Lowering the activation energy of the ES_2 transition state in the three-state form of Fig. 19 a, or lowering the free energy of the ES_2 form in the model of Fig. 19 b, will increase selectively the net transport rate in the 1 to 2 direction, by increasing the flow out of the ES form in the former case or by reducing the back flow from ES_2 in the latter case. These properties are shared by the simple pore model discussed earlier. Thus, the simple carrier can yield asymmetric forms as a result of modification of relative energies of carrier states, either of the free carrier or of carrier–substrate complexes, depending on what transitions are rate limiting. In this it shares properties with the simple pore or with the exchange-only models, which appear, in this respect, as limiting cases of the carrier. Again, for the simple carrier (in net experiments), asymmetry appears only as the substrate concentrations is raised. A highly asymmetric carrier will appear symmetric at low substrate concentrations. In infinite-*trans* situations the reverse is the case, with asymmetry at low, and symmetry at high *cis* concentrations. The simple carrier in net flow experiments has a low affinity for substrate at that face of the membrane from which its maximum velocity is greatest.

II. Energetics of Countertransport Systems

The heart of the efficiency problem in coupled transport systems is this: if we assume that a gradient exists of the driving substrate or of chemical reaction, we have to show how this gradient can be used so as to speed up selectively the rate of transport in the forward direction of the coupled transport. In any event, the equilibrium distribution of the driven substrate is given by the gradient – but how can its flow be speeded up? Consider the classical countertransport model of Fig. 11. If P is the driving substrate, we take it that a good gradient of P exists, P_2 being far higher than P_1. How are we to ensure that the flow of S from 1 to 2 is as fast as possible? One could, perhaps, manipulate the energetics of the system so that the affinity of E_1 for S would be low. Then much of the time, E would flow from 1 to 2 loaded with P rather than S. This wastes no energy since P returns to side 2 to be available, once again, to drive carrier to side 1. But this movement wastes time and, in the competition against parallel leak systems, efficiency will be reduced. Hence, the affinity of E for S at side 1 should be maximalized, so that E always returns to side 2 loaded with the driven substrate. How can this be arranged? We can understand this from our previous discussion of Fig. 16 and of the "exchange-only" carrier. For a high affinity of S at side 1, relative to side 2, E_1 must be of high energy with respect to E_2 (Fig. 20). Indeed, it is an advantage if E_1 $(+S_1)$ is of higher energy than ES_1, ES_1 higher than SE_2, and ES_2 higher than E_2 $(+S_2)$. Flow of S will then be maximized in the 1 to 2 direction, giving a maximum rate of pumping of the driven substrate. But clearly, this situation where E_1 is of higher energy than E_2 is precisely the condition also for a high rate of flow of the driving substrate in the 1 to 2 direction. However, for efficiency, it must flow rather in the 2 to 1 direction. This difficulty is fundamental to all coupled systems and is ineluctable. It is only by virtue of the high gradient of the driving substrate in the 2 to 1 direction that the system will work.

Consider Fig. 20a. This depicts the energetics of a countertransport system, with S the driven and P the driving substrate. In the figure, the carrier affinity at side 1 for S is greater than that for P, so S will bind preferentially and be carried in the (desired) 1 to 2 direction. This is achieved by raising the energies of the intermediate states in the case of P. But if the EP states are raised with respect to the free carrier at side 1, they must be so raised with respect to the free carrier at side 2. Hence, the carrier E_2 binds P with poor affinity with respect to S. Return of S from 2 to 1 would result (with a waste of time but not of energy), were it not for the high concentration of P at side 2, which allows effective competition for E_2. Indeed, the countertransport system can be built with an additional subtlety which allows for flow from 1 to 2 to be of the driven substrate, while making use even more efficiently of the gradient of the driving substrate. The affinity of P for carrier at side 2 can be effectively reduced by raising the energy state of EP_2 (Fig. 20b). This has the effect of thereby confining flow of P to the 2 to 1 direction. In the insightful analysis by JENCKS (1980), the substrate P does not make use of all its possible binding energy when it forms EP_2. Only on the transition to EP_1 are additional carrier–substrate bonds made which lower the energy of EP_1 with respect to EP_2. The affinity of E_2 for P is lower than it might have been were not some of the possible bonds held in reserve for the stabilization of EP_1 with respect to EP_2.

In particular, we can approach chemiosmotic coupling in such energetic terms. In Fig. 20b we depict a system where the flow of substrate S is coupled to the counterflow of a chemical reaction, the hydrolysis of ATP to ADP and to in-

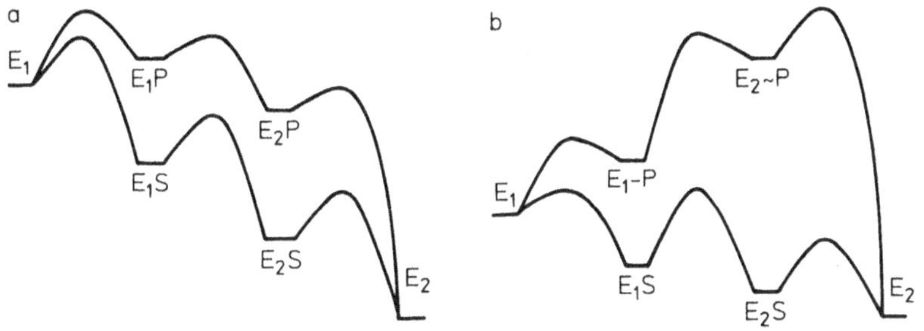

Fig. 20 a, b. Energy levels for countertransport, two-state complex. **a** osmotic-osmotic coupling, with two substrates, S and P; **b** chemiosmotic coupling, where P_1 is ATP, P_2 is ADPi, and E_1-P represents a low energy state while $E_2 \sim P$ is a high energy state

organic phosphate, Pi. All the arguments previously given for osmotic-osmotic flow by the model of Fig. 20a apply. In particular, phosphorylation of the transport enzyme can ensure that the EP_2 and EP_1 forms differ markedly in free energy. EP_2 possesses a "high energy" phosphate bond, and EP_1 a "low energy" bond, this energy difference channeling the transformation of the P-loaded carier enzyme in the 1 to 2 direction. Once again, this is done at the expense of a relatively poor affinity of the E_2 form for its substrate ATP, as compared with the affinity of E_2 for the transportable substrate S. The ATP, however, is itself a compound of high standard state free energy, compared with ADP and Pi, so that a low concentration of ATP has a large combining power for enzyme. This model demonstrates another important point stressed by JENCKS (1980). The fact that the form of the transport enzyme which transforms from state 1 to state 2 with transfer of substrate is unphosphorylated, whereas that which returns from 2 to 1 is phosphorylated, allows a simple mechanism for efficient coupling. What are really two quite different proteins, the free and the phosphorylated forms, can easily have quite different free energy relations between 2-facing and 1-facing states and, hence, two opposing asymmetries. The free transport enzyme can be designed so as to be relatively more stable in the 2-facing state, whereas the phosphorylated protein can be more stable in the opposite form. In this way, channeling of the transformations which bring about coupling of substrate flow and chemical reaction can be efficiently directed.

Finally, a most important aspect of the efficiency design of such countertransport systems is that the flow of *free* carrier or transport enzyme, unlinked to substrate flow or to chemical reaction, must be minimized and, preferably, reduced to zero. Presumably this is done by erecting huge energy barriers along the path for the $E_1 \rightarrow E_2$ interconversion. What is the nature of these energy barriers and how does binding of substrate or chemical intermediate remove these barriers so as to allow fast transport, are two of the key questions that remain to be investigated in carrier kinetics and thermodynamics.

III. Energetics of Cotransport

Let us consider Figs. 12 and 16 where cotransport models are depicted. There are four different cases which we will discuss in turn: (1) where the driving substrate,

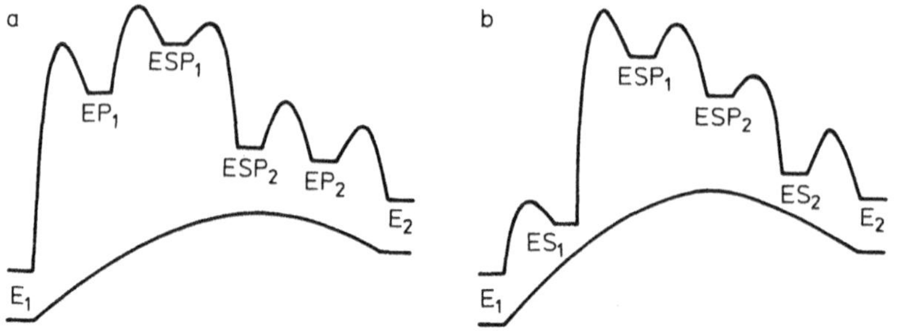

Fig. 21 a, b. Energy levels for cotransport. Two-state ternary complex. **a** driving substrate binds first at both faces; **b** driven substrate binds first at both faces. The energy levels of the free forms must be thought of as on a different plane, since they are drawn without addition of substrates S and P

here P, is the first to bind at both membrane faces; (2) where P is the second to bind at both faces; (3) where P binds first at face 1 and second at face 2; and (4) the reverse case.

For case (1), the driven substrate S binds to EP_1 or EP_2 at each membrane face, so that for S, the form EP is equivalent to being its carrier. Many of the arguments of the previous section dealing with the simple carrier apply here. Pumping of S will be efficient if the operative affinity of the "carrier" for S at side 1 is high, while that at side 2 is low. Such will be the case if the free energy of the form EP_1 is higher than that of EP_2, when it is the pathway $EP_2 \rightarrow E_2 \rightarrow E_1 \rightarrow EP_1$, that is slow compared with the pathway $EP_1 \rightarrow ESP_1 \rightarrow ESP_2 \rightarrow EP_2$. Alternatively, if the route through the ternary complex is the slower step, the transition steps between ESP_1 and ESP_2 must be such that the ESP_1 is of higher energy. Figure 21 a depicts the free energy profile of an efficient pumping system for case (1). The higher energy of EP_1 (or its subsequent transition state) compared with EP_2 (or its transition state) can arise only from a poorer affinity for the driving substrate at side 1, as compared with side 2. Once again, the situation in which the driving substrate is at a high relative concentration (at side 1 compared with side 2) must be *used* to overcome the reduced binding potential. The relative free energies of the free carrier forms, E_1 and E_2, are of critical importance to efficient coupling. The transition between E_2 and E_1 must be favored and fast. However, the $EP_1 \rightarrow EP_2$ intertransformation must be "forbidden." In chemiosmotic coupling (Fig. 14), EP_1 will be a "high energy" form, as will EPS_1. The form EPS_2 and, hence, EP_2 will be "low energy" (Fig. 21 a). Once again, the phosphorylation of the transport enzyme ensures that a large free energy difference can be found between forms of the transport enzyme bound to the driving substrate. The "forward" and "return" forms of the transport enzyme are different chemical entities and therefore can have very different asymmetries across the membrane.

In one important respect, this cotransport case differs from a simple carrier, as far as flow of the driven substrate is concerned. The affinity of carrier for substrate must be high at the membrane face from which pumping is occurring, but here this can be accompanied by a high maximum rate of pumping. For the carrier, a high affinity leads to a low maximum velocity (in zero-*trans* conditions).

For the coupled transport, this rate reduction is overcome by the presence of high concentrations of the driving substrate which draws the equilibrium between carrier forms over into that form which favors transport of S from side 1, namely, EP_1. This driving of the equilibrium, of course, requires the presence of the high gradient of the driving substrate. The high affinity of transport enzyme for the driven substrate arises as a result of the poor relative affinity of the driving substrate ans, as JENCKS pointed out, the total binding energy of the driving substrate and enzyme can be released in the formation of the stabilized forms further along the reaction path.

For case (2), as Fig. 21 b depicts, the required high affinity of S at side 1 (as compared with side 2) is achieved by the setting of the free carrier E_1 at lower energy than E_2. The binding of S to E_2 at side 2 is competed for by the flow of E from 2 to 1. But in order that the overall reaction should be cotransport in the 1 to 2 direction, ESP_1 must be of higher energy than ESP_2. Thus, the driving substrate must bind relatively poorly at side 1. Once again, a high affinity for the driven substrate is at the expense of the driving substrate. In chemiosmotic coupling, EPS_1 and EPS_2 can be high and low energy forms, respectively, so that the fact of phosphorylation is once again used to ensure oppositely directed asymmetries for the two different chemical entities, EPS and E. The $ES_1 \rightarrow ES_2$ transition is an internal leak and must be "forbidden," while the $E_1 \rightarrow E_2$ transformation needs to be rapid for efficient pumping.

Cases (3) and (4) possess some interesting features in that the chemical species that combine with the driven substrate on either side of the membrane are different. On one side of the membrane it is the ligand carrier or phosphorylated protein, and on the other the free or dephosphorylated form, that so combines. Such features must allow additional subtleties of energetic relations. For such systems in the case of a chemiosmotic coupling, where ATP splitting is the driving chemical reaction, once again the asymmetries across the membrane can be easily arranged to be different in the two directions, since the chemical species involved in these transitions are free protein and phosphorylated protein in the two situations.

While it has hardly ever been clearly demonstrated for any coupled system which, precisely, is the order in which driving and driven substrates bind to the pump enzyme, it can already be seen how the carrier lends itself to exploitation in the interests of efficient pumping. It will be important in the years to come to pursue the further analysis of the molecular details of such coupled systems and thereby to reach an understanding of the details of intestinal transport.

References

Alvarado F (1965) The relationship between Na^+ and the active transport of arbutin in the small intestine. Biochim Biophys Acta 109:478–494

Aronson PS (1978) Energy dependence of phloridzin binding to isolated renal microvillus membranes. J Membr Biol 142:81–98

Baker GF, Widdas WF (1973) The asymmetry of the facilitated transfer system for hexoses in human red cells and the simple kinetics of a two component model. J Physiol (Lond) 231:143–165

Beauge LA, Glynn IM (1979) Occlusion of K ions in the unphosphorylated sodium pump. Nature 280:510–512
Bihler I, Crane RK (1962) Studies on the mechanism of intestinal absorption of sugars V. The influence of several cations and anions on the active transport of sugars in vitro, by various preparations of hamster small intestine. Biochim Biophys Acta 58:78–93
Britten HG (1977) Calculation of steady-state rate equations and the fluxes between substrates and products in enzyme reactions. Biochem J 161:517–526
Cabantchik ZI, Ginsburg H (1977) Transport of uridine in human red cells. Demonstration of a simple carrier-mediated process. J Gen Physiol 69:75–96
Cass CE, Gaudette LA, Paterson ARP (1974) Mediated transport of nucleosides in human erythrocytes. Specific binding of the inhibitor nitrobenzethioinosine to nucleoside transport sites in the erythrocyte membrane. Biochim Biophys Acta 345:1–10
Christensen HN, Riggs TE, Ray NE (1952) Concentrative uptake of amino acids by erythrocytes in vitro. J Biol Chem 194:41–51
Cleland WW (1963) The kinetics of enzyme-catalysed reactions with two or more substrates or products. Biochim Biophys Acta 67:104–187
Crane RK (1960) Intestinal absorption of sugars. Physiol Rev 40:789–825
Crane RK (1962) Hypothesis of mechanism of intestinal active transport of sugars. Fed Proc 21:891–895
Crane RK, Forstner G, Eichholz A (1965) Studies on the mechanism of the intestinal transport of sugars. X. An effect of Na^+ concentration on the apparent Michaelis constants for intestinal sugar transport in vitro. Biochim Biophys Acta 109:467–477
Csáky TZ, Thale M (1960) Effect of ionic environment on intestinal sugar transport. J Physiol (Lond) 151:59–65
Csáky TZ, Zollicoffer L (1960) Ionic effect on intestinal transport of glucose in the rat. Am J Physiol 198:1056–1058
Csáky TZ, Hartzog HG, Fernald GW (1961) Effect of digitalis on active intestinal sugar transport. Am J Physiol 200:459–460
Danielli JF (1954) The present position in the field of facilitated diffusion and selective active transport. Proc Symp Colston Res Soc 7:1–4
Davson H, Danielli JF (1943) The permeability of natural membranes. Cambridge University Press, Cambridge
Deves R, Krupka RM (1978) A new approach in the kinetics of biological transport. The potential of reversible inhibition studies. Biochim Biophys Acta 510:186–200
Deves R, Krupka RM (1979) A simple experimental approach to the determination of carrier transport parameters for unlabeled substrate analogs. Biochim Biophys Acta 556:524–532
Edwards PAW (1972) Evidence for the carrier model in red cell glucose and choline transport. J Physiol (Lond) 225:36–37p
Edwards PAW (1973a) The inactivation by fluorodinitrobenzene of glucose transport across the human erythrocyte membrane. The effect of glucose inside or outside the cell. Biochim Biophys Acta 307:415–418
Edwards PAW (1973b) Evidence for the carrier model of transport from the inhibition by N-ethylmaleimide of choline transport across the human red cell membrane. Biochim Biophys Acta 311:123–140
Edwards PAW (1974) A test for non-specific diffusion steps in transport across cell membranes and its application to red cell glucose transport. Biochim Biophys Acta 345:373–386
Glynn IM, Karlish SJD (1975) The sodium pump. Ann Rev Physiol 37:13–55
Goldner AM, Schultz SG, Curran PF (1969) Sodium and sugar fluxes across the mucosal border of rabbit ileum. J Gen Physiol 53:362–383
Heinz E, Geck P, Wilbrandt W (1972) Coupling in active transport. Activation of transport by co-transport and/or counter-transport with the fluxes of other solutes. Biochim Biophys Acta 225:442–461
Höber R (1945) Physical chemistry of cells and tissues. Churchill, London
Höber R, Höber J (1937) Experiments on the absorption of organic solutes in the small intestine of rats. J Cell Comp Physiol 10:401–422

Honig B, Stein WD (1978) Design principles for active transport systems. J Theor Biol 75:299–305
Hopfer U, Groseclose R (1980) The mechanism of Na^+-dependent D-glucose transport. J Biol Chem 255:4453–4462
Jencks WP (1980) The utilisation of binding energy in coupled vectorial processes. Adv Enzymol 51:75–106
Jung CY (1974) Inactivation of glucose carriers in human erythrocyte membranes by 1-fluoro-2,4-dinitrobenzene. J Biol Chem 249:3568–3573
Kessler M, Tannenbaum V, Tannenbaum C (1978) A simple apparatus for performing short-time (1–2 seconds) uptake measurements in small volumes. Its applications to D-glucose transport studies in brush border vesicles from rabbit jejunum and ileum. Biochim Biophys Acta 509:348–359
Koefoed-Johnsen V, Ussing HH (1958) Nature of the frog skin potential. Acta Physiol Scand 42:298–308
Krupka RM (1971) Evidence for a carrier conformational change associated with sugar transport in erythrocytes. Biochemistry 10:1143–1148
LeFevre PG (1948) Evidence of active transfer of certain non-electrolytes across the human red cell membrane. J Gen Physiol 31:505–527
Lieb WR (1982) A kinetic approach to transport studies. In: Ellory JC, Young JD (eds) Red cell membranes – a methodological approach. Academic, London, pp 135–164
Lieb WR, Stein WD (1974a) Testing and characterising the simple pore. Biochim Biophys Acta 373:165–177
Lieb WR, Stein WD (1974b) Testing and characterising the simple carrier. Biochim Biophys Acta 373:178–196
Lieb WR, Stein WD (1976) Testing the simple carrier using irreversible inhibitors. Biochim Biophys Acta 455:913–927
Mitchell P (1966) Chemiosmotic coupling in oxidative and photosynthetic phosphorylation. Biol Rev 41:445–502
Mitchell P (1967) Translocations through natural membranes. Adv Enzymol 29:33–88
Mitchell P (1977) Vectorial chemisomotic processes. Ann Rev Biochem 46:996–1005
Murer H, Kinne R (1977) Sidedness and coupling of transport processes in small intestine and renal epithelia. In: Semenza G, Carafoli E (eds) Biochemistry of membrane transport. Springer, Berlin Heidelberg New York, pp 292–304
Murer H, Hopfer U, Kinne-Saffran E, Kinne R (1974) Glucose transport in isolated brush-border and lateral-basal plasma-membrane vesicles from intestinal epithelial cells. Biochim Biophys Acta 345:170–179
Park CR, Post RL, Kalman CF, Wright JH Jr, Johnson LH, Morgan HE (1956) Transport of glucose and other sugars across cell membranes and the effects of insulin. Ciba Foundation Coll Endocrinol 9:240–249
Post RL, Hegevary C, Kume S (1972) Activation by adenosine triphosphate in the phosphorylation kinetics of sodium and potassium ion transport adenosine triphosphatase. J Biol Chem 247:6530–6540
Rosenberg T (1954) Concept and definition of active transport. Symp Soc Exp Biol 8:136–144
Rosenberg T, Wilbrandt W (1957) Uphill transport induced by counterflow. J Gen Physiol 41:289–296
Schultz SF, Zalusky R (1964) Ion transport in isolated rabbit ileum II. The interaction between active sodium and active sugar transport. J Gen Physiol 47:1043–1059
Semenza G (1967) Rate equations of some cases of enzyme inhibition and activation-their application to sodium-activated membrane transport systems. J Theor Biol 15:145–176
Stein WD (1967) Movement of molecules across cell membranes. Academic, New York
Stein WD (1977a) How the kinetic parameters of the simple carrier are affected by an applied voltage. Biochim Biophys Acta 467:376–385
Stein WD (1977b) Testing and characterising a simple carrier model for co-transport. In: Kramer M, Lauterbach F (eds) Intestinal permeation. Excerpta Medica, Amsterdam, pp 262–273

Stein WD, Honig B (1977) Models for the active transport of cations ... the steady-state analysis. Mol Cell Biochem 15:27–45

Toggenburger G, Kessler M, Rothstein A, Semenza G, Tannenbaum C (1978) Similarity in effects of Na^+ gradients and membrane potentials on D-glucose transport by, and phloridzin binding to, vesicles derived from brush borders of rabbit intestinal mucosal cells. J Membrane Biol 40:269–290

Widdas WF (1952) Inability of diffusion to account for placental glucose transfer in the sheep and consideration of the kinetics of a possible carrier transfer. J Physiol (Lond) 118:23–39

Widdas WF (1954) Facilitated transfer of hexoses across the human erythrocyte membrane. J Physiol (Lond) 125:163–180

Wilbrandt W (1977) The asymmetry of sugar transport in the red cell membrane. In: Semenza G, Carafoli E (eds) Biochemistry of membrane transport. Springer, Berlin Heidelberg New York, pp 204–211

Wilbrandt W, Laszt LA (1933) Untersuchungen über die Ursachen der selektiven Glukoseresorption aus dem Darm. Biochem Ztschr 259:398–417

CHAPTER 8

Energetics of Intestinal Absorption

D. S. PARSONS

A. Introduction

The small intestine exhibits unusual features with respect to tissue energy metabolism. First, it is the major portal of entry of energy-providing nutrients of carnivorous and omnivorous animals. The fact that in omnivorous and carnivorous animals large quantities of energy-yielding nutrients are absorbed relative to the actual requirements of the absorbing tissue has implications with respect to the segregation of these nutrients from the cellular metabolism of the intestine. For an adult human with an intake of 2,500 kcal (10.5 MJ) per day and equivalent to 9×10^5 kcal (3.8 GJ) a year, it has been calculated that the requirements of the intestinal mucosa are not more than about 450 kJ per day (164 MJ per year) (PARSONS 1975). The energy requirements of the mucosa are therefore probably less than 5% of the energetic value of the nutrients handled by the tissue during digestion and absorption.

A second feature characteristic of the intestine is that fuels are available to the cells of the epithelium not only directly from the blood, but also from the intestinal lumen. A third, but related, feature is that the metabolism of the fuel available to the tissue from the intestinal lumen may be different when the same is available to the epithelium from the blood.

In ruminants and caecal-fermenting herbivores the major route for the intake of energy-providing nutrients is, in the former, the rumen and in the latter, the caecum and large intestine. In these cases the nutrients are short-chain volatile fatty acids, the products of microbial and protozoal fermentation of the diet (see ANNISON and LEWIS 1959; WRONG et al. 1981). It is an interesting question as to whether in, for example, human subjects, volatile fatty acids formed in the colon contribute significantly to the energy intake. They can certainly be absorbed (MCNEIL et al. 1978) and can sustain the metabolism of the colonic mucosa (ROEDIGER 1979).

B. Special Fuels as Sources of Energy

Steam engines, electric motors, internal combustion engines, muscles and the mucosa of the small intestine have a common feature: they must be supplied with energy in order to do work; furthermore the energy has to be derived from a special fuel. In the case of the steam engine the energy of, usually, fossil fuel is released by combustion and caused to generate steam pressure which is then converted by means of mechanical linkages into the energy of rotation of the crank-shaft. An

Table 1. Some definitions

Electrochemical gradient ($\Delta\bar{\mu}$)

For a monovalent cation

$$\Delta\bar{\mu} = RT \ln \Delta a + F\Delta E$$

where $a = a_{out}/a_{in}$, a = activity

and sign of the membrane potential, ΔE, is inside-negative

For a monovalent anion

$$\Delta\bar{\mu} = RT \ln \Delta a - F\Delta E$$

Energy: ability to do work

Flux: J = quantity, Q (mol), moved in unit time

$J = Q/t$

Work: W = quantity (Q mol) moved against the gradient multiplied by the gradient

$W = Q\Delta\bar{\mu}$

Power: $\boldsymbol{P}$ = rate of doing work

Power output of a pump: $\boldsymbol{P} = Q\Delta\bar{\mu}/t$

$\boldsymbol{P} = J\Delta\bar{\mu}$

electric motor converts electrial energy into the energy of rotation of the armature. For the reciprocating variety of internal combustion engine, the energy of a refined fossil fuel is converted by combustion into the energy of a gas under pressure which in turn is converted by means of mechanical linkages into the energy of rotation of the crank-shaft; in a jet engine the energy of a refined fossil fuel is converted by combustion into the energy of a rapidly moving stream of hot gases, which is used directly to propel the vehicle to which the jet engine is attached (Table 1).

In animal tissues, in contrast, a fundamental concept is that the combustion in these tissues of the major energy foodstuffs, i.e. the fuels derived immediately from the diet, leads to the formation of a special form of chemical energy. This dogma, first clearly proposed by LIPMANN in 1941, is that the first stage of energy transduction in living tissues is the conversion of the free energy of the fuels of tissue metabolism into the free energy of the terminal pyrophosphate bond of ATP. This process seems to occur with an overall efficiency as high as about 70%, higher than that of machines (KREBS and KORNBERG 1957).

The second stage of energy transduction in animal tissues is the translation of the free energy present in the ATP into work, i.e. muscle contraction or the pumping of ions across biological membranes. Another important use of ATP is as an energy source for biosynthetic reactions: synthesis of nucleic acids, of proteins, of fatty acids, of glycogen, etc.

It must be pointed out that in living cells generally, in addition to and independently of ATP utilization, two other sources of energy are in fact available to drive membrane transport processes. These other sources are, first the direct coupling of energy dissipated by ions running down their electrochemical gradient across a membrane to the "uphill" movement of a solute across the same membrane, this will be further considered in Sect. J. The second source is the capture of the energy of light. In *Halobacterium halobium* the energy of light is used directly to pump H^+ ions from inside the bacteria out into the medium. This proton pumping is mediated by the membrane-bound purple pigment bacteriorhodopsin (see, e.g. MACDONALD and LANYI 1977; EISENBACH and CAPLAN 1979).

C. Membrane Transport and Oxidative Phosphorylation

More recently, it has become appreciated that the oxidative biosynthesis of ATP (oxidative phosphorylation) itself involves energy transduction during the operation of membrane transport processes. According to the chemiosmotic theory, the principles of which now appear to be generally accepted, the functioning and arrangement of electron and hydrogen carriers located within biological membranes, e.g., the inner mitochondrial membrane, drive directly a proton pump, an electrochemical potential gradient of H^+ ions thus being established across the membrane (GREVILLE 1969; MITCHELL and MOYLE 1974; SIMONI and POSTMA 1975). In the case of mitochondria, the protons are pumped outwards across the inner mitochondrial membrane; according to the chemiosmotic theory, during oxidative phosphorylation it is the energy dissipated by the re-entry of the protons into the mitochondria along a separate special channel, and down their electrochemical gradient, that is directly coupled to the synthesis of ATP from ADP. In other words a "redox pump" establishes an electrochemical gradient of protons, i.e. the energy released by oxidation is transduced into the energy of an electrochemical gradient. The energy of this gradient is then itself transduced into that of the terminal pyrophosphate bond of ATP.

It has been suggested that redox pumps may be present in the *plasma* membranes of animal cells, but there is as yet no direct evidence that the electrochemical potential gradient of protons established by the functioning of such pumps can be used to drive directly any membrane transport process (LOW and CRANE 1978).

D. General Features of Energy Utilization

Tissues utilize energy in two ways; there is a continuing basal utilization of energy by all tissues and an additional utilization incurred in working tissues. The basal energy requirements are those necessary to sustain the organization and operation of the tissue – for example, to provide energy for ion pumping to maintain cell volume (PARSONS 1976; MACKNIGHT and LEAF 1977) and for the synthesis of cell constituents including components of membranes such as glycoproteins and phospholipids.

The additional energy requirements are those incurred during the physiological operations performed by the tissue. In the case of the intestinal epithelium, these additional working loads are those associated with the uptake, translocation and secretion of organic molecules and of ions across the epithelium. This work may include the requirements for the synthesis and assembly of macromolecules – for example, the synthesis of the triglyceride and the lipoprotein incorporated into chylomicrons during the absorption of long-chain fatty acids.

In addition to these requirements for the absorptive processes of the epithelium, the energy requirements during intestinal absorption overall will also include those necessary to sustain the contractions of the gastrointestinal musculature that are responsible for propulsion of the intestinal contents along its length.

E. Basal Energy Requirements of Tissues

It appears that ion pumping processes account for more than half of the basal energy requirements of tissues, while the energy that has to be provided to sustain protein synthesis and growth may be about 15% of the total basal requirements (WHITTAM and WHEELER 1970; MILLIGAN 1971). In this connection, the efficiency of energy utilization is of importance. For both basal and working conditions, this efficiency can be defined as the quotient (power output)/(power input) and can be called the machine efficiency. For processes underlying ion pumping across membranes (membrane transport), the machine efficiency seems to be about 60% (MILLIGAN 1971; KUSHMERICK and DAVIES 1969; KUSHMERICK 1977).

For membrane transport, it is possible to estimate the energy requirements from a knowledge of the rate of transport and the electrochemical gradient of a transported ion or molecule that exists across the membrane. In the case of epithelial transport, a valid estimate is at present impossible because, as shown in Sect. F, epithelial transport is a multistep process. For a valid calculation of the energy requirement for epithelial transport of a particular substrate, it is necessary to know the route (or routes) of that substrate across the epithelium and the magnitude and direction of the relevant electrochemical gradient across each step of membrane transport that lies in the pathway (or pathways) of translocation. A knowledge of the electrochemical gradient that exists across the whole epithelium is of no help in this regard, and indeed can be positively misleading. A further complication in the small intestine is that some organic molecules that are absorbed may undergo significant metabolism within the epithelium and be converted into another, different, substance which is secreted into the blood (see Sect. H). A fuller consideration of some of these points has been given elsewhere (PARSONS 1975). It must be concluded that it is not yet possible to obtain satisfactory estimates of the machine efficiency of the epithelial transport of organic substance, ions or water.

F. The Energetics of Absorption Are the Energetics of Movement Along a Multistep Pathway

Intestinal absorption, the translation of substances from the intestinal lumen into the circulation in vivo or into artificial fluids in vitro, is a sequential, multistep process, and the movement through any single step may be rate limiting to absorption. It is often difficult to identify which step is rate limiting to the transfer of a particular substrate for any given set of conditions for absorption. Indeed, depending upon the procedures employed to investigate the absorption, different steps may be rate limiting to the translation of a particular substrate (Table 2).

Table 2. The pathway of the cellular route of intestinal epithelial absorption. Which one is rate limiting to the overall transport of your favourite substrate by your favoured preparation? The pathway is seen as containing five bridges each of which requires, usually, more than one step for the crossing. The arrangement of the analogous pathway for the paracellular route is suggested as an exercise for the reader. After PARSONS (1972)

Bridge	Nature of bridge	Step	Nature of step	Driving forces
I	Delivery systems	1	Move from stomach into lumen from small intestine, movement along length of small intestine	Motility of gastrointestinal muscles
		2	Move in radial direction from bulk phase in lumen across unstirred layer to absorbing surface at brush border membranes	Diffusion
II	Entry systems Phase of cellular entry. Hydrolysis of some oligomers of dietary polymers may occur here	3	Attach to transport channel	Na, along downhill gradient, the movement coupled to accumulative entry of amino acids, hexoses and sometimes Cl
		4	Move through transport channel	
		5	Detach from transport channel and enter cell interior	
III	Transcellular transport Metabolic transformations may occur here, e.g. transamination reactions and hydrolysis of dipeptides	6	Move across cell interior through permeable organelles and passing around impermeable organelles to basolateral membrane	Diffusion Cytoplasmic movement (?)
IV	Output systems	7	Attach to transport channel	For sugars and amino acids: chemical gradient; for Na: ATP hydrolysis
		8	Move through transport channel	
		9	Detach from transport channel and enter extracellular (intercellular) space	
V	Clearance system	10	Move along and across extracellular (including intercellular) space	Diffusion
		11	Enter blood capillary or lymphatics or, in vitro, move across serosa	

The movement of a substrate, or of its products of metabolism, though any step implies energy changes. These changes may involve passive movements of the substrate down gradients of concentration or of electrochemical potential during which the gradient is dissipated, unless work is done elsewhere in renewing it. The energy to drive movements through a step where the gradient is "uphill" has to be derived from some source of power coupled directly to the movement.

There are two routes through the epithelium: through the cells (cellular route) and through the paracellular shunt pathway (paracellular route) and the nature of the pathway of the *cellular* route of intestinal epithelial transport is shown in Table 2. Movement along the *paracellular* pathway is considered in Sect. K, N and O.

G. Variable Patterns of Fuels Available to the Small Intestine

Because the input of energy into animals is episodic, yet its expenditure by the tissues is continuous, systems for transporting and storing energy exist. The cost and efficacy of storage of some common fuels is shown in Table 3. The nature of the fuels being metabolized by a tissue at any moment therefore depends upon the immediate nutritional history of the animal. During the phase of intestinal absorption, fuels in the diet will be present in the intestinal lumen, while at the same time fuels that have been absorbed are being stored in the tissues. During this phase glucose is the principal circulating fuel in the blood that is available to all tissues, including the intestinal mucosa. However, at this time blood-borne glutamine is also an important respiratory fuel of the mucosa.

In the later post absorptive and fasting states, amino acids are mobilized, chiefly from the muscle proteins as glutamine and alanine, and transported to the liver where the latter enters the gluconeogenic pathway and thence supplies the

Table 3. Cost and efficiency of metabolic fuels (MILLIGAN 1971; PARSONS 1973)

Precursors		Product	Cost of storage[a]	Efficiency of storage[b]
Substrate (mol)	ATP (mol)	(mol)		
Average amino acid (1)	4	Protein (100 g)	11	89
Glucose (1) + glycogen ($n-1$)	2	Glycogen (n)	3	97
Glucose (2)	2	Lactose (1)	2	98
Glucose (12.5)	34	Triglyceride (tripalmitin) (1)	17	83
Acetate (8)	43	Palmitate (1)	29	71
Palmitate (3) + glycerol (1)	8	Tripalmitin (1)	3	97

[a] Calculated as $\frac{\text{(precursor free energy)} - \text{(product free energy)}}{\text{precursor free energy}} \times 100$

[b] Calculated as 100 − cost of storage

blood glucose. The predominant fuels circulating in the later stages of fasting and in starvation are nonesterified fatty acids mobilized from the stores in adipose tissue, and the ketone bodies that are formed in the liver from these fatty acids. All these fuels are available to the intestine from the blood, but blood-borne glutamine continues to be an important fuel for this thissue during fasting (HANSON and PARSONS 1977, 1980; WINDMUELLER and SPAETH 1980). The possible pathways of glutamine metabolism by enterocytes of rat intestine are discussed by HANSON and PARSONS (1980).

H. Intestinal Metabolism of Nutrients During Absorption

The small intestine does not simply pump nutrients from the intestinal lumen into the portal blood and mesenteric lymphatics. In practice nutrients are often subjected to some form of metabolism during their passage across the epithelium from the intestinal lumen. Thus, fatty acids of chain length greater than C_{12} that enter the intestinal mucosa as micelles, either in the form of free fatty acids, as monoglyceride or as cholesterol ester, are secreted as the triglyceride of the very low density lipoprotein of the chylomicrons (see BRINDLEY 1977). The extent to which long-chain fatty acids entering the epithelium from the lumen are oxidized as fuels is not yet clear.

Although most of the amino acids are metabolized only to a minor extent during absorption, the dicarboxylic amino acids, L-glutamate and L-aspartate, are almost completely transaminated during absorption in many animals. This results in the amino nitrogen of these two amino acids appearing in portal blood as the amino nitrogen of L-alanine (Table 4). This transfer of the amino nitrogen is achieved by the operation of transamination reactions within the epithelial cells,

Table 4. Transamination of glutamate, aspartate or glutamate and aspartate together during absorption by rat jejunum and ileum in vitro. Appearance of alanine, aspartate and glutamate in the fluid transported across the serosal surface of jejunal segments of rat intestine in the presence in the luminal fluid of glucose (28 m*M*) and: (1) glutamate (10 m*M*); (2) aspartate (10 m*M*); or (3) glutamate (10 m*M*) + aspartate (10 m*M*). Values are corrected for the appearance of amino acids in the absence of glutamate or aspartate in the luminal fluid. Values are of mean ± standard error of four (Glu) or five (Asp), (Asp + Glu) experiments. After VOLMAN-MITCHELL and PARSONS (1974)

Amino acid appearing	Rate of appearance of amino acid in serosal fluid (μmol/h per gram dry weight)		
Jejunum	(1) Glu	(2) Asp	(3) Asp + Glu
Alanine	34.8 ± 1.8	43.4 ± 6.6	56.2 ± 8.6
Aspartate	0.8 ± 0.0	6.6 ± 1.4	6.0 ± 1.2
Glutamate	11.0 ± 1.6	3.0 ± 1.0	11.6 ± 0.6
Ileum			
Alanine	45.4 ± 4.0	58.4 ± 1.2	83.0 ± 12.0
Aspartate	1.4 ± 0.0	7.4 ± 1.0	6.8 ± 1.4
Glutamate	9.2 ± 2.0	1.8 ± 0.2	7.2 ± 0.6

Table 5. Soluble glutamate–pyruvate transaminase of mammalian intestinal mucosa. Specific activity of glutamate–pyruvate transaminase in high speed supernatants of homogenates of mucosal tissues of gastrointestinal tract and liver of fed animals. In all these species at least 90% of the activity of this enzyme is in the soluble fraction of the homogenates. Specific activity values are mean ± standard error; figures in parentheses are numbers of experiments. Units of specific activity are nmol substrate transaminated per milligram protein per minute. After VOLMAN-MITCHELL and PARSONS (1974)

Tissue	Rat	Mouse	Guinea-pig	Hamster
Liver	184 (2)	278 (2)	46 (2)	237 ± 14 (4)
Stomach	189 ± 7 (4)	123 (2)	52 ± 6 (4)	14 ± 0 (4)[a]
				45 ± 3 (4)[b]
Duodenum	415 ± 2 (4)	130 (2)	50 ± 3 (4)	89 ± 11 (4)
Jejunum	453 ± 37 (4)	264 (2)	73 ± 6 (4)	71 ± 10 (3)
Ileum	292 ± 20 (4)	202 (2)	96 ± 2 (4)	40 ± 7 (3)
Caecum	62 ± 5 (3)	40 (2)	0	12 ± 1 (3)
Proximal colon	58 ± 4 (3)	41 (2)	0	19 (1)

[a] Nonglandular portion
[b] Glandular (acid-secreting) portion

the carbon skeleton of the alanine being derived from the pyruvate that is formed during the metabolism of glucose (NEAME and WISEMAN 1957; VOLMAN-MITCHELL and PARSONS 1974; PARSONS and VOLMAN-MITCHELL 1974). The relevant transaminases have been reported in a wide variety of species (Table 5). The corresponding dicarboxylic keto acids that are formed during transamination reactions are largely oxidized by the epithelium during absorption (NEAME and WISEMAN 1958; VOLMAN-MITCHELL 1973).

The quantities of transaminase enzymes that are present within the epithelial cells of rat intestine do not appear to be a rate-limiting factor in the transfer of dicarboxylic acid amino nitrogen to alanine; rather it appears to be the uptake of the dicarboxylic amino acids from the intestinal lumen into the epithelium that is limiting to the reactions. Thus it has been found in the case of the rat that, when the dipeptide LGlu-L-Glu is absorbed, alanine is secreted from the tissue at faster rates than when an equivalent concentration of L-Glu is present in the lumen (PARSONS and VOLMAN-MITCHELL 1975–1976, unpublished work).

It is of interest that, when L-glutamine is absorbed, very little glutamate appears in the portal venous effluent from vascularly perfused intestine of the rat, although significant quantities of L-glutamine, up to one-third of that absorbed, are transferred. The rest of the amino nitrogen appears in the portal effluent, largely as alanine together with some ammonia (PARSONS and HANSON 1978, unpublished work). Because dietary proteins contain significant quantities of glutamine these findings suggest that, at least in the rat, the small intestine can contribute significant amounts of NH_3 to the portal venous blood. It remains to be discovered whether asparagine is treated in the same sort of way as glutamine during absorption, and also how these derivatives of the dicarboxylic amino acids are metabolized during absorption by human intestine.

The widespread distribution of transaminases in the intestinal mucosae of different species has relevance to the composition of the mixtures of amino acids used in parenteral nutrition of human subjects. Evidently the mixtures that are infused ought to be deficient in the dicarboxylic amino acids, but enriched with alanine (see PARSONS 1979).

J. Energetics of Brush Border Transport Processes

The hydrolysis of the terminal pyrophosphate bond of ATP by enzyme systems located in the plasma membrane drives the pumping of Na and K ions across the plasma membrane (see SCOU and NØRBY 1979). This pumping, Na outwards and K inwards, which incidentally need not be electrically neutral (i.e. *n*Na exchanging with *m*K) and may therefore be electrogenic (HODGKIN 1951; THOMAS 1972), will result in charging up a store of electrochemical potential energy across the plasma membranes of the cell. In practice, this store seems largely to consist of the electrochemical gradient of Na ions. However, in an asymmetrical cell such as a small intestinal mucosal epithelial cell, where the membranes at opposite poles of the cell have differing structures and properties and the outside faces of which are exposed to differing environments, the potential energy of the store across one part of the plasma membrane, e.g. the brush border, may differ from that across another, different, region of the plasma membrane, e.g. the basolateral membrane. This follows because not only may the local activity of Na ions differ outside the cell at the two sites, but the local membrane potential may also be different because the permeability of the membranes, particularly with respect to small anions and cations, may differ at the two sites.

Using modern ion-selective microelectrodes, it is now possible to measure the activity of the intracellular Na in intact cells, in situ within the epithelium. Also, using standard electrophysiological methods for intracellular recording, the potentials existing across the brush border membrane between the environment in the lumen and the cell interior can be determined. On the assumption that such measurements are valid estimates of the ionic activities and potentials relevant to the systems of transduction present in the brush border membranes, it is found for bullfrog small intestine that the energy inherent in the electrochemical potential gradient from Na across these membranes in the steady state is more than adequate to account for the work done in concentrating galactose in the epithelium during transport (ARMSTRONG et al. 1979). The efficiency of the coupling of the energy transduction is not easy to assess in these experiments because the galactose being transported across the cells leaks out across the basolateral membranes and maximum concentrations of the sugar cannot be obtained.

However, even these elegant and ingenious experiments on the intestinal mucosa are not able to provide unequivocal estimates of the energy changes involved when Na enters (or leaves) the cells. The reasons for this are first that the Na activity inside (*trans* side) the microvilli may differ from that measured inside the bulk cytoplasm by the probing microelectrode. Indeed it has been suggested that the Na activity is not uniform across the cells in the direction normal to the plane of the epithelium (ZEUTHEN 1976). Second, the ionic environment outside the microvilli (*cis* side) must be influenced by any fixed charges present on this surface

Table 6. Energy released or absorbed[a] at 38 °C by ions or molecules moving through boundaries across which differences of concentration and voltage exist

Concentration ratio	Energy (KJ/mol) (uncharged molecule or, for ions, $\Delta\Psi=0$)	$\Delta\Psi$ Potential difference (mV)	Energy (KJ/mol) (charge = 1)
1.1	0.23	5	0.48
1.5	0.89	10	0.97
2.0	1.75	20	1.93
2.5	2.34	30	2.90
3.0	2.79	40	3.86
4.0	3.50	50	4.82
5.0	4.08	60	5.80
10.0	5.75	80	7.72
15.0	6.87	100	9.65
20.0	7.58		

[a] For an ion carrying unit charge, the potential difference will, depending on the sign, either increase or decrease the energy dissipated or expended compared with the movement of an uncharged molecule. Thus 1 mol sodium moving into a cell down a concentration ratio of 10:1 and through a potential difference of 50 mV (outside-positive) would liberate $5.75+4.82=10.57$ KJ, which is also the minimum amount of energy which has to be expended to expel sodium from the cell. For 1 mol chloride ions moving into a cell down a concentration gradient of 10:1 and through a potential difference of 50 mV (outside-positive) the energy liberated would be $5.75-4.82=0.93$ KJ, which is also the minimum amount of energy which has to be expended to expel the same quantity of chloride from the cell. Note that if the fractional efficiency of any biochemical process coupled with such movements is e ($e<1$) then the real metabolic cost of solute pumping, e.g. of extruding sodium, is C/e, where C is the theoretical energy requirement. Similarly the maximum energy which could be made available from coupling to solute movements occurring in the *downhill* direction is $e \cdot C$. Strictly speaking, the $\Delta\Psi$ tabulated is not the membrane potential, but the difference between the membrane potential and the equilibrium (Gibbs–Donnan) potential, however, the latter is usually only a few millivolts

of the membrane. Such charges (e.g. "fixed" anions) will be expected to be associated with the surface glycoproteins that compose the glycocalyx. While it is easy to calculate the effects on the local Na activity of the presence of such surface charges, the results of such calculations are speculative in the absence of knowledge of the density of the charges. However, if the net charge on the surface is negative the local (*cis*) activity of Na will be increased and hence will alter the magnitude of the electrochemical gradient for Na. In addition the effects of the presence of such fixed surface charges on the local membrane potential have to be considered.

Nevertheless, in spite of such local complications it seems true that the *minimum* energy required to move a molecule or ion uphill (or liberated by an ion or molecule moving downhill) from the external bulk phase to the cell interior will be that given by the difference in electrochemical potential between the bulk phase in the lumen and the cell interior. An indication of the energy changes involved is given in Table 6.

The application of current techniques for subcellular fractionation has enabled reliable preparations of vesicles formed from brush border membranes to be made. The use of such vesicles has allowed an even more direct experimental approach to the question as to whether the electrochemical potential gradient of Na ions across the brush border membrane is sufficient to account for the work done in pumping organic molecules such as glucose or amino acids across it (SACTOR 1977; SACHS et al. 1980; MURER and KINNE 1980; WEST 1980).

In experiments with a very stable preparation of such membrane vesicles, derived from rabbit intestine, KESSLER and SEMENZA (1979) have now shown that the magnitude of the electrochemical gradient for Na is adequate to perform the work that is required to account for the concentration of glucose that is achieved inside the vesicles in these experiments. The efficiency of the coupling of the two inward fluxes, the "downhill" movement of sodium with the "uphill" movement of glucose seems to be rather high, possibly as great as 80%. These and other similar experiments (see e.g. MURER and HOPFER 1977) have now demonstrated unequivocally that the driving force contains an electrogenic component and is accordingly dependent upon the magnitude and direction of the membrane potential existing across the brush border membrane. Evidence at present available seems to indicate that the ratio between the two fluxes J is unity, i.e. that

$$J_{\text{in}}(\text{Na})/J_{\text{in}}(\text{glucose}) = 1 .$$

A question of some interest is: what happens to Na entry across the brush border from the lumen when no appropriate organic substrate is available in the intestinal lumen for cotransport? One possibility is that Na would still enter, but now in exchange for H ions. Indeed, such an exchange has been observed in brush border vesicles (MURER and HOPFER 1977). An exchange leading to the establishment of an electrochemical potential gradient of protons could, given appropriate buffering, form the basis of an additional energy store also derived, as in the case of the electrochemical gradient for Na ions across the same membrane, at the expense of ATP hydrolysis. When fully charged, i.e., when the necessary buffers present are fully titrated, the store could be used in such a way that the movement becomes reversed and the inward flux of H ions used either to pump intracellular Na out across the brush border or to drive an inward flux of an organic solute. The answer to such questions requires more experimental evidence on proton-coupled exchanges across the brush border membrane. Further experiments are also required to provide evidence on the extent to which the rate of outward pumping of Na by the Na^+-K^+-ATPase enzyme system that is located in the basolateral membranes of the mucosal epithelial cells is altered by the movement inwards of nonmetabolized substrates such as 3-*O*-methylglucose across the brush border membranes. If the rate is found, for example, to be increased, then evidence is required on the time course of the increase in relation to that of the inward movements across the brush border.

K. Influence of Circulation on Epithelial Transport: General Principles

Consideration of the energetics of epithelial transport processes such as those of intestinal absorption usually neglect the influence of the circulation. After all, most experiments on epithelial transport in the intestine in vitro are conducted on sheets or tubes of the tissue, while in studies on intestinal absorption undertaken in vivo the blood flow is assumed to be constant, so that with but few exceptions (see WINNE 1979; LOVE 1976) its influence is neglected. However, with the advent of reasonably satisfactory preparations for the perfusion of the vascular bed it has now become possible to investigate the influence of the mesenteric circulation on intestinal transport and metabolism (see PARSONS and PRICHARD 1968; BOYD et al. 1975; HANSON and PARSONS 1976). The presence of a functioning mesenteric circulation can influence the movement of substances across the epithelium and can enable metabolic fuels to be delivered directly to the epithelium at physiological concentrations.

Mesenteric blood flow can influence the translation of substrate from the intestinal lumen, in theory at any rate, by influencing two processes: convective transport and cellular transport. These processes are in fact closely related. There are corresponding influences on the energy requirements.

I. Convective Transport

In water-absorbing epithelia there occurs a convective translation of substrate. This depends upon the substrate being entrained in the stream of water moving out of the lumen and presumably (the route is at present controversial) extracellularly. The convective flux J_{con} is given by

$$J_{con} = J_v \phi \bar{c},$$

where J_v is the volume flow, $\bar{c}$ the mean concentration of the substrate at the input to the convective route out of the lumen and ϕ is a filtration coefficient (values $1 > \phi > 0$) equivalent to $1 - \sigma$ where σ is the effective reflection coefficient for that substrate at the epithelium.

The work done on the convected molecules during their translation is derived from the energy inherent in the volume flux J_v, and is expended in overcoming the frictional resistances acting on the convected molecules during their passage along this route. The primary source of energy for such convective flow is thus that responsible for establishing the local forces within the epithelium, hydraulic, osmotic, etc. that drive the inward net volume flux.

One influence of mesenteric blood flow on the convective flow of substrate across the epithelium, if it occurs at all, may be by influencing J_v, although by virtue of other influences of flow on the rate of absorption there may in theory be effects on $\bar{c}$. Evidently direct measurement of fluxes through the convective route at differing rates of mesenteric flow are required (but see PARSONS and WADE 1982b).

II. Cellular Transport: Influence of Vascular Flow on Power Requirements

The second way in which mesenteric vascular flow can influence the translation of substrates from the intestinal lumen across the epithelium is by direct effects on the clearance of absorbed substrate away from the tissue, thereby significantly influencing the rate of flux through and the energetics of the cellular route.

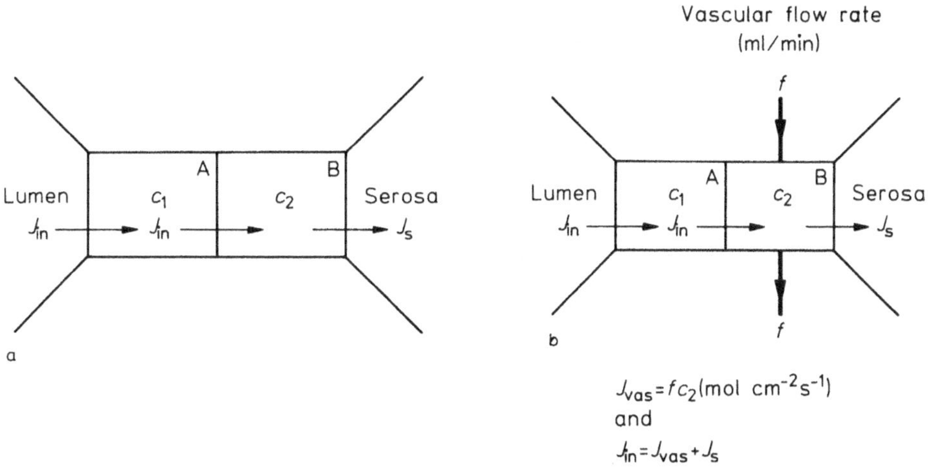

Fig. 1. a Model of intestinal mucosal epithelium in vitro. In the steady state of transfer the flux J_{in} across the brush border membranes into the cellular compartment A is equal to the flux J_s from the extracellular compartment B across the serosal membrane into the serosal compartment. For further details see text. **b** Model of vascularly perfused intestinal mucosal epithelium. In the steady state of transfer the flux J_{in} across the brush border membranes into the cellular compartment A is equal to the efflux J_{vas} in the portal effluent, c_2f, where c_2 is the concentration of transported substrate in compartment B and f the rate of portal outflow, supposed to be equal to that of the substrate-free arterial inflow, plus J_s. At very low rates of vascular flow J_s may become significant. For further details see text

III. A Simple Model

Consider the following very simplified model (Fig. 1 a). A and B are respectively the well-stirred cellular and extracellular mucosal compartments of an absorbing small intestine. During the steady state of absorption of a species of small uncharged organic molecules (e.g. hexose) maintained in the lumen at concentration c_m, it is assumed that pumping occurs across the brush border at a constant rate J_{in} that is independent of the concentration of the absorbed substrate within A, c_1. The absorbed substrate leaves compartment A (e.g. the epithelial cells) across the boundary separating compartments A and B. For simplicity it is assumed that this boundary has a permeability of P_1 (dimensions of volume/time). Under in vitro conditions the substrate moves out of B, where the concentration is c_2, across the serosal boundary, into the fluid bathing the serosal surface and in which the concentration is maintained at a constant level of c_s. If the permeability of the serosal boundary is P_2, then

$$J_{in} = P_1(c_1 - c_2) = P_2(c_2 - c_s)$$

and

$$c_1 = J_{in}(1/P_1 + 1/P_2) + c_s .$$

Because the work done in unit time by the substrate pump in the brush border, i.e. the power required to derive the concentration c_1, is given by the product of the flux and the work done in moving and concentrating 1 mol substrate at concentration c_m in the lumen to a concentration of c_1, the power $\boldsymbol{P}$, required is

$$\boldsymbol{P}(\text{in vitro}) = J_{in} RT \ln\left(\frac{c_1}{c_m}\right)$$

or

$$\boldsymbol{P}(\text{in vitro}) = J_{in} RT \ln\left[\frac{J_{in}}{c_m}\left(\frac{1}{P_1} + \frac{1}{P_2}\right) + \frac{c_s}{c_m}\right] \tag{1}$$

or, if c_s is negligibly small,

$$\boldsymbol{P}(\text{in vitro}) = J_{in} RT \ln\left[\frac{J_{in}}{c_m}\left(\frac{1}{P_1} + \frac{1}{P_2}\right)\right]. \tag{2}$$

In vivo, the serosal fluid does not normally exist and absorbed substrate delivered to compartment B is removed by the mesenteric circulation. This model can be converted into a model of an intestine absorbing in vivo (Fig. 1 b). Let the rate of blood flow into B be f units of volume per unit time. On the assumption that the rate of net absorption of fluid is negligible when compared with f, and if it is further supposed that the substrate concentration is zero in the arterial inflow (single-pass flow) and that the venous outflow is in equilibrium with the substrate present in B, then

$$J_{in} = P_1(c_1 - c_2) = fc_2 + P_2c_2\,,$$

where the term P_2c_2 represents the "leak" over into the peritoneal cavity, so

$$c_1 = J_{in}\left[\frac{1}{P_1} + \frac{1}{(f+P_2)}\right]$$

and the power required is given by

$$\boldsymbol{P}(\text{in vitro}) = J_{in} RT \ln \frac{J_{in}}{c_m}\left[\frac{1}{P_1} + \frac{1}{(f+P_2)}\right]. \tag{3a}$$

If the blood flow is high compared with P_2 this reduces to

$$\boldsymbol{P}(\text{in vitro}) = J_{in} RT \ln \frac{J_{in}}{c_m}\left(\frac{1}{P_1} + \frac{1}{f}\right) \tag{3b}$$

and if the blood flow is very high this becomes

$$\boldsymbol{P}(\text{in vitro}) = J_{in} RT \ln\left(\frac{J_{in}}{P_1 c_m}\right). \tag{4}$$

Comparing Eq. (2) with Eqs. (3) and (4) it can be seen that the rate of vascular flow can be regarded as a permeability constant, and if the flow is sufficiently high, the permeability constant P_1 that determines the movement between compartment A and compartment B becomes the major factor in determining the work done at a given rate of pumping into A from any particular value of c_m.

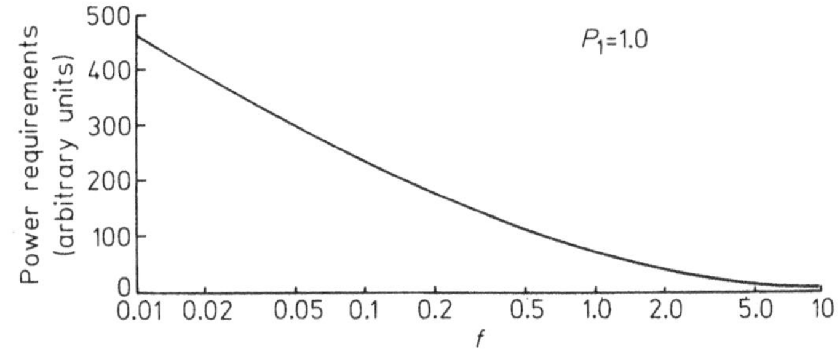

Fig. 2. Power requirements for solute transport into vascular effluent at different rates of vascular flow for the model depicted in Fig. 1 b. The permeability coefficient P_1 for the membrane separating compartments A and B is assumed to have unit value. Note logarithmic scale of abscissa. For the model of absorption in vitro (Fig. 1 a) the values of f can be directly substituted by corresponding values of P_2, the permeability coefficient of the barrier separating compartment B from the serosal compartment. For further details see text

The effects of varying the rate of vascular flow f or the equivalent effects of varying the permeability coefficient, P_2, on the power required by the tissue to maintain a constant rate of transport are shown in Fig. 2. It must be pointed out that Eq. (3 a) indicates that, at very low rates of vascular flow, exit from B across the serosal border will start to occur at significant rates, in accord with Eqs. (1) and (2). In this case substrate will leave compartment B at a rate $c_2(P_2+f)$.

Two assumptions implicit in this model must be considered. First, in the model it is supposed that the exit from compartment A can be considered in terms of a simple permeability coefficient P_1 which has the dimensions of flux per unit concentration difference, i.e. those of volume per unit time and of a constant value, i.e. independent of c_1. But there is clear evidence that the exit of certain monosaccharides (Boyd and Parsons 1979) and also of some amino acids (Parsons and Sanderson 1980) from the epithelium of, at least, frog small intestine is not by simple diffusion, but exhibits a selectivity and thus implies the existence of specialized transport systems for exit. Nevertheless, until the special system for exit is saturated the rate of exit from compartment A will increase with c_1 up to its maximum rate. The second assumption is that for a given value of c_m the rate of pumping inward across the brush border membranes J_{in} is constant and independent of c_1. Although there is no firm evidence in the case of real brush borders whether this is so or not, very high values of c_1 would be expected to inhibit the dissociation of substrate from the "inside" end of the pump (i.e. inside A) and hence reduce the magnitude of J_{in}.

The average concentration of absorbed substrate within the tissue wall is

$$(c_1 v_a + c_2 v_b)/(v_a + v_b) ,$$

where v_a and v_b are the respective volumes of compartments A and B. Values of the quotient (concentration in tissue water)/(concentration in lumen fluid) (i.e. the so-called T/M ratio) of greater than unity have sometimes been used as tests of the occurence of active transport in in vitro preparations. The question arises here as to whether values greater than unity are found for the ratio T/M or, in the

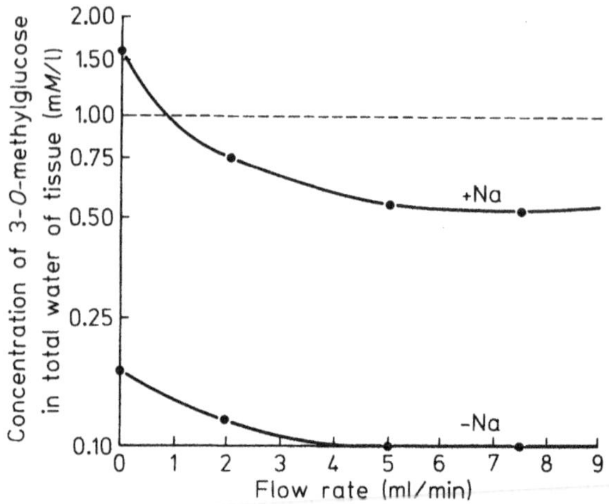

Fig. 3. Influence of rate of vascular flow on average concentration (m*M*) in tissue water of 3-*O*-methylglucose during absorption in the steady state by small intestine of *Rana ridibunda*. Concentration of 3-*O*-methylglucose in the lumen maintained at 1 m*M*. +Na; Na ions present in lumen, −Na; Na ions replaced by K ions in lumen. Note logarithmic scale of ordinate. After BOYD and PARSONS (1978)

model

$$(c_1 v_a + c_2 v_b)/c_m(v_a + v_b)$$

during the steady state of absorption with mesenteric blood flow occurring.

BOYD and PARSONS (1978) have shown that in the small intestine of *Rana ridibunda* the concentration of the sugar 3-*O*-methylglucose, within the tissue during absorption, is markedly dependent upon the rate of vascular perfusion. With what are thought to be physiological rates of flow and above, the mean concentration in the tissues is about half that within the lumen, whereas at zero flow, i.e. under classical in vitro conditions, the mean concentration in the tissue water is nearly double that in the lumen. With Na in the lumen replaced by K ions, the 3-*O*-methylglucose concentration in the tissue is very low at all vascular flow rates (Fig. 3). Similar results have been obtained for the amino acid cycloleucine (PARSONS and SANDERSON 1980).

L. Effects of Circulation on Epithelial Transport in the Steady State

In experiments on the epithelial transport of the nonmetabolized sugar, 3-*O*-methylglucose, BOYD (1977) and BOYD and PARSONS (1978) examined the effects of changing the rate of mesenteric blood flow through the absorbing segment on the rates of transport in the steady state. They found that, with Na ions present in the lumen, increasing the rate of blood flow only slightly increased the rate of transport, so that there was a relatively high rate of transport of 3-*O*-methylglucose at low rates of vascular perfusion. The relationship between transport from the lumen into the vascular bed and the rate of vascular perfusion was linear, and extrapolation of the regression line indicated that a significant transfer would occur at zero flow. The transfer was inhibited in the presence of other sugars in the intestinal lumen, and was almost completely inhibited by phlorhizin in the lumen. With Na ions replaced in the lumen by K ions the transfer was markedly dependent upon the rate of vascular flow. Extrapolation of the regression line relating these data back to the intercept of zero flow indicates that no transfer would be expected in the absence of circulation. However, even at high rates of vascular flow in the absence of Na ions rate of transfer of 3-*O*-methylglucose from lumen to blood were always less than when Na ions were present.

Experiments with cycloleucine show exactly analogous features (PARSONS and SANDERSON 1980). Thus with sodium present in the lumen, the transport of cycloleucine from the lumen into the blood is only slightly dependent upon vascular flow; the transport occurs at high rates even at low rates of vascular perfusion and it is inhibited by the presence in the lumen of another amino acid (leucine). When the Na ions in the lumen were replaced by K, it was found that at low rates of vascular flow the transport of cycloleucine occurs only very slowly,

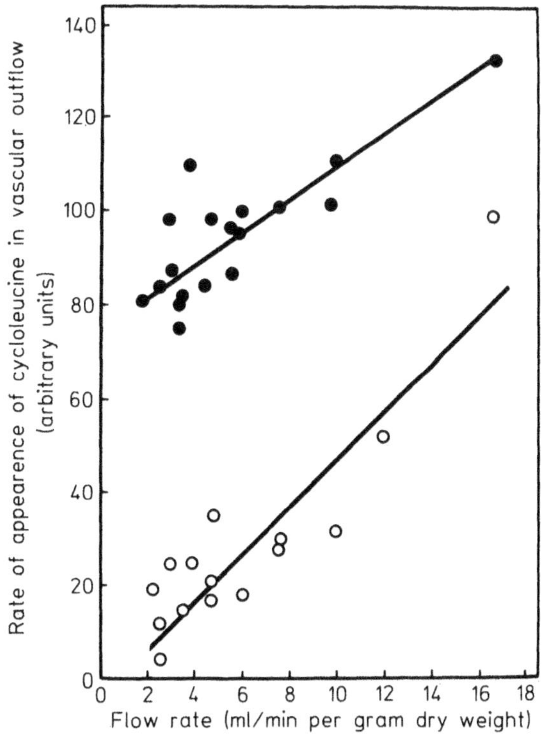

Fig. 4. Influence of rate of vascular flow on steady state rate of transfer of cycloleucine from lumen into vascular effluent of *Rana ridibunda*. With Na ions present in the lumen *full circles*, appearance $= 3.42 \pm 0.58 \cdot$ (flow rate) $+ 75.8$ (19). With Na ions replaced by K ions in the lumen *open circles*, appearance $= 5.09 \pm 0.7 \cdot$ (flow rate) $- 2.04$ (16). In both cases, for significance of regression coefficient, $P < 0.001$. After PARSONS and SANDERSON (1980)

but increases substantially as the rate of mesenteric blood flow increases. However, as was found for 3-*O*-methylglucose, at all rates of vascular flow the rates of transport of cycloleucine from the lumen into the blood were always less than the values found with sodium present (Fig. 4).

These observations help to account for the lack of agreement between experiments using brush border membranes or the intestinal mucosal epithelium in vitro (e.g. everted sacs) where Na ions in the lumen are certainly required for the uphill transport of monosaccharides and amino acids, and the findings for the intestine in vivo where the dependence of amino acid and monosaccharide transport upon Na can be less marked (FORDTRAN 1975; FÖRSTER 1972). Also CHEESEMAN and PARSONS (1976) have shown that transport of L-leucine and glycine from lumen to blood in vascularly perfused frog intestine was reduced, but not abolished, when Na ions in the lumen fluid were replaced by K.

These apparent differences between in vivo and in vitro conditions with respect to the requirement for Na ions for sugar and amino acid uptake can be explained if Na ions are required only for accumulative uptake, but not for entry, across the brush border membranes. In this case all steps in the translation of substrate from the intestinal lumen into the blood would have to be "downhill", i.e. down the electrochemical gradient; clearly these experiments throw no light on whether this is so or not. An alternative explanation would be that the microscopic environment of the brush border membrane in the lumen is not after all Na free in the vascularly perfused experiments. It is possible that, with a functioning mesenteric circulation, Na enters the "unstirred layer" region from the extracellular fluid of the tissue via the paracellular route, to be taken up across the brush border. Any Na recycling in such a fashion would not be "seen" in the bulk phase in the lumen. The Na moving in such a fashion would, of course, be accompanied by an anion (Cl or HCO_3) or exchanged for another cation (e.g. K).

M. Influence of Circulation on Wash-out from Epithelium

Another effect of blood flow on epithelial transport of monosaccharides has been described by BOYD and PARSONS (1978). Previously absorbed 3-*O*-methylglucose is washed out from the epithelium into the blood in a biexponential fashion; the rate constant of the "fast" component of the wash out for 3-*O*-methylglucose is related to the blood flow such that the faster the flow, the bigger the rate constant. A similar effect has also been found for cycloleucine (PARSONS and SANDERSON 1980). The wash-out of this amino acid into the vasculature can be described as a biexponential function and the "fast" rate constant, which accounts for about 80% of the wash-out, is flow dependent; the second rate constant is flow independent (see PARSONS 1975).

It appears that the processes underlying the exit of amino acids from the epithelium distinguish between α-aminoisobutyric acid (AIB) and cycloleucine, the latter being discharged during wash-out from the epithelium with biexponential kinetics, while AIB is discharged at lower rates, and in a monoexponential fashion. Some of these features for the two amino acids are analogous to the cases of 3-*O*-methylglucose and α-methylglucoside (BOYD and PARSONS 1978). Thus the

Table 7. Apparent diffusion coefficient D' for exit along path of length of 25 or 50 μm from small intestine of *Rana ridibunda* perfused at rate of 5 ml per gram dry weight through the vascular bed. *K*, observed rate constant of exit into plasma. After BOYD and PARSONS (1978) and PARSONS and SANDERSON (1980)

			Path length (μm) 25		50	
	$10^3 \times K$ (s^{-1})	$10^6 \times D$ (cm^2/s)	$10^9 \times D'$ (cm^2/s)	D/D'	$10^9 \times D'$ (cm^2/s)	D/D'
Urea	2.52	12	6.38	1,880	25	480
3-*O*-methylglucose	2.08	6	5.26	1,140	21	288
Cycloleucine	2.50	7	6.33	1,110	25	280

exit of 3-*O*-methylglucose exhibits biexponential kinetics, while for α-methylglucoside the exit is monoexponential in form, and from a very large pool.

In the experiments on the transport of cycloleucine, and in those reported earlier for 3-*O*-methylglucose (BOYD and PARSONS 1978), altering the vascular flow rate produces changes in the rate constant for exit into the vasculature of the bulk of previously absorbed substrate. One way of interpreting this effect is in terms of changes in the diffusive pathway between the cells and the vasculature. Thus if D' is the effective diffusion coefficent and the mean path length over which diffusion is occuring is L, then

$$D' = 4kL^2/\pi^2 \ ,$$

where k is the rate constant for the final two-thirds of the wash-out. (HILL 1928 Eq. (42); see also KEYNES 1954; CALDWELL and KEYNES 1969).

In Table 7 are shown values for D' calculated from observed values of the apparent rate constant, for two different values of L, the mean path length of exit from the epithelium into the capillaries of the intestinal wall. Depending upon the path length assumed, the apparent diffusion coefficent D' in the exit pathway appears to be around 1/250–1/2,000 of that for diffusion in free solution. Thus, because increasing the rate of vascular perfusion increases the value of the rate constant, the effective permeability of the exit processes is increased, e.g. by making the apparent diffusion coefficient larger, or by reducing the length of the diffusive pathway, by increasing the area available for diffusion, or by changing all these variables. These conclusions are in accord with the predictions derived from the simple model described in Sect. K. III.

It can be concluded that exit of some amino acids and monosaccharides from the epithelium into the blood of the vascularly perfused preparation involves exit from the epithelial cells followed by a diffusive movement along a relatively restricted pathway. At some step, presumably at the basolateral membrane, the exit process exhibits high specificity; for example, the amino acid cycloleucine is much more permeable that AIB, while for monosaccharides 3-*O*-methylglucose is much more permeable than α-methylglucoside. The effects of increasing the rate of mesenteric blood flow include an increase in the apparent permeability of the exit path. However, all stages of the movements of these substances are along the direction of the chemical gradient, i.e. "downhill" from the epithelium into the vasculature.

N. Influence of Circulation on Sodium Fluxes Across Vascularly Perfused Intestine

In experiments in our laboratory, Dr. S. A. WADE has measured the magnitude of the unidirectional fluxes of sodium across the small intestine and colon of frogs and has examined the effects of changing the rate of vascular flow upon these fluxes. The findings are of interest in connection with current views on the importance of a low resistance pathway that forms a "paracellular" shunt across the intestinal epithelium. The existence of this shunt has been deduced from findings obtained in experiments on the small intestine using electrophysiological procedures such as short-circuit procedures and microelectrodes to measure membrane potentials and intracellular ionic activities (see e.g. SCHULTZ 1977).

I. Na Fluxes Across the Small Intestine

In early experiments, the individual unidirectional fluxes were measured separately using ^{24}Na. The pooled values of these fluxes seemed to indicate no net Na movement in either direction across the small intestine of *R. ridibunda*, over the rates of vascular flow employed. Using both ^{22}Na and ^{24}Na to measure the unidirectional fluxes simultaneously, the mean of the difference between the paired fluxes also revealed no net Na movement across the small intestine of both *R. ridibunda* and *R. pipiens* for similar rates of vascular flow. The undirectional and net Na fluxes measured simultaneously across the small intestine of *R. ridibunda* and *R. pipiens* are shown in Table 8.

Table 8. Unidirectional and net fluxes of Na across vascularly perfused small intestine of *Rana ridibunda*.[a] After D. S. PARSONS and S. A. WADE (1980, unpublished work) and PARSONS and WADE (1981)

	Glucose concentration in lumen	Sodium flux		
		Lumen–blood	Blood–lumen	Net flux
Series I	0	8.73 ± 1.18	8.73 ± 1.15	$+0.01 \pm 0.13$[b]
	0	9.22 ± 1.51	9.35 ± 1.49	-0.13 ± 0.11[b]
Series II	10	11.0 ± 1.72	11.0 ± 1.62	$+0.02 \pm 0.18$[b]
Glucose-induced increase		1.77 ± 0.38[c]	1.66 ± 0.32[c]	$+0.11 \pm 0.21$[b]

[a] In all cases butyrate (1 m*M*) was present as substrate in the vascular inflow. In series I (7 frogs) glucose was absent throughout the experiments. In series II (5 frogs) in each frog the fluxes were measured simultaneously first before and then after the addition of glucose to the fluid passing through the lumen. Values are µmol per square centimetre serosal surface per hour (mean ± standard error). Plus sign indicates net absorption from lumen

[b] For significance of net absorption, $P > 0.1$

[c] For significance of glucose-induced increase in flux, $0.01 > P > 0.001$

Table 9. Values of the unidirectional and net fluxes across the vascularly perfused colon of frogs.[a] After D. S. PARSONS and S. W. WADE (1980, unpublished work) and PARSONS and WADE (1982a)

Frog	Sodium flux		
	Lumen–blood	Blood–lumen	Net flux
R. ridibunda	3.21 ± 0.42	1.44 ± 0.30	+ 1.77 ± 0.45 (10)[b]
R. pipiens	5.28 ± 1.30	2.03 ± 0.46	+ 3.25 ± 0.97 (6)[c]

[a] Unidirectional and net fluxes measured simultaneously across the colon. In all cases, butyrate (1 m*M*) was present as substrate in vascular inflow. Values are of μmol per square centimetre serosal surface per hour (mean ± standard error; figures in parentheses indicate numbers of frogs). Plus sign indicates net absorption from lumen

[b] $0.01 > P > 0.001$

[c] $0.05 > P > 0.02$

The magnitude of these fluxes is greater than has been found from numerous studies on intestine in vitro. Thus, they are up to five times higher than found in rat ileum in Ussing chambers (CURRAN 1960) and up to ten times higher than reported by ARMSTRONG (1976) for the in vitro jejunum of the bullfrog *R. catesbeiana*. The fluxes are also of the same order of magnitude as those found across the intestine in vivo, and are at least two orders of magnitude greater than values reported for the unidirectional Na flux across the plasma membrane of animal cells (CEREIJIDO and ROTUNNO 1968; PARSONS 1976). The findings are in accord with the view that in these frogs a large proportion of the total unidirectional Na flux in either direction across the small intestine occurs largely by diffusion, possibly via extracellular pathways.

II. Na Fluxes Across the Colon

In contrast to the case for the small intestine in these species, simultaneous measurement of unidirectional Na fluxes using ^{22}Na and ^{24}Na across the colon of *R. ridibunda* and *R. pipiens* shows that there is marked net absorption (Table 9). The lumen-blood Na flux for both species is at least twice the blood-lumen flux, giving a significant net Na absorption. The magnitudes of the unidirectional fluxes are lower than those across the small intestine (Table 8), but similar to those reported for isolated amphibian and mammalian colon (COOPERSTEIN and HOGBEN 1959; FRIZZELL et al. 1976). Thus, although the magnitude of the unidirectional Na fluxes across the colon may be lower than across the small intestine, the colon is an important site of Na absorption from the intestine of *R. ridibunda* and *R. pipiens*.

III. Factors Affecting Na Fluxes Across Frog Intestine

1. Glucose

Actively transported sugars have varying effects on fluid and electrolyte movement across the small intestine. Thus, in 1953 FISHER and PARSONS showed that while glucose stimulates water transport across rat jejunum galactose is unable to do so. Surprisingly, acetate, pyruvate and short-chain fatty acids are not able to support NaCl transport and hence water absorption in this tissue under aerobic conditions. On the other hand while glucose, but not galactose, also stimulates fluid transport in rat ileum, the transport is stimulated by the presence of acetate, pyruvate and lower fatty acids (see e.g. PARSONS 1967).

Although the presence of glucose in the intestinal lumen enhances the net flux of Na across the small intestine of a wide variety of species the effects on the magnitudes of the individual unidirectional fluxes of Na is ambiguous. SCHULTZ and ZALUSKY (1964) found that although glucose induced a decrease in the magnitude of serosa–mucosa flux of Na across rabbit ileum in vitro there was no effect on the flux in the mucosa–serosa direction. Similar results were found by QUAY and ARMSTRONG (1969) using isolated small intestine of the bullfrog. In contrast, in other studies (e.g. FIELD et al. 1970) it has been found that glucose stimulates Na flux in the direction mucosa–serosa but is without effect on the flux in the opposite direction.

We have now found that the addition of 10 m*M*-glucose to the lumen of the small intestine of *R. ridibunda* produces a significant increase in both the lumen–blood and the blood–lumen Na fluxes (Table 8). Moreover, both fluxes are stimulated to the same degree (mean 1.7 ± 0.1 μmol $cm^{-2}h^{-1}$) so that, in the presence of glucose, there is no significant net Na transport. Measurement of transepithelial glucose influx across *R. ridibunda* small intestine gave values of approximately 1 μmol $cm^{-2}h^{-1}$ which are similar to those found by PARSONS and PRICHARD (1970, unpublished work) using isolated, vascularly perfused small intestine of *R. pipiens*. In contrast, the influx of 3-*O*-methylglucose, from a luminal concentration of 1 m*M*, is about 40 nmol $cm^{-2}h^{-1}$. Because most of the monosaccharide that is absorbed by *R. ridibunda* and *R. pipiens* seems to be phlorhizin sensitive, and hence to pass through the cellular route (as opposed to, for example, convective flow through a paracellular route PARSONS and PRICHARD 1971; BOYD and PARSONS 1978), our findings indicate that some, but not all, of the stimulation by glucose of the Na flux in the direction lumen–blood could be accounted for in terms of a glucose-coupled cellular influx of Na.

2. Vascular Flow Rate

It has been shown in Sect. L , that there is a significant linear relationship between the vascular flow rate and the net flux of some sugars and amino acids across the anuran small intestine. For both the amino acids and the sugars, increasing the rate of vascular flow slightly increases the net absorption in the presence of Na in the lumen, while the increase in net absorption is marked when Na ions are replaced by K ions in the lumen. In all cases the relationship between flow and net flux is linear.

In experiments on Na movements, a significant positive linear correlation between the unidirectional fluxes and the rates of vascular flow has been found for both the lumen–blood and the blood–lumen fluxes (PARSONS and WADE 1982b). Interestingly, LOVE (1976) has also found that the rate of mucosal blood flow through the small intestine of dogs in vivo can influence Na movement. In the dog, the bidirectional fluxes of Na were both reduced with reduced rates of mesenteric blood flow.

O. Effects of Vascular Flow on Size of Tissue Fluid Compartments

These findings raise the question as to why changing the vascular flow rate alters the Na fluxes. It has already been shown that increasing the vascular flow increases the permeability of the exit path from the epithelium to the blood for some amino acids and saccharides. Since it appears that a high proportion of the Na flux is a passive transfer, it is possible that changing the vascular flow rate alters in some way the accessibility of these pathways for Na transfer to and from the blood. This might be reflected by change in the volume occupied by the interstitial fluid of the mucosal epithelium.

I. Measurement of Extracellular and Interstitial Space

A nondestructive method for estimating the total extracellular and vascular volume has been devised. The procedure involves the simultaneous introduction of two markers into arterial inflow to the intestine. From measurement on the time course of the concentration changes of the markers in the venous effluent, volumes of distribution can be calculated. As a marker for extracellular space sucrose ^{14}C is suitable (even in the intestinal lumen, for the frog lacks sucrose). To measure the intravascular volume, a convenient marker is the erythrocyte. Frog blood is not easily available in sufficient quantities so we have used washed erythrocytes of bovine origin. These cells have a diameter (7 μm) considerably less than that of the frog capillary (15 μm). The concentration of red cells in the vascular effluent is determined by measuring the haemoglobin in solution after lysis.

In estimating the space occupied by each of the two markers the following assumptions are made.

a) The system is in an hydraulic steady state i.e. the rate of vascular flow in, f (volume per unit time), equals the rate of flow out.
b) Fluid transfer by absorption or secretion into or from the vascular bed occurs at a rate that is negligible compared with f.
c) The volume V of the compartment is constant.
d) The compartment is well stirred so that the concentration of marker c in the venous effluent is identical with that within the compartment.
e) The volume of the dead space V_d is constant.

If the concentration of marker in the inflow is c_i, then it can be shown that

$$\ln(1-c/c_i)=\frac{V_d}{V}-\frac{f}{V}t\,.$$

By plotting $\ln(1-c/c_i)$ against t, the slope $(-f/V)$ and intercept (V_d/V) can be determined and hence V can be calculated. The volume of the interstitial space is given by the difference between the values of the extracellular and vascular spaces.

Pooled data from a series of experiments using red cells and sucrose as markers show that there is a positive linear correlation between the extracellular space and the rate of vascular flow (Parsons and Wade 1982b). Although the extracellular space increases significantly with increasing vascular flow rate, the total tissue water appears to be independent of the flow rate.

II. Influence of Vascular Flow on Permeability of the Pathway Between Epithelium and Blood

The increase in extracellular space with increasing vascular flow seems to be largely accounted for by an increase in the volume occupied by the interstitial fluid. Furthermore, there is a positive correlation between the size of the extracellular space and the influx of Na ($r=0.81$, $P<0.01$, $n=8$). Thus it seems that altering the vascular flow rate increases the size of the interstitial portion of the extracellular space, which may enhance the accessibility of the low resistance, paracellular pathway for Na.

The permeability coefficient P (volume per unit time) for exit through the extracellular space, from the epithelium into the circulation for a segment of intestine of unit dry weight (or unit length or unit serosal area), is given by

$$P=DA/l$$

(see also Sect. K.III) where D is the diffusion coefficient within the extracellular space; A is the area in the plane parallel to the epithelium across which the diffusion is occurring and l the apparent path length in the direction normal to the plane of the epithelium. The relationship can also be written as $P=DV/l^2$ where V is the volume of the extracellular space.

Our experiments have shown that increasing the vascular flow: (1) increases the apparent permeability for exit of amino acids and hexose from the epithelium into the blood: (2) increases the magnitude of the unidirectional fluxes of Na in both directions between the intestinal lumen and blood, these fluxes being largely movements through extracellular pathways, and (3) increases the volume of the extracellular fluid of the intestinal wall.

An increase in extracellular volume associated, at least in part, with an increase in the volume of the interepithelial cellular extracellular space would reconcile all three of these findings; the increased separation of the epithelial cells would allow a larger area in the plane parallel to that of the epithelium across which diffusion occurs, but without increase in the path length. Further experiments are required to throw more light on these ideas.

P. Conclusions

Intestinal absorption, the translation of substances from the intestinal lumen into the circulation in vivo or into artificial fluids in vitro, is a sequential, multistep process, any step of which may be rate limiting to absorption. The steps of absorption can be classified into three sorts in sequence: (1) those of delivery to the epithelium; (2) those of epithelial transport; and (3) those of clearance from the epithelium into the mesenteric circulation. The forces underlying the movements across the first and third sorts of step, those of delivery and clearance, are those of diffusion down chemical concentration gradients in the direction perpendicular to the plane of the epithelium. In vivo, energy-consuming physiological systems external to the epithelium have important influences in stimulating these diffusive movements. Delivery to the epithelium in vivo can be assisted by the gastrointestinal movements, including villus pumping, the energy for these movements being derived from the metabolism of the intrinsic musculature of the intestine. In vitro, the delivery to the intestinal epithelium of a substrate present in the lumen will be dependent upon the extent to which energy is supplied to stir the bulk contents of the lumen by mechanical means, e.g. by pumping fluid through the intestinal lumen or across the surface of a sheet of the epithelium.

Clearance into the blood away from the epithelium of substrate, or its derivatives originally present in the lumen, is also by diffusion. It can be shown that, for Na and for some hexoses and amino acids, increasing the rate of the mesenteric circulation has the effect of increasing the apparent permeability of the extracellular phase of the exit pathway from the epithelium into the blood. This has the effect that, for a given rate of transfer, the local concentration gradients along which diffusion occurs are reduced, leading in turn to a reduction in the work done by the epithelium in driving the transfer at that rate. The energy for maintaining the circulation is, of course, derived from the work done by the heart at the expense of the metabolism of the cardiac muscle.

Under in vitro conditions, i.e. in the absence of a mesenteric circulation, additional work therefore has to be done by the epithelium for a given rate of transfer of a substrate or its metabolic derivatives. This extra work is undertaken at the expense of an increased metabolism of the tissue, an increased tissue content of substrate and, at least in the case of most amino acids and monosaccharides, an increase in the local concentration of substrate.

The second series of steps in intestinal absorption, those of epithelial transport, can be subdivided into two parallel routes, those for the cellular route and those for the paracellular (or shunting) route. In the case of the cellular route the steps comprise at least two steps of membrane transport, one a translation of substrate from the luminal fluid adjacent to the brush border into the epithelial cells by passing across the brush border membrane and the other a translation of the original substrate, or of products derived from it, from the interior of the epithelial cells into extracellular tissue fluid of the epithelium. These movements through membranes involve interaction with specific proteins that span the membranes (transport channels; transporter proteins) and may be of two sorts: downhill or passive and uphill or active.

Passive movement occurs down the electrochemical gradient of the substrate across the membrane (downhill), the energy of the movement being derived from the dissipation of this gradient; examples of such passive movements are currently thought to include Na entry across the brush border and monosaccharide and amino acid exit across the basolateral membranes.

All uphill or active movements require a power supply; ultimately the energy for these movements is derived from the hydrolysis of the terminal pyrophosphate bond of ATP. The free energy of hydrolysis of ATP can be used directly to pump for example, Na ions actively outwards across the basolateral membranes. This free energy of hydrolysis may also be used indirectly, by coupling the downhill flux of sodium ions across the brush border membranes into the cell, with the up-

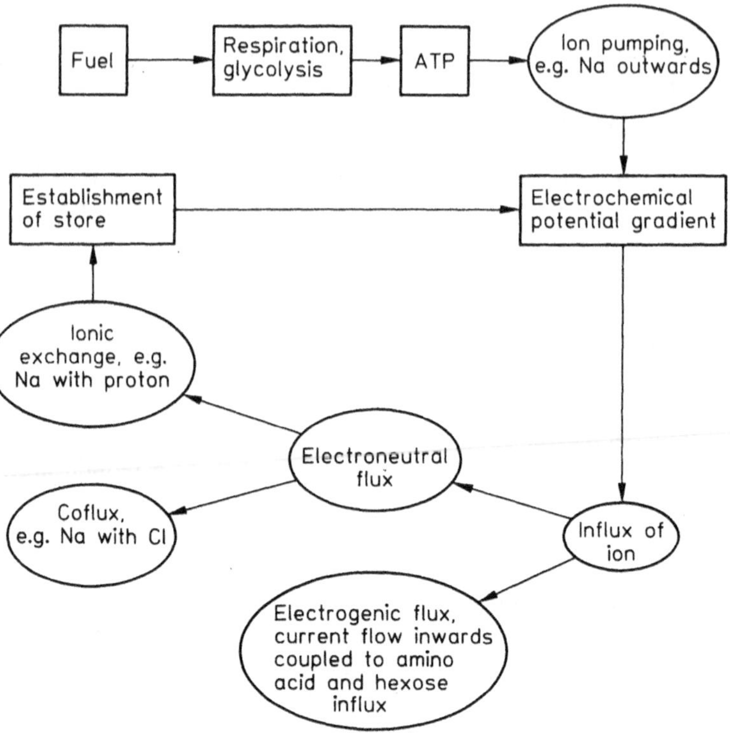

Fig. 5. Flow diagram summarizing interrelationships between energy sources (*rectangles*) and fluxes (*ovals*) across plasma membran of small intestinal mucosal epithelial cell. The outward pumping of Na (*top right-hand corner*) occurs across the basolateral membrane. All the other fluxes occur across the brush border membrane. All the steps are now well documented except for the concept of the generation across the brush border membrane of an electrochemical gradient of protons: this is a speculation of the author's

hill flux of some sugars or amino acids or anions in the same direction across these membranes.

Movement through the paracellular shunt route across the zonulae occludentes is dependent upon the establishment by cellular transport of local hydraulic, osmotic and electrochemical gradients and so too depends ultimately upon ATP hydrolysis. The notion that the oxidative generation of ATP from ADP (oxidative phosphorylation) is itself a consequence of the functioning of membrane processes is now securely established. However, it is only recently that attention has been directed to the fuels that are metabolized by mammalian small intestinal epithelium to provide the ATP required to drive the processes of epithelial transport.

The mucosa of the intestine is unusual because fuels are available to it not only directly from the blood, but also from the intestinal lumen. The spectrum of nutrients available at any moment to the mucosa of the small intestine is accordingly different in fed and fasted animals. Important fuels of the fed intestine and originating from the lumen are glucose and 2-oxoglutarate derived from glutamic acid. A major blood-borne fuel of the intestine in both fed and fasted states is glutamine derived from muscle. Ketone bodies and to some extent glucose are also blood-borne fuels of the fasting intestine.

An interesting feature of the energy metabolism of the small intestine of omnivores and carnivores is the fact that this organ is the portal of entry of the majority of the energy-providing nutrients of these animals. The fact that the energetic value of these nutrients must be at least 20 times the energy requirements of the epithelium upon which the entry depends raises questions concerning the possible segregation of the nutrients from the cellular metabolism of the intestine during the transport. A scheme summarizing some of the energy relations of solute fluxes across the plasma membrane of the small intestinal epithelial cell is shown in Fig. 5.

Acknowledgements. I wish to thank Dr. RICHARD BOYD, Dr. PETER HANSON, Dr. IAN SANDERSON, Mrs. HETTY VOLMAN-MITCHELL and Dr. SIMON WADE, who have been responsible for much of the work in my laboratory that is described here. I have benefitted greatly from their lively and critical discussion of the experiments and the ideas derived from the findings. The work has been supported by various grants from the Medical Research Council, to which body I am grateful.

References

Annison EF, Lewis D (1959). Metabolism in the Rumen, Ch 6. Methuen, London, pp 142–177

Armstrong W McD (1976) Bioelectric parameters and sodium transport in bullfrog small intestine. In: Robinson JWL (ed) Intestinal Ion Transport. MTP Press, Lancaster, England, pp 19–40

Armstrong W MCD, Garcia-Diaz JF, O'Doherty J, O'Regan MG (1979) Transmucosal Na^+ electrochemical potential difference and solute accumulation in epithelial cells of the small intestine. Fed Proc 38:2722–2728

Boyd CAR (1977) Vascular flow and compartmental distribution of transported solutes within the small intestinal wall. In: Kramer M, Lauterbacher F (eds) Intestinal permeation, Workshop conferences Hoechst 4. Excerpta Medica, Amsterdam, pp 41–47

Boyd CAR, Parsons DS (1978) Effects of vascular perfusion on the accumulation, distribution and transfer of 3-O-methyl-D-glucose within and across the small intestine. J Physiol (Lond) 274:17–36

Boyd CAR, Parsons DS (1977) Movements of monosaccharides between blood and tissues of vascular perfused small intestine. J Physiol (Lond) 287:371–391

Boyd CAR, Cheeseman CI, Parsons DS (1975). Amino acid movement across the wall of the avian small intestine perfused through the vascular bed. J Physiol (Lond) 250:409–429

Brindley DN (1977) Absorption and transport of lipids in the small intestine. In: Kramer M, Lauterbach F (eds) Intestinal permation. Workshop conferences Hoechst 4. Excerpta Medica, Amsterdam, pp 350–360

Caldwell PC, Keynes RD (1969) The exchange of ^{22}Na between frog sartorious muscle and the bathing medium. In: Passow H, Stämpfeli R (eds). Laboratory techniques in membrane biophysics. Springer, Berlin Heidelberg New York, pp 63–68

Cereijido M, Rotunno CA (1968) Fluxes and distribution of sodium in frog skin. A new model. J Gen Physiol 51:280–289S

Cheeseman CI, Parsons DS (1976) The role of some small peptides in the transfer of amino nitrogen across the wall of vascular perfused intestine. J Physiol (Lond) 262:459–476

Cooperstein IM, Hogben CAM (1959) Ionic transfer across the isolated frog large intestine. J Gen Physiol 42:461–473

Curran PF (1960) Na, Cl and water transport by rat ileum in vitro. J Gen Physiol 43:1137–1148

Eisenbach M, Caplan SR (1979) The light-driven proton pump of Halobacterium halobium: mechanism and function. Curr Top Membr Transp 12:166–249

Field M, Fromm D, McColl I (1970) Ion transport in rabbit ileal mucosa. I. Na and Cl fluxes and short circuit current. Am J Physiol 220:1388–1396
Fisher RB, Parsons DS (1953) Galactose absorption by the surviving small intestine of the rat. J Physiol (Lond) 119:224–232
Fordtran JS (1975) Intestinal absorption of sugars in the human in vivo. In: Csaky TZ (ed) Intestinal absorption and malabsorption. Raven, New York, pp 229–234
Förster H (1972) Views dissenting with the "gradient hypothesis". Intestinal sugar absorption, studies in vivo and in vitro. In: Heinz E (ed) Na-linked Transport of organic solutes, Springer, Berlin Heidelberg New York, pp 134–139
Frizzell RA, Koch MJ, Schultz SG (1976) Ion transport by rabbit colon. I. Active and passive components. J Membr Biol 27:297–316
Greville GD (1969) A scrutiny of Mitchell's chemiosmotic hypothesis of respiratory chain and photosynthetic phosphorylation. Curr Top Bioenergetics 3:1–78
Hanson PJ, Parsons DS (1976) The utilization of glucose and production of lactate by in vitro preparation of rat small intestine: Effects of vascular perfusion. J Physiol (Lond) 255:775–795
Hanson PJ, Parsons DS (1977) Metabolism and transport of glutamine and glucose in vascularly perfused small intestine of the rat. Biochem J 166:509–519
Hanson PJ, Parsons DS (1980) The interrelationship between glutamine and alanine in the intestine. Biochem Soc Trans 8:506–509
Hill AV (1928) The diffusion of oxygen and lactic acid through tissues. Proc R Soc Lond [Biol] 104:39–96
Hodgkin AL (1951) The ionic basis of electrical activity in nerve and muscle. Biol Rev 26:339–409
Kessler M, Semenza G (1979) On the efficiency of energy conversion in sodium-driven D-glucose transport across small intestinal brush border membrane vesicles: an estimation. FEBS Lett 108:205–208
Keynes KD (1954) The ionic fluxes in frog muscle. Proc R Soc Lond [Biol] 142:359–382
Krebs H, Kornberg HL (1957) A survey of the energy transformations on living matter. Ergeb Physiol 49:212–298
Kushmerick MJ (1977) Energy balance in muscle contraction: a biochemical approach. Curr Top Bioenergetics 6:137
Kushmerick JM, Davies RE (1969) The chemical energetics of muscle contraction. II. The chemistry, efficiency and power of maximally working sartorious muscles. Proc R Soc Lond [Biol] 174:315–353
Lipmann F (1941) Metabolic generation and utilization of phosphate bond energy. Adv Enzymol 1:97–102
Love AMG (1976) Intestinal blood flow and sodium exchange. In: Robinson JWL (ed) Intestinal ion transport. MTP Press, Lancaster, England, pp 261–265
Low H, Crane FL (1978) Redox functions in plasma membranes. Biochim Biophys Acta 515:141–161
MacDonald RE, Lanyi JK (1977) Light-activated amino acid transport in Halobacterium halobium envelope vesicles. Fed Proc 36:1828–1832
MacKnight ADC, Leaf A (1977) Regulation of cellular volume. Physiol Rev 57:510–573
Mc Neil NI, Cummings JH, James WPT (1978) Rectal absorption of short fatty acids in the absence of chloride. Gut 20:400–403
Milligan LP (1971) Energetic efficiency and metabolic transformations. Fed Proc 30:1454–1461
Mitchell P, Moyle J (1974) The mechanism of protein translocation in reversible proton-translocating adenosine triphosphatase. In: Bronk JP (ed) Membrane adenosine triphosphatases and transport processes. Biochem Soc Sp Publ 4:91–111
Murer H, Hopfer U (1977) The functional polarity of the intestinal epithelial cell; studies with isolated plasma membrane vesicles. In: Kramer M, Lauterbach F (eds) Intestinal permeation. Workshop conference Hoechst 4. Excerpta Medica, Amsterdam, pp 294–311
Murer H, Kinne R (1980) The use of isolated membrane vesicles to study epithelial transport processes. J Membr Biol 55:81–95

Neame KD, Wiseman G (1957) The transamination of glutamic and aspartic acids during absorption by the small intestine of the dog in vivo. J Physiol 135:442–450
Neame KD, Wiseman G (1958) The alanine and oxo-acid concentrations in mesenteric blood during the absorption of L-glutamic acid by the small intestine of the dog, cat and rabbit in vivo. J Physiol (Lond) 140:148–155
Parsons DS (1967) Salt and water absorption by the intestinal tract. Br Med Bull 23:252–257
Parsons DS (1972) Summary. In: Burland WL, Samuel PD (eds) Transport across the intestine. Chap 24, Churchill-Linvingstone, London, pp 253–278
Parsons DS (1973) Energy foods. In: Hollingsworth D, Russell M (eds) Nutritional problems in a changing world, Chap 15, Applied Science Publishers, London, pp 161–172
Parsons DS (1975) Energetics of intestinal transport. In: Csaky TZ (ed) Intestinal absorption and malabsorption. Raven Press, New York, pp 9–36
Parsons DS (1976) Closing summary. In: Robinson JWL (ed) Intestinal Transport. MTP Press, Lancaster, England, pp 407–430
Parsons DS (1979) Fuels of the small intestinal mucosa. In: Truelove SC, Willoughby CP (eds) Topics in Gastroenterology vol 7: Blackwell Scientific Publications, Oxford, pp 253–271
Parsons DS, Prichard JS (1968) A preparation of perfused small intestine for the study of absorption in amphibia. J Physiol 198:405–434
Parsons DS, Prichard JS (1971) Relationship between disaccharide hydrolysis and sugar transport in amphibian small intestine. J Physiol (Lond) 212:299–319
Parsons DS, Sanderson IR (1980) Influence of vascular flow on amino acid transport across frog small intestine. J Physiol 309:447–460
Parsons DS, Volman-Mitchell HBJM (1974) The transamination of glutamate and aspartate during absorption in vitro by small intestine of chicken, guinea-pig and rat. J Physiol 239:677–694
Parsons DS, Wade SA (1981). Sodium fluxes across vasculary perfused intestine of the frog. In: MacKnight ADC, Leader JP (eds) Epithelial water transport. Raven, New York, pp 211–219
Parsons DS, Wade SA (1982a) Sodium movements across the vascularly perfused anuran small intestine and colon. Quart J exp Physiol 67:121–131
Parsons DS, Wade SA (1982b) Influence of vascular and lumen flow on sodium movements across anuran intestine in vitro. Quart J exp Physiol 67:323–334
Quay JF, Armstrong W McD (1969) Sodium and chloride transport by isolated bullfrog small intestine. Am J Physiol 217:694–702
Roediger WEW (1979) Nutrition of the colonic mucosa. In: Truelove SC, Willoughby CP (eds) Topics in Gastroenterology, Blackwell Scientific Publications, Oxford, pp 281–290
Sachs GR, Jackson J, Rabon EC (1980) Use of plasma membrane vesicles. Am J Physiol G151–G169
Sactor B (1977) Transport in membrane vesicles from brush borders of kidney and intestine. Curr Top bioenergetics 6:39–81
Schultz SG (1977) Some properties and consequences of low resistance paracellular pathways across the small intestine: the consequence of being "leaky". In: Kramer M, Lauterbach F (eds) Intestinal permeation, Workshop conferences Höchst 4. Excerpta Medica, Amsterdam, pp 382–391
Schultz SG, Zalusky R (1964) Ion transport in isolated rabbit ileum. II. The interaction between active sodium and active glucose transport. J Gen Physiol 47:1043–1059
Simoni RD, Postma PW (1975) Energetics of bacterial transport. Ann Rev Biochem 44:523–554
Skou JC, Nørby JG (eds) (1979) Na, K-ATPase structure and Kinetics. Academic, London, p 549
Thomas RC (1972) Electrogenic sodium pump in nerve and muscle cells. Physiol Rev 52:563–594
Volman-Mitchell HBJM (1973) Metabolism of amino acids by intestinal mucosal cells. Thesis, Oxford University

Volman-Mitchell HBJM, Parsons DS (1974) Distribution and activities of dicarboxylic amino acid transaminases in gastrointestinal mucosa of rat, mouse, hamster, guinea pig, chicken and pigeon. Biochem Biophys Acta 334:316–327
West IC (1980) Energy coupling in secondary active transport. Biochem Biophys Acta 604:91–126
Whittam R, Wheeler KP (1970) Transport across cell membranes. Ann Rev Physiol 32:21–60
Windmueller HG, Spaeth AE (1980) Respiratory fuels and nitrogen metabolism in vivo in small intestine. J Biol Chem 255:107–110
Winne D (1979) Influence of blood flow on intestinal absorption of drugs and nutrients. Pharmacol Ther 6:333–393
Wrong OM, Edmonds CJ, Chadwick VS (1981) The large intestine. MTP Press, Lancaster, p 217
Zeuthen T (1976) Microelectrode recording of ultracellular gradients of electrical and chemical potential in secretory epithelia. J Physiol (Lond) 263:113P

CHAPTER 9

Polarity of Intestinal Epithelial Cells: Permeability of the Brush Border and Basolateral Membranes

G. Esposito

A. Introduction

Before discussing in detail the function of the intestinal epithelial cell in general, and the characteristics of its polarity in particular, a brief mention of the importance and of the general function of the plasma membrane should be made. The cell plasma membrane is not a passive barrier separating the cell compartment from the surrounding media, but is an active structure which participates in maintaining the difference in composition between the intracellular and extracellular milieux. Besides holding cell components, the plasma membrane is also the place where several enzymes are located and where many enzymatic reactions take place; the enzymes thus have a support for their action. In addition, some enzymes span the plasma membrane in well-defined spots so that a substrate can be picked up from one side and the product released to the other.

The plasma membrane is also asymmetric in shape and chemical composition as far as the cytoplasmic and external surfaces are concerned (Rothman and Lenard 1977; Singer 1977). Glycoproteins, for instance, are almost exclusively located outwardly. Some proteins are asymmetrically distributed on the outer and the inner surface of the membrane, while others are embedded or span the lipid matrix. Also, phospholipids are placed in a different array between the two surfaces. These observations lead to the conclusion that biologic membranes are vectorial structures providing a molecular basis for functional polarity.

Finally, besides the anatomic and biochemical functions, the plasma membrane also develops a physiologic function, i.e., it constitutes a selective barrier regulating the movement of different substances with or without utilizing metabolic energy. With regard to these three functions (anatomic, biochemical, and physiologic), it is possible to study the plasma membrane from different viewpoints and with different methods in order to have as complete a model as possible.

B. Functionally Polarized and Unpolarized Cells

Depending on their special functions, the cells can be divided into functionally polarized and unpolarized. The first kind of cell includes those transport mechanisms are symmetrically distributed along the whole plasma membrane. These cells perform an activity consisting of moving solutes and water in and out of the cell across the plasma membrane. For instance, blood, muscle, and nerve cells behave in this way. On the contrary, functionally polarized cells perform a net transfer of solutes and water from one side to the other. In order to do that, such cells must possess transport mechanisms asymmetrically distributed in the two opposite plasma membranes. Cells behaving in this way are, for instance, the epithelial cells of many organs such as the epithelia of the gastrointestinal tract, of kidney tubules, of amphibian bladder, and so on. For example, if we consider net active transport of sodium ion from the lumen of the intestine to the blood, we observe that during its transcellular movement this ion has to cross two in-series membranes, namely the brush border and the basolateral membrane of the enterocyte.

In order to achieve a net absorption, two asymmetrically distributed mechanisms of crossing these membranes have to be postulated, one in the apical and the other in the contraluminal aspect of the absorbing cell. In fact we now know that Na^+ mainly enters the cell from the lumen by a carrier-mediated mechanism down an electrochemical potential gradient, while it leaves the cell towards the blood by an active extrusion mechanism located in the basolateral membrane, against an electrochemical potential gradient.

C. The Epithelial Layer as a Selective Barrier

As previously mentioned, the plasma membrane does not behave as a passive structure separating two compartments; it selectively allows the passage of substances and maintains the differences between the internal and external milieux. As long as an organism develops, its organs which now possess many cells, are in contact with extracellular spaces. In this case, the internal milieu is separated from the external one by more complicated barriers. Since we are now dealing with more developed organisms, these barriers cannot be made by simple plasma membranes but by layers of contiguous cells, similar to fences. this layer has been named "epithelium", which has the same function, but now related to the entire organism, as that of plasma membrane related to the single cell; in other words, it has a cohesive, biochemical and physiologic function, that is to say it holds together materials and cells of the organism and it is able to transform substances coming from the outside, in order to neutralize or destroy them if dangerous, or to modify them in a way useful to the organism. Finally, it selects, absorbs, or secretes solutes and fluids as needed.

The epithelial layer, held together by junctional complexes, rests on a basal membrane made of reticulofibrillar connective tissue, mucopolysaccharide in nature, with large meshes (of the order of a few tens of nm). This basal membrane does not seem to be a selective barrier, but it probably functions as a support for the epithelium in order to ensure mechanical stability.

Since epithelial cells are arranged like a fence, their plasma membranes cannot be considered uniform and with the same function in all their parts. On the contrary, one pole of the cell faces the external compartment; this part of the plasma membrane is commonly named apical, external, luminal, or mucosal. The other part faces the internal compartment of the organism and is commonly named serosal, internal, contraluminal, or basolateral. Without going into further detail it is sufficient to say that the eptithelial cells are sealed, i.e., encircled and held together around their apical region by means of two peculiar structures: the zonula occludens or tight junction (externally) and the zonula adherens or intermediate junction. The tight junction, 100–200 nm long, is the place where the plasma membranes of two adjacent cells seem to fuse, resulting in a pentalaminar structure. Actually, they do not completely fuse but close up to few Å; they are also linked by protein bridges crossing the lipid bilayer of the two adjacent plasma membranes. Among the network of these bridges there are empty spaces, allowing communication between the lumen of the gut and the intercellular spaces (STAEHELIN and HULL 1978). At first it was assumed that these junctions were closed, thus preventing transepithelial fluxes of water and solutes. It has been subsequently demonstrated that only large molecules are excluded, but that water, small ions, and small solute molecules can cross these structures (FRÖMTER and DIAMOND 1972; MACHEN et al. 1972; CLAUDE and GOODENOUGH 1973; DIAMOND 1974). Therefore, they behave in a way as a passive selective barrier.

A second structure contributing to the adhesion among the cells is called the desmosome, which is arranged in such a way as to assure stability to the epithelial layer. Desmosomes do not select molecules when crossing the epithelial barrier. A third structure connecting cells along their lateral plasma membrane is named the gap junction. These junctions are very important because they allow communication between adjacent cells since they are provided by small channels in which small molecules (up to a molecular weight of 1,000) can move. Therefore, important solutes like ions, amino acids, monosaccarides, vitamins, and some important messengers such as cyclic AMP (cAMP) and steroid hormones can cross these junctions. This structure has been postulated by LOEWENSTEIN et al. (1965) during studies on electrical measurements where it was concluded that cells must have electrical connections at low resistance. More detailed information on this topic is reported by LOEWENSTEIN (1978, 1981).

From this discussion it follows that underneath the zonulae occludentes et adherentes the adjacent cells are relatively free to widen their separating spaces, depending on different physiologic conditions. These spaces are commonly named intercellular spaces, lateral intercellular spaces, or intercellular channels. These channels, at the base of the cell, end at and open through the meshes of the connective basal membrane.

It must be briefly mentioned that the epithelial layer is not exclusively composed of columnar absorbing cells (also named enterocytes), but other cell types are present, even if in a much lower proportion, e.g., goblet cells (29% by volume of the mucosa in the upper small intestine, GEBAUER 1969; 10% of the jejunal epithelium, DE WOLFF 1973) or several other cells present in the crypts of villi. Finally, the epithelial organization can be visualized as a "six-pack of beer extended indefinitely in two dimensions" (DIAMOND 1977).

As a conclusion, the epithelial layer can be regarded as a selective barrier with specific transport mechanisms asymmetrically distributed in the apical and/or in the basolateral membrane which allow a transcellular movement of water and solutes. Moreover, this barrier is also able to permit the movement of water and small ions and solutes along a path which bypasses the cell, commonly named the paracellular pathway (SCHULTZ 1977).

D. Brush Border Membrane: Morphology, Chemical Composition, and Biochemical Characteristics

As already mentioned, the plasma membrane of the enterocyte consists mainly of two different regions: the brush border and the basolateral membrane which are morphologically, structurally, and functionally different.

I. Morphology

First of all the microvillous membrane is about 10 nm thick (SJÖSTRAND 1963; ROBERTSON 1964; SACKTOR 1977) while the basolateral membrane is 7.5 nm thick MILLINTON and FINEAN 1963; ROBERTSON 1964; DOUGLAS et al. 1972). The apical pole of the enterocyte is characterized by peculiar structures that increase the intestinal surface: the microvilli. They are coated with plasma membrane and are approximately 1–2 μm high and 0.1–0.2 μm wide. Their number is variable, but it ranges from few units per μm^2 to 70–80 per μm^2. Within the core they contain a few protein filaments (6.0 nm in diameter) which, at the microvillus base, are linked to the terminal web. Both core microfilaments and terminal web are made of F actin (molecular weight 43,000), similar to that present in the muscle cell. At the level of the terminal web the microfilaments are in contact with molecules of heavy meromyosin (molecular weight 200,000); other proteins similar to those of muscle cell are also present (MOOSEKER 1976). All these proteins allow the microvillus to contract. The terminals web is laterally linked to the tight junctions and the desmosomes of the upper part of the lateral plasma membrane; therefore, the upper part of the enterocyte, consisting of the terminal web, the junctional complex, and the microvilli, forms a mechanically very steady compact unit. This unit is protected externally, against mechanical damage and friction, by highly hydrated glycosaminoglycans and glycoconjugates which entirely cover the microvilli. The glycoconjugates form the fuzzy coat with long filaments on the top of the microvilli; these filaments cross each other in order to make a structure (the enteric surface coat) separating the luminal compartment from the villi (ITO 1969). All these structures form the glycocalyx, mainly made of glycoproteins and glycolipids. As a conclusion, the apical aspect of the enterocyte is morphologically very different from the basolateral membrane. The major difference is due to the presence of the microvilli, while the contraluminal membrane possesses many folds, almost exclusively, in the lateral part of this membrane, irregular in shape and without core filaments.

II. Chemical Composition

From the structural and chemical point of view, the apical pole of the enterocyte differs from the basolateral membrane. Without going into detail it is worth pointing out some chemical features of the plasma membrane in general and of the apical pole of the enterocyte in particular.

1. Lipids and Glycolipids

The lipids present in plasma membranes are of different kinds, but the amphipathic in nature predominate; for this reason they are mostly phospholipids, but

Table 1. Lipid composition of the apical and basolateral membranes of the enterocyte

	Apical membrane		Basolateral membrane	
Total lipids	0.60	FORSTNER et al. (1968a)	0.95	KAWAI et al. (1974)
(mg per milligram protein)	0.61	KAWAI et al. (1974)		
	0.49	MAX et al. (1978)		
	0.50	HAUSER et al. (1980)		
Neutral lipids (mg per milligram protein)	0.16	KAWAI et al. (1974)	0.24	KAWAI et al. (1974)
Cholesterol [a]	55.4%	KAWAI et al. (1974)	47.4%	KAWAI et al. (1974)
	58.0%	HAUSER et al. (1980)		
Free fatty acids	25.8%	KAWAI et al. (1974)	28.7%	KAWAI et al. (1974)
Triglycerides	6.9%	KAWAI et al. (1974)	10.7%	KAWAI et al. (1974)
Cholesterol esters	12.0%	KAWAI et al. (1974)	13.3%	KAWAI et al. (1974)
Phospholipids [b]	0.16	TAKESUE and SATO (1968)	0.70	DOUGLAS et al. (1972)
(mg per milligram protein)	0.13	FORSTNER et al. (1968a, b)		
	0.11	LOUVARD et al. (1973)		
	0.16	KAWAI et al. (1974)	0.59	KAWAI et al. (1974)
	0.19	HAUSER et al. (1980)		
Phosphatidylethanolamine [b]	49.0%	KAWAI et al. (1974)	27.4%	KAWAI et al. (1974)
	39.0%	HAUSER et al. (1980)		
Phosphatidylcholine	25.1%	KAWAI et al. (1974)	51.0%	KAWAI et al. (1974)
	33.3%	HAUSER et al. (1980)		
Phosphatidylinositol	11.6%	KAWAI et al. (1974)	8.6%	KAWAI et al. (1974)
	8.2%	HAUSER et al. (1980)		
Sphingomyelin	8.3%	KAWAI et al. (1974)	9.9%	KAWAI et al. (1974)
	10.3%	HAUSER et al. (1980)		
Phosphatidylserine	6.0%	KAWAI et al. (1974)	3.1%	KAWAI et al. (1974)
	7.4%	HAUSER et al. (1980)		
Cholesterol:phospholipid	1.11:1	FINEAN et al. (1966)		
(molar ratio)	1.26:1	FORSTNER et al. (1968a)	0.50:1	DOUGLAS et al. (1972)
	0.87:1	BRASITUS and SCHACTER (1980)	0.62:1	BRASITUS and SCHACTER (1980)
Cholesterol:phospholipid: glycolipid (molar ratio)	2:1:1	FORSTNER and WHERRETT (1973)		
	1:1:1	KAWAI et al. (1974)	1:2.5:0.3	KAWAI et al. (1974)
Fatty acids [c]				
16:0	15.6%	FORSTNER et al. (1968a)		
	13.6%	KAWAI et al. (1974)	19.7%	KAWAI et al. (1974)
	26.3%	HAUSER et al. (1980)		
16:1	0.8%	FORSTNER et al. (1968a)		
	3.4%	HAUSER et al. (1980)		
18:0	29.5%	FORSTNER et al. (1968a)		
	28.0%	KAWAI et al. (1974)	22.7%	KAWAI et al. (1974)
	16.9%	HAUSER et al. (1980)		
18:1	5.8%	FORSTNER et al. (1968a)		
	7.6%	KAWAI et al. (1974)	7.5%	KAWAI et al. (1974)
	16.1%	HAUSER et al. (1980)		
18:2	14.4%	FORSTNER et al. (1968a)		
	28.4%	KAWAI et al. (1974)	31.6%	KAWAI et al. (1974)
	24.4%	HAUSER et al. (1980)		

Table 1 (continued)

	Apical membrane		Basolateral membrane	
18:3	1.3%	FORSTNER et al. (1968 a)		
	3.7%	HAUSER et al. (1980)		
20:3	2.3%	FORSTNER et al. (1968 a)		
20:4	22.0%	FORSTNER et al. (1968 a)		
	9.1%	KAWAI et al. (1974)	7.6%	KAWAI et al. (1974)
22:0	2.3%	KAWAI et al. (1974)	2.6%	KAWAI et al. (1974)
24:0	5.5%	KAWAI et al. (1974)	4.0%	KAWAI et al. (1974)
% saturated	51.7%	KAWAI et al. (1974)	51.2%	KAWAI et al. (1974)

[a] Percentage of neutral lipid fraction
[b] Percentage of total lipid phosphorus
[c] Data from KAWAI et al. (1974) refer to fatty acid composition of phospholipids; other data refer to fatty acid composition of total lipids

not triglycerides; cholesterol, but not sterids. The phospholipids are represented mainly by lecithins and cephalins; their fatty acids differ from one membrane to another, especially in the length of the aliphatic chain, the presence of branched chains, and the degree of unsaturation. This is very important in assigning different properties to different membranes.

It is presumed that a plasma membrane is tight and poorly permeable if it contains a high proportion of cholesterol and long-chain saturated fatty acids. On the contrary, a plasma membrane should be more permeable if it contains a low proportion of cholesterol and many short-chain, branched and unsaturated fatty acids (O'BRIEN 1967). All these properties have been verified experimentally by using black lipid membranes. In general, plasma membranes may differ from one another in the tightness of the packing of their constituent lipids and consequently in their efficiency as permeability barriers.

The chemical composition of the luminal pole of the enterocyte has not been completely elucidated yet, but several works on this topic are available. Such composition differs remarkably from that of basolateral membrane (Table 1). The lipid content of the microvillus membrane is approximately 0.6 mg per milligram protein (FORSTNER et al. 1968). The molar ratio between cholesterol, phospholipids, and glycolipids of the rat microvillus membrane is 2:1:1 (FORSTNER and WHERRETT 1973). Free cholesterol represents approximately 70% of the neutral lipid fraction of the microvillus membrane; the remaining fraction is almost all diglycerides and free fatty acids. The cholesterol:phospholipid molar ratio is 1.26:1 (FORSTNER et al. 1968a) while in the basolateral membrane it is 0.5:1 (DOUGLAS et al. 1972); in the latter case the lower ratio is due to the major increase of phospholipid content.

The glycolipids (Table 2), which are typical components of the plasma membrane of nervous tissue, are surprisingly abundant here. It is also interesting to observe that glycolipids extracted from dog intestine are mainly cerebrosides, gangliosides, and ceramides and, to a lesser extent, sulfatides (MCKIBBIN 1969).

Table 2. Glycolipid, glycoprotein, and protein composition of the apical and basolateral membranes of the enterocyte

	Apical membrane		Basolateral membrane	
Glycolipids (mg per milligram protein)	0.290	KAWAI et al. (1974)	0.124	KAWAI et al. (1974)
Neutral glycolipids	0.135	KAWAI et al. (1974)	0.069	KAWAI et al. (1974)
Globosides	0.155	KAWAI et al. (1974)	0.055	KAWAI et al. (1974)
Gangliosides	0.001	KAWAI et al. (1974)	0.002	KAWAI et al. (1974)
Glycoproteins (mg carbohydrate per milligram protein)	0.075 0.095	JONAS et al. (1977) COOPER and KENT (1978)		
Hexose : hexosamine : neuraminic acid (molar ratio)	23 : 12 : 1	ROBINSON (1975)		
Membrane proteins [a]	66%	FORSTNER et al. (1968 b)		

[a] Percentage of total proteins

Interestingly, a ganglioside is present in the plasma membrane of the apical pole of the enterocyte which should represent the specific membrane receptor for cholera toxin (CUATRECASAS 1973; WALKER et al. 1974; HOLMGREN et al. 1975).

The lipoidal fraction of the membrane represents a barrier for the rapid diffusion of large, water-soluble solutes because the occasional aqueous channels (the dynamic pores) have an approximate radius of 0.4–0.5 nm (LINDEMAN and SOLOMON 1962; FORDTRAN et al. 1965), too small to allow them to cross the plasma membrane. Owing to the semifluid nature of this lipid bilayer (WIDDAS 1963) there is a continuous formation and disappearance of holes (dynamic pores) so that, at any moment, there is always, statistically, a certain number of pores present in the membrane having a proper mean equivalent radius. On the contrary, lipid-soluble substances (such as the products of lipid digestion) may readily move across the lipid bilayer by simple diffusion.

2. Proteins and Glycoproteins

Plasma membranes contain proteins and lipids, but generally more proteins than lipids. The microvillus membrane contains approximately 50% proteins (EICHHOLZ 1967), mostly enzymes. Membrane proteins are extrinsic (peripheral) and intrinsic (integral) according to whether they are on the external part of the lipid bilayer or are partially embedded in or spanning the lipid interior of the membrane (SINGER 1977). Integral proteins can be of different types, but are usually globular and amphipathic molecules. They are probably responsible for the structured hydrophilic pores through which small water-soluble solutes can diffuse. Others are enzymes or constitute part of the carrier molecules.

Many studies on membrane proteins have been performed electrophoretically. The electrophoretic patterns on polyacrylamide gel of brush border and its subfraction of jejunum and ileum have shown the presence of at least 25–30 protein bands and about 10 glycoprotein bands (MAESTRACCI et al. 1973; STARITA-GERIBALDI et al. 1977; SIGRIST-NELSON et al. 1977). Their molecular weights range from 25,000 to over 400,000; many of these proteins and glycoproteins are related to enzymic activity. The presence of predominant bands with high molecular weight seems to be peculiar to the brush border membrane, unlike other plasma membranes.

A different protein pattern has also been found in jejunum and ileum brush border which has been ascribed to the different distribution of some enzymes and transport activities in these two regions. Interestingly, when using an iodinating procedure, it has ben shown that iodonaphtylazide nonspecifically labels the portion of membrane proteins inserted into the lipid bilayer matrix of the brush border membrane (SIGRIST-NELSON et al. 1977). Recently, it has been shown that several brush border proteins and enzymes undergo variations during postnatal development (SEETHARAM et al. 1977). In any case, many differences are observed when comparing brush border with basolateral membranes; the former possesses rather large molecules most of which are also periodic acid–Schiff reagent positive, while in the latter there are no protein components with corresponding molecular weights and the dominant band of the electrophoretic pattern is periodic acid-Schiff reagent negative (FUJITA et al. 1973).

As already mentioned, on the plasma membrane covering microvilli there is a surface coat of proteins and glycoconjugates; this sialic acid-containing glycoproteinaceous fibrillar layer, approximately 10 nm thick (ITO 1965) is an integral part of the membrane and not a layer of mucus produced by goblet cells. It seems that glycoproteins of the fuzzy coat are synthesized in the Golgi apparatus and then they migrate towards the apical cell surface where they contribute to the surface charge of the membrane. Most probably, this fuzzy coat is able to adsorb pancreatic enzymes, thus contributing to intestinal digestion. It is interesting to observe that, unlike the plasma membrane of other cells such as kidney brush border (QUIRK and ROBINSON 1972), liver cells, and lymphocytes (GLICK 1976), a low sialic acid content seems to be a peculiarity of the small intestinal brush border (COOPER and KENT 1978). However, it has recently been found that the sialic acid content of glycocalyx glycoproteins shows a species-specific difference; rat enterocytes have about ten times as much sialic acid as human absorptive cells (BLOK et al. 1980).

In negative stained preparations, the external part of the microvillus membrane appears to be studded with knobs approximately 6.0 nm in diameter (TAKESUE and SATO 1968; JOHNSON 1969). These particles seem to be hydrolytic enzymes such as invertase and maltase. Therefore, both particles and enzymic activities are located in the fuzzy coat, hence external to the plasma membrane of the microvilli. This interpretation fits well with CRANE's concept of the digestive–absorptive function of the brush border (CRANE 1968) as well as with UGOLEV's views on contact digestion (UGOLEV 1965, 1968; UGOLEV et al. 1977, 1979).

3. Brush Border Enzymes

Whether the enzymes of the brush border are attached to or inserted within the outer surface of the microvillus membrane has not been completely defined (UGOLEV et al. 1979). For the purposes of this chapter it is sufficient to report a ten-

Table 3. Enzyme activities localized in the brush border membrane of the enterocyte

Maltase	LOJDA (1965), MILLER and CRANE (1961), DAHLQVIST (1964), EICHHOLZ (1967), BENSON et al. (1971), FORSTNER et al. (1968 b), SEMENZA (1976), TSUBOI et al. (1979)
Lactase	EICHHOLZ (1967), FORSTNER et al. (1968 b), SEMENZA (1976), TSUBOI et al. (1979)
Sucrase	MILLER and CRANE (1961), LOJDA (1965), FORSTNER et al. (1968 b), TAKESUE and SATO (1968), BENSON et al. (1971), SEMENZA (1976), OLSEN and KORSMO (1977)
Isomaltase	EICHHOLZ (1967), FORSTNER et al. (1968 b), BENSON et al. (1971), SEMENZA (1976)
Trehalase	FORSTNER et al. (1968 b), SACKTOR (1968), BENSON et al. (1971), SASAJMA et al. (1975), SEMENZA (1976)
Cellobiase	FORSTNER et al. (1968 b)
Glucoamylase	MALATHI and CRANE (1968), SEMENZA (1976)
Phlorhizin hydrolase (glycosylceramidase)	DIEDRICH (1968), MALATHI and CRANE (1969), LEESE and SEMENZA (1973), SEMENZA (1976)
Alkaline phosphatase	HOLT and MILLER (1962), FORSTNER et al. (1968 b), MIRCHEFF and WRIGHT (1976), BOUHOURS (1978)
Ca^{2+}-ATPase	MIRCHEFF and WRIGHT (1976), GHIJSEN and VAN OS (1979)
Anion-ATPase	HUMPHREYS and CHOU (1979), HUMPHREYS et al. (1980)
HCO_3^--ATPase	JACKSON et al. (1977)
Dipeptidase	WOJNAROWSKA and GRAY (1975)
Oligopeptidase	HOLT and MILLER (1962), RHODES et al. (1967), PETERS (1970), ARVANITAKIS et al. (1976)
Ca^{2+}-activated phospholipase A	HAUSER et al. (1980)
Enterokinase	HOLMES and LOBLEY (1970), NORDSTROM and DAHLQVIST (1970), SCHMITZ et al. (1974)
γ-Glutamyltransferase	COHEN et al. (1969)
Guanylate cyclase	DE JONGE (1975), QUILL and WEISER (1975)
Cholesterol ester hydrolase	DAVID et al. (1966)
Retinol ester hydrolase	MALATHI (1967)

The references reported are only indicative and are not necessarily the earliest or the only reports of brush border enzyme activities

tative list of brush border enzyme activities (Table 3). Since the typical marker enzyme for this membrane is represented by sucrase, any enzyme that during purification of microvillus membrane undergoes a specific activity increase parallel to that of sucrase over the tissue homogenate probably belongs to the brush border membrane.

III. The Brush Border as a Selective Membrane

Without going into further chemical and biochemical detail, but taking into consideration the physiologic function of the brush border, it is possible to make the following remarks. The brush border plays the major role in the digestive–absorptive function, first of all because many pancreatic enzymes are adsorbed on it where they can easily exert their function. In addition, some hydrolytic enzymes are directly involved in transport activities of substrates derived from digestive processes. In fact the brush border region can be divided into an outer digestive surface and an inner region containing specific carriers (Crane et al. 1961; Crane 1977). The outer region could be the site where hydrolytic enzymes can act, while the inner region, where specific transport inhibitors can act, seems to have mainly a transport activity function.

As to simple diffusion of solutes across the apical membrane, it is known that this membrane is rather selective in nature. As previously mentioned, besides structural pores, there are occasional aqueous channels, allowing the passage of water molecules (under a concentration or hydrostatic pressure difference) and of small watersoluble substances (with a molecular weight not greater than 100–130) together with small ions. With regard to charged molecules and ions, it is important to point out that the inner walls of the pore channels are probably coated by fixed charges that can hinder or facilitate the movement of these solutes. It is probable that the electrical charges coating the structured pores of the small channels of tight junctions are negative charges due, for instance, to carboxyl, phosphate, or carbonyl groups. The presence of negative charges has been mainly postulated on the existence of streaming potentials (Smyth and Wright 1966).

As far as pore dimension is concerned, it is difficult at present to find a uniform average value, especially for a leaky epithelium like the intestine; this is mainly due to a contemporaneous presence of different pore routes existing in the transcellular and paracellular pathways and to the different methods used to determine it. Anyway, in the case of the small intestine, an approximate value is around 0.4–0.5 nm in radius, if movement takes place via the transcellular pathway, and around 1.0–1.5 nm in radius, if movement is via the larger, but far less numerous routes called paracellular pathways (Höber and Höber 1937; Lindeman and Solomon 1962; Fordtran et al. 1965, 1968; Levitt et al. 1969; Schultz 1977).

Some larger molecules that would not move through these pathways do nevertheless cross the apical pole of the enterocyte. By studying the kinetics of this passage, the effect of the inhibitors and of structural analogs on the transport, it seems reasonable to accept the existence of a carrier-mediated transport mechanism. The details and the modalities of movement of these substances is beyond the scope of this chapter, but they will be discussed in Chapter 7. The external surface of the plasma membrane of the luminal pole of the enterocyte contains some binding proteins with specific binding sites for ions such as Ca^{2+} (Wasserman et al. 1966; Bredderman and Wasserman 1974), Zn^{2+} (Kowarsky et al. 1974), iron (Greenberger et al. 1969; Huebers and Rummel 1977), some molecules such as folate (Leslie and Rowe 1972), very large molecule like intrinsic factor vitamin B_{12} complex (Toskes and Deren 1973; Mathan et al. 1974; Donaldson 1977) and γ-globulins, at least in the newborn (Walker and Isselbacher 1974). Part of these binding proteins are integral membrane proteins while others are peripheral membrane proteins.

Concerning the problem of water permeability across the intestinal epithelium, some complications arise because we are dealing with a "leaky epithelium"; therefore, it is difficult to ascertain which of the two in-series membranes is more permeable to water since the permeability feature of the paracellular shunt pathway is very high. By considering the hydraulic conductivity L_p it was shown some years ago (LINDEMAN and SOLOMON 1962) that L_p of the luminal border of the mucosal cells of rat small intestine has a value of 6×10^{-6} cm s^{-1} atm^{-1}, very similar to that found for the whole epithelium (7.7×10^{-6} cm s^{-1} atm^{-1}) by SMYTH and WRIGHT (1966).

This seems to mean that the apical plasma membrane of the enterocyte is much less permeable than the basolateral membrane. For instance, in the kidney collecting duct (which possesses however a tight epithelium) the rate-limiting barrier to osmotic flow is represented by the luminal border of the cells while the peritubular border is relatively permeable to water (GRANTHAM et al. 1969). This fact does not necessarily mean that the epithelium has asymmetric permeability characteristics for water. Evidence for that, however, has been obtained in other leaky epithelia. At present it seems that the paracellular shunt pathway accounts not only for the major route of transepithelial ionic diffusion, but also for the major role of the transepithelial hydraulic conductivity (SCHULTZ 1977). Finally, it is known that in many epithelia there exists the phenomenon named rectification of volume flow or nonlinear osmosis (a nonlinear relationship between net volume flux and osmotic pressure gradient). One possible explanation for this phenomenon is based on the assumption that epithelia behave like double-membrane systems with asymmetric water permeabilities.

E. Basolateral Membrane: Chemical and Biochemical Organization

I. Chemical Composition

Studies of the chemical composition, the biochemical organization, and the precise physiologic function of the basolateral membrane of the enterocyte are rather recent and unfortunately incomplete. It has been demonstrated that the thickness of the basolateral membrane is less than the corresponding apical one: 7.5 nm vs 10.0–11.5 nm (see Sect. D. I). Contrary to the basolateral membrane of the proximal tubular cells, that of the enterocyte does not possess basal infoldings; unlike the brush border, the basolateral membrane is devoid of fuzzy coat and is sharply delineated when observed in the electron microscope.

As already mentioned, the luminal membrane is characterized by possessing components with rather large apparent molecular weights, up to 400,000, most of which are also periodic acid–Schiff reagent positive. On the contrary, the contraluminal membrane has no protein components with such large molecular weights. Most of these studies have been performed by using sodium dodecylsulfate polyacrylamide gel electrophoresis which has shown that the electrophoretic profile of basolateral membrane components is very simple and that the predominant band has a molecular weight of 101,000, periodic acid–Schiff reagent negative, so that no major components are shared by the two membranes (FUJITA et al. 1973).

The molar ratio between cholesterol and phospholipid, which is 1.26 : 1 for the brush border, is only 0.5:1 here; the lower ratio is due to the major increase in phospholipid content (DOUGLAS et al. 1972). This value is comparable to that found by other authors for many other plasma membranes (STECK and WALLACH 1970).

The glycolipid content of the basolateral membrane is 42% of the total membrane lipids, a value significantly higher than that found in other plasma membranes. Both brush border and basolateral membranes of the enterocyte are rich in cholesterol and sphingolipids; however, the major part of the sphingolipids in the contraluminal membrane are tri- and tetrahexosylceramides. On the contrary, as already mentioned, the brush border sphingolipids are mono-, di-, and trihexosylceramides and gangliosides. It has been recently found (BOUHOURS 1978) that the ceramide content of the basolateral membrane is much higher than that of the brush border. Therefore, owing to glycosphingolipids and sphingomyelin, the outer aspect of the lipid bilayer in the basolateral and brush border surfaces is very different as far as outward-facing lipid polar head groups are concerned.

II. Enzyme Content

The enzymic pattern of the basolateral membrane behaves very differently from that of the brush border. It is now well established that one of the most characteristic enzymes present almost exclusively in the basolateral membrane is Na^+, K^+-ATPase which is involved in many transport activities of the enterocyte. This enzyme has been located in this membrane by physiologic (SCHULTZ and ZALUSKY 1964; CSÁKY and HARA 1965) and morphological studies (by radioautography, STIRLING 1972) as well as by a biochemical isolation procedure (QUIGLEY and GOTTERER 1969; FUJITA et al. 1971, 1972; FAELLI et al. 1976) and it has been identified as the "sodium pump". Traces of this enzymic activity in other membrane fractions would mean a basolateral membrane contamination. It has also been reported that cells of the villus tip possess the highest specific activity of Na^+, K^+-ATPase in comparison with cells of the crypts (CHARNEY et al. 1974).

Other enzymes have been found in this membrane, i.e., a K^+-stimulated phosphatase, a 5′-nucleotidase, and a F^--activated adenylate cyclase (MURER et al. 1976a). Contrary to most previous literature, alkaline phosphatase has also been found in the basolateral membrane (MIRCHEFF and WRIGHT 1976) together with a Ca^{2+}-ATPase and some acid phosphatase. The enzyme adenylate cyclase which

Table 4. Enzyme activities localized in the basolateral membrane of the enterocyte

Adenylate cyclase	MURER et al. (1976a), FIELD (1978)
Acid phosphatase	MIRCHEFF and WRIGHT (1976)
Alkaline phosphatase	MIRCHEFF and WRIGHT (1976), DOUGLAS et al. (1972)
Ca^{2+}-ATPase	MIRCHEFF and WRIGHT (1976), GHIJSEN and VAN OS (1979)
Na^+, K^+-ATPase	QUIGLEY and GOTTERER (1969), FUJITA (1971, 1972), STIRLING (1972), MIRCHEFF and WRIGHT (1976), MURER and HOPFER (1977), BOUHOURS (1978)
5′-Nucleotidase	MURER and HOPFER (1977)
Glycosyltransferase	WEISER et al. (1978)
K^+-stimulated PNPase	JACKSON et al. (1977)

The references reported are only indicative and are not necessarily the earliest or the only reports of basolateral membrane enzyme activities

is involved in the formation of cAMP, is located in the basolateral membrane (PARKINSON et al. 1972; MURER et al. 1976a). A list of enzymes thought to be localized in the basolateral membrane of the enterocyte is reported in Table 4.

F. Permeability of Brush Border and Basolateral Membranes

As discussed in Sect. A, the enterocyte is able to perform a net transport of solutes and water from one aqueous compartment to another, in the absence or even against a chemical, electrical, or electrochemical potential difference. In order to achieve this purpose, the characteristics of the luminal and contraluminal membranes must differ both morphologically and physiologically. In the preceding sections some examples have been reported in order to support this concept. However, it is difficult to present a detailed description of the solutes that permeate one membrane of the enterocyte more easily than the other. This is mainly due to the rather recent observation that, in addition to a transcellular pathway for solutes and water, there is also a paracellular pathway; thus, besides distinguishing and characterizing the permeability properties of the brush border and the basolateral membranes, one should also describe the permeability properties of the tight junctions, since some solutes and even water can cross both the luminal pole of the cell and the junctional complex before reaching the subepithelial compartment. I think a good compromise would be the description of permeability of the luminal and contraluminal membranes to solutes whose mechanisms of transport have been extensively studied and elucidated, together with the well-defined and differently localized enzymic systems involved in transport phenomena.

The role of sodium ion has been thought to be of primary importance in biologic transport (MCHARDY and PARSONS 1957; RIKLIS and QUASTEL 1958; CSÁKY and THALE 1960; for a comprehensive review see SCHULTZ and CURRAN 1970). It is known that Na^+ enters the intestinal absorbing cell from the lumen, down its electrochemical potential gradient since the cytoplasmic side of the apical membrane is negatively charged and cell Na^+ concentration is lower than outside. Entry through the luminal membrane is supposed to be a neutral NaCl influx mechanism, showing typical carrier-mediated kinetics (NELLANS et al. 1973). Another possible means of entry is a carrier mechanism responsible for a Na^+–H^+ exchange (TURNBERG et al. 1970; MURER et al. 1976b). Therefore, in the absence of actively transported solutes, Na^+ can move across the brush border via two routes: one coupled to Cl^- and the other which is Cl^- independent but coupled with an H^+ extrusion mechanism. The presence of actively transported solutes stimulates Na^+ entry into the cell by a formation of a ternary complex at the level of the brush border membrane. On the contrary, the basolateral membrane is essentially impermeable to Na^+; only in this membrane has an active extrusion mechanism, responsible for the exit of Na^+ from the cell towards the subepithelial spaces, been demonstrated. This mechanism was identified with an ATP–ATPase system (the sodium pump); as a matter of fact, as already seen, Na^+, K^+-ATPase has been found predominantly in the basolateral membrane. Ouabain, a potent inhibitor of this ATPase, is effective only if acting on the contraluminal plasma membrane (SCHULTZ and ZALUSKY 1964; CSÁKY and HARA 1965; STIRLING 1972).

Another inhibitor of active Na^+ transport is ethacrynic acid which is more effective when placed in the mucosal compartment than on the serosal side (CHEZ et al. 1969). This inhibitor, however, does not prevent Na^+ entry into the cell from the lumen; its effect is probably due to an impairment of Na^+, K^+-ATPase and/or to a negative effect on cell metabolism.

It is also known that the small intestine develops only a small transepithelial electrical potential difference (a few millivolts, serosal side positive), since this epithelium is characterized by low resistance intercellular shunts (FRIZZEL and SCHULTZ 1972). Therefore, the shunt pathway strongly reduces the difference between the electromotive forces through the apical and basolateral membranes of the enterocyte; consequently this epithelium is characterized by a low transepithelial electrical potential difference (PD). By using microelectrodes, measurements of apical and basolateral membrane PDs have been made. Also, this parameter shows an asymmetry between the two opposite membranes. More precisely, the PD across the apical membrane (cell interior negative) is lower than PD across the basolateral membrane (cell interior negative) (ROSE and SCHULTZ 1971). Finally, there is evidence that active Na^+ extrusion is a rheogenic process since the rate of extrusion seems to exceed the rate of coupled active K^+ uptake (ROSE and SCHULTZ 1971; SCHULTZ 1973).

Concerning the net transintestinal Cl^- movement, it seems that here too we are dealing with two different mechanisms asymmetrically distributed; the first one, responsible for Cl^- influx from the lumen, is an Na^+-coupled mechanism (as discussed earlier in this section), while the Cl^- movement towards the serosal compartment seems due to passive diffusion.

As far as potassium ion is concerned it appears that the apical plasma membrane of the enterocyte is practically impermeable and that in the basolateral membrane there is a pump–leak system (coupled with active Na^+ extrusion) that maintains a steady state cell K^+ concentration. A complete description of this behavior is reported by SCHULTZ (1978).

One of the most paradigmatic examples of permeability difference of the two enterocyte membranes is represented by the different mechanisms shared by some actively transparted solutes, such as sugars and amino acids, mechanisms that are differently localized in the two opposite plasma membranes. Without going into detail, it is enough to say that the D-glucose entry mechanism into the cell differs widely from the exit one. The permeability of brush border membrane to glucose mainly depends on the presence of Na^+ in the lumen and on the electrochemical potential gradient of this ion across this membrane as well as on the presence, in the apical membrane, of a carrier molecule which specifically binds glucose. This binding process is strongly inhibited by phlorhizin, but not by its aglycone, phloretin. The coupled interaction between Na^+ and D-glucose influx across the brush border is not affected either by ouabain or metabolic inhibitors, thus indicating that this process of sugar entry is not an active one (SCHULTZ and CURRAN 1970). Many experiments have proved that D-glucose movement (as well as that of some amino acids) from the cell to the serosal compartment across the basolateral membrane is a passive, carrier-mediated diffusion, since this membrane is practically impermeable to glucose and some amino acids (HAJJAR et al. 1972; BIHLER and CIBULSKY 1973; MURER et al. 1974). An interesting feature of this process is that it is Na^+ independent and specifically inhibited by phloretin (KIMMICH and RANDLES 1975; MURER and HOPFER 1977). Therefore, also in this case, in order to have a net transintestinal solute transport, two different mechanisms located in two distinct regions of the enterocyte must exist. The possibility of an active sugar extrusion at the level of the basolateral membrane has also been postulated (ESPOSITO et al. 1973a).

Also, some small water-soluble nonelectrolytes, known to cross the intestinal barrier by simple diffusion, display different permeability as far as apical and basolateral plasma membranes are concerned. For instance, acetamide can passively diffuse through the intestinal epithelium; however, it has been observed that the brush border possesses a higher permeability to this solute than the basolateral membrane, i.e., the resistance to diffusion is due to a greater extent to the contraluminal membrane than to the brush border (ESPOSITO et al. 1972).

Another phenomenon which can influence the differences of the two opposite membranes of the enterocyte, is the presence of unstirred water layers close to these membranes. These layers, owing to their possibly different size, can differently affect the movement of solutes of different molecular weights in these two regions, external to the cell, thus modifying the concentration profile at the opposite poles of the cells. This topic, however, will be treated in Chap. 21.

It is also possible that a microclimate is present in the two regions close to the opposite membranes. These environments could strongly affect the passage of strong and weak electrolytes because of pH changes observed in these regions (BLAIR et al. 1975; LUCAS 1976; LUCAS and BLAIR 1978). It has been demonstrated, by pH microelectrodes, that the apical region of the enterocyte has a pH lower than that of the lumen. This pH is further lowered by the presence of glucose in the mucosal fluid while aminophylline has a reverse effect. This latter effect is much more evident in the mucosal rather than in the serosal aspect of the absorbing cell. This microclimate is another factor responsible for the polarity of the intestinal epithelial cells. Whatever the mechanism of establishing this microclimate is, it results in an important influence on the movement of electrolytes through the intestinal barrier.

Even if not directly involved in the polarity of the enterocyte, it is interesting to note that a compartment system composed by three spaces seems to account for the transport of weak electrolytes by the intestine. This system is formed by two in-series barriers separating three aqueous compartments: the mucosal, the intermediate, and the serosal compartment. The first barrier is represented by the epithelial layer whereas the second barrier may be associated with a connective tissue layer. The main driving force responsible for transport of weak electrolytes is due to a pH difference between the intermediate compartment (the subepithelial extracellular space) and the other two bulk phases. The vectorial characteristics of such a system are based on the different permeabilities of the two barriers (JACKSON and KUTCHER 1977).

It is known that, at least in in vitro preparations, the intestinal mucosal cells produce large amounts of lactic acid anaerobically (DICKENS and WEIL-MALHERBE 1941; WILSON 1956b; PORTEOUS 1977). The lactate produced appears in higher concentration in the serosal than in the mucosal compartment. This permeability asymmetry has been ascribed to a different chemical composition of the two opposite plasma membranes. As a matter of fact if a lipid-soluble, nonmetabolizable substance such as phenylacetate is used, it has been demonstrated that brush border permeability to this substance is higher than the contraluminal membrane. On the contrary, if water-soluble, nonmetabolizable substances such as urea, thiourea, or lactate are used, they move preferentially towards the serosal compartment across the basolateral membrane. These observations have also been interpreted on the basis of different chemical composition (and consequently of different permeability characteristics) of the two opposite membranes of the enterocyte (LIPPE et al. 1965, 1966).

G. Factors Affecting Membrane Permeability

Many physical, chemical, and physiologic factors can affect the permeability of the intestinal epithelium, but it is difficult to assess which of the two plasma membranes of the enterocyte is influenced. In general, among the physical factors, temperature seems to play an important role. It can, for instance, modify the physical state of membrane lipids. Membrane components are supposed to exist in a liquid crystalline state where the fluidity is greatest in the midplane occupied by the acyl chains and the lowest in the belt region near each polar face. A variation of temperature, especially in the range of the gel-liquid crystalline phase transition, can provoke a great change in microviscosity and in the underlying molecular motions. More generally, an increase in temperature is associated with a decrease of microviscosity (THOMPSON and HUANG 1978). It is also known that dissociation of membrane proteins could be increased by temperature and therefore modifications of permeability can thus result.

Finally, it has been observed that hydrostatic pressure can differentially affect net transintestinal water transport if applied to the mucosal or to the serosal side of the intestinal barrier (WILSON 1956a; SMYTH and TAYLOR 1957; HAKIM and LIFSON 1969). More precisely, if a hydrostatic pressure of 5–10 cmH_2O is applied to the serosal side, net water transport is abolished, or even a net secretion takes place; on the contrary, such pressure when applied to the mucosal side failed to increase the net water flow. This asymmetric effect has been interpreted as follows: even a small serosal pressure can enlarge the intercellular channels and the consequent distension of the spaces may damage the tight junctions between the enterocytes. This interpretation could explain the failure of mucosal pressure to produce an increase of net water absorption (mucosa to serosa) since distension of the intercellular spaces probably does not occur.

Among the chemical factors, the concentration and ionic composition of fluids bathing the enterocytes can strongly and differentially affect the two membranes of the intestinal cell. For instance, H^+ concentration can modify the degree of dissociation of membrane proteins and the acidic microclimate close to the enterocyte. These modifications can influence accordingly the permeability characteristics of the membrane. In addition, the concentrations of several ions present in the physiologic fluids can affect the conditions of hydration of membrane colloids which in turn modify membrane permeability. It has been demonstrated that lowering the Na^+ concentration in the incubating fluid results in a decrease of the noncarrier-mediated transport of passive diffusing substances across the intestinal wall (ESPOSITO et al. 1970, 1972). More specifically, it seems that low concentrations of Na^+ could affect the physicochemical properties mainly of the brush border membrane because of, for instance, the varied $Na^+:Ca^{2+}$ ratio.

As to the physiologic factors affecting membrane permeability, we can distinguish between endogenous factors, such as hormones, and exogenous factors, such as drugs. However, to list all substances that in some way modify membrane permeability is beyond the aim of this chapter. I will briefly mention the influence on permeability of those substances that have been extensively studied and whose mechanisms of action have been mostly elucidated. It is known that cAMP preferentially influences permeability of one of the two membranes of the enterocyte. It has been previously mentioned that the brush border membrane possesses a higher permeability to small uncharged and water-soluble solutes, such as acetamide, than the basolateral membrane. cAMP placed in the serosal side of an in vitro intestinal preparation increases brush border permeability to these solutes (FAELLI et al. 1972; ESPOSITO et al. 1973b). It is also known that substances able to increase the intracellular level of cAMP, modify membrane permeability as well. cAMP seems to inhibit the coupled NaCl influx through the brush border. Theophylline, a phosphodiesterase inhibitor, which is known to raise the intracellular level of cAMP, produces the same effect. Therefore, the mucosa to serosa unidirectional fluxes of NaCl are reduced while the opposite fluxes are not. Under these conditions a net NaCl and water secretion occurs. However, the effect of cAMP on ion movements across the brush border membrane seems to be specific for a coupled Na^+–Cl^- mechanism and not for other Na^+-coupled processes such as, for instance, those coupled with D-glucose and amino acids. In addition it seems that cAMP induces, in the crypt cell, an active anion secretion. Most of these data are reported in two recent reviews (SCHULTZ 1974; FIELD 1978).

Several bacterial enterotoxins cause diarrhea; in this process, the increase of cellular cAMP is in some way involved. Cholera toxin is, among the toxins, the best studied; it is a complex molecule with a molecular weight of approximately 86,000. It has been found that the brush border membrane contains a glycolipid (a monosialoganglioside) which seems to be the principal cell membrane receptor for cholera toxin (HOLMGREN et al. 1973; KING and VAN HEYNINGEN 1973). When the toxin specifically binds to this receptor, a subunit of the toxin penetrates the cell and activates the enzyme adenylate cyclase located in the basolateral membrane of the enterocyte which in turn raises the cell level of cAMP and consequently a modification of membrane permeability occurs.

Also, prostaglandins and vasoactive intestinal peptide (VIP) seem to stimulate intestinal adenylate cyclase and consequently intestinal secretion (PIERCE et al. 1971; SCHWARTZ et al. 1974; FIELD 1974).

Acetylcholine increases, in a transient way, the cAMP level (ISAACS et al. 1976) and catecholamines enhance active intestinal Na^+ and Cl^- absorption (FIELD and MCCOLL 1973). The latter compounds seem to inhibit the sodium–anion efflux process located in the brush border membrane, thus enhancing net Na^+ and Cl^- absorption. For the action of other hormones on the intestinal transport phenomena see LEVIN (1969).

Among the drugs, amphotericin B seems to increase luminal permeability, probably by inducing cation-selective and hydrophilic pores in the plasma membrane so that the main leak pathway seems to be transcellular rather than paracellular. This antibiotic interacts with sterol groups in artificial membranes (Holz and Finkelstein 1970; Andreoli 1974), but the increase in permeability has been demonstrated in many epithelia (Lichtenstein and Leaf 1965; Bentley 1968) including the intestine (Chen et al. 1973). In general, ionophores, substances that facilitate the transfer of ions across lipid membranes, form lipid-soluble complexes with ions which can cross lipid barriers owing to their apolar nature. Therefore, these molecules are able to modify the permeability of plasma membrane to ions.

Several antiinflammatory drugs, such as aspirin (Farris et al. 1976; Powell et al. 1979), indomethacin (Wald et al. 1977), and methylprednisolone (Charney and Donowitz 1976) seem to stimulate intestinal fluid absorption; it appears that the mechanism is a cAMP-independent one. Both indomethacin and aspirin are known to inhibit prostaglandin synthesis (Vane 1971) while methylprednisolone increases Na^+, K^+-ATPase of the enterocyte.

Dimethylsulfoxide (DMSO) is a substance that strongly and reversibly increases D-glucose (Csáky and Ho 1966), but not 3-*O*-methyl-D-glucose absorption. It seems that the increased absorption is based on the formation of an apolar glucose–DMSO complex which is easily membrane soluble and thus bypasses the glucose–carrier system. Bile acids are known to lower the permeability of the intestinal epithelium (Nell et al. 1972); most probably, the site of action of these substances is at the level of tight junctions.

Cytochalasin-B, a fungal metabolite, is able to inhibit the energy-independent facilitated sugar transport in many types of mammalian cells. It has been recently shown that, in the intestine, this molecule specifically affects basolateral transport of sugars which utilize a Na^+-independent transport system (Bihler 1977; Kimmich and Randles 1979).

H. Concluding Remarks

In most animals, vertebrates and invertebrates, the intestinal epithelial cells are organized in such a way as to constitute a barrier separating the internal milieu from the outside. Through this barrier, fluxes of water, electrolytes, and nonelectrolytes continuously occur. We know that this barrier is selective in nature and is able to perform net transport of matter. The epithelial cell must possess mechanisms asymmetrically distributed in its two opposite and in-series plasma membranes in order to achieve this purpose. In addition, it has to display different permeability characteristics as far as the two membranes are concerned. Such differences are mainly due to different chemical composition and biochemical organization of the brush border and basolateral membranes. That is why factors affecting one or both plasma membranes can modify their permeabilities, which in turn affect transport processes. Finally, we must remember that the regions of the intercellular connections – the tight junctions – play an important role in the whole function of the intestine, an organ which is of the utmost importance in the maintenance of the homeostasis of the entire organism.

References

Andreoli TE (1974) The structure and function of amphotericin B-cholesterol pores in lipid bilayer membranes. Kidney Int 4:337–345

Arvanitakis, C, Ruhlen J, Folscroft J, Rhodes JB (1976) Digestion of tripeptides and disaccharides: relationship with brush border hydrolases. Am J Physiol 231:87–92

Benson RL, Sacktor B, Greenawalt JW (1971) Studies on the ultrastructural localization of intestinal disaccharidases. J Cell Biol 48:711–716

Bentley PJ (1968) Action of Amphotericin-B on the toad bladder: evidence for sodium transport along two pathways. J Physiol (Lond) 196:703–711

Bihler I (1977) Sugar transport at the basolateral membrane of the mucosal cell. In: Kramer M, Lauterbach F (eds) Intestinal Permeation. Excerpta Medica, Amsterdam, p 85

Bihler I, Cybulsky R (1973) Sugar transport at the basal and lateral aspect of the small intestinal cell. Biochem Biophys Acta 298:429–437

Blair JA, Lucas ML, Matty AJ (1975) Acidification in the rat proximal jejunum. J Physiol (Lond) 245:333–350

Blok J, Mulder-Stapel AA, Ginsel LA, Daems WT (1980) Binding of cationized ferritin to the cell-coat glycoproteins of human and rat small intestinal absorptive cells. Histochemistry 69:131–135

Bouhours JF (1978) Glicosphingolipids and ceramide distribution in brush border and basolateral membranes of the rat mature intestinal cells. Arch Int Physiol Biochim 86:847–849

Brasitus TA, Schacter D (1980) Lipid dynamics and lipid-protein interactions in rat enterocyte basalateral and microvillus membranes. Biochemistry 19:2763–2769

Bredderman PJ, Wasserman RH (1974) Chemical composition, affinity for calcium and some related properties of the vitamin D dependent calcium-binding protein. Biochemistry 13:1687–1694

Charney AN, Donowitz M (1976) Prevention and reversal of cholera toxin-induced intestinal secretion by methylprednisolone induction of Na^+-K^+-ATPase. J Clin Invest 57:1590–1599

Charney AN, Gots RE, Giannella RA (1974) (Na^+-K^+)-stimulated adenosine triphosphatase in isolated intestinal villus tip and crypt cells. Biochim Biophys Acta 367:265–270

Chen LC, Guerrant RL, Rohde JE, Casper AGT (1973) Effect of amphotericin B on sodium and water movement across normal and cholera toxin-challenged canine jejunum. Gastroenterology 65:252–258

Chez RA, Horger EO, Schultz SG (1969) The effect of ethacrynic acid on sodium transport by isolated rabbit ileum. J Pharmacol Exp Ther 168:1–5

Claude P, Goodenough DA (1973) Fracture faces of zonulae occludentes from "tight" and "leaky" epithelia. J Cell Biol 58:390–400

Cohen MI, Gartner LM, Blumenfeld OO, Arias IM (1969) Gamma glutamyl transpeptidase: measurement and development in guinea pig small intestine. Pediatr Res 3:5–11

Cooper JR, Kent PW (1978) The composition and biosynthesis of the glycoproteins and glycolipids of the rabbit small intestinal brush border. Biochim Biophys Acta 513:364–381

Crane RK (1968) A concept of the digestive-absorptive surface of the small intestine. In: Code F (ed) Alimentary Canal. Digestion. American Physiological Society, Washington DC, p 2535 (Handbook of Physiology, Sect 6, vol V

Crane RK (1977) Digestion and absorption: water-soluble organics. Int Rev Physiol 12:325–365

Crane RK, Miller D, Bihiler I (1961) The restrictions on the possible mechanisms of intestinal active transport. In: Kleinzeller A, Kotyk A (eds) Membrane transport and metabolism, Academic Press, New York, p 439

Csáky TZ, Hara Y (1965) Inhibition of active intestinal sugar transport by digitalis. Am J Physiol 209:467–472

Csáky TZ, Ho PM (1966) Effect of dimethylsulfoxide on the intestinal sugar transport. Proc Soc Exp Biol Med 122:860–865

Csáky TZ, Thale M (1960) Effect of ionic environment on intestinal sugar transport. J Physiol (Lond) 151:59–65

Cuatrecasas P (1973) Gangliosides and membrane receptors for cholera toxin. Biochemistry 12:3558–3566

Dahlqvist A (1964) Intestinal disaccharidases. In: Durand P (ed) Il Pensiero Scientifico, Rome, p 7. Disorders due to intestinal defective carbohydrate digestion and absorption

David JSK, Malathi P, Ganguly J (1966) Role of the intestinal brush border in the absorption of cholesterol in rats. Biochem J 98:662–668

De Jonge HR (1975) The localization of guanylate cyclase in rat small intestinal epithelium. FEBS Lett 53:237–243

De Wolff FA (1973) Drug effects on intestinal epithelium. PhD Thesis, University of Leiden

Diamond JM (1974) Tight and leaky junctions of epithelia: a perspective on kisses in the dark. Fed Proc 33:2220–2224

Diamond JM (1977) The epithelial junction: bridge, gate and fence. Physiologist 20:10–18

Dickens F, Weil-Malherbe H (1941) Metabolism of normal and tumor tissue. 19. The metabolism of intestinal mucous membrane. Biochem J 35:7–15

Diedrich DF (1968) Is phloretin the sugar transport inhibitor in intestine? Arch Biochem Biophys 127:803–812

Donaldson RM Jr (1977) Intestinal transport of cobalamine. In: Kramer M, Lauterbach F (eds) Intestinal Permeation. Excerpta Medica, Amsterdam, p 363

Douglas AP, Kerley R, Isselbacher KJ (1972) Preparation and characterization of the lateral and basal membranes of the rat intestinal epithelial cell. Biochem J 128:1329–1338

Eichholz A (1967) Structural and functional organization of the brush border of intestinal epithelial cells. III. Enzymic activities and chemical composition of various fractions of tris-disrupted brush borders. Biochim Biophys Acta 135:475–482

Esposito G, Faelli A, Capraro V (1970) Effect of sodium on passive permeability of non-electrolytes through the intestinal wall. In: Bolis I, Katchalsky A, Keynes RD, Loewenstein WR, Pethica BA (eds) Permeability and function of biological membranes. North-Holland, Amsterdam, p 74

Esposito G, Faelli A, Capraro V (1972) A sodium-dependent, non-carrier mediated transport of a passive diffusing substance across the intestinal wall. In: Heinz E (ed) Sodium-linked transport of organic solutes, Springer, Berlin Heidelberg New York, p 170

Esposito G, Faelli A, Capraro V (1973a) Sugar and electrolyte absorption in the rat intestine perfused in vivo. Pflugers Arch 340:335–348

Esposito G, Faelli A, Capraro V (1973b) Cyclic AMP and passive permeability of the intestinal brush-border. Atti Accad Naz Lincei 54:813–815

Faelli A, Esposito G, Garotta G, Parotelli R, Capraro V (1972) Relationship between passive permeability and active transport of the isolated rat intestine. Possible involved mechanisms. Atti Accad Naz Lincei 52:102–106

Faelli A, Esposito G, Simonetta M, Capraro V (1976) (Na^+, K^+)-activated ATPase and transintestinal transport in rat intestine incubated in vitro at different temperatures. Atti Accad Naz Lincei 61:518–529

Farris RK, Tapper EJ, Powell DW, Morris SM (1976) Effect of aspirin on normal and cholera toxin-stimulated intestinal electrolyte transport. J Clin Invest 57:916–924

Field M, McColl I (1973) Ion transport in rabbit ileal mucosa. III. Effects of catecholamines. Am J Physiol 225:852–857

Field M (1974) Intestinal secretion. Gastroenterology 66:1063–1084

Field M (1978) Cholera toxin, adenylate cyclase and the process of active secretion in the small intestine: the pathogenesis of diarrhea in cholera. In: Andreoli TE, Hofman JF, Fanestil DD (eds) Physiology of membrane disorders. Plenum Medical Book, New York, pp 877–899

Finean JB, Coleman R, Green WA (1966) Studies of isolated plasma membrane preparations. Ann NY Acad Sci 137:414–420

Fordtran JS, Rector FC Jr, Ewton MF, Soter N, Kinney J (1965) Permeability characteristics of the human small intestine. J Clin Invest 44:1935–1944

Fordtran JS, Rector FC Jr, Carter NW (1968) The mechanisms of sodium absorption in the human small intestine. J Clin Invest 47:884–900

Forstner GG, Wherrett JR (1973) Plasma membrane and mucosal glycosphingolipids in the rat intestine. Biochim Biophys Acta 306:446–459

Forstner GG, Tanaka K, Isselbacher KJ (1968 a) Lipid composition of the isolated rat intestinal microvillus membrane. Biochem J 109:51–59

Forstner GG, Sabesin SM, Isselbacher KJ (1968 b) Rat intestinal microvillus membrane. Purification and biochemical characterization. Biochem J 106:381–390

Frizzell RA, Schultz SG (1972) Ionic conductances of extracellular shunt pathway in rabbit ileum: influence of shunt on transmural sodium transport and electrical potential differences. J Gen Physiol 59:318–346

Frömter E, Diamond JM (1972) Route of passive ion permeation in epithelia. Nature 235:9–13

Fujita M, Matsui H, Nagano K, Nakao M (1971) Asymmetric distrubition of ouabain-sensitive ATPase in rat intestinal mucosa. Biochim Biophys Acta 233:404–408

Fujita M, Ohta H, Kawai K, Matsui H, Nakao M (1972) Differential isolation of microvillous and basolateral plasma membranes from intestinal mucosa: mutually exclusive distribution of digestive enzymes and ouabain-sensitive ATPase. Biochim Biophys Acta 274:336–347

Fujita M, Kawai K, Asano S, Nakao M (1973) Protein components of two different regions of an intestinal epithelial cell membrane. Regional singularities. Biochim Biophys Acta 307:141–151

Gebauer G (1969) Quantitative Bestimmungen am Darmkanal der weißen Ratte. PhD Dissertation University of Homburg Saar

Ghijsen WEJM, van OS CH (1979) Ca-stimulated ATPase in brush border and basolateral membranes of rat duodenum with high affinity sites for Ca ions. Nature 279:802–803

Glick MC (1976) Isolation of surface membranes from mammalian cells. In: Jamieson GA, Robinson DM (eds) Mammalian cell membranes, Vol II. Butterworths, London pp 45–77

Grantham JJ, Ganote CE, Burg MB, Orloff J (1969) Paths of transtubular water flow in isolated renal collecting tubules. J Cell Biol 41:562–576

Greenberger NJ, Balcerzak SP, Ackerman GA (1969) Iron uptake by isolated intestinal brush borders: changes induced by alterations in iron stores. J Lab Clin Med 73:711–721

Hajjar JJ, Khuri RN, Curran PF (1972) Alanine efflux across the serosal border of turtle intestine. J Gen Physiol 60:720–734

Hakim AA, Lifson N (1969) Effects of pressure on water and solute transport by dog intestinal mucosa in vitro. Am J Physiol 216:276–284

Hauser H, Howell K, Dawson RMC, Bowyer DE (1980) Rabbit small intestinal brush border membrane. Preparation and lipid composition. Biochim Biophys Acta 602:567–577

Höber R, Höber J (1937) Experiments on the absorption of organic solutes in the small intestine of rats. J Cell Comp Physiol 10:401–422

Holmes R, Lobley RW (1970) The localization of enterokinase to the brush border membrane of the guinea-pig small intestine. J Physiol (Lond) 211:50P–51P

Holmgren J, Lönnroth J, Svennerholm L (1973) Tissue receptor for cholera exotoxin. Postulated structure from studies with G_{ml} ganglioside and related glycolipids. Infect Immun 8:208–214

Holmgren J, Lönnroth J, Mannson JE, Svennerholm L (1975) Interaction of cholera toxin and membrane G_{MI} ganglioside of small intestine. Proc Natl Acad Sci USA 72:2520–2524

Holt JH, Miller D (1962) The localization of phosphomonoesterase and aminopeptidase in brush borders isolated from intestinal epithelial cells. Biochim Biophys Acta 58:239–243

Holz R, Finkelstein A (1970) The water and non electrolyte permeability induced in thin lipid membranes by the polyene antibiotics nystatin and amphotericin B. J Gen Physiol 56:125–145

Huebers H, Rummel W (1977) Iron binding proteins: mediators in iron absorption. In: Kramer M, Lauterbach F (eds) Intestinal permeation. Excerpta Medica, Amsterdam, p 377

Humphreys MH, Chou LYN (1979) Anion-stimulated ATPase activity of brush-border from rat small intestine. Am J Physiol 236:E70–E76

Humphreys MH, Kaysen GA, Chou LY, Watson JB (1980) Anion-stimulated phosphohydrolase activity of intestinal alkaline phosphatase. Am J Physiol 238:G3–G9

Isaacs PET, Corbett CL, Riley AK, Hawker PC, Turnberg LA (1976) In vitro behaviour of human intestinal mucosa: the influence of acetyl choline on ion transport. J Clin Invest 58:535–542

Ito S (1965) The enteric surface coat on cat intestinal microvilli. J Cell Biol 27:475–491

Ito S (1969) Structure and function of the glycoacolix Fed Proc 28:12–25

Jackson MJ, Kutcher LM (1977) The three-compartment system for transport of weak electrolytes in the small intestine. In: Kramer M, Lauterbach F (eds) Intestinal Permeation. Excerpta Medica, Amsterdam, p 65

Jackson RJ, Stewart HB, Sachs G (1977) Isolation and purification of normal and malignant colonic plasma membranes. Cancer 40:2487–2496

Johnson CF (1969) Hamster intestinal brush-border surface particles and their function. Fed Proc 28:26–29

Jonas A, Flanagan PR, Forstner GG (1977) Pathogenesis of mucosal injury the blind loops syndrome. Brush border enzyme activity and glycoprotein degradation. J Clin Invest 60:1321–1330

Kawai K, Fujita M, Nakao M (1974) Lipid components of two different regions of an intestinal epithelial cell membrane of mouse. Biochim Biophys Acta 369:222–233

Kimmich GA, Randles J (1975) A Na^+-independent, phloretin sensitive monosaccharide transport system in isolated intestinal epithelial cells. J Membrane Biol 23:57–76

Kimmich GA, Randles J (1979) Energetics of sugar transport by isolated intestinal epithelial cells: effects of cytochalasin B. Am J Physiol 237:C56–C63

King CA, Van Heyningen WE (1973) Deactivation of cholera toxin by a sialidase-resistant monosialoganglioside. J Infect Dis 127:639–647

Kowarsky S, Blair-Stanek CS, Schachter D (1974) Active transport of zinc and identification of zinc binding protein in rat jejunal mucosa. Am J Physiol 226:401–407

Leese HJ, Semenza G (1973) On the identity between the small intestinal enzymes phlorizin hydrolase and glycosylceramidase. J Biol Chem 248:8170–8173

Leslie GI, Rowe PB (1972) Folate binding by the brush border membrane proteins of small intestinal epithelial cells. Biochemistry 11:1696–1703

Levin RJ (1969) The effects of hormones on the absorptive, metabolic and digestive functions of the small intestine. J Endocrinol 45:315–348

Levitt DG, Hakim AA, Lifson N (1969) Evaluation of components of transport of sugars by dog jejunum in vivo. Am J Physiol 217:777–783

Lichtenstein NS, Leaf A (1965) Effect of amphotericin B on the permeability of toad bladder. J Clin Invest 44:1328–1342

Lindemann B, Solomon AK (1962) Permeability of luminal surface of intestinal mucosal cells. J Gen Physiol 45:801–810

Lippe C, Bianchi A, Cremaschi D, Capraro V (1965) Different types of asymmetric distribution of hydrosoluble and liposoluble substances at the two sides of a mucosal intestinal preparation. Arch Int Physiol Biochim 73:43–54

Lippe C, Cremaschi D, Capraro V (1966) Asymmetric distribution of lactic acid in epithelial tissues. Rev Roum Biol Zool 11:129–135

Loewenstein WR (1978) Cell-to-cell communication: permeability, formation, genetics and functions of the cell-cell membrane channel. In: Andreoli TE, Hoffman JF, Fanestil DD (eds) Physiology of membrane disorders. Plenum Medical Book Co, New York, p 335

Loewenstein WR (1981) Junctional intercellular communication: the cell-to-cell membrane channel. Physiol Rev 61:829–913

Loewenstein WR, Socolar SJ, Higashino S, Kanno Y, Davidson N (1965) Intercellular communication: renal, urinary bladder, sensory and salivary gland cells. Science 149:295–298

Lojda Z (1965) Some remarks concerning the histochemical detection of disaccharides and glucosidases. Histochemie 5:339–345

Louvard D, Maroux S, Baratti J, Desnuelle P, Mutaftschiev S (1973) On the preparation and some properties of closed membrane vesicles from hog duodenal and jejunal brush border. Biochim Biophys Acta 291:747–763

Lucas ML (1976) The association between acidification and electrogenic events in the rat proximal jejunum. J Physiol (Lond) 257:645–662

Lucas ML, Blair JA (1978) The magnitude and distribution of the acid microclimate in proximal jejunum and its relation to luminal acidification. Proc R Soc Lond (Biol) 200:27–41

Machen TE, Erlij D, Wooding FBP (1972) Permeable junctional complexes: The movement of lanthanum across rabbit gallbladder and intestine. J Cell Biol 54:302–312

Maestracci D, Schmitz J, Preiser H, Crane RK (1973) Proteins and glycoproteins of the human intestinal brush border membrane. Biochim Biophys Acta 323:113–124

Malathi P (1967) Localization of cholesteryl and retinyl ester hydrolases in the microvillous membrane of brush-borders isolated from intestinal epithelial cells. Gastroenterology 52:1106 (abstract)

Malathi P, Crane RK (1968) Spatial relationship between intestinal disaccharides and the active transport system for sugars. Biochim Biophys Acta 163:275–277

Malathi P, Crane RK (1969) Phlorizin hydrolase: a β-glucosidase of hamster intestinal brush-border membrane. Biochim Biophys Acta 173:245–256

Mathan VI, Babior BM, Donaldson RM Jr (1974) Kinetics of the attachment of intrinsic factor bound cobamides to ileal receptors. J Clin Invest 54:598–608

Max EE, Goodman DBP, Rasmussen H (1978) Purification and characterization of chick intestine brush border membrane. Effects of 1, 25 (OH) vitamin D_3 treatment. Biochim Biophys Acta 511:224–239

McHardy GJR, Parsons DS (1957) The absorption of water and salts from the small intestine of the rat. Q J Exp Physiol 42:33–48

McKibbin JM (1969) The composition of the glycolipids in dog intestine. Biochemistry 8:679–685

Miller D, Crane RK (1961) The digestive function of the epithelium of the small intestine. II. Localization of disaccharide hydrolysis in the isolated brush border portion of intestinal epithelial cells. Biochim Biophys Acta 52:293–298

Millington PF, Finean JB (1963) Studies on the structural integrity of the brush border of rat intestinal epithelial cells. In: Prazer AC (ed) Biochemical problems of lipids. Elsevier Publishing Co, Amsterdam, p 116

Mircheff AK, Wright EM (1976) Analytical isolation of plasma membranes of intestinal epithelial cells: identification of Na, K-ATPase rich membranes and the distribution of enzyme activities. J Membr Biol 28:309–333

Mooseker MS (1976) Brush border motility. Microvillar contraction in tryton-treated brush borders isolated from intestinal epithelium. J Cell Biol 71:417–433

Murer H. Hopfer U (1977) The functional polarity of the intestinal epithelial cell; studies with isolated plasma membrane vesicles. In: Kramer M, Lauterbach F (eds) Intestinal Permeation. Excerpta Medica, Amsterdam, p 294

Murer H, Hopfer U, Kinne-Saffran E, Kinne R (1974) Glucose transport in isolated brush-border and basal-lateral plasma membrane vesicles from intestinal epithelial cells. Biochim Biphys Acta 345:170–179

Murer H, Ammann E, Biber J, Hopfer U (1976a) The surface membrane of the small inestinal epithelial cell. I. Localization of adenyl cyclase. Biochim Biphys Acta 433:509–519

Murer H, Hopfer U, Kinne R (1976b) Sodium/proton antiport in brush border membrane vesicles isolated from rat small intestine and rat kidney. Biochem J 154:597–604

Nell G, Forth W, Rummel W, Wanitschke R (1972) Abolition of the apparent Na^+ impermeability of the colon mucosa by deoxycholate. In: Back P, Gerok W (eds) Proceedings of the 2nd Bile Salt Meeting. Freiburg/Brg 1972. Schattauer, Stuttgart, p 263

Nellans HL, Frizzell RA, Schultze SG (1973) Coupled sodium-chloride influx across the brush-border of rabbit ileum. Am J Physiol 225:467–475

Nordstrom C, Dahlqvist A (1970) The cellular localization of enterokinase. Biochim Biophys Acta 198:621–622

O'Brien JS (1967) Cell membranes – Composition: structure: function. J Theor Biol 15:307–324

Olsen WA, Korsmo H (1977) The intestinal brush border membrane in diabetes. Studies of sucrase-isomaltase metabolism in rats with streptozotocin diabetes. J Clin Invest 60:181–188

Parkinson DK, Ebel H, Dibona DR, Sharp GWG (1972) Localization of the action of cholera toxin on adenylate cyclase in mucosal epithelial cells of rabbit intestine. J Clin Invest 51:2292–2298

Peters TJ (1970) The subcellular localization of di- and tripeptide hydrolase activity in guinea pig small intestine. Biochem J 120:195–203

Pierce NF, Carpenter CHCJ, Elliot HL, Greenough WB (1971) Effect of prostaglandins, theophyllin and cholera exotoxin upon transmucosal water and electrolyte movement in the canine jejunum. Gastroenterology 60:22–21

Porteous JW (1977) The regulation of glucose metabolism during its oxigen-dependent translocation through the columnar absorptive cells of rat jejunum. In: Kramer M, Lauterbach F (eds) Intestinal Permeation. Excerpta Medica, Amsterdam, p 240

Powell DW, Tapper EJ, Morris SM (1979) Aspirin-stimulated intestinal electrolyte transport in rabbit ileum in vitro. Gastroenterology 76:1429–1437

Quigley JP, Gotterer GS (1969) Distribution of (Na^+–K^+)-stimulated ATPase activity in rat intestinal mucosa. Biochim Biophys Acta 173:456–468

Quill H, Weiser MM (1975) Adenylate and guanylate cyclase activities and cellular differentiation in rat small intestine. Gastroenterology 69:470–478

Quirk SJ, Robinson GB (1972) Isolation and characterization of rabbit kidney brush borders. Biochem J 128:1319–1328

Rhodes JB, Eichholz A, Crane RK (1967) Studies on the organization of the brush border in intestinal epithelial cells. IV. Aminopeptidase activity in microvillus membranes of hamster intestinal brush borders. Biochim Biophys Acta 135:959–965

Riklis E, Quastel JH (1958) Effects of cations on sugar absorption by isolated surviving guinea pig intestine. Can J Biochem Physiol 36:347–362

Robertson JD (1964) Unit membranes: a review with recent new studies of experimental alterations and a new subunit structure in synaptic membranes. In: Locke M (ed) Cellular membranes in development. Academic, New York, p 1

Robinson GB (1975) The isolation and composition of membranes. In: Parsons DS (ed) Biological membranes. Clarendon Oxford, p 8

Rose RC, Schultz SG (1971) Studies on the electrical potential profile across ileum: effects of sugars and amino acids on transmural and transmucosal electrical potential differences. J Gen Physiol 57:639–663

Rothman JE, Lenard J (1977) Membrane asymmetry. Science 195:743–753

Sacktor B (1968) Trehalase and the transport of glucose in the mammalian kidney and intestine. Proc Natl Acad Sci USA 60:1007–1014

Sacktor B (1977) Transport in membrane vesciles isolated from the mammalian kidney and intestine. In: Sanadi R (ed) Current topics in bioenergetics, vol VI. Academic, New York, p 39

Sasajima K, Kawachi T, Sato S, Sugimura T (1975) Purification and properties of α, α-trehalase from the mucosa of rat small intestine. Biochim Biphys Acta 403:139–146

Schmitz J, Presider H, Maestracci D, Crane RK, Troesch V, Hadorn B (1974) Subcellular localization of enterokinase in human small intestine. Biochim Biophys Acta 343:435–439

Schultz SG (1973) Shunt pathway, sodium transport and the electrical potential profile across rabbit ileum. In: Ussing HH, Thron NA (eds) Transport in epithelia. Munksgaard, Copenhagen, p 281

Schultz SG (1974) Ion transport by mammalian small intestine. Ann Rev Physiol 35:51–91

Schultz SG (1977) The role of paracellular pathways in isotonic fluid transport. Yale J Biol Med 50:99–113

Schultz SG (1978) The double-membrane model for transepithelial ion transport: are homocellular and transcellular ion transport related? In: Solomon AK, Karnowsky M (eds) Molecular specialization and asymmetry in membrane function, Harvard University Press, Cambridge, p 253

Schultz SG, Curran PF (1970) Coupled transport of sodium and organic solutes. Physiol Rev 50:637–718

Schultz SG, Zahlusky R (1964) Ion transport in isolated rabbit ileum. II. The interaction between active sodium and active sugar transport. J Gen Physiol 47:1043–1059

Schwartz CJ, Kimberg DV, Sheerin HE, Field M, Said SI (1974) Vasoactive intestinal peptide stimulation of adenylate cyclase and active electrolyte secretion in intestinal mucosa. J Clin Invest 54:536–544

Seetharam B, Yeh KY, Moog F, Alpers DH (1977) Development of intestinal brush border membrane proteins in the rat. Biochim Biophys Acta 470:424–436

Semenza G (1976) Small intestinal disaccharidases: their properties and role as sugar translocators across natural and artificial membranes. In: Martonosi A (ed) The enzymes of biological membranes, vol 3. Membrane transport. Plenum, New York, p 349

Sigrist-Nelson K, Sigrist H, Bercovici T, Gitler C (1977) Intrinsic proteins of the intestinal microvillus membrane iodonaphtylazide labeling studies. Biochim Biophys Acta 468:163–176

Singer SJ (1977) The proteins of membranes. J Colloid Interface Sci 58:452–458

Sjöstrand FS (1963) The fine structure of the columnar epithelium of the mouse intestine with special reference to fat absorption. In: Frazer AC (ed) Biochemical problems of lipids. Elsevier, Amsterdam, p 91

Smyth DH, Taylor CB (1957) Transfer of water and solutes by an in vitro intestinal preparation. J Physiol (Lond) 136:632–648

Smyth DH, Wright EM (1966) Streaming potentials in the rat small intestine. J Physiol (Lond) 182:591–602

Staehelin LA, Hull BE (1978) Junctions between living cells. Sci Am 238(5):141–152

Starita-Geribaldi M, Fehlmann M, Sudaka P (1977)Etudes des protéines de la bordure en brosse des entérocytes du chien. Arch Int Physiol Biochim 85:245–254

Steck TL, Wallach DFH (1970) The isolation of plasma membranes. Methods Cancer Res 5:93–153

Stirling CE (1972) Radioautographic localization of sodium pump sites in rabbit intestine. J Cell Biol 53:704–714

Takesue Y, Sato R (1968) Biochemical and morphological characterization of microvilli isolated from intestinal mucosal cells. J Biochem 64:885–893

Thompson TE, Huang C (1978) Dynamics of lipids in biomembranes. In: Andreoli TE, Hoffman JF, Fanestil DD (eds) Physiology of membrane disorders. Plenum, New York, p 27

Toskes PP, Deren JJ (1973) Vitamin B_{12} absorption and malabsorption. Gastroenterology 65:662–683

Tsuboi KK, Schwartz SM, Burrill PH, Kwong LK, Sunshine P (1979) Sugar hydrolases of the infant rat intestine and their arrangement on the brush border membrane. Biochim Biophys Acta 554:234–248

Turnberg LA, Bieberdorf FA, Morawsky SG, Fordtran JS (1970) Interrelationship of chloride, bicarbonate, sodium and hydrogen transport in the human ileum. J Clin Invest 49:557–567

Ugolev AM (1965) Membrane (contact) digestion. Physiol Rev 45:555–595

Ugolev AM (1968) Physiology and pathology of membrane digestion. Plenum, New York

Ugolev AM, De Laey P, Iezuitova NN (1977) Adsorption of enzymes by cell membrane structures (on the example of enterocytes) under normal and pathological conditions. In: Enzymology and its clinical use. Acta Univ Carol Med 12:5–19

Ugolev AM, Smirnova LF, Iezuitova NN, Timofeeva NM, Mityushova NM, Egorova VU, Parshkov EM (1979) Distribution of some adsorbed and intrinsic enzymes between the mucosal cells of the rat small intestine and the apical glycocalyx separated from them. FEBS Lett 104:35–38

Vane JR (1971) Aspirin. Possible action through inhibition of synthesis of prostaglandines. Nature 231:232–234

Wald A, Gotterer GS, Rajendra GR, Turjman NA, Hendrix TR (1977) Effect of Indomethacin on cholera-induced fluid movement, unidirectional sodium fluxes, and intestinal cAMP. Gastroenterology 72:106–110

Walker WA, Isselbacher KJ (1974) Uptake and transport of macromolecules in the intestine. Possible role in clinical disorders. Gastroenterology 67:531–550

Walker WA, Field M, Isselbacher KJ (1974) Specific binding of cholera toxin to isolated intestinal microvillus membranes. Proc Natl Acad Sci USA 71:320–324

Wasserman RH, Taylor AN, Kallfelz FA (1966) Vitamin D and transfer of plasma calcium to intestinal lumen in chiks and rats. Am J Physiol 211:419–423

Weiser MM, Neumeier MM, Quaroni A, Kirsch K (1978) Synthesis of plasmalemmal glycoproteins in intestinal epithelial cells. Separation of Golgi membranes from villus and crypt cell surface membranes; glycosyltransferase activity of surface membrane. J Cell Biol 77:722–734

Widdas WF (1963) Permeability. In: Creese R (ed) Recent advances in physiology, Churchill, London, p 1

Wilson TH (1956a) A modified method for study of intestinal absorption in vitro. J Appl Physiol 9:137–140

Wilson TH (1956b) The role of lactic acid production in glucose absorption from the intestine. J Biol Chem 222:751–763

Wojnarowska F, Gray GM (1975) Intestinal surface peptide hydrolases: identification and characterization of three enzymes from rat brush border. Biochim Biophys Acta 403:147–160

CHAPTER 10

Electrical Phenomena and Ion Transport in the Small Intestine

W. McD. Armstrong and J. F. Garcia-Diaz

A. Introduction

The absorption of water, electrolytes, and nutrient substances by the small intestine has been a central concern of gastrointestinal physiology for many years. Beginning as early as the mid-seventeenth century, there is a more or less continuous history of experimental investigation in this field (Parsons 1968). In this area, as in many other areas of experimental science, the first half of this century witnessed a tremendous intensification of effort. This increase in the number of investigations designed to uncover the fundamental mechanisms of salt and water transport resulted in a concomitant proliferation of published results and the elaboration of a variety of ingenious hypotheses (see, e.g., Höber 1946; Schultz and Curran 1968). This activity has increased, in volume and intensity, until the present time and seems likely (given the survival of a reasonably supportive socioeconomic milieu) to continue increasing for many years to come. Despite all this, it is a salutory thought that, as pointed out by Schultz and Curran (1968), modern theories of intestinal absorption can still be described, in general terms, by Heidenhain's (1894) hypothesis. That is, that the absorption process results from a combination of physicochemical (osmotic) driving forces and the intrinsic driving force (*Triebkraft*) generated by the absorptive cells. Thanks, in large part, to the development of much more sophisticated investigative methods, the specific driving forces have been better defined, the transport pathways have been more clearly identified, and progress has been made towards unraveling the molecular mechanisms of intestinal absorption. Nevertheless, in terms of fundamental concepts, the notion that net transport across the intestine involves the interplay of two kinds of flows, passive flows (that is, flow down a gradient of chemical or electrochemical potential) and active flows (i.e., flows that, because of coupling to metabolism or other extrinsic energy sources, can be driven against the appropriate thermodynamic gradient) remains paramount.

In retrospect, the late 1950s and early 1960s appear as a kind of watershed in the history of intestinal transport. During that time a number of noteworthy developments, theoretical and experimental, began. Many of these were sparked by the reemergence, following a period of relative eclipse, of in vitro methods for the study of intestinal absorption and secretion. The development and refinement of new ideas and techniques have made the last two decades or so particularly exciting and significant in terms of the physiology of intestinal function. Prominent among these developments are the following:

1. The discovery of specific coupling between the transepithelial transport, by the small intestine, of Na^+ and that of organic nonelectrolytes such as sugars and amino acids (Csáky 1961, 1963, 1968; Crane 1962, 1965, 1977).
2. The demonstration of coupled ionic transport in the small intestine (Quay and Armstrong 1969; Nellans et al. 1973; Frizzell et al. 1979)
3. The emergence of the idea that fluid and electrolyte transport in the small intestine occurs via two separate pathways, a transcellular pathway and an extracellular or paracellular "shunt" pathway (Clarkson 1967); White and Armstrong 1971; Frizzell and Schultz 1972), and that the paracellular pathway modulates, in important respects, the bioelectric and transporting properties of this organ.
4. The realization that transcellular Na^+ transport plays a unique role in the energetics of intestinal transfer (Csáky 1968; Armstrong et al. 1979 b).

On the experimental side, the "coming of age" of intestinal electrophysiology contributed greatly to our understanding of the specific properties of the cellular and paracellular transport pathways and to the definition of the driving forces for individual ions across the apical and basolateral membranes of the intestinal absorptive cell. In addition to the study of the transepithelial electrical characteristics of isolated sheets of intestinal tissue, this approach now includes the measurement, with appropriate microelectrodes, of apical cell membrane potentials and intracellular ionic activities (Armstrong 1977). The development of methods for preparing viable suspensions of isolated enterocytes (Kimmich 1970) and for isolating apical and basolateral cell membrane vesicles that retain all or most of the transport properties of their parent membranes (Kessler et al. 1978; Wright et al. 1979) has greatly clarified and extended our knowledge of specific transport mechanisms and of the sites where these occur. In this respect, the study of radiotracer fluxes in vesicular systems has been particularly useful. In addition to their value for studying the kinetics of intestinal transport, membrane vesicles have helped to clarify the electrophysiologic correlates of membrane transport processes. For example, exposure of these vesicles to agents that either hyperpolarize or depolarize their membranes (e.g., valinomycin, amphotericin B), has provided information about the role of the membrane potential in the Na^+-dependent transport of organic solutes such as hexose sugars and neutral amino acids across the brush border membrane of the absorptive cell (Kinne and Mürer 1976). Because vesicular membrane potentials are not accessible to measurement with microelectrodes, much of this electrophysiologic information has been, so far, inferential rather than direct. The rapidly increasing use of chemical and optical probes for measuring membrane potentials (Waggoner 1979; Leader 1981) will, hopefully, permit quantitative information about the electrical behavior of membrane vesicles to be routinely obtained in the near future. To date, very little appears to have been done in the way of direct electrophysiologic studies with isolated enterocytes. This is an area of investigation that deserves systematic study. Finally, one may note that similar and concurrent developments with other epithelia have, by highlighting the commonality of epithelial transport mechanisms in different organ systems (e.g., the intestine, the kidney, and the gallbladder), exerted an important synergistic effect on the study of intestinal transport and led to the recognition of "epitheliology" as a distinct subdiscipline in physiology. In this regard, the emergence of methods for culturing cells in the form of flat sheets (CEREJIDO et al. 1981) holds great promise for future investigations with the intestine and other epithelial systems.

This chapter will attempt to summarize the major advances that resulted from these new ideas and techniques. It will focus particularly on the role of electrical forces in intestinal transport. Because of the very large number of publications in this area during recent years, no attempt will be made at encyclopedic coverage of the pertinent literature. Furthermore, because of space limitations, the present account will deal mainly with in vitro studies. Fortunately, the role of electrical potentials in the intestinal transport of various solutes, and the electrical phenomena associated with specific transport processes have been discussed in a number of reviews during the last decade or so (e.g., SCHULTZ and CURRAN 1970; SCHULTZ et al. 1974; SCHULTZ 1979, 1981; KIMMICH 1973, 1981 b; AMSTRONG 1975, 1976; ARMSTRONG et al. 1979). The reader is referred to these for a more comprehensive listing of pertinent publications than is feasible within the limitations of the present survey. Excellent summaries of the more "classical" studies that led to recent developments in the general area of the present discussion will be found in the reviews by CRANE (1968) and by SCHULTZ and CURRAN (1968).

Finally, it seems appropiate at this point to sound a note of caution. In terms of its cellular make up, the mucosa of the small intestine, in mammals at least, is a complex epithelium (TRIER and MADARA 1981). In addition to absorptive cells there are, in the villous region, goblet cells, though these are relatively few in number. In the crypt, which is the site of cell proliferation, there are, in addition to goblet cells, Paneth cells, enterochromaffin cells, and undifferentiated cells. There is strong evidence that all four of these cell types have secretory functions. During the "classical" phase of gastrointestinal physiology, when the absorptive function of the small intestive was of paramount interest, and when the techniques available permitted only the overall assessment of transport by large numbers of cells, the specific contributions of individual cell types to intestinal transport as a whole were not amenable to experimental definition. As modern studies focus more and more on the behavior of single cells and of isolated cell membranes, and as the specific sites of individual transport processes are progressively identified, the cellular heterogeneity of the intestinal mucosa assumes an increasing critical importance. For example, as discussed more fully in Sect. F, it has been suggested that the net cAMP-induced secretion of Cl^- in vitro preparation of mammalian small intestine is mediated by crypt cells rather than by the absorptive cells (FRIZZELL et al. 1979). At the present time this hypothesis rests largely on indirect evidence. Again, in *Amphiuma* intestine, which appears to lack true crypts, significant functional differences have been identified in villous and intervillous regions (GUNTER-SMITH and WHITE 1979 a). These examples underline the need, in future studies, for increasingly critical differentiation between the specific functional roles, in intact intestinal tissue, of different cell types.

B. Transepithelial Electrical Parameters and Ionic Fluxes in the Small Intestine

In this section, the application of the classical Ussing chamber technique (Ussing and Zerahn 1951) to the measurement of transepithelial electrical parameters and transepithelial ionic fluxes in the small intestine will be discussed. In its original form, and as it is still frequently used, this technique permits experimental measurements and interventions to be made only in the external media that bathe the intestinal or other epithelial preparation and requires that events within the epithelial cell layer be, to a large extent, inferred rather than directly observed. For this reason it is often referred to as a "black box" approach. However, despite the somewhat deprecatory flavor of this appellation, it should be emphasized that the technique has played a crucial role in the development of modern epithelial electrophysiology and is still the method of choice for measuring, under precisely controlled conditions, the transepithelial fluxes of ions and other solutes. In modified form, it is an essential component of contemporary systems for microelectrode studies on intact sheets of epithelial tissue, and has been adapted to measure the influx (J^{j}_{mc}) of various solutes from the mucosal bathing solution to the cell interior[1]. It seems appropriate, therefore, to give an account of the Ussing chamber technique as it applies to studies with the small intestine.

In this technique, the tissue is mounted vertically as a flat sheet between the two sides of a divided chamber. Usually, the solutions in each half-chamber are identical, except when relatively small amounts of transported solutes, e.g., sugars or amino acids, or other agents such as metabolic inhibitors, secretagogues, etc., are added to either the mucosal or the serosal solution only. A simple chamber of this type, designed by Quay and Armstrong (1969) for studies with amphibian small intestine, is shown schematically in Fig. 1. Modified Ussing chambers designed for microelectrode studies and for mucosal influx measurement are illustrated in Figs. 2 and 3, respectively. As in Fig. 1, the chamber shown in Fig. 3 was specifically designed for studies with amphibian (bullfrog) small intestine (White and Armstrong 1971). However, aside from arrangements to maintain the temperature of the system at levels different from the ambient temperature, chambers designed for studies with mammalian intestine are essentially similar to these.

It is apparent from Fig. 1 that the volume of solution in each half-chamber can easily be adjusted so that there is no hydrostatic pressure difference across the intestinal sheet. In addition to appropriate arrangements for oxygenating and circulating the bathing solutions in both half-chambers, provision is made for the insertion of salt bridges that make contact with external electrodes. Two of these bridges are positioned as close as possible to the tissue, without actually touching it, and serve to monitor the transepithelial potential, V_T. For this purpose they

1 It is interesting that, although the Ussing chamber was not applied to the study of the small intestine until the late 1950s (Ussing and Andersen 1955), and did not come into general use for this purpose until several years later, a divided chamber of essentially similar design to that of Ussing (Ussing and Zerahn 1951) was applied by Reid to the study of intestinal fluid absorption in vitro well before the turn of the century (Reid 1892; see also Parsons 1968).

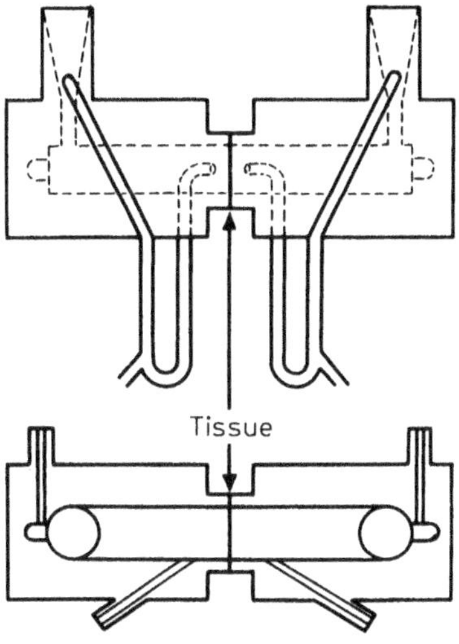

Fig. 1. Apparatus for measuring transepithelial potential, short-circuit current, and transepithelial fluxes in the small intestine in vitro

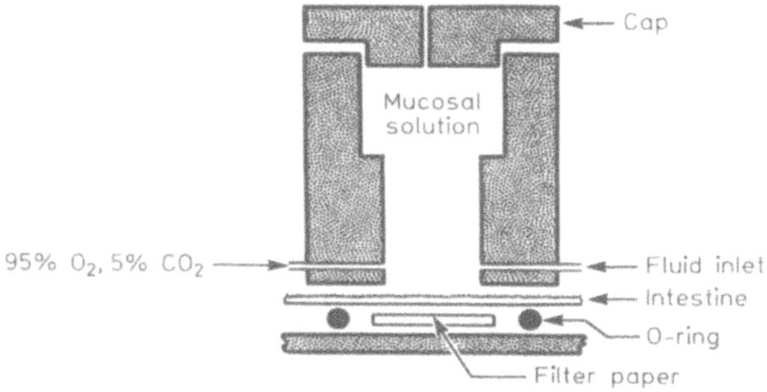

Fig. 2. Experimental arrangement for measuring mucosal influxes in the isolated small intestine

are connected through reversible electrodes (e.g., calomel or Ag/AgCl electrodes) to a suitable voltage recording device. The other two bridges are connected, through appropriate elctrodes, to a current source from which a current of known strength can be passed across the tissue, either in brief pulses or continuously. Since all known physicochemical driving forces across the epithelial sheet can be precisely controlled, it is clear that, with this technique, unidirectional mucosal to serosal and serosal to mucosal fluxes J^j_{ms}, J^j_{sm} for any solute *j*, and their difference, the net flux J^j_{net} can be obtained, under known conditions, by adding a radiolabeled form of *j* to each half-chamber in turn and measuring its rate of appearance in the contralateral fluid compartment.

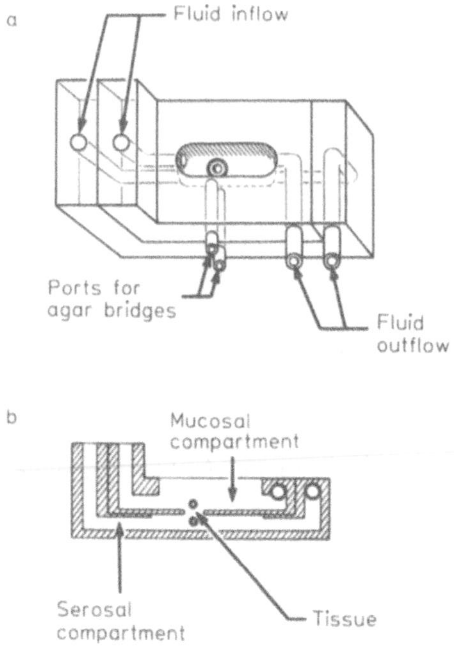

Fig. 3 a, b. A modified Ussing chamber apparatus that permits the measurement of apical membrane potentials and intracellular ionic activities in the small intestine and other epithelia. **a** top view; **b** side view

A number of studies (e.g., Schultz and Zalusky 1964a; Quay and Armstrong 1969) in which V_T was measured as a function of the applied current I_T across the intestine have shown that, at least over a range of V_T values from $+50$ to -50 mV or so, the small intestine behaves as a simple ohmic resistor. Thus, by passing a current pulse of known strength across the tissue and measuring the resulting change in V_T, transepithelial resistance R_T or its reciprocal, transepithelial conductance G_T is readily obtained.

Two parameters are of particular interest from an electrophysiologic viewpoint. One is the open-circuit potential V_{TO}, that is, the spontaneous value of V_T in the absence of an applied current. The demonstration, without the uncertainties inherent in contemporaneous in vivo recordings, that the in vitro small intestine, when bathed on both sides by identical Ringer's solutions, maintains a finite steady state V_{TO}, and that this potential is generated by the epithelial cell layer, and not by underlying structures such as the external smooth muscle layers (Ussing and Andersen 1955; Cooperstein and Hogben 1959), focused attention on the role of electrical forces in the transport of ions by this tissue.

The second parameter that is of special interest from the standpoint of epithelial transport and electrophysiology is the short-circuit current, I_{sc}. This is the external current required to bring V_{TO} to zero when the tissue is mounted between identical bathing solutions and all known net physicochemical driving forces across it are eliminated. Under these conditions, the transepithelial electrochemical potential difference for each ionic species in the bathing media is abolished. Therefore, I_{sc} corresponds to the algebraic sum of net fluxes of those ions that are actively transported, i.e.,

$$I_{sc} = \sum_{j=1}^{j=n} z_j F J^j_{net} . \quad (B.1)$$

where z_j is the valence of the ion $_j$ and F the Faraday's constant. By measuring J^j_{ms} and J^j_{sm} for individual ions under short-circuit conditions, I_{sc} can be dissected into its component parts.

In applying the short-circuit technique to the small intestine, some important modifications of the original technique of USSING and ZERAHN (1951) are necessary. First, because the small intestine is a relatively highly conducting epithelium, and because the salt bridges leading to the reversible electrodes used to monitor V_T must terminate at a finite, though small distance from the surface of the tissue, it is necessary, during short-circuiting to compensate for the drop in electrical potential (*IR* drop) due to current flow across the layers of solution between the ends of the bridges and the tissue surface. Manual (CLARKSON and TOOLE 1964) and automatic (ROTHE et al. 1969) methods for accomplishing this *IR* compensation have been described. Clearly, with chambers similar to that shown in Fig. 1, an *IR* drop will occur, regardless of the specific epithelial tissue under investigation. With highly resistive tissues such as frog skin and toad urinary bladder (Table 1), one can easily show that, unless the bathing solutions have extremely low electrolyte concentrations, the *IR* drop is negligible. With tissue like the small intestine, the resistance of the fluid layers outside the tissue will, in virtually all circumstances, account for a significant fraction of the total resistance between the end of the potential-sensing bridges (ROTHE et al. 1969).

A second complication in short-circuiting the small intestine arises from the existence, on the serosal side of the tissue, of relatively massive layers of smooth muscle. Two effects of these layers on the electrical and transporting properties of this tissue have been reported. WHITE (1977a) has shown that, in certain circumstances at least, the electrical resistance of the muscle layers can contribute significantly to total tissue resistance. Thus, with unstripped intestinal preparations, even though adequate allowance may have been made for the external solution resistance, the condition $V_T = 0$ may deviate significantly from the true short-circuited state and the current when $V_T = 0$ may not correspond to I_{sc}. Equally important, there is convincing evidence (FRIZZELL et al. 1974) that, in the conventional Ussing chamber, unstripped preparations of mammalian small intestine may not receive adequate oxygenation.

Because of these complexities, contemporary studies with intestinal preparations mounted in Ussing chambers are usually performed with tissues from which the external muscle layers have been removed, either by blunt dissection (FIELD et al. 1971) or by carefully separating them from the mucosa with a glass microscope slide (SCHULTZ et al. 1966). Under histologic examination, such preparations are found to consist of the epithelial cell layer together with the structures adjacent thereto, i.e., the basement membrane, lamina propria, and muscularis mucosae. There is no doubt that stripping greatly ameliorates the difficulties discussed in the preceding paragraphs. Whether or not it completely abolishes them

Table 1. Spontaneous transepithelial potential V_{TO}, transepithelial conductance G_T, and the value of paracellular shunt conductance G_S divided by G_T in the small intestine and other epithelia

Tissue	V_{TO} (mV)[a]	G_T (Ω^{-1}cm^{-2}10^{-3})[a]	G_S/G_T
Small intestine			
Rabbit ileum 1)	2–3	25.0	>0.90
Rabbit jejunum 2)	1–2	27.0	
Rat jejunum 3)	1–2	25.0	>0.85
Guinea pig ileum 4)	7	16.0	
Human ileum 5)	4–6	11.0	
Flounder 6)	−3 to −4	24.0	
Bullfrog 7)[b]	1	8.0	
Bullfrog 8)[c]	0 to −1	20.0	
Colon			
Rabbit 9)	10–50	2–5	
Rat 10), 11)	10–15	9	
Human 12)	10–20	6	
Bullfrog 13)	15–60	2	
Proximal tubule 14)			
Rat	1	200.0	>0.95
Necturus	15	14.0	>0.95
Gallbladder 14)			
Rabbit	0	33.0	0.95
Necturus	3	3.0	0.96
Frog skin	20–100	0.1–1	0.5
Toad urinary bladder	60	0.3	0.25

[a] V_{TO} and G_T values are rounded averages
[b] Unstripped
[c] Stripped
1) Field et al. (1971); 2) Fromm (1973); 3) Munck and Schultz (1974); 4) Powell et al. (1972); 5) Grady et al. (1967); 6) Frizzell et al. (1979); 7) Quay and Armstrong (1969); 8) Armstrong and Youmans (1980); 9) Schultz et al. (1977); 10) Edmonds and Marriott (1968); 11) Edmonds and Marriott (1970); 12) Grady et al. (1970); 13) Cooperstein and Hogben (1959); 14) see Schultz (1979) for detailed references

is a matter for conjecture. For example, no quantitative study has yet been made on the resistive properties of the tissue components that remain after stripping. The development of methods for culturing epithelial cells in the form of flat sheets that are suitable for use in the Ussing chamber (Misfeldt et al. 1976) should help to resolve this and related problems[2].

I. Ionic Conductance and its Structural and Functional Correlates

The values of V_{TO} and G_T reported in vitro preparations of the small intestine from a number of animal species are summarized in Table 1. For comparative purpose, corresponding values for the large intestine and for a number of nonintestinal epithelia are included in this table. Considering first the V_{TO} values listed, one sees that, in the small intestine, this parameter, though usually finite, is small relative to its value in some other epithelia (e.g., frog skin, toad urinary bladder). Also in the small intestine, the orientation of V_{TO} in different animal species is quite variable. In mammals, it is usually oriented so that the luminal medium is negative with respect to the serosal fluid. In marine teleosts, the opposite orientation has been found. In amphibian intestine, the orientation of V_{TO} may depend on the presence of HCO_3^- in the external medium. Table 1 includes examples of these variations. Their probable origin is discussed in Sects. B. II. 2 and 3.

Turning to the G_T values listed in Table 1 it is apparent that certain epithelia, e.g., the small intestine, proximal renal tubule, and gallbladder, have G_T values that are about two orders of magnitude higher than those of some other epithelial systems such as frog skin and toad urinary bladder. In this respect, the large intestine occupies an intermediate position (Table 1).

The values for V_{TO} and G_T shown in Table 1 reflect the fact that, as pointed out by CLARKSON (1967), epithelia can be divided, on the basis of their transepithelial electrical characteristics, into two contrasting groups, those with high G_T and low V_{TO} values and those that display the opposite characteristics. In vivo, members of the former group transport large amounts of fluid and electrolytes and are bathed by solutions of roughly similar composition. By contrast, epithelia of the latter kind separate solutions that differ widely in composition and ionic strength. This dichotomous classification of epithelial systems was further developed by FRÖMTER and DIAMOND (1972) who coined the terms "tight" and "leaky" for epithelia that displayed low and high G_T values, respectively. While this remains a useful operational basis for distinguishing between obviously "tight" epithelia (e.g., frog skin, toad urinary bladder) and epithelia that are clearly "leaky" like the small intestine, there are instances where V_{TO} and G_T do not, by themselves, permit unequivocal classification. Two examples are the large intestine (Table 1) and the distal renal tubule. For such tissues, other criteria, e.g., their ability to effect net transport against large gradients of chemical or electrochemical potential, must be invoked to justify their inclusion in the category of "tight" epithelia (FRÖMTER and DIAMOND 1972; USSING et al. 1974; ERLIJ and MARTINEZ-PALOMO 1979).

CLARKSON (1967) correctly surmised that the overall transport properties of leaky epithelia such as the rat ileum could be explained by postulating the exis-

2 The complexities under present discussion may be the reason for a number of apparent discrepancies in the literature, e.g., the different values reported in two studies under apparently identical conditions, for J_{net}^{Na} in the short-circuited small intestine of the bullfrog (QUAY and ARMSTRONG 1969; ARMSTRONG and YOUMANS 1980). In the earlier study, unstripped segments of intestinal tissue were used. In the later one, the external muscle layers were surgically removed before the tissue was mounted in the Ussing chamber. One may note, however, that intestinal Na^+ and Cl^- absorption in another amphibian *Amphiuma*, is apparently unaffected by anoxia (WHITE 1977a). In experiments where V_{TO} and its response to various experimental manipulations is the primary focus of interest, the everted sac preparation (WILSON and WISEMAN 1954) offers a viable alternative to the Ussing chamber (see, e.g., SMYTH 1968). Although this preparation can be short-circuited (CLARKSON and TOOLE 1964), the technique involved is cumbersome and this approach does not permit the use of stripped preparations.

tence of a highly permeable extracellular or paracellular shunt pathway in parallel with the transcellular transport pathway. He suggested that, in rat ileum, the shunt pathway could be accounted for by the transient "channels" opened up by cell exfoliation at the tips of the villi (Ritter 1957; Bertalannfy and Lau 1962). The possibility that such cellular exfoliation does contribute to paracellular shunt conductance G_S in the small intestine, particularly in vivo, cannot be totally discounted. However, for the following reasons, it seems highly unlikely that it can be the major determinant of the in vitro transporting and electrical properties of this tissue. There is now ample evidence for the existence of paracellular shunt pathways, not only in the small intestine (White and Armstrong 1971; Rose and Schultz 1971; Frizzell and Schultz 1972; Munck and Schultz 1974), but also in a diversity of epithelia where cell exfoliation cannot be invoked as a causative factor. These epithelia include frog skin (Ussing and Windhager 1964), proximal renal tubule (Boulpaep 1972), gallbladder (Frömter 1972), toad urinary bladder (Reuss and Finn 1975a), etc. These and many other studies have clearly shown that the differences in G_T between tight and leaky epithelia are, in large part, due to differences in G_S. The conductances of the transcellular pathway for ionic transfer (i.e., the series resistances of the apical and basolateral cell membranes) appear to be comparable for a wide variety of epithelial systems (Erlij and Martinez-Palomo 1979). G_S/G_T for several epithelia is shown in Table 1; it is apparent that it exceeds 0.9 in leaky epithelia like the small intestine, whereas, in tight epithelia like frog skin and toad bladder, G_S accounts for no more than 10%–50% or so of G_T.

Numerous studies have established the fact that the shunt pathway in transporting epithelia is located in the junctional–intercellular space complexes rather than in specialized cells with highly conducting membranes. In some instances, this has been directly demonstrated by electrophysiologic (Frömter 1972) and histochemical studies (Whittenbury and Rawlins 1971; Machen et al. 1972; Tischer and Yarger 1973). Although several attempts have been made to correlate the relative "tightness" or "leakiness" of several epithelia with ultrastructural differences in their tight junctions (Claude and Goodenough 1973; Pricam et al. 1974; Martinez-Palomo and Erlij 1975), the precise morphological and molecular determinants of these characteristics remain undefined.

II. Ionic Fluxes

Table 2 summarizes the unidirectional and net Na^+ and Cl^- fluxes, under short-circuit conditions, in the small intestine of a number of animal species. The corresponding I_{sc} values are also shown. Historically, Na^+ and Cl^- have been the most intensively studied ionic species under these conditions. The probable reasons for this are as follows. First, although there has been a resurgence of interest, during recent years, in secretion by the small intestine (Binder 1979), most of the early electrophysiologic studies with this tissue were concerned with the process of fluid and electrolyte absorption. As the principal ionic components of the intestinal absorbate, Na^+ and Cl^- were, naturally, the major centers of attention. Second, the pioneering studies of Ussing and his collaborators with isolated frog

Table 2. Undirectional serosal to mucosal (J_{sm}) and net (J_{net}) fluxes of sodium and chloride across the small intestine of different animals, together with corresponding short-circuit currents (I_{sc})[a]

	J_{sm}^{Cl}	J_{net}^{Cl}	J_{sm}^{Na}	J_{net}^{Na}	I_{sc}
Animal					
Rabbit (ileum)	8	2	11	4	4 1)
Rabbit (jejunum)	10	0	15	−2	1 2)
Guinea pig (ileum)	7	−1	8	0	4 4)
Human (ileum)	9	0	7	3	2–3 15)
Flounder	2	4	11	2	−2 to −4 6)
Bullfrog	3	0	5	0	0 8)
Bullfrog[b]	9	5	9	0	−1 to −2 8)

[a] All values in μequiv.cm^{-2} h^{-1} rounded to nearest integer. Negative numbers indicate net secretory fluxes and net mucosal to serosal flow of negative charge
[b] HCO_3^- in external medium
15) AL-AWQATI et al. (1973); other references as in Table 1.
Note that J_{ms} can be obtained as $J_{sm} + J_{net}$

skin (USSING 1960) clearly established that, in this tissue, under normal circumstances, I_{sc} was fully accounted for by J_{net}^{Na} and that, under these conditions, Na^+ was the only ion actively transported across the skin. Equally clearly, active transepithelial Na^+ transport was implicated as the primary source of V_{TO}. Shortly thereafter, a similar relationship between J_{net}^{Na}, I_{sc} and V_{TO} was found to hold for the isolated toad urinary bladder (see LEAF 1982). Indeed, in these tissues, I_{sc} can often be employed as a reliable and virtually instantaneous measure of active Na^+ transport and of changes in this parameter (see, e.g., NAGEL et al. 1981).

These findings focused attention on J_{net}^{Na} as a possible determinant of I_{sc} and V_{TO} in other epithelial systems, including the small intestine. However, as the data in Table 2 show, it soon became apparent that the pristine simplicity of the relationship between J_{net}^{Na} and I_{sc} observed with frog skin and toad bladder does not apply to the small intestine[3]. In this tissue, J_{net}^{Na} may be less than, equal to, or greater than I_{sc}. In the remainder of this section, the relationship between I_{sc} and the corresponding transepithelial ionic fluxes will be examined in some intestinal preparations that have been rather extensively studied in this regard.

1. Mammalian Small Intestine

The most intensively studied preparation of mammalian small intestine to date has been the terminal ileum of the New Zealand white rabbit. Early studies by SCHULTZ and ZALUSKY (1964a) utilized intact intestinal sheets. Under control conditions (i.e., in bathing solutions without any source of metabolic energy, e.g., glucose), J_{net}^{Na} was 2.8 μequiv. cm^{-2} h^{-1}. This did not differ significantly from the I_{sc}, i.e., the net mucosal to serosal flow of positive charge (2.6 μequiv. cm^{-2} h^{-1}) ob-

3 A similar situation exists in the colon where I_{sc} may be larger than, equal to, or less than J_{net}^{Na}, depending on the animal species involved (POWELL 1979)

served in the same experiments, suggesting that Na^+ was the only ion that was actively transported across the tissue under these conditions. These results were supported by further studies (SCHULTZ et al. 1964) in which J_{net}^{Cl} was found to be zero under short-circuit conditions. Furthermore, when V_T was clamped at non-zero values, Cl^- fluxes were consistent with a purley passive transepithelial movement of this ion. CLARKSON and TOOLE (1964) reported that in isolated rat ileum exposed to Ringer's solutions containing glucose, the relationship $J_{net}^{Na} = I_{sc}$ was valid within the limits of experimental error.

The conclusions of SCHULTZ and ZALUSKY for rabbit ileum were challenged by the findings of FIELD et al. (1971; see also FIELD 1971). In addition to net Na^+ absorption these authors reported that, under short-circuit conditions, there was also a net absorption of Cl^-. Since I_{sc} exceeded the sum of these, it was concluded that a further "residual" net ionic flux J_R was also occurring. Several lines of evidence (e.g., the fact that J_R is greatly reduced when HCO_3^- is omitted from the external medium and that there was no demonstrable net flux of K^+) suggest that this residual flux reflects a net secretion of HCO_3^-. These experiments were performed with mucosal sheets from which the external smooth muscle layers had been surgically removed. FIELD et al. (1971) suggested that the discrepancy between their results and those of SCHULTZ and ZALUSKY (1964a) might be attributable to this. As already mentioned, it has been found (FRIZZELL et al. 1974) that the oxygen consumption of mucosal scrapings or of stripped mucosal sheets of rabbit ileum exceeds that of intact ileal segments. This raises the possibility that, in the experiments of SCHULTZ and ZALUSKY (1964a), the tissue was inadequately oxygenated and that its transport functions were therefore impaired. Suffice it to say that the results of FIELD et al. (1971) for stripped ileal mucosa have been amply confirmed in subsequent studies (see, e.g., SCHULTZ et al. 1974)

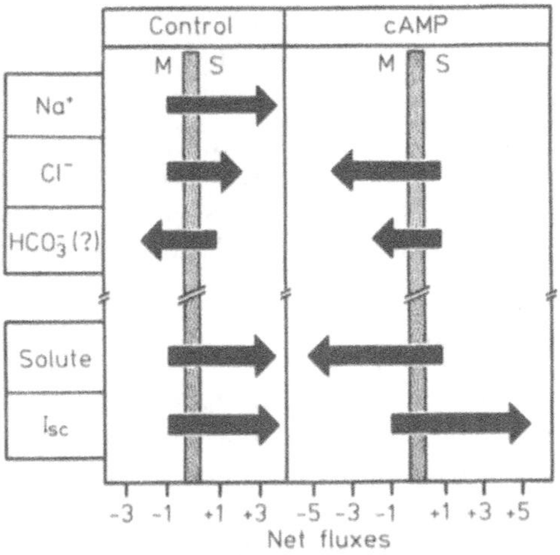

Fig. 4. Short-circuit current I_{sc} and net ionic fluxes in rabbit ileal mucosa under control conditions and following exposure of the tissue to cAMP. Absorptive (M→S) and secretory (S→M) fluxes respectively indicated by positive and negative numbers on the abscissa. For further discussion, see text. After FIELD (1971)

and that they serve to underline the complex nature of the ionic fluxes that contribute to the I_{sc} in the mammalian small intestine. Moreover, the magnitude of the I_{sc} under a given set of conditions and the changes in this parameter that result from specific experimental interventions, cannot, in the small intestine, readily be related to events involving the transepithelial flux of an individual ion, e.g., Na^+. The data of FIELD (1971), shown in Table 2 and summarized schematically in Fig. 4, illustrate this point. In these experiments, I_{sc} and J_{net}^{Na} were numerically equal under control conditions, but, as shown in Fig. 4, active Cl^- absorption and a residual net flux, assumed to be a net secretion of HCO^-, also occurred. However, in the example shown, these two processes, taken together, did not result in any net charge transfer across the epithelial cell layer. Therefore, they did not contribute to the observed I_{sc}. Furthermore, although addition of adenosine-3′,5′-monophosphate (cAMP) to the serosal bathing medium caused a marked increase in I_{sc}, this increase was not due to enhanced Na^+ absorption. It was, rather, the result of an *inhibition* of Na^+ absorption together with a changeover from net Cl^- absorption to net Cl^- secretion. This secretion exceeded in magnitude the net Cl^- absorption observed under control conditions.

2. Amphibian Intestine

In intact segments of isolated bullfrog small intestine bathed by normal HCO_3^- -free Ringer's solutions, QUAY and ARMSTRONG (1969) found a net absorption of both Na^+ and Cl^- under short-circuit conditions. Na^+ absorption was larger than that of Cl^-. In these experiments, I_{sc} was fully accounted for by the sum of J_{net}^{Na} and J_{Net}^{Cl}. When Cl^- in the bathing media was completely replaced by SO^{2-}, I_{sc} and V_{TO} increased and I_{sc} was identical to J_{net}^{Na}. Since no net flux of K^+ or of SO_4^{2-} was observed, it was concluded that, under these conditions, Na^+ was the only ion actively transported.

Although I_{sc} was larger in Na_2SO_4 than in NaCl media, the opposite was true for J_{net}^{Na}, in fact, the latter parameter was only about one quarter as large in the absence of Cl^- as in the presence of this ion. This suggested that Na^+ transport in this tissue is coupled in some way to that of Cl^-. Similarly, in Na^+-free media, J_{net}^{Cl} was greatly reduced (see also ARMSTRONG et al. 1972). These findings led QUAY and ARMSTRONG (1969) to propose the existence, in the apical membrane of the absorptive cell, of a coupled NaCl entry process. Subsequent events have confirmed the existence of coupled transapical NaCl entry as an important component of trancellular Na^+ and Cl^- transport in a variety of epithelia (see Sect. C. I. 2.).

Subsequently, ARMSTRONG and YOUMANS (1980) reported that, in stripped segments of bullfrog small intestine, net Na^+ and Cl^- absorption was very small or nonexistent in the absence of external HCO_3^-. Similarly, under these conditions, the average I_{sc} was negligible, indicating the absence of any significant residual net flux J_R. The possible origins of the discrepancy between these results and those reported earlier by QUAY and ARMSTRONG (1969) have already been discussed (see footnote 2). In media containing 25 mM HCO_3^-, there was no change in J_{net}^{Na}. However, J_{net}^{Cl} increased sharply, largely because of an increase in J_{ms}^{Cl}. At the same time, V_{TO} assumed a significant serosal negative value. However, when the preparation was short-circuited, the observed I_{sc} was much smaller than J^{Cl}_{net}. Thus there was a sizeable J_R that was consistent with net secretion of an anion (or anions). Since J_R was completely dependent on the presence of HCO_3^- in the external medium it was assumed to represent HCO_3^- secretion.

Mechanistically, the apparent secretion of HCO_3^- observed in these experiments was considered to be consistent with the existence, in the basolateral cell membrane, of a Cl^-/HCO_3^- exchange mechanism which, in the presence of a high external HCO_3^- concentration, serves to effect net HCO_3^- movement from the serosal medium to the cell interior. Confirmatory evidence for such an exchange mechanism was obtained in experiments with 4-acetamido-4′-isothiocyano-2,2′-stilbene disulfonate (SITS), an agent that is known to inhibit Cl^-/HCO_3^- exchange in a variety of cell types (Ehrenspeck and Brodsky 1976; Cabantchik et al. 1978). When added to the serosal medium, SITS abolished the HCO_3^--induced I_{sc}.

To account for the serosal negative V_{TO} developed in the presence of HCO_3^-, and the corresponding I_{sc} when the preparation was short-circuited, it was proposed that the basolateral Cl^-/HCO_3^- exchange mechanism was electrogenic, i.e., that, under the conditions studied, the Cl^-/HCO_3^- exchange ratio was greater than unity (Armstrong and Youmans 1980). However, in terms of the model proposed by Field (See Frizzell et al. 1979) to account for the serosal negative V_{TO} and corresponding I_{sc} observed in flounder intestine (see Sec. C. II. 2), it is entirely possible that Cl^-/HCO_3^- exchange in bullfrog small intestine is an electroneutral 1/1 coupled process.

It is of interest to note that cAMP, added to the serosal medium, significantly reduced the HCO_3^--induced J^{Cl}_{net} observed in the experiments of Armstrong and Youmans (1980). This inhibition reflected a decrease in J^{Cl}_{ms} in the presence of cAMP. At the same time there was a significant decrease in J^{Cl}_{ms}. These findings are consistent with the well-known inhibitory effect of cAMP on coupled transapical NaCl entry in a variety of epithelia. This effect is discussed more fully in Sect. F. I; cAMP had no effect on J_R.

A somewhat similar pattern of transepithelial ionic fluxes and transepithelial electrial characteristics to that found in stripped segments of bullfrog small intestine (Armstrong and Youmans 1980) emerged from studies with the proximal small intestine of *Amphiuma* (Gunter-Smith and White 1979 b). When Cl^- and HCO_3^- were present in the bathing media, a serosal negative V_{TO} was observed. When Cl^- or HCO_3^- were replaced or omitted, V_{TO} was reduced in magnitude and usually reversed in sign. The carbonic anhydrase inhibitor acetazolamide virtually abolished V_{TO}. Theophylline reversed the sign of V_{TO} and increased I_{sc}. These effects were dependent on external Na^+ and HCO_3^- concentrations. In Cl^--free media, the theophylline-induced increase in I_{sc} was not due to enhanced Na^+ absorption and was attributed to a residual ion flux. This flux was inhibited by acetazolamide. Subsequently, it was identified as a net secretion of HCO_3^- (White and Imon 1981).

3. Teleost Intestine

Field et al. (1978 b) reported that in stripped intestinal segments from the winter flounder, *Pseudopleuronectes americanus*, I_{sc} corresponds to a net mucosal to serosal transfer of negative charge. Under short circuit conditions, both Na^+ and Cl^- are absorbed, but the rate of Cl^- absorption exceeds that of Na^+. Na^+ absorption was not affected by external HCO_3^-. However, this ion increased Cl^- absorption, e.g., in media containing 20 m*M* HCO_3^- J_{ms}^{Cl} was about 70% higher than in media containing 5 m*M* HCO_3^-. J_{sm}^{Cl} was the same in both media. The sum of J_{net}^{Na} and J_{net}^{Cl} differed only slightly from the I_{sc}, suggesting that net HCO_3^- transport is slight or absent in this species. The effect of HCO_3^- on Cl^- absorption by this tissue was further studied by FIELD et al. (1978 a). Stripped segments of intestine, mounted in Ussing chambers, were allowed to reach an electrical steady state in identical mucosal and serosal media containing 20 m*M* HCO_3^-. The fluid in one or other of these compartments was then replaced by a medium containing 2 m*M* HCO_3^-. Mucosal replacement had little effect on transepithelial Cl^- fluxes. Reduction of serosal HCO_3^- lowered J_{ms}^{Cl} to about one-half of its initial value, but had little effect of J_{sm}^{Cl}. Because of this, Cl^- absorption was drastically reduced. Measurements of the mucosal uptake of ^{36}Cl indicated that serosal HCO_3^- levels did not affect the rate of Cl^- influx across the brush border membrane. It was concluded that serosal HCO_3^- affects Cl^- transfer across the basolateral cell membrane.

In summary, it appears that the small intestine of several species displays a complex pattern of ionic transfer processes in the short-circuited state. In mammalian, amphibian, and teleost intestine, both Na^+ and Cl^- are actively absorbed under normal conditions. A net secretory movement of HCO_3^- is also frequently observed. Furthermore, apart from its role as a component of active intestinal ion transport, HCO_3^- exerts a profound influence on Cl^- absorption. A considerable body of evidence points to a Cl^-/HCO_3^- exchange mechanism in the basolateral cell membrane as an important component of net Cl^- absorption. Although Cl^-/HCO_3^- exchange across the brush border membrane may be a significant factor in the intestinal transport of these ions (see Sect. C. I. 2. c), its role, if any, in net HCO_3^- secretion remains to be established.

C. Pathways of Ion Transport in the Small Intestine

As already discused (Sec. B. I), there is now compelling evidence that ion transport in the small intestine, and other epithelia, occurs via two parallel routes. These are: (1) a transcellular route that involves movement of the transported species across two functionally different membranes (the apical and basolateral cell membranes) in series; and (2) an extracellular route located in the junctional intercellular spaces between adjacent cells. A detailed knowledge of the transport characteristics of these two routes, and of the ways in which each of them can influence the transporting properties of the other is, therefore, an essential prerequisite to an understandig of transepithelial transport in intact tissues. It is, therefore, not surprising that recent years have witnessed intensive efforts to identify the individual transport processes that are located in the apical and basolateral membranes, respectively, and the specific properties of the extracellular transport route. The results of these studies will be reviewed in this section.

I. The Cellular Pathway

In recent years, a number of techniques have contributed significantly to the analysis of transcellular ion transport in the small intestine. Mucosal influx and microelectrode studies have permitted the identification of the specific transport steps that are associated with the apical and basolateral cell membranes, respectively, and the precise definition of the transmembrane driving forces for ions. The development of methods for preparing membrane vesicles has allowed individual transport processes, in one or other of the limiting cell membranes, to be isolated and characterized in the absence of complications arising from cellular metabolism or of interference arising from events occuring elsewhere in the intact cellular system.

1. Definition of Transmembrane Driving Forces

Under the usual conditions of biologic investigation, i.e., at constant temperature and in the absence of large hydrostatic pressure differences across the cell membrane, the transmembrane driving force for an ion j is given by the equation

$$\Delta\tilde{\mu}_j/zF = RT\ln(a_j^c/_j^o) + V_m\,, \qquad \text{(C.I. 1)}$$

where $\Delta\tilde{\mu}_j$ is the electrochemical potential difference across the membrane for j; F, R, and T have their usual meanings; a_j^c and a_j^o are the activities of j in the cell interior and the extracellular medium respectively, z is the valence, and V_m is the membrane potential. Since F and R are universal constants, and T and z are known for any specific instance, the determination of $\Delta\tilde{\mu}_j/F$ reduces to the measurement of a_j^o, a_j^c, and V_m; a_j^o is readily determined by standard physicochemical techniques (ROBINSON and STOKES 1965). The measurement of V_m with microelectrodes, though already a venerable technique with certain cell types (THOMAS 1978) is of comparatively recent vintage in epithelial electrophysiology. The direct determination, with ion-selective microelectrodes, of intracellular ionic activities (a_j^c) is, in all respects, comparatively new (LEV and ARMSTRONG 1975). Some account of these two techniques, and particularly of their application to epithelial cells of the small intestine, seems appropriate.

a) Apical Cell Membrane Potentials

First, one may note that, in epithelial cells, there are two membrane potentials. These are the apical V_a and the basolateral V_s membrane potentials. Except for the condition $V_T=0$, these will not, in general, be equal but, in the small intestine, the difference between them, which is clearly equal to V_T, is usually small in the open-circuit state (Table 1). Since $V_T = V_s - V_a$ it is apparent that any one of these three parameters is readily obtained if the other two are known. Because direct impalement with microectrodes of the basolateral membrane is technically difficult, even in stripped intestinal preparations, it is customary to measure V_T and V_a and calculate then V_s.

Early studies with the small intestine of the Greek tortoise and the hamster (GILLES-BAILLIEN and SCHOFFENIELS 1965, 1968; WRIGHT 1966) clearly established that the absorptive cell interior is negative with respect to the mucosal so-

Table 3. Apical membrane potentials V_a in the small intestine

Animal	V_a (mV)[a]	Reference
Aplysia	−68	GERENCSER and WHITE (1980)
Sole	−32	ZEUTHEN et al. (1978)
Flounder	−69	DUFFEY et al. (1978)
Tortoise	−7	WRIGHT (1966)
	−28	GILLES-BAILLIEN and SCHOFFENIELS (1965)
Amphiuma	−33[b]	WHITE (1977b)
Necturus	−35	GARCIA-DIAZ et al. (1978) WARD and BOYER (1980)
	−40	GUNTER-SMITH et al. (1982)
Bullfrog	−24	ARMSTRONG et al. (1977)
	−34	ARMSTRONG et al. (1979a)
	−45[c]	WHITE and ARMSTRONG (1971)
Rabbit (ileum)	−35	ROSE and SCHULTZ (1971)
	−19	HIRSCHORN and FRAZIER (1973)
	−5 to −32	DE JESUS et al. (1975)
	−5 to −34	ZEUTHEN and MONGE (1976)
Rat (jejunum)	−9	LYON and SHEERIN (1971) BARRY and EGGENTON (1972a)
	−55	OKADA et al. (1976)

[a] All values are with respect to an external reference electrode in the mucosal solution and are rounded to the nearest mV
[b] Summer animals
[c] Na_2SO_4 medium

lution, i.e., on penetrating the brush border membrane there is a sharp negative deflection of the potential recorded by the microelectrode. Although some of the V_a values recorded in these early studies were unacceptably low by present standards (Table 3), they did establish the fact that V_a is numerically greater than V_T. Therefore, in open-circuit or short-circuit conditions, the electrical potential profile across the cell in shaped like a well, i.e., both the mucosal and serosal bathing solutions are electrically positive with respect to the cell interior. Thus, the electrical moiety of the thermodynamic driving force across each membrane $\Delta\tilde{\mu}_j/F$ acts to enhance electrodiffusive entry of absorbed cations into the cell across the brush border membrane and to oppose their exit from the cell across the basolateral membrane. The opposite is true for anions.

In recent years, significant progress has been made towards the establishment of reliable, objective criteria for evaluating the acceptability of microelectrode impalements in epithelial cells of the small intestine and other tissues. The data summarized in Table 3 emphasize the need for such criteria.

At the outset, it may be noted that, in those instances where the distribution of the V_a values summarized in Table 3 was analyzed in detail (e.g., WHITE and ARMSTRONG 1981; ROSE and SCHULTZ 1971) this distribution was unimodal. There seems, therefore, little reason to believe that the scatter in the results shown in this table rises from the inclusion, within them, of V_a values measured in different cell types. Hence the lack of agreement in the reported V_a values, particularly in the same tissue (e.g., rat jejunum, tortoise intestine) under identical conditions, seems to argue strongly in favor of the idea that early measurements of this parameter in the small intestine were compromised by a number of technical shortcomings. Detailed discussions of the technical difficulties involved in obtaining accurate recordings of membrane potentials from relatively small cells such as those of the intestinal mucosa, and recommended procedures for circumventing these difficulties can be found elsewhere (Armstrong 1975, 1976; Nelson et al. 1978; Armstrong and Garcia-Diaz 1981). In summary, the problems encountered stem from two sources. These are the small size of the cells themselves and the correspondingly small microelectrode tip diameters required to impale them successfully. If microelectrodes with inappropriately large tips[4] are used, a frequent complication in impaling cells of dimensions similar to those of intestinal absorptive cells in the occurrence of excessive membrane damage, that is, disruption of the membrane to an extent that cannot be compensated by spontaneous resealing around the glass wall of the microelectrode. The resulting low resistance pathway across the cell membrane leads to rapid depolarization. In isolated cells, and, in extreme cases, in the small intestine (Hirschorn and Frazier 1973), this causes complete dissipation, within a short time, of the membrane potential. Therefore, in early studies with the small intestine, the attainment, following impalement, of a microelectrode potential that was constant within ± 1–2 mV was frequently taken as a sufficient criterion of acceptability (Wright 1966, Lyon and Sheerin 1971; Barry and Eggenton 1972a). However, as emphasized empirically by White and Armstrong (1971) and as discussed more explicitly by Armstrong and Garcia-Diaz (1981), it is not unusual to find, with the intestine, impalements which, following an initial partial depolarization, V_a attains a steady or quasisteady state that may persist for many minutes (see, e.g., Fig. 2A in Armstrong and Garcia-Diaz 1981). The occurrence of such low but finite and relatively stable potential differences in epithelial system no doubt reflects the existence of transverse electrical coupling between adjacent cells (Loewenstein 1981).

A second factor that may give rise to anomalously low values of V_a in the small intestine is leakage of the filling solution from the tip of the microelectrode to the cell interior. This factor, which has been discussed in detail by Nelson et al. (1978) and by Fromm and Schultz (1981) again depends of the size of the microelectrode tip and is particularly serious when filling solutions containing high concentrations of K^+ (e.g., 3 M KCl) are used. This problem can be eliminated or at least significantly reduced by using high resistance microelectrodes and more dilute filling solutions (Armstrong and Garcia-Diaz 1981). Recently, a most ingenious solution to it has been devised (Thomas and Cohen 1981). This consists in using, for the determination of membrane potentials, liquid membrane

4 A useful and easily measured index of microelectrode tip size is the tip resistance. Microelectrodes with tip resistances about 20 MΩ (filled with 1 M KCl and immersed in Ringer's solution) have tip diameters of approximately 1 µm. In the author's laboratories, these have been found satisfactory for impaling the epithelial cells of *Necturus* gallbladder. In studies with isolated frog skin, acceptable impalements were routinely obtained in the range 20–30 MΩ (Nagel et al. 1981). These use of microelectrodes with significantly smaller tips (i.e., with tip resistances not less than 50 MΩ) is strongly recommended for studies with the small intestine (White and Armstrong 1971)

microelectrodes of the type originally developed by WALKER (1971) for measuring intracellular K^+ and Cl^- activities (see Sect. C.I. 1.). In these microelectrodes, the tip contains a lipophilic anion or cation, dissolved in a droplet of a hydrophobic solvent. The selectivity of these microelectrodes for different cations or anions is determined, almost exclusively, by the properties of the nonaqueous solvent (ARMSTRONG 1981). By using an appropriate combination of lipophilic anion and solvent, THOMAS and COHEN (1981) were able to construct microelectrodes in which the responses to cytoplasmatic K^+ and Na^+ respectively "cancel out" and do not significantly affect the measured membrane potential. These microelectrodes do not permit leakage of the filling solution into the cell interior and, although they are more difficult to construct and, because of their high resistances, have longer response times than conventional open-tip microelectrodes, can be used to evaluate the effect of microelectrode leakage on the membrane potentials measured under a given set of conditions.

A complication that can lead to artifactually high, rather than anomalously low membrane potentials arises when the microelectrode tip is partially occluded by structural components of the cell. This is particularly likely to occur with ultrafine-tip microelectrodes such as those recommended for studies with the small intestine. Artifacts of this kind have been reported for both tight and leaky epithelia (ARMSTRONG and GARCIA-DIAZ 1981), and are, in all probability, included in some of the V_a values in the upper part of the ranges reported by WHITE and ARMSTRONG (1971), ROSE and SCHULTZ (1971), and OKADA et al. (1975), and summarized in Table 3. Fortunately, such artifacts are almost always accompanied by significant increases in microelectrode resistance R_{me} which disappear when the microelectrode is withdrawn from the cell [5]. They are readily detected by continuously monitoring R_{me} and can sometimes be eliminated by adjusting, by a few μm, the position of the microelectrode tip within the cell (ARMSTRONG and GARCIA-DIAZ 1981).

In view of this discussion it is, clearly, very difficult, at this time, to suggest a truly "representative" value for V_a in the small intestine. The most recent studies (WHITE 1976; ARMSTRONG et al. 1979a; WARD and BOYD 1980; GUNTER-SMITH et al. 1982) indicate a probable value, under normal conditions, of about −35 mV for amphibian intestine.

b) Ionic Activities and Concentrations in Epithelial Cells

The development by WALKER (1971) of liquid ion exchanger microelectrodes, in which the specific ion sensor is a droplet of ion exchanger solution held in the tip

5 This observation is particularly relevant to the V_a values for the rat intestine reported by OKADA et al. (1975, 1976, 1977a, b), since these authors found that the apparent resistances of their microelectrodes increased by about 20% following cell impalement. In *Necturus* gallbladder, a leaky epithelium that shows many analogies, in its ion transport and electrophysiological properties, to the small intestine, one can calculate from FROMTER's (1972) results that, because of intercellular coupling, the expected increase in microelectrode resistance, under these circumstances, should not exceed 2 MΩ or thereabouts (ARMSTRONG and GARCIA-DIAZ 1981). Admittedly, data similar to those reported by FROMTER (1972) for *Necturus* gallbladder are not yet available for rat jejunum. Nevertheless, the possibility that artifactually high V_a values are included in the results reported by OKADA et al. (Table 3) remains strong

of a conventional microelectrode, stimulated a rapid expansion in the application of this technique to the measurement of intracellular activities. Before this development, these measurement had involved the fabrication and use of microelectrodes made from special ion-selective glasses. Despite the reassurance of electrophysiologic virtuosi like R. C. Thomas (1978), this process remains, for many investigators, a difficult one. As a result, before the appearance of Walker's (1971) paper, intracellular activity measurements were restricted to a relatively small number of cell types. Most of these cells were fairly large (Lev and Armstrong 1975). The introduction by Walker of liquid ion exchanger microelectrodes, and the subsequent development of liquid membrane microelectrodes in which highly selective neutral carrier molecules form the basis of the ion-sensitive element (Simon and Morf 1973; Steiner et al. 1979; O'Doherty et al. 1979, 1980) significantly extended both the range of application and the simplicity of preparation of these devices. As a result, the measurement of intracellular ionic activities in relatively small cells such as those of transporting epithelia is now a fairly routine procedure (Armstrong 1981).

The technical problems encountered in the fabrication of the very fine tipped liquid membrane microelectrodes (tip diameters ≤ 1 μm) required for successful impalements in the intestinal mucosa and similar epithelial systems have been discussed in detail elsewhere (Thomas 1978; Armstrong and Garcia-Diaz 1980). In the present context, one may note that avoidance of excessive membrane damage during impalement is equally important whether one is using conventional or ion-selective microelectrodes. This is because, if one assumes the simplest situation,[6] i.e., that the ion-selective microelectrode responds exclusively to one ionic species j, the voltage change observed when this microelectrode penetrates the cell membrane is given by equation

$$\Delta V = (V_{\text{in}} - V_{\text{out}}) = V_a + S \log(a_j^c / a_j^o) \qquad \text{(C.I. 2)}$$

where V_a is the membrane potential and S is the voltage change recorded by the microelectrode for a tenfold change in a_j^c/a_j^o.

The most frequently used method for measuring intracellular ionic activities is the so-called method of averaging. In this technique, representative samples of impalements are made separately with a conventional and an ion-selective microelectrode. The average values of V_a and of ΔV obtained are then inserted in Eq. (C.I. 2). It is clear that the validity of this procedure requires that impalements made with both microelectrodes must meet the same criteria. Even when double-barreled microelectrodes (i.e., microelectrodes with one conventional and one ion-selective barrel) are used, together with differential recording of the potential difference between them (whereby V_a is eliminated as a measured component of ΔV in Eq. (C.I. 2); see, e.g., de Jesus et al. 1975; White 1976) it is essential to avoid excessive membrane damage, since this could cause relatively rapid changes in V_a. In addition, with small cells like the absorptive cells of the small intestine, mem-

---

6 The more complex, and, in practice, more usual situation in which the ion-selective microelectrode displays some selectivity for ionic species other than the one to which it responds primarily, is discussed in detail by Armstrong and Garcia-Diaz (1981)

Table 4. Intracellular ionic concentrations and activities (C^c, a^c) in the small intestine

Animal	Reference	Cl^-			K^+		Na^+	
		C^c (mM)	a^c	a^c/a^{eq}	C^c (mM)	a^c	C^c (mM)	a^c
Aplysia	1)		10	0.4				
Sole	2)		35	1.2				
Flounder	3)		24	3.4				
Goldfish	4)	66			133		67	
Tortoise	5)				103		51	
Amphiuma	6), 7)	53	28 [a]	1.3 [a]	146	41		6
Necturus	8), 9), 10)		33	1.7		108		9
Bullfrog	11)	51	33	1.7	105	80	52	18
	12)		71	2.2				
	13)					85 [b]		14 [b]
Rabbit (ileum)	14)	67			130		61	
	15)		30–80	1				
	16)				116		31	
	17)		60–80	0.6–0.3		30–120		
Rat (jejunum)	18)	61			121		73	
	19)				129		44	

[a] Summer animals
[b] Na_2SO_4 medium.
a^{eq} is the intracellular Cl^- activity that corresponds to a passive distribution of this ion across the apical membrane of the absorptive cell
1) Gerencser and White (1980); 2) Zeuthen et al. (1978); 3) Duffey et al. (1978); 4) Albus et al. (1979); 5) Hajjar et al. (1972); 6) White (1976); 7) White (1977b); 8) Garcia-Diaz et al. (1978); 9) Garcia-Diaz and Armstrong (1980), (1981, unpublished work); 10) O-Doherty et al. (1979); 11) Armstrong et al. (1979a); 12) Armstrong et al. (1977); 13) Lee and Armstrong (1972); 14) Frizzell et al. (1973); 15) de Jesus et al. (1975); 16) Simmons and Naftalin (1976); 17) Zeuthen and Monge (1976); 18) Okada et al. (1976); 19) Barry and Eggenton (1972a)

brane damage could result in significant and rapid changes in intracellular ionic activities. Obviously, when double-barreled microelectrodes are used, it is also important to avoid other causes of artifactual potentials such as leakage of the filling solution from the open-tipped barrel or partial blockade of the open tip.

Available date for K^+, Na^+, and Cl^- activities in absorptive cells of the small intestine are shown in Table 4. When these activities are divided by the appropriate activity coefficients (e.g., 0.75 for mammalian and 0.78 for amphibian tissues) the equivalent intracellular concentrations are obtained. For Cl^-, the ratio a^c/a^{eq} is also shown in Table 4. a^{eq} is obtained from the Nernst equation

$$a^{eq} = a^o \exp(FV_a/RT) \tag{C.I.3}$$

and is the value of a^c that corresponds to an equilibrium distribution of Cl^- across the brush border membrane. Finally, the table includes the apparent intracellular concentrations, determined by conventional chemical analyses, of K^+, Na^+, and Cl^- in the intestinal mucosa of several animal species.

Considering first the Cl^- activities shown in Table 4, it is clear that, with a few exceptions, a^c_{Cl}/a^{eq}_{Cl} is greater than unity, i.e., a^c_{Cl} exceeds the value that corresponds to an equilibrium distribution of this ion across the apical cell membrane. Since V_{TO} in the small intestine is usually small (see Table 1), one can show that, in general, a^c_{Cl} also exceeds the value that corresponds to electrochemical equilibrium across the basolateral cell membrane. A similar Cl^- distribution has been found in other leaky epithelia such as the gallbladder and proximal renal tubule (FRIZZELL et al. 1979) and for isolated frog skin (NAGEL et al. 1981). The significance of this finding is discussed later in this section. First, however, the apparent exceptions to it that are shown in Table 4 deserve comment. One of these is the value of a^c_{Cl} reported for the intestine of the marine invertebrate Aplysia (GERENCSER and WHITE 1980). Although similarities between transcellular Cl^- transport in this tissue and the corresponding process in vertebrate intestine have been reported (GERENCSER et al. 1976), it not yet clear whether in fact the underlying mechanisms are identical. The other two examples shown in Table 4 are the studies of DE JESUS et al. (1975) and the in vivo measurements of ZEUTHEN and MONGE (1975, 1976) with rabbit ileum. In isolated sheets of rabbit ileum bathed by Ringer's solutions containing the normal amount of Cl^- (145 mM), DE JESUS et al. reported that a^c_{Cl}, over a wide range of V_a values, was rather consistently below the value that corresponds to electrochemical equilibrium. However, the V_a values recorded by these authors were not only low, but, on the author's own admission, frequently unstable. Indeed, in a number of instances, two values of V_a and a^c_{Cl} were reported for a single impalement. When this was done, the apparent value of a^c_{Cl} early in the impalement tended to exceed the corresponding value for a^{eq}_{Cl}. Later in the impalement, the opposite was true. In the light of the previous discussion (Sect. C.I. 1) concerning criteria for the acceptance of microelectrode impalements in absorptive cells of the small intestine, it would appear that the results of DE JESUS et al. (1975) are open to serious question on technical grounds.[7]

Similar comments would seem to apply to the results reported by ZEUTHEN and MONGE (1975, 1976). In these studies, a^c_{Cl} was measured with double-barreled microelectrodes during two in vivo experiments on rabbit ileum. Double-barreled K^+-selective microelectrodes were used to obtain a number of estimates of a^c_K under the same conditions. From the description given by the authors, these experiments might be termed heroic. From the results obtained, ZEUTHEN and MONGE claimed that, in the absorptive cells of rabbit ileum, there were gradients, along the major axis of the cells, in electrical potential, a^c_{Cl}, and a^c_K. Thus, V_a near the apical cell membrane was -5 mV and increased in magnitude to -30 mV in the neighborhood of the basolateral membrane. Along the same axis, a^c_{Cl} decreased from 60 to 8 mM and a^c_K increased from 30 to 120 mM (Table 4).

The status of these results remains controversial. The electron microprobe studies of GUPTA et al. (1978) disclosed the existence of gradients for Na^+, K^+, and Cl^-, along the major axis of the cytoplasm, that were qualitatively similar

7 It is interesting to note that, in this study, a^c_{Cl} in rabbit ileum immersed in Ringer's solutions containing 20 mM Cl^- was reported to be consistently *above* the value corresponding to electrochemical equilibrium

to those reported by ZEUTHEN and MONGE. However, the data of GUPTA et al. (1978) relate to the total ionic content, rather than the ionic concentration of the cytoplasm. The probability discussed later in this section that there is significant compartmentation of cytoplasmic Na^+ and Cl^- in the absorptive cells of the small intestine complicates any direct comparison between electron microprobe analyses of these ions and measurements, with ion-selective microelectrodes, of their intracellular activities. Furthermore, the effect of diffusion artifacts during specimen preparation on the final ionic distributions observed with the electron microprobe remains, in this and other studies, somewhat ill defined. It should be emphasized, however, that GUPTA et al. (1978) contend that such effects could only reduce the magnitude of preexisting gradients and could not, de novo, generate such gradients. Moreover, ZEUTHEN's subsequent claim (1977) that similar gradients of electrical potental occur in the epithelial cells of *Necturus* gallbladder has been directly and rather convincingly challenged by SUZUKI and FRÖMTER (1977). Finally, careful and extensive measurements of V_a and of ionic activities in this tissue (see, e.g., GARCIA-DIAZ and ARMSTRONG 1980) have failed to yield any evidence that supports ZEUTHEN's position. On the contrary, as already mentioned (Sect. C. I. 1; see also ARMSTRONG and GARCIA-DIAZ 1981) they have uncovered the existence of impalement artifacts that may, in part at least, account for the apparent intracellular gradients postulated by ZEUTHEN.

In brief, there appears to be convincing evidence, for vertebrate intestine at least, that steady state intracellular Cl^- levels exceed those that correspond to an equilibrium distribution of this ion across either the brush border or the basolateral cell membrane. In terms of the overall energetics of intestinal Cl^- absorption, this clearly pinpoints the brush border membrane as the locus of the uphill step in transcellular Cl^- transport. Equally clearly, this finding rules out the possibility that net Cl^- transport across the brush border membrane can occur by simple electrodiffusion and underlines the need for a continuous input of external energy to effect such transport. The mechanisms by which transapical Cl^- transport is believed to occur are discussed in Sects. C.I. 2 and C.I. 3.

To date, there have been relatively few reports concerning a_K^c and a_{Na}^c in the intestine. As in other animal cells, K^+ appears to be the major osmotically active ion in intestinal absorptive cells. In general, a_K^c values ranging from 80 to about 100 m*M* have been reported (Table 4). An exception is *Amphiuma* intestine where a_K^c was reported to be about 40 m*M* (WHITE 1976). This result is intriguing in view of the chemically determined intracellular K^+ concentration (146 m*M*) reported in the same paper and the relatively high apparent activity coefficient for K^+ ($a_K^c/C_K^c \sim 0.7$) observed in a wide variety of cell types (LEV and ARMSTRONG 1975). The origin of the striking differences between the a_K^c value reported for *Amphiuma* intestine and those observed in intestinal preparations from other amphibia, e.g., the bullfrog and *Necturus* (Table 4), is not clear. Similar low a_K^c/C_K^c values were reported by KHURI (1976) for rat kidney proximal and distal tubule cells and for *Necturus* proximal tubule. However, later studies (EDELMAN et al. 1978; GRAF and GIEBISCH 1979) have not confirmed these findings. The possibility exists that the low a_K^c values reported by WHITE (1976) may be related to the well-known phenomenon of seasonal variation in amphibia. Recently, in one of the authors' laboratory, low and extremely variable a_K^c values have been observed in *Necturus* gallbladder during the summer months. It is not yet known if these are associated with unusually low C^c_K values.

With the exception of the data reported by White (1976) for *Amphiuma* intestine, the results summarized in Table 4 indicate that most, if not all, of the cytoplasmic K^+ in intestinal absorptive cells is osmotically active, i.e., little, if any, K^+ is sequestered in intracellular regions or in physical states that are inaccessible to K^+-selective microelectrodes. This agrees with the results reported for the majority of cell species in which a^c_K and C^c_K have been directly compared (Lev and Armstrong 1975; Walker and Brown 1977).

So far, the only species for which a^c_{Na} and C^c_{Na} have been directly compared under identical conditions is the bullfrog (Table 4). The a^c_{Na}/C^c_{Na} values observed (0.3–0.5) are, again, in good agreement with those reported for a variety of cell types (Lev and Armstrong 1975; Walker and Brown 1977). However, they lead to conclusions concerning the distribution of intracellular Na^+ that are quite different from those advanced herein for cellular K^+. As an example, one may consider the data reported for isolated bullfrog small intestine bathed in normal frog Ringer's solution (Armstrong et al. 1979a). The a^c_{Na}/C^c_{Na} value observed in these experiments (0.31) is far below the value (0.77) predicted on the assumption that all, or virtually all, the chemically determined intracellular Na^+ is osmotically active. Even if one allows for the very considerable uncertainties inherent in the determination of intracellular ionic concentrations by classical chemical methods (Lev and Armstrong 1975), this observation strongly supports the idea that a large fraction of the intracellular Na^+ exists in a state or states where its thermodynamic activity is not accessible to measurement with Na^+-selective microelectrodes.

The situation with respect to intracellular Cl^- is less clear. The results obtained by Armstrong et al. (1979a) with bullfrog small intestine yield an estimate of 0.63 for a^c_{Cl}/C^c_{Cl}. Although this is considerably smaller than the value of 0.77 predicted by a free solution model for cytoplasmic Cl^-, and suggests some intracellular binding or compartmentation of this ion, the uncertainties involved in the determination of C_{Cl} make such a conclusion highly tentative for this particular study. The results of White (1977b) for *Amphiuma* intestine are less equivocal. His data (Table 4) give a value of 0.53 for a^c_{Cl}/C^c_{Cl}.

It is noteworthy that Frizzell et al. (1973) found that about 10% of the apparent intracellular Cl^- in the mucosal layer of rabbit ileum did not exchange with ^{36}Cl in the bathing medium. Thus, on balance, the available evidence favors the existence of some degree of heterogeneity in Cl^- distribution within the absorptive cells of the small intestine. Further studies are, however, required to clarify this point.

To conclude this section, we have attemted in Fig. 5 to illustrate, in schematic form, the information, relative to transcellular ion transport in the small intestine, that can be obtained by measuring V_a and steady state intracellular ionic activities. For this purpose we chose our data for *Necturus* small intestine (Table 4). There were two reasons for this choice. First, all the data shown in Fig. 5 were obtained under identical experimental conditions. Second, because the absorptive cells in *Necturus* intestine are larger than those in the small intestine of many other

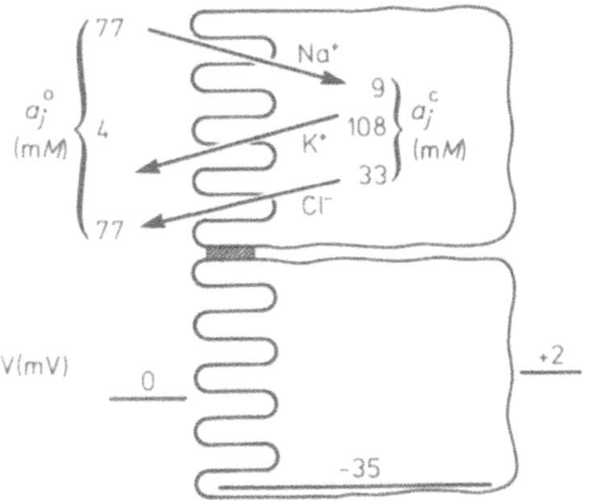

Fig. 5. Intracellular ionic activities and potential profile of absorptive cells in *Necturus* small intestine

species, impalement artifacts are less likely to compromise the electrophysiologic data obtained.

The data in Fig. 5 show that the intracellular Na^+ electrochemical potential is considerably lower than that of the mucosal or serosal bathing medium. Thus, electrodiffusive forces tend to drive Na^+ into the cell. By contrast, a_K^c and a_{Cl}^c are higher than their respective equilibrium values, calculated from the Nernst equation. Therefore, the appropriate differences in electrochemical potential between the cell interior and the bathing media tend to drive both K^+ and Cl^- out of the cell. Thus, Na^+ exit from the cell and K^+ and Cl^- entry into the cell are all active processes in ROSENBERG's (1948) original sense, i.e., all these processes, if they are to function continuously, require coupling to an external energy source. Nowadays, the term "active" is often reserved for transport processes that are directly linked to an input of metabolic energy, e.g., the Na^+-pump. As discussed in the following section, Cl^- entry, across the brush border membrane, appears to be an example of "secondary" active transport for which the driving force is the transapical Na^+ gradient.

2. Mucosal Entry Processes

Since Na^+ entry from the mucosal medium to the interior of intestinal absorptive cells occurs down a favorable gradient of electrochemical potential (Fig. 5), it is unnecessary, in principle, to invoke any mechanism, aside from a purely electrodiffusive process, to account for this entry. However, recent investigations have disclosed the presence, in the brush border membrane, of two carrier-mediated mechanisms that are involved, under physiologic conditions, in net Na^+ transport from the mucosal medium to cell interior. When actively transported organic solutes, such as sugars or amino acids, are present in the mucosal bathing solution, additional carrier-mediated pathways for Na^+ entry come into play. These pathways will be discussed in Sect. E. At this point, two mechanisms will be considered. These are: (a) electroneutral Na^+/H^+ exchange (antiport); and (b) coupled NaCl entry (symport). In passing, it is worth noting that both these processes are examples of transport mechanisms that appear to be common to many, if not all, leaky epithelia (FRIZZELL et al. 1979).

a) Na^+/H^+ Exchange

MURER et al. (1976) clearly demonstrated the existence of an electroneutral Na^+/H^+ exchange mechanism in brush border vesicles isolated from rat small intestine and renal cortex. Following the imposition of an inwardly directed Na^+ concentration gradient, an ejection of protons from the interior of the vesicles was observed. Similarly, in the presence of an outwardly directed proton gradient, a transient increase in Na^+ uptake was noted. The essentially electroneutral nature of the Na^+/H^+ exchange process was demonstrated by the finding that, in the presence of cation gradients, altering the vesicular membrane potential (e.g., with valinomycin) did not affect the rate of Na^+/H^+ exchange. Thus a Na^+/H^+ stoichiometry of 1/1 may be assumed. In these experiments, a very small rheogenic entry of Na^+ into the vesicles was also observed.

KINSELLA and ARONSON (1980, 1981 a, b) studied Na^+/H^+ exchange in more detail. In their experiments, brush border vesicles from rabbit kidney were used. Na^+ uptake was found to be saturable and was inhibited by Li^+ and NH_4^+, but not by K^+, Rb^+, Rb^+, Cs^+, or choline. Li^+ was able to substitute for Na^+ in the exchange process. No rheogenic entry of Na^+ was observed in these studies. In addition, since replacement of Cl^- by other anions had no effect on Na^+ uptake, it was concluded that, if NaCl cotransport occurs at the mucosal membrane of this tissue, its rate must be slow compared with that of Na^+/H^+ exchange. In the experiments of KINSELLA and ARONSON, Na^+/H^+ exchange was inhibited by harmaline and amiloride. It was not inhibited by furosemide, acetazolamide, or SITS.

b) Coupled NaCl Entry

The experiments of QUAY and ARMSTRONG (1969) on transepithelial Na^+ and Cl^- transport by isolated bullfrog small intestine prompted these authors to propose the existence of a coupled NaCl entry process across the brush border membrane of the absorptive cells of this tissue. Shortly thereafter, the existence of a correlation between J_{net}^{Na} and J_{net}^{Cl} in short-circuited rabbit ileum was noted by FIELD et al. (1971).

Direct evidence for the existence of a coupled mucosal NaCl entry mechanism in the small intestine was obtained by NELLANS et al. (1973) using the mucosal influx technique (cf. Fig. 2). Their experiments established the fact that mucosal Na^+ or Cl^- influx (J_{mc}^{Na}, J_{mc}^{Cl}) in rabbit ileum was reduced when Cl^- or Na^+ respectively was omitted from the mucosal bathing medium. The extent to which the mucosal influx of each ion was inhibited by the absence of the other was the same. This suggested an obligatory 1/1 coupled entry of these ions. Theophylline, an agent that was known to inhibit Na^+ and Cl^- absorption (FIELD 1971) inhibited J_{mc}^{Na} and J_{mc}^{Cl} to the same extent. This is consistent with the inhibition by theophylline of a 1/1 coupled NaCl entry process. NELLANS et al. (1973) proposed a kinetic model for coupled NaCl entry. This featured a random combination of both transported ions with a carrier located in the brush border membrane of the absorptive cell. Experiments in which the effects of ionic replacements on transepithelial Na^+ and Cl^- fluxes were studied (NELLANS et al. 1974) confirmed the fact that coupled mucosal NaCl entry is responsible for the net Cl^- absorption observed in the rabbit ileum in vitro. Replacement of external Na^+ by choline abolished net Cl^- absorption, indicating an absolute dependence of this process on Na^+.

Chemical determinations of C^c_{Cl} in rabbit ileum (FRIZZELL et al. 1973) showed that, in the steady state, C^c_{Cl} exceeded the equilibrium value expected from the measured V_a in this tissue (ROSE and SCHULTZ 1971). Exposure of the tissue to theophylline caused C^c_{Cl} to decline towards its equilibrium value. This prompted the suggestion (FRIZZELL 1976) that coupled mucosal NaCl entry could effect intracellular Cl^- accumulation and that the energy required for this purpose could be derived from the simultaneous dissipation of the Na^+ gradient between the luminal medium and the cell interior. This could be accomplished by a mechanism similar to that which is believed to be responsible for Na^+-dependent sugar and amino acid transport by the intestine (SCHULTZ and CURRAN 1970; see also Sect. E). In principle, such a mechanism alone could account, in energetic terms, for net transcellular Cl^- absorption, since the exit of Cl^- from the cell interior to the serosal medium would be a downhill process and, as such, would not require an input of external energy.

As already discussed (Sect. C.I. 1), ionic activity measurements in the absorptive cells of several intestinal preparations have confirmed that a^c_{Cl} does indeed exceed the value corresponding to electrochemical equilibrium. Electrophysiologic studies have also established that Na^+ and Cl^- transport across the apical cell membrane are energetically linked. Many of these studies were performed with the gallbladder which exhibits a coupled transapical NaCl transport similar to that found in the brush border membrane of the intestinal absorptive cell. Thus, in the gallbladder of the rabbit (DUFFEY et al. 1978) and *Necturus* (REUSS and GRADY 1979; GARCIA-DIAZ and ARMSTRONG 1980), and in the proximal renal tubule of *Necturus* (SPRING and KUMURA 1978), complete removal of Na^+ from the mucosal bathing solution causes a^c_{Cl} to decline to its equilibrium value across the apical cell membrane. Similarly, when Cl^- is absent from the mucosal bathing solution, a^c_{Na} falls to a very low value (ARMSTRONG et al. 1981). A number of substances have been found to inhibit coupled NaCl transport. These include cAMP and the diuretics furosemide and bumetanide. During cAMP inhibition of coupled NaCl in *Necturus* gallbladder a^c_{Cl} declined to a value that did not differ significantly from that corresponding to electrochemical Cl^- equilibrium across the apical cell membrane. Simultaneously, a^c_{Na} decreased to a level that corresponded to its value in a Cl^--free medium (ARMSTRONG et al. 1981). The essential electroneutrality of the coupled NaCl entry processes is supported by the finding that maneuvers such as replacement of Cl^- or of Na^+ in the mucosal medium by nontransported anions or cations and inhibition of the NaCl cotransport process by cAMP have no measurable effect on V_a (HENIN and CREMASCHI 1975; ARMSTRONG et al. 1981). It should be noted that, since the entry process is electroneutral, the appropriate driving force for net NaCl transport is $(\Delta\mu_{Na} + \Delta\mu_{Cl})$.

c) Na^+ and Cl^- Transport Across the Brush Border Membrane: Single Symport or Parallel Antiports?

In the preceding section, it was assumed that coupled NaCl entry across the brush border membrane of the intestinal absorptive cell occurs via NaCl symport on single carrier. However, an alternative model has been proposed for this process. This alternative stems from a suggestion originally made by TURNBERG et al. (1970) to explain some of their in vivo observations on electrolyte transfer by the human ileum. It postulates the existence, in the brush border membrane, of separate carriers for Na^+ and Cl^-. The Na^+ carrier is the Na^+/H^+ exchange system discussed in Sect. C.I. 2. a). The Cl^- carrier exchanges Cl^- for HCO_3^- (or OH^-). With both these processes operating in parallel across the brush border membrane,[8] the overall entry of Na^+ and Cl^- into the absorptive cell would be electroneutral.

To date, little direct electrophysiologic evidence has emerged that would permit one to discriminate between these two hypotheses. In fact, with whole cell preparations, such discrimination is difficult because experimental manipulations that affect the influx of Na^+ have concomitant effects on the influx of Cl^- and vice versa. Studies with isolated brush border vesicles have yielded more explicit information. LIEDKE and HOPFER (1977), working with brush border vesicles prepared from rat small intestine found that at least 60% of vesicular Cl^- uptake was mediated by an electroneutral mechanism, but stated that their experiments could not distinguish between a simple NaCl symport or a combination of a Na^+/H^+ antiport with a HCl symport. Na^+/H^+ antiport in brush border vesicles from rat small intestine was reported by MURER et al. (1976). More recent experiments by LIEDKE and HOPFER (1982a, b) have dealt more explicitly with the detailed mechanism of NaCl cotransport in this preparation. In the first of these papers (LIEDKE and HOPFER 1982a), the prediction of the NaCl symport model that, under appropriate conditions, the rate of Na^+ or Cl^- transport should increase with increasing concentrations of the counterion was found not to hold. On the contrary, the velocity of Na^+ or of Cl^- exchange was constant regardless of the ambient Cl^- or Na^+ concentration. Minimally, 70% of Cl^- exchange and 40% of Na^+ exchange proceeded by way of the pathways involved in net NaCl movement. Cl^- transport was saturable ($K_m = 255$ mM). These findings were interpreted to be consistent with a double exchange of Na^+ for H^+ and Cl^- for OH^- (or HCO_3^-).

In a subsequent paper (LIEDKE and HOPFER 1982b), Cl^-/OH^- exchange was demonstrated by the observation that concentrative Cl^- uptake could be driven by a pH gradient (extravesicular pH < intravesicular pH). A Cl^- conductance pathway was demonstrated by showing that concentrative Cl^- uptake could be driven by a K^+ diffusion potential (extravesicular K^+ concentration < intravesicular K^+ concentration). Furosemide and SITS strongly inhibited Cl^-/OH^- exchange (this accounted for about 63% of Cl^- transport) but did not affect Cl^- conductance, Na^+/Na^+ exchange, or Na^+-dependent glucose transport.

8 It should be emphasized that TURNBERG et al. (1970) did not specify the actual site of their putative double exchange system, and, indeed, their data did not permit this

In summary, although it has been rather generally assumed (FRIZZELL et al. 1979) that, in intact sheets of intestine and other epithelia, NaCl cotransport involves direct coupling, via a common carrier, between the transport of Na^+ and that of Cl^-, studies with membrane vesicles appear to challenge this view. These studies tend to support the concept that Na^+ and Cl^- entry into the epithelial cells involve separate, parallel pathways and that the coupling between Na^+ and Cl^- is indirect. According to this view, the H^+ gradient generated by Na^+/H^+ exchange is the coupling factor for NaCl cotransport.

Some recent experiments with intact sheets of *Necturus* gallbladder are of interest in the present context. WEINMAN and REUSS (1982) have presented evidence for an amiloride-inhibitable apical Na^+/H^+ exchange in this tissue, but have not determined if this is a significant component of overall NaCl cotransport. In a careful study of volume regulation by gallbladder epithelial cells and its response to changes in the external ionic milieu, specific transport inhibitors, etc., SPRING and ERICSON (1982) concluded that Na^+/H^+ and Cl^-/HCO_3^- exchange serve to mediate apical entry of Na^+ and Cl^- during regulatory increases in cell volume. During steady state transepithelial fluid absorption (i.e., when cell volume is constant), transapical entry of Na^+ and Cl^- is mediated by NaCl cotransport. Clearly, at this time, further experiments, particularly with intact epithelial preparations, and designed specifically to evaluate conflicting viewpoints concerning transapical Na^+ and Cl^- transport, are a crucial requirement in studies with the small intestine and other epithelial system.

3. Serosal Exit Processes

a) The Basolateral Na^+/K^+ Exchange Pump

As in virtually all animal cells, a^c_{Na} in absorptive cells of the small intestine is far below the level that corresponds to electrochemical equilibrium across either of the limiting cell membranes. Net Na^+ transfer from the cell interior to the serosal bathing medium is, therefore, an energy-requiring process. This situation, which is common to all vertebrate epithelia so far studied, was explicitly addressed by KOEFOED-JOHNSON and USSING (1958) in their model for transcellular Na^+ transport by the isolated frog skin, a model that rapidly established itself as the archetypal concept of transepithelial transport. A cardinal feature of this model is that the ubiquitous Na^+, K^+-ATPase pump, which is responsible for the maintenance of relatively low a^c_{Na} levels in virtually all animal cells, is, in frog skin, confined to the basolateral cell membrane. Therefore, in addition to its usual role in the regulation of a^c_{Na}, it serves, in this tissue, as a major mediator of net transepithelial Na^+ transport.

The applicability of this idea to transcellular Na^+ transport in the small intestine is supported by a number of observations. Autoradiographic studies (STIRLING 1972) and enzymatic analyses of intestinal cell fractions (QUIGLEY and GOTTERER 1969; FUJITA et al. 1972; DOUGLAS et al. 1972; MURER et al. 1974) have localized ouabain-binding sites and Na^+, K^+-ATPase activity to the basolateral cell membrane. Little or no Na^+, K^+-ATPase activity has been found in the brush border membrane. SAWADA and ASANO (1963) reported that ouabain abolished net transepithelial Na^+ transport by rat small intestine only when it was present in the serosal bathing medium. When added to the mucosal medium, the glycoside had no effect on Na^+ transport. This observation was confirmed for intact sheets of rabbit ileum (Schultz and Zalusky 1964a) and bullfrog small intestine (Gerencser and Armstrong 1972). Thus, the location of the Na^+, K^+-ATPase pump and the fact that the action of a powerful pump inhibitor is associated with cessation of net transepithelial Na^+ transport strongly suggest that the pump mechanism is a major component of transcellular Na^+ transport by the small intestine. However, the assumption that net transepithelial Na^+ transport and homocellular (i.e., intracellular) Na^+ and K^+ regulation are controlled by the same mechanism has been challenged by Nellans and Schultz (1976). These authors studied the relationship between transepithelial Na^+ transport and K^+ uptake (J^K_{sc}) across the basolateral cell membrane in a stripped preparation of rabbit ileum. Their results may be summarized as follows. In the presence of serosal ouabain or when Na^+ is absent from both the mucosal and the serosal bathing solutions, active Na^+ absorption is abolished and C^c_K decreases. In addition, J^c_{sc} is significantly inhibited. These results are consistent with a Na^+/K^+ exchange mechanism that subserves both transcellular Na^+ transport and homocellular Na^+ and K^+ regulation. However, when active Na^+ absorption is abolished by removing Na^+ from the mucosal medium only, J^c_{sc} and C^K_{sc} are not affected. Similarly, stimulation of Na^+ absorption by adding L-alanine or glucose to the mucosal medium does not affect J^K_{sc}.

Nellans and Schultz (1976; see also Schultz 1979 for a thorough discussion) argue that the "uncoupling" of net transepithelial Na^+ transport from J^K_{sc} demonstrated by their results, though not incompatible with the mediation of net transepithelial transport by a Na^+/K^+ exchange process in the basolateral cell membrane, does run counter to the notion that transepithelial transport and homocellular regulation are controlled by the same process. One interpretation of these results, which in Schultz's (1979) view finds considerable indirect support in the literature, is that the Na^+/K^+ exchange process involved in transepithelial Na^+ transport occurs between the serosal medium and a very small cellular Na^+ compartment, or "transport pool." Since the size of this putative pool is such that it is, by definition, below the detection limits of current methods for measuring cellular Na^+ and K^+ levels, its direct experimental demonstration will undoubtedly present a challenge.

Whatever the ultimate explanation may be for the "dissociation," in the experiments of Nellans and Schultz, between the mechanisms that mediate transepithelial Na^+ transport and those responsible for homocellular Na^+ and K^+ regulation, the available evidence is entirely consistent with the idea that net Na^+ exit across the basolateral membrane of the intestinal absorptive cell is, for all practical purposes, regulated by a ouabain-sensitive Na^+/K^+ exchange pump that is directly coupled to metabolic energy through the terminal phosphate bond of ATP. The question of the rheogenicity of this basolateral Na^+-pump, i.e., the extent to which it can contribute to V_T, is discussed in Sect. E.III.

b) Cl^- Transport Across the Basolateral Cell Membrane

The mechanism (or mechanisms) of net Cl^- exit across the basolateral membrane of the intestinal absorptive cell remains, to a large extent, poorly defined. In a strict thermodynamic sense, that is, if one considers the Cl^- ion only as a component of the transport process, basolateral Cl^- exit is an energetically downhill process. In principle, therefore, it could occur by simple electrodiffusion. It seems unlikely, however, that the Cl^- conductance of the basolateral membrane is sufficiently high to account for net Cl^- movement under steady state conditions (FRIZZELL et al. 1979). This is certainly so in the gallbladder where the ionic permeabilities of the apical and basolateral cell membranes have been more critically measured than in the small intestine (REUSS 1979). It also appears to be true for *Necturus* proximal tubule (SHINDO and SPRING 1981; GUGGINO et al. 1982). It seems reasonable to suppose that in the small intestine, as in the gallbladder, a major fraction of net Cl^- exit across the basolateral membrane of the absorptive cell occurs, under normal conditions, via mechanisms that involve the coupling of Cl^- transport to that of other ions.

Currently, two mechanisms for coupled Cl^- transport from the cell interior to the serosal medium appear to be supported by a number of observations in the literature. A considerable body of evidence suggests a role for HCO_3^- in this process. FIELD et al. (1978a) found that, in stripped intestinal preparation from the winter flounder *Pseudopleuronectes americanus,* maintained under short-circuit conditions, the rate of active Cl^- absorption depended directly on the external HCO_3^- concentration. This dependence was entirely mediated by changes in J_{ms}^{Cl}. GUNTER-SMITH and WHITE (1979b) observed that replacement, by other anions, of Cl^- or HCO_3^- in the solution bathing isolated segments of stripped *Amphiuma* intestine reversed the sign of the normally serosal positive V_T. They suggested the possible existence of a Cl^-/HCO_3^- exchange mechanism in this tissue. This conclusion has been well supported by subsequent studies, (e.g., WHITE and IMON 1981).

ARMSTRONG and YOUMANS (1980) examined the effect of external HCO_3^- on Cl^- transport by stripped preparations of bullfrog small intestine. In these experiments, V_T and I_{sc}, in HCO_3^--free media, did not differ significantly from zero. Following the addition of 25 m*M* HCO_3^- to the bathing solution, V_T and I_{sc} became serosal negative, and assumed values that differed significantly from zero. Radiotracer flux measurements, under short-circuit conditions showed that in the presence of external HCO_3^-, J_{ms}^{Cl} was substantially increased. There was no corresponding change in J_{sm}^{Cl} so that a large absorption of Cl^- was induced. At the same time, a highly significant residual flux, consistent with a net serosal to mucosal flow of negative charge, appeared. Because of its absolute dependence on the presence of HCO_3^- in the external medium, this was construed as a net secretion of HCO_3^-, reminiscent of that found in *Amphiuma* intestine (GUNTER-SMITH and WHITE 1979b).

These results were interpreted as indicating the presence, in the basolateral membrane of the absorptive cell, of a coupled Cl^-/HCO_3^- exchange mechanism that, in the presence of external HCO_3^-, facilitates the exit of Cl^- from the cells. In agreement with this idea, the HCO_3^--induced absorption of Cl^- appeared to be blocked by SITS, a known inhibitor of Cl^-/HCO_3^- exchange in other systems (CABANTCHIK et al. 1978). Because Cl^- absorption was accompanied by the development of a serosal negative V_T, ARMSTRONG and YOUMANS (1980) concluded that basolateral Cl^-/HCO_3^- exchange in bullfrog small intestine was rheogenic.

The model proposed by FIELD (see Sect. C.II.2) for Na^+ and Cl^- absorption in the flounder intestine offers an alternative explanation for this serosal negative V_T. The net secretion of HCO_3^- suggested by the experiments of ARMSTRONG and YOUMANS (1980), of which the putative basolateral Cl^-/HCO_3^- exchange mechanism forms a part, require a net movement of HCO_3^- from the cell interior to the mucosal medium. The nature of this transport process remains unknown.

An alternative proposal for coupled Cl^- movement from the cell interior to the serosal fluid in leaky epithelia such as the gallbladder and the small intestine was advanced by REUSS (1979). According to this proposal, Cl^- exits across the basolateral membrane of the gallbladder epithelial cell by an electroneutral KCl coupled symport. The driving force for this movement is given by $(\Delta\mu_K^{cs}+\Delta\mu_{Cl}^{cs})$. Although direct evidence in support of this hypothesis is still lacking, some indirect observations, particularly in the gallbladder, suggest that coupled KCl cotransport may be an important component of transcellular Cl^- transport by a number of epithelial systems (REUSS et al. 1980; DIEZ DE LOS RIOS et al. 1981; GUNTER-SMITH and SCHULTZ 1982). Further investigation of this possibility is clearly warranted at this time.[9]

4. Ionic Permeabilities of the Absorptive Cell Membranes

In addition to an estimate of the appropriate transmembrane electrochemical potential differences, the complete description of electrodiffusive ionic transfer across cell membranes requires a knowledge of individual ionic permeabilities. With many cell types, these are easily derived from the corresponding partial ionic conductances. These, in turn, are obtained from the change in the cell membrane potential that occurs when the ion in question is replaced, in the external solution, by a nonpermeant ion (HODGKIN and HOROWICZ 1959; STRICKHOLM and WALLIN 1967; FRÖMTER et al. 1971). However, in the small intestine and other leaky epithelia, this procedure does not yield unequivocal results. This is because the transcellular route for ion permeation is shunted by a highly conducting paracellular pathway (see Sect. C.II). Therefore, in general, measurements of V_a and V_s, in these systems, do not provide direct estimates of the intrinsic electromotive forces (emfs) across the apical and basolateral cell membranes. The same uncertainty applies to measured *changes* in V_a and V_s. Furthermore, since the paracellular shunt pathway shows marked ionic permselectivity (Sect. C.II.1), unilateral replacement of a given ion may generate a transepithelial diffusion potential across this pathway. This can also affect the observed change in V_a or V_s. As discussed later (Sect. D and Fig. 6), the electrical behavior of the small intestine and

9 It is interesting to reflect that the increasing evidence for coupled ionic transfer processes (i.e., processes in which the transmembrane chemical or electrochemical potential difference for an ion energizes the uphill movement of another ion or of an uncharged species) in the small intestine and other epithelial systems highlights, to a progressively greater degree, the role of the Na^+-pump as a "prime mover" in the energetic sense, of transepithelial transport. It is, au fond, the Na^+-pump that, to a great extent, conserves the other ionic gradients needed for the sustained operation of coupled epithelial transport systems. This view was clearly and articulately outlined a good many years ago by CSÁKY (1968). Probably because it was not, at that time, supported by specific models for coupled ionic transfer, CSÁKY's (1968) suggestion received rather scant attention. In retrospect, it appears as a remarkably prescient conclusion

other leaky epithelia can be analyzed in terms of a simple equivalent electrical circuit. With certain assumptions, and providing that the numerical values of the resistive elements in this circuit are known, one can calculate changes in the emf of the apical or basolateral cell membrane from observed changes in V_T and in the appropriate cell membrane potential. For a homogeneous flat epithelium, cable analysis can be used to calculate the magnitudes of the resistive elements in the equivalent electrical circuit model (EISENBERG and JOHNSON 1970; SHIBA 1971). This approach has been applied with some success to *Necturus* gallbladder (FRÖMTER 1972; REUSS and FINN 1975a, b). However, the complex geometry of the intestinal villi, together with the presence of different cell types, precludes this approach to the equivalent circuit analysis of the small intestine. A further difficulty in analyzing ionic conductances across the basolateral cell membrane arises from the existence of large unstirred layer effects. These effects are greatly enhanced, even in stripped intestinal preparations, by the presence of subserosal connective and muscular tissue elements. Therefore, one can obtain qualitative estimates only of relative ionic conductance across the apical and basolateral membranes in absorptive cells of the small intestine.

To date, only a few studies of the effect on V_a of ionic substitutions in the mucosal medium have been reported. Unfortunately, all of these are open to question, because of the complexities already outlined and because, in most of them, no account was apparently taken of a technical shortcoming that, if uncorrected, can attenuate, or completely mask changes in V_a induced by changes in the ionic composition of the external medium. This is the fact that, when the ionic composition of only one of the bathing media is changed, an asymmetric junction potential may be generated at the tip of the external electrode in that solution. This potential may be quite large, e.g., in a recent study with *Necturus* gallbladder (CORCIA et al. 1982), junction potentials of 9–10 mV were recorded when 90 m*M* Na gluconate was substituted for the same concentration of NaCl in the bathing medium. Methods for reducing, measuring, and correcting for such junction potentials are discussed by FRIZZELL and SCHULTZ (1972).

ROSE and SCHULTZ (1971) found that V_a in the rabbit ileum hyperpolarized when mucosal Na^+ was replaced by Tris [tris(hydroxymethyl)aminomethane] or by choline. Restoring Na^+ to the mucosal medium depolarized V_a. Replacement of mucosal Na^+ by K^+ did not appreciably affect V_a. Similarly, removal of external HCO_3^- or replacement of Cl^- by SO_4^{2-} did not significantly change V_a. It was concluded that the major ions contributing to the conductance of the brush border membrane are K^+ and Na^+ and that the membrane is about equally permeable to each of these ions.

BARRY and EGGENTON (1972a, b) studied the effects of mucosal ionic substitutions on V_a and V_T in rat jejunum. Their results may be summarized as follows. Substitution of KCl or LiCl for NaCl in the mucosal medium had little effect on V_a or V_T. Replacement of mucosal Na^+ by Tris-Cl or mannitol hyperpolarized V_a and decreased the serosal positive V_T to such an extent that V_s remained unchanged. Following ionic substitutions in the serosal medium, V_s and V_T changed in parallel so that V_a remained unaltered. The observed changes in V_a during ionic substitutions in the mucosal medium were analyzed in terms of the Goldman constant field equation (GOLDMAN 1943; HODGKIN and KATZ 1949). In this analysis

Cl^- was neglected since replacement of mucosal Cl^- by SO_4^{2-} had no apparent effect on V_a. Chemical estimates of C^c_{Na} were used in analyzing the results obtained. From this analysis, P_K/P_{Na} for the brush border membrane was calculated to be about 1.26.

It is difficult to assign more than a broadly qualitative significance to the results of BARRY and EGGENTON. The reasons for this are as follows. First, as discussed in Sect. C.I.1, the low V_a values recorded by these authors and the instability of their recordings strongly indicate severe membrane damage during their impalements. This alone would seriously compromise the results of their ionic substitution experiments. Second, there are no indications in their paper that the effects of asymmetric junction potentials on the observed changes in V_T were considered. Finally, the independent behavior of V_a and V_s in this study is surprising. It suggests that there is no electrical coupling between V_a and V_s, i.e., that the paracellular pathway has a much higher resistance than the transcellular route for ionic conductance. In other words, it suggests that the rat small intestine is a tight epithelium. BARRY and EGGENTON (1972b) apparently concluded that this was so and that the low R_T values exhibited by this preparation are entirely accounted for by the properties of the transcellular pathway. This runs counter to virtually every other electrophysiologic study of vertebrate small intestine yet published. Specifically, it contradicts the conclusions of CLARKSON (1967) and of MUNCK and SCHULTZ (1974) for the rat small intestine. MUNCK and SCHULTZ (1974) estimated that at least 85% of the total ionic conductance of the rat jejunum occurs via the paracellular pathway.

OKADA et al. (1975, 1976) reinvestigated the effects of mucosal ionic substitutions on V_a and V_T in rat jejunum. Their approach was as follows. Cells were impaled under control conditions and following a specific ionic substitution. The average V_a value was then calculated for each experimental condition. This procedure eliminates uncertainties arising from the generation of junction potentials during cell impalement with microelectrodes. It does, however, lead to considerable scatter in the data obtained. Moreover, there is reason to suspect that the V_a values recorded by OKADA et al. may have been affected by "pretip" potential artifacts (Sect. C.I.1). Nevertheless, they appear, on the whole, to be technically superior to those of BARRY and EGGENTON (1972b). When the ionic strength of the mucosal medium was maintained constant with Tris-Cl, OKADA et al. (1975) found that elevation of mucosal $[K^+]$, at constant mucosal $[Na^+]$, depolarized V_a. When mucosal $[K^+]$ was less than 50 mM, the relationship between $\log[K^+]$ and V_a was a straight line with a slope of 61.5 mV per decade. When mucosal $[K^+]$ was less than 40 mM, reducing mucosal $[Na^+]$, at constant $[K^+]$, hyperpolarized V_a. In a later paper, OKADA et al. (1976) showed that replacement of 65 mM Na^+, in the mucosal medium, by K^+ depolarized V_a from -52 to -28 mV. The concomitant change in V_T was less than 2 mV.

Using the Goldman equation and assuming that V_a represented "the effective emf of the duodenal epithelial cell membrane," OKADA et al. (1975, 1976) calculated that P_{Na}/P_K ranged from virtually zero at high mucosal K^+ concentrations to about 0.09 when mucosal $[K^+]$ was less than 10 mM. However, in their analysis, the shunting effect of the paracellular pathway was ignored, ionic concentrations instead of ionic activities were used and it was assumed that R_a, the resistance of the mucosal membrane, remained constant. If, however, the mucosal membrane has, as OKADA et al. concluded, a much higher conductance for K^+ than for Na^+, replacement of Na^+ by K^+ should cause R_a to decrease. As outlined explicitly in Sect. D, equivalent circuit analysis shows that such a decrease, aside from any change in the intrinsic emf across the mucosal membrane, can result in a depolarization of V_a. The apparent variability of P_{Na}/P_K reported by OKADA et al. could, in part at least, arise from this cause.

In summary, one may say that the studies just reviewed on the ionic permeability of the mucosal membrane in absorptive cells of the small intestine permit the qualitative conclusion that $P_K > P_{Na}$. The contribution of Cl^- to mucosal membrane conductance appears to be much less[10] than that of K^+ or Na^+. For reasons that have been sufficiently elaborated, current estimates of the numerical relationship between P_K and P_{Na} are highly questionable. It is doubtful if the few measurements available so far permit even qualitative conclusions to be drawn concerning ionic permeabilities in the basolateral cell membrane. From an energetic viewpoint one might surmise that P_{Na} in this membrane is very low. This would favor efficient operation of the basolateral Na^+ pump by preventing a "backleak" of Na^+ into the cells via a conductive pathway in the basolateral membrane. This appears to be true for the gallbladder where P_{Na} for the basolateral cell membrane seems to be close to zero (REUSS 1979). Moreover, it has been claimed (SCHULTZ et al. 1974) that, in rabbit ileum, J_{sm}^{Na} is mediated entirely by the paracellular pathway so that little or no recycling of Na^+ occurs through the basolateral cell membrane.

In conclusion, it might seem that, from the paucity of the experimental data available and the uncertainties inherent in the conclusions derived from them the rather detailed discussion of ionic permeabilities in the small intestine presented herein is, at best, marginally justified. The authors' intent, however, is to draw attention to the fact that this is, at present, one of the most poorly defined areas in intestinal electrophysiology and to emphasize the need for further, more carefully conceived experiments. Until reasonably accurate estimates of passive ionic permeabilities in the brush border and basolateral membranes of the intestinal absorptive cell become available, many aspects of intestinal ionic transfer will remain obscure.

II. The Paracellular Pathway

As already indicated (Sect. B and Table 1), the paracellular pathway is the major route for passive ionic permeation in the small intestine and other leaky epithelia. It is, therefore, scarcely surprising to find that, in these systems, the paracellular pathway plays an important regulatory role in the ion transport and bioelectric

10 The studies of LIEDKE and HOPFER (1982a) with brush border vesicles suggest that Cl^- conductance in the mucosal membrane of rat intestine may be higher than one might suppose from the electrophysiologic studies reviewed in this section. Aside from the uncertainties involved in the electrophysiologic measurements, the question whether brush border vesicles have the same ionic permeabilities as the parent membranes from which they are derived, or whether, during isolation, they become more leaky to ions remains open

properties of the tissue as a whole. In the present section, the consequences of this role are analyzed.

1. Ionic Permeabilities

The relative ionic permeabilities of the paracellular pathway in a number of small intestinal preparations and in other leaky epithelia have been explored in some detail. Basically, two approaches have been used in these studies. These are: (1) to determine the effect of unilateral ionic substitutions on V_T and to analyze the ΔV_T values obtained in terms of the Goldman–Hodgkin–Katz constant field equation (HODGKIN and KATZ 1949); (2) to measure the effect of an imposed V_T on unidirectional or net ionic fluxes. When both these approaches are applied to the same preparation under the same conditions, they yield essentially similar results (FRIZZELL and SCHULTZ 1972).

Table 5 summarizes the relative P_K, P_{Na}, and P_{Cl} values for the shunt pathway obtained in a number of studies with the small intestine. For comparative purposes, data for some other leaky epithelia are included.[11] The salient findings that emerge from these results are as follows. The relative ionic permeabilities of the shunt pathway are strikingly similar in a number of epithelia. Under normal physiologic conditions, this pathway is cation selective, e.g., the P_K/P_{Cl} value therein is significantly larger than the value in free solution (Table 5). This suggests that the shunt pathway presents a predominately negatively charged environment to diffusing ions. However, a number of findings are not consistent with the idea that this pathway behaves as a simple ion exchanger. For example, the conductance of ion exchangers is virtually independent of the ionic concentrations in the bathing solution until saturation of the ion exchanging sites is approached. In epithelia, the conductance is a linear function of concentration over a wide range (WRIGHT et al. 1971; WRIGHT 1972; FRIZZELL and SCHULTZ 1972).

Similarly, consideration of the shunt pathway as a neutral pore, i.e., a channel lined with electronegative sites that lack a net charge (e.g., carbonyl groups), though compatible with some features of cation permeability (BARRY et al. 1971), also encounters difficulties. One of these concerns the effect of pH and of polyvalent cations on shunt permeability. In rabbit gallbladder (WRIGHT and DIAMOND 1968), and rat jejunum (SMYTH and WRIGHT 1966), reduction of the external pH to about 3 changes the shunt from a cation-selective to an anion-selective pathway. A similar reversal of selectivity has been observed when rabbit gallbladder is exposed to La^{3+} (WRIGHT and DIAMOND 1968) or Th^{4+} (MACHEN and DIAMOND 1972). Such observations suggest the presence, in the shunt pathway, of fixed negative charges (e.g., carboxyl and/or phosphoryl groups) with a pK_a of 3–4. Reduction of the external pH would titrate these groups and permit the selectivity of the shunt pathway to be dominated by positively charged groups. FRIZZELL and SCHULTZ (1972) suggested that the channels in the shunt pathway

11 More comprehensive tabulations, including relative permeabilities for Cs^+, Rb^+, and Li^+ are given by ERLIJ and MARTINEZ-PALOMO (1979) and by SCHULTZ (1979). A very comprehensive survey of current knowledge and ideas concerning the structure and properties of the paracellular pathway will be found in a recent collection of papers edited by BRADLEY and PURCELL (1982)

Table 5. Relative ionic permeabilities of the shunt pathway in leaky epithelia

	P_K	P_{Na}	P_{Cl}
Rabbit ileum 1)	1.14	1.0	0.55
Rat jejunum 2)	1.6	1.0	0.2
Rat jejunum 3)	1.2	1.0	0.1
Rat ileum 4)		1.0	0.8
Human ileum 5), 6)	1.2	1.0	0.3
Frog jejunum 7)	1.47	1.0	0.25
Rabbit gallbladder 8)	1.7	1.0	0.33
Rat proximal tubule 9)	1.1	1.0	0.65
Frog choroid plexus 7)	1.27	1.0	0.69
Free solution 10)	1.47	1.0	1.52

1) FRIZZELL and SCHULTZ (1972)
2) MUNCK and SCHULTZ (1974)
3) WRIGHT (1966)
4) CLARKSON (1967)
5) TURNBERG et al. (1970)
6) TURNBERG (1971)
7) WRIGHT (1972)
8) BARRY et al. (1971)
9) FROMTER et al. (1971)
10) ROBINSON and STOKES (1965)

are lined with oppositely charged groups in approximately equal numbers. These are equivalent to a complex of zwitterions. Thus, overall, these channels behave, in many respects, like neutral pores. Cation selectivity could be explained by postulating that the anionic groups are aligned in such a way that they restrict the entry of anions into and/or the mobility of anions within the channels. This is an attractive suggestion but, to date, the data available do not permit an unequivocal choice between a number of competing models for the ionic permeability of the shunt pathway (ERLIJ and MARTINEZ-PALOMO 1979).

The relative permeabilities of the shunt pathway in leaky epithelia to alkali metal cations show a very similar pattern to the relative mobilities of these ions in free solution (ERLIJ and MARTINEZ-PALOMO 1979; SCHULTZ 1979). This strongly suggests that the shunt pathway presents a predominantly aqueous environment to permeating ions. In rabbit and rat small intestine, the shunt pathway is impermeable to tetramethylammonium ions (SCHULTZ 1979). This suggests an effective diameter of about 10–15 Å for the channels within the shunt. Similar dimensions have been estimated for the diameters of the conducting channels in the shunt pathway of rabbit and frog gallbladder (MORENO and DIAMOND 1975a, b).

2. Ion Transport

a) Na^+ Transport

FRIZZELL and SCHULTZ (1972) showed that diffusional Na^+ movement through a functionally neutral shunt pathway conforms to the Goldman constant field equation (Goldman 1943). On this basis, and assuming that the partial ionic conductance G_{Na} is independent of V_T, diffusional Na^+ movement through the shunt pathway can be analyzed as follows (Schultz and Curran 1974; Schultz 1979). The net diffusional Na^+ flux via the shunt pathway (dJ^{Na}_{net}) may be written as the sum of two unidirectional terms, i.e.,

$$dJ^{Na}_{net} = dJ^{Na}_{ms} - dJ^{Na}_{sm} , \qquad \text{(C.II.2a-1)}$$

when V_T is in the range ± 10 mV, the two terms on the right-hand side of Eq. (C.II.2a-1) can be approximated by

$$dJ^{Na}_{ms} = P_{Na}[Na^+]_m \exp(-FV_T/2RT) , \qquad \text{(C.II.2a-2)}$$

$$dJ^{Na}_{sm} = P_{Na}[Na^+]_s \exp(FV_T/2RT) . \qquad \text{(C.II.2a-3)}$$

Inserting Eqs. (C.II.2a-2) and (C.II.2a-3) in Eq. (C.II.2a-1) and putting $[Na^+]_m = [Na^+]_s$, one obtains as a first approximation

$$dJ^{Na}_{net} = -P_{Na}[Na^+]FV_T/RT . \qquad \text{(C.II.2a-4)}$$

It is apparent that Eq. (C.II.2a-2) or Eq. (C.II.2a-3) can be used to obtain an estimate of P_{Na}. When $V_T = O$, this is defined by the equation

$$P_{Na} = dJ^{Na}_{sm}/[Na^+]_s = dJ^{Na}_{ms}/[Na^+]_m . \qquad \text{(C.II.2a-5)}$$

P_{Na} may be estimated as follows (Frizzell and Schultz 1972). One may assume that the total unidirectional Na^+ flux (J^{Na}_{ms} or J^{Na}_{sm}) is the sum of a diffusive and a nondiffusive (cellular) component (cJ^{Na}). If it is further assumed that the cellular component is independent of V_T, one may write, taking J^{Na}_{ms} as an example,

$$J^{Na}_{ms} = cJ^{Na}_{ms} + P_{Na}[Na^+]_m \exp(-FV_T/2RT) . \qquad \text{(C.II.2a-6)}$$

If J^{Na}_{ms} is measured over an appropriate range of V_T values, Eq. (C.II.2a-6) predicts that the measured flux should be a linear function of $\exp(-FV_T/2RT)$ and should have an intercept, on the y-axis, of cJ^{Na}_{ms}.

From studies of this kind, Frizzell and Schultz (1972) determined the shunt permeability P^s_{Na} in rabbit ileum to be 0.035 cm h^{-1}. Insertion of this value, together with $V_T = 3$ mV and $[Na^+]_m = 140$ mM in Eq. (C.II.2a-4) gives -0.6 μequiv. cm^{-2} h^{-1} for dJ^{Na}_{net}. Since the rate of net Na^+ absorption under these conditions was only 2.3 μequiv. cm^{-2} h^{-1}, it is evident that, even at low V_T values, backflux through the paracellular shunt pathway can greatly modify the rate of Na^+ absorption by leak epithelia such as the small intestine.

An equation analogous to Eq. (C.II.2a-6) can be written for J^{Na}_{sm}. Schultz and Zalusky (1964b) and Nellans and Schultz (1976) showed that $cJ^{Na}_{sm} = 0$, i.e., the entire serosal to mucosal flux of Na^+ is paracellular. Desjeux et al. (1974) have contested this claim. In the same tissue under identical conditions they obtained a nonzero intercept when J^{Na}_{sm} was plotted as a function of $\exp(FV_T/2RT)$ and concluded that about 20% of J^{Na}_{sm} occurs via the cellular pathway. This discrepancy is not yet resolved (Schultz 1979). However, the conclusion that, in rabbit ileum, and presumably in the small intestine of other animal species, the greater part at least of J_{sm}^{Na} is paracellular seems well warranted.

b) Cl^- Transport

There is evidence that, at neutral or near-neutral pH, Cl^- movement through the paracellular shunt pathway occurs via a different route than the one that mediates the movement of Na^+ and other cations (BARRY et al. 1971). The most direct evidence for this emerges from the studies of MORENO (1974, 1975 a, b) and MORENO and DIAMOND (1975 a, b), who have shown that certain polyamines, notably triaminopyridinium (TAP), which in its monoprotonated from has strong hydrogen bonding activity, reversibly reduces P_{Na} in rabbit, bullfrog, and *Necturus* gallbladder, rabbit and bullfrog small intestine, and bullfrog choroid plexus. In every case TAP increased R_T and reduced P_{Na} without affecting P_{Cl}. Unlike the Na^+ pathway which is highly cation selective, the Cl^- pathway seems to be best described as a free solution shunt (BARRY et al. 1971; MORENO and DIAMOND 1975b).

c) Paracellular Shunt Selectivity and V_{TO}

In the final analysis, V_{TO} in epithelial systems has its origin in the emfs that exist across the apical and basolateral cell membranes. These, in turn, are determined by the ionic transfer properties of the cellular pathway. However, in leaky epithelia, the presence of a highly conducting pathway in parallel with the transcellular route for ionic movements would be expected to reduce or attenuate V_{TO} significantly. There is compelling evidence that this is so. This "conductive" effect of the paracellular shunt pathway on V_{TO} is most conveniently analyzed in terms of equivalent electrical circuit models for the small intestine and other leaky epithelia, as shown in Sect. D. In the present section, some consequences of the cation selectivity of the paracellular shunt for V_{TO} and for Na^+ and Cl^- absorption in leaky epithelia will be discussed. Initially, the effects to be described arose from an ingenious proposal to explain the fact that, in rabbit gallbladder, V_{TO}, though small (< 1 mV) is normally serosal negative, even though Na^+ and Cl^- absorption by this tissue appears to be electrically neutral (MACHEN and DIAMOND 1969). According to this proposal, Na^+ and Cl^- are accumulated, in accordance with the predictions of the "standing osmotic gradient" hypothesis (DIAMOND and BOSSET 1967) in the lateral intercellular spaces. There they attain steady state concentrations in excess of those in the mucosal bathing solution. This concentration difference generates a driving force for the backdiffusion of NaCl into the mucosal media. Since the paracellular pathway is more permeable to Na^+ than to Cl^-, a mucosal positive V_{TO} is thereby generated.

FIELD (1981) has invoked a similar model for the isolated intestine of the winter flounder, *Pseudopleuronectes americanus*. In this model, the normally serosal negative V_{TO} observed with this preparation (see Table 1) and the fact that, under short-circuit conditions, $J_{net}^{Cl} > J_{net}^{Na}$ are accounted for by a "recycling" of Na^+ through the paracellular pathway. The serosal negative V_{TO} observed in isolated bullfrog small intestine when HCO_3^- is present in the bathing medium, and the enhanced Cl^- absorption seen under these conditions when this preparation is short-circuited (ARMSTRONG and YOUMANS 1980; see Table 1 and Sect. C.I.3), also appear to be consistent with this model.

D. Analysis of Intestinal Electrical Parameters in Terms of Electrical Equivalent Circuits

It will be apparent from earlier sections of this chapter that analysis of the electrical characteristics of epithelia, particularly leaky epithelia, presents a number of difficulties. These arise from two major sources. First, unlike symmetric cells, e.g., those of nerve and muscle, epithelial cells have a definite polarity. This means that specific transport properties and specific ionic permeabilities are asymmetrically distributed between the apical and basolateral cell membranes. Second, the conductive paracellular pathway permits electrical communication between these morphologically and functionally distinct membranes, i.e., the two cell membranes are electrically coupled through this pathway. This is particularly important in leaky epithelia like the small intestine. In analyzing the electrophysiologic behavior of epithelial systems it is, therefore, necessary to utilize conceptual models that take account of these facts.

Figure 6 shows a "lumped" electrical equivalent circuit that has been widely used for the electrophysiologic analysis of the small intestine (White and Armstrong 1971; Rose and Schultz 1971; Armstrong et al. 1975; Okada et al. 1976) and other leaky epithelia (Boulpaep 1971; Frömter 1972; Reuss and Finn 1975a). Slightly different representations of this circuit are given by various authors, but all of them can be reduced to the form shown in Fig. 6. In this figure, V_a and V_T are measured with respect to a grounded mucosal solution. E_a and E_s are the intrinsic emfs of the mucosal and serosal cell membranes, and R_a and R_s are the corresponding lumped transmembrane resistances. The paracellular pathway is represented by an emf E_j and a lumped resistance R_j. This representation of the total resistance across the junctional intercellular space complexes assumes that this resistance is localized, i.e., that the resistances of the intercellular spaces are negligible compared with those of the tight junctions. This may not be strictly true for leaky epithelia such as the small intestine. If it is not, then one must consider a distributed resistance model, such as the one discussed by Boulpaep and Sackin (1980), for the paracellular pathway. The implications of this are discussed in the closing paragraphs of this section.

E_j in Fig. 6 is a diffusion potential across the paracellular pathway. Because of the permselectivity of this pathway, E_j may be quite high when the mucosal and serosal bathing solutions have different ionic compositions. However, even when these solutions are identical, the accumulation of salt in the intercellular

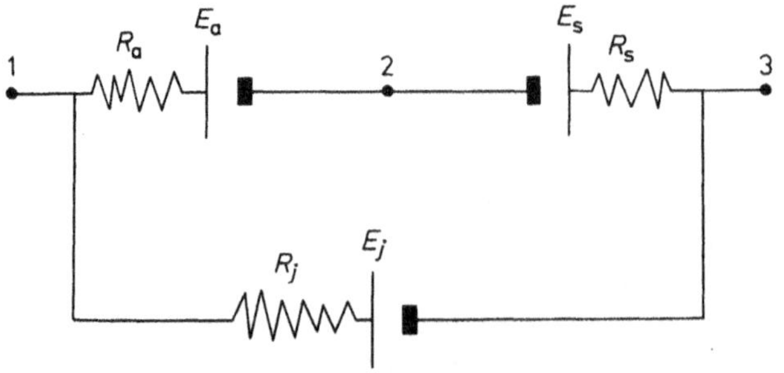

Fig. 6. An equivalent electrical circuit model for the small intestine

spaces owing to active Na^+ and Cl^- absorption (DIAMOND and BOSSERT 1967) can generate a diffusion potential of 1–2 mV across the shunt pathway (MACHEN and DIAMOND 1969; GARCIA-DIAZ and CORCIA 1977). Since, in this pathway, $P_{Na} > P_{Cl}$ (Table 5), the orientation of E_j will be as shown in Fig. 6, i.e., E_j will be serosal negative. The orientation of E_s is assumed to be the same as that of the measured membrane potential V_s, i.e., the cell interior is negative with respect to the serosal solution. This is consistent with the fact (Sect. C.I.4) that P_{Na} in the basolateral cell membrane is probably much smaller than P_K. Furthermore, as discussed in Sect. E.III, the active Na^+ transport mechanism in this membrane may be rheogenic and contribute to a serosal positive E_s.

There has been some controversy concerning the orientation of E_a in the small intestine. As will appear from the analysis to be presented, the orientation of the measured V_a does not necessarily coincide with the orientation of E_a. This is because E_s, through the paracellular pathway, can modify V_a. The uncertainty about the real orientation of E_a in the small intestine stems from the lack of fully convincing data concerning the ionic permeabilities of the mucosal cell membrane (Sect. C.I.4). Nevertheless, the orientation shown in Fig. 6 seems probable. From the data of OKADA et al. (1975, 1976), P_{Na} in this membrane, appears to be much smaller than P_K. If one takes the a^c_K and a^c_{Na} values for *Necturus* intestine shown in Fig. 5 as representative of the small intestine in general, application of the Goldman equation shows that for any value of P_{Na}/P_K less than unity, E_a will have the orientation shown in Fig. 6. The experiments of ARMSTRONG et al. (1975) with isolated bullfrog intestine provide additional evidence in favor of this orientation. These authors showed that, if one assumes that, in essence, the only effect of changes in external osmolality is to alter R_j, the observed changes in V_a following alterations in the osmolality of the bathing media are consistent with the orientation of E_a shown in Fig. 6. However, the assumption underlying these experiments requires further experimental examination since REUSS and FINN (1977) reported that, in *Necturus* gallbladder, hyperosmolality of the mucosal bathing solution decreased R_a, in addition to causing an increase in R_j. In any event is should be emphasized that the following analysis of the electrical equivalent circuit shown in Fig. 6 does not depend on the actual orientation of E_a. For an orientation opposite to that shown, it is necessary only to change the sign of E_a in the appropriate equations.

Assume that a current I is passed through the circuit in the serosal to mucosal direction. Then, since the voltages across the cellular and paracellular pathways must be equal, one may write

$$-E_a + E_s + I_c(R_a + R_s) = -E_j + I_j R_j \,. \tag{D.1}$$

In this equation I_c and I_j are the fractions of I that flow through the cellular and paracellular pathways, respectively. Rearranging Eq. (D.1) and substituting $I_j = (I - I_c)$ one obtains

$$I_c = (E_a - E_s - E_j + IR_j)/(R_a + R_s + R_j) \tag{D.2}$$

V_a, V_s, and V_T are obtained from the expressions

$$V_a = -E_a + I_c R_a\,; \quad V_s = E_s + I_c R_s\,; \quad V_T = -E_j + (I - I_c)\,R_j \tag{D.3}$$

and are readily calculated to be as follows:

$$V_a = [-E_a(R_s + R_j) - (E_s + E_j) R_a + IR_jR_a]/R_t \,, \tag{D.4}$$

$$V_s = [E_s(R_a + R_j) + (E_a - E_j) R_s + IR_jR_s]/R_t \,, \tag{D.5}$$

$$V_T = [-E_j(R_a + R_s) + (E_s - E_a) R_j + IR_j(R_a + R_s)]/R_t \,. \tag{D.6}$$

In these equations $R_t = R_a + R_s + R_j$. Under open-circuit conditions (ARMSTRONG et al. 1975), $I = 0$ and the third term inside the brackets disappears from Eqs. (D.4), (D.5), and (D.6). When small current pulses of amplitude ΔI are passed through the epithelium, the corresponding changes in V_a, V_s, and V_T are readily obtained from these equations as follows

$$\Delta V_a = \Delta I(R_jR_a/R_t) \,; \quad \Delta V_s = \Delta I(R_jR_s/R_t) \,; \quad \Delta V_T = \Delta I[R_j(R_a + R_s)/R_t] \,. \tag{D.7}$$

The transepithelial resistance is given by

$$R_T = \Delta V_T/\Delta I = R_j(R_a + R_s)/R_t \,. \tag{D.8}$$

Furthermore,

$$\Delta V_a/\Delta V_T = R_a/(R_a + R_s) = FR_a \,; \; \Delta V_s/\Delta V_T = R_s/(R_a + R_s) = FR_s \tag{D.8 a, b}$$

Eqs. (D.8 a) and (D.8 b) define the fractional resistance of the mucosal and serosal cell membranes, respectively. These are the fractions of the total transcellular resistance contributed by each of these membranes. Note that, in this analysis, FR_a and FR_s are independent of the magnitude of R_j.

These relationships are of practical use in microelectrode studies with epithelial systems (see Sect. C.I.1). Thus, by applying transepithelial current pulses of known amplitude while a microelectrode is inside a cell, one can monitor R_T and FR_a in addition to V_a and V_T. Since $V_s = V_T - V_a$ and $FR_s = 1 - FR_a$, these parameters can also be obtained. The use of FR_a as a criterion for assessing the quality of microelectrode impalements with flat sheets of epithelial cells has already been discussed (Sect. C.I.1; see also ARMSTRONG and GARCIA-DIAZ 1981).

By setting $V_T = 0$ in Eq. (D.6), the short-circuit current I_{sc} is obtained [12] as

$$I_{sc} = (E_j/R_j) + (E_a - E_s)/(R_a + R_s) \,. \tag{D.9}$$

Equation (D.9) predicts that, if $E_j = 0$, I_{sc} does not depend on the properties of the shunt pathway. In other words, if the shunt pathway has the properties of a simple ohmic resistor, any change in R_j will affect V_T and R_T to the same proportionate degree. Thus, I_{sc} will remain unchanged. On the other hand, if $E_j \neq 0$, a change in R_j will not affect V_T and R_T equally and will give rise to a concomitant change in I_{sc}.

This prediction was used by ARMSTRONG et al. (1975) to examine the significance of E_j in the steady state electrical behavior of the isolated small intestine when both the mucosal and serosal bathing solutions have the same ionic composition. Earlier analyses (WHITE and ARMSTRONG 1971; ROSE and SCHULTZ 1971) had assumed that E_j is significant only when the small intestine is bathed by ionically asymmetric solutions. When these solutions are symmetric, it was assumed that E_j is negligible, i.e., the paracellular pathway could be modeled as a simple

12 Note that I_{sc} can be obtained from Eqs. (D.5) and (D.6) by means of the equation $I_{sc} = -(V_T/R_T)$

resistor. ARMSTRONG et al. (1975) simultaneously changed the osmolality of the mucosal and serosal media that bathed sheets of isolated bullfrog small intestine. This was done without altering their ionic composition. It was assumed in these experiments that the predominant, if not the sole effect of these changes was on R_j, i.e., that lowering the external osmolality increased R_j and vice versa. In agreement with the predictions of Eq. (D.9), it was found that, when the external osmolality was changed, I_{sc} also changed and that the change in I_{sc} was in the opposite direction to the presumptive change in R_j.

These results indicate that, even when the solutions bathing both sides of the small intestine have identical ionic compositions, E_j must be taken into account in any attempt to analyze the electrical behavior of this tissue. However, some comments are in order. First, as already mentioned, the assumption that the electrical responses of the small intestine to changes in the osmolality of the external media can be accounted for exclusively, or virtually exclusively, by corresponding changes in R_j, although it forms a consistent basis for a number of observations by ARMSTRONG et al. (1975), as yet lacks confirmation from other studies. Second, the experiments of ARMSTRONG et al. (1975) were performed in a sodium sulfate medium. Since it is highly likely that P_{Na}/P_{SO_4} in the shunt pathway is significantly greater than the corresponding value of P_{Na}/P_{Cl}, it might be argued that the use of a sulfate medium amplifies the relative importance of changes in R_j when the external osmolality is varied. However, the osmotically induced electrical effects reported by GARCIA-DIAZ and CORCIA (1977) for the isolated rat jejunum bathed by NaCl media suggest that the results of ARMSTRONG et al. (1975) may be rather generally applicable to the small intestine in vitro.

Under voltage clamp conditions, (V_T = constant), the equivalent electrical circuit model shown in Fig. 6 yields simpler expressions for V_a and V_s than those given by Eqs. (D.4) and (D.5). Rewriting Eq. (D.1) in the form

$$V_T = -E_a + E_s + I_c(R_a + R_s)\,, \tag{D.10}$$

where V_T is now the external command voltage, one obtains for the current I_c through the cellular pathway

$$I_c = (V_T + E_a - E_s)/(R_a + R_s)\,. \tag{D.11}$$

If, now, one inserts this value for I_c in the expressions for V_a and V_s given by Eq. (D.3), one obtains

$$V_a = -[(E_a R_s + E_s R_a)/(R_a + R_s)] + FR_a V_T \tag{D.12}$$

and

$$V_s = [(E_a R_s + E_s R_a)/(R_a + R_s)] + FR_s V_T\,, \tag{D.13}$$

where FR_a and FR_s are defined by Eqs. (D.8 a, b). Under short-circuit conditions $V_T = 0$ and

$$-V_a^{sc} = V_s^{sc} = (E_a R_s + E_s R_a)/(R_a + R_s)\,. \tag{D.14}$$

Note that Eq. (D.14) states that, under short-circuit conditions, V_a and V_s do not depend on the properties of the shunt pathway.

So far, the equivalent circuit analysis presented herein rests on the assumption that the resistance of the intercellular space to the flow of electric current is small enough to be neglected. In other words, it has been assumed that the total resistance of the paracellular pathway is, effectively, confined to the tight junction. If this is not so, and the resistance of the intercellular space is significant, relative to that of the tight junction, the "lumped" model for R_j shown in Fig. 6 is no longer appropriate. Instead, a distributed model must be employed. A simple calculation suggests that this may be true for leaky epithelia like the small intestine. If one assumes that R_j is approximately equal to R_T, then R_j falls in the range 30–100 Ω cm^2 for a number of leaky epithelia. BOULPAEP and SACKIN (1980) estimated that the resistances of the lateral intercellular spaces may lie between 6 and 60 Ω cm^2. Thus there is a strong possibility that these spaces could contribute significantly to R_j in the small intestine.

A distributed equivalent circuit model such as that analyzed in detail by BOULPAEP and SACKIN (1980) has important implications for the measurement of electrical parameters in epithelia. For example, this model predicts that, for any finite value of the ratio between the intercellular space resistance and the total shunt resistance (R_j of Fig. 6), the relationship $\Delta V_a/\Delta V_T = FR_a$ (Eq. 8a) will not hold. On the contrary, under these conditions, $\Delta V_a/\Delta V_T < R_a/(R_a+R_s)$. For a given value of R_a/R_j, the amount by which $R_a/(R_a+R_s)$ exceeds $\Delta V_a/\Delta V_T$ will increase as the intercellular space resistance increases relative to R_j. Thus, in leaky epithelia, the apparent value of FR_a obtained by measuring $\Delta V_a/\Delta V_T$ may be significantly smaller than its true value. It should be noted however that, as long as the ratio of the intercellular space resistance to R_j remains essentially constant, the use of $\Delta V_a/\Delta V_T$ as an empirical criterion for the acceptability of microelectrode impalements (Sect. C.I.1) is entirely legitimate.

E. Na^+-Coupled Transport of Organic Solutes by the Small Intestine

It is now clear that active transepithelial Na^+ transport by the small intestine plays an essential role in the transfer, across this tissue, of a wide variety of solutes. This role can be direct or indirect. Indirect coupling between the transport of Na^+ and that of other solutes arises from the enhancing effect of this ion on water absorption. There is convincing evidence that increased water absorption by the small intestine is associated with a widening of the lateral intercellular spaces and an increase in the permeability of the shunt pathway to ions and low molecular weight nonelectrolytes. Thus, diffusive and convective (i.e., solvent drag) movements of low molecular weight solutes across the intestinal wall may be enhanced. Conversely, decreased water absorption, or secretion of water, has opposite effects. This indirect coupling between the intestinal transport of Na^+, water, and other solutes is discussed in Chap. 12. Direct coupling, through interactions with putative carrier systems in the apical or basolateral cell membrane, between the transport of Na^+ and that of a variety of other solutes has been demonstrated. Some examples, e.g., coupling between the transport of Na^+ and that of other ions (K^+, Cl^-) have already been described (Sect. C.I). In this section we will discuss the coupled transport of Na^+ and certain organic solutes. Hexose sugars and amino acids will be mainly considered, since these are the examples that have been most extensively studied. It should be noted, however, that there is evidence for a direct involvement of Na^+ in the transport of other solutes, e.g., oligopeptides (MATTHEWS 1975) and biotin (BERGER et al. 1972) by the intestine.

Moreover, it appears that the phenomenon of Na^+-coupled transport is of very wide occurrence throughout the plant and animal kingdoms (SCHULTZ and CURRAN 1970; HEINZ 1972). In the present discussion the major emphasis will be on the effects of actively transported sugars and amino acids on Na^+ transport and its electrical correlates. The converse question, i.e., the effect of Na^+ on sugar and amino acid uptake by the small intestine is most appropriately considered in the context of sugar or amino acid uptake per se (Chap. 16).

I. Transepithelial Effects: The Na^+ Gradient Hypothesis

Although the stimulation, by Na^+, of intestinal sugar transport had been noted by Wayland Reid as early as 1900 (see SCHULTZ and CURRAN 1968) and became the subject of intensive study following its rediscovery in the late 1950s (RIKLIS and QUASTEL 1958; CSÁKY and THALE 1960), there was, for some time, considerable uncertainty about the exact nature of this phenomenon. Specifically, it was for a time unclear whether the uphill absorption of sugars, and other organic solutes, merely required the presence, in the mucosal medium, of Na^+ (which might function as some kind of activator for solute transfer without being itself transported) or whether there was a direct coupling between the transport of Na^+ and that of sugars. If the latter is the mechanism involved, the reciprocity principle requires that those solutes whose transport is Na^+ dependent should, in turn, enhance Na^+ absorption. The first clear indication that this might be so stemmed from the observation (CLARKSON et al. 1961); that the addition of glucose to the solution bathing the mucosal surface of the small intestine induced a rapid, sustained increase in V_T. Initially, it was suggested that the glucose-induced increase in V_T was due to the fact that exogenous glucose provided additional metabolic energy for transepithelial Na^+ transport (CLARKSON et al. 1961). However, it soon became apparent (SCHACTER and BRITTEN 1961; BARRY et al. 1962) that hexose-induced increases in V_T were correlated with the ability of sugars to undergo uphill (i.e., active) transport rather than with their utility as metabolic fuels. Actively transported amino acids were also found to induce rapid and sustained increases in V_T (BAILLIEN and SCHOFFENIELS 1962). This finding was confirmed by KOHN et al. (1966) who also observed that some dipeptides and disaccharides exert similar effects.

SCHULTZ and ZALUSKY (1963a) showed that the glucose-induced increase in V_T is abolished by anoxia, KCN, or serosal ouabain. The first two of these findings indicate that this increase depends on the oxidative metabolism of the absorptive cell. In an extensive series of studies with rabbit ileum (SCHULTZ and ZALUSKY 1963b; 1964a, b; 1965) these authors established, inter alia, that sugar- and amino acid-evoked increases in V_T were accompanied by and dependent upon concomitant changes in active mucosal to serosal Na^+ transport. It will be recalled (Sect. B.II) that, in their experiments, net mucosal to serosal Na^+ transport under short-circuit conditions corresponded to I_{sc}. The changes in V_T and I_{sc} induced by sugars and amino acids were saturable functions of mucosal Na^+ concentration. Moreover, they were equivalent, i.e., solute-induced Na^+ transport had no measurable effect on R_T. However, the changes in V_T induced by sugars and amino acids were additive. This suggests the involvement of separate mechanisms in the stimulation of Na^+ transport by each of these two classes of solute. Similar results were obtained with the isolated rat intestine by SAWADA and ASANO (1963), ASANO (1965), and BARRY et al. (1965).

R. J. C. BARRY and his colleagues examined the relationship between hexose-induced increases in V_T, hexose transfer, and hexose metabolism in the rat intestine. Their studies showed that both glucose and an actively transported but poorly metabolized sugar, galactose, induced sustained increaes in V_T under aerobic conditions. Under anaerobic conditions, glucose only was effective. Phlorhizin, in concentrations that were known to prevent sugar entry into the absorptive cells, but not to inhibit sugar metabolism (NEWEY et al. 1959) abolished hexose-induced increases in V_T.

CRANE and his associates (see, e.g., BOSAKOVA and CRANE 1965a, b; LYON and CRANE 1966a, b) studied in detail the effect of actively transported sugars on V_T in the rat intestine. These and other studies led CRANE (1962, 1965) to formulate a model for Na^+-coupled sugar transport that, under the sobriquet "the sodium gradient hypothesis" has become a cornerstone of contemporary interpretations of Na^+-coupled transport processes in general (ARMSTRONG et al. 1979b). The essential features of this model are as follows. The primary event underlying the stimulatory effect of actively transported sugars (and other solutes) on Na^+ transport (and, in a reciprocal sense, the stimulatory effect of Na^+ on the transport of these solutes – see Chap. 16) is a coupled entry, via a mobile carrier in the brush border membrane, of Na^+ and sugar into the absorptive cell. The carrier is supposed to be a "bifunctional" entity, that is, it is supposed to possess two specific binding sites, one for Na^+ and one for sugar. It is well established (see Chap. 8) that sugar transport via this carrier mechanism is accumulative, i.e., the steady state intracellular concentration exceeds that of the mucosal medium. Since the movement of sugar is coupled to that of Na^+; sugar accumulation does not, in principle, require an input of external energy. It could be, as CRANE (1962, 1965) proposed, energized by the transapical Na^+ gradient. However, since the operation of the coupled carrier mechanism involves dissipation of this gradient, there is an indirect requirement for external energy. This is required to conserve or restore the Na^+ gradient and allow the coupled transport process to function continuously. In the intact living cell, this is accomplished by the basolateral Na^+/K^+ exchange pump. The model does not specifically address the question of sugar exit across the basolateral membrane of the absorptive cell. This is a downhill process in the energetic sense and could be accomplished either by diffusive transport or via a carrier.

CRANE's model accounts satisfactorily, in a qualitative manner, for the effects of actively transported sugars on V_T and I_{sc} already noted. In addition, it readily explains the observed correlation between these effects and the ability of a given sugar to be actively transported rather than its utility as a metabolic substrate. At the same time it explains the need for a supply of metabolic energy to sustain, over extended time periods, the effect of transported sugars on V_T and I_{sc} and accounts for the inhibition of these effects by phlorhizin which blocks sugar transport across the brush border membrane. It is not too surprising, therefore, that this model stimulated intensive investigations of the interrelationships between the intestinal transport of Na^+ and that of sugars (see, e.g., BIHLER 1968; SMYTH

1968; SCHULTZ and CURRAN 1970; KIMMICH 1973, for useful reviews of these studies). Extension of the Na^+-gradient hypothesis to the coupled transport of Na^+ and amino acids by the small intestine (SCHULTZ and CURRAN 1970) aroused a similar interest in Na^+–amino acid interactions at the brush border membrane of the absorptive cell. Nevertheless, many pertinent questions remained unanswerable by the "black box" approach involved in measuring transepithelial electrical parameters and transepithelial Na^+ fluxes. For example, as pointed out by CURRAN (1965), sugar- and amino acid-induced changes in V_T could not be analyzed unequivocally by these methods, because their site of origin (the brush border membrane, the basolateral membrane, or both of these) remained obscure. Further progress in understanding the mechanisms of these coupled transfer processes required the use of techniques such as intracellular recording and studies with isolated membrane vesicles. The application of these techniques to the study of Na^+-coupled transport in the small intestine is reviewed in the following sections.

II. Intracellular Effects: The Electrical Potential Profile of the Absorptive Cell

The results of early studies on the effects of actively transported organic solutes on the transcellular potential profile in the small intestine were conflicting. Studies by GILLES-BAILLIEN and SCHOFFENIELS (1965) and by WRIGHT (1966) with intestinal preparations from the Greek tortoise, as well as WRIGHT's (1966) experiments with hamster intestine, suggested that the addition of actively transported sugars or amino acids to the mucosal medium had no effect on V_a. Consequently, V_T and V_s hyperpolarized to the same extent. Similar results were later reported for rat and rabbit intestine (LYON and SHEERIN 1971; BARRY and EGGENTON 1972a; HIRSCHORN and FRAZIER 1973). By contrast, in contemporaneous studies with bullfrog small intestine (WHITE and ARMSTRONG 1971) and rabbit ileum (ROSE and SCHULTZ 1971), it was found that actively transported sugars and amino acids depolarize V_a. This depolarization is uniquely dependent on the presence of Na^+ in the mucosal medium (ROSE and SCHULTZ 1971) and is elicited only by those sugars and amino acids that display a Na^+-dependent entry into the absorptive cell (WHITE and ARMSTRONG 1971; ROSE and SCHULTZ 1971). At the same time, V_T hyperpolarizes, but this hyperpolarization is significantly smaller than the concomitant depolarization of V_a (i.e., $\Delta V_a/\Delta V_T > 1$). Therefore, V_s must also depolarize, but to a smaller extent than V_a. As can be seen from Sect. D and as discussed in more detail in Sect. E.III, this response pattern is easily understood in terms of a relatively low resistance paracellular shunt that electrically couples the apical and basolateral membranes of the absorptive cell.

These conflicting findings point to two different sites for the transepithelial electrical effects of sugars and amino acids. Furthermore, they lead to conflicting conclusions concerning the rheogenicity, or otherwise, of the coupled Na^+ entry process. If V_s and V_T, but not V_a are affected, one must conclude that Na^+-coupled solute entry into the cell is electroneutral. On the other hand, depolarization of V_a clearly indicates a rheogenic Na^+ entry process. In terms of CRANE's (1962, 1965) carrier hypothesis, either conclusion is acceptable. This author suggested a counterflow of K^+, via the Na^+–sugar carrier, from the cell interior to the mucosal medium. This could result in the coupled entry process being, in the overall sense, electroneutral. However, from the standpoint of the Na^+-gradient hypothesis the rheogenicity or otherwise of the coupled entry process has important energetic connotations. For electroneutral entry involving 1/1 Na^+/K^+ exchange, the appropriate driving force would be the algebraic sum of the transmembrane chemical potential differences for the ions involved ($\Delta\mu_{Na}+\Delta\mu_K$). For rheogenic entry, the driving force is the transmembrane electrochemical potential difference for Na^+ ($\Delta\tilde{\mu}_{Na}$). In the first instance, one would not expect V_a to influence the rate of entry of Na^+ or sugars vie the coupled mechanism. In the second case, V_a would be expected to influence strongly the rate of coupled entry. Quantitatively, however, the influence of V_a on entry rates may be difficult to predict because movement of the charged complex across the cell membrane could be coupled to other nonconjugate driving forces (SCHULTZ 1979).

At this time there seems to be fairly compelling evidence that sugar and amino acid-coupled Na^+ entry across the brush border membrane is rheogenic (with electroneutrality being conserved by anion movement through a separate pathway) and that the pattern of electrical responses observed by WHITE and ARMSTRONG (1971) and by ROSE and SCHULTZ (1971) is correct. This evidence can be summarized as follows. In the first place, as pointed out by ARMSTRONG (1976) and by SCHULTZ (1979), it seems likely that the results of those studies that failed to disclose any effect of actively transported solutes on V_a are compromised by the existence of significant membrane damage during impalement. This is indicated by the fact that the V_a values reported were, in general, low (see Table 3) and lacked temporal stability. Few, if any of the criteria currently considered essential for evaluating membrane potential measurements in epithelial cells (ARMSTRONG and GARCIA-DIAZ 1981; see also Sect. C.I.1.a) were applied. It is easily seen that, if the mucosal membrane of a single absorptive cell in an intact intestinal sheet is severely damaged during impalement, the only observable response to an actively transported solute will be a change in V_T, since this is measured as a signal average from a large number of cells. Furthermore, the depolarization of V_a reported by WHITE and ARMSTRONG (1971), and by ROSE and SCHULTZ (1971) has been confirmed in the small intestine of the rat (OKADA et al. 1975) and in the intestine of *Amphiuma* (GUNTER-SMITH and WHITE /1979 a), *Necturus* (WARD and BOYD 1980; GUNTER-SMITH et al. 1982), and *Ascaris* (GRADY and REUSS 1981). Similar results have been reported for the proximal renal tubule, an epithelium that also exhibits Na^+-coupled sugar and amino acid transport (MARUYAMA and HOSHI 1972; FRÖMTER and LUER 1973; SAMARZIYA and FRÖMTER 1975). WARD and BOYD (1980) also showed that the addition of dipeptides to the solution bathing the mucosal surface of *Necturus* intestine depolarized V_a.

Further evidence for the rheogenicity of coupled Na^+ entry emerges from a number of studies with isolated brush border membrane vesicles and isolated enterocytes. Using brush border vesicles isolated from rat intestine, MURER and HOPFER (1974) and SIGRIST-NELSON et al. (1975) showed that the uptake of D-glucose and L-alanine can be stimulated by imposing an inside-negative potential difference across the vesicular wall. This was done by establishing a cation (e.g.,

K^+, H^+) gradient between the inside and the outside of the vesicle and adding an appropriate ionophore (e.g., valinomycin, carbonyl cyanide *p*-trifluoromethoxyphenylhydrazone) to the outside solution. This generated a diffusion potential across the vesicular membrane, and this diffusion potential was shown to act as a driving force for the coupled transport of Na^+ and the organic solute. KIMMICH and CARTER-SU (1978) and CARTER-SU and KIMMICH (1980) induced a diffusion potential across the cell membrane of isolated chick enterocytes by adding valinomycin to the solution bathing K^+-loaded cells. Both the initial rate of entry and the steady state inside/outside distribution of 3-O-methylglucose (an actively transported sugar analog) were found to increase as the magnitude of the imposed K^+ diffusion potential increased. Similar experiments were performed by BECK and SACTOR (1975, 1978) with isolated brush border vesicles from renal proximal tubule.

Thus, many studies clearly establish the rheogenicity of the Na^+–sugar and Na^+–amino acid entry mechanisms in the small intestine. Therefore, effects of V_a on kinetic (K_T and V_{max}) and thermodynamic parameters of transport can be anticipated. From a thermodynamic viewpoint, the effect of V_a as a driving force for solute accumulation is relatively straightforward since, thermodynamically, V_a and $\Delta\mu_{Na}$ are completely interchangeable (ARMSTRONG et al. 1979b). Therefore, in the presence of Na^+ ions, a similar effect on the transport of sugars and amino acids can be predicted whether the immediate driving force is a chemical Na^+ gradient ($\Delta\mu_{Na}$) or a numerically equivalent V_a. On the other hand, as discussed by GECK and HEINZ (1976), the effects of V_a on the kinetics of Na^+-coupled solute transfer depend on factors such as the specific nature of the kinetic process and the electrical charge carried by the unloaded carrier. Therefore, system-dependent variations in the kinetic effects of V_a may be anticipated. This seems to be borne out by experimental findings. For example, CARTER-SU and KIMMICH (1980) found that, in isolated chick enterocytes, the effect of the membrane potential on the kinetics of 3-O-methylglucose transport is greater than that of an energetically equivalent $\Delta\mu_{Na}$. The opposite result was found for the effect of these two driving forces on initial sugar influx rates in renal brush border vesicles (BECK and SACTOR 1978). Moreover, in chick enterocytes, the membrane potential increased V_{max} for sugar transport, leaving K_T unaffected (CARTER-SU and KIMMICH 1980) whereas, in renal brush border vesicles, both $\Delta\mu_{Na}$ and the membrane potential stimulated sugar transport by lowering the K_T (ARONSON and SACTOR 1975; ARONSON 1978).

III. Equivalent Circuit Analysis: Is the Na^+/K^+ Exchange Pump Rheogenic?

In terms of the electrical equivalent circuit shown in Fig. 6, the observed effects of actively transported sugars and amino acids on the transcellular potential profile (that is, a decrease in V_a together with a numerically smaller increase in V_T) can be accounted for, in a qualitative sense, by assuming that the only effect of these solutes is to depolarize E_a (the emf of the mucosal membrane). Under open-circuit conditions, one can show this as follows (WHITE and ARMSTRONG 1971; ROSE and SCHULTZ 1971). Under these conditions ($I=0$), Eqs. (D.4) and (D.6) may be written

$$V_T=[R_j(E_s-E_a)-E_j(R_a+R_s)]/R_t\ , \tag{E.III.1}$$

$$V_a=-[E_a(R_s+R_j)+R_a(E_s+E_j)]/R_t\ . \tag{E.III.2}$$

With the assumption that the only effect of actively transported solutes is to decrease E_a, one obtains the following relationships from these equations,

$$\Delta V_T=-(R_j/R_t)\,\Delta E_a\ , \tag{E.III.3}$$

$$\Delta V_a=-[(R_s+R_j)/R_t]\,\Delta E_a \tag{E.III.4}$$

from which it is clear that

$$\Delta V_T/\Delta V_a=1/(1+R_s/R_j)\ . \tag{E.III.5}$$

It is apparent from Eq. (E.III.5) that, for any finite value of R_s/R_j, ΔV_T will be smaller than ΔV_a.

This analysis is, at first glance, consistent with the changes in V_a and V_T observed by WHITE and ARMSTRONG (1971), ROSE and SCHULTZ (1971), and OKADA et al. (1977b). Moreover, taken at face value, it suggests that the increased rate of transepithelial Na^+ transport induced by actively transported sugars and amino acids might not necessarily involve any change in E_s, the emf of the basolateral membrane. In other words, in terms of this analysis, the basolateral Na^+/K^+ exchange pump, in the small intestine might be electroneutral or at most very weakly rheogenic. On closer examination, however, this conclusion encounters significant difficulties.

First, it should be stressed that a merely qualitative agreement between the predictions of Eq. (E.III.5) and the changes in V_a and V_T observed experimentally does not exclude the possibility that a hyperpolarization of E_s, arising from an increased rate of rheogenic Na^+ pumping across the basolateral cell membrane, contributes to the latter. Quantitative agreement between Eq. (E.III.5) and the observed results would constitute a much stronger argument in this respect. Second, in view of the fact that the Na^+/K^+ exchange pump in a wide variety of tissues is rheogenic, i.e., the Na^+/K^+ coupling ratio exceeds unity (FLEMING 1980), the existence of an electroneutral pumping mechanism in the small intestine would be surprising. For these reasons, evidence pointing to the existence of a rheogenic basolateral Na^+/K^+ exchange pump in the small intestine will now be examined.

Early efforts in this direction were indirect and beset by a number of uncertainties. Two main approaches to the problem were attempted. First, by inserting experimentally observed values of ΔV_T and ΔV_a in Eq. (E.III.5), one obtains corresponding estimates of R_s/R_j. For example, the average values of $\Delta V_a/\Delta V_T$ obtained with three different intestinal preparations when glucose was added to the mucosal medium were 2.7 for bullfrog small intestine (WHITE and ARMSTRONG 1971), 3.1 for rabbit ileum (ROSE and SCHULTZ 1971), and 1.07 for rat ileum (OKADA et al. 1977b). The corresponding R_s/R_j values obtained from Eq. (E.III.5) are 1.7, 2.1, and 0.07. Assuming that G_S/G_T in the small intestine is about 0.9 (see Table 1), it is clear from the G_T values reported for a variety of intestinal preparations (see Table 1) that, if Eq. (E.III.5) and its underlying assumptions truly reflect the realities of intestinal electrophysiology, R_s in the small intestine must lie in the approximate range 60–200 Ω cm^2. Until very recently, this would have been regarded as an improbably low estimate of R_s, and therefore as an indirect argument that the major assumption underlying Eq. (E.III.5) (i.e., that ΔV_T and ΔV_a are the results of a change in E_a only) is incorrect. For example, in *Necturus* gallbladder, where G_S/G_T is about 0.95, R_s was estimated by several investigators to be about 3 KΩ cm^2 (FRÖMTER 1972; REUSS and FINN 1975a, 1977; REUSS and GRADY 1979). Similarly, R_s/R_j was calculated to be in the range 6 (REUSS and FINN 1975a) to 9 (FRÖMTER 1972). Recently, however, using a different technique, FRÖMTER et al. (1981) have reported average values of 202 and 127 Ω cm^2 for R_s, with corresponding R_s/R_j values of 2.2 and 1.4, respectively. The reason for the discrepancy between these and FRÖMTER's (1972) earlier estimates is not yet clear.

ROSE and SCHULTZ (1971) sought to clarify the rheogenicity or otherwise of the basolateral Na^+/K^+ exchange pump by another approach based on the equivalent electrical circuit of Fig. 6. This approach was as follows. If, in addition to decreasing E_a, actively transported sugars and amino acids, by stimulating a rheogenic Na^+/K^+ exchange pump, cause E_s to increase, and if the remaining parameters of the circuit shown in Fig. 6 remain essentially unchanged, then Eq. (E.III.2) yields the following expression

$$\Delta V_T = [R_j(\Delta E_s - \Delta E_a)]/R_t \, . \qquad \text{(E.III.6)}$$

Equation (E.III.6) shows that a depolarization of E_a and a hyperpolarization of E_s will contribute additively to an observed change in V_T. Therefore, if the response of E_s to an actively transported sugar or amino acid were blocked (e.g., by exposing the tissue to the Na^+/K^+ exchange pump inhibitor, ouabain or to metabolic inhibitors), the observed change in V_T should be smaller than the corresponding change under control conditions. In tissues poisoned with ouabain and/or cyanide, ROSE and SCHULTZ (1971) found that the ΔV_T induced by alanine was only about 20% of the corresponding change observed in unpoisoned tissues. By contrast, ΔV_a in poisoned and in normal tissues was essentially the same. This was interpreted as evidence for a rheogenic (pump) component in the overall response of the small intestine to actively transported solutes. However, this conclusion must be regarded as tentative since it rests on the somewhat unlikely possibility that ouabain and cyanide specifically block the solute-induced change in E_s and do not significantly affect the basic electrical parameters of the tissue.

A major limitation of the electrical equivalent circuit analyses of the effects of transported solutes so far presented is that they do not take account of the fact that rheogenic Na^+ entry across the brush border membrane, whether this entry is coupled or not, will not only depolarize E_a but will also reduce R_a. From Eqs. (E.III.1) and (E.III.2) one can see that a decrease in R_a will increase V_T and depolarize V_a. Recent studies with the intestine of *Ascaris* (GRADY and REUSS 1981) and *Necturus* (GUNTER-SMITH et al. 1982) in which R_a/R_s was measured continuously by passing current pulses across the tissue have shown that the addition of actively transported sugars and amino acids to the mucosal bathing solution decreases this ratio by approximately 40%. This decrease is most probably due to a decrease in R_a. The arguments already given in favor of a contribution by E_s

to the overall tissue response to these solutes are therefore compromised since they rest on the assumption that R_a remains constant.

Direct evidence for a role of the basolateral cell membrane in the electrical response of intestinal epithelium to actively transported solutes was presented by Gunter-Smith et al. (1982). These authors found that, in *Necturus* intestine, the response of V_a to alanine or galactose (added to the mucosal medium) was biphasic. Initially, there was a rapid depolarization of the mucosal membrane that, in some instances, reversed the polarity of V_a. At the same time, R_a/R_s decreased. Subsequently, and more slowly, V_a repolarized and R_a/R_s increased so that both approached their initial values. V_T and I_{sc} increased in phase with the repolarization of V_a. In metabolically poisoned tissues, the initial rapid depolarization of V_a and the concomitant decrease in R_a/R_s were, essentially, the only electrical responses observed. The subsequent slow increases in V_T and I_{sc} were very small. Phlorhizin, added simultaneously with galactose, inhibited the response of the tissue to the sugar. When phlorhizin was added in the presence of galactose, and after V_a had repolarized, V_a increased still further and R_a/R_s increased above its initial value in the absence of galactose and phlorhizin. These observations suggest that the increase in R_a/R_s, following its initial decline, is due to a metabolism-dependent decrease in R_s.

As yet, the reason for the biphasic response of *Necturus* intestine, in contrast to the intestines of other species studied, is unknown. Gunter-Smith et al. (1982) suggested that it might reflect the relatively large size of the intestinal absorptive cells in *Necturus*. Whatever the reason, these observations are important in that they permit temporal resolution of the electrical events that occur following the addition, to the mucosal bathing solution, of an actively transported sugar or amino acid. That is to say events occurring at the mucosal cell membrane can be separated in time from those that occur at the basolateral membrane. Further exploitation of this finding should yield important new insights into the electrophysiologic correlates of sugar and amino acid transport by the small intestine.

The evidence for a solute-induced increase in E_s that emerges from the experiments of Gunter-Smith et al. (1982) is as follows: If one assumes that the orientation of E_a is as shown in Fig. 6 (which, in the light of the arguments summarized in Sect. D seems to be the most plausible assumption), it is clear from Eq. (D.14) that, once the initial electrical changes at the apical membrane have occurred, a decrease in R_s alone would not repolarize V_a. On the contrary, it would cause V_a to depolarize still further. To account for the observed *repolarization* of V_a one has, under these conditions, to postulate an increase in E_s. On the other hand, if E_a has the opposite orientation to that shown in Fig. 6 [i.e., E_a in Eq. (D.14) is negative], a decrease in R_s alone would be sufficient to account for the observed repolarization of V_a. In any event, whether the electrical response that occurs at the basolateral membrane involves a decrease in R_s only, or a decrease in R_s together with an increase in E_s, the fact that this response depends upon the availability of metabolic energy argues strongly in favor of the involvement of the Na^+-pump.

These results support the idea of "electrochemical feedback" in the absorptive cell as formulated by Schultz (1977). Transapical entry of Na^+ coupled to that of sugars or amino acids could stimulate the basolateral Na^+-pump by lowering the gradient of Na^+ electrochemical potential against which it must work. This would most likely be accomplished by a depolarization of V_s since a^i_{Na} appears to remain almost constant in the presence of actively transported sugars (LEE and ARMSTRONG 1972; ARMSTRONG 1975). In turn, the response generated by the Na^+ pump under these circumstances would tend to counteract the depolarizing effect, on V_a, of coupled transapical Na^+ entry. This would assist in maintaining a favorable gradient for Na^+ entry across the brush border membrane. It is important to recall that, in opencircuit, such electrical interactions between the apical and basolateral membranes of the absorptive cell are allowed by the existence in the small intestine of a low resistance paracellular shunt pathway.

Finally, one other consequence of the rheogenic nature of Na^+-coupled sugar and amino acid influx across the brush border membrane should be noted. Because they depolarize V_a, these processes reduce $\Delta\tilde{\mu}_{Na}$ across this membrane. Thus, the onset of any one of them immediately reduces the driving force for transapical Na^+ entry by the same or by any other rheogenic route. This, in turn, will reduce the driving force for the entry and intracellular accumulation of any uncharged solute that moves into the cell via an Na^+-coupled mechanism. Many observations have established the existence of mutual or cross inhibitions between the intestinal absorption of sugars and amino acids when both kinds of solute are present in the mucosal medium (see, e.g., SMYTH 1968; KIMMICH 1973; Chap. 16). A number of explanations have been proposed for these findings. These include competition for entry via a "polyfunctional" carrier that can transport sugars and amino acids together with Na^+ (ALVARADO 1975), competition for a common energy supply (NEWEY and SMYTH 1964; SMYTH 1968), and reduction of the chemical component of the transmucosal Na^+ gradient due to an increase in the Na^+ content of the absorptive cell (CHEZ et al. 1966; READ 1967; FRIZZELL and SCHULTZ 1972; SEMENZA 1971). As already indicated, the effect of sugars and amino acids on $\Delta\tilde{\mu}_{Na}$ in intact intestinal cells frequently appears to involve dissipation of its electrical rather than its chemical component (LEE and ARMSTRONG 1972; CARTER-SU and KIMMICH 1980; ARMSTRONG et al. 1981). This dissipation, which is reflected in the depolarizing effect of these solutes on V_a, offers a simple explanation for cross-inhibition between Na^+-coupled sugar and amino acid transport and is, most probably, an important contributory factor to this. Whether or not it can, by itself, account quantitatively for the inhibitory interactions involved remains to be determined.

IV. Transapical Sugar Transport: Energetics and Stoichiometry

As outlined in the preceding sections, there now seems to be compelling evidence that the transapical Na^+ gradient plays a major role in the active transport of sugars, amino acids, and other organic solutes by absorptive cells of the small intestine. Similarly, the Na^+-gradient model for Na^+-coupled entry of these solutes across the mucosal cell membrane originally proposed by CRANE (1962, 1965) has succeeded, in a virtually unmodified form, in accounting satisfactorily for many recent electrophysiologic and other observations concerning Na^+-coupled solute transfer. Because intracellular accumulation of actively transported sugars and amino acids depends completely on the presence of Na^+ in the mucosal solution, the Na^+-gradient hypothesis, in its pristine form requires that the transapical Na^+ gradient be the *sole* source of energy for the accumulation of these solutes. A necessary, though not sufficient, prerequisite for this requirement is that the energy available from the movement of Na^+ from the mucosal medium to the cell interior be adequate to account for the degree of solute accumulation observed. In recent years, several studies have addressed this question, particularly with respect to Na^+-coupled hexose accumulation by intestinal absorptive cells. These studies are reviewed in this section. It should be noted, however, that the general principles discussed herein apply, mutatis mutandis, to other neutral solutes whose uphill movement, across the brush border membrane, is coupled to transapical Na^+ transport.

As already stressed, if Na^+ and a neutral solute are the only transported species directly involved in the coupled entry process, then regardless of the specific nature of this process or of the exact stoichiometry involved, it necessarily results in a net transfer of positive charge across the mucosal cell membrane. Therefore V_a, in addition to the transmembrane activity ratio, contributes to the overall thermodynamic driving force for transport. This fact, though clearly enunciated by Parsons (1967) was largely ignored in early discussions of the Na^+-gradient hypothesis (e.g. Schultz and Curran 1970; Kimmich 1973), possibly because, until the advent of microelectrode studies with the small intestine, the rheogenicity or otherwise of coupled Na^+ entry remained a matter for speculation.

If one takes account of V_a, the maximal inside/outside accumulation value, across the apical cell membrane for a neutral solute S is given (Armstrong et al. 1979b) by the equation

$$\Delta\mu_S^a \leqq -\nu\Delta\tilde{\mu}_{Na}^a \, . \qquad \text{(E.IV.1)}$$

In this equation, ν is the coupling or stoichiometric relationship between Na^+ and S, i.e., the number of Na^+ ions that necessarily accompany each molecule of S transported. Equation (E.IV.1) may be written more explicitly as

$$RT \ln a_s^c/a_s^m \leqq -\nu(RT \ln a_{Na}^c/a_{Na}^m + FV_a) \, . \qquad \text{(E.IV.2)}$$

At first glance it might appear that the determination of the energetic adequacy of $\Delta\tilde{\mu}_{Na}$ for solute accumulation under a given set of conditions is, in principle, a relatively simple matter that involves only the measurement of (a_s^c/a_s^m), (a_{Na}^m/a_{Na}^m), ν, and V_a for the appropriate conditions and their insertion into Eq. (E.IV.2).

However, it is important to recognize that Eq. (E.IV.2) corresponds to the so-called static head situation in which there is no significant efflux of accumulated solute from the cell. Clearly, under normal conditions, this is not so. Therefore, in the steady state, a_s^c/a_s^m may correspond to the requirements of Eq. (E.IV.2), but this correspondence may be fortuitous because efflux of S may be occurring through the mucosal membrane, the basolateral membrane, or both of these. As pointed out by Kimmich and Randles (1979), a valid test of Eq. (E.IV.2) can be obtained only under conditions where efflux of S is completely inhibited, or virtually so. Early attempts to evaluate the applicability of Eq. (E.IV.2) to Na^+-coupled sugar accumulation by the small intestine (e.g., ARMSTRONG et al. 1973) did not take into account possible effects of sugar efflux on the steady state a_s^c/a_s^m values observed.

In the small intestine, sugar efflux appears to occur largely via a high capacity carrier-mediated facilitated diffusion process in the basolateral cell membrane (KIMMICH and RANDLES 1976). The discovery (KIMMICH and RANDLES 1979) that a_s^c/a_s^m for actively transported sugars could be increased in the presence of inhibitors of this basolateral exit process (e.g., phloretine, cytochalasin-B) sparked a careful reevaluation by KIMMICH and his co-workers of the energetic adequacy of the transapical Na^+ gradient for sugar accumulation by absorptive cells of the small intestine. Using isolated enterocytes from chick intestine, these workers (KIMMICH and RANDLES 1979) showed that, in the presence of cytochalasin-B, the a_s^c/a_s^m value for 3-*O*-methylglucose could be as high as 70. The equivalent steady state transapical driving force (obtained by dividing the left-hand side of Eq. (E.IV.2) by F) is approximately 110 mV. If one assumes a_{Na}^c in chick enterocytes to be about the same as the value measured with Na^+-selective microelectrodes in *Necturus* intestine (Fig. 5) and that V_a in this species is approximately −35 mV, $\Delta\tilde{\mu}_{Na}/F$ in this tissue is about −95 mV. Thus, if one assumes $\nu = 1$ for Na^+-coupled sugar transport (GOLDNER et al. 1969) $\Delta\tilde{\mu}_{Na}$ is apparently not sufficient to account for the steady state a_s^c/a_s^m value.

These calculations are open to question. First, the actual values of a_{Na}^c and V_a in chick enterocytes could differ significantly from those assumed in the calculation. In particular, either or both of these parameters could differ substantially in the presence of cytochalasin-B, from its value under control conditions. Direct measurements, under the conditions of the experiments of KIMMICH and RANDLES (1979), of a_{Na}^c and V_a in isolated chick erythrocytes are required to resolve these questions.[13]

More recently, KIMMICH and his co-workers (KIMMICH 1981 b) have reported data for steady state sugar accumulation ratios in chick enterocytes that appear to be free from the uncertainties inherent in their earlier experiments with cytochalasin-B. In these cells, α-methylglucoside appears to enter via the mucosal Na^+-coupled sugar transport process, but is not transported by the serosal facilitated diffusion carrier. With this solute, a_s^c/a_s^m values of nearly 100 have been observed, even though a (relatively minor) diffusional "leak" pathway for α-methylglucoside was not controlled. Clearly, such large accumulation ratios are not compatible with the Na^+-gradient hypothesis if ν in Eq. (E.IV.2) has a value of unity. The accurate evaluation of ν for a given sugar thus becomes of prime importance.

GOLDNER et al. (1969) measured the influxes of Na^+ and of several actively transported sugars across the brush border membrane of isolated rabbit ileum.

---

13 A puzzling and as yet unresolved question relative to these results is the observation (MAK et al. 1974) that cytochalasin-B failed to alter the uptake of 3-*O*-methylglucose by everted rings of hamster intestine. Even more puzzling is the fact that, under identical conditions to those employed by KIMMICH and RANDLES (1979), cytochalasin-B did not affect the steady state accumulation of 3-*O*-methylglucose by intact segments of chick intestine (DIEZ DE LOS RIOS et al. 1980)

They found that Na^+ influx was linearly related to that of 3-*O*-methylglucose when the mucosal concentration of the sugar analog was varied at constant $[Na^+]_m$. At the three levels of $[Na^+]_m$ tested, there was a 1/1 relationship between 3-*O*-methylglucose influx and the sugar-dependent Na^+ influx. Hence, a kinetic model was proposed for Na^+–sugar symport that involved a 1/1 binding of Na^+ and sugar to the membrane carrier.

Although the kinetic model of Goldner et al. (1969) was in fairly good agreement with their experimental data, there are grounds for believing that, in their studies, the Na^+–sugar stoichiometry was underestimated. First, their sugar influx data were not corrected for the fraction of sugar influx that is independent of Na^+. Since this fraction depends on $[S]_m$ it will be larger at higher than at lower values of total sugar influx. Second, at the time when the experiments of Goldner et al. (1969) were performed, the depolarizing effect of actively transported sugars on V_a was not known. As pointed out by Kimmich and Randles (1981), this depolarization reduces the transapical driving force for that fraction of the total Na^+ influx that is independent of the transport of sugar. Therefore, the observed difference between the influx of Na^+ in the presence and absence respectively of the sugar is less than the true value of sugar-dependent Na^+ influx. Once again, the extent of this discrepancy will increase with increasing values of $[S]_m$. Thus, failure to take these two factors into account will lead respectively to an overestimate of Na^+-dependent sugar influx and an underestimate of sugar-dependent Na^+ influx, and both these errors will tend to reduce ν in Eq. (E.IV.2) below its true value.

Kimmich and Randless (1981) approached the measurement of ν in the following way. To offset the depolarizing effect of the coupled entry of Na^+ and 3-*O*-methylglucose, ATP-depleted chick enterocytes were equilibrated with a high external K^+ concentration in the presence of valinomycin. In this way the membrane potential was "clamped" at a near zero value. The high P_K of the membrane under these conditions permits K^+ to move outwards in response to an inward movement of Na^+, thus "neutralizing" the depolarizing effect of Na^+ on V_a. Two parallel sets of experiments were performed, a control set and one in which the coupled entry process was inhibited by phlorhizin. The difference between the influx found under control conditions and that observed in the presence of phlorhizin was taken as a measure of the coupled influx for Na^+ and 3-*O*-methylglucose. The ratio between the coupled influxes of Na^+ and of sugar, measured in this way, did not differ significantly from 2. Inserting a value of 2 for ν in Eq. (E.IV.2) and calculating the theoretical maximum for a_s^c/a_s^m as before, one obtains a value of about 400 for this parameter (Kimmich 1981). On this basis, the energetic adequacy of $\Delta\tilde{\mu}_{Na}$ to sustain even the highest values of a_s^c/a_s^m so far observed appears to be amply demonstrated.

There are other reports that support a stoichiometry of 2/1 for the coupled transport of Na^+ and organic solutes. Smith and Sepulveda (1979) found that when alanine influxes in rabbit ileum (Schultz et al. 1967) are corrected for the Na^+-independent moiety, a Na^+/alanine influx ratio close to 2 is obtained under conditions where the uncorrected value was about 1. Results consistent with $\nu = 2$ were obtained for Na^+-dependent phenylalanine uptake by renal brush border vesicles (Evers et al. 1976) and for transepithelial Na^+-coupled glucose transport across cultured monolayers of the kidney LLC-PK_1 cell line (MISFELDT and SANDERS 1981).

A Na^+/sugar stoichiometry of 2/1 raises some intriguing kinetic possibilities. Unlike the situation where $\nu = 1$, a Na^+/sugar stoichiometry of 2/1 is compatible with a free carrier that carries a single negative charge. The quaternary (2Na^+) complex would then possess a single positive charge. In this situation, V_a would facilitate the movement of the positively charged complex towards the inside surface of the apical cell membrane and at the same time assist the movement of the free carrier towards the outside of the membrane. Such an effect of V_a on the movement of the carrier within the membrane could explain the dependence on V_a of phlorhizin binding observed by ARONSON (1978) in renal brush border vesicles.

Finally, in a situation where ternary (1 Na^+) or quaternary (2 Na^+) complexes between Na^+, solute, and carrier can be formed and where both forms of complex are capable of translocation through the membrane, the system may exhibit variable stoichiometry. The value of ν observed will depend on the relative fractions of the total coupled transport that occur via the ternary or quaternary complex, respectively. These fractions could be a function of the transmembrane driving forces for coupled Na^+–solute transfer. This point has not been considered in the studies reviewed in this section. Rather, it has generally been assumed that ν, whatever its numerical value, is fixed for a given cotransport process. This assumption implies that the transport of Na^+ and organic solutes is completely coupled, i.e., the degree of coupling as defined by KEDEM and CAPLAN (1965) is unity. There is no real evidence that this is so. If the degree of coupling can be less than unity, then Eq. (E.IV.1) is no longer valid and one must use the equation

$$J_S \Delta\mu_S^a \leqq -J_{Na} \Delta\tilde{\mu}_{Na}^a \,, \qquad \text{(E.IV.3)}$$

where J_S and J_{Na} are the *coupled* net fluxes of S and Na^+ across the mucosal membrane. In this situation, the flux ratio J_{Na}/J_S, which, in Eq. (E.IV.3) corresponds to ν is no longer constant, i.e., independent of the driving forces $\Delta\mu_S^a$ and $\Delta\tilde{\mu}_{Na}^a$. On the contrary, as shown by KEDEM and CAPLAN (1965), the flux ratio becomes a function of the ratio of the driving forces. Thus, it is not too surprising to find, as SCHULTZ et al. (1967) reported for Na^+-coupled alanine influx in rabbit ileum, that J_{Na}/J_S can vary when the experimental conditions are changed.

F. The Regulation of Ion Transport in the Small Intestine

It will be apparent from the previous sections of this chapter that any agent, or any change in external conditions, that alters the electrophysiologic and ion transporting properties of the small intestine may do so in a variety of ways. These include changes in the permeability characteristics of the tissue (transcellular or paracellular) without alterations in the driving forces, a change in driving forces without alteration of permeability characteristics, or a combination of these. In addition, factors that influence transcellular transport may act specifically at the apical or the basolateral cell membrane. Clearly, then, the interpretation of the modes of action of substances that regulate or modulate intestinal ion transport and electrophysiology can be a complex problem requiring for its solution a variety of approaches in which the properties of the intact epithelial cell layer and those of isolated membrane vesicles must be studied.

A comprehensive survey of the extensive and rapidly growing literature that exists on the effects of drugs, enzyme and metabolic inhibitors, secretagogues, gastrointestinal hormones, etc., on the electrical and transport properties of the small intestine is outside the scope of this chapter. Much useful information in this area is summarized in a symposium volume edited by Binder (1979) and in a recent review by Field (1981). As an example of the physiologic regulation of ion transport and electrophysiology in the small intestine, we will discuss the effects of cAMP. This example is chosen because: (1) considerable insight has already been gained into the nature of the specific events, at the membrane level, by which the overall response of the intestinal mucosa to cAMP are mediated; (2) cAMP acting through, or in parallel with, changes in cytosolic Ca^{2+} concentrations has been implicated as a regulatory factor for stimulus/secretion coupling in many cell types (Berridge 1979). Hence, the mode of action of cAMP on the small intestine is of interest in a much wider physiologic context.

I. Cyclic Nucleotides and Intestinal Transport: Secretion

Cyclic nucleotides, particularly cAMP, have been implicated in salt and water secretion by a wide variety of epithelia, including the small intestine (Nellans et al. 1974; Berridge 1979). There is considerable evidence that the secretory response to cAMP and other secretagogues is mediated by changes in cytosolic Ca^{2+} levels. However, the exact nature of the interactions that occur between cAMP, other secretagogues, and cytosolic Ca^{2+} is as yet unclear. It seems safe to say that the study of these interactions will continue, for some time to come, to be a central preoccupation of investigators interested in the mechanism of stimulus/secretion coupling in a wide variety of cellular systems.

Interest in the effects of cAMP and related secretagogues, e.g., theophylline and prostaglandins (both of which are known to increase cAMP levels in the intestine) on intestinal ion transport was stimulated by the similarities between their effects and those elicited by cholera toxin and other bacterial enterotoxins. Cholera toxin mimics the effects of cAMP on intestinal transport in vitro, and increases intestinal cAMP levels. Moreover, infusion of theophylline or of prostaglandins into the mesenteric artery induces a cholera-like secretion of water and electrolytes by canine jejunum in vivo. These and other findings suggested that cAMP is a key factor in the secretory responses induced by cholera toxin and other bacterial enterotoxins in the in vivo intestine. These responses underlie the massive losses of water and electrolytes from the gastrointestinal tract that characterize a number of enterobacterial infections. Therefore, cAMP has been considered to play a central role in the pathophysiology of a number of gastrointestinal disorders.

In vitro experiments with short-circuited preparations of the small intestine have uncovered interesting variations in their response to external cAMP and related secretagogues. In mammalian (rabbit) small intestine, cAMP and agents that increase intracellular cAMP levels (theophylline, cholera and heat-labile *Escherichia coli* enterotoxins, vasoactive intestinal peptide, and prostaglandins

Table 6. Effect of cAMP on Na^+ and Cl^- fluxes across rabbit ileal mucosa

	J^{Na}_{ms}	J^{Na}_{sm}	J^{Na}_{net}	J^{Cl}_{ms}	J^{Cl}_{sm}	J^{Cl}_{net}	I_{sc}	J_r
Control	10	9	1	8	7	1	3	−3
cAMP	7	9	−2	5	9	−4	5	−3

Ion fluxes and I_{sc}, expressed in μequiv. $cm^{-2}h^{-1}$, are rounded values based on those given by FIELD (1979). I_{sc} is expressed as a net mucosal to serosal movement of *positive* charge. J_r is the difference between I_{sc} and $(J^{Na}_{net}+J^{Cl}_{net})$ and represents net HCO_3^- secretion

E_1, E_2, and F) all produce effects on transepithelial Na^+ and Cl^- fluxes similar to those shown in Table 6 (FIELD 1979). These changes are consistent with two effects of cAMP on intestinal ion transport. These are: (1) an antiabsorptive effect due to an inhibition of transapical coupled NaCl entry (note that both J^{Na}_{ms} and J^{Cl}_{ms} in Table 6 are reduced by cAMP); and (2) a direct stimulation of Cl^- secretion (cf. the changes in J^{Na}_{net} and J^{Cl}_{net}, Table 6). Together, these two effects contribute to an overall secretory response of the tissue to cAMP. Note that the residual flux J_R found in rabbit ileum under control conditions and which has been ascribed to a net secretion of HCO_3^- (DIETZ and FIELD 1973) is not affected by cAMP.

The inhibitory effect of cAMP on coupled NaCl entry into the absorptive cells of rabbit ileum has been confirmed by direct measurement of Na^+ and Cl^- influxes across the brush border membrane (NELLANS et al. 1973). This effect of the nucleotide appears to be rather general. It has been observed in the intestine of the flounder (FRIZZELL et al. 1979; FIELD et al. 1980) and the bullfrog (ARMSTRONG and YOUMANS 1980) as well as in mammalian and amphibian (*Necturus*) gallbladder (FRIZZELL et al. 1975; DIEZ DE LOS RIOS et al. 1981). In keeping with the electroneutral nature of coupled transapical NaCl transport, inhibition of this process by cAMP does not affect V_a (ARMSTRONG and YOUMANS 1980; DIEZ DE LOS RIOS et al. 1981).

The cAMP-stimulated Cl^- secretion found in mammalian small intestine is not seen in the intestine of the bullfrog or the flounder, nor is it observed in the gallbladder. Since these tissues do not appear to possess functional crypts of Lieberkühn, it has been suggested (FIELD 1979, 1981; FIELD et al. 1980) that cAMP-stimulated anion secretion in mammalian intestine is mediated by the crypt cells rather than the villous absorptive cells. Indeed, a specific model for Cl^- secretion based on this idea has been proposed (see, e.g., FIELD 1979). According to this model, Cl^- enters the secretory cell against a gradient of electrochemical potential via a coupled NaCl transport mechanism located in the *basolateral* cell membrane. Electrogenic Cl^- secretion is initiated by a cAMP-induced increase in the Cl^- conductance of the luminal membrane.

The idea that different cell types are implicated in the antiabsorptive and secretory responses respectively of the mammalian small intestine to cAMP is supported by a number of findings. For example, following brief exposure of rat intestine to cholera toxin, villous, but not crypt adenylate cyclase was stimulated. Salt and water absorption were inhibited, but secretion was not stimulated. More prolonged exposure stimulated crypt as well as villous adenylate cyclase and elicited secretion (De Jonge 1975). Furthermore, selective destruction of villous cells by osmotic shock did not diminish the secretory activity induced by cholera toxin (Roggin et al. 1972). Despite these findings, the suggestion that the antiabsorptive and secretory responses to cAMP are mediated by villous and crypt cells respectively, remains somewhat tentative, as does the specific model for cAMP-induced secretion that is based on this idea. Several facets of the action of cAMP on intestinal ion transport still pose intriguing questions. For example, in mammalian small intestine in vivo, HCO_3^- and not Cl^- is the major anion involved in the secretory response to cAMP and related secretagogues (Schultz et al. 1974). In the isolated intestine of *Amphiuma,* in which the presence of functional crypts has not been clearly established, theophylline elicits a secretory response. Moreover, in this preparation, HCO_3^- is the secreted anion (Gunter-Smith and White 1979 b). Finally, the net secretion of Na^+ observed in isolated rabbit ileum under short-circuit conditions and in the presence of cAMP and related secretagogues (Table 6) is not readily explained by the model for Cl^- secretion outlined previously. It has been suggested (Field 1979) that the apparent secretion of Na^+ observed under these conditions may be an artifact arising from incomplete short-circuiting of the crypt lumen when intact sheets of intestinal mucosa are short-circuited by conventional methods.

Involvement of Ca^{2+} in the response of the small intestine to cAMP is strongly indicated by the fact that addition of the Ca^{2+} ionophore A23187 to the solution bathing rabbit ileal mucosa produces changes in transepithelial Na^+ and Cl^- fluxes that are similar to, but smaller than those elicited by cAMP. Unlike cAMP, the ionophore exerts these effects only when the external medium contains Ca^{2+} (Bolton and Field 1977). The fact that A23187 does not increase the cAMP or cGMP content of the intestinal mucosa (Bolton and Field 1977; Field 1979) suggests that cytosolic Ca^{2+} may be the immediate effector of intestinal secretion and that cAMP may exert its secretory effect by eliciting an increase in cytosolic free Ca^{2+} concentrations. Much additional work is required to unravel the specific roles of Ca^{2+} and cAMP in this regard. In particular, the use of Ca^{2+}-selective microelectrodes (O'Doherty et al. 1980) to monitor changes in cytosolic Ca^{2+} concentrations that may be associated with the onset of secretion by the samll intestine whould provide new and significant findings. In the present context, it is interesting to note that A23187 also mimics the action of cAMP in the large intestine (Frizzell 1977).

A number of recent studies, notably the investigations of Field and his associates (Field 1979) strongly suggest that cGMP can stimulate intestinal secretion, or at least inhibit the active absorption of electrolytes. For example, a heat-stable peptide that is a component of *E. coli* enterotoxin stimulates guanyl cyclase and increases intestinal cGMP levels. This peptide inhibits the absorption of Na^+ and Cl^- by the in vitro ileum. Its inhibitory effect does not require external Ca^{2+}. This peptide has no effect on intestinal cAMP levels. However, the role, if any, of cGMP in regulating intestinal ion transport remains ambiguous, since there are a number of substances that can increase intestinal cGMP levels without significantly affecting ion transport, or for which increases in cGMP and changes in ion transport are not well correlated. Examples of these are insulin, cholecystokinin, and α-adrenergic agents, e.g., epinephrine (Brasitus et al. 1976). Finally, it may be noted that LÜCKE et al. (1979) have reported that, during in vivo perfusion of rat small intestine with Ringer's solutions containing dibutyryl-cAMP or theophylline, the absorption of 3-*O*-methylglucose was enhanced whereas that of Na^+ and water was significantly inhibited. Brush border vesicles isolated from rats that had been perfused with these agents showed enhanced Na^+-dependent glucose uptake compared with vesicles isolated from animals perfused with control solutions.

G. Conclusion

This chapter has attempted to summarize recent progress in those areas of investigation that have contributed most significantly to a fuller understanding of the cellular and molecular basis of intestinal ion transport and electrophysiology. An effort has been made to identify specific areas and problems that, in the author's opinion, urgently require further work and in which additional studies seem likely to yield new and incisive insights. The sheer bulk of the literature, relevant to these goals, that has appeared during the last 20 years or so, precluded any attempt at a complete survey. Therefore, a somewhat arbitrary choice of topics for detailed discussion has been made. This choice inevitably reflects, to some degree, the personal preoccupations and prejudices of the authors. Consequently, certain topics that, in the opinion of many investigators, are of equal interest and importance to those treated at length herein, are mentioned only briefly or even omitted. An effort has been made to rectify this in the references cited. However, in the final analysis, the authors take comfort in the thought that encyclopedias, like museums, often tend to be little more than monuments to past accomplishments. If this chapter, despite its shortcomings, plays a role in stimulating *future* studies in the field of intestinal ion transport, its authors will be well content.

Acknowledgments. The support of the United States Public Health Service (USPHS Grants AM 12715; HL 23332) in the preparation of this chapter is most gratefully acknowledged. Our sincere thanks are also due to Ms. Marsha Hunt, Department of Physiology, Indiana University, School of Medicine, who, with patience, good humor, and skill, produced order and legibility from the pristine chaos of this manuscript.

References

Al-Awqati Q, Cameron JL, Greenough WB (1973) Electrolyte transport in human ileum: Effect of purified cholera toxin. Am J Physiol 224:818–823

Albus H, Groot JA, Siegenbeck van Heukelom J (1979) Effects of glucose and ouabain on transepithelial electrical resistance and cell volume in stripped and unstripped goldfish intestine. Pflugers Arch 383:55–66

Alvarado F (1975) Sodium-driven transport. A re-evaluation of the sodium-gradient hypothesis. In: Robinson JWL (ed) Intestinal ion transport. MTP, Lancaster, pp 117–154

Armstrong WMcD (1975) Electrophysiology of sodium transport by epithelial cells of the small intestine. In Csaky TZ (ed) Intestinal absorption and malabsorption. Raven, New York, pp 45–66

Armstrong WMcD (1976) Bioelectric parameters and sodium transport in bullfrog small intestine. In: Robinson JWL (ed) Intestinal ion transport. MTP, Lancaster, England, pp 19–40

Armstrong WMcD (1977) Ionic activities and solute transfer in epithelial cells of the small intestine. In: Jungreis AM, Kleinzeller A, Schultz SG (eds) Water relations in membrane transport in plants and animals. Academic, New York, pp 215–231

Armstrong WMcD (1981) The use of ion-selective microelectrodes to measure intracellular ionic activities. In: Macknight ADC, Leader JP (eds) Epithelial ion and water transport. Raven, New York, pp 85–96
Armstrong WMcD, Garcia-Diaz JF (1980) Ion-selective microelectrodes: theory and technique. Fed Proc 39:2851–2859
Armstrong WMcD, Garcia-Diaz JF (1981) Criteria for the use of microelectrodes to measure membrane potentials in epithelial cells. In: MacKnight ADC, Leader JP (eds) Epithelial ion and water transport. Raven, New York, pp 43–53
Armstrong WMcD, Youmans SJ (1980) The role of bicarbonate ions and of adenosine 3′5′ monophosphate (cAMP) in chloride transport by epithelial cells of bullfrog small intestine. Ann NY Acad Sci 341:139–155
Armstrong WMcD, Suh TK, Gerencser GA (1972) Stimulation by anoxia of active chloride transfer in insolated bullfrog small intestinal epithelia. Biochim Biophys Acta 255:647–662
Armstrong WMcD, Byrd BJ, Hamang PM (1973) Energetic adequacy of Na^+ gradients for sugar accumulation in epithelial cells of small intestine. Biochim Biophys Acta 330:237–241
Armstrong WMcD, Byrd BJ, Cohen ES, Cohen SJ, Hamang PM, Myers CJ (1975) Osmotically induced electrical changes in bullfrog small intestine. Biochim Biophys Acta 401:137–151
Armstrong WMcD, Wojtkowski W, Bixenman WR (1977) A new solid state microelectrode for measuring intracellular chloride activities. Biochim Biophys Acta 465:165–170
Armstrong WMcD, Bixenman WR, Frey KF, Garcia-Diaz JF, O'Regan MG, Owens JL (1979 a) Energetics of coupled Na and Cl entry into epithelial cells of bullfrog small intestine. Biochim Biophys Acta 551:207–219
Armstrong WMcD, Garcia-Diaz JF, O'Doherty J, O'Regan MG (1979 b) Transmucosal Na^+ electrochemical potential difference and solute accumulation in epithelial cells of small intestine. Fed Proc 38:2722–2728
Armstrong WMcD, Garcia-Diaz JF, Diez de los Rios A (1981) Energetics of coupled sodium chloride entry in absorptive cells of leaky epithelia. In: Schutz SG (ed) Ion transport by epithelia. Raven, New York, pp 151–162
Aronson PS (1978) Energy-dependence of phlorizin binding to isolated renal microvillus membrane. J Membr Biol 42:81–98
Aronson PS, Sactor B (1975) The Na-gradient-dependent transport of D-glucose in renal brush border membranes. J Biol Chem 250:6032–6039
Asano T (1965) Effect of sugars on potential difference across wall of small intestine of rodents. Proc Soc Exp Biol Med 119:189–192
Baillien M, Schoffeniels E (1962) Action des acides amines sur le difference de potential electrique et sur le courant de court circuitage au niveau de l'epithelium isolé de l'intestine grele de la tortue greque. Arch Int Physiol Biol 70:140–142
Barry PH, Diamond JM, Wright EM (1971) The mechanism of cation permeation in rabbit gallbladder. Dilution potentials and bi-ionic potentials. J Membr Biol 4:358–394
Barry RJC, Eggenton J (1972 a) Membrane potentials of epithelial cells in rat small intestine. J Physiol (Lond) 227:201–216
Barry RJC, Eggenton J (1972 b) Ionic basis of membrane potentials in epithelial cells of rat intestine. J Physiol (Lond) 227:217–231
Barry RJC, Matthews J, Smyth DM, Wright EM (1962) Potential difference and intestinal transport of solutes and water. J Physiol (Lond) 161:17P–18P
Barry RJC, Smyth DH, Wright EM (1965) Short circuit current and solute transfer by rat jejunum. J Physiol (Lond) 181:410–431
Beck JC, Sactor B (1975) Energetics of the Na^+-dependent transport of D-glucose in renal brush border membrane vesicles. J Biol Chem 250:8674–8680
Beck JC, Sactor B (1978) The sodium electrochemical potential-mediated uphill transport of D-glucose in renal brush-border membrane vesicles. J Biol Chem 253:5531–5535
Berger E, Long E, Semenza G (1972) The sodium activation of biotin absorption in hamster small intestine in vitro. Biochim Biophys Acta 255:873–887

Berridge MJ (1979) Relationship between calcium and the cyclic nucleotides in ion secretion. In: Binder HJ (ed) Mechanisms of intestinal secretion. Liss, New York, pp 65–81
Bertalannfy FD, Lau C (1962) Cell renewal. Int Rev Cytol 13:357–366
Bihler I (1968) Intestinal sugar transport: Ionic activation and chemical specificity. In: Armstrong WMcD, Nunn AS Jr (eds) Intestinal transport of electrolytes, amino acids, and sugars. Thomas, Springfield, IL, pp 144–162
Binder HJ (1979) Mechanisms of intestinal secretion. Liss, New York
Bolton J, Field M (1977) Ca ionophore-stimulated ion secretion in rabbit ileal mucosa: Relation to action of cyclic AMP and carbamylcholine. J Membr Biol 35:159–174
Bosakova J, Crane RK (1965a) Cation inhibition of active sugar transport and Na^{22} influx into hamster small intestine in vitro. Biochim Biophys Acta 102:423–435
Bosakova J, Crane RK (1965b) Intracellular sodium concentrations and active sugar transport by hamster small intestine in vitro. Biochim Biophys Acta 102:436–441
Boulpaep EL (1972) Electrophysiological properties of the proximal tubule: Importance of cellular and intercellular transport pathways. In: Giebisch G (ed) Electrophysiology of epithelial cells. Schattauer, Stuttgart, pp 91–112
Boulpaep EL, Sackin H (1980) Electrical analysis of intraepithelial barriers. In: Bronner F, Kleinzeller A (eds) Current topics in membranes and transport, vol 13. Academic, New York, pp 169–197
Bradley SE, Purcell EF (eds) (1982) The paracellular pathway. Josiah Macy Jr. Foundation, New York
Brasitus TA, Field M, Kimberg DV (1976) Intestinal mucosal cyclic GMP: Regulation and possible role in ion transport. Am J Physiol 231:275–282
Cabantchik ZI, Knauf PA, Rothstein A (1978) The anion transport system of the red blood cell. The role of membrane protein evaluated by the use of "probes." Biochim Biophys Acta 515:239–302
Carter-Su C, Kimmich GA (1980) Effect of membrane potential on Na^+-dependent sugar transport by ATP-depleted intestinal cells. Am J Physiol 238:C73–C80
Cerejido M, Meza I, Martinez-Palomo A (1981) Occluding junctions in cultured epithelial monolayers. Am J Phys 240:C96–C102
Chez RA, Schulz SG, Curran PF (1966) Effects of sugars on transport of alanine in intestine. Science 153:1012–1013
Clarkson TW (1967) The transport of salt and water across isolated rat ileum. Evidence for at least two distinct pathways. J Gen Physiol 50:695–727
Clarkson TW, Toole SR (1964) Measurement of short-circuit current and ion transport across the ileum. Am J Physiol 206:658–668
Clarkson TW, Cross AC, Toole SR (1961) Dependence on substrate of the electrical potential across the isolated gut. Nature 191:501–502
Claude P, Goodenough DA (1973) Fracture faces of zonulae occludentes from "tight" and "leaky" epithelia. J Cell Biol 58:390–400
Cooperstein IL, Hogben CAM (1959) Ionic transfer across the isolated frog large intestine. J Gen Physiol 42:461–473
Corcia A, Garcia-Diaz JF, Armstrong WMcD (1982) Removal of luminal Cl^- alters K^+ permeability in *Necturus* gallbladder. Fed Proc 41:1495
Crane RK (1962) Hypothesis for mechanism of intestinal active transport of sugars. Fed Proc 21:891–895
Crane RK (1965) Na^+-dependent transport in the intestine and other animal tissues. Fed Proc 24:1000–1006
Crane RK (1968) Absorption of sugars. In: Code CF (ed) Handbook of physiology, Section 6, vol III. Williams and Wilkins, Baltimore, pp 1323–1351
Crane RK (1977) The gradient hypothesis and other models of carrier-mediated active transport. Rev Physiol Biochem Pharmacol 78:101–119
Csaky TZ (1961) Significance of sodium ions in active intestinal transport of non-electrolytes. Am J Physiol 201:999–1001
Csaky TZ (1963) A possible link between active transport of electrolytes and non-electrolytes. Fed Proc 22:3–7

Csaky TZ (1968) Physiological consideration of the relationship between intestinal absorption of electrolytes and nonelectrolytes. In: Armstrong WMcD, Nunn AS Jr (eds) Intestinal transport of electrolytes, amino acids and sugars. Thomas, Springfield, IL. ch 10, pp 188–212

Csaky TZ, Thale M (1960) Effect of ionic environment on intestinal sugar transport. Am J Physiol 198:1056–1058

Curran PF (1965) Ion transport in intestine and its coupling to other transport processes. Fed Proc 24:993–999

De Jesus CH, Ellory JC, Smith MW (1975) Intracellular chloride activities in the mucosal epithelium of rabbit terminal ileum. J Physiol (Lond) 244:31P–32P

De Jonge HR (1975) The response of small intestinal villus and crypt epithelium to cholera toxin in rat and guinea pig. Evidence against a specific role of the crypt cells in choleragen-induced secretion. Biochim Biophys Acta 381:128–143

Desjeux JF, Tai YH, Curran PF (1974) Characteristics of sodium flux from serosa to mucosa in rabbit ileum. J Gen Physiol 64:274–292

Diamond JM, Bossert WH (1967) A mechanism for coupling of water and solute transport in epithelia. J Gen Physiol 50:2061–2083

Diez de los Rios A, Baxendale LM, Armstrong WMcD (1980) Cytochalasin-B does not stimulate sugar uptake into small intestine of *Necturus* or chick. Biochim Biophys Acta 603:207–210

Diez de los Rios A, De Rose NE, Armstrong WMcD (1981) Cyclic AMP and intracellular ionic activities in *Necturus* gallbladder. J Membr Biol 63:25–30

Dietz J, Field M (1973) Ion transport in rabbit ileal mucosa. IV. Bicarbonate secretion. Am J Physiol 225:858–861

Douglas AP, Kerley R, Isselbacher KJ (1972) Preparation and characterization of the lateral and basal plasma membranes of the rat intestinal epithelial cell. Biochem J 128:1329–1338

Duffey ME, Turnheim K, Frizzell RA, Schultz SG (1978) Intracellular chloride activities in rabbit gallbladder: Direct evidence for the role of the sodium-gradient in energizing "uphill" chloride transport. J Membr Biol 42:229–245

Edelman A, Curci S, Samarzija I, Frömter E (1978) Determination of intracellular K activity in rat kidney proximal tubular cells. Pflugers Arch 378:37–45

Edmonds GJ, Marriott JC (1968) Electrical potential and short circuit current of an in vitro preparation of rat colonic mucosa. J Physiol (Lond) 194:479–494

Edmonds CJ, Marriott JC (1970) Sodium transport and short-circuit current in rat colon in vivo; effect of aldosterone. J Physiol (Lond) 210:1021–1039

Ehrenspeck G, Brodsky WA (1976) Effects of 4-acetamido-4′-isothiocyano-2-2′ disulfonic stilbene on ion transport in turtle bladder. Biochim Biophys Acta 419:555–558

Eisenberg RS, Johnson EA (1970) Three-dimensional electrical field problems in physiology. Prog Biophys Mol Biol 20:1–64

Erlij D, Martinez-Palomo A (1979) Role of tight junctions in epithelial function. In: Giebisch G (ed) Membrane transport in biology, vol III, Transport across multi-membrane systems. Springer, New York, pp 27–54

Evers J, Murer H, Kinne R (1976) Phenyl-alanine uptake in isolated renal brush border vesicles. Biochim Biophys Acta 426:598–615

Field M (1971) Ion transport in rabbit ileal mucosa. II. Effects of cyclic 3′5′-AMP. Am J Physiol 221:992–997

Field M (1979) Intracellular mediators of secretion in the small intestine. In: Binder HJ (ed) Mechanisms of intestinal secretion. Liss, New York, pp 83–91

Field M (1981) Secretion of electrolytes and water by mammalian small intestine. In: Johnson LR (ed) Physiology of the gastrointestinal tract, vol 2. Raven, New York, pp 963–982

Field M, Fromm D, McColl I (1971) Ion transport in rabbit ileal mucosa. I. Na and Cl fluxes and short-circuit current. Am J Physiol 220:1388–1396

Field M, Smith PL, Clayton DA, Frizzell RA (1978a) Role of HCO_3 in the regulation of Cl transport by flounder intestine. Mount Desert Island Biol Lab Bull 18:44–45

Field M, Karnaky KJ Jr, Smith PL, Bolton JE, Kinter WB (1978b) Ion transport across the isolated intestinal mucosa of winter flounder, *Pseudopleuronectes Americanus*. I. Functional and structural properties of cellular and paracellular pathways for Na^+ and Cl^-. J Membr Biol 41:265–293

Field M, Smith PL, Bolton JE (1980) Ion transport across the isolated intestinal mucosa of the winter flounder, *Pseudopleuronectes Americanus*. II. Effects of cyclic AMP. J Membr Biol 55:157–163

Fleming WW (1980) The elctrogenic Na^+, K^+-pump in smooth muscle. Physiologic and pharmacologic significance. Ann Rev Pharmacol Toxicol 20:129–149

Frizzell RA (1976) Coupled sodium-chloride transport by small intestine and gallbladder. In: Robinson JWL (ed) Intestinal ion transport. MTP, Lancaster, England, pp 101–109

Frizzell RA (1977) Active chloride secretion by rabbit colon. Calcium-dependent stimulation by ionophore A23187. J Membr Biol 35:175–187

Frizzell RA, Schultz SG (1972) Ionic conductances of extracellular shunt pathway in rabbit ileum: Influence of shunt on transmural sodium transport and electrical potential differences. J Gen Pyhsiol 59:318–346

Frizzell RA, Nellans HN, Rose RC, Markscheid-Kaspi L, Schultz SG (1973) Intracellular Cl concentration and influxes across the brush border of rabbit ileum. Am J Physiol 224:328–337

Frizzell RA, Markscheid-Kaspi L, Schultz SG (1974) Oxidative metabolism of rabbit ileal mucosa. Am J Physiol 226:1142–1148

Frizzell RA, Dugas MC, Schultz SG (1975) Sodium chloride transport by rabbit gallbladder. Direct evidence for a coupled NaCl influx process. J Gen Physiol 65:769–795

Frizzell RA, Field M, Schultz SG (1979) Sodium-coupled chloride transport by epithelial tissues. Am J Physiol 236:F1–F8

Fromm D (1973) Na and Cl transport across proximal small intestine of the rabbit. Am J Physiol 224:110–116

Fromm M, Schultz SG (1981) Some properties of KCl-filled microelectrodes: Correlation of potassium "leakage" with tip resistance. J Membr Biol 55:213–222

Frömter E (1972) The route of passive ion movement through the epithelium of *Necturus* gallbladder. J Membr Biol 8:259–301

Frömter E, Diamond JM (1972) Route of passive ion permeation in epithelia. Nature 255:9–13

Frömter E, Luer K (1973) Electrical studies on sugar transport kinetics of rat proximal tubule. Pflügers Arch 343:R47

Frömter E, Müller CW, Wick T (1971) Permeability properties of the proximal tubular epithelium of the rat kidney studied with electrophysiological methods. In: Giebisch G (ed) Electrophysiology of epithelial cells. Schattauer, Stuttgart, pp 119–148

Frömter E, Suzuki K, Kottra G, Kampmann L (1981) The paracellular shunt conductance of *Necturus* gallbladder epithelium: Comparison of measurements obtained by cable analysis with measurements obtained by a new approach based on intracellular impedance analysis. In: MacKnight ADC, Leader JP (eds) Epithelial ion and water transport. Raven, New York, pp 73–83

Fujita M, Ohta H, Kawai K, Matsui H, Nakao M (1972) Differential isolation of microvillus and basolateral membranes from intestinal mucosa: Mutually exclusive distribution of digestive enzymes and ouabain-sensitive ATPase. Biochim Biophys Acta 274:336–344

Garcia-Diaz JF, Armstrong WMcD (1980) The steady-state relationship between sodium and chloride transmembrane electrochemical potential differences in *Necturus* gallbladder. J Membr Biol 55:213–222

Garcia-Diaz JF, Corcia A (1977) Electrical changes in isolated rat jejunum produced by hypertonicity. Biochim Biophys Acta 465:177–187

Garcia-Diaz JF, O'Doherty J, Armstrong WMcD (1978) Potential profile, K^+ and Na^+ activities in *Necturus* small intestine. Physiologist 21:41

Geck P, Heinz E (1976) Coupling in secondary transport: Effect of electrical potential on the kinetics of ion-linked cotransport. Biochim Biophys Acta 443:49–63

Gerencser GA, Armstrong WMcD (1972) Sodium transfer in bullfrog small intestine: Stimulation by exogenous ATP. Biochim Biophys Acta 255:663–674

Gerencser GA, White JF (1980) Membrane potentials and chloride activities in epithelial cells of *Aplysia* intestine. Am J Physiol 239:R445–R449

Gerencser GA, Hong SK, Malvin G (1976) Metabolic dependence of active chloride transport in isolated *Aplysia* intestine. Fed Proc 35:464

Gilles-Baillien M, Schoffeniels E (1965) Site of action of L-alanine and D-glucose on the potential difference across the intestine. Arch Int Physiol Biochem 73:355–357

Gilles-Baillien M, Schoffeniels E (1968) Amino acids and bioelectric potentials in the small intestine of the Greek tortoise. Life Sci 7:53–63

Goldman DE (1943) Potential, impedance and rectification in membranes. J Gen Physiol 27:37–60

Goldner AM, Schultz SG, Curran PF (1969) Sodium and sugar fluxes across the mucosal border of rabbit ileum. J Gen Physiol 53:362–383

Grady GF, Madoff MA, Duhamel RC, Moore EW, Chalmers TC (1967) Sodium transport by human ileum in vitro and its response to cholera toxin. Gastroenterology 53:737–744

Grady GF, Duhamel RC, Moore EW (1970) Active transport of sodium by human colon in vitro. Gastroenterology 59:583–588

Grady TP, Reuss L (1981) Intracellular microelectrode studies in *Ascaris* intestine. Fed Proc 40:371

Graf J, Giebisch G (1979) Intracellular sodium activity and sodium transport in *Necturus* gallbladder epithelium. J Membr Biol 47:327–355

Guggino WB, Boulpaep EL, Giebisch C (1982) Electrical properties of chloride transport across the *Necturus* proximal tubule. J Membr Biol 65:188–196

Gunter-Smith PJ, Schultz SG (1982) Potassium transport and intracellular potassium activities in rabbit gallbladder. J Membr Biol 65:41–47

Gunter-Smith PJ, White JF (1979a) Contribution of villous and intervillous epithelium to intestinal transmural potential difference and response to theophylline and sugar. Biochim Biophys Acta 557:425–435

Gunter-Smith PJ, White JF (1979b) Response of *Amphiuma* small intestine to theophylline: Effect on bicarbonate transport. Am J Physiol 236(6):E775–E783

Gunter-Smith PJ, Grassett E, Schultz SG (1982) Sodium-coupled amino acid and sugar transport by *Necturus* small intestine. An equivalent electrical circuit analysis of a rheogenic co-transport system. J Membr Biol 66:25–39

Gupta BL, Hall TA, Naftalin RJ (1978) Microprobe measurement of Na, K, and Cl concentration profiles in epithelial cells and intercellular spaces of rabbit ileum. Nature 272:70–73

Hajjar JJ, Khuri RN, Curran PF (1972) Alanine efflux across the serosal border of the turtle intestine. J Gen Physiol 60:720–734

Heidenhain R (1894) Neue Versuche über die Aufsaugung im Dünndarm. Arch Ges Physiol 56:579–631

Heinz E (ed) (1972) Na-linked transport of organic solutes. Springer, Berlin

Henin S, Cremaschi D (1975) Transcellular ion route in rabbit gallbladder. Electric properties of the epithelial cells. Pflügers Arch 335:125–139

Hirschorn N, Frazier HS (1973) The electrical profile of stripped, isolated rabbit ileum. Johns Hopkins Med J 132:271–281

Höber R (1946) Intestinal absorption. In: Höber R (ed) Physical chemistry of cells and tissues, ch 34. Blackiston, Philadelphia, pp 531–552

Hodgkin AL, Horowicz P (1959) The influence of potassium and chloride ions on the membrane potential of single muscle fibres. J Physiol (Lond) 148:127–160

Hodgkin AL, Katz B (1949) The effect of sodium ions on the electrical activity of the giant axon of the squid. J Physiol (Lond) 108:37–77

Kedem O, Caplan SR (1965) Degree of coupling and its relation to efficiency of energy conversion. Trans Faraday Soc 61:1897–1911

Kessler M, Acuto O, Storelli C, Murer H, Müller M, Semenza G (1978) A modified procedure for the rapid preparation of efficiently transporting vesicles from small intestinal brush border membranes. Biochim Biophys Acta 506:136–154

Khuri RN (1976) Intracellular potassium in single cells of renal tubules. In: Kessler M, Clark LC Jr, Lübbers DW, Silver IA, Simon W (eds) Ion and enzyme electrodes in biology and medicine. Urben u. Schwartzenberg, Berlin, pp 364–371

Kimmich GA (1970) Active sugar accumulation by isolated cells. A new model for sodium-dependent metabolite transport. Biochemistry 9:3669–3677

Kimmich GA (1973) Coupling between Na and sugar transport in small intestine. Biochim Biophys Acta 300:31–78

Kimmich GA (1981 a) Intestinal absorption of sugar. In: Johnson LR (ed) Physiology of the gastrointestinal tract, vol 2. Raven, New York, pp 1035–1061

Kimmich GA (1981 b) The Na^+-dependent sugar carrier as a sensor of the cellular electrochemical Na^+ potential. In: Dinno MA, Callahan AB (eds) Membrane biophysics: Structure and function in epithelia. Liss, New York, pp 129–142

Kimmich GA, Carter-Su C (1978) Membrane potentials and the energetics of intestinal Na^+-dependent transport systems. Am J Physiol 235:C73–C81

Kimmich GA, Randles J (1976) 2-Deoxy-glucose transport by intestinal epithelial cells isolated from the chick. J Membr Biol 27:363–379

Kimmich GA, Randles J (1979) Energetics of sugar transport by isolated intestinal epithelial cells: Effects of cytochalasin-B. Am J Physiol 237:C56–C63

Kimmich GA, Randles J (1981) Evidence for an intestinal Na^+: Sugar coupling stoichiometry of 2.0. Biochim Biophys Acta 596:439–444

Kinne R, Mürer H (1976) Polarity of epithelial cells in relation to transepithelial transport in kidney and intestine. In: Robinson JWL (ed) Intestinal ion transport. MTP, Lancaster, England, pp 79–95

Kinsella JL, Aronson PS (1980) Properties of the Na^+-H^+ exchanger in renal microvillus membrane vesicles. Am J Physiol 238:F461–F469

Kinsella JL, Aronson PS (1981 a) Amiloride inhibition of the Na^+-H^+ exchanger in renal microvillus membrane vesicles. Am J Physiol 241:F374–F379

Kinsella JL, Aronson PS (1981 b) Interaction of NH_4^+ and Li^+ with the renal microvillus membrane Na^+-H^+ exchanger. Am J Physiol 241:C220–C226

Koefoed-Johnsen V, Ussing HH (1958) The nature of the frog skin potential. Acta Physiol Scand 42:298–308

Kohn PG, Smyth DH, Wright EM (1966) Effects of dipeptides and disaccharides on the electrical potential across the rat small intestine. J Physiol (Lond) 185:47P–48P

Leader JP (1981) Alternative methods for the measurement of membrane potentials. In: MacKnight ADC, Leader JP (eds) Epithelial ion and water transport. Raven, New York, pp 55–62

Leaf A (1982) From toad bladder to kidney. Am J Physiol 242:F103–F111

Lee CO, Armstrong WMcD (1972) Activities of sodium and potassium ions in epithelial cells of small intestine. Science 175:1261–1264

Lev AA, Armstrong WMcD (1975) Ionic activities in cells. In: Kleinzeller A, Bronner F (eds) Current topics in membranes and transport, vol 6. Academic, New York, pp 59–123

Liedke CM, Hopfer U (1977) Anion transport in brush border membranes isolated from rat small intestine. Biochim Biophys Res Commun 76:579–585

Liedke CM, Hopfer U (1982a) Mechanism of Cl^- translocation across small intestinal brush-border membrane. I. Absence of Na^+-Cl^- cotransport. Am J Physiol 242:G263–G271

Liedke CM, Hopfer U (1982b) Mechanism of Cl^- translocation across small intestinal brush-border membrane. II. Demonstration of Cl^--OH^- exchange and Cl^- conductance. Am J Physiol 242:G272–G280

Loewenstein WR (1981) Junctional intercellular communication: The cell-to-cell membrane channel. Physiol Rev 61:829–913

Lücke H, Kinne R, Mürer H (1979) Effect of cellular cyclic AMP on the transport of sugars by the jejunum in vivo and by brush border membrane vesicles in vitro. In: Binder H (ed) Mechanisms of intestinal secretion. Liss, New York, pp 111–116

Lyon I, Crane RK (1966a) Studies on transmural potentials in vitro in relation to intestinal absorption. I. Apparent Michaelis constants for Na^+ dependent sugar transport. Biochim Biophys Acta 112:278–291

Lyon I, Crane RK (1966b) Studies on transmural potentials in vitro in relation to intestinal absorption. II. An effect of ouabain on glucose-dependent increment of transmural potential of rat small intestine. Biochim Biophys Acta 125:146–153

Lyon I, Sheerin HE (1971) Studies on transmural potentials in vitro in relation to intestinal absorption. VI. The effect of sugars on electrical potential profiles in jejunum and ileum. Biochim Biophys Acta 249:1–14

Machen TE, Diamond JM (1969) An estimate of the salt concentration in the lateral intercellular spaces of rabbit gallbladder during maximal fluid transport. J Membr Biol 1:194–213

Machen TE, Diamond JM (1972) The mechanisms of anion permeation in thorium-treated gallbladder. J Membr Biol 8:63–96

Machen TE, Erlij D, Wooding FBP (1972) Permeable tight junction complexes. The movement of lanthanum across rabbit gallbladder and intestine. J Cell Biol 54:302–312

Mak KM, Trier JS, Serfilippi D, Donaldson RM Jr (1974) Resistance of adult mammalian intestinal mucosa to cytochalasin-B. Exp Cell Res 86:325–332

Martinez-Palomo A, Erlij D (1975) Structure of tight junctions in epithelia with different permeability. Proc Nat Acad Sci USA 72:4487–4491

Maruyama T, Hoshi T (1972) The effects of D-glucose on the electrical potential profile across the proximal tubule of newt kidney. Biochim Biophys Acta 282:214–225

Matthews DM (1975) Intestinal absorption of peptides. Physiol Rev 55:537–608

Misfeldt DS, Sanders MJ (1981) Transepithelial Na^+: D-glucose stoichiometry is two. Ann NY Acad Sci 372:465–467

Misfeldt DS, Hanamoto ST, Pitelka DR (1976) Transepithelial transport in cell culture. Proc Nat Acad Sci USA 73:1212–1216

Moreno JH (1974) Blockage of cation permeability across the tight junctions of gallbladder and other leaky epithelia. Nature 251:150–151

Moreno JH (1975a) Blockage of gallbladder tight junction cation-selective channels by 2,4,6-triaminopyrimidinium. J Gen Physiol 66:97–115

Moreno JH (1975b) Routes of nonelectrolyte permeability in gallbladder. Effects of 2,4,6-triaminopyrimidinium. J Gen Physiol 66:117–128

Moreno JH, Diamond JM (1975a) Cation permeation mechanism, and cation selectivity in "tight" junctions of gallbladder epithelium. In: Eisenman G (ed) Membranes. Dekker, New York, pp 383–497

Moreno JH, Diamond JM (1975b) Nitrogenous cations as probes of permeation channels. J Membr Biol 21:197–259

Munck BG, Schultz SG (1974) Properties of the passive conductance pathway across in vitro rat jejunum. J Membr Biol 16:163–174

Mürer H, Hopfer U (1974) Demonstration of electrogenic Na^+-dependent D-glucose transport in intestinal brush border membranes. Proc Nat Acad Sci USA 71:484–488

Mürer H, Hopfer U, Kinne-Saffran E, Kinne R (1974) Glucose transport in isolated brush-border and lateral basal plasma membrane vesicles from intestinal epithelial cells. Biochim Biophys Acta 345:170–179

Mürer H, Hopfer U, Kinne R (1976) Sodium/proton antiport in brush-border-membrane vesicles isolated from rat-small intestine and kidney. Biochem J 154:597–604

Nagel W, Garcia-Diaz JF, Armstrong WMcD (1981) Ionic activities in frog skin. J Membr Biol 61:127–134

Nellans HN, Schultz SG (1976) Relations among transepithelial sodium transport, potassium exchange and cell volume in rabbit ileum. J Gen Physiol 68:441–463

Nellans HN, Frizzell RA, Schultz SG (1973) Coupled sodium-chloride influx across the brush border of rabbit ileum. Am J Physiol 25:467–475

Nellans HN, Frizzell RA, Schultz SG (1974) Brush border processes and transepithelial Na and Cl transport by rabbit ileum. Am J Physiol 226:1131–1141

Nelson DJ, Ehrenfeld J, Lindemann B (1978) Volume changes and potential artifacts of epithelial cells of frog skin following impalement with microelectrodes filled with 3M KCl. J Membr Biol 40:91–119

Newey H, Smyth DH (1964) Effects of sugars on intestinal transport of amino acis. Nature 202:400–401

Newey H, Parsons BJ, Smyth DH (1959) The site of action of phlorhizin in inhibiting intestinal absorption of glucose. J Physiol (Lond) 148:83–92

O'Doherty J, Garcia-Diaz JF, Armstrong WMcD (1979) Sodium-selective liquid ion-exchange microelectrodes for intracellular measurements. Science 203:1349–1351

O'Doherty J, Youmans SJ, Armstrong WMcD, Stark RJ (1980) Calcium regulation during stimulus-secretion coupling: Continuous measurement of intracellular calcium activities. Science 209:510–513

Okada Y, Sato T, Inouye A (1975) Effects of potassium ions and sodium ions on membrane potential of epithelial cells in rat duodenum. Biochim Biophys Acta 413:104–115

Okada Y, Irimajiri A, Inouye A (1976) Permeability properties and intracellular ion concentrations of epithelial cells in rat duodenum. Biochim Biophys Acta 436:15–24

Okada Y, Irimajiri A, Inouye A (1977a) Electrical properties and active solute transport in rat small intestine. II. Conductive properties of transepithelial routes. J Membr Biol 31:221–232

Okada Y, Tsuchiya W, Irimajiri A, Inouye A (1977b) Electrical properties and active solute transport in rat small intestine. I. Potential profile changes associated with sugar and amino acid transport. J Membr Biol 31:205–219

Parsons DS (1967) Sodium chloride absorption by the small intestine and the relationships between the absorption of H_2O and some organic molecules. Proc Nutr Soc 26:46–54

Parsons DS (1968) Methods for investigation of intestinal absorption. In: Code CF (ed) Handbook of physiology, Section 6, vol III. Williams and Wilkins, Baltimore, pp 1177–1216

Powell DW (1979) Transport in large intestine. In: Giebisch G (ed) Membrane transport in biology, vol IV.B, Transport organs. Springer, New York, pp 781–809

Powell DW, Binder HJ, Curran PF (1972) Electrolyte secretion by the guinea pig ileum in vitro. Am J Physiol 223:531–537

Pricam C, Humbert F, Perrelet A, Orci L (1974) A freeze-etch study of the tight junctions of the rat kidney tubules. Lab Invest 30:286–291

Quay JF, Armstrong WMcD (1969) Sodium and chloride transport by isolated bullfrog small intestine. Am J Physiol 217:694–702

Quigley JP, Gotterer GS (1969) Distribution of (Na+K)-stimulated ATPase activity in rat intestinal mucosa. Biochim Biophys Acta 173:456–468

Read CP (1967) Studies on membrane transport: 1. A common transport system for sugars and amino acids. Biol Bull 133:630–642

Reid EW (1892) Preliminary report on experiments upon intestinal absorption without osmosis. Br Med J 1:1133–1134

Reuss L (1979) Electrical properties of the cellular transepithelial pathway in *Necturus* gallbladder: III. Ionic permeability of the basolateral cell membrane. J Membr Biol 51:15–31

Reuss L, Finn AL (1975a) Electrical properties of the cellular transepithelial pathway in *Necturus* gallbladder: I. Circuit analysis and steady-state effects of mucosal solution ionic substitutions. J Membr Biol 25:115–139

Reuss L, Finn AL (1975b) Electrical properties of the cellular transepithelial pathway in *Necturus* gallbladder. II. Ionic permeability of the apical cell membrane. J Membr Biol 25:141–161

Reuss L, Finn AL (1977) Effects of luminal hyperosmolality on electrical pathways of *Necturus* gallbladder. Am J Physiol 232:C99–C108

Reuss L, Grady TP (1979) Effects of external sodium and cell membrane potential on intracellular chloride activity in gallbladder epithelium. J Membr Biol 51:15–31

Reuss L, Weinman SA, Grady TP (1980) Intracellular K^+ activity and its relation to basolateral membrane ion transport in *Necturus* gallbladder epithelium. J Gen Physiol 76:33–52

Riklis E, Quastel JH (1958) Effects of cations on sugar absorption by isolated surviving guinea-pig intestine. Can J Biochem Physiol 36:347–362

Ritter U (1957) Histophysiologische Untersuchungen am Darmepithel während der Verdauung. Gastroenterologia 88:133–171

Robinson RA, Stokes RH (1965) Electrolyte solutions, 2nd ed. Butterworths, London, pp 174–222

Roggin GM, Banwell JG, Yardley JH, Hendrix TH (1972) Unimpaired response of rabbit jejunum to cholera toxin after selective damage to villus epithelium. Gastroenterology 63:981–989

Rose RG, Schultz SG (1971) Studies on the electrical potential profile across rabbit ileum. Effects of sugars and amino acids on transmural and transmucosal electrical potential differences. J Gen Physiol 51:639–663

Rosenberg T (1948) On accumulation and active transport in biological system. I. Thermodynamic considerations. Acta Chem Scand 2:14–33

Rothe CF, Quay JR, Armstrong WMcD (1969) Measurement of epithelial electrical characteristics with an automatic voltage clamp device with compensation for solution resistance. IEEE Trans Biomed Eng BME-16:160–164

Samarziya I, Frömter E (1975) Electrical studies on amino acid transport across brush border membrane of Na^+ proximal tubule in vivo. Pflügers Arch 359:R119

Sawada M, Asano T (1963) Effects of metabolic disturbance on potential difference across intestinal wall of rat. Am J Physiol 204:105–108

Schacter D, Britten JS (1961) Active transport of non-electrolytes and the potential gradients across intestinal segments in vitro. Fed Proc 20:137

Schultz SG (1977) Sodium-coupled solute transport by the small intestine: A status report. Am J Physiol 233:E249–E254

Schultz SG (1979) Transport across small intestine. In: Giebisch G (ed) Membrane transport in biology, vol IV.B, Transport organs. Springer, New York, pp 749–780

Schultz SG (1981) Salt and water absorption by mammalian small intestine. In: Johnson R (ed) Physiology of the gastrointestinal tract, vol 2. Raven, New York, pp 983–989

Schultz SG, Curran PF (1968) Intestinal absorption of sodium chloride and water. In: Code CF (ed) Handbook of physiology, Section 6, vol III. Williams and Wilkins, Baltimore, pp 1245–1277

Schultz SG, Curran PF (1970) Coupled transport of sodium and organic solutes. Physiol Rev 50:637–718

Schultz SG, Curran PF (1974) Sodium and chloride transport across isolated rabbit ileum. In: Kleinzeller A, Bronner F (eds) Current topics in membranes and transport, vol 5. Academic, New York, pp 225–281

Schultz SG, Zalusky R (1963a) The interaction between active sodium transport and active sugar transport in the isolated rabbit ileum. Biochim Biophys Acta 71:503–505

Schultz SG, Zalusky R (1963b) Transmural potential difference, short circuit current and sodium transport in isolated rabbit ileum. Nature 198:894–895

Schultz SG, Zalusky R (1964a) Ion transport in isolated rabbit ileum. I. Short-circuit current and Na^+ fluxes. J Gen Physiol 47:567–584

Schultz SG, Zalusky R (1964b) Ion transport in isolated rabbit ileum. II. The interaction between active sodium and active sugar transport. J Gen Physiol 48:375–378

Schultz SG, Zalusky R (1965) Interactions between active sodium transport and active amino acid transport in isolated rabbit ileum. Nature 205:292–294

Schultz SG, Zalusky R, Gass AE (1964) Ion transport in isolated rabbit ileum. III. Chloride fluxes. J Gen Physiol 48:375–378

Schultz SG, Fuisz RE, Curran PF (1966) Amino acid and sugar transport in rabbit ileum. J Gen Physiol 49:849–866

Schultz SG, Curran PF, Chez RA, Fuisz RE (1967) Alanine and sodium fluxes across mucosal border of rabbit ileum. J Gen Physiol 50:1241–1260

Schultz SG, Frizzell RA, Nellans HN (1974) Ion transport by mammalian small intestine. Ann Rev Physiol 36:51–91
Schultz SG, Frizzell RA, Nellans HN (1977) Sodium transport and the electrophysiology of rabbit colon. J Membr Biol 33:351–384
Semenza G (1971) On the mechanism of mutual inhibition among sodium-dependent transport systems in the small intestine: A hypothesis. Biochim Biophys Acta 241:637–649
Shiba H (1971) Heaviside's " Bessell cable" as an electric model for flat simple epithelial cells with low resistive junctional membranes. J Theor Biol 30:59–68
Shindo T, Spring KR (1981) Chloride movement across the basolateral membrane of proximal tubule cells. J Membr Biol 58:35–42
Sigrist-Nelson K, Murer H, Hopfer U (1975) Active alanine transport in isolated brush border membranes. J Biol Chem 250:5674–5680
Simmons NL, Naftalin RJ (1976) Factors affecting the compartmentalization of sodium ion within rabbit ileum in vitro. Biochim Biophys Acta 448:411–425
Simon W, Morf WE (1973) Alkali cation specificity of carrier antibiotics and their behavior in bulk membranes. In: Eisenman G (ed) Membranes, vol 2. Dekker, New York, pp 329–375
Smith MW, Sepulveda FV (1979) Sodium dependence of neutral amino acid uptake into rabbit ileum. Biochim Biophys Acta 555:374–378
Smyth DH (1968) Energetics of intestinal transfer. In: Armstrong WMcD, Nunn AS Jr (eds) Intestinal transport of electrolytes, amino acids and sugars. Thomas, Springfield, IL, pp 52–75
Smyth DH, Wright EM (1966) Streaming potentials in the rat small intestine. J Physiol (Lond) 182:591–602
Spring KR, Ericson AC (1982) Epithelial cell volume modulation and regulation. J Membr Biol 69:167–176
Spring KR, Kimura G (1978) Chloride reabsorption by renal proximal tubules of *Necturus*. J Membr Biol 38:233–254
Steiner RA, Oehme M, Amman D, Simon W (1979) Neutral carrier sodium ion-selective microelectrode for intracellular studies. Anal Chem 51:351–353
Stirling ES (1972) Radioautographic localization of Na pumps in rabbit intestine. J Cell Biol 53:704–714
Strickholm A, Wallin BG (1967) Relative ion permeabilities in the crayfish giant axon determined from rapid external ion changes. J Gen Physiol 50:1929–1953
Suzuki K, Frömter E (1977) The potential and resistance profile of *Necturus* gallbladder cells. Pflügers Arch 371:109–117
Thomas RC (1978) Ion-sensitive microelectrodes: How to make and use them. Academic, New York
Thomas RC, Cohen CJ (1981) A liquid ion-exchanger alternative to KCl for filling intracellular reference microelectrodes. Pflügers Arch 390:96–98
Tisher CC, Yarger WE (1973) Lanthanum permeability of the tight junction (zonula occludens) in the renal tubule of the rat. Kidney Int 3:328–350
Trier JS, Madara JL (1981) Functional morphology of the mucosa of the small intestine. In: Johnson LR (ed) Physiology of the gastrointestinal tract, vol 2. Raven, New York, pp 925–961
Turnberg LA (1971) Potassium transport in the human small bowel. Gut 12:811–818
Turnberg LA, Bieberdorf FA, Morawski SG, Fordtran JS (1970) Interrelationships of chloride, bicarbonate, sodium, and hydrogen transport in the human ileum. J Clin Invest 49:557–567
Ussing HH (1960) The alkali metal ions in isolated cells and tissues. In: Ussing HH, Kruhoffer P, Hess Theysen J, Thorn NA (eds) Alkali metal ions in biology. Springer, Berlin, pp 1–195
Ussing HH, Andersen B (1955) The relation between solvent drag and active transport of ions. Proc Third International Congress of Biochemistry, Brussels, pp 434–440
Ussing HH, Windhager EE (1964) Nature of shunt path and active sodium transport path through frog skin epithelium. Acta Physiol Scand 61:484–504
Ussing HH, Zerahn K (1951) Active transport of sodium as the source of electric current in the short-circuited isolated frog skin. Acta Physiol Scand 23:110–127

Ussing HH, Erlij D, Lassen U (1974) Transport pathways in biological membranes. Ann Rev Physiol 36:17–49

Waggoner AS (1979) Dye indicators of membrane potential. Ann Rev Biophys Bioeng 8:47–68

Walker JL Jr (1971) Ion specific liquid ion-exchanger microelectrodes. Anal Chem 43:89A–93A

Walker JL, Brown HL (1977) Intracellular activity measurements in nerve and muscle. Physiol Rev 57:729–778

Ward MR, Boyd CAR (1980) Intracellular study of ionic events underlying intestinal membrane transport of oligopeptides. Nature 287:157–158

Weinman SA, Reuss L (1982) Na^+-H^+ exchange at the apical membrane of *Necturus* gallbladder. Extracellular and intracellular pH studies. J Gen Physiol 80:299–321

White JF (1976) Intracellular potassium activities in *Amphiuma* small intestine. Am J Physiol 231:1214–1219

White JF (1977a) Alterations in electrophysiology of isolated amphibian small intestine produced by removing the muscle layers. Biochim Biophys Acta 467:91–102

White JF (1977b) Activity of chloride in absorptive cells of *Amphiuma* small intestine. Am J Physiol 232:E553–E559

White JF, Armstrong WMcD (1971) Effect of transported solutes on membrane potentials in bullfrog small intestine. Am J Physiol 221:194–201

White JF, Imon MA (1981) Intestinal bicarbonate secretion in *Amphiuma* intestine measured by pH stat in vitro: Relationship with metabolism and transport of sodium and chloride ions. J Physiol (Lond) 314:429–443

Whittenbury G, Rawlins FA (1971) Evidence of a paracellular pathway for ion flow in the kidney proximal tubule: Electromicroscopic demonstration of lanthanum precipitate in the tight junction. Pflügers Arch 330:302–309

Wilson TH, Wiseman G (1954) The use of sacs of everted small intestine for the study of the transference of substances from the mucosal to the serosal surface. J Physiol (Lond) 123:126–130

Wright EM (1966) The origin of the glucose dependent increase in the potential difference across the tortoise small intestine. J Physiol (Lond) 185:486–500

Wright EM (1972) Mechanisms of ion transport across the choroid plexus. J Physiol (Lond) 226:545–571

Wright EM, Diamond JM (1968) Effect of pH and polyvalent cations on the selective permeability of the gall-bladder epithelium to monovalent ions. Biochim Biophys Acta 163:57–74

Wright EM, Barry PH, Diamond JM (1971) The mechanism of cation permeation in rabbit gallbladder: Conductances, the current-voltage relation, concentration dependence of anion-cation discrimination and the calcium competition effect. J Membr Biol 4:331–357

Wright EM, Mircheff AK, Hanna SD, Harms V, van Os EH, Walling MW, Sachs G (1979) The dark side of the intestinal epithelium: The isolation and characterization of basolateral membranes. In: Binder HJ (ed) Mechanisms of intestinal secretion. Liss, New York, pp 117–130

Zeuthen T (1977) Intracellular gradients of electrical potential in the epithelial cells of the *Necturus* gallbladder. J Membr Biol 33:281–309

Zeuthen T, Monge C (1975) Intra- and extracellular gradients of electrical potential and ionic activities of epithelial cells of the rabbit ileum in vivo recorded with microelectrodes. Philos Trans R Soc Lond (Biol) 71:277–281

Zeuthen T, Monge C (1976) Electrical potentials and ion activities in the epithelial cell layer of the rabbit ileum in vivo. In: Kessler M, Clark LC Jr, Lübbers DW, Silver IA, Simon W (eds) Ion and enzyme electrodes in biology and medicine. Urban u. Schwartzenberg, Berlin, pp 345–350

Zeuthen T, Ramos M, Ellory JC (1978) Inhibition of active chloride transport by piretanide. Nature 273:678–680

CHAPTER 11

Intestinal Permeation of Water

K. TURNHEIM

A. Introduction

Water is the main constituent of the human body. The weight fraction in males varies between 59% at age 10–16 years and 52% above 60 years; in females the water content is a few percent lower (EDELMAN and LEIBMAN 1959). Several basic data of water homeostasis in the human under normal conditions of body temperature regulation are compiled in Table 1. In comparison with other mammals such as dog, beef, elephant, rabbit, and rat the daily water intake of the human is low when expressed as a percentage of body weight (FITZSIMONS 1979). Clearly, over extended periods of time, intestinal water absorption and the water recovered from the metabolism of nutrients have to be equal to the combined water loss via the kidneys, intestine, lung, and skin. Whereas renal mechanisms are known as regulatory systems which preserve the dynamic water equilibrium of the organism, for example the effect of antidiuretic hormone (ADH) on the distal nephron, little is known of feedback systems between water demand and intestinal water absorption. Up to enormously high amounts of daily oral water intake, for instance in the case of diabetes insipidus, practically all the water ingested is absorbed. Hence, the amount of intestinal water absorption appears to be primarily determined by the rate of oral water intake. Oral water intake, in turn, is controlled by our consciousness, specifically by thirst. Considerable progress has been made in elucidating the factors coupling water homeostasis and the sensation of thirst, as reviewed by FITZSIMONS (1979) and PETERS (1980).

However, the amount of water absorbed in the gastrointestinal tract is much larger than the normal daily oral water intake of approximately 2.5 l, since about 8 l/day is secreted into the gut lumen in the form of salivary, gastric, biliary, pan-

Table 1. External turnover of water in a healthy human in moderate climate, data of SCHNEIDER (1964) and FITZSIMONS (1979)

Water intake (ml/day)		Water output (ml/day)	
Water drunk	1,200–1,300	Urine	1,500
Water in food	1,000	Respiration	300– 550
Metabolic water	300– 350	Skin	600– 450
		Feces	100– 150
Total	2,500–2,650	Total	2,500–2,650

creatic, and small intestinal juices. Hence, the intestinal water absorption averages 10 l in 24 h, so that the daily turnover of water in the gastrointestinal tract represents three times the volume of blood plasma water or 25% of total body water. However, the maximum capacity for intestinal fluid absorption is considerably higher. LOVE et al. (1968) estimated the absorptive capacity of the entire human intestinal tract to be approximately 21 l in 24 h, but this value appears to represent a lower limit, since the curvilinear relation between water intake and water absorption was still rising at the highest rates of water intake tested. From the studies of FORDTRAN et al. (1961) the absorptive capacity of the small bowel may be calculated to be about 22 l in 24 h, and DEBONGNIE and PHILLIPS (1978) reported that the normal human colon is capable of absorbing up to 6 l in 24 h. Therefore, the total intestinal capacity for fluid absorption can be estimated to be approximately 28 l in 24 h. This remarkable absorptive work is accomplished by an epithelium, the surface of which is approximately 10 m^2 because of folds and villi. When the enlargement due to microvilli is included, the absorptive area is increased up to 300 m^2.

Although water transport is clearly the dominant function of the intestine in quantitative terms, surprisingly little space is assigned in textbooks of physiology to the discussion of intestinal water absorption in comparison with the space devoted to the absorption of solutes such as sugars, amino acids, and inorganic electrolytes, probably because the mechanism of intestinal water transport is still not totally resolved. The difficulty in analyzing transepithelial water transport stems in part from the fact that water is the primary solvent of the organism. Hence it was not possible to employ kinetic methods for the investigation of intestinal water transport such as the study of the concentration dependence of permeation rates, a technique that has helped immensely to clarify solute transfer mechanisms. It was not until KEDEM and KATCHALSKY (1958) developed the formal description of transport in terms of irreversible thermodynamics, that the modern era in the investigation of water transport began.

Intestinal water absorption is only one facet of the general problem of water permeation across membranes. In fact, many of the basic investigations on water transport were performed by use of membranes of other origin such as amphibian epithelia or artificial lipid bilayers. Insofar as data from these membranes help to understand intestinal water permeation, they will be briefly dealt with. One epithelium with the same phylogenetic and ontogenetic origin as the intestinal epithelium, that from gallbladder, commands special attention, since its functional properties have been most extensively studied.

B. Historical Concepts of Intestinal Fluid Absorption

The early physiologists did not differentiate between the absorptive mechanisms of the individual constituents of food, but were concerned with the fate of the total chyle. For instance, in 1874 the Vienna physiologist BRÜCKE explained the absorption of intestinal fluids by filtration into the lacteals; the blood vessels were considered totally unfit to play a major role in absorption, since their hydrostatic pressure exceeds that in the intestinal lumen. The filtration pressure was assumed to be provided by the pumping action of the villi, pressing the absorbate into the lacteals, in which many valves were taken to prevent backflux. Relaxation of the villi would result in a decrease in the intravillus pressure, thereby causing fluid permeation across the epithelium. The problem of transepithelial permeation was accounted for the BRÜCKE (1874) as follows (all translations are fairly literal).

> The fact that granules of fat and the other substances enter the cells is not mysterious, because there is no cell membrane on the luminal side, only the rod-apparatus (brush border) which is an extension of the protoplasm. From the epithelial cells the granules migrate into the stroma of the villi. Obviously the epithelial cells have to possess an opening at the stroma side similar to the opening at the luminal side across which the droplets enter and leave the cells.

Only a few years later HEIDENHAIN (1888) reported that the rate of lymph flow was only increased by 60 ml when 756 ml 0.3% NaCl solution was absorbed from then small intestine. HEIDENHAIN therefore concluded that most of the water absorbed is taken up by the blood capillaries of the villi rather than by the lacteals. This notion was also supported by the finding of REID (1900) that intestinal absorption of fluid is not altered when the mesenteric lymph vessels are ligated. REID agreed with BRÜCKE insofar as he showed that the hydrostatic pressure in the mesenteric veins was 13.5–18.4 mmHg, whereas the pressure in the intestinal lumen was only 4–6 mmHg, but was careful to conclude only that absorption is not brought about by filtration from the intestinal lumen into the blood.

The fundamental experiments of HEIDENHAIN (1894) exclude diffusion and transepithelial osmosis from being responsible for absorption, since dogs totally absorbed dog serum. This important paper also reports that water is absorbed even from hypertonic solutions, and NaCl is absorbed from solutions having a NaCl concentration far lower than that of blood plasma. "Both phenomena point with necessity to other forces (other than osmosis and diffusion) whose origin can only be in the living gut wall." Because of the notion that the driving force for absorption resides in the epithelium itself, HEIDENHAIN was accused of "vitalistic" conceptions.

Simultaneously to HEIDENHAIN in Breslau, REID in Dundee rejected the theory of "osmotic absorption" in favor of "vital absorption." REID conducted pioneering experiments on isolated tissues in vitro, because "to prove that living intestine can absorb when osmotic action is absent, the fluids on the two sides of the epithelial barrier must be of identical composition, a condition that can only be realized by using exsected gut, and taking advantage of the post mortem life of the tissue." When a disc of rabbit ileum was mounted as a separating membrane between the two sides of a horizontally placed cylindrical glass chamber, the volume of fluid on the serosal side increased and that on the luminal side decreased. This effect originated in the epithelium, since scraping of the luminal surface of the gut abolished the absorptive stream (REID 1892, 1901). Thus, "the cells of the gut wall appear to be capable of sucking up fluid and passing it over to the blood. [These phenomena] are as distinctly opposed to a simple physical explanation as are those previously studied in the absorption of serum" (REID 1902). However, the epithelial driving force was still doubted, the finding of REID on isolated gut walls being interpreted by pumping of the villi, although isolated frog skin also generated an asymmetric water flow (REID 1901), proving beyond reasonable doubt "that an absorbing membrane can function as a motor even without an effective muscular apparatus" (HÖBER 1907).

Further important observations were made by GUMILEWSKI and COHNHEIM late in the nineteenth century. Distilled water is absorbed to a lesser extent from the intestine than are solutions containing NaCl, whereas solutions containing Na_2SO_4 were not absorbed faster than distilled water, prompting GUMILEWSKI (1886) to not that "the salutary effect of certain table-salt-containing wells is brought nearer to our comprehension." COHNHEIM (1898, 1899) reported a peculiar asymmetry of the intestinal permeability. NaCl was found to permeate only to a small extent from blood plasma into the intestinal lumen, whereas it readily permeated in the direction lumen to blood. This striking phenomenon was later explained by INGRAHAM and VISSCHER (1938) by a fluid circuit mechanism, according to which, in essence, the selective transport of materials against concentration gradients is a result of the circulation of fluid through differentially permeable membranes. Water is conceived to move continuously across the intestinal epithelium into the gut lumen through structures completely impermeable (or nearly so) to all electrolytes and simultaneously to move in the reverse direction from the gut lumen to the blood through other structures which are permeable to the solutes in question. Hence, in effect, the solutes would be trapped on one side of the epithelium. According to this concept water flow has to be produced by a primary active transport system, on which INGRAHAM and VISSCHER (1938) preferred not to speculate: "The nature of the force driving the fluid through the membrane is a separate problem." The mechanism of active water transport has puzzled physiologists to this day, and only recently has the question been resolved whether active water transport by epithelia is primary or secondary (CURRAN and SOLOMON 1957).

From this brief historical survey of some of the earlier work on the mechanism of intestinal fluid transport one should deduce a certain amount of skepticism towards today's dogmas concerning intestinal transport. A detailed account of the work on intestinal absorption up to 1920, focusing especially on the controversy between the "vitalistic" theory and that based on purely physicochemical forces, was given by GOLDSCHMIDT (1921).

C. Formal Description of Water Transfer

In order to understand the experimental data given in the later sections and to make this chapter self-sufficient it is necessary to give a short theoretical introduction. For detailed formal descriptions of membrane transport the reader is referred to the excellent accounts of KEDEM and KATCHALSKY (1958), SNELL et al (1965), KATCHALSKY and CURRAN (1965), STEIN (1967), LAKSHMINARAYANAIAH (1969), HOUSE (1974), GLASER (1976), and SCHULTZ (1980). The theoretical basis of membrane permeation is also discused by CAPRARO in Chap. 3.

In principle, the permeation of water across a membrane should be treated exactly like the permeation of any other compound. There are two formal approaches to the analysis of transmembrane fluxes: a kinetic approach and a thermodynamic approach. Contrary to most other compounds, water flux data are exclusively treated thermodynamically, that is by analyzing the driving forces. However, these forces not only cause water movement, the water in turn affects all molecules dispersed in it. This interaction is a consequence of resistive or frictional forces, or in other words, a consequence of the viscosity of water.

I. General Principles

Without going into the intricacies of irreversible thermodynamics it is intuitively clear that transport represents a change of state of the system under consideration. Basically, any thermodynamic force F acting on a molecular species i is capable of generating a flow, which usually is vectorial, but which may also be nonvectorial (for example chemical flow, production of a substance). Vectorial flow of matter is also referred to as flux, defined as the number of molecules of the permeant species crossing a unit area per unit time. The thermodynamic force is equal to the rate of decrease (or the negative gradient) in potential energy E with respect to distance, therefore

$$F_i = -\frac{\mathrm{d}E_i}{\mathrm{d}x}. \tag{C.1}$$

In three-dimensional space the potential energy would dissipate in all directions, however in the case of a driving force for transmembranous transport, the gradient of potential energy may be assumed to exist perpendicular to the membrane.

The flux J_i is not only proportional to the driving force F_i, but also to the number of particles per unit volume on which this driving force is exerted, c_i. Hence

$$J_i = \omega_i c_i F_i. \tag{C.2}$$

ω_i, which is termed mobility, is a proportionality factor relating F_i and c_i to J_i. Clearly, ω_i is dependent upon the nature of the permeant species i, its molecular size and shape, and the properties of the membrane, and is a result of resistive or frictional forces within the membrane medium. The product $\omega_i F_i$ is termed velocity, so that Eq. (C.2) may also be understood to express flux as the product of concentration and velocity; c_i and ω_i may be combined in the coefficient L_i so that

$$J_i = L_i F_i. \tag{C.3}$$

L_i is the flux of substance i per unit driving force and has the dimensions of conductance. L_i is assumed to be independent of F_i. This is usually the case with relatively low flux rates, i.e., when the system is not too far from equilibrium, however, when F_i is very high the relation between J_i and F_i may no longer be linear.

Equation (C.3) expresses the relation between a flux and its direct driving force. For instance, the direct driving force for the displacement of volume is a pressure gradient, whereas the direct driving force for the movement of electrical charge is a gradient of electrical potential. In the language of thermodynamics, properties of the system such as volume or charge are termed extensive properties, which are displaced by gradients in their conjugate intensive properties, in our case pressure and electrical potential, respectively. Since the proportionality coefficients relating fluxes to their conjugate driving forces do not imply a particular molecular mechanism of interaction of the permeant species with the membrane or a particular route of passage across the membrane, these coefficients are termed phenomenological coefficients.

According to Eq. (C.1), the driving force is given by the rate of decrease of potential energy; therefore fluxes as defined by Eq. (C.3) can occur only downhill. This is certainly the case when an isolated process is considered, consisting of a single flow driven by its conjugate driving force. However, when several flows, each driven by its conjugate driving force, occur in a system simultaneously, there may be interaction between flows such that there is coupling between a flow and a nonconjugate driving force. When n flows are coupled, it is possible that an individual flow occurs against its conjugate driving force, as long as the sum of the products of the fluxes and their conjugate driving forces

$$\sum_{i=1}^{n} (J_i F_i)$$

yields a loss of potential energy, where

$$\sum_{i=1}^{n} (J_i F_i)$$

equals the co-called dissipation function. Examples of transmembrane fluxes of a substance driven by a nonconjugate driving force are solvent drag, which will be discussed later, and transport coupled to the flow of a chemical reaction (primary active transport).

If the relation between a flow and the nonconjugate driving forces is also assumed to be linear, then the phenomenological equations relating fluxes to conjugate and nonconjugate driving forces are

$$\begin{aligned} J_i &= L_{ii}F_i + L_{ij}F_j + L_{ik}F_k + \ldots + L_{in}F_n \\ J_j &= L_{ji}F_i + L_{jj}F_j + L_{jk}F_k + \ldots + L_{jn}F_n \\ J_k &= L_{ki}F_i + L_{kj}F_j + L_{kk}F_k + \ldots + L_{kn}F_n \\ &\vdots \\ J_n &= L_{ni}F_i + L_{nj}F_j + L_{nk}F_k + \ldots + L_{nn}F_n \,. \end{aligned} \tag{C.4}$$

In this matrix of linear flux equations, L_{ii}, L_{jj}, ..., L_{nn} are the direct (straight-) coefficients which relate the flows to their corresponding conjugate driving forces, whereas the L_{ij} $(i \neq j)$ and so forth relate flows to nonconjugate driving forces and are therefore termed coupling (cross-) coefficients. Since in isothermal systems the sum of the products of the flows and their conjugate driving forces must equal the dissipation function, the cross coefficients must satisfy the relation

$$L_{ij} = L_{ji} \,. \tag{C.5}$$

Equation (C.5) is usually referred to as the Onsager reciprocal relation. Therefore, we do not need n^2 independent coefficients to describe the interaction of n driving forces on n flows according to Eq. (C.4), but only $n(n+1)/2$. For example, only three phenomenological transport coefficients are necessary to formulate the fluxes of a solvent and a solute across a membrane. Further, it is intuitively clear that the degree of coupling between two flows cannot surpass 100%. When two flows are driven by two conjugate driving forces, then

$$L_{ii}L_{jj} \geqq L_{ij}^2 \, . \tag{C.6}$$

The degree of coupling may be expressed according to KEDEM and CAPLAN (1965) by

$$q_{ij} = \frac{L_{ij}}{\sqrt{L_{ii}L_{jj}}} \, . \tag{C.7}$$

q_{ij} can vary between 0 and 1; when there is no coupling between flows, $q=0$, whereas in the case of tight coupling q will approach 1.

After these general considerations we will attempt to illustrate and give examples for the phenomenological transport coefficients, starting with the simplest cases that there is no coupling between flows ($L_{ij}=0$).

II. Diffusion

Since water is a nonelectrolyte we will deal only with the formalisms describing diffusion of uncharged compounds.

1. Diffusion of Uncharged Compounds Across Homogeneous Membranes

The laws of diffusion apply to water as to any other compound. In the case of diffusion of an uncharged substance across a homogeneous barrier the conjugate driving force is the negative gradient of the chemical potential across the membrane and may be expressed as

$$F_i = -\frac{d\mu_i}{\mathrm{d}x} = -\frac{d}{\mathrm{d}x}(\mu_i^0 + RT \ln c_i) \, , \tag{C.8}$$

where c_i is the concentration of substance i. Solving this differential equation according to conventional rules, we arrive at

$$F_i = -\frac{RT}{c_i}\frac{\mathrm{d}c_i}{\mathrm{d}x} \, . \tag{C.9}$$

More correctly, the driving force is not a concentration gradient, but one in activity, $a_i = \gamma_i c_i$, where γ_i is the activity coefficient. For the sake of simplicity we will assume that we are dealing with ideal solutions, $\gamma_i = 1$.

Substituting Eq. (C.9) into the general flux equation for a single flow, Eq. (C.2), we can write

$$J_i = -\omega_i RT \frac{\mathrm{d}c_i}{\mathrm{d}x} \, . \tag{C.10}$$

The quantity $\omega_i RT$ is defined as the diffusion coefficient D_i, which has the dimensions $\mathrm{cm}^2\,\mathrm{s}^{-1}$. Thus, Eq. (C.10) reduces to

$$J_i = -D_i \frac{\mathrm{d}c_i}{\mathrm{d}x} \tag{C.11}$$

which is Fick's law of diffusion.

If the potential gradient is assumed to be uniform across the membrane or when the system is in a steady state so that J_i is the same at all points within the membrane, it is justified to express dc_i and dx as Δc_i and Δx, the concentration difference between the two surfaces of the membrane and the thickness of the membrane, respectively. Hence

$$J_i = -D_i \frac{\Delta c_i}{\Delta x}. \tag{C.12}$$

Experimentally, it is very difficult to measure D_i because Δx and the concentrations of the diffusing compound just within the two limiting surfaces of the membrane are, in general, not known. These concentrations are not only a function of the bulk phase concentrations but also of the partition coefficient K_i of the permeant species between the membrane medium and the limiting solutions. Both Δx and K_i may be experimentally accessible in artificial membranes composed of well-defined chemical components. However, in biologic membranes such as epithelia which are composed of complex cellular and extracellular structures in series and parallel and containing various lipids and proteins, it is almost impossible to obtain correct values of these parameters. Therefore, these factors are conveniently lumped together in the term P_i, the permeability coefficient, which is defined as

$$P_i = \frac{K_i D_i}{\Delta x}. \tag{C.13}$$

P_i has the dimensions of velocity, cm s^{-1}.

P_i is usually determined from tracer flux measurements across membranes in equilibrium with the permeant under conditions of zero volume flow

$$P_i = -\frac{J_i}{c_{i2}^* - c_{i1}^*}. \tag{C.14}$$

where c_{i1}^* and c_{i2}^* denote the concentration of the labeled substance on the two sides of the membrane. In the case of water diffusion, the flux may be expressed in volume per unit time and membrane area, from which the water permeability coefficient of the membrane under investigation, P_w, follows.

2. Diffusion of Uncharged Compounds Across Porous Membranes

In the preceding section, a phenomenological description of diffusion of uncharged compounds across a homogeneous membrane was given. However, the properties of most biologic membranes suggest that they are heterogeneous. According to the fluid mosaic model of cell membranes given by SINGER and NICOLSON (1972), proteins are embedded in a fluid lipid bilayer. From thermodynamic considerations and from permeability measurements of small hydrophilic compounds, it was concluded that there exist membrane proteins which form continuous water-filled pores or channels across membranes (SINGER 1974). For instance, for human erythrocytes and equivalent pore radius of 4 Å was calculated (PAGANELLI and SOLOMON 1957; BARTON and BROWN 1964), whereas certain synthetic membranes have pores of radius 2–4 nm (DURBIN 1960; GINZBURG and

KATCHALSKY 1963). In cell layers such as epithelia, additional water-filled channels appear to be formed by the lateral intercellular spaces which have their narrowest part in the zonula occludens.

When we consider a membrane separating two aqueous phases and possessing uniform cylindrical water-filled pores, and when we further assume that the permeant can pass the membrane via the aqueous route only, it is clear that the permeability with respect to the permeant species is related to the number of pores per unit membrane area and to the molecular size of the permeating compound in relation to the diameter of the pores. In this case of "restricted diffusion" Eq. (C.12) can be modified according to PAPPENHEIMER et al. (1951) as follows

$$J_i = -D_{is} A_i \frac{\Delta c_i}{\Delta x}, \tag{C.15}$$

where D_{is} is the diffusion coefficient of the permeant in the aqueous phase (solution) and A_i is a factor representing the restriction imposed by the membrane on the diffusion of the permeating compound. Therefore the diffusional flux of labeled water across a porous membrane equals

$$J_w^* = -D_w A_w \frac{c_w^*}{\Delta x} \tag{C.16}$$

(MAURO 1957). In the case of diffusion across a porous membrane, P_i can also be determined according to Eq. (C.14), but P_i is no longer expressed by Eq. (C.13), rather

$$P_i = \frac{D_{is} A_i}{\Delta x}. \tag{C.17}$$

III. Filtration

In the presence of a hydrostatic pressure difference across a membrane, $-\Delta p$, but at zero concentration difference, the rate of volume flow is related to its conjugate driving force by

$$J_v = -L_p \Delta p\,. \tag{C.18}$$

This relation is intuitively obvious. It may also be derived thermodynamically, since the chemical potential of an uncharged compound i under isothermal conditions is

$$\mu_i = \mu_i^0 + RT \ln c_i + \bar{v}_i p\,, \tag{C.19}$$

where $\bar{v}_i$ is the partial molar volume of the compound. Since the conjugate driving force for a flux of an uncharged compound is the rate of change of the chemical potential along the x-axis of the flux, we may write

$$F_i = -\frac{\mathrm{d}(\mu_i^0 + RT \ln c_i + \bar{v}_i p)}{\mathrm{d}x} \tag{C.20}$$

or

$$F_i = -\frac{RT}{c_i} \frac{\mathrm{d}c_i}{\mathrm{d}x} - \bar{v}_i \frac{\mathrm{d}p}{\mathrm{d}x}. \tag{C.21}$$

When there is no concentration gradient across the membrane, the rate of volume flow driven by a hydrostatic pressure gradient is

$$J_v = -\lambda \bar{v}_i \frac{\mathrm{d}p}{\mathrm{d}x}, \tag{C.22}$$

λ being the proportionality factor relating the hydrostatic pressure gradient to volume flow. When the pressure gradient is constant across the width of the membrane,

$$J_v = -\lambda \bar{v}_i \frac{\Delta p}{\Delta x}. \tag{C.23}$$

The term $(\lambda \bar{v}_i / \Delta x)$ is referred to as L_p. Hence Eq. (C.23) reduces to Eq. (C.18). L_p is commonly termed hydraulic conductivity, hydraulic permeability coefficient, mechanical filtration coefficient, hydrostatic filtration coefficient, or pressure filtration coefficient.

IV. Osmosis

One of the basic properties of most membranes found in living organisms is that they are selective, implying that some chemical substances readily penetrate them, whereas others penetrate poorly. Thus, biologic membranes are usually semipermeable. When a membrane is completely impermeable for one substance but permeable for another, it is termed "ideally semipermeable," a condition approached by some artificial membranes. One of the consequences of selective permeability of membranes is the phenomenon of osmosis.

The rational basis for understanding osmosis is the concept of the chemical potential. As we have seen in the preceding sections, a gradient in chemical potential of a compound between two compartments separated by a membrane causes a diffusional flux across the membrane, if its permeability with respect to the permeating species is finite. In the case of simple diffusion, this flux is not associated with volume displacement because simultaneously there is a flux of solvent in the opposite direction. This solvent flux results from a gradient of chemical potential which is oppositely directed to the solute gradient.

Now let us consider a system in which an ideally semipermeable membrane separates two solutions, implying that only the solvent is able to cross the membrane. In this case only a transmembranous flux of solvent along its gradient will be possible. Since this solvent flux is not balanced by a solute flux in the opposite direction, there will be net volume flow, or osmotic flow, towards the compartment containing the higher concentration of the impermeant solute. Net volume flow will cease, i.e., the system will be in equilibrium, when the hydrostatic pressure difference between the two compartments is identical to the driving force for the solvent flux. This pressure difference, or, more correctly, the pressure difference that must be applied to prevent net volume flow is defined as the osmotic pressure difference, $\Delta\pi$. In thermodynamic terms, the osmotic pressure is defined as the increase in pressure required to raise the chemical potential of the solvent in the solution to that of the pure, i.e., undiluted, solvent.

When certain simplifying assumptions are made (the membrane is ideally semipermeable, the solvent is absolutely incompressible, and the solution is dilute so that the mole fraction of solvent approaches unity), the osmotic pressure difference is given by

$$\Delta\pi = RT\Delta c_i \,, \tag{C.24}$$

where Δc_i is the concentration difference of the impermeant solute. This equation was derived empirically by van't Hoff. For descriptions of the theoretical basis of the van't Hoff equation the reader is referred to SNELL et al. (1965), LAKSHMINARAYANAIAH (1969), GLASER (1976), and SCHULTZ (1980). Since $R = 0.0821$ atm mol^{-1} K^{-1}, $\Delta\pi$ at 37 °C and a concentration difference of the impermeant solute of 1 M across the membrane is 25.42 atm.

The osmotic volume flow is again linearly related to its driving force, the osmotic pressure difference due to an impermeant solute. When there is no other driving force, then

$$J_v = L_{\mathrm{os}} \Delta\pi \,. \tag{C.25}$$

The proportionality factor L_{os} is the osmotic conductivity or the osmotic permeability coefficient and has the dimensions cm s^{-1} atm^{-1}. Ideally, L_{os} is identical to L_p, the hydraulic conductivity of the membrane. That this is not always the case in biologic membranes will be shown in Sect. D.IV. But since according to the van't Hoff equation it should be irrelevant whether a volume flow is driven by Δp or $RT\Delta c_i$, frequently the term L_p is used to relate osmotic flow to an osmotic pressure difference.

J_v is related to J_s, the flux of the solvent in terms of mol cm^{-2} s^{-1}, by

$$J_v = \bar{v}_s J_s \,, \tag{C.26}$$

where $\bar{v}_s$ is the partial molar volume of the solvent in the solution, which in the case of water is approximately 18 cm^3 mol^{-1}.

In principle, L_{os} may be determined experimentally according to Eq. (C.25) by measuring the volume flux in the presence of a known concentration difference of a completely impermeable solute. However, the volume flow may alter the solute concentration gradients across the membrane and thereby cause time-dependent changes in the apparent osmotic conductivity of the membrane. This serious experimental problem, which has not been solved satisfactorily to this day, will be dealt with in more detail in Sect. D.II.

Equation (C.25) holds if the membrane under investigation is indeed perfectly semipermeable, i.e., the resistance against solute permeation is infinite. However, when we return to the real world and consider a membrane with a finite resistance against permeation of the solute, less hydrostatic pressure will have to be applied to compensate the osmotic pressure, hence $\Delta p < \Delta\pi$. In other words, the transmembrane volume flow observed for a given Δc_i will be less than if the solute were completely impermeant or if we imposed a pressure difference calculated according to the van't Hoff equation. If $J_{v(ip)}$ is the osmotic flow observed in the presence of a given concentration gradient of a permeant solute ip and $J_{v(ii)}$ is the osmotic flow for the same gradient of the impermeant solute ii, the reflection coefficient σ is defined by

$$\sigma_{ip} = \frac{J_{v(ip)}}{J_{v(ii)}} = \frac{\Delta\pi'}{RT\Delta c_{i(\mathrm{p\,or\,i})}}, \tag{C.27}$$

i.e., the value of the apparent osmotic pressure difference, $\Delta\pi'$, divided by that predicted by the van't Hoff equation.

The term σ_i was introduced by STAVERMAN (1952) in order to relate solute and solvent permeabilities; σ_i can be determined from

$$\sigma_i = \frac{\Delta p}{RT\Delta c_i}, \tag{C.28}$$

where Δp is the hydrostatic pressure difference necessary to prevent osmotic volume flow. Alternatively, σ_i may be taken to represent the proportion of solute particles reflected by the membrane

$$\sigma_i = 1 - \frac{c_{if}}{c_{io}}. \tag{C.29}$$

Equation (C.29) is used to calculate σ_i from ultrafiltration experiments. A solution containing solute i at concentration c_{io} is forced across a membrane by applying hydrostatic pressure. Owing to a difference in the permeability of the membrane for solvent and solute the concentration of the solute in the filtrate, c_{if}, will differ from that in the original solution, and σ_i may be derived from Eq. (C.29). This procedure is not suited for most biologic membranes, because the permeability may not be independent of the applied pressure. However, it illustrates the properties of the membrane as a molecular sieve. The quantity σ_i is a dimensionless number, varying under most conditions between 0 and 1, and may be used to estimate the equivalent pore radius of membranes (DURBIN 1960; SOLOMON 1968; WRIGHT and DIAMOND 1969; HOLZ and FINKELSTEIN 1970).

From Eq. (C.27) it is clear that for a nonideally semipermeable membrane

$$J_{v(ip)} = \sigma_{ip} J_{v(ii)} = \sigma_{ip} L_{os} \Delta\pi \tag{C.30}$$

and generally

$$\Delta\pi' = \sigma_i RT\Delta c_i\,. \tag{C.31}$$

Conversely, the solute permeability of a membrane may be derived from the efficiency with which the solute generates osmotic flow. Thus, the osmometric approach is useful not only to assess the osmotic conductivity, but also to derive estimates for the solute permeability coefficient and reflection coefficient.

V. Interaction Between Solute and Solvent Fluxes

When a membrane separates two solutions with different concentrations of solute i, the fluxes of solute and solvent across the membrane will interact, as discussed in general terms in Sect. C.I, see Eq. (C.4). The total volume flow will be

$$J_v = \bar{v}_s J_s + \bar{v}_i J_i\,, \tag{C.32}$$

$\bar{v}_s$ and $\bar{v}_i$ being the partial molar volume of solvent s and solute i, respectively. The velocity of solute relative to that of solvent is defined as

$$J_D = \frac{J_s}{c_s} - \frac{J_i}{c_i}, \tag{C.33}$$

where c_s and c_i are the respective concentrations of solvent and solute in the region of interest. The interaction of solvent and solute fluxes is described by the following two phenomenological equations, which were originally formulated by KEDEM and KATCHALSKY (1958)

$$\begin{aligned} J_v &= L_p \Delta p + L_{p\mathrm{D}} RT \Delta c_i \\ J_\mathrm{D} &= L_{\mathrm{D}p} \Delta p + L_\mathrm{D} RT \Delta c_i \,. \end{aligned} \tag{C.34}$$

The physical meaning of Eqs. (3.34) is that we have two flows, each driven by its conjugate driving force, J_v by Δp and J_D by Δc_i, but in addition there is interdependence of the flows such that Δc_i may produce a volume flow even when $\Delta p = 0$. This phenomenon is referred to as osmotic flow and was discussed in Sect. C.IV. On the other hand, Δp may not only cause a volume flow, but may also influence J_D, the velocity of solute relative to that of solvent. This phenomenon is known as ultrafiltration. These interdependences are quantitatively expressed by the cross-coefficients $L_{p\mathrm{D}}$ and $L_{\mathrm{D}p}$. According to the Onsager reciprocal relation $L_{p\mathrm{D}} = L_{\mathrm{D}p}$, therefore the permeability of a membrane towards a solution of an uncharged compound is characterized by three coefficients. When $\Delta c_i = 0$, L_p can be determined experimentally from $L_p = J_v / \Delta p$. Further, under condition $\Delta c_i = 0$, $J_\mathrm{D} = L_{\mathrm{D}p} \Delta p$, hence an ultrafiltration experiment will give us $L_{\mathrm{D}p}$, the ultrafiltration coefficient.

When we assume that our system is in equilibrium so that $J_v = 0$, then

$$L_p \Delta p + L_{p\mathrm{D}} RT \Delta c_i = 0 \,. \tag{C.35}$$

As we have pointed out earlier, the hydrostatic pressure difference necessary to offset an osmotic flux across an ideally semipermeable membrane is $\Delta p = RT \Delta c_i$, in which case $-L_{p\mathrm{D}} / L_p = 1$. From Eq. (C.35) it is clear that $L_{p\mathrm{D}}$ is identical to L_os as used in Sect. C.IV. In other words, the osmotic conductivity, L_os, is a cross-coefficient.

However, $L_p = L_\mathrm{os}$ only in ideally semipermeable membranes. When the solute permeability of the membrane is finite, it follows from Eq. (C.28) that

$$\sigma_i = -\frac{L_{p\mathrm{D}}}{L_p} \,. \tag{C.36}$$

According to this definition the reflection coefficient equals the negative ratio of the ultrafiltration coefficient to the hydraulic conductivity, since $L_{p\mathrm{D}} = L_{\mathrm{D}p}$. The fact that σ_i contains a cross-coefficient is to be expected, since σ_i is a measure of the coupling between the transmembraneous fluxes of solvent and solute.

1. Solvent Drag

The flow of a solute that is brought about by friction between solvent and solute is commonly termed solvent drag, i.e., the solute flux that is due to J_v when $\sigma \neq 1$ and $\Delta c_i = 0$. This flux may be envisaged as entrainment of the solute molecules in the stream of solvent. Thus, movement of the solute may be either accelerated or retarded by solvent drag. When a solute is driven by both a concentration gradient and a volume flow,

$$J_i = (1 - \sigma_i) \bar{c}_i J_v + D_i \Delta c_1 \,, \tag{C.37}$$

where $\bar{c}_i$ is the mean concentration of the ith solute in the transmembrane solvent permeation pathway and the term $(1-\sigma_i)\bar{c}_i J_v$ expresses the coupling of solvent and solute flows within the membrane. Hence solvent flow will have a large effect on solute movement when the reflection coefficient for the solute in question is low, whereas solvent flow will not affect solute movement when the reflection coefficient is 1. For instance, in the human upper jejunum, σ for NaCl was determined to be 0.45, therefore the filtrate should contain 55% of the NaCl concentration in the parent solution. Indeed, when a hypertonic solution of mannitol was perfused through the gut, the concentration of Na in the filtrate pulled from blood plasma into the intestinal lumen was approximately 60 mM, whereas in the lower ileum, where σ_{NaCl} approached 1, the concentration of Na in the filtrate was only 10 mM (FORDTRAN et al. 1965).

However, the convective flux may cause a "sweeping away" effect on the solute such that the solute concentration is increased on the side of the membrane from which volume flow originates. Consequently, the concentration gradient of solute across the membrane may not be equal to the concentration gradient between the bulk phases of the solutions on the two sides of the membrane. To distinguish the true solvent drag phenomenon, i.e., coupling of solvent and solute fluxes within the membrane, from changes in the diffusional component of solute produced by volume flow-dependent changes in the transmembrane solute concentration, ANDREOLI et al. (1971) developed an equation, which will not be discussed here, for the sum of diffusive and convective solute fluxes across a porous membrane in series with unstirred layers.

2. Electroosmosis

Charged compounds may be driven across a membrane by an electromotive force which is proportional to the gradient in electrochemical potential. Since it can be reasonably assumed that water moves across the membrane in the undissociated form, the transfer of water will not be directly affected by a difference in electrical potential across the membrane. However, together with charged particles, water will move across the membrane as solvent. This phenomenon, which is another example of coupling between solute and solvent fluxes within the membrane, is termed electroosmosis. Since the gradient of the electrochemical potential for the charged solute is a nonconjugate driving force for water flux, J_v is related to the transmembrane gradient of the electrochemical potential by a phenomenological cross-coefficient, L_{pE}.

The coupling between an electrical current and water flow includes the water of the hydration shells of the ions. In the inner region of hydration, in which water molecules are immobilized adjacent to the ion (FRANK and WEN 1957), only a very small amount of water appears to be bound. According to CONWAY (1952) the first hydration shells of Na and Cl contain four and three molecules of water, respectively. Hence, the daily intestinal absorption of 1 mol NaCl in the adult human would be accompanied by only 0.13 l water, whereas in fact the daily intestinal water absorption averages 10 l. However, the amount of water transferred per Na or Cl ion may be considerably larger than four or three molecules, since the electrical field of the ions reaches beyond the inner region of immobilized water, as is apparent from the altered structure of water in this secondary zone of hydration (FRANK and WEN 1957). Since electroosmosis is defined as water flux due to coupling to an electrical current, the mechanism of coupling not only implies electrostatic forces, but also frictional forces between water and ions. From the water flow due to electroosmosis in rabbit gallbladder reported by WEDNER and DIAMOND (1969), HOUSE (1974) calculated that electroosmotic coupling may achieve a flux of up to 20 water molecules per ion transported.

If an applied difference in electrical potential can produce water movement in a solution of charged particles, it is also possible to produce a transmembrane electrical potential difference, the "streaming potential," by pressure-driven volume flow. The phenomenological equations describing the electrokinetic effects arising from coupling of solvent and current fluxes are special cases of Eq. (C.4) as discussed by KEDEM and KATCHALSKY (1963).

Similar to other examples of solute–solvent coupling, the quantitative expressions of electrokinetic phenomena are complicated by changes in ion concentration in the vicinity of the membrane (WEDNER and DIAMOND 1969; BARRY and HOPE 1969a, b). These ionic gradients in the unstirred layers next to the membrane not only give rise to a polarization potential difference across the membrane, but also to an osmotic water flow which may obscure the water flow due to electroosmosis. Indeed, from experiments in rabbit gallbladder, WEDNER and DIAMOND (1969) concluded that the major fraction of ion-transport-coupled water flow is driven by the ionic concentration gradients in the unstirred layers and not by true electroosmosis. Thus, the biologic significance of electroosmosis remains doubtful (HOUSE 1974). On the other hand, electroosmosis appears to be involved in volume flow in wide channels such as phloem in plants (BOWLING 1969).

D. Passive Water Transport

Measurements of the permeability of epithelia to water are basic to any discussion of possible mechanisms of transepithelial water transport. Usually two kinds of measurements of water permeability are made. The rate of water transfer is determined in the absence or presence of an imposed osmotic pressure gradient, yielding the diffusional and osmotic permeability coefficients. In addition to osmotic pressure gradients, the effect of hydrostatic pressure gradients on the rate of water transfer has been determined in several instances. Each of these permeabilities will be dealt with separately. From a comparison of the effects of the various driving forces on water transfer, certain conclusions concerning the structure of epithelia and the route of water permeation can be made.

I. Diffusional Water Permeability

For the determination of the diffusional permeability to water, radiolabeled water is introduced on one side of the membrane separating identical solutions, and the rate of appearance on the other side of the membrane is measured. Care should be taken that there is no net volume flow across the membrane, so that the exchange of water is indeed being measured. However, it is not always possible to ascertain that there is really no net volume flow, especially under in vivo conditions, but an even larger problem for the determination of passive permeability coefficients in both in vivo and in vitro studies is that caused by unstirred layers. As discussed in more detail in Chap. 21. Vol. 2, there are regions adjacent to the membrane where the convective fluid flow of the well-stirred bulk phase of the bathing solution decreases gradually as the distance to the membrane surface decreases until there is a layer of static fluid in the immediate vicinity of the membrane. Hence, the role of convection will decrease and that of diffusion will increase in importance for the movement of a molecular species with decreasing distance from the membrane. Unstirred layers may be especially prominent in epithelia in which mucus and the fuzzy coat on one side and connective tissue (and possibly even muscle layers in cases of intestinal preparations without vascular perfusion) on the other side separate the bathing solutions from the epithelium, the permeability properties of which are intended to be studied. Thus, the tracer exchange method does not in fact determine the flux across the epithelium, but across a complex system consisting of the epithelium itself plus two or more series resistances.

Unstirred layers have caused a great deal of confusion among investigators of membrane transport and rendered many of the reported values of passive permeability of epithelia doubtful, or, as HILL (1980) states, "to the outsider [the field of epithelial transport] must seem a rather treacherous jungle at the moment, where if he is not careful he is likely to be severely bitten by an unstirred layer." However, it appears that scaring epitheliologists is not the only function of unstirred layers, more importantly, these regions seem to be essential for the coupling of solute and water transport, as will be discussed in Sect. E.II.

As a consequence of the unstirred layers, the concentration of a permeating species at the membrane–solution interface may be different from the concentration in the bulk phase of the bathing solution. This phenomenon is especially pronounced with small molecules for which the membrane is highly permeable, in which case the transfer across the unstirred layers may become rate limiting for permeation. Although the diffusion coefficient of water in an aqueous medium is usually much higher than that in biologic membranes, the diffusional permeability coefficient of water in the unstirred layer may be low in comparison with that of the membrane, if the combined thickness of the unstirred layers on the two sides of the membrane is larger than that of the membrane, since according to Eq. (C.13) P_i is inversely proportional to the thickness of the diffusion layer. Under these conditions, an imposed concentration gradient between the bulk phases of the two bathing solutions will be attenuated by the unstirred layers (for a typical concentration profile across a membrane with unstirred layers see Fig. 1 of DAINTY and HOUSE 1966a) and P_i will be estimated spuriously low.

Since the relation of the diffusive and osmotic permeability coefficients has important repercussions concerning the possible route of transepithelial permeation, numerous attempts were made to correct for the unstirred layer effect in order to obtain "true" values of P_i for the membrane. These correction procedures include vigorous stirring (DAINTY and HOUSE 1966b), measurement of the thickness of the unstirred layers by analysis of the time course of diffusion potentials after changes in the Na or K concentration of the bathing solutions (DAINTY and HOUSE 1966a; SMULDERS and WRIGHT 1971), measurement of the P_i of highly lipid-soluble compounds the overall permeability of which is almost exclusively determined by the movement across the unstirred layers (HOLZ and FINKELSTEIN 1970; VAN OS and SLEGERS 1973; VAN OS et al. 1974), or by performing flux measurements of the whole thickness of the epithelium and the underlaying stroma separately (PARISI et al. 1980). In isolated cells, the use of nuclear magnetic resonance spectroscopy has lately provided another approach to differentiate between the turnover of extracellular and intracellular water (CONLON and OUTHRED 1978; LIPSCHITZ-FARBER and DEGANI 1980).

Besides the unstirred layer problem the determination of the diffusional water permeability, P_w, of epithelia in vivo by use of radiolabeled water is complicated by the fact that the rate of the intestinal absorption of small molecules may not be limited by the permeability of the epithelium, but by the mucosal blood flow. WINNE (1966, 1972) and DOBSON (1979) have shown that the absorption rate of tritiated water from rat jejunum or sheep rumen increases in a curvilinear relation with intestinal blood flow. Hence the intestinal absorption of tritiated water is clearly blood flow limited as are compounds for which the epithelial permeability is high (OCHSENFAHRT and WINNE 1969; WINNE and REMISCHOVSKY 1971a, b). Vasoactive agents such as 5-hydroxytryptamine (LEMBECK et al. 1964), adenosine (GRANGER et al. 1980), or CO_2 (DOBSON 1979) change the absorption rate of tritiated water parallel to their effects on intestinal blood flow.

Estimates of P_w derived from the absorption rate of tritiated water in vivo are therefore not only contaminated by unstirred layer effects, but also by the blood flow limitation of the exchange of label. The values of P_w of various intestinal epithelia which are compiled in Table 2 have to be regarded with these reservations in mind. Therefore they represent only lower limits. For reasons of comparison estimates of P_w of nonintestinal epithelia, single cell membranes, and artificial lipid membranes are listed in Tables 3–5. Whenever a value has been corrected for unstirred layer effects, this is indicated in the tables. Additional values of P_w of single cell membranes and artificial membranes of older studies are given by STEIN (1967) and HOUSE (1974).

In order to illustrate the resistance of membranes against the movement of water, the diffusional permeability coefficients of water in layers of water of comparable thickness to that of single cell membranes or epithelia are given in Table 6. These values were calculated according to

$$p_w = \frac{D_w}{\Delta x}. \tag{D.1}$$

Equation (D.1) is a special case of Eq. (C.13), since the partition coefficient is naturally 1 at the water–water interface. The free diffusion coefficient of water, D_w, is taken to be 0.24×10^{-4} cm^2 s^{-1} at 25 °C and 0.30×10^{-4} cm^2 s^{-1} at 36 °C (WANG et al. 1953). For instance, when the thickness of a cell membrane is 7.5 nm, P_w of a water layer of equal thickness will be $325\,500 \times 10^{-4}$ cm s^{-1} at room temperature, whereas the estimates of P_w of the cell membranes of various cell types are 4–5 orders of magnitude lower (see Table 4). In contrast, the values of

Table 2. Water permeability coefficients of intestinal epithelia. P_w = diffusional water permeability coefficient, P_{os} = osmotic permeability coefficient, ms = mucosa to serosa, sm = serosa to mucosa, the temperature (°C) is given in parentheses

	P_w (10^{-4} cm s^{-1})	P_{os}	P_{os}/P_w	Reference
Small intestine				
Human (37)				
Jejunum	0.14	48	343	SOERGEL et al. (1968)
		89[b]		FORDTRAN et al. (1965)
Ileum	0.17	23	135	SOERGEL et al. (1968)
		18[b]		FORDTRAN et al. (1968)
Dog (37)				
Duodenum	0.15			GRIM (1962)
Jejunum	0.13			GRIM (1962)
Ileum	0.18			GRIM (1962)
	0.30			VISSCHER et al. (1944)
Cat (37)		21– 41[c]		HALLBÄCK et al. (1980)
Jejunum	0.26	49	189	HALLBÄCK et al. (1979 b)
Ileum	0.18	31	172	HALLBÄCK et al. (1979 b)
Guinea pig (37)	0.60[d]			LAUTERBACH (1977)
Rat (37)		26[e]		SMYTH and WRIGHT (1966)
Duodenum		28[f]		MILLER et al. (1979)
Jejunum	0.20–0.41[g]			WINNE (1966)
	0.20[h]			BERGER et al. (1970)
	0.51[j]	15[j]	30	WINNE (1972)
Ileum	0.25			CURRAN and SOLOMON (1957)
	0.18[h]			BERGER et al. (1970)
		24[f]		MILLER et al. (1979)
Frog (22)				
ms		148–165		LOESCHKE et al. (1970)
sm		19– 23		
Large intestine				
Dog (37)	0.63			GRIM (1962)
Rat (37) sm		30		LÜCKHOFF and HORSTER (1981)
Hen (39)	0.83	20– 31	24–37	SKADHAUGE (1967)
	1.24[a]			SKADHAUGE (1967)
ms		35		BINDSLEV and SKADHAUGE (1971)
		61[k]		
sm		19		BINDSLEV and SKADHAUGE (1971)
		22[k]		
Colon ms		6		BINDSLEV (1981)
		42[k]		BINDSLEV (1981)
Colon sm		6[k]		BINDSLEV (1981)
Coprodeum ms		5		BINDSLEV (1981)
		17[k]		BINDSLEV (1981)
Coprodeum sm		4		BINDSLEV (1981)
		3[k]		BINDSLEV (1981)

Table 2 (continued)

	P_w (10^{-4} cm s^{-1})	P_{os}	P_{os}/P_w	Reference
Total intestine				
Eel	0.67		70	SKADHAUGE (1974)
ms		46		SKADHAUGE (1974)
sm		116		SKADHAUGE (1974)
Stomach				
Dog (37)	0.40	10	25	ALTAMIRANO and MARTINOYA (1966)
		11– 26		MOODY and DURBIN (1969)
Mouse (37)	0.15–0.19			ÖBRINK (1956)
Frog (22)	0.49	12	24	DURBIN et al. (1956)
		22		VILLEGAS (1963)
ms		6		MAKHLOUF (1972)
sm		11		MAKHLOUF (1972)

[a] Corrected for unstirred layer effects

[b] FORDTRAN et al. (1965) report an osmotic flow of 0.044 ml min^{-1} per mosm/l per 20-cm test segment of upper jejunum, the corresponding value in lower ileum was 0.005 ml/min per mosm/l. Assuming a surface area of the small intestinal mucosa of 7.2 m^2, a diameter of 4.5 cm of the upper jejunum, one of 2.5 cm of the lower ileum, and 4 m total length of the small intestine (SIEGELBAUER 1958), a ratio of mucosal to serosal surface area of 16:1 may be calculated. By use of these anatomic data, the values of FORDTRAN et al. (1965) may be transformed into those given in the table. Similar values are obtained when the estimates of 243 cm^2 mucosal surface area per centimeter serosal length jejunum and 195 cm^2 per centimeter ileum are used, as reported by SOERGEL et al. (1968)

[c] With collapsed and dilated lateral intercellular spaces, respectively

[d] Measured in an in vitro preparation consisting only of the epithelium with almost no submucosa

[e] The value of 0.015 ml/hr per mosm/l per 24-cm^2 serosal surface area reported by SMYTH and WRIGHT (1966) can be transformed into units of cm s^{-1} by assuming a ratio of mucosal to serosal surface area of 3.7:1, as reported by FISHER and PARSONS (1950) for rat small intestine

[f] The values of 0.016 and 0.008 ml/hr per mosm/l per gram segment of duodenum and ileum, respectively, reported by MILLER et al. (1979) can be transformed into those given in the table by assuming 8.2 cm^2 mucosal surface area per centimeter serosal length duodenum and 4.4 cm^2 per centimeter ileum (FISHER and PARSONS 1950), a total length of the small intestine of 100 cm (WOOD 1944), and a total weight of 9.3 g

[g] For male and female animals, respectively. WINNE (1966) gives his data in units of µl/min per milligram dry weight, which can be converted into cm s^{-1} by assuming that 22.7 mg dry weight is equal to 1 cm serosal length (BERGER et al. 1970) which in turn corresponds to 6.3 cm^2 mucosal surface area (FISHER and PARSONS 1950)

[h] BERGER et al. (1970) give their results in units of ml/h per 100 g dry tissue weight, which can be transformed into those of the table by using the relation 22.7 mg dry weight = 1 cm serosal length, as reported by these authors and a mucosal surface area per centimeter serosal length of rat small intestine of 6.3 cm^2 (FISHER and PARSONS 1950). LINDEMANN and SOLOMON (1962) reported a value of 28.8 mg/cm serosal length for rat small intestine

[j] WINNE (1972) gives P_w in units of ml/min per gram wet weight and P_{os} in ml^2 min^{-1} mol^{-1} per gram wet weight and reports that 1 g wet weight corresponds to 128 cm^2 serosal surface area

[k] In the presence of ADH

Table 3. Water permeability coefficients of nonintestinal epithelia. Symbols as in Table 2; bl = blood to lumen, lb = lumen to blood

	P_w (10^{-4} cm s^{-1})	P_{os}	P_{os}/P_w	Reference
Gallbladder				
Dog (37)	0.92			GRIM (1962)
Rabbit (35)	2.1	64	33	VAN OS and SLEGERS (1973)
	19.4 [a]		3.5	VAN OS and SLEGERS (1973)
	15.9 [a]			VAN OS et al. (1974)
ms (22)		47		WRIGHT et al. (1972)
sm (22)		14		WRIGHT et al. (1972)
	2.0 [a]			WRIGHT and PIETRAS (1974)
(20)		93		VAN OS et al. (1979)
		500 [a]		VAN OS et al. (1979)
Frog (23)	6.8 [a]	150	22	MORENO (1975)
Fish (22)		66		DIAMOND (1962c)
Nephron				
Rabbit (25)				
Cortical collecting tubules	4.7	6	1.3	SCHAFER and ANDREOLI (1972)
	14.2 [e]	186 [e]	13 [e]	
lb		20		SCHAFER et al. (1974b)
bl		88		SCHAFER et al. (1974b)
Proximal straight tubules		5,160		ANDREOLI and SCHAFER (1979)
Proximal convoluted tubules		3,560		ANDREOLI and SCHAFER (1979)
Rat (37)				
Proximal tubules	56.4	2,085	37	PERSSON and ULFENDAHL (1970)
Distal tubules	15.7	222	14	PERSSON (1970)
	32.7 [e]	848 [e]	26 [e]	PERSSON (1970)
Necturus (22)				
Proximal tubules		21		WHITTEMBURY et al. (1959)
		45		BENTZEL et al. (1968)
Distal tubules		5.6		MAUDE et al. (1966)
Urinary bladder				
Dog (37)	0.63			GRIM (1962)
Toad (22)	0.94	5	5	HAYS and LEAF (1962)
	1.59 [e]	192 [e]	120 [e]	HAYS and LEAF (1962)
	1.19 [a]			HAYS and FRANKI (1970)
	2.40 [b]			HAYS and FRANKI (1970)
	10.80 [c]	236 [c]	23 [c]	HAYS and FRANKI (1970)
	1.3 [e]			WRIGHT and PIETRAS (1974)
	> 13.0 [a,e]			PIETRAS and WRIGHT (1975)

Table 3 (continued)

	P_w (10^{-4} cm s^{-1})	P_{os}	P_{os}/P_w	Reference
Amphibian skin				
Frog (21)	0.69–1.16 [d]			HEVESY et al. (1935)
	0.73			GARBY and LINDERHOLM (1953)
	0.65	3.2	5	DAINTY and HOUSE (1966a)
	1.54 [a]		2	DAINTY and HOUSE (1966a)
Toad (21)	1.03	6.8	7	KOEFOED-JOHNSON and
	1.16 [e]	14.9 [e]	13 [e]	USSING (1953)
		1.9		BENTLEY (1961)
Choroid plexus				
Frog (22)	0.68 [a]			WRIGHT and PIETRAS (1974)
		38.9		WRIGHT (1970)
Corneal epithelium				
Rabbit (35)		83 [a]		KLYCE and RUSSEL (1979)
Toad (20)	6.17 [a]			PARISI et al. (1980)
Corneal endothelium				
Rabbit (37)		88		FISCHBARG et al. (1977)
		221 [a]		FISCHBARG et al. (1977)
		572 [a]		KLYCE and RUSSEL (1979)
Tracheal epithelium				
Cow (37)		64		DURAND et al. (1981)

[a] Corrected for unstirred layer effects
[b] P_w of the epithelium without supporting layers of muscle, collagen, and blood vessels
[c] In the presence of ADH, otherwise conditions as described in footnote b
[d] Calculated from the observation that 1 l heavy water passed across 1 cm^2 frog skin in 100–107 days
[e] In the presence of ADH

Table 4. Water permeability coefficients of cell membranes. Symbols as in Table 2

	P_w (10^{-4} cm s^{-1})	P_{os}	P_{os}/P_w	Reference
Intestinal epithelium				
Hog, gastric epithelial cell membrane		1		RABON et al. (1980)
Rat, jejunum (37) luminal surface		83		LINDEMANN and SOLOMON (1962)
Guinea pig, small intestine (37)				
Luminal surface	1.4			LAUTERBACH (1977)
Serosal surface	1.3			LAUTERBACH (1977)

Table 4 (continued)

	P_w (10^{-4} cm s^{-1})	P_{os}	P_{os}/P_w	Reference
Goldfish intestine luminal surface (20)		140		SIEGENBECK van HEUKELOM et al. (1981)
Gallbladder epithelium				
Necturus (25)				
Luminal surface		550[a]		PERSSON and SPRING (1982)
Serosal surface		1,200[a]		PERSSON and SPRING (1982)
Nephron				
Rabbit, peritubular membrane (37)				
Proximal straight tubules		1,380[a]		GONZALES et al. (1982)
Proximal convoluted tubules		2,300[a]		CARPI-MEDINA et al. (1983)
Frog skin				
Outer membrane		< 1		MACROBBIE and USSING (1961)
Inner membrane		24		MACROBBIE and USSING (1961)
Red blood cells				
Human (21–25)	53		2.5	PAGANELLI and SOLOMON (1957)
		127		SIDEL and SOLOMON (1957)
	21[a]			FABRY and EISENSTADT (1978)
	24			CONLON and OUTHRED (1978)
	24			BRAHM (1982)
		200		MLEKODAY et al. (1983)
(37)		144		KUTCHAI et al. (1980)
Dog (21)	44	199	4.5	RICH et al. (1967)
	57			REDWOOD et al. (1974)
Novikoff hepatoma cells (20)	9.7[a]	8.2	0.9	POLEFKA et al. (1981 a, b)
Ovary egg				
Frog (22)	1.3	89	69	PRESCOTT and ZEUTHEN (1953)
(20)	1.7[a]	1.8	1	HANSSON-MILD et al. (1974)
Neurolemma (23)	1.4	10.6	7.4	VILLEGAS and VILLEGAS (1968)
		8		VARGAS (1968)
Amoeba				
Chaos Chaos (22)	0.23	0.37	1.6	PRESCOTT and ZEUTHEN (1953)
Algae				
Dunaliella (25)		15–18		DEGANI and AVRON (1982)

[a] Corrected for unstirred layer effects

Table 5. Water permeability coefficients of artificial lipid membranes. Symbols as in Table 2

	P_w (10^{-4} cm s^{-1})	P_{os}	P_{os}/P_w	Reference
Brain lipids (36)	10.6[a]	11.4	1.1	CASS and FINKELSTEIN (1967)
plus cholesterol (25)	2.0[a]	2.0	1	HOLZ and FINKELSTEIN (1970)
plus cholesterol and nystatin (25)	12.0[a]	40.0	3.3	HOLZ and FINKELSTEIN (1970)
Sheep red cell phospholipids plus cholesterol (27)	13.8[a]	16.8	1.2	ANDREOLI and TROUTMAN (1971)
plus amphotericin B	107.5[a]	405	3.8	ANDREOLI and TROUTMAN (1971)
Phospholipid : cholesterol (36) molar ratio				
1:0		42		FINKELSTEIN and CASS (1967)
1:2		19		
1:4		8		FINKELSTEIN and CASS (1967)
1:8		6		
1:2		18		HANAI and HAYDON (1966)
Glycerol monoolein-*n*-hexadecane (25)	40.4[a]			PETERSEN (1980)
Egg phosphatidylcholine (25)	29.1[a]			LIPSCHITZ-FARBER and DEGANI (1980)

[a] Corrected for unstirred layer effects

Table 6. Diffusional water permeability (P_w) of water layers of varying thickness

Thickness (μm)	Temperature (°C) 25	36
	P_w (10^{-4} cm s^{-1})	
500	4.9	6
100	24.4	30
50	49	60
10	244	300
0.0075	325,000	400,000

P_w of epithelia are only 1–2 orders of magnitude lower than those of water layers of comparable thickness. This fact may be explained by the relatively large content of aqueous compartments in epithelia in comparison with the primary lipid composition of cell membranes.

The diffusional water permeability of mammalian small intestine ranges between 0.13 and 0.63×10^{-4} cm s^{-1} with surprisingly little variation among species and different gut segments. However, it has to be noted that most of these values are not corrected for unstirred layer effects. With the exception of the studies of ÖBRINK (1956) and DURBIN et al. (1956) on mouse and frog stomach and the investigation of LAUTERBACH (1977) on guinea pig small intestine, all of the reported values of P_w for intestinal epithelia were obtained from in vivo experiments with intact blood supply, but the dependence of P_w on mucosal blood supply was not evaluated except in the study of WINNE (1972).

The intestine is clearly more resistent to water diffusion than the gallbladder or the nephron. Whereas the unstirred layers were reported to be of minor importance in the nephron (PERSSON and ULFENDAHL 1970; SCHAFER and ANDREOLI 1972), in rabbit gallbladder the "true" P_w corrected for unstirred layer effects is almost ten times higher than the apparent P_w (VAN OS and SLEGERS 1973).

In contrast to whole epithelia, for which many estimates of P_w are given in the literature, there are almost no reports on the diffusional water permeability of the individual cell membranes of the enterocytes. Although work with isolated membrane vesicles from various epithelial cells has become quite popular in recent years, surprisingly P_w of these membrane vesicles has not been measured (H. MURER 1981, personal communication). LAUTERBACH (1977) has estimated P_w of the luminal and the basolateral cell membrane of guinea pig small intestine from transepithelial fluxes and intracellular concentrations under steady state conditions and from unidirectional influxes of tritiated water acros the two membranes. P_w for both the luminal and the basolateral cell membrane was found to be approximately equal, ranging between 1.2 and 1.5×10^{-4} cm s^{-1}. This finding is somewhat unexpected, since usually the luminal or apical membrane is considered to be much less permeable to small hydrophilic nonelectrolytes than the basolateral or contraluminal membrane (LEAF 1959; LIPPE et al. 1965). As will be discussed later, there is also evidence that the osmotic water permeability of the apical membrane is lower than that of the basolateral membrane.

Generally, the deduction of cell membrane permeability coefficients from flux measurements in epithelia may be compromised by the following problems:

1) Especially in leaky epithelia a clearcut differentiation between luminal and basolateral water influx is hard achieve.

2) Epithelial cells are not water-filled bags with only two diffusional barriers in series, the apical and the basolateral cell membrane. Rather, there may be intracellular constraints to diffusion. SCHAFER and ANDREOLI (1972) discussed the possibility that the resistance of the cell interior to water diffusion in cortical collecting tubules might be substantially greater than that of an equivalent layer of water. This notion was based on the finding that the diffusional resistance of the collecting tubules for several lipophilic solutes was found to be 12–25 times greater than predicted for an equivalent layer of water, and SCHAFER and ANDREOLI (1972) suggested that water diffusion is similarly retarded. This intracellular constraint to diffusion may be due to the cytoplasmic viscosity, as indicated by FENICHEL and HOROWITH (1963) and DICK (1964), or, alternatively, it may be that water and other small molecules traverse selective, restricted pathways in the cell cytoplasm. Whatever the mechanism of the diffusive resistance of the cell interior is, clearly transepithelial fluxes or unidirectional influxes into epithelia can only yield overall permeability coefficients and not that of individual cell membranes.

II. Osmotic Water Permeability

According to the van't Hoff equation, osmotic flow is linearly related to the osmotic pressure difference across a membrane, L_{os} being the proportionally factor see Eq. (C.25). The osmotic permeability coefficient or osmotic conductance is expressed in many different units, very much to the dismay of the reader. In order to facilitate comparison of the osmotic permeability of a membrane with its diffusional water permeability, we will use the coefficient P_{os} with the dimensions cm s^{-1}, since

$$P_{os} = \frac{L_{os} RT}{\bar{v}_w} . \tag{D.2}$$

A very useful conversion table of the various units found in the literature for the osmotic permeability coefficients is given by STEIN (1967).

Tables 2–5 contain estimates of P_{os} for intestinal and nonintestinal epithelia, cell membranes, and artificial membranes. These values suffer from the following inaccuracies. In order to arrive at permeability coefficients, water flow has to be expressed as volume or number of moles transferred per unit driving force and unit area membrane. Precise measurement of the membrane area may be possible with artificial membranes, but is very difficult if not impossible with biologic membranes. For instance, osmotic flow across intestinal epithelia in vivo is frequently given as volume per unit serosal length of the intestinal loop or per unit serosal surface area. In these cases, fluxes were converted to volume per unit luminal surface area by use of anatomic data which are specified in the footnotes of Table 2, since the values of P_w listed in Tables 2 and 3 are also given per unit luminal surface area. Hence the values of P_{os} of intestinal epithelia given in Table 2 permit comparison of the osmotic permeability coefficient of different intestinal segments and different species. However, it has to be stressed that these data are only rough estimates based on average ratios of luminal to serosal surface areas or luminal surface area per milligram wet or dried tissue weight. The enlargement of the luminal surface by the microvilli of the epithelial cells is disregarded.

Another source of error in determining P_{os} is the existence of unstirred layers. Since the permeability of the membrane for the solute is low compared with that of the solvent, the osmotic volume flow will cause an accumulation of solute in the unstirred layer on the side of the membrane from which volume flow originates, whereas the solute will be diluted in the unstirred layer on the side of then membrane towards which volume flow occurs. In other words, when there are unstirred layers on the two sides of the membranes, net water flow will sweep solute towards the membrane on the dilute solution side and sweep solute away from the membrane on the hypertonic solution side. Hence, these effects will reduce the effective osmotic gradient across the membrane. The concentration of solute i at the membrane surface c_{im} is related to the solute concentration in the bulk phase of the bathing solution c_{ib}, the transmembrane volume flow J_v, the thickness of the unstirred layer δ, and the diffusion coefficient of the solute in the bathing solution D_i according to

$$c_{im} = c_{ib} \exp(-J_v \delta / D_i) . \tag{D.3}$$

Thus, c_{im} will be changed in exponential relation to J_v and the term δ/D_i, which is the diffusional resistance $1/P_i$ of the unstirred layer. Since J_v is proportional to the osmotic permeability of the tissue, it is clear that the error in estimating P_{os} is especially large in leaky epithelia. Equation (D.3) was given by DAINTY (1963) and DIAMOND (1966b) and in similar terms by BRODSKY and SCHILB (1965). Obviously δ has to be known in order to calculate c_{im}.

Although nobody questions the existence of unstirred layers, it remains highly controversial what quantitative corrections should be applied to the apparent values of P_{os}. PEDLEY and FISCHBARG (1978) made a theoretical analysis of the errors involved in estimating the osmotic permeability coefficient of a semipermeable membrane with a region of thickness δ near the membrane where the spread of solute takes place largely by diffusion. The steady state of c_{im}/c_{ib} was shown to depend on a singly parameter β which is equal to the osmotic flow driven by the bulk phase solute concentration ($=L_{os}RTc_{ib}$) divided by the permeability of the unstitted layer ($=D_i/\delta$). Hence

$$\beta = L_{os}RTc_{ib}\delta/D_i\,. \qquad \text{(D.4)}$$

When numerical example for typical cell membranes and very leaky epithelia, i.e., membranes with low and high values of P_{os}, are calculated assuming high and low osmotic gradients, it is found that for cell membranes the error in estimating P_{os} is negligible, but in leaky epithelia P_{os} may be underestimated by as much as 80%.

It should be emphasized that these correction factors were calculated by PEDLEY and FISCHBARG (1978) for an ideally semipermeable membrane. Further, the solute was assumed to be present on only one side of the membrane, hence only the sweeping away effect was considered, or in other words, the unstirred layer on only one side of the membrane was taken to attenuate the osmotic gradient. Biologic membranes, however, especially epithelia, are not ideally semipermeable, therefore the reflection coefficient has to be introduced into the flux equation, and since the solute permeability of the membrane is nonzero, the solute concentration on the hypotonic side of the membrane will be significant. Therefore, the effective osmotic gradient will not only be reduced by an unstirred layer effect on the hypertonic side, but also on the hypotonic side. Thus, the effective concentration gradient of the solute across the membrane is

$$c_{im}^1 - c_{im}^2 = c_{ib}^1 \exp(-J_v\delta_1/D_i) - c_{ib}^2 \exp(J_v\delta_2/D_i)\,, \qquad \text{(D.5)}$$

where 1 and 2 denote the two sides of the membrane.

An additional factor that is not included in the analysis of PEDLEY and FISCHBARG (1978) is that epithelia are usually incubated in physiologic saline, to which a solute (the osmotic probe) is added on one side of the tissue to generate an osmotic flow. Hence, in addition to the unstirred layer effects on the osmotic probe, the volume flow effects on other solutes in the incubation media on both sides of the tissue have to be considered. Salts will be swept away from the epithelium on the side to which the osmotic probe was added, whereas salts will be swept toward the epithelium on the side from which volume flow originates. For each solute an effective transepithelial concentration gradient will be established according to Eq. (D.5). The existence of these salt gradients, which are opposite in direction to the gradient of the osmotic probe, is not only apparent from streaming potentials

(MACHEN and DIAMOND 1969), but also from a reversed osmotic flow occurring immediately after removal of the osmotic probe (WRIGHT et al. 1972). Since the salt concentrations in the incubation media usually exceed the concentration of the osmotic probe, salt polarization may cause even larger errors in estimating P_{os} than the sweeping away of the osmotic probe itself (DIAMOND 1979).

Equation (D.3) expresses the influence of an unstirred layer and volume flow on the solute concentration at the membrane surface under steady state conditions. In other words, Eq. (D.3) corrects the time-independent error caused by an unstirred layer, but unstirred layers are also responsible for a time-dependent error in osmotic water flow measurements. When the solution bathing a membrane is suddenly changed to one with a different solute concentration, the unstirred layers will cause a time delay until the osmotic gradient becomes effective across the membrane interface. This time delay again is due to the fact that concentration changes in the unstirred layers are brought about primarily by diffusion. When the solute reaches the membrane surface, an osmotic flow will be initiated, which will further slow down the rate at which the solute approaches its steady state concentration profile across the membrane and adjacent unstirred regions.

A theoretical analysis of osmotic transients with numerical solutions for the case of rabbit cortical collecting tubules was given by SCHAFER et al. (1974a), and PEDLEY and FISCHBARG (1978) derived a general equation for the time transient of the solute concentrations in the unstirred layer. Without going into the details of the mathematical treatment of PEDLEY and FISCHBARG (1978) it should be noted that the time period in which the steady state concentration profile is reached is again a function of β. For the two limiting cases of a cell membrane with a low P_{os} and a leaky epithelium with a high P_{os}, the time periods for the establishment of the steady state are in the range 74–215 s, which is short compared with the time scale of most osmotic flow experiments.

In contrast to the reported values of P_w, of which a large fraction is corrected for unstirred layer effects (see Tables 2–5), only a few attempts have been made up to now to correct P_{os} values for solute polarization. VAN OS et al. (1979) corrected the apparent P_{os} of rabbit gallbladder epithelium by estimating the flow-induced solute polarization from streaming potentials. Their "true" P_{os} is five times higher than the apparent P_{os}. This correction factor is somewhat higher than the factor of three or four given in the theoretical treatment of PEDLEY and FISCHBARG (1978) for a very leaky epithelium. FISCHBARG et al. (1977) reported values of P_{os} of rabbit corneal endothelium corrected for unstirred layer effects by use of Eq. (D.3) and by extrapolating initial rates of osmotic flow to time zero. The extrapolated P_{os} value derived from the osmotic transient was 2.5 times higher than the apparent P_{os} calculated from steady state osmotic fluxes. Similarly, values of P_{os} corrected for unstirred layer effects were calculated by KLYCE and RUSSEL (1979) from osmotic flow transients in rabbit corneal endothelium and epithelium.

The values of intestinal osmotic water permeability presently available (Table 2) do not account for solute polarization. Hence, these values most likely represent underestimates. Since the absolute value of the osmotic permeability has important consequences with respect to the plausibility of the theories of water absorption based on local osmosis (see Sect. E), it is necessary to discuss the possible magnitude of the error of the apparent P_{os} values.

Frequently the data of WRIGHT et al. (1972) are cited to argue that, in a leaky epithelium, the true P_{os} is at least one order of magnitude higher than the apparent P_{os}. In the experiments reported by WRIGHT et al. (1972) the osmotic water permeability of rabbit gallbladder was determined by suspending a cannulated everted or noneverted gallbladder in a beaker of saline and measuring net water flow by weighing the sac at 5 or 15 min intervals. The osmotic water flow in the direction serosa to mucosa measured by this technique in everted sac preparations was high initially, but declined within 15–30 min to a steady state value of about one-tenth the initial rate of flow. However, when the osmotic water permeability is not measured gravimetrically, but by using a chamber preparation with continuous volumetric recording, no osmotic flow transients are observed between 5 s and 20 min after introducing the hypertonic solution on the luminal side of the epithelium (VAN OS et al. 1979). The discrepancy between the results of WRIGHT et al. (1972) and those of VAN OS et al. (1979) obviously is due to methodological differences. With the volumetric method the volumes of the bathing fluids are monitored; changes in these volumes reflect transmural flows. The gravimetric method, on the other hand, cannot distinguish between weight changes of the sac due to transmural water flow or due to shrinkage or swelling of the tissue. Indeed, VAN OS et al. (1979) showed that the tissue wet weight changes with the osmotic gradient imposed across it. Mucosal hypertonicity reduced tissue wet weight, while serosal hypertonicity increased it. These observations are in agreement with the effects of osmotic gradients on the morphology of gallbladders as described by SMULDERS et al. (1972). Thus, the apparent osmotic flow transients reported by WRIGHT et al. (1972) do not seem to be due to solute polarization, but rather to changes in the water content of the tissue. The slow time course of the osmotic transient of 15–30 min observed by WRIGHT et al. (1972) is inconsistent with solute polarization, because according to VAN OS et al. (1979) streaming potentials reach their steady state within 5 s in this tissue. The notion that the transients observed by WRIGHT et al. (1972) are indeed due to alterations in tissue water content is supported by the finding that the changes in wet weight of the gallbladders during osmosis have time courses which correlate very well with the osmotic flow transients (VAN OS et al. 1979). The results of WRIGHT et al. (1972) were also subjected to a theoretical examination by use of the mathematical treatment of the unstirred layer effects on solute concentration profiles and time transients described by PEDLEY and FISCHBARG (1978). This analysis showed that when reasonable estimates for unstirred layer thickness and solute diffusion coefficients are used, a difference of only about 10%, not tenfold, would be predicted between the initial and the steady state osmotic flows (PEDLEY and FISCHBARG 1980). However, the theoretical analysis of PEDLEY and FISCHBARG may underestimate the error in conventional P_{os} measurements, as discussed previously. Further, the predicted time period until the steady state is established is only 2 min, considerably less than the 15–30 min transient observed by WRIGHT et al. (1972). Also, in rabbit cortical collecting tubules, no transients in osmotic flow were detectable 20–30 s after initiating osmosis (SCHAFER et al. 1974a).

In summary, it can be stated that at present there is no experimental evidence that the apparent values of P_{os} are in error by more than a factor of five. The underestimation of P_{os} increases with increasing leakiness of the membrane and unstirred layer thickness. Hence, in tight epithelia, such as amphibian skin and urinary bladder, or epithelia with thin unstirred layers, such as the nephron, the values of P_{os} given in Tables 2 and 3 may be viewed with more confidence than those of leaky epithelia with thick unstirred layers, such as the gallbladder. The intestinal epithelia probably occupy an intermediate position.

Generally, the osmotic permeability seems to be higher in jejunum than in ileum, whereas the diffusional water permeability is practically indistinguishable (Table 2). In contrast to the distal nephron, urinary bladder, and amphibian skin there is no evidence that ADH increases the P_{os} of intestinal epithelia (HELLER and SMIRK 1932) with the exception of hen coprodeum (BINDSLEV and SKADHAUGE 1971; BINDSLEV 1981). ADH also fails to influence intestinal Na transport (GREEN and MATTY 1966). If anything, ADH appears to diminish the absorption of Na, Cl, and water in rat jejunum, ileum, and colon in vivo (DENHARDT 1976). ADH was also shown not to affect P_{os} of fish and frog gallbladder (DIAMOND 1962c). For a review of the ADH effects on water flow in ADH-sensitive epithelia see ANDREOLI and SCHAFER (1976).

In contrast to the abundance of P_{os} estimates for epithelia, only scarce information is available on the P_{os} values of the individual cell membranes. In epithelia in which ADH regulates water flow through the tissue, it is generally accepted that the rate-limiting barrier for water transfer is at the luminal border (LICHTENSTEIN and LEAF 1966; GRANTHAM et al. 1969; JARD et al. 1971; HEBERT and ANDREOLI 1982). A lower osmotic permeability of the apical cell membrane in comparison with that of the basolateral cell membrane may also be inferred from the following reasoning: Addition of the polyene antibiotic amphotericin B increases the Na and K permeability of the luminal cell membrane of toad urinary bladder, rabbit descending colon, and rabbit gallbladder, whereas the basolateral cell membrane is not affected (LICHTENSTEIN and LEAF 1965; ROSE and NAHRWOLD 1976; FRIZZELL and TURNHEIM 1978). This selectivity of the amphotericin action suggests that the luminal cell membrane contains far more sterols than the basolateral membrane, because the presence of sterols in the membrane was shown to be a prerequisite for the incorporation of amphotericin B in natural and artificial membranes (ANDREOLI and MONAHAN 1968; CASS et al. 1970; for a review see NORMAN et al. 1976). On the other hand, FINKELSTEIN and CASS (1967) demonstrated in artificial phospholipid membranes that P_{os} decreases with increasing sterol content in the membrane (see Table 5). All these findings taken together suggest that P_{os} of the luminal cell membrane may be expected to be lower than that of the basolateral cell membrane.

Further, there is circumstantial morphological evidence indicating that P_{os} of the apical cell membrane is lower than that of the basolateral cell membrane: MACROBBIE and USSING (1961) used microscopic measurements of the epithelial thickness to monitor osmotically induced volume changes in frog skin epithelium. Decreasing the tonicity of the solution bathing the inner side of isolated frog skin caused an increase in cell volume which was reversible on return to a more concentrated solution. Changes in the tonicity of the outside bathing solution were without detectable effects on cell volume. Analogous results were obtained in toad skin (DÖRGE et al. 1981), toad urinary bladder (DIBONA et al. 1969), and *Necturus* proximal tubules (BENTZEL et al. 1969). From their microscopic observations MACROBBIE and USSING (1961) estimated P_{os} of the inner membrane to be 24×10^{-4} cm s^{-1}, whereas the upper limit of P_{os} of the outer membrane was only 1×10^{-4} cm s^{-1}. Basically similar observations were also made in intestinal and gallbladder epithelia: luminal hypertonicity decreases the width of the lateral intercellular spaces, whereas serosal hypertonicity dilates these spaces (TORMY and DIAMOND 1967; LOESCHKE et al. 1970; SMULDERS et al. 1972; WRIGHT et al. 1972). Thus, the cell volume appears to decrease with serosal hypertonicity, whereas it is unchanged (LOESCHKE et al. 1970) or may even increase with luminal hypertonicity (SMULDERS et al. 1972), hence P_{os} of the luminal membrane must be low compared with that of the basolateral membrane.

Recently, PERSSON and SPRING (1982) have used a microscope-video system to monitor the rate of changes in cell colume of *Necturus* gallbladder epithelium in response to osmolality changes of the solutions bathing either the luminal or the serosal surface of the tissue. P_{os} of the basolateral membrane was found to be more than twice as high as that of the apical membrane (Table 4).

LINDEMANN and SOLOMON (1962) determined P_{os} of the luminal surface of rat small intestine by gravimetrically measuring the initial rate of cell volume changes in response to alterations in tonicity of the solution bathing the luminal side of the tissue. By this procedure a value of 83×10^{-4} cm s^{-1} was obtained, which is not too far below that of red blood cells (see Table 4). The fact that P_{os} of the entire epithelium of rat small intestine was estimated to be only $24–26 \times 10^{-4}$ cm s^{-1} (Table 2) may indicate that there is an osmotic or hydraulic barrier in addition to the apical membrane. This conclusion is at odds with the suggestion made by HOUSE (1974) that the P_{os} for the apical membrane is practically identical to that for the total epithelium, and that consequently there would be only a single barrier for osmotic water flow. HOUSE (1974) based his suggestion on the similar P_{os} values reported by LINDEMANN and SOLOMON (1962) for the luminal surface of rat small intestine and by SMYTH and WRIGHT (1966) for the entire tissue (83×10^{-4} and 96×10^{-4} cm s^{-1}, respectively). However, these values cannot be compared, since LINDEMANN and SOLOMON (1962) gave their value with respect to luminal surface area, whereas SMYTH and WRIGHT (1966) gave their value with respect to serosal surface area of the tissue. When the value of SMYTH and WRIGHT (1966) is also expressed per unit luminal surface area (this is the value given in Table 2), the resulting P_{os} for the entire tissue, which is in excellent agreement with that given by MILLER et al. (1979), is considerably lower than that of the luminal barrier. Hence, these experimental findings are consistent with the notion that the epithelium consists of at least two osmotic or hydraulic barriers arranged in series. A model with two hydraulic barriers is also basic to the currently acceptable explanations of osmotic flow rectification, as discussed in Sect. D.III.

III. Rectification of Osmotic Water Flow

The direct proportionality between osmotic water flow and the osmotic pressure gradient predicted by the van't Hoff equation is observed experimentally when small osmotic pressure gradients are imposed (DIAMOND 1962c; VAN OS et al. 1976; MILLER et al. 1979). However, when the osmotic gradients are large (>150 mosm/l), the relation between osmotic water flow and its driving force has been shown to be markedly nonlinear in toad urinary bladder (BRODSKY and SCHILB 1965), frog skin (HOUSE 1965; FRANZ and VAN BRUGGEN 1967), rabbit gallbladder (DIAMOND 1966 a), and rat colon (LÜCKHOFF and HORSTER 1981). The curvilinear relation between osmotic flow and the osmotic gradient is also reflected by a parallel dependence of the streaming potential on the osmotic gradient. As a consequence of nonlinear osmosis the apparent P_{os} of several epithelia is not equal when obtained from osmotic water flow in opposite directions across the tissue. For example, in frog small intestine P_{os} determined from osmotic water flow in the direction mucosa to serosa was up to nine times higher than that determined from osmotic water flow in the direction serosa to mucosa (LOESCHKE et al. 1970). This asymmetry or rectification of osmotic water flow was also observed in rabbit gallbladder, in which P_{os} for water flow from mucosa to serosa was measured to be approximately three times larger than that for flow in the reverse direction (WRIGHT et al. 1972). Osmotic flow rectification was also reported for the proximal tubules of *Necturus* kidney (BENTZEL et al. 1968, 1969), although the asymmetry was less pronounced in this tissue than in frog small intestine or rabbit gallbladder. Intimately associated with this type of osmotic flow rectification is the finding that hypertonicity of the luminal solution reduces the epithelial permeability for both ions and hydrophilic nonelectrolytes, whereas hypertonicity of the serosal solution causes no discernible effects (SMULDERS et al. 1972).

Rectified and nonlinear osmosis is not only observed in epithelia, but also in single cell membranes such as red blood cells and algae. We will deal in this chapter solely with possible mechanisms for osmotic flow rectification in epithelia. For a discussion of the mechanism of this phenomenon in single cell membranes the reader is referred to HOUSE (1974).

Theoretically, osmotic flow rectification can be caused by an asymmetry of the unstirred layers on the two sides of the epithelium, since according to Eq. (D.3) the concentration of the osmotic probe at the membrane surface is negatively correlated with the thickness of the unstirred layer. In gallbladder epithelium, for instance, the unstirred layer on the serosal side is estimated to be approximately 400–800 μm thick, primarily because adherent connective tissue impedes convective flow, whereas the luminal unstirred layer is only 100 μm thick (SMULDERS and WRIGHT 1971; SMULDERS et al. 1972). Therefore, the effective osmotic gradient will be reduced considerably more when the hypertonic solution is placed on the serosal side of the epithelium than when it is placed on the luminal side. Consequently, this type of unstirred layer asymmetry would be expected to cause osmotic flow rectification such that the apparent P_{os} would be lower for osmotic water transfer in the direction mucosa to serosa than in the direction serosa to mucosa. Experimentally, the opposite type of osmotic flow rectification is observed in this tissue; hence the asymmetry of unstirred layer thickness cannot be responsible for the higher osmotic water permeability in the direction mucosa to serosa. Similarly, unstirred layer effects have also been excluded to account for osmotic flow rectification in frog small intestine (LOESCHKE et al. 1970).

PEDLEY and FISCHBARG (1980) carried out a numerical evaluation of the effect of asymmetric unstirred layer thickness on osmotic permeability for the case of rabbit gallbladder and concluded that P_{os} derived from steady state osmotic flows in the direction serosa to mucosa is underestimated by a factor of 1.1–1.2, whereas

P_{os} derived from flows in the direction mucosa to serosa is underestimated by a factor of 1.6–20. Thus, the discrepancy between the osmotic permeabilities for flow in the two directions across the epithelium is probably much greater than that measured.

Of the theories advanced to explain rectification of osmotic water flow, two appear to be most plausible at present, one is based on changes in the morphology of the epithelium with different osmotic gradients, the other is the so-called asymmetric double-membrane model. According to the morphological theory, the transepithelial route for osmotic water transfer is dependent on the direction of the osmotic gradient. BRODSKY and SCHILB (1965) suggested that changes in the dimensions of water-filled channels may be responsible for the decrease in P_{os} with increasing osmotic gradients. Indeed, in rabbit gallbladder, frog small intestine, and *Necturus* proximal tubules, osmotic water flow toward the luminal solution is accompanied by a collapse of the lateral intercellular spaces and other extracellular compartments of the epithelium, whereas osmotic flow in the opposite direction causes these spaces to dilate (BENTZEL et al. 1969; LOESCHKE et al. 1970; SMULDERS et al. 1972; WRIGHT et al. 1972). Concomitantly with the collapse of the lateral intercellular spaces owing to luminal hypertonicity the electrical resistance of rabbit gallbladder increases (SMULDERS et al. 1972). Osmotically induced changes in electrical resistance have also been observed by FRÖMTER and LÜER (1969) in proximal tubules of rat kidney and by SMULDERS et al. (1972) in frog gallbladder, frog choroid plexus, and rabbit ileum. Thus, there is good evidence that the lateral intercellular spaces play an important role in transepithelial osmotic water transfer and that the resistance for both water and electrolyte flow is increased when these spaces collapse. Simplified, the overall resistance to water flow may be envisaged as being composed of two series resistances, one constituted by the luminal cell membrane–tight junction complex and the other by the lateral intercellular spaces. Since conductance is the reciprocal value of resistance, the overall conductance of the system L_p is

$$\frac{1}{L_p} = \frac{1}{L_p^1} + \frac{1}{L_p^2}, \tag{D.6}$$

where L_p^1 and L_p^2 are the conductances of the apical barrier and the lateral intercellular spaces, respectively. Hence

$$L_p = \frac{L_p^1 L_p^2}{L_p^1 + L_p^2}. \tag{D.7}$$

Provided that net water flow in the lateral intercellular spaces may be described by Poiseurille's law, the flow through n channels of radius r is given by

$$J_v = -\frac{n\pi r^4 \Delta p}{8\eta \Delta x}, \tag{D.8}$$

where η is the viscosity of the solution in the channels. Equation (D.8) expresses filtration across pores or channels and is only a special case of Eq. (C.18). We may therefore write

$$L_p^2 = \frac{n\pi r^4}{8\eta \Delta x}. \tag{D.9}$$

Clearly, the conductance of the lateral intercellular spaces is primarily determined by the channel radius. For instance, a 16% reduction of r will decrease L_p^2 by a factor of 2. Hence osmotically induced changes in the dimensions of the lateral intercellular spaces may profoundly affect L_p^2 and consequently L_p. The conductance of the dilated lateral intercellular spaces may be assumed to be large compared with that of the apical barrier, so according to Eq. (D.7) the overall conductance will be practically equal to that of the barrier with the lower conductance. However, when the conductance of the lateral intercellular spaces decreases because of a collapse of these spaces, L_p^2 may approach L_p^1, and the overall conductance will decrease. From similar models SMULDERS et al. (1972) also calculated that transfer through the lateral intercellular spaces becomes rate limiting as these spaces decrease in width. Although these authors emphasize that several sources of uncertainty surround the attempt to relate epithelial structure quantitatively to conductance, the morphological changes observed with oppositely directed osmotic gradients provide a satisfactory explanation for osmotic flow rectification.

For the alternative explanation of osmotic flow rectification, the asymmetric double-membrane model, consider two membranes in series, bathed on both sides by an identical solution. If both membranes are permeable for the solvent and solute, but differ in their reflection coefficients, a volume flow across the double-membrane system will produce either depletion or accumulation of the solute in the middle compartment, depending on the direction of the volume flow. In other words, owing to the difference in the reflection coefficients of the two membranes, the solvent drag effect at each membrane will be dissimilar, thereby decreasing or increasing the solute concentration in the middle compartment. This effect will cause an asymmetric relation between volume flow and the driving force and hence an asymmetry of the apparent L_p. It is irrelevant for the phenomenon of flow rectification in this system whether the driving force for volume flow is a hydrostatic pressure gradient or an osmotic pressure gradient, created by an impermeant solute. PATLAK et al. (1963) have given a formal description of the transfer properties of the asymmetric double-membrane model. An application of this theoretical scheme to explain osmotic flow rectification in rabbit gallbladder was discussed by HOUSE (1974). In that analysis, the lateral intercellular spaces were assumed to constitute the middle compartment, the epithelial cells with their tight junctions were taken to represent the barrier with the high reflection coefficient, and a hydraulic barrier on the serosal side of the epithelial cells (the basement membrane or the subserosal connective tissue) was assumed to be the porous membrane. Although no quantitative estimates of the water and solute permeabilities of the two barriers are available, the model qualitatively mimics the experimental results of WRIGHT et al. (1972) in rabbit gallbladder.

It should be noted that both explanation for osmotic flow rectification, the morphological theory and the asymmetric double-membrane model, ascribe a dominant role to the lateral intercellular spaces and require two hydraulic barriers: the apical membrane with its tight junctions plus either the lateral intercellular spaces or some other hydraulic barrier on the serosal side of the epithelium.

However, in rabbit cortical collecting tubules, which is a tissue with high transepithelial electrical resistance, there is osmotic flow rectification favoring the reverse direction. According to SCHAFER et al. (1974b), P_{os} was approximately four times higher when osmotic flow was generated in the direction blood to lumen than when it was produced in the opposite direction. In order to explain this "reverse rectification" of osmotic flow by the asymmetric double-membrane model one would have to assign different anatomic structures the functions of the membranes with high and low reflection coefficients. The morphological theory for osmotic flow rectification, on the other hand, is also consistent with the asymmetry in osmotic permeability favoring the direction blood to lumen, since typical morphological changes appear to be associated with this type of osmotic flow rectification; in other high resistance epithelia for which morphological data are available, frog skin and toad urinary bladder, luminal or outside hypertonicity causes formation of blisters in the tight junctions, presumed to represent widening of these structures (ERLIJ and MARTINEZ-PALOMO 1972; WADE et al. 1973; DIBONA and CIVAN 1973; BINDSLEV et al. 1974). Conceivably, these deformations are responsible for the increase in P_{os}.

SCHAFER et al. (1974b) proposed that the direction of osmotic flow rectification is another functional difference of tight and leaky epithelia. According to the terminology of FRÖMTER and DIAMOND (1972), leaky epithelia such as gallbladder, small intestine, and proximal tubules may be distinguished from tight epithelia such as amphibian skin and urinary bladder by their lower transepithelial electrical resistance, lower spontaneous transepithelial electrical potential difference, and inability to maintain steep salt gradients across the tissue; further, leaky epithelia perform isotonic fluid transport, whereas in tight epithelia the transported fluid is usually hypertonic relative to the bathing solution. As pointed out earlier in this section, an additional common feature of leaky epithelia seems to be a characteristic response to luminal hypertonicity: the lateral intercellular spaces collapse, the transepithelial electrical resistance increases, and the permeability to electrolytes and hydrophilic nonelectrolytes decreases. In these tissues, osmotic flow rectification favors the direction mucosa to serosa (LOESCHKE et al. 1970; SMULDERS et al. 1972; WRIGHT et al. 1972; BENTZEL et al. 1969). In tight epithelia, on the other hand, luminal or outside hypertonicity causes opening of the tight junctions, decreases the transepithelial electrical resistance (LINDLEY et al. 1964; ERLIJ and MARTINEZ-PALOMO 1972; WADE et al. 1973; DIBONA and CIVAN 1973; BINDSLEV et al. 1974), and increases the permeability for hydrophilic nonelectrolytes (USSING 1966; FRANZ and VAN BRUGGEN 1967; SCHAFER et al. 1974b). In addition, contrary to leaky epithelia P_{os} was found in frog gastric mucosa (MAKHLOUF 1972) and rabbit cortical collecting tubules (SCHAFER et al. 1974 b), both high resistance epithelia, to be lower in the direction lumen to blood than in the reverse direction. However, in other tight epithelia this type of osmotic flow rectification is not found. In frog skin, osmosis was reported to be nonlinear (FRANZ and VAN BRUGGEN 1967), but the sigmoidal relation between water flow and the osmotic gradient appears to be symmetric with positive and negative osmotic gradients (HOUSE 1965). In toad urinary bladder, water transfer down an osmotic gradient was reported to be more rapid toward the serosal side than toward the luminal side (BENTLEY 1961), similar to the type of osmotic flow rectification observed in leaky epithelia, but objections may be raised against the data from the study with toad urinary bladder, since active transport toward the serosal side was not blocked or ADH was present. In any case, rectification of osmotic water flow favoring the direction blood to lumen or inside to outside does not seem to be a consistent feature of tight epithelia. However, the other responses to luminal or outside hypertonicity, changes in the morphology of the extracellular transepithelial pathway, in the transepithelial electrical resistance, and in the permeability to small hydrophilic solutes, are apparently opposite in leaky and tight epithelia, which is in accordance with the proposition of SCHAFER et al. (1974b).

IV. Route of Diffusional and Osmotic Water Flow

For a homogeneous lipid membrane without pores, the mechanism of water permeation driven by an osmotic gradient may be expected to be diffusion, i.e., water enters into the lipid phase of the membrane on the dilute solution side, diffuses across the lipid membrane phase, and redissolves into the aqueous phase on the hypertonic solution side. For such a membrane P_w and P_{os} should be identical. However, as is clear from Tables 2–4, P_{os}/P_w exceeds unity in most biologic membranes. PAPPENHEIMER et al. (1951) and KOEFOED-JOHNSON, and USSING (1953) showed in a formal analysis that P_{os}/P_w is a function of membrane structure. The P_{os}/P_w value may be expected to be unity only for the limiting case that water passes the membrane solely by dissolving in the membrane phase, whereas for a porous membrane the permeability as measured by osmotic flow is larger than the permeability calculated from the diffusion of water. This effect is primarily a result of a lower resistance for laminar water flow across cylindrical pores or channels, which is assumed to follow Poiseuille's law. Accordingly, osmotic water flow is a bulk flow, the resistance of the membrane varying inversely with the fourth power of the radius of the membrane channels. The diffusional water movement across a porous membrane, on the other hand, will depend on the solubility of water in the lipid membrane phase and on the cross-sectional area of the pores, which of course varies with the second power of the radius. Since the other membrane properties such as membrane thickness and the number of pores will equally affect both the diffusional and the osmotic water permeability, the difference between P_{os} and P_w is a function of only the pore radius. Consequently, a deviation of the P_{os}/P_w value from unity has been taken to indicate the existence of aqueous pores in a membrane (PAPPENHEIMER et al. 1951; KOEFOED-JOHNSON and USSING 1953; PRESCOTT and ZEUTHEN 1953; SOLOMON 1968). Indeed, it has been shown experimentally in homogeneous artificial lipid membranes that P_{os} is identical to P_w, but that formation of aqueous pores in these membranes by use of the polyene antibiotics nystatin or amphotericin B will increase P_{os}/P_w above unity (HOLZ and FINKELSTEIN 1970; ANDREOLI and TROUTMAN 1971).

On the tentative assumption that water moves exclusively via aqueous pores across the membrane the diffusive water permeability is

$$P_w = n\pi r^2 \frac{D_w}{\Delta x}, \qquad \text{(D.10)}$$

whereas L_{os} is identical to the conductivity of a tube for hydrodynamic flow as expressed by Eq. (D.9). Hence, dividing L_{os} by P_w and rearranging gives an equation for the calculation of the "equivalent pore radius" (PAPPENHEIMER et al. 1951; ROBBINS and MAURO 1960; KEDEM and KATCHALSKY 1961)

$$r^2 = 8\eta D_w \frac{L_{os}}{P_w}. \tag{D.11}$$

However, many questions surround the calculation of equivalent pore sizes by this method: what is the actual shape of the pores, is Poiseuille's law applicable to describe bulk flow through very narrow channels, to what extent is permeation through the channels restricted when the radius of the permeating species approaches that of the pore, is it justified to assume that water diffuses exclusively across the pores and not across the lipid phase of the membrane? Despite these uncertainties, the pore radii calculated by Eq. (D.11) seem reasonable, since similar values were obtained from the determination of the reflection coefficients of a series of hydrophilic molecules with different molecular dimensions (see for instance RENKIN and PAPPENHEIMER 1957; DURBIN et al. 1956; GOLDSTEIN and SOLOMON 1961; RICH et al. 1967).

Recently, an alternative explanation for the difference in P_{os} and P_w was proposed by SCHÖNERT (1980). The basic feature of this theory is reversible association of water molecules in the form of clusters. Accordingly, water exists in the form of monomers, dimers, and so on, each with a different diffusion coefficient. In contrast to the conventional concept that osmotic flow is a quasilaminar one, SCHÖNERT assumes that osmotically induced volume flow is purely diffusional. According to the cluster model the difference between P_{os} and P_w is due to the fact that during osmotic flow all species move together, as clusters, through the membrane, whereas tracer diffusion comes about by exchange from cluster to cluster; hence, water molecules do not permeate independently during osmotic flow. Another form of transmembrane permeation whereby the rate of transfer depends on the interaction of several molecules of the permeant species is single-file diffusion (HODGKIN and KEYNES 1955). Under these conditions the ratio P_{os}/P_w may also exceed unity (see HEBERT and ANDREOLI 1982).

According to the theory of PAPPENHEIMER et al. (1951) and KOEFOED-JOHNSON and USSING (1953) it seems obvious that there are water-filled pores in intestinal epithelia when we consider the high P_{os}/P_w values for these tissues given in Table 2, if we were not confronted again with the ever present spoiler of epitelial physiology, the unstirred layer. As we have discussed in Sect. D.I, unstirred layers may cause a significant underestimation of P_w. Hence the true values of P_{os}/P_w may be much smaller than the apparent ones. Indeed, the P_{os}/P_w ratios of frog skin and rabbit gallbladder fall markedly when P_w is corrected for unstirred layer effects (DAINTY and HOUSE 1966b; VAN OS and SLEGERS 1973), but in both epithelia the P_{os}/P_w values remain well above unity, even after correcting P_w for unstirred layer effects (see Table 3).

The P_{os}/P_w values for intestinal epithelia are very large. Even when it is assumed that the P_w values are underestimated by a factor of ten (this is the upper limit of the increase in P_w after correction for unstirred layer effects in gallbladder), the P_{os}/P_w values remain well above unity. Additionally, it has to be taken into account that the reported values of P_{os} also represent underestimates, as discussed in Sect. D.II. Therefore, insofar as values of P_{os}/P_w greater than unity indicate the existence of pores, we have to conclude that there are aqueous pores in the intestinal epithelium. This notion is also supported by the finding that the reflection coefficients for small hydrophilic solutes are less than unity. From the permeation rates of probing molecules and their molecular radii, DURBIN et al. (1956) concluded that the frog gastric mucosa may be represented operationally by an equivalent membrane composed of two groups of pores, with 93% of the pore area contributed by pores of 2.5 Å and 7% by pores of 60 Å radius. ALTAMIRANO and MARTINOYA (1966) used the same method and also found that there are at least two populations of pores in dog gastric mucosa, with 89% of the pores having a pore radius of 2.4 Å and 11% one of 95 Å. However, when Eq. (D.11) was used to calculate the equivalent pore radius, values of 17–19 Å were obtained.

These studies substantiate the earlier work of HÖBER and HÖBER (1937), who correlated the absorption rates of lipid-insoluble substances in rat small intestine with their molecular size. Since molecules above a molecular weight of approximately 180, which corresponds to a molecular radius of about 4 Å, were not absorbed, HÖBER and HÖBER concluded that this tissue contains small water-filled channels. LINDEMANN and SOLOMON (1962) calculated the same equivalent pore radius for the luminal barrier of rat jejunum from the reflection coefficients of a number of lipid-insoluble nonelectrolytes. Using a modification of Eq. (D.11), CURRAN and SOLOMON (1957) arrived at a value of 36 Å for the equivalent pore radius of rat ileum. These authors also calculated an equivalent pore radius of 40 Å from the results of VISSCHER et al. (1944) obtained in dog ileum. For the human jejunum and ileum, equivalent pore radii of 7–8.5 Å and 3–3.8 Å, respectively, were derived from the reflection coefficients of a series of lipid-insoluble small molecules (FORDTRAN et al. 1965).

The existence of aqueous pores in epithelia is also apparent from the relation between the diffusive permeability coefficients of a series of compounds and their oil–water partition coefficients (Fig. 1). In agreement with OVERTON's rule (1902) that the permeability of biomembranes is proportional to the lipid solubility of the permeant compound, there is a linear relation in epithelia between P_i and the oil–water partition coefficient. This observation corresponds with the old empirical knowledge that highly lipid-soluble drugs are in general rapidly absorbed from the gastrointestinal tract, while decidedly lipid-insoluble drugs are usually poorly absorbed (HOGBEN et al. 1959), but, similar to the finding of COLLANDER and BÄRLUND (1933) in *Chara* plant cells that in addition to lipid solubility the cellular permeability of solutes is related to their molecular size, small water-soluble compounds penetrate epithelia more rapidly than predicted on the basis of their oil–water partition coefficients (Fig. 1). This phenomenon indicates that these small molecules do not (only) cross the membrane by dissolving in the lipid phase of the membrane, but (in addition) by diffusing across an aqueous pathway. The relation between P_i and the molecular weight for small molecules is similar to that found in the red cell membrane doped with the pore-forming antibiotics nystatin and amphotericin B (SOLOMON and GARY-BOBO 1972), suggesting that the steric hindrance offered to the small molecules in these diverse systems is rather similar (WRIGHT and PIETRAS 1974). Additional evidence for the presence of aqueous pores in epithelia stems from an analysis of the temperature depen-

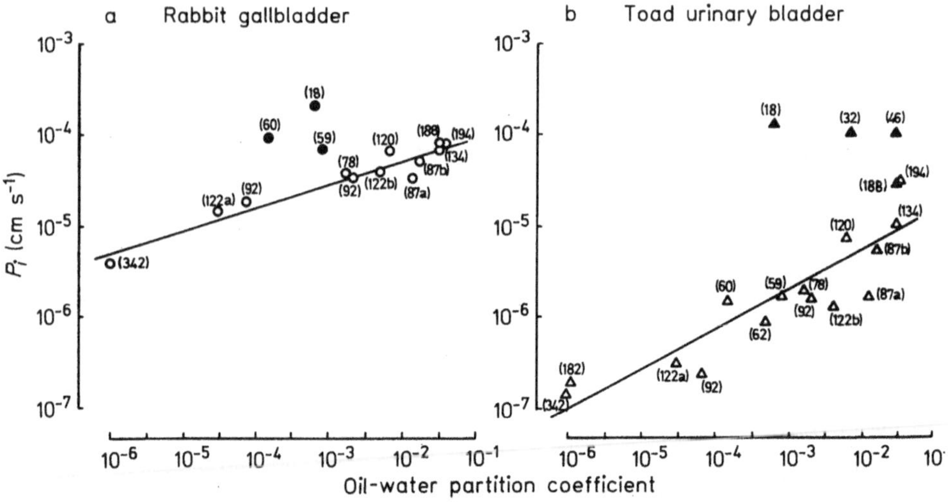

Fig. 1 a, b. Relation between the diffusive permeability of rabbit gallbladder (**a**) and toad urinary bladder (**b**) for a series of compounds and their respective olive oil–water partition coefficients. The linear regressions were calculated for all data points except the *full symbols*. The numbers in parentheses give the molecular weights of the tested compounds: (18) Water; (32) methanol; (46) ethanol; (59) acetamide; (60) urea; (62) ethylene glycol; (78) 1,2-propanediol; (78a) *n*-butyramide; (78b) isobutyramide; (92) 1,4-butanediol; (120) 1,6-hexanediol; (122a) erythritol; (122b) nicotinamide; (134) 1,7-heptanediol; (188) antipyrine; (194) caffeine. SMULDERS and WRIGHT (1971), WRIGHT and PIETRAS (1974), and WRIGHT (1977)

dence of P_i. In rabbit gallbladder, the apparent activation energy for transepithelial permeation of urea, acetamide, and sucrose was found to range between 5 and 7.5 kcal mol^{-1}, values very similar to the activation energy for diffusion of urea and mannitol in aqueous solution (4.5 kcal mol^{-1}). In contrast, the apparent activation energies for 1,4-butanediol and antipyrine, 12 and 15 kcal mol^{-1}, are approximately twice those expected for diffusion in aqueous solutions. These results suggest that small water-soluble solutes permeate via a more polar route than solutes which are expected to permeate by virtue of their lipid solubility alone (SMULDERS and WRIGHT 1971).

In fact, SMULDERS and WRIGHT (1971) postulated the existence of two separate polar pathways in rabbit gallbladder epithelium, one for small molecules such as urea and acetamide and one for large molecules such as sucrose and inulin. The evidence for the large pores is that $P_{\text{sucrose}}/P_{\text{inulin}} = 6$, which is close to the ratio of their diffusion coefficients in free solution. Further, as pointed out previously, the apparent activation energy for sucrose permeation is very similar to that for sucrose diffusion in aqueous solution. Hence SMULDERS and WRIGHT (1971) concluded that there is a "free solution shunt" across the tissue permeable for inulin and sucrose. Edge damage due to clamping of the tissue between the two sides of the chamber was excluded from being responsible for this shunt, since a reduction of the edge : surface area ratio by changing the exposed area of the tissue did not influence P_{sucrose}. A transepithelial permeation pathway for sucrose and inulin was also found by VAN OS et al. (1974). These pores may correspond to the large pores described by DURBIN et al. (1956) and ALTAMIRANO and MARTINOYA (1966) in frog and dog stomach, respectively. Inulin, a rod-shaped molecule of 50 Å length and 6 Å diameter (PHELPS 1965) was also found to penetrate guinea pig small intestine (TURNHEIM and LAUTERBACH 1977), and polyethylene glycol of similar molecular weight was reported to cross rat jejunum (MUNCK and RASMUSSEN 1977). Hence an extracellular permeation pathway for molecules the size of inulin seems to be a general feature of intestinal and gallbladder epithelia.

Large pores were also detected in rabbit small intestine by measuring the plasma clearance of water-soluble molecules of different molecular weight (LOEHRY et al. 1970). These investigators found a linear relation between the logarithm of molecular weight and clearance, which holds for molecular weights between 60 and 80,000; it was therefore concluded that there is a continuous spectrum of pore sizes with very many small pores and very few large pores.

It should be noted that small hydrophilic solutes and water diffuse primarily across the small pores, since their P_i values are much larger than those of sucrose and inulin. The number of large pores is so small that the reflection coefficient of gallbladder epithelium for sucrose is indistinguishable from unity (SMULDERS and WRIGHT 1971), but during osmotic volume flow a significant amount of fluid transfer may occur through the few large pores, because the frictional resistance against hydrodynamic flow in tubes decreases with the fourth power of the radius, as pointed out earlier. Therefore, many small pores will resist volume flow much more than a few large pores of the same aggregate cross-sectional area.

Now that we have established the existence of aqueous pores in epithelia from a host of independent evidence, let us turn to the question of whether passive water permeation occurs via a transcellular or an extracellular route. In leaky epithelia, the tight junctions have been shown to represent the high ionic conductance pathway arranged in parallel with the low conductance cellular route; in these tissues, as much as 85%–95% of the passive transepithelial flux of electrolytes such as Na, K, or Cl occurs through the tight junctions (WINDHAGER et al. 1967; BARRY et al. 1971; FRÖMTER 1972; FRÖMTER and DIAMOND 1972; FRIZZEL and SCHULTZ 1972; FRIZZELL et al. 1976). In other words, the transepithelial electrical resistance is primarily determined by the resistance of the extracellular shunt pathway. In order to examine whether this extracellular pathway is also of importance for passive water transfer, the relation between P_w and P_{os} and the transepithelial electrical resistance R_e of a wide variety of epithelia is plotted in Fig. 2. Clearly, there is no dependence of P_w on R_e, whereas P_{os} appears to decrease with increasing R_e. The results are consistent with the notion that diffusive water permeation is primarily transcellular, while osmotic water flow at least in part uses the extracellular shunt pathway for passive ion permeation.

The transcellular route for water diffusion is also obvious from the following simple calculation given by ÖBRINK (1956). P_w of mouse stomach is 0.19×10^{-4}, cm s^{-1}, determined from the rate of exchange of $H_2{}^{18}O$. Since the thickness of mouse stomach is given by ÖBRINK to be 0.05 cm, and the diffusion coefficient of $H_2{}^{18}O$ is taken to be 0.365×10^{-4} cm^2 s^{-1}, the P_w of a disc of water of 0.05 cm thickness can be calculated from Eq. (3.13) to be 7.3×10^{-4} cm s^{-1}. Because the measured value of P_w of mouse stomach is aproximately 3% of that of a water

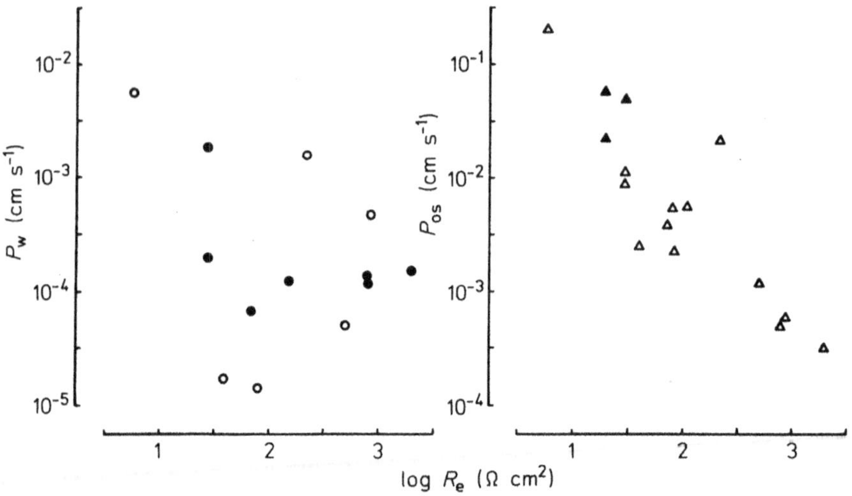

Fig. 2. Relation between the diffusive water permeability coefficient P_w and the osmotic permeability coefficient P_{os} of various epithelia and their corresponding transepithelial electrical resistance R_e. The *full symbols* represent values corrected for unstirred layer effects. The R_e values of the individual epithelia were taken from FRÖMTER and DIAMOND (1972), USSING et al. (1974), CORBETT et al. (1977), FISCHBARG et al. (1977), and BINDSLEV (1981); the values of P_w and P_{os} are those of Tables 2 and 3

layer of equal thickness, about 3% of the mucosal area would have to be water-filled pores. This large pore area can hardly be extracellular, since for instance the fractional pore area of muscle capillaries is only 0.2% of the total surface area (PAPPENHEIMER et al. 1951). It is therefore concluded that water penetrates not only via an extracellular route, but also via a transcellular route.

Transcellular water permeation may occur across the small aqueous pores described by HÖBER and HÖBER (1937), DURBIN et al. (1956), LINDEMANN and SOLOMON (1962), FORDTRAN et al. (1965), ALTAMIRANO and MARTINOYA (1966), LOEHRY et al. (1970), SMULDERS and WRIGHT (1971), and VAN OS et al. (1974). However, in recent years it has become increasingly clear that water also permeates across the lipid phase of the biological membranes with remarkable speed. For instance in Novikoff hepatoma cells the P_{os}/P_w value was found to be close to unity and the apparent activation energy for osmotic water transfer was significantly greater than that for diffusion in water (POLEFKA et al. 1981a, b). These data are interpreted as evidence for water movement across the lipid phase of the membrane rather than through aqueous pores. Consistent with this concept are the remarkably high values for P_w and P_{os} found in homogeneous artificial lipid bilayers (see Table 6). Similarly, P_w and the apparent activation energy for water transfer in chromaffin granule membrane are comparable to the corresponding values in simple lipid belayers (SHARP and SEN 1982). A simple model, the liquid hydrocarbon or solubility diffusion model, has been used to predict the water permeability of unmodified lipid bilayers (HANAI and HAYDON 1966; CASS and FINKELSTEIN 1967; FINKELSTEIN and CASS 1968; DIAMOND et al. 1974; FINKELSTEIN 1976).

The liquid hydrocarbon model views the lipid bilayer as simply a thin slice of the appropriate bulk hydrocarbon. Water passes through the membrane by dissolving into the hydrocarbon, diffusing across it, and redissolving into the aqueous phase on the other side. Hence, the diffusional permeability coefficient of such a membrane can be predicted from Eq. (C.13) if data on the partition coefficient of water into the hydrocarbon and the diffusion coefficient of water in the hydrocarbon are available. Indeed, at least for artificial lipid membranes, the liquid hydrocarbon model gives reasonable predictions of diffusional water permeability (HANAI and HAYDON 1966; PETERSEN 1980; LIPSCHITZ-FARBER and DEGANI 1980). Hence, it is clear that in principle water is capable of permeating cell membranes across their lipid phase. However, the quantitative importance of this permeation route for the specific case of the apical cell membrane of intestinal epithelium is obscure. As already pointed out, there is circumstantial evidence that the apical cell membrane contains more cholesterol than the basolateral membrane. Since, both in artificial lipid membranes (FINKELSTEIN and CASS 1967) and membranes of human erythrocytes (KUTCHAI et al. 1980), water permeability decreases as the cholesterol content of the membrane increases, it is questionable whether water permeation across the lipid phase of the membrane is quantitatively as important as permeation across aqueous pores in the apical cell membrane. DURBIN and HELANDER (1978) calculated that water permeation across the lipid phase of the basolateral cell membrane of rabbit gallbladder may account for the observed rates of water absorption in this tissue. Further, RABON et al. (1980) found the apparent energy of activation for water permeation in membrane vesicles from hog gastric mucosa to be 14 kcal/mol, which is characteristic for water diffusion through a lipid membrane, and concluded that there is no aqueous permeation pathway in these vesicles. Hence, the lipid pathway for water permeation across cell membranes deserves increased attention in the future.

In contrast to diffusional water permeation, which takes primarily a transcellular route, osmotic volume flow may take an extracellular route as suggested by the negative correlation between P_{os} and R_e illustrated in Fig. 2. For frog gastric mucosa, which is composed of large and small pores, DURBIN et al. (1956) calculated that osmotic flow passes primarily through the large pores, although they contribute only 7% to the total pore area. These pores are most likely extracellular and possibly reside in the tight junctions (SMULDERS and WRIGHT 1971). Also, DIBONA and CIVAN (1973) suggested that the tight junctions of toad urinary bladder are highly conductive for osmotic flow. Further, BENTZEL et al. (1969) considered the tight junction–lateral intercellular space complex to accommodate a large part of the transepithelial osmotic flow in *Necturus* proximal tubule. FISCHBARG et al. (1977) attributed osmotic flow totally to net water flow across the tight junctions in rabbit corneal endothelium, because the junctional width calculated from the measured P_{os}, assuming that the junctions are water-filled slits allowing laminar flow, was practically identical to the junctional width estimated from anatomic studies and from the observation that horseradish peroxidase passes the junctions.

However, VAN OS et al. (1974) are of the opinion that only a small fraction of osmotically induced volume flow crosses the tight junctions. These authors estimated the equivalent radius of the junctional pores to be approximately 40 Å with 5×10^7 pores per square centimeter of gallbladder epithelium. The length of the channels through the zonula occludens was taken to be 2,000 Å. Assuming that bulk flow across the channels follows Poiseuille's law, the osmotic flow in response to a 100 mosm/l gradient of an impermeant solute was calculated to be 80% of the osmotic flow observed experimentally in response to a gradient of 100 mosm/l sucrose. But there is general agreement that the reflection coefficient of the large pores is significantly less than unity; VAN OS et al. (1974) derived a σ_{sucrose} of 0.2. Taking this value, the contribution of the extracellular shunt to osmotic flow would be only 16% of the total flow. Hence, these investigators concluded that osmotic flow induced by sucrose passes the epithelium mainly by a transcellular route. The calculations of VAN OS et al. (1974) are similar to those of WRIGHT et al. (1972) who assumed an equivalent junctional pore radius of 12 Å and attributed maximally 10% of the osmotic flow to transjunctional flow. These authors also noted that the reflection coefficients for all sugars with more than three carbon atoms have been shown to be unity in rabbit gallbladder. This finding can be reconciled with a junctional pore radius of 12 Å only if almost all the water passes through an entirely different set of much smaller pores. In order for osmotic volume flow to penetrate across such smaller pores there must be an enormous number of them to explain the measured P_{os}. The tight junctions are not sufficiently extensive to accommodate this large number of small pores. This is taken as additional evidence that the pathway for osmotic flow is predominantly transcellular. In accordance with this notion is the finding that 2,4,6-triaminopyrimidinium (TAP), which obstructs the junctional channels for cations, does not affect P_{os} in gallbladder (MORENO 1975).

In conclusion, there is no definite answer to the question of the predominant route of transepithelial osmotic volume transfer. There is general agreement that the lateral intercellular spaces constitute the final common pathway, irrespective of whether water reaches the spaces via the cells or via the tight junctions. All the arguments for a predominance of either one of these two routes are conjectural. There is evidence that P_{os} is related to the passive ion permeability of the extracellular shunt pathway, but the relative contribution of the extracellular pathway for osmotic volume flow remains to be measured directly. How this can be done is not yet clear. However, two simple arguments render it doutbful that the tight junctions are of major importance for transepithelial osmotic flow: (1) the tight junctions occupy only a very minute fraction of the total epithelial surface area (0.004% according to WRIGHT 1977), hence the osmotic permeability of the junctions would have to be enormous to account for the observed large osmotic volume flows; (2) the reflection coefficients of the extracellular pathway for those compounds which are usually employed to generate osmotic flow (e.g., sucrose, urea, NaCl) are negligible. Even for inulin and polyethylene glycol, they are well below unity. Hence, these compounds will not be able to maintain sizeable osmotic gradients across the tight junctions.

V. Water Flow Driven by a Hydrostatic Pressure Gradient

Theoretically it should be irrelevant whether the hydraulic permeability of a membrane is determined by an osmotic pressure gradient or by a hydrostatic pressure difference $\Delta p = \sigma_i RT \Delta c_i$. Therefore, the term hydraulic permeability coefficient or hydraulic conductivity is frequently used indiscriminately to denote the membrane permeability for net water flow induced osmotically or by a hydrostatic pressure gradient. However, when we compare the hydraulic permeability coefficient measured with an imposed hydrostatic pressure difference given in Table 7 (this type of permeability coefficient will be termed "hydrostatic filtration coefficient" to make it perfectly clear which driving force we are referring to) with the osmotic permeability coefficients of Tables 2–4, it is obvious that the conductivity of most epithelia is not identical for osmosis and filtration. In contrast, no difference exist between osmotic and hydrostatic driving forces for water transfer in artificial membranes such collodion, cellophane, or dialysis tubing (MESCHIA and SETNIKAR 1958; DURBIN 1960). An equivalence between hydrostatic and colloid osmotic pressures as driving forces for fluid exchange across the capillary wall is also implicit in the STARLING hypothesis (1896). Indeed, in capillaries of the hindleg of cat and dog, the intravascular hydrostatic pressure necessary to prevent net fluid movement across the capillary wall is almost identical to the colloid osmotic pressure of the plasma proteins (PAPPENHEIMER and SOTO-RIVERA 1948), indicating that the hydraulic conductivity of the capillary wall is similar for both driving forces.

Of the epithelia for which data with both driving forces are available, an identity of the osmotic permeability coefficient and the hydrostatic filtration coefficient was reported only for rabbit corneal endothelium (FISCHBARG et al. 1977); it was therefore suggested that in this tissue osmotic and hydrostatic water flows pass across the same high conductance pathway, possibly the tight junctions. In intestinal and gallbladder epithelia, the hydrostatic filtration coefficients, measured for water flows in the direction serosa to mucosa, are 2–3 orders of magnitude larger than the corresponding osmotic permeability coefficients (see Tables 2, 3, and 7). A difference in response to osmotic and hydrostatic pressure gradients is not unique to epithelia, but is also observed in cell membranes, for instance squid axon in which the hydrostatic filtration coefficient was found to be 100 times larger that P_{os}(VARGAS 1968); this difference was explained by osmotic dehydration of the cell membrane, thereby making it tighter.

A detailed description of the relation between hydrostatic pressure gradients and transepithelial fluid transfer was given for in vitro dog small intestine by HAKIM and LIFSON (1969). Excess serosal hydrostatic pressure of 2–6 cmH_2O reduced fluid absorption to zero, and further elevations of serosal pressure produced fluid secretion at a rate of 60 $\mu l\ h^{-1}\ cm^{-2}$ per cmH_2O serosal pressure, but excess luminal pressure up to 22 cmH_2O did not noticeably affect fluid transfer. This finding is in agreement with the earlier observation of FISHER (1955) in isolated small intestine of the rat that intraluminal pressure increases had little effect on fluid absorption, SWABB et al. (1982) even reported a decrease in fluid absorption with increased intraluminal hydrostatic pressure in rabbit small intestine in vivo. Also, in isolated guinea pig gallbladder, excess intraluminal pressure did not cause a sustained increase in fluid absorption (HEINTZE et al. 1978). However, in dog and frog stomach (MOODY and DURBIN 1969; VILLEGAS 1978) and in rabbit gallbladder (VAN OS et al. 1979), excess luminal pressure was shown to be capable of producing a filtrate; nevertheless, from the studies in which the effects of hy-

Table 7. Hydrostatic filtration coefficients of epithelia, capillaries, neurolemma, and artifical membranes. Symbols as in Tables 2 and 3

	Filtration coefficient (10^{-4} cm s^{-1})	Reference
Small intestine		
Dog (37) sm	30,300 [b]	HAKIM and LIFSON (1969)
sm	2,400 [c]	YABLONSKI and LIFSON (1976)
Rat (37) sm	1,200– 2,900 [d]	LEE (1973)
Large intestine		
rat (37) sm	14,300 [e]	WANITSCHKE et al. (1977)
Gallbladder		
Rabbit (20) ms	1,500	VAN OS et al. (1979)
sm	45,000	VAN OS et al. (1979)
Stomach		
Dog (37) ms	3,000	MOODY and DURBIN (1969)
Frog (22) ms	161	VILLEGAS (1978)
Nephron		
Rat proximal tubule bl	88,000	SATO (1975)
Corneal endothelium		
Rabbit (37)	83	FISCHBARG et al. (1977)
	114 [a]	FISCHBARG et al. (1977)
Capillaries		
Cat intestinal villus (37)		
Rest	3,200	BIBER et al. (1973)
Maximal vasodilation	6,250	BIBER et al. (1973)
Frog mesentary (24)	7,780	LANDIS (1927)
Arterial part	6,700	MICHEL (1980)
Venous part	11,000	MICHEL (1980)
Cat and dog muscle (37)	350 [f]	RENKIN and PAPPENHEIMER (1957)
Mammalian kidney glomerulum (37)	41,700–83,400	RENKIN and PAPPENHEIMER (1957)
Neurolemma		
Squid (23)	1,030	VARGAS (1968)
Artifical membranes		
Cellophane	872 [f]	DURBIN (1960)
Dialysis tubing	230 [f]	DURBIN (1960)

[a] Corrected for unstirred layer effects

[b] Calculated from a fluid transfer of 0.4 ml hr^{-1} cm H_2O^{-1} per 6.4-cm^2 serosal surface area, assuming a ratio of mucosal to serosal surface area of 8 : 1 (WARREN 1939)

[c] Composite hydraulic permeability of the series resistances between the intravascular space and the intestinal lumen. YABLONSKI and LIFSON's (1976) value of 0.045 ml min^{-1} cm H_2O^{-1} per 100 g wet tissue was converted into cm s^{-1} by assuming a loop diameter of 2.5 cm with a ratio of mucosal to serosal surface area of 8 : 1 (WARREN 1939); YABLONSKI and LIFSON (1976) report that 3–4 cm dog small intestine weights approximately 5 g

[d] Composite hydraulic permeability of the series resistances between the intravascular space and the intestinal lumen measured with imposed hydrostatic pressure differences of 20 and 40 mmHg, respectively. A conversion factor of 6.3 cm^2 mucosal surface area per centimeter serosal length (FISHER and PARSONS 1950) was used to transform the data of LEE (1973)

[e] WANITSCHKE et al. (1977) use flow units of ml/h per gram dry weight, which were converted into cm s^{-1} by use of the relation 3.5 mg dry weight = 1 cm^2 serosal surface (WANITSCHKE et al. 1977) and a ratio of mucosal to serosal surface area of 1 : 1, as reported by WOOD (1944) for rat colon

[f] The hydraulic permeability coefficient is identical with imposed hydrostatic or osmotic (oncotic) pressure gradients

drostatic pressure gradients were tested in both directions across the epithelium, it is clear that the conductivity of small intestine and gallbladder for fluid filtration is markedly larger in the secretory than in the absorptive direction (HAKIM and LIFSON 1969; VAN OS et al. 1979). Thus, the asymmetry of the hydrostatic filtration coefficients is just the opposite from that of the osmotic permeability coefficients in these epithelia.

The relation between urea and glucose movements and pressure-induced fluid secretion in dog small intestine is consistent with the occurrence of solvent drag through channels with little or no sieving. Also, the permeability of the tissue for inulin, Evans blue, and ferritin was increased, even erythrocytes were seen entering the luminal fluid when a serosal pressure of 10 cmH_2O was maintained (HAKIM and LIFSON 1969). These observations indicate that excess serosal hydrostatic pressure widens existing channels, opens new ones, or both, thereby causing an increase in hydraulic water permeability.

The asymmetry in response to excess serosal and luminal hydrostatic pressure was explained by PARSONS (1968) by the fact that the epithelial cells are attached only at their apical ends, whereas below this region the cells are separate. An excess serosal hydrostatic pressure could cause the cell to separate upward from the bases, eventually to involve the region of the tight junctions so that a leak of fluid into the lumen could occur between the cells. Indeed, dilatation of the lateral intercellular spaces in response to increases in serosal hydrostatic pressure has been observed in *Necturus* gallbladder (SPRING and HOPE 1978). On the other hand, when the intraluminal pressure is in excess of that on the serosal side, there is no tendency of the cells to separate since the tight junctions are located at the very apical end of the cells so that the luminal surface of the epithelium is a flat continuum. In other words, the lateral intercellular spaces in combination with the tight junctions would, in effect, function as valves, offering less resistance to filtration in the direction serosa to mucosa than in the direction mucosa to serosa.

HAKIM and LIFSON (1969) also considered the possibility that defects in the epithelium left by the continuous shedding of cells are a potential route for filtration. But these areas of denudation are usually located at the villus tips, and LEE (1973) has shown by use of Evans blue that the secretory filtrate originates primarily from the intervillous spaces between the bases of the villi. Further, gallbladder epithelium exhibits a similar asymmetry in response to hydrostatic pressure gradients (VAN OS et al. 1979), although this tissue does not have distinct areas of exfoliation of cells such as villus tips. Hence, it seems reasonably safe to conclude that the route of filtration is primarily across the lateral intercellular space–tight junction complex.

Consistent with an increase in junctional conductance is the observation of VAN OS et al. (1979) in rabbit gallbladder that excess serosal hydrostatic pressure caused an enormous increase in epithelial permeability to large molecules such as ethylene glycol and inulin, whereas an excess luminal hydrostatic pressure did not change or even decreased the permeability for these compounds. An increase in epithelial permeability for inulin and plasma proteins was also observed in vivo after venous pressure elevation (YABLONSKI and LIFSON 1976), but only a small number of tight junctions appear to rupture during hydrostatic water filtration because the transepithelial electrical resistance was practically unchanged by excess serosal hydrostatic pressure (VAN OS et al. 1979). In *Necturus* gallbladder

SPRING and HOPE (1978) observed small dilatations of the lateral intercellular spaces or "lakes" of fluid in these spaces particularly at the junctions of three epithelial cells. Hence these junctions between three cells may be the locus minoris resistentiae for excess serosal pressure. VAN OS et al. (1979) calculated that the large secretory flows produced by excess serosal pressure can be accounted for when less than 0.01% of the junctions between three joining cells dilate to form pores of 0.5 μm diameter. It is clear that the reflection coefficient of such large pores for sucrose or NaCl will be near zero, hence these compounds cannot be expected to generate osmotic flow through these pores. It follows that water flows driven by osmotic and hydrostatic pressure gradients cross the epithelium on different routes, therefore equality of the osmotic permeability coefficient and the hydrostatic filtration coefficient cannot be expected.

Hydrostatic fluid secretion into the intestine may also be caused by perturbations of the equilibrium of the Starling forces regulating extravascular fluid exchange, as will be discussed in Sect. F.

Possibly related to the asymmetric hydrostatic water permeability is the finding that the intestinal permeability for compounds that are usually employed as extracellular markers, e.g., mannitol, inulin, or polyethylene glycol, is higher in the direction serosa to mucosa than in the reverse direction. This appears to be a general property of intestinal and gallbladder epithelia, since it has been observed in a wide variety of tissues and species, for instance bullfrog small and large intestine (CHALFIN et al. 1958), hamster small intestine (BIHLER and CRANE 1962), guinea pig jejunum (TURNHEIM and LAUTERBACH 1977; LAUTERBACH 1977), rat small intestine (MUNCK and RASMUSSEN 1977), and rabbit gallbladder (VAN OS et al. 1979). In all these studies, isolated epithelial preparations were mounted between two half-chambers except in the work of CHALFIN et al. (1958), who used everted and noneverted sacs of intestine. In all cases, the incubation medium was agitated by a stream of oxygen, thereby causing small oscillations in hydrostatic pressure gradients across the tissue. Although the magnitude of these small pressure differences will be equal in the two directions across the tissue over an extended period of time, the pressure gradients in the direction serosa to mucosa will cause a larger amount of the extracellular markers to permeate across the tissue, since the hydrostatic filtration coefficient is larger in this direction and consequently bulk flow of fluid is higher than in the reverse direction. The observation that the asymmetry in the permeability of the tissue for mannitol, inulin, and polyethylene glycol was abolished when active transport was inhibited, either by omitting glucose from the incubation medium (MUNCK and RASMUSSEN 1977) or by serosal addition of ouabain (VAN OS et al. 1979), can be reconciled with the presented explanation of the asymmetry of permeability, since blockade of active fluid absorption is associated with a collapse of the lateral intercellular spaces (BLOM and HELANDER 1977; SPRING and HOPE 1979). Hence, it is conceivable that the hydrostatic filtration coefficient is identical in both directions under these conditions. Incidentally, in guinea pig jejunum, anaerobiosis did not completely abolish the asymmetry in tissue permeability for inulin (TURNHEIM and LAUTERBACH 1977).

A different explanation for the observed rectification of the transepithelial permeability of solutes which are not actively transported by the tissue was proposed by MUNCK and RASMUSSEN (1977). The basis of their explanation is not an asymmetry in the hydrostatic filtration coefficients, but rather a fluid circuit mechanism. According to this concept transcellular solute-linked net water transport causes a distension of the lateral intercellular spaces. The increased hydrostatic pressure in these spaces drives the absorbed water to the serosal side of the epithelium, but in addition may create a water flow across the tight junctions to the luminal side. Hence, for solutes confined to the extracellular space, there will be a solvent drag effect in the direction serosa to mucosa, but not in the direction mucosa to serosa, since their reflection coefficient at the cell membrane is close to unity. According to this hypothesis, the asymmetry in the tissue permeability for extracellular markers has to be abolished by a blockade of active fluid absorption. This is not always the case, as already pointed out. It could well be that both the asymmetry in hydrostatic filtration coefficients and a fluid circuit mechanism contribute to the observed rectification of passive solute fluxes across intestinal and gallbladder epithelia.

E. Active Water Transport

Net water flow produced by gradients of chemical potential, due to a difference in either hydrostatic pressure or solute concentration, is referred to as passive transport. In the absence of such gradients net water flow may also occur which is defined as active transport and presumed to arise from metabolic processes occurring in the membrane (USSING 1949). In this sense the term "active transport" is analogous to the "vital" or "physiologic force" ascribed by some of the physiologists of the late nineteenth century to the epithelium. The old controversy between vitalistic concepts and those based on purely physicochemical principles has long been settled, since researchers have begun to unravel the mechanisms of active transport itself in terms of physicochemical forces.

From the fundamental experiments of HEIDENHAIN, REID, GUMILEWSKI, and COHNHEIM briefly reviewed in Sect. B it is clear that: (1) intestinal water absorption occurs in the absence of external osmotic gradients; (2) water is absorbed even against osmotic gradients; (3) distilled water is not as readily absorbed as water containing NaCl; (4) in contrast to NaCl, Na_2SO_4 does not stimulate water absorption; (5) the permeability of the intestinal epithelium for NaCl is larger in the direction mucosa to serosa than in the opposite direction; (6) NaCl is absorbed against a concentration gradient; and (7) destruction of the epithelial cells abolishes these phenomena. Later studies substantiated the dependence of water absorption on metabolic energy supply: small intestine in vitro absorbs water only in the presence of glucose (FISHER 1954) and oxygen, and water absorption is prevented by various metabolic inhibitors (SMYTH and TAYLOR 1957). Epithelial water transport against osmotic gradients has been verified repeately (MCHARDY and PARSONS 1957; VISSCHER 1957; VAUGHAN 1960, PARSONS and WINGATE 1961; GRIM 1962; DIAMOND 1962c; WHEELER 1963; DIETSCHY 1964; DIAMOND 1964a; SKADHAUGE 1967, 1969; LÜCKHOFF and HORSTER 1981). All these findings together make it inevitable to conclude that intestinal water absorption is an active transport process.

The next question is whether water transport is a primary or secondary active transport process, or in other words, are the water molecules themselves a substrate for an active transport system, or is water transport somehow coupled to the active transport of one or more other compounds? For instance, NaCl and glucose were repeately shown to be essential for intestinal water absorption, as pointed out previously. For some time, the question whether solute transport is coupled to primary active water transport or vice versa was unresolved. Among others GRIM (1962) was of the opinion that "it appears that during absorption of sodium chloride solutions from dog ileum, the net flux of sodium and chloride is due entirely to diffusion and bulk flow and none is transported by active processes. Water is actively transported as such across the wall of the intestine." The same position was taken by VISSCHER (1957).

The controversy over primary or secondary active water transport was finally decided by CURRAN and SOLOMON (1957) and WINDHAGER et al. (1959), who showed unequivocally that water movement across intestinal and renal epithelia is a secondary process due to primary active solute transport. The evidence for this conclusion is simple. Net water transport depends directly on the rate of NaCl absorption, the linear relation passing through the origin. The rate of NaCl absorption was varied in these experiments by altering the NaCl concentration in the incubation medium. Since isotonicity was maintained at all times, mannitol replacing NaCl isosmotically, there was no gradient in the chemical activity of water across the epithelium. The linear relation between NaCl transport and net water transport, which was confirmed in numerous studies (CURRAN 1960; CURRAN and SCHWARTZ 1960; CLARKSON and ROTHSTEIN 1960; BARRY et al. 1965; FORDTRAN et al. 1968; HALLBÄCK et al. 1979 b) demonstrates therefore that water movement depends on salt transport rather than on differences in water activity. Additionally, the hypertonicity of the luminal solution necessary to stop water absorption (i.e., the so-called turning point) was found to increase linearly with the rate of NaCl transport (SKADHAUGE 1974). When there is no NaCl transport there is no water transport, indicating that there is no primary active water transport system. Na, on the other hand, is transported across the epithelium in the absorptive direction against an electrochemical gradient (CURRAN and SOLOMON 1957; WINDHAGER et al. 1959; CURRAN 1960; CURRAN and SCHWARTZ 1960; CLARKSON and ROTHSTEIN 1960). Water absorption secondary to active NaCl transport was also shown by similar evidence in gallbladder of fish (DIAMOND 1962 a, b, c) and rabbit (WHEELER 1963; DIAMOND 1964 a, b).

The coupling between solute and water transport must be extremely tight, since the osmolality of the absorbed fluid approaches that of the luminal fluid of small intestine and gallbladder; in some experiments, the osmolality of the absorbate was even found to be indistinguishable from that of the luminal solution (Table 8). Similar results were obtained in proximal tubules of kidney (WINDHAGER et al. 1959; KOKKO et al. 1971; SCHAFER et al. 1974c). In fact, the absorbed fluid was also found to be isotonic to the luminal solution when the osmolality of the luminal solution was varied over a wide range from hypotonic to hypertonic by changing the NaCl concentration or by adding nonelectrolytes (RABINOVITCH 1927; DIAMOND 1964 b; LEE 1968; HILL and HILL 1978 a). The problem that next confronted epitheliologists therefore concerned the coupling mechanism

Table 8. Osmolality of absorbed fluid, expressed as the fraction of the osmolality of the luminal bathing solution

		Reference
Intestine		
Human		
Jejunum	1.2	SOERGEL et al. (1968)
Ileum	1.8	SOERGEL et al. (1968)
Rat		
Jejunum	1.1	CURRAN and SOLOMON (1957)
	1.0	CURRAN (1960)
	1.0	CLARKSON and ROTHSTEIN (1960)
	1.0–1.1	LEE (1968)
	1.1	POWELL and MALAWER (1968)
Ileum	1.3	POWELL and MALAWER (1968)
Colon	1.6	POWELL and MALAWER (1968)
Eel	1.6–1.8	SKADHAUGE (1974)
Gallbladder		
Rabbit	1.2	WHEELER (1963)
	1.0	DIAMOND (1964b)
Necturus	1.0	HILL and HILL (1978a, b)

by which active solute transport causes net water transport. To be more precise, what was most puzzling was the efficacy of the salt–water transport coupling, i.e., that at least in leaky epithelia such as small intestine and gallbladder, the transported fluid is virtually isotonic. Hence, when NaCl solution isotonic with blood plasma is absorbed, each Na and Cl ion has to drag along close to 185 molecules of water. Osmotic equilibration of the absorbate somehow seems to be connected to the "leakiness" of the tissue, since the absorbate is hypertonic in tight epithelia (FRÖMTER and DIAMOND 1972). Also, in the more aboral regions of rat intestine, which are characterized by increasing transepithelial electrical resistance, fluid absorption becomes increasingly hypertonic (POWELL and MALAWER 1968).

Several theories and models have been proposed to account for the coupling of salt and water transport.

I. The Series Membrane Model

WINDHAGER et al. (1959) and CURRAN and SCHWARTZ (1960) have pointed out that in order for water flux to be passive, movement must take place down a gradient of water activity. If the passage of NaCl from lumen to blood creates a region, however small, in which the osmotic pressure is greater than on the luminal side of the epithelium, water transport will be passive. CURRAN (1960) has suggested a model which is capable of explaining the experimental findings that: (1) water is absorbed from a hypertonic solution (this observation constituted the strongest argument for primary active water transport); and (2) a hydrostatic pressure gradient in the direction mucosa to serosa has only a slight effect on water transport, but a low hydrostatic pressure gradient in the direction serosa to

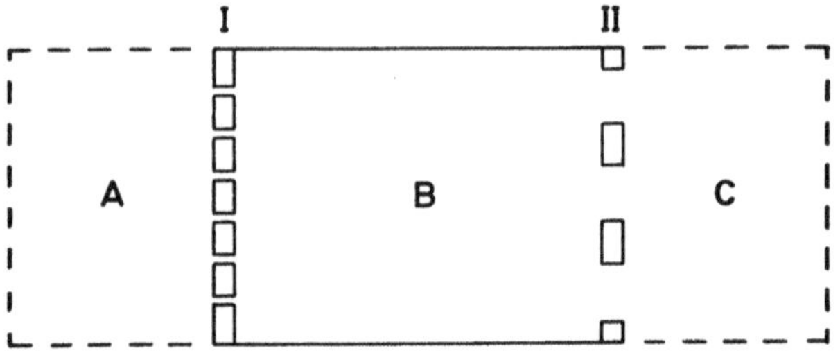

Fig. 3. Series membrane model for water transport. *A* and *C* represent the external solutions, *B* the middle compartment. I and II denote the two membranes with small and large pores, respectively. After CURRAN (1960)

mucosa abolishes water absorption. CURRAN's model consists of three compartments arranged in series, where the external compartments are open (Fig. 3). Compartment A is separated from compartment B by a membrane with small pores (membrane I), whereas a membrane with large pores separates compartments B and C (membrane II). Compartments A and C contain solutions of equal composition. In the intestine in vitro, the barrier with the small pores may be one of the membranes of the epithelial cells, while the other may be the submucosal or muscle layers. Active solute transport across membrane I is taken to increase the solute concentration in compartment B. The resulting concentration gradient across the two limiting membranes generates osmotic influx only across the membrane with the small pores, but not across the membrane with the large pores, since the reflection coefficient of this membrane for the solute will be close to zero. The influx of water from compartment A into compartment B causes an increase in hydrostatic pressure in compartment B, producing net water flow primarily to compartment C because according to Poiseuille's law the hydrostatic filtration coefficient of the membrane with the large pores exceeds that of the membrane with the small pores. The net result would be movement of volume from compartment A to compartment C without requiring primary active water transport.

The experimental observation of fluid absorption from a hypertonic solution can be easily explained by CURRAN's series membrane model: water transport from compartment A to compartment C could occur even if the solute concentration in A is greater than in C as long as active solute transport is sufficient to maintain the solute concentration in B greater than in A. Consequently, the hypertonicity of the solution in compartment A at which net water movement stops (the turning point) would be a measure of the hypertonicity in compartment B. The experimental finding that a small excess hydrostatic pressure on the serosal side abolishes net water flow whereas excess luminal pressure has a much smaller effect on net water transfer is also consistent with the model, since a small excess hydrostatic pressure in C could balance the hydrostatic pressure increase due to osmotic flow in B, whereas an excess hydrostatic pressure applied to A would only have a small effect because of the low hydrostatic filtration coefficient of membrane I.

The similarity of CURRAN's series membrane model with the asymmetric double-membrane model discussed in Sect. D.III is evident. Hence, this system is not only capable of accounting for osmotic flow rectification in epithelia, but can also explain qualitatively solute-coupled water transport. It should be mentioned that, in the original scheme, CURRAN (1960) pictured the membrane with the small pores to be thin, whereas the membrane with the large pores was taken to be thicker. However, this is not a critical point for the system to function as described.

CURRAN's series membrane hypothesis was tested in an artificial model, consisting of a cylinder separated into three compartments by two membranes, one being cellophane dialysis tubing and the other a sintered glass disc. Similar to Fig. 3, the two external compartments were open, but the middle compartment was closed. When a hypertonic sucrose solution was placed in the middle compartment, net water flow was generated across the series membrane system in accordance with the predictions. It was even possible to produce net water flow from a hypertonic solution, as long as the osmolality of the middle compartment was higher (CURRAN and MACINTOSH 1962). The important point is that this inanimate system is capable of generating net water transport, although no gradients in potential energy exist between the two external solutions, or, as pointed out, net water transport is possible even against an osmotic gradient between the external solutions. Hence, without a detailed knowledge of the structure of the system, the differences in the reflection coefficients and the hydrostatic filtration coefficients of the individual barriers, and the osmotic pressure of the middle compartment in relation to the osmotic pressure of the external compartments, one could erroneously arrive at the conclusion that the system is equipped with a primary active transport process for water.

II. Hypertonic Interspace Mechanisms (Local Osmosis Theories)

In the years after CURRAN's pioneering studies, the structure of epithelia was analyzed for possible hypertonic compartments. Morphological studies of gallbladder epithelium suggested that the lateral intercellular spaces play a major role in water absorption (HAYWARD 1962; JOHNSON et al. 1962; DIAMOND 1964b; WHITLOCK and WHEELER 1964), and KAYE et al. (1966) considered the possibility that the lateral intercellular spaces may constitute the middle compartment of CURRAN's series membrane model. DIAMOND (1964b) advanced the concept of "local osmosis" which is a special case of the series membrane model; this theory was later refined to the "standing gradient" hypothesis (DIAMOND and BOSSERT 1967).

Basic to the standing gradient hypothesis is the finding that the lateral intercellular spaces appear to be the route of fluid absorption in gallbladder, since these spaces are dilated when maximal fluid transport occurs, but are collapsed under all conditions which inhibit transport (KAYE et al. 1966; TORMEY and DIAMOND 1967). This notion was substantiated by the later studies of BLOM and HELANDER (1977) and SPRING and HOPE (1979). Characteristically, epithelia that produce an isotonic absorbate have very long lateral intercellular channels. Further, the size of the apical cell surface seems to be smaller in isotonically absorbing

a

b

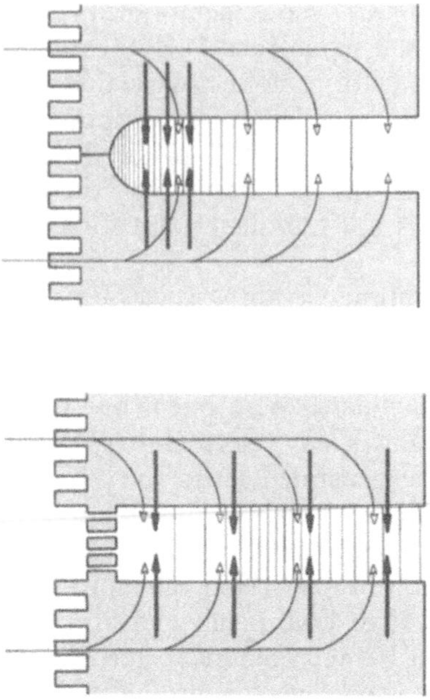

Fig. 4 a, b. Schematic illustration of the hypertonic interspace models for epithelial water absorption. *Thick arrows* represent active solute transport, *thin arrows* denote osmotically driven water flow. The density of the *vertical lines* in the lateral intercellular spaces reflects the hypertonicity of the solution in these spaces. **a** model of DIAMOND and BOSSERT (1967) with impermeable tight junctions and active solute transport confined to the closed end of the lateral intercellular spaces; **b** model of SACKIN and BOULPAEP (1975) with permeable tight junctions and a uniform distribution of active solute transport along the length of the lateral intercellular spaces

epithelia than in hypertonically absorbing epithelia. As a consequence of this observation, there are more lateral intercellular spaces per unit epithelial surface area in epithelia producing an isotonic absorbate than in those producing a hypertonic absorbate (DIBONA and MILLS 1979). All these findings substantiate the importance of the lateral intercellular spaces for isotonic fluid absorption.

According to the standing gradient hypothesis, NaCl is actively pumped from the cells into the lateral intercellular spaces, making these spaces hypertonic (Fig. 4a). Water is pulled into the lateral intercellular spaces osmotically. Whereas active electrolyte transport is generally taken to be transcellular, the route by which water enters the lateral intercellular spaces is unclear. TORMEY and DIAMOND (1967) suggested that water traverses primarily the cells and not the tight junctions to reach the lateral intercellular spaces, because these investigators assumed a maximal diameter of the pores in the tight junctions of 6 Å with a total area of 0.02% of the mucosal surface. Under these conditions, a pressure difference of several hundred atmospheres would be required to drive fluid across the tight junctions at the rate of fluid absorption observed experimentally.

The important point of DIAMOND and BOSSERT's model is that the geometry of the lateral intercellular spaces provides the explanation for isotonic water–

solute transport coupling. If solute were transported across a flat membrane, it would diffuse away, yielding a grossly hypertonic absorbate, since only incomplete osmotic equilibration could take place, but when the solute is transported across the lateral cell membranes into the spaces between the cells, the length and structure of these channels could retard the loss of solute by diffusion. Osmotic equilibration would take place along the entire length of the channels, resulting in a virtually isotonic fluid at the basement membrane. Since a high osmolality is assumed to be maintained in the lateral intercellular spaces by active solute transport, with the highest osmolality of the fluid at the closed end near the tight junctions and a decline in hypertonicity towards the open serosal end of the spaces, that is the "standing osmotic gradient," the system is capable of time-independent water absorption. Clearly, a precondition for local osmosis to function is the existence of unstirred layers between or near the cells in which standing osmotic gradients can be maintained. Hence, the impression one could get from Sect. D that unstirred layers are nothing but a nuisance to epitheliologists may need correction.

DIAMOND and BOSSERT (1967) gave a quantitative appraisal of the standing gradient osmotic flow model. The osmolality of the absorbed fluid was calculated to depend on channel properties such as length, radius, and water permeability, and on solute properties such as its active transport rate and diffusion coefficient. The osmolality of the absorbed fluid will deviate less from that of the luminal solution as the channel radius or the solute diffusion coefficient is decreased, or as channel length or water permeability is increased. However, in the analysis of DIAMOND and BOSSERT (1967), the emergent fluid is only near isotonicity when active solute transport is confined to the closed end of the channels, but becomes progressively hypertonic as solute input is spread over a greater fraction of the channel length toward the open end. These authors also indicate the possibility that standing osmotic gradients in epithelia performing solute-linked water transport may be maintained in long narrow channels other than the lateral intercellular spaces, for instance basal infoldings, brush border microvilli, or intracellular canaliculi.

Aside from the problem of the osmotic permeability of epithelia, which will be dealt with later, the standing gradient model was criticized for two reasons: DIAMOND and BOSSERT (1967) assumed that: (1) the lateral intercellular spaces are closed at their luminal ends; and (2) active solute transport is confined to the luminal tenth of the channel length. As was discussed in Sect. D.IV, there is ample evidence that the tight junctions are permeable to both water and inorganic monovalent electrolytes. Also, the second assumption of DIAMOND and BOSSERT that active electrolyte transport takes place exclusively at the apical end of the lateral intercellular spaces is doubtful. KAYE et al. (1966) did in fact find most of the ATPase activity in the apical and middle portion of the lateral cell membrane of rabbit gallbladder, but most investigators report a uniform distribution of the ATPase along the lateral and basal cell membranes of various epithelia (STIRLING 1972; KYTE 1976; MILLS and DIBONA 1978; DIBONA and MILLS 1979; MØLLGÅRD and ROSTGAARD 1980). However, a uniform distribution of the ATPase does not exclude the possibility that the solute transport rate is higher at the apical end of the lateral intercellular spaces, for example if the substrate concentration for active transport is higher in this cell region than in the basal region of the cell. Indeed, KAYE et al. (1966) report that Na, visualized by pyroantimonate precipitation, was preferentially localized along the intracellular side of the supranuclear portion of the lateral cell membrane.

SACKIN and BOULPAEP (1975) modified the standing gradient model to account for permeable tight junctions and for uniform active solute transport along the entire length of the lateral intercellular spaces. In the Diamond–Bossert model the solute concentration decreases continuously from the closed end to the mouth of the channel, whereas according to the modification of SACKIN and BOULPAEP the solute concentration increases somewhat from the permeable tight junctions towards the central part of the lateral intercellular spaces (Fig. 4 b). Thus, the standing osmotic gradient characteristic of the Diamond–Bossert model is replaced by more or less uniformly hypertonic lateral intercellular spaces. Since the uniform solute input along the entire channel length produces a hypertonic absorbate at the serosal end of the channels, SACKIN and BOULPAEP proposed that there is an unstirred layer beyond the serosal end of the epithelial cells and that isotonicity is only reached in the capillaries. Thus, in contrast to the Diamond–Bossert model, osmotic equilibration is not achieved by the time the fluid reaches the serosal end of the lateral intercellular channels. Alternatively, SACKIN and BOULPAEP (1975) discuss the possibility that isotonicity of the absorbate is a consequence of nonzero salt reflection coefficients of the basement membrane or subsequent barriers. A mathematical assessment of a standing gradient model of the lateral intercellular space including a basement membrane of finite solute permeability was recently presented by WEINSTEIN and STEPHENSON (1981 a, b).

A formal analysis of the hypertonic interspace models, including permeable tight junctions, was also given by KING-HELE and PAULSON (1977), according to which the overall hydrodynamic resistance of the lateral intercellular spaces is determined primarily by the geometric properties of the tight junctions. Also the fraction of solute leaking back through the tight junctions is influenced by the structure of the lateral intercellular spaces. These authors agree with the earlier criticism of HILL (1975 a) that the geometric parameters used by DIAMOND and BOSSERT in their numerical analysis of the standing gradient model are unrealistic. If "realistic" values are used, the influence of diffusion is greatly increased and the osmolality of the emergent fluid is very hypertonic, contrary to observations. The Diamond–Bossert model can be made to yield a quasi-isotonic absorbate when the osmotic permeability of the epithelium is increased and/or the diffusion coefficient of the actively transported solute is decreased. In other words, after the theroretical framework of local osmosis had been advanced, the question of primary concern was whether the properties of epithelia and actively transported solutes are such that local osmosis can be realistically expected to account for epithelial fluid absorption. This question has been a matter of great controversy to this day, primarily because of the difficulty of obtaining "true" osmotic permeability coefficients for the individual epithelial barriers as discussed in Sect. D.II.

Common to the models of CURRAN, DIAMOND and BOSSERT, and SACKIN and BOULPAEP is the existence of a distinctly hypertonic compartment in the epithelium. What was needed after these models had been proposed was experimental proof that there are hypertonic regions in epithelia. MACHEN and DIAMOND (1969) concluded from theoretical considerations that local osmotic gradients should give rise to diffusion potentials because of the permselective properties of epithelia, i.e., $P_{Na} > P_{Cl}$ in the case of rabbit gallbladder. Indeed, in this tissue which has a neutral NaCl pump MACHEN and DIAMOND measured small transepithelial electrical potential differences which changed in parallel with the rates of fluid transport. From these potentials and diffusion potentials resulting from known NaCl concentration differences, the mean NaCl concentration in the lateral intercellular spaces was estimated to be approximately 10 m*M* above that in the external bathing solutions. Further indirect evidence for the existence of a hypertonic compartment in epithelia was reported by SIOMMONS and NAFTALIN (1976), who concluded from the kinetics of Na efflux from isolated rabbit ileum that there is an extracellular pool containing Na at a concentration of 180 m*M*, whereas the bathing solutions contained 140 m*M*. The extracellular high Na pool was dependent on the Na concentration in the bathing solutions and was abolished by ouabain, but augmented by galactose.

The first direct confirmation that the lateral intercellular spaces contain hypertonic fluids was provided by WALL et al. (1970) for insect rectal pads. Rectal pads are thickenings of the epithelium composed of tall columnar cells with lateral intercellular spaces large enough to permit collection of fluid samples from them by micropuncture. Samples collected from the spaces were 31–300 mosm/l more concentrated than the fluid in the rectal lumen.

GUPTA et al. (1978) used electron microprobe X-ray analysis to measure the concentration profiles of several electrolytes in rabbit ileal mucosa. The Na and K concentrations in the lateral intercellular spaces were significantly higher than the respective concentrations in the external bathing solutions and in the capillary fluid. Also, the Cl concentrations were elevated, but this effect was less clear-cut. The Na, K, and Cl concentrations increased from the tight junctions to a plateau in the central part of the lateral intercellular spaces, where the osmolality was found to be as much as 100 mosm/l hypertonic to the external solutions, when the measured electrolytes are assumed to be in free solution. In a later publication the same group of investigators reported a hypertonicity of the lateral intercellular spaces of 40–70 mosm/l in rabbit ileum (GUPTA and HALL 1981). The increase in the ion concentrations from the tight junctions to the central part of the lateral intercellular spaces was interpreted as resulting from osmotic flow of water across the tight junctions (or backflux of electrolytes across the tight junctions). Consistent with this interpretation is the finding that in the dead-end canaliculus of insect salivary glands the hypertonicity was largest near the closed end of the channels and decreased towards the open end (GUPTA and HALL 1979), in agreement with the standing gradient hypothesis of DIAMOND and BOSSERT. However, the concentration profiles obtained by electron microprobe analysis in rabbit ileum are consistent with the predictions of the model of SACKIN and BOULPAEP (1975) insofar as the electrolyte concentration was lowest near the tight junctions. Also in agreement with the model of SACKIN and BOULPAEP, GUPTA et al. (1978) did not find total osmotic equilibration at the serosal end of the lateral intercellular spaces, rather the fluid in the submucosa was still hypertonic, isotonicity being only approached in the capillaries. Ouabain markedly reduced the hypertonicity of the lateral intercellular spaces, although this result may be uncertain since the channels collapsed and the resolution of the method may limit the differentiation of extracellular and intracellular concentrations.

The methodological problems involved in electron microprobe analysis are also illustrated by the finding of GUPTA et al. (1978) that the measured K concentration in the lateral intercellular spaces of up to 50 m*M* markedly exceeds that in the external bathing solutions of 15 m*M*. This observation may possibly be due to the fact that the lateral intercellular spaces are interrupted by a large number of foldings of the lateral cell membranes (see following paragraphs), hence in fact the sampling area of the electron beam may include both extracellular and intracellular spaces. In fact, when the data are corrected for cytoplasmic contamination using the microprobe phosphate signal, the maximum K concentration in the lateral intercellular spaces is reduced to 23 m*M* (GUPTA and HALL 1981). CURCI and FRÖMTER (1979) measured K activities in the lateral intercellular spaces of *Necturus* gallbladder by use of a K-selective microelectrode and found them only slightly higher than the K activity of the external bathing solutions. Further, also employing ion-selective microelectrodes SIMON et al. (1981) detected only small elevations of the Na and Cl concentrations in the lateral intercellular spaces in comparison to the external bathing solutions, the hypertonicity of the lateral intercellular spaces amounting to only 15 mosm/l.

If indeed osmolality profiles exist in the lateral intercellular spaces, the question arises how these concentration gradients can be maintained in the apparent absence of significant diffusion constraints in these spaces. The maintenance of solute concentration gradients in the lateral intercellular spaces may be a consequence of the tortuosity of these spaces. WELLING and WELLING (1979) illustrated the complex three-dimensional folding of the lateral cell membranes of rabbit kidney proximal tubules by morphometric means. The cells in this region of the nephron are 7.5 μm high and have a diameter of the apical surface of 9.8 μm. With respect to these dimensions the cells have a surprisingly large circumference which increases from 80 μm near the lumen to approximately 1,400 μm near the basement membrane. This enormous enlargement of the cell circumference is brought about by elongations and dichotomous divisions of radiating cell processes. Also in rabbit and *Necturus* gallbladder, the lateral intercellular spaces were shown to be interrupted by numerous finger-like evaginations of leaflets projecting from the lateral cell surfaces, and immediately above the basement membrane the channels become very narrow (BLOM and HELANDER 1977; SCHIFFERDECKER and FRÖMTER 1978). Alternatively, the geometrical constraints concerning the lateral intercellular spaces could be considerably relaxed, if the fluid in these spaces had the properties of a gel (KLYCE and RUSSEL 1980). However, at present there is no experimental evidence for elevated viscosity of the fluid in the lateral intercellular spaces.

The theory that quasi-isotonic water absorption is brought about by osmotic gradients within the epithelium was challenged, at least for epithelia that exhibit high rates of isotonic fluid absorption, primarily on the grounds that the osmotic permeability coefficients of the apical and the basolateral cell membrane are too low to permit the formation of an isotonic absorbate (HILL 1975a; HILL 1980). In other words, theories based on local osmosis are qualitatively capable of explaining the coupling of salt and water transport, however, owing to the problems in the determination of the permeability properties of epithelia and the paucity of osmolality measurements in the various tissue compartments, the feasibility of the local osmosis theories remains highly controversical in quantitative terms. For instance, DIAMOND (1964b) calculated that the P_{os} of rabbit gallbladder would have to be $1{,}600 \times 10^{-4}$ cm s^{-1} in order to obtain an absorbate which is 1% hypertonic to a 300 mosm/l bathing solution, whereas with the range of P_{os} measurements given in Table 3 (14–93×10^{-4} cm s^{-1}) and the same solute transport rate as used by DIAMOND (1964b), the osmolality of the absorbate would be between 20% and 87% above that of the bathing solution. Thus, the measured P_{os} values are grossly insufficient to permit complete osmotic equilibration of the transported fluid. Similarly, from the rate of active solute transport and the P_{os} reported for rat small intestine, the predicted osmolality of the absorbed fluid would be 116 mosm/l higher than the osmolality of the bathing solution; the corresponding values for proximal tubules would be 20 mosm/l and that for frog stomach 95 mosm/l (DIAMOND 1964b). All these tissues actually transport fluid isotonically. In order to reconcile the enormous discrepancy of up to two orders of magnitude between the measured P_{os} values and the P_{os} values necessary to account for isotonic absorption, it was argued that indeed such large osmotic permeabilities do exist, but that unstirred layers cause serious underestimations of P_{os} (DIAMOND 1978). In fact, when the value of P_{os} corrected for unstirred layer effects by use of streaming potentials (VAN OS et al. 1979; see Table 3) is employed to calculate the osmolality of the absorbed fluid in rabbit gallbladder, it may be predicted to be only 4% hypertonic to the bathing fluid.

DURBIN and HELANDER (1978) attempted a numerical analysis of the relation between the osmotic permeability of the basolateral cell membrane of rabbit gallbladder and observed rates of fluid absorption in this tissue. From the morphometric study of BLOM and HELANDER (1977), the surface area of the basolateral membrane was taken to be 173 cm^2 for every 1 cm^2 macroscopic epithelial surface area, and the P_{os} of the transporting membrane was assumed to be 18×10^{-4} cm s^{-1} as determined in artificial lipid bilayers containing phospholipids and cholesterol in a molar ratio of 1:2 (HANAI and HAYDON 1966; FINKELSTEIN and CASS 1967). From these data and experimentally determined rates of water absorption, DURBIN and HELANDER calculated that the osmolality of the solution on the serosal side of the transporting membrane would have to be only 1.3% in excess of the luminal solution to generate the observed rates of net water flow. It should be noted that DURBIN and HELANDER (1978) assumed water transport across the lipid phase of the membrane, a route of water permeation discussed in Sect. D.IV; pores in the cell membranes are not necessary if the water permeability of the lipid phase of the cell membrane is as high as that of artificial lipid bilayers. The basic feature of this concept is that, owing to an anormous enlargement of the basolateral cell membrane, the osmotic gradient within the epithelium required to drive net water transport is minimized.

Taking into account that, according to BLOM and HELANDER (1977), the surface area of the basolateral membrane is approximately two orders of magnitude larger than the macroscopic epithelial surface area, P_{os} of the basolateral membrane expressed with respect to apical surface area should be approximately $1{,}800 \times 10^{-4}$ cm s^{-1} when the osmotic permeability of the basolateral membrane is assumed to be equal to that of an artificial lipid bilayer. In excellent agreement with this prediction is the value of $1{,}200 \times 10^{-4}$ cm s^{-1} determined by PERSSON and SPRING (1982) for the basolateral membrane of *Necturus* gallbladder epithelium. From this high osmotic permeability and the rate of fluid absorption in this tissue it can be calculated that the osmotic gradient across the basolateral membrane would have to be only 1.1 mosm/l in order to generate the observed rate of fluid absorption. Using the P_{os} of the apical membrane it was estimated that the cell interior must be 2.4 mosm/l hypertonic to the luminal solution, hence the total osmotic gradient across both membranes would be 3.5 mosm/l (PERSSON and SPRING 1982; SPRING and ERICSON 1982). An absorbate hypertonicity of 3.5 mosm/l or 1.8% above isoosmolality is within the measurement error of current methods for osmolality determinations, and the transported fluid may be considered isotonic.

However, when indeed P_{os} of the cell membranes is high enough to account for isotonic fluid absorption, then the tissue may no longer be capable of transporting water against an adverse osmotic gradient. WEINSTEIN and STEPHENSON (1981 a, b) calculated for physiologically relevant parameters that the ability for uphill water transport, which in this assessment depends on the solute permeability of the basement membrane, is diminished by cell membrane water permeability. Hence one of the dilemmas that confronts the local osmosis theories, besides the lack of "true" P_{os} values for the individual epithelial barriers, is that they must be able to explain both the experimental observations of isotonic fluid absorption and fluid absorption against osmotic gradients. In order to settle the question of the quantitative feasibility of the local osmosis theories for solute-water transport coupling, novel experimental techniques may be necessary to obtain P_{os} values uncontaminated by unstirred layer effects (DIAMOND 1979). In addition, more direct measurements of the hypertonicity and the concentration profiles in the lateral intercellular spaces and other channels that may play a role in water absorption are needed. The technique of electron microprobe analysis raises some hopes of providing sound data in this respect, although this approach is still the subject of methodological controversies.

The concept of osmotic coupling of solute and water transport within the epithelium is not only attractive because it is founded on a wealth of both experimental and theoretical work, but also because it is difficult to account for the observed rates of net water transport by nonosmotic mechanisms. For example, HILL (1975 b) proposed fluid transport by electroosmosis. This mechanism would of course not necessitate concentration gradients in the lateral intercellular spaces. However, HILL later retracted this theory on the grounds that the relation of water molecules to ions transported necessary to account for the observed rates of water absorption would be far too great to be conceivable, especially for absorption from dilute solutions (HILL and HILL 1978 a; HILL 1980).

Another possible mechanism for coupled salt-water absorption is single-file diffusion through narrow channels such that one ion permeating through the channel moves the water molecules contained in it. Indeed, interaction of water molecules during passage across cell membranes in the form of single-file diffusion is consistent with the observations that the permeability coefficients calculated from rates of net water movement are higher than those obtained from exchange studies with labeled water (HODGKIN and KEYNES 1955), or, with other words, that the P_{os}/P_w ratio exceeds unity (see HEBERT and ANDREOLI 1982). For example, in ADH-responsive epithelial water transport across the apical membrane was reported to occur by single-file diffusion through narrow channels containing approximately 6 water molecules per channel (HEBERT and ANDREOLI 1982). But a relation between the transport of water molecules and ions of 6 to 1 would result in a grossly hypertonic absorbate, hence transport pathways containing much more water molecules but still exhibiting the properties of single-file diffusion would have to be assumed. Under these conditions the stoichiometry between the transport of water and ions and consequently the osmolality of the absorbate would be determined by the number of ions migrating across the transport pathway at a time. However, of the various epithelial transport processes for ions, evidence for a channel mechanism has been obtained only for electrogenic apical Na entry (VAN DRIESSCHE and LINDEMANN 1979), and it is totally unclear whether water and ions permeate through the same channels. Clearly, more information on the epithelial transport pathways for actively transported electrolytes is needed to evaluate the possible significance of this nonosmotic mechanism for coupled salt-water absorption.

Pinocytosis is clearly inadequate to explain water absorption as HILL and HILL (1978 a) and HILL (1980) point out, since it would not only require a specific rejection mechanism for solutes not transported, but also because the number of vesicles necessary would have to be vast, requiring an enormous amount of membrane material owing to the high surface to volume ratio of small vesicles. PARSONS (1963) estimated that to absorb fluid at 7 l/day from the human small intestine entirely by pinocytosis, a rate of vesicle formation of the order of 1,000 vesicles per second for each epithelial cell would be required for the whole 24 h, assuming a vesicle diameter of 60 nm.

HILL and HILL (1978 a) report findings which are difficult to reconcile with osmotic coupling of solute and solvent transport. These investigators observed in *Necturus* gallbladder that fluid absorption is isotonic with the bathing fluid over a range of bathing solution osmolalities of 400 mosm/l down to 1 mosm/l. Fluid transport was reported to be inhibited by ouabain, even with the low bathing solution osmolalities. From these findings the authors concluded that fluid transport cannot be produced by local osmosis across the lateral cell membranes for the following reasons. Either the cells remain intact during exposure to the low osmolality bathing solutions, then the cytoplasm is hypertonic to the bathing medium, in which case the transported fluid must be hypertonic to the bathing solution because osmotic equilibration along the lateral intercellular spaces can only produce an absorbate of higher or maximally equal tonicity compared with that of the cell interior. Or, alternatively, the cell membranes have ruptured owing to osmotic swelling, in which case the reflection coefficient for the actively transported solutes will be low and consequently no osmotic volume flow can be generated. Further, HILL and HILL (1978 b) reported that the absorbate contained sucrose at practically the same concentration as that added to the luminal solution. If it is accepted that sucrose permeates the tissue across an extracellular pathway, this finding indicates convective water flow across this pathway, moving sucrose by solvent drag. Since the convective flow necessary to account for the observed sucrose permeation was estimated to amount to almost the entire epithelial water absorption, it was concluded that water absorption is accomplished by flow across the tight junctions and not by transcellular flow driven by an osmotic gradient in the lateral intercellular spaces. These studies were criticized mainly because of the extremely unphysiologic conditions under which they were performed. The sucrose permeability was investigated over an extremely long incubation period of 12–14 h in a 50 mosm/l salt solution, whereas *Necturus* plasma has 200 mosm/l. Conceivably, the hypotonic incubation medium may alter the permeability properties of the tissue. Another problem is the low Ca concentration in the low osmolality bathing solutions used. It is commonly known that epithelia become very leaky when incubated in a low Ca solution, in fact the transepithelial electrical resistance may practically vanish. Hence the results obtained by HILL and HILL (1978 a, b) may not apply to normal gallbladders with intact permeability barriers (DIAMOND 1979).

Further, the possibility of fluid absorption via an extracellular pathway was rejected for *Necturus* gallbladder epithelium since P_{os} of the apical membrane is 550×10^{-4} cm s^{-1}; in order to account for the observed rates of fluid absorption P_{os} of the tight junctions would have to be an unrealistic $5 \times 10^{+2}$ cm s^{-1}, because the available area of the tight junctions is only 1/10,000th of the total apical surface area (SPRING and ERICSON 1982). Also in rabbit gallbladder epithelium the tight junctions do not seem to play a significant role in fluid absorption, since the polyvalent cationic dye Alcian-blue causes an almost complete collaps of the intercellular spaces apical of the tight junctions and an increase in transepithelial resistance, but this agent does not alter net mucosa to serosa fluid transport (FREDERIKSEN et al. 1979). Additional evidence for transcellular water absorption in ADH-responsive epithelia was recently summarized by HEBERT and ANDREOLI (1982).

Although the experimental basis for the existence of transjunctional water absorption, at least in gallbladder, is fragmentary at best, and HILL did not provide a sound explanation for the mechanism of extracellular fluid absorption – there is not the least experimental evidence for the nonosmotic mechanisms for water absorption discussed by HILL (1980) such as electrokinetic phenomena similar to phloem transport or peristalsis of the lateral cell membranes – the possibility of transjunctional water absorption in some epithelia cannot be excluded. In kidney proximal tubules, for instance, a large fraction of fluid absorption appears to proceed via the tight junctions. BERRY and BOULPAEP (1975) observed that there was no net flux of sucrose across *Necturus* proximal tubules in the absence of net water flow, whereas during solute-coupled water absorption, there was a striking asymmetry in the unidirectional fluxes of sucrose, resulting in net sucrose efflux from the lumen to the blood side of the tubule. ANDREOLI et al. (1979) also concluded that a major fraction of fluid absorption in isolated rabbit superficial straight tubules occurs via an extracellular pathway. Since previous experiments indicated that Cl absorption is entirely passive, Cl crossing the epithelium on an extracellular route, solvent drag was implicated to be the nondiffusional mechanism of Cl transfer. From the rates of water and Cl transfer and the Cl reflection coefficient of proximal straight tubules ANDREOLI et al. (1979) calculated that about 86% of the fluid absorption occurs via an extracellular route.

According to ANDREOLI and SCHAFER (1979), the driving forces for transjunctional fluid absorption in proximal tubules are small differences in the effective osmotic pressures of the external solutions. P_{os} of the proximal tubules was reported to be extremely large, so that small transepithelial osmotic gradients may be sufficient to account for the observed rates of fluid absorption. With the P_{os} value given by ANDREOLI and SCHAFER (1979) for proximal tubules (see Table 3) effective transepithelial osmotic pressure differences of only 1.6–6.4 mosm/l can account for the experimentally determined rates of fluid absorption. In contrast to the hypertonic interspace models ANDREOLI and SCHAFER (1979) argued that the lateral intercellular spaces are in osmotic equilibrium with the peritubular space because of the high osmotic permeability of this tissue. Additionally, the very low transepithelial electrical resistance of $5\,\Omega\,cm^2$ indicates a low diffusive resistance of the lateral intercellular spaces for ions, so that it is unlikely that osmotic gradients can be maintained in these spaces. ANDREOLI and SCHAFER (1979) proposed that the effective transepithelial osmotic gradient could be generated by preferential HCO_3 absorption along the length of the proximal tubules. If the reflection coefficient for HCO_3 is higher than that for Cl, an effective osmotic driving force would be established, although isotonicity of both external bathing solutions is preserved. Alternatively, active Na absorption could render the luminal solution slightly hypotonic.

Let us evaluate this interesting model, which in fact represents a return to classical osmosis inasmuch as the osmotic gradient is not assumed to be established within the epithelium, but rather between the external solutions, by making a few simple calculations. The only basic restriction which we have to impose on the system is that the epithelium is impermeable to inulin, a rod of 50 Å length and 6 Å diameter (PHELPS 1965). SCHAFER et al. (1975) found that the isethionate : Cl permeability ratio in superficial proximal straight tubules is 0.03 : 1, prompting the conclusion that the effective pore radius required for such selectivity is less than 15 Å (ANDREOLI et al. 1979). Clearly, the pores would have to be small enough to result in relatively high reflection coefficients for Na and/or HCO_3, a prerequisite for osmotic gradients to be established. Most likely the equivalent pore radius would have to approach 5 Å.

Assuming that volume flow through the junctional pores may be described by Poiseulle's law, the number of pores per unit area required to account for the observed rates of fluid absorption can be calculated from

$$n=\frac{8J_v\eta l}{\pi r^4 \Delta p}, \tag{E.1}$$

where J_v is the rate fluid absorption ($4.8\times10^{-5}\,ml\,cm^{-2}\,s^{-1}$ according to ANDREOLI and SCHAFER 1979), η is the viscosity of the absorbed fluid (0.01 poise), l is the length of the junctional complex (2×10^{-5} cm), r is the equivalent pore radius, and Δp is the pressure gradient, 0.16 atm, calculated from a transepithelial osmotic gradient of 6.4 mosm/l (ANDREOLI and SCHAFER 1979) using the van't Hoff equation. Further, the electrical resistance R_e of an epithelium with n pores per unit area of radius r may be derived from

$$R_e=\frac{\varrho l}{n\pi r^2}, \tag{E.2}$$

where ϱ is the specific electrical resistance of Ringer's solution ($100\,\Omega$ cm).

Table 9. Relationship between the equivalent pore radius r and the number of pores n per unit area, necessary to account for a given volume flow J_v driven by an osmotic pressure gradient of 6.4 mosm/l. R_e is the electrical resistance. The values were calculated according to Eqs. (E.1) and (E.2) with a pore length $l = 2 \times 10^{-5}$ cm

r (10^{-8} cm)	n (pores/cm^2)	R_e ($\Omega\, cm^2$)	J_v (10^{-5} ml cm^{-2} s^{-1})
5	2×10^{13}	0.01	4.8
15	3×10^{11}	0.1	4.8
15	6×10^{9}	5.0	0.1
110	1×10^{8}	5.2	4.8

The results of the calculations of the number of pores per unit area as a function of the equivalent pore radius for the conditions defined are compiled in Table 9 which also gives the resulting electrical resistances. Clearly, the number of pores is enormous when small pore radii of 15 Å or less are assumed, and the resulting electrical resistances are much lower than the measured value of $5\,\Omega\, cm^2$. With $r = 15$ Å and $R_e = 5\,\Omega\, cm^2$, only 2% of the experimentally observed fluid absorption would pass via the route that determines R_e in this leaky tissue, i.e., the extracellular pathway. On the other hand, in order to reconcile the observed rates of fluid absorption with the measured electrical resistance of $5\,\Omega cm^2$ the pores would have to be very large, thereby precluding that Na or HCO_3 could establish an osmotic gradient across them. In calculating the values given in Table 9, the length of the junctional complex was assumed to be 2×10^{-5} cm as reported by TORMEY and DIAMOND (1967) for gallbladder epithelium. It should be noted that from Eqs. (E.1) and (E.2) it is obvious that a decrease of l to a minimum of 50 Å, the equivalent of a single lipid bilayer, decreases n but does not affect R_e since l and n are linearly related.

In summary, the calculated values given in Table 9 cast some doubt on the notion that a major fraction of volume absorption occurs via the extracellular route, primarily because the junctional pore radii would have to be very small in order for Na or HCO_3 to become osmotically effective. This fact in turn would require a very large number of pores, which not only may be difficult to accomodate in the tight junctions, but which would also render the electrical resistance of the epithelium much lower than actually observed.

The concept of small effective osmotic gradients between the external solutions can hardly account for the phenomenon of water absorption against large osmotic gradients of up to 400 mosm/l observed in intestinal epithelia. But one feature of the concept of ANDREOLI and SCHAFER (1979) could have wider applicability. An effective osmotic gradient may be produced across an epithelium by the asymmetric distribution of solutes with different reflection coefficients. The theory that an effective osmotic gradient may result from transport-dependent asymmetries in fluid composition between the absorbate and the luminal solution and differences in the reflection coefficients of the asymmetrically distributed solutes has also been formulated by FRÖMTER (1974) and in fact follows from STAVER-

MAN's (1952) work. Hence osmotic volume flow may ensue, although the cryoscopic osmolalities of the external solutions on the two sides of the epithelium are identical.

III. Countercurrent Exchanger Model

In the models discussed up to now, the epithelium constitutes the functional unit which is responsible for fluid absorption. HALJAMÄE et al. (1973), on the other hand, proposed that the intestinal villus is the functional unit which produces fluid absorption; they found in cat jejunum in vivo that the Na concentration per unit weight of protein is 3–4 times higher in the villus tip than at the villus base. This concentration gradient was increased by luminal addition of glucose, while ischemia, intense vasodilation, or intraarterial infusion of ouabain reduced the Na concentration gradient from villus tip to villus base. These findings were explained by the existence of a countercurrent exchange system in the villus, based on the anatomy of the villus vasculature. Each villus of cat small intestine is supplied by one or two central arteries running to the villus tip, where they branch into a network of capillaries beneath the epithelium. The distance between the arteries and the subepithelial capillary network is only 10–20 μm. Finally, the capillaries collect into veins which run in the central portion of the villus (see HALJAMÄE et al. 1973; HALLBÄCK et al. 1978). Hence there are hairpin vascular loops which are consistent with countercurrent exchange diffusion. This system appears to be responsible for the observation that oxygen, antipyrine, and possibly urea are extravascularly shunted from the central arteries to the capillary network at the villus base. On the other hand, substances entering the capillaries across the epithelium from the gut lumen may be "trapped" in the countercurrent exchanger, and consequently absorption of these compounds could be delayed (see LUNDGREN 1974; HALLBÄCK et al. 1978). A rigorous discussion of the countercurrent exchanger and its influence on intestinal absorption and excretion was given by WINNE (1975).

The absorption of water may be enhanced by the countercurrent exchanger system, if it functions to establish a hypertonic region within the villus. According to this concept the actively absorbed solutes render the capillary blood slightly hypertonic. Shunting of these solutes from the subepithelial capillary network to the central artery or of water in the reverse direction would also increase the tonicity of the arterial blood. If this process is repeated along the villus length, the interstitial fluid may become increasingly hypertonic toward the tip. From their data on the Na concentrations in the villlus tissue, HALJAMÄE et al. (1973) estimated the osmolality of the interstitial fluid to range between 575 and 1,600 mosm/l at the villus tip. According to these investigators, the hypertonic villus core represents the anatomic counterpart of the middle compartment of CURRAN's series membrane model where the osmotic coupling of solute and water transport takes place.

In an attempt to obtain direct evidence for the existence of a hypertonic villus core, JODAL et al. (1978) developed a cryoscopic technique by which they determined the tissue osmolality along the villus of cat small intestine in vivo. The principle of this method is slowly to thaw frozen tissue sections 10–15 μm thick under observation through a microscope and to monitor the fraction of tissue that is thawed at each temperature increment by taking photographs. The cryoscopic method is calibrated by measuring the melting points of salt solutions of different osmolalities or by observing the melting process of sections of intestine which had been incubated for 60 min in Krebs solution varying in osmolality between 300 and 1,000 mosm/l by addition of mannitol. Undoubtedly some bias is introduced into the method since the proportion of villus tissue melted at each temperature is determined by inspecting the photographs, and difficulties were reported in visualizing the melting process of ice crystals in tissue sections in comparison with salt solutions (KOKKO 1978).

According to JODAL et al. (1978), thawing of the intestinal wall always starts at the villus tips and proceeds to the base as the temperature is increased in a step-wise manner. By this technique the osmolality of the villus tips was determined to be approximately 1,100 mosm/l with a quasiexponential decline to the villus base. Using the same method, villus tip osmolality in human small intestine was estimated to be approximately 700 mosm/l (HALLBÄCK et al. 1978). Replacing Na in the luminal solution by choline markedly reduced villus tip osmolality (JODAL et al. 1978; HALLBÄCK et al. 1978). When intestinal blood flow was increased fivefold by intraarterial infusion of isoproterenol, the hypertonicity of the villus tips of cat jejunum was reduced from 1,100 to 709 mosm/l (JODAL et al. 1978). All these results are in agreement with the countercurrent exchanger hypothesis. Clearly, an osmotic gradient of approximately 800 mosm/l across that part of the villus which is in the most intimate contact with the luminal contents would represent an enormous driving force for water absorption, even if the effective osmotic gradient is attenuated by solute reflection coefficients below unity. Indeed, water absorption was shown to be positively correlated with villus tip osmolality (HALLBÄCK et al. 1979b, 1980). The finding of LEE (1969) that water is absorbed primarily at the tips of the villi is also consistent with a maximum in driving force for water absorption in this region of the villus.

Further support for the existence of a countercurrent exchanger in the intestinal villi was inferred by HALLBÄCK et al. (1978) from the washout kinetics of intraarterially injected ^{85}Kr from the small and large intestine. The elimination of label from the intestine was a composite exponential curve, which HALLBÄCK et al. (1978) subjected to a compartmental analysis by use of a curve-stripping technique. By this procedure the authors claim to resolve the washout curve from the small intestine into four components, whereas they find only three components in the washout curve from the colon. Since the compartment with the shortest half-time of washout was observed only in the small intestine, this fast component of elimination was interpreted to reflect exchange diffusion between the two limbs of the hairpin vascular loops of the villi. However, it has to be stated that the evidence for the fast component with the shortest half-time is rather weak, since it is based on two or three points of the washout curve at most. No indication is given whether the model with four exponential functions indeed exhibits a better fit to the experimental data than a model with three experimental functions. In addition, with washout curves composed of as many as four exponential functions, it is very difficult to assign the individual components to specific components of blood flow. As KOKKO (1978) stresses, the washout technique is not optimal to evaluate the properties of villus blood flow.

At present the experimental evidence for the involvement of the villus vasculature in generating a gradient of solute concentrations from tip to base may be summed up as follows: (1) vasodilation greatly reduces the villus tip hypertonicity; (2) villus tip osmolality of cat jejunum is approximately 1,100 mosm/l under in vivo conditions, but only 520 mosm/l under in vitro conditions; and (3) no tissue hypertonicity is found in cat gallbladder which is a flat epithelium (HALJAMÄE et al. 1973; JODAL et al. 1978; HALLBÄCK et al. 1978).

DOBSON (1979) derived additional indirect evidence for the existence of an intestinal countercurrent exchanger from the curvilinear relation between the absorption of tritiated water and blood flow discussed in Sect. D.I. DOBSON fitted the clearance of tritiated water from sheep rumen as a function of blood flow by use of model equations given by WINNE (1978). The model which gave the best fit to the experimental data was one in which the clearance depends not only on epithelial and capillary permeability and blood flow, but in addition on an extravascular shunt between arterioles and venules. However, DOBSON himself indicated that recruitment of additional capillaries with an increase in blood flow would affect water absorption in a manner similar to extravascular shunting of tritiated water between arterioles and venules.

HALJAMÄE et al. (1973) and HALLBÄCK et al. (1978) compare the function of the villus vasculature to the countercurrent multiplication system of the loops of Henle in the renal medulla, although such a comparison is probably not warranted. The thick ascending limb of Henle, which is impermeable to water, actively transports solute into the interstitium which thereby becomes somewhat hypertonic. Owing to the hairpin arrangement of the two limbs of the loop of Henle, the fluid in the descending limb will also increase in osmolality. Therefore, a somewhat hypertonic solution will reach the thick ascending limb, where again a small osmotic gradient is superimposed. Since this process is repeated along the length of the loop of Henle, the interstitial osmolality is continuously increased towards the kidney papilla. The basic prerequisite for this countercurrent multiplier mechanism is, aside from the hairpin arrangement and different water permeabilities of the two limbs, active solute transport in the ascending limb. The hairpin blood vessels of the intestinal villi do not actively transport solutes, therefore they cannot function as a countercurrent multiplier. Rather, the function of the villus blood vessels may be compared to that of the vasa recta of the kidney medulla which serve to maintain the osmotic gradient in the medulla by preventing solute loss from it by countercurrent exchange. The hypertonicity of the villus tip is therefore not produced by the blood vessels, but by the epithelial cells. In order for the blood vessels to trap the absorbed solutes in the villus, the two limbs of the hairpin vessels have to be highly permeable to solutes and water. This may be expected for the capillaries of the subepithelial network, but is unclear in the case of the central villus arteries. In addition, the surface area of the arteries most likely is small compared with the surface area of the subepithelial capillary network, hence the permeability × surface area product of the villus arteries may be the limiting factor of the intestinal countercurrent exchanger system.

When indeed the villus vasculature effectively traps solutes and a standing osmotic gradient is established in the villus core, it follows that the concentration gradient against which solute has to be transported by the epithelial cells increases from villus base to tip, whereas the countercurrent exchanger would decrease the oxygen supply to the villus tip. Hence, those epithelial cells would get the least oxygen which are pumping solute against the highest concentration gradient. Another problem that renders the role of the countercurrent exchanger model for intestinal water absorption dubious is the fact that up to now experimental evidence for the existence of countercurrent exchange is available only for the cat small intestine, but not for the small intestine of other species such as rabbit or rat, possibly because the rabbit and the rat small intestine have a different structure of the villous vasculature which may not be favorable for countercurrent exchange (WINNE 1975). In short, although several uncertainties still surround the countercurrent exchanger theory for intestinal water absorption, it certainly is an attractive possible mechanism for water absorption in epithelia equipped with villi.

Clearly, the countercurrent exchanger concept for intestinal water absorption differs markedly from the models based on osmotic gradients within the epithelium. Whereas the local osmosis theories require a very large osmotic permeability of the epithelium, in fact the "true" P_{os} has to be orders of magnitude higher than the values of P_{os} actually measured in order to yield an isotonic absorbate, the countercurrent exchanger concept necessitates a low osmotic permeability of the epithelium, otherwise the large villous hypertonicities could not be maintained. In contrast to the isotonic fluid which emerges from the lateral intercellular spaces according to the standing gradient model, the fluid transported by the epithelium would be very hypertonic, at least at the villus tips, according to the countercurrent exchanger model. In fact, standing osmotic gradients in the lateral intercellular spaces as proposed by DIAMOND and BOSSERT are not compatible with the countercurrent exchanger model, rather a high solute concentration on the serosal side of the epithelium is expected. Consequently, the gradient in the lateral intercellular spaces would be, if anything, opposite in direction to the one proposed by DIAMONG and BOSSERT (1967). Hence, we are again confronted with the fundamental unsolved questions of intestinal and epithelial water transport in general: what are the osmotic permeability coefficients of epithelia; what are the osmotic pressures in the different parts of an epithelium and the rest of the mucosa under in vitro and under in vivo conditions, i.e., with intact blood supply; what are the reflection coefficients of the solutes distributed symmetrically or asymmetrically across the individual barriers of an epithelium; and what is the route of transepithelial water transport?

Clearly, the countercurrent exchanger model is not capable of accounting for fluid absorption in flat epithelia such as gallbladder, colon, or the nephron, but why should there be a single mechanism of water absorption in epithelia of different organs and species? We have general agreement that there is no primary active transport of water across epithelia, but passive transport processes such as local osmosis, classical osmosis due to transepithelial osmotic gradients, electroosmosis, filtration, and possibly other mechanisms may operate alone or in combination to produce net water transport in different tissues. In other words, there is no reason to assume that one unifying explanation can account for water absorption across all epithelia. Just as there are several different mechanisms for transepithelial Na transport such as neutral and electrogenic mechanisms, and Na transport coupled to the transport of certain sugars and amino acids (SCHULTZ et al. 1974; FRIZZELL and SCHULTZ 1979), a number of different mechanisms may also be operative to secure the vital function of fluid absorption.

F. Relation Between Intestinal Blood Flow and Water Absorption

The term absorption implies uptake of a substance into the bloodstream. Hence, we will finally consider briefly the factors regulating the exchange of fluid between intestinal capillaries and the interstitial space. According to STARLING (1896) the direction and rate of fluid transfer between the intravascular and extravascular space is determined by the hydrostatic and oncotic pressures on the two sides of the capillary wall and the permeability of the capillary membrane. The Starling theory was substantiated for amphibian and mammalian capillaries by LANDIS (1927) and PAPPENHEIMER and SOTO-RIVERA (1948), respectively, who demonstrated that transcapillary fluid exchange is a linear function of the difference between the hydrostatic capillary pressure and the effective osmotic pressure of the plasma proteins.

Generally, transcapillary fluid exchange, J_v^C, is related to the hydrostatic and osmotic pressure differences across the capillary wall according to

$$J_v^C = L_p^C A_C (p_C - p_T - \sigma_M \pi_p + \sigma_M \pi_T) , \tag{F.1}$$

where L_p^C is the hydraulic permeability coefficient of the capillary wall, A_C is the capillary surface area, p_C and p_T are the capillary and tissue hydrostatic pressures, and π_P and π_T are the oncotic pressure of blood plasma and tissue interstitial fluid, respectively. σ_M stands for the reflection coefficient of the capillary wall for the macromolecules of blood plasma and interstitial fluid. Under physiologic conditions without intestinal fluid absorption or secretion, the sum of the transcapillary pressures (the net effective filtration pressure) generates a capillary filtrate which is identical to the lymph flow of the tissue (LIFSON 1979).

GRANGER and TAYLOR (1978) picture the following scenario for fluid removal from the interstitial space of the intestine. During water absorption, the interstitial fluid volume increases (GRANGER et al. 1980) and the interstitial oncotic pressure decreases, as reflected by a decrease in the lymph oncotic presssure (LEE 1981). Consequently, the hydrostatic pressure in the tissue increases, and therefore lymph flow is enhanced, but capillary filtration decreased. The driving forces for fluid removal via the capillaries are the hydrostatic pressure gradient plus the oncotic pressure gradient across the capillary wall, whereas the driving force for fluid drainage via the lymphatic vessels is only the hydrostatic pressure gradient. Therefore, fluid is preferentially removed by the blood capillaries. Although intestinal lymph flow is increased during fluid absorption compared to the nonabsorptive state (GRANGER and TAYLOR 1978; LEE 1981) and may be accelerated by rhythmic contractions of the intestinal villi (LEE 1974), there is no clear correlation between intestinal lymph flow and fluid absorption. Moreover, obstruction of the mesenteric lymph vessels causes no change in fluid absorption, indicating that lymphatic drainage is not obligatory for fluid absorption (REID 1900; LEE 1981). Similarly, absorption studies using labeled water have shown that only 2% of the absorbed label is found in the lymph (WINNE 1979).

Aside from the Starling forces intestinal water absorption may be influenced by the countercurrent exchanger mechanism of the villi discussed in Sect. E.III. It is unclear whether the rate of blood flow in the capillaries represents an additional factor for removal of intestinal fluid by a mechanism analogous to the suction developed by a jet of fluid according to the law of Bernoulli.

The quantitative efficiency of the mechanism for fluid removal from the intestine is considerable. In dog, volume absorption from the intestine amounts to approximately 20% of the absorptive site blood flow under control conditions (MAILMAN 1980).

Clearly, perturbations of the equilibrium of the Starling forces as expressed by Eq. (F.1) will affect transcapillary fluid exchange and therefore intestinal water absorption. An increase in capillary filtration will lead to a rise in tissue hydrostatic pressure which may decrease intestinal fluid absorption or may even reverse fluid absorption to fluid secretion because of the high hydrostatic filtration coefficient of the intestinal epithelium in the secretory direction (see Sect. D.V).

One of the primary buffering mechanisms of the intestine to prevent an excessive rise in tissue hydrostatic pressure is a high reflection coefficient of its capillaries for plasma proteins. Although the intestinal capillaries are fenestrated (HAMMERSEN 1971), they appear to restrict the movement of macromolecules to a larger extent than capillaries of other organs (GRANGER et al. 1979; GRANGER and TAYLOR 1980). Measurements of the permeability properties of mesenteric capillaries for macromolecules, the transcapillary oncotic pressure difference plays a dominant role in preventing interstitial edema subsequent to venous pressure elevation (RICHARDSON et al. 1980). Intestinal capillary pressure has to rise above that fluid uptake into the bloodstream may be highly effective in the venous portion of the capillaries. As a result of the high reflection coefficient of the intestinal capillaries for macromolecules, the transcapillary oncotic pressure difference plays a dominant role in preventing interstitial edema subsequent to venous pressure elevation (RICHARDSON et al. 1980). Intestinal capillary pressure has to rise above a threshold of 30–35 cmH_2O to produce net capillary filtration into the intestinal lumen (YABLONSKI and LIFSON 1976; MORTILLARO and TAYLOR 1976), above this threshold the rate of secretion is linearly related to the increase in capillary pressure. In excellent agreement with these results is the finding of DUFFY et al. (1978) that a decrease in plasma oncotic pressure of 11–15 cmH_2O, produced by plasma volume expansion, causes intestinal secretion, the relation between plasma protein concentration and transepithelial volume flow being linear. Also LEE (1973) demonstrated in vascularly perfused rat rejunum that fluid is secreted when the oncotic pressure of the arterial perfusate is decreased or when the arterial perfusion pressure is increased. The ability to prevent intestinal secretion is not specific for certain plasma proteins, but a general property of all macromolecules as shown with dextran, bovine serum albumin, blood plasma, and whole blood (LEE 1973).

Other possibilities of producing a secretory filtrate into the intestinal lumen include negative intraluminal pressures (WELLS 1931; HAKIM et al. 1977), obstruction of the lymphatic drainage (RUSZNYAK et al. 1967), and reduction of the reflection coefficient of the capillary wall for plasma proteins, for instance due to intestinal inflammation. Thus, any cause that raises the tissue hydrostatic pressure above the luminal hydrostatic pressure may cause fluid secretion. This behavior appears to be a more or less general pathophysiologic response of transporting epithelia to elevated transepithelial pressure differences (LIFSON 1979).

An additional factor that may facilitate intestinal secretion is an increase in the hydraulic conductivity of the tight junctions, for example brought about by deoxycholate or oxyphenisatin (WANITSCHKE et al. 1977).

Interestingly, diarrhea does not seem to be a prominent feature in portal hypertension. Patients with portal venous pressures of 14–75 cmH_2O (normal values are 0–11 cmH_2O) exhibited no consistent signs of intestinal secretion or impaired absorption (NORMAN et al. 1980). Perhaps the slowly progressive nature of portal hypertension, for instance during the course of chronic liver disease, permits adaptive changes such as increased lymphatic drainage, decreased capillary permeability, and increased epithelial resistance to secretory filtration, thereby maintaining the absorptive function and preventing intestinal secretion (YABLONSKI and LIFSON 1976).

Clearly, mucosal blood flow is essential for intestinal water absorption, not only because it removes interstitial fluid, but also because it supplies the oxygen and substrates necessary for the generation of metabolic energy driving active solute transport. There are mechanisms for autoregulation of blood flow in the intestine, i.e., local vasoregulatory control systems which maintain blood flow at a fairly constant level, despite changes in arterial blood pressure. This phenomenon is not as intense as in other organs, but becomes pronounced when the metabolic rate is stimulated by placing transportable nutrients into the intestinal lumen (SHEPHERD 1980). Autoregulation of intestinal blood flow is unaffected by chronic denervation or sympatholytic agents and appears to be mediated by both hormonal and metabolic factors (GRANGER and KVIETYS 1981).

When arterial blood pressure is lowered from 100 to 30 mmHg, total blood flow of the small intestine decreases, but villous blood flow remains practically unaltered (LUNDGREEN and SVANVIK 1973), indicating that a larger fracton of intestinal blood flow is diverted to the absorptive cells during arterial hypotension than under control conditions. Hence, the autoregulatory capacity of the villous vasculature seems to be larger than that of the other blood vessels of the small intestine. Similarly, subepithelial blood flow is very well autoregulated in the colon, but total blood flow is not (GRANGER et al. 1980). In both small intestinal and colonic mucosa, venous pressure elevation decreases total blood flow and increases vascular resistance, but reduces absorptive site blood flow considerably less (LUNDGREN and SVANVIK 1973; GRANGER et al. 1980). Also β-adrenergic agents dilate primarily villous blood vessels (BIBER et al. 1973).

Maintenance of subepithelial blood flow when arterial blood pressure decreases may preserve intestinal absorption, despite a decreased total intestinal blood flow. Indeed, GRANGER et al. (1980) showed that net absorptive water transport in canine colon was unchanged when mean arterial blood pressure was reduced from 115 to 15 mmHg, although the unidirectional water fluxes were significantly decreased. Adenosine is a possible mediator of the metabolic regulation of mucosal vascular resistance, since this nucleoside was found to increase absorptive site and total intestinal blood flow and did not significantly change net water absorption, although both the unidirectional absorptive and secretory water fluxes were markedly increased. This result is not in contrast to those of WINNE (1966, 1972) and DOBSON (1979), who reported that the absorption of tritiated water is enhanced by an increase in blood flow (see Sect. D.I), because these authors do not claim that net water absorption depends similarly on blood flow. As a matter of fact, WINNE (1966), although he did not monitor the effect of mucosal blood flow on net water absorption, states that there is evidence that the secretory flux of tritiated water is blood flow dependent, just like the absorptive flux of tritiated water. This finding is in total agreement with the results of GRANGER et al. (1980). The important point of the studies of LUNDGREN and SVANVIK (1973) and of GRANGER et al. (1980) is that autoregulation of subepithelial blood flow appears to be associated with autoregulation of intestinal absorption.

G. Conclusion

The resolution of the mechanism of intestinal water permeation is dominated by the fact that water is the main solvent in living systems. Water deviates from other nonelectrolytes in that its rate of diffusion across epithelia and cell membranes is higher than predicted by its lipid solubility. This phenomenon indicates permeation of the small water molecule (molecular diameter 1.5Å) across water-filled pores or channels. The presence of water-filled channels in intestinal epithelia is also apparent from the fact that the osmotic water permeability exceeds the diffusional water permeability. The quantitative importance of water permeation across the lipid phase of epithelial cell membranes is unclear.

Although water transport is the main task of the intestine in quantitative terms, the picture we have of water absorption is less clear than that of most solutes. Obviously, the structure of the intestinal epithelium plays a dominant role in water absorption. Water transport was unequivocally shown to be secondary to active solute transport, hence the pharmacology of intestinal water transport is the pharmacology of active solute transport, either in the absorptive or secretory direction. The effects of bacterial toxins, hormones, laxatives, or secretagogue drugs on intestinal salt and water transport are dealt with in other chapters of this handbook. Additionally, the extent and direction of net intestinal water movement is dependent on the Starling forces which regulate capillary fluid exchange.

The concept that the coupling of solute and water transport is due to local osmosis, i.e., that a region within the epithelium is made hypertonic by active solute transport and water follows passively, has been substantiated in the last few years by direct and indirect evidence showing that indeed such hypertonic compartments exist in epithelia. However, more direct experimental confirmation is needed to render the local osmosis theories quantitatively tenable. We need to take a new close look at epithelia to find out what the transepithelial route of water transport is, morphometric data may tell us more about the structure and dimensions of the channels involved in water absorption. An interesting proposition in this regard was made by MØLLGARD and ROSTGAARD (1978, 1981) who described a transcellular tubular transport system in epithelial cells capable of isotonic fluid transport. Elements of a variety of the agranular endoplasmic reticulum were found to be abundant in the narror 1 µm wide band of peripheral cytoplasm which was implicated by GUPTA et al. (1978) to be involved in fast transcellular fluxes of solutes and water. Certainly, the statement of HÖBER made in his review on the physiology of intestinal absorption in 1907 is as true today as it was then: "As things stand right now, one has to be inclined to consider the absorptive process to be even more complicated than it already seems."

References

Altamirano M, Martinoya C (1966) The permeability of gastric mucosa of dogs. J Physiol (Lond) 184:771–790

Andreoli TE, Monahan M (1968) The interaction of polyene antibiotics with thin lipid membranes. J Gen Physiol 52:300–325

Andreoli TE, Schafer JA (1976) Mass transport across cell membranes: The effect of antidiuretic hormone on water and solute flows in epithelia. Annu Rev Physiol 38:451–500

Andreoli TE, Schafer JA (1979) External solution driving forces for isotonic fluid absorption in proximal tubules. Fed Proc 38:154–160

Andreoli TE, Troutman SC (1971) An analysis of unstirred layers in series with "tight" and "porous" lipid bilayer membranes. J Gen Physiol 57:464–478

Andreoli TE, Schafer JA, Troutman SL (1971) Coupling of solute and solvent flows in porous lipid bilayer membranes. J Gen Physiol 57:479–493

Andreoli TE, Schafer JA, Troutman SL, Watkins ML (1979) Solvent drag component of Cl^- flux in superficial proximal straight tubules: evidence for a paracellular component of isotonic fluid absorption. Am J Physiol 237:F455–F462

Barry PH, Hope AB (1969a) Electroosmosis in membranes: effects of unstirred layers and transport numbers. I. Theory. Biophys J 9:700–728

Barry PH, Hope AB (1969b) Electroosmosis in membranes: effects of unstirred layers and transport numbers. II. Experimental. Biophys J 9:729–757

Barry RJC, Smyth DH, Wright EM (1965) Short-circuit current and solute transfer by rat jejunum. J Physiol (Lond) 181:410–431

Barry PH, Diamond JM, Wright EM (1971) The mechanism of cation permeation in rabbit gallbladder. Dilution potentials and biionic potentials. J Membr Biol 4:358–394

Barton TC, Brown DAJ (1964) Water permeability of the fetal erythrocyte. J Gen Physiol 47:839–849

Bentley PJ (1961) Directional differences in the permeability to water of the isolated urinary bladder of the toad, Bufo marinus. J Endocrinol 22:95–100

Bentzel CJ, Davies M, Scott WN, Zatzman M, Solomon AK (1968) Osmotic volume flow in the proximal tubule of Necturus kidney. J Gen Physiol 51;517–533

Bentzel CJ, Parsa B, Hare DK (1969) Osmotic flow across proximal tubule of Necturus: correlation of physiological and anatomical studies. Am J Physiol 217:570–580

Berger EY, Pecikyan R, Kanzaki G (1970) Water flux across the rat jejunum and ileum. J Appl Physiol 29:130–132

Berry CA, Boulpaep EL (1975) Nonelectrolyte permeability of the paracellular pathway in Necturus proximal tubule. Am J Physiol 228:581–595

Biber B, Lundgren O, Svanvik J (1973) Intramural blood flow and blood volume in the small intestine of the cat as analyzed by an indicator dilution technique. Acta Physiol Scand 87:391–403

Bihler I, Crane RK (1962) Studies on the mechanism of intestinal absorption of sugars. V. The influence of several cations and anions on the active transport of sugars, in vitro, by various preparations of hamster small intestine. Biochim Biophys Acta 59:78–93

Bindslev N, Skadhauge E (1971) Salt and water permeability of the epithelium of the coprodeum and large intestine in the normal and the dehydrated fowl (Gallus domesticus). In vivo perfusion studies. J Physiol (Lond) 216:735–751

Bindslev N (1981) Water and NaCl transport in the hen lower intestine during dehydration. In: Ussing HH, Bindslev N, Lassen NA, Sten-Knudsen O (eds) Water transport across epithelia. Alfred Benzon symposium 15. Munksgaard, Copenhagen, pp 468–481

Bindslev N, Tormey JMcD, Pietras RJ, Wright EM (1974) Electrically and osmotically induced changes in permeability and structure of toad urinary bladder. Biochim Biophys Acta 332:286–297

Blom H, Helander HF (1977) Quantitative electron microscopical studies on in vitro incubated rabbit gallbladder epithelium. J Membr Biol 37:45–61

Bowling DJF (1969) Evidence for the electroosmosic theory of transport in the phloem. Biochim Biophys Acta 183:230–232

Brahm J (1982) Diffusional water permeability of human erythrocytes and their ghosts. J Gen Physiol 79:791–819

Brodsky WA, Schilb TP (1965) Osmotic properties of isolated turtle bladder. Am J Physiol 208:46–57

Brücke E (1874) Vorlesungen über Physiologie. Braumüller, Wien

Carpi-Medina P, Gonzales E, Whittembury G (1983) Cell osmotic water permeability of isolated rabbit convoluted tubules. Am J Physiol 244:F554–F563

Cass A, Finkelstein A (1967) Water permeability of thin lipid membranes. J Gen Physiol 50:1765–1784

Cass A, Finkelstein A, Krespi U (1970) The ion permeability induced in thin lipid membranes by the polyene antibiotics nystatin and amphotericin B. J Gen Physiol 56:100–124

Chalfin D, Cooperstein IL, Hogben AM (1958) Fluid and electrolyte movement across intestinal wall of bullfrog. Proc Soc Exp Biol Med 99:746–748

Clarkson TW, Rothstein A (1960) Transport of monovalent ions by the isolated small intestine of the rat. Am J Physiol 199:898–906

Cohnheim O (1898) Über Dünndarmresorption. Z Biol 36:129–153

Cohnheim O (1899) Über die Resorption im Dünndarm und der Bauchhöhle. Z Biol 37:443–482

Collander R, Bärlund H (1933) Permeabilitätsstudien an Chara cerata phylla. II. Die Permeabilität für Nichtelektrolyte. Acta Bot Fenn 11:1–114

Conlon T, Outhred R (1978) The temperature dependence of the erythrocyte water diffusion permeability. Biochim Biophys Acta 511:408–418

Conway BE (1952) Electrochemical data. Elsevier, Amsterdam

Corbett CL, Isaacs PET, Riley AK, Turnberg LA (1977) Human intestinal ion transport in vitro. Gut 18:136–140

Curci S, Frömter E (1979) Micropuncture of lateral intercellular spaces of Necturus gallbladder to dertermine space fluid K^+ concentration. Nature 278:355–357

Curran PF (1960) Na, Cl, and water transport by rat ileum in vitro. J Gen Physiol 43:1137–1148

Curran PF, MacIntosh JR (1962) A model system for biological water transport. Nature 193:347–348

Curran PF, Schwartz GF (1960) Na, Cl, and water transport by rat colon. J Gen Physiol 43:255–268

Curran PF, Solomon AK (1957) Ion and water fluxes in the ileum of rats. J Gen Physiol 41:143–168

Dainty J (1963) Water relations of plant cells. Adv Bot Res 1:279–326

Dainty J, House CR (1966a) Unstirred layers in frog skin. J Physiol (Lond) 182:66–78

Dainty J, House CR (1966b) An examination of the evidence for membrane pores in frog skin. J Physiol (Lond) 185:172–184

Debongnie JC, Phillips SF (1978) Capacity of the human colon to absorb fluid. Gastroenterology 74:694–703

Degani H, Avron M (1982) The diffusional water permeability in the halotherant alga *Dunaliella* as measured by nuclear magnetic resonance. Biochim Biophys Acta 690:174–177

Denhardt R (1976) Effect of ADH on intestinal electrolyte and water absorption. In: Robinson JWL (ed) Intestinal ion transport. MTP Press, Lancaster, pp 183–186

Diamond JM (1962a) The reabsorptive function of the gallbladder. J Physiol (Lond) 161:442–473

Diamond JM (1962b) The mechanism of solute transport by the gallbladder. J Physiol (Lond) 161:474–502
Diamond JM (1962c) The mechanism of water transport by the gallbladder. J Physiol (Lond) 161:503–527
Diamond JM (1964a) Transport of salt and water in rabbit and guinea pig gallbladder. J Gen Physiol 48:1–14
Diamond JM (1964b) The mechanism of isotonic water transport. J Gen Physiol 48:15–42
Diamond JM (1966a) Non-linear osmosis. J Physiol (Lond) 183:58–82
Diamond JM (1966b) A rapid method for determination voltage – concentration relations across membranes. J Physiol (Lond) 183:83–100
Diamond JM (1978) Solute-linked water transport in epithelia. In: Hoffman JF (ed) Membrane transport processes. Raven, New York, pp 257–276
Diamond JM (1979) Osmotic water flow in leaky epithelia. J Membr Biol 51:195–216
Diamond JM, Bossert WH (1967) Standing – gradient osmotic flow. A mechanism for coupling of water and solute transport in epithelia. J Gen Physiol 50:2061–2083
Diamond JM, Szabo G, Katz Y (1974) Theory of nonelectrolyte permeation in a generalized membrane. J Membr Biol 17:148–152
Dibona DR, Civan MM (1973) Pathways for movement of ions and water across toad urinary bladder. I. Anatomical site of transepithelial shunt pathways. J Membr Biol 12:101–128
Dibona DR, Mills JM (1979) Distribution of Na^+ pump sites in transporting epithelia. Fed Proc 38:134–143
Dibona DR, Civan MM, Leaf A (1969) The cellular specificity of the effect of vasopressin on toad urinary bladder. J Membr Biol 1:79–91
Dick DA (1964) The permeability coefficient of water in the cell membrane and the diffusion coefficient in the cell interior. J Theor Biol 7:504–531
Dietschy JM (1964) Water and solute movement acros the wall of the everted rabbit gallbladder. Gastroenterology 47:395–408
Dobson A (1979) The choice of models relating tritiated water absorption to subepithelial blood flow in the rumen of the sheep. J Physiol (Lond) 297:111–121
Dörge A, Rick R, Katz U, Thurau K (1981) Determination of intracellular electrolyte concentrations in amphibian epithelia with the use of electron microprobe analysis. In: Ussing HH, Bindslev N, Lassen NA, Sten-Knudsen O (eds) Water transport across epithelia, Alfred Benzon Symposium 15. Munksgaard, Copenhagen, pp 36–46
Duffy PA, Granger DN, Taylor AE (1978) Intestinal secretion induced by volume expansion in the dog. Gastroenterology 75:413–418
Durand J, Durand-Arczynska W, Haab P (1981) Volume flow, hydraulic conductivity and electrical properties across bovine tracheal epithelium: effect of histamin. Pflügers Arch 392:40–45
Durbin RP (1960) Osmotic flow of water across permeable cellulose membranes. J Gen Physiol 44:315–326
Durbin RP, Helander HF (1978) Distribution of osmotic flow in stomach and gallbladder. Biochim Biophys Acta 513:179–181
Durbin RP, Frank H, Solomon AK (1956) Water flow through frog skin mucosa. J Gen Physiol 39:535–551
Edelman IS, Leibman J (1959) Anatomy of body water and electrolytes. Am J Med 27:256–277
Erlij D, Martinez-Palomo A (1977) Opening of tight junctions in frog skin by hypertonic solutions. J Membr Biol 9:229–240
Fabry ME, Eisenstadt M (1978) Water exchange across red cell membranes: II. Measurement by nuclear magnetic resonance T_1, T_2, and T_{12} hybrid relaxation. The effects of osmolarity, cell volume, and medium. J Membr Biol 42:375–398
Fenichel IR, Horowitz SB (1963) The transport of non-electrolytes in muscle as a diffusional process in cytoplasm. Acta Physiol Scand 60 (Suppl 221):1–63
Finkelstein A (1976) Water and nonelectrolyte permeability of lipid bilayer membranes. J Gen Physiol 68:127–135

Finkelstein A, Cass A (1967) Effect of cholesterol on the water permeability of thin lipid membranes. Nature 216:717–718

Finkelstein A, Cass A (1968) Permeability and electrical properties of thin lipid membranes. J Gen Physiol 52:145s–171s

Fischbarg J (1978) Pathways for water permeation across epithelia. In: Bourguet J, Chevalier J, Parisi M, Ripoche P (eds) Contrôle hormonal des transports epitheliaux, INSERM, vol 85. INSERM, Paris, pp 323–334

Fischbarg J, Warshavsky CR, Lim JJ (1977) Pathways for hydraulically and osmotically – induced water flow across epithelia. Nature 266:71–74

Fisher RB (1954) The absorption of water and some non-electrolytes from the surviving small intestine of the rat. J Physiol (Lond) 124:21P–22P

Fisher RB (1965) The absorption of water and some small solute molecules from the isolated small intestine of the rat. J Physiol (Lond) 130:655–664

Fisher RB, Parsons DS (1950) The gradient of mucosal surface area in the small intestine of the rat. J Anat 84:272–282

Fitzsimons JT (1979) The physiology of thirst and sodium appetite. Cambridge University Press, Cambridge

Fordtran JS, Levitan R, Bikerman V, Burrows BA, Ingelfinger FJ (1961) The kinetics of water absorption in the human intestine. Trans Assoc Am Physicians 74:195–205

Fordtran JS, Rector FC Jr, Ewton MF, Soter N, Kinney J (1965) Permeability characteristics of the human small intestine. J Clin Invest 44:1935–1944

Fordtran JS, Rector FC, Carter NW (1968) The mechanism of sodium absorption in the human small intestine. J Clin Invest 47:884–900

Frank HS, Wen WY (1957) Structural aspects of ion – solvent interaction in aqueous solutions; a suggested picture of water structure. Discuss Faraday Soc 24:133–140

Franz TJ, Van Bruggen TJ (1967) Hyperosmolarity and net transport of non-electrolytes in frog skin. J Gen Physiol 50:933–949

Frederikson O, Møllgård K, Rostgaard J (1979) Lack of correlation between transepithelial transport capacity and paracellular pathway ultrastructure in Alcian blue-treated rabbit gallbladders. J Cell Biol 83:383–393

Frizzell RA, Schultz SG (1972) Ionic conductance of the extracellular shunt pathway in rabbit ileum: Influence of the shunt on transmural sodium transport and electrical potential difference. J Gen Physiol 59:318–346

Frizzell RA, Schultz SG (1979) Models of electrolyte absorption and secretion by gastrointestinal epithelia. In: Crane RK (ed) International review of physiology, vol 19, gastrointestinal physiology III. University Park Press, Baltimore, pp 205–225

Frizzell RA, Turnheim K (1978) Ion transport by rabbit colon. II. Unidirectional sodium influx and the effects of amphotericin B and amiloride. J Membr Biol 40:193–211

Frizzell RA, Koch MJ, Schultz SG (1976) Ion transport by rabbit colon. I. Active and passive components. J Membr Biol 27:297–316

Frömter E (1972) The route of passive ion movement through the epithelium of Necturus gallbladder. J Membr Biol 8:259–301

Frömter E (1974) Electrophysiology and isotonic fluid absorption of proximal tubules of mammalian kidney. In: Thurau K (ed) Kidney and urinary tract physiology. MTP International Review of Science, Physiology, Ser 1, vol 6. Butterworth, London; University Park Press, Baltimore, pp 1–36

Frömter E, Diamond JM (1972) Route of passive ion permeation in epithelia. Nature, New Biology 235:9–11

Frömter E, Lüer K (1969) Konzentration und isoelektrischer Punkt der Festladungen im proximalen Konvolut der Ratenniere. Pflügers Arch 307:R76

Garby L, Linderholm H (1953) The permeability of frog skin to heavy water and to ions, with special reference to the effect of some diuretics. Acta Physiol Scand 28:336–346

Ginzburg BZ, Katchalsky A (1963) The frictional coefficients of the flows of non-electrolytes through artificial membranes. J Gen Physiol 47:403–418

Glaser R (1976) Einführung in die Biophysik. Gustav Fischer, Jena

Goldschmidt S (1921) On the mechanism of absorption from the intestine. Physiol Rev 1:421–453

Goldstein A, Solomon AK (1961) Determination of equivalent pore radius for human red cells by osmotic pressure measurement. J Gen Physiol 44:1–17
Gonzales E, Carpi-Medina P, Whittembury G (1982) Cell osmotic water permeability of isolated rabbit proximal straight tubules. Am J Physiol 242:F321–F330
Granger DN, Kvietys PR (1981) The splanchnic circulation: intrinsic regulation. Annu Rev Physiol 43:409–418
Granger DN, Taylor AE (1978) Effects of solute-coupled transport on lymph flow and oncotic pressures in cat ileum. Am J Physiol 235:E429–E436
Granger DN, Taylor AE (1980) Permeability of intestinal capillaries to endogeneous macromolecules. Am J Physiol 238:H457–H464
Granger DN, Granger JP, Brace RA, Parker RE, Taylor AE (1979) Analysis of the permeability characteristics of cat intestinal capillaries. Circ Res 44:335–344
Granger DN, Kvietys PR, Mailman D, Richardson PDI (1980) Intrinsic regulation of functional blood flow and water absorption in canine colon. J Physiol (Lond) 307:443–451
Granger DN, Mortillaro NA, Kvietys PR, Rutili G, Parker JC, Taylor AE (1980) Role of the interstitial matrix during intestinal volume absorption. Am J Physiol 238:G138–G189
Grantham JJ, Ganote CE, Burg MB, Orloff J (1969) Path of transtubular water flow in isolated renal collecting tubules. J Cell Biol 41:562–576
Green K, Matty AJ (1966) Effects of vasopressin on ion transport across intestinal epithelia. Life Sci 5:205–209
Grim E (1962) Water and electrolyte flux rates in the duodenum, jejunum, ileum, and colon, and effects of osmolarity. Am J Dig Dis 7:17–27
Gumilewski D (1886) Über Resorption im Dünndarm. Pflügers Arch 39:556–592
Gupta BL, Hall TA (1979) Quantitative electrone probe X-ray microanalysis of electrolyte elements within epithelial tissue compartments. Fed Proc 38:144–153
Gupta BL, Hall TA (1981) Microprobe analysis of fluid-transporting epithelia: evidence for local osmosis and solute recycling. In: Ussing HH, Bindslev N, Lassen NA, Sten-Knudsen O (eds) Water transport across epithelia, Alfred Benzon Symposium 15. Munksgaard, Copenhagen, pp 17–31
Gupta B, Hall TA, Naftalin RJ (1978) Microprobe measurement of Na, K, and Cl concentration profiles in epithelial cells and intercellular spaces of rabbit ileum. Nature 272:70–73
Hakim AA, Lifson N (1969) Effects of pressure on water and solute transport by dog intestinal mucosa in vitro. Am J Physiol 216:276–284
Hakim AA, Papeleux CB, Jane JB, Lifson N, Yablonski ME (1977) Mechanism of production of intestinal secretion by negative luminal pressure. Am J Physiol 233:E416–E421
Haljamäe H, Jodal M, Lundgren O (1973) Countercurrent multiplication of sodium in intestinal villi during absorption of sodium chloride. Acta Physiol Scand 89:580–593
Hallbäck DA, Hultén L, Jodal M, Lindhagen J, Lundgren O (1978) Evidence for the existence of a countercurrent exchanger in the small intestine in man. Gastroenterology 74:683–690
Hallbäck DA, Jodal M, Lundgren O (1979a) Importance of sodium and glucose for the establishment of a villus tissue hyperosmolality by the intestinal countercurrent multiplier. Acta Physiol Scand 107:89–96
Hallbäck DA, Jodal M, Sjöquist A, Lundgren O (1979b) Villus tissue osmolality and intestinal transport of water and electrolytes. Acta Physiol Scand 107:115–126
Hallbäck DA, Jodal M, Lundgren O (1980) Villous tissue osmolality, water and electrolyte transport in the cat small intestine at varying luminal osmolalities. Acta Physiol Scand 110:95–100
Hammersen S (1971) Anatomie der terminalen Strombahn. Urban and Schwarzenberg, München
Hanai T, Haydon DA (1966) The permeability of water of bimolecular lipid membranes. J Theor Biol 11:370–382
Hansson-Mild K, Carlson L, Løvtrup S (1974) The identity of filtration and diffusion permeability coefficients in frog egg membrane. J Membr Biol 19:221–228

Hays RM, Franki N (1970) The role of water diffusion in the action of vasopressin. J Membr Biol 2:263–276

Hays RM, Leaf A (1962) Studies on the movement of water through the isolated toad bladder and its modification by vasopressin. J Gen Physiol 45:905–919

Hayward AF (1962) Aspects of the fine structure of the gallbladder epithelium of the mouse. J Anat 96:227–236

Hebert SC, Andreoli TE (1982) Water permeability of biological membranes. Lessons from antidiuretic hormone-responsive epithelia. Biochim Biophys Acta 650:267–280

Heidenhain R (1888) Beiträge zur Histologie und Physiologie der Dünndarmschleimhaut. Pflügers Arch Ges Physiol 43 (Suppl) 1–103

Heidenhain R (1894) Neue Versuche über die Aufsaugung im Dünndarm. Pflügers Arch Ges Physiol 56:579–631

Heintze K, Petersen KU, Busch L (1978) Effects of hydrostatic pressure on fluid transfer by the isolated gallbladder. Pflügers Arch 373:9–13

Heinz E (1978) Mechanics and energetics of biological transport. Springer, Berlin Heidelberg New York

Heller H, Smirk FH (1932) Studies concerning the alimentary absorption of water and tissue hydration in relation to diuresis. J Physiol (Lond) 76:283–292

Hevesy GV, Hofer E, Krogh A (1935) The permeability of the skin of frogs to water as determined by D_2O and H_2O. Scand Arch Physiol 72:199–214

Hill AE (1975a) Solute – solvent coupling in epithelia: a critical examination of the standing gradient osmotic flow theory. Proc R Soc Lond [Biol] 190:99–114

Hill AE (1975b) Solute – solvent coupling in epithelia: an electroosmotic theory of fluid transfer. Proc R Soc Lond [Biol] 190:115–134

Hill A (1980) Salt – water coupling in leaky epithelia. J Membr Biol 56:177–182

Hill BS, Hill AE (1978a) Fluid transfer by Necturus gall bladder epithelium as a function of osmolarity. Proc R Soc Lond [Biol] 200:151–162

Hill AE, Hill BS (1978b) Sucrose fluxes and junctional water flow across Necturus gall bladder epithelium. Proc R Soc Lond [Biol] 200:163–174

Höber R (1907) Die physikalische Chemie in der Physiologie der Resorption, der Lymphbildung und der Sekretion. In: Korányi A, Richter PF (Hrsg) Physikalische Chemie und Medizin, vol I. Thieme, Leipzig, pp 294–419

Höber R, Höber J (1937) Experiments on the absorption of organic solutes in the small intestine of rats. J Cell Comp Physiol 10:401–422

Hodgkin AL, Keynes RD (1955) The potassium permeability of a giant nerve fibre. J Physiol (Lond) 128:61–88

Hogben CAM, Tocco DJ, Brodie BB, Schanker LS (1959) On the mechanism of intestinal absorption of drugs. J Pharmacol Exp Ther 125:275–282

Holz R, Finkelstein A (1970) The water and nonelectrolyte permeability induced in thin lipid membranes by the polyene antibiotics nystatin and amphotericin B. J Gen Physiol 56:125–145

House CR (1965) Rectification of water flow across frog skin. Biophys J 5:987–988

House CR (1974) Water transport in cells and tissues. Arnold, London

Ingraham RC, Visscher MB (1938) Further studies on intestinal absorption with the performance of osmotic work. Am J Physiol 121:771–785

Jard S, Bourquet J, Favard P (1971) The role of the intercellular channel in the transepithelial transfer of water and sodium in the frog urinary bladder. J Membr Biol 4:124–147

Jodal M, Hallbäck DA, Lundgren O (1978) Tissue osmolality in intestinal villi during luminal perfusion with isotonic electrolyte solutions. Acta Physiol Scand 102:94–107

Johnson FR, McMinn RMH, Birchenough RF (1962) The ultrastructure of the gallbladder epithelium of the dog. J Anat 96:477–487

Katchalsky A, Curran PF (1965) Nonequilibrium thermodynamics in biophysics, 1st edn. Harvard University Press, Cambridge

Kaye GI, Wheeler HO, Whitlock RT, Lane N (1966) Fluid transport in the rabbit gallbladder. A combined physiological and electron microscopic study. J Cell Biol 30:237–268

Kedem O, Caplan SR (1965) Degree of coupling and its relation to efficiency of energy conversion. Trans Farad Soc 61:1897–1911

Kedem O, Katchalsky A (1958) Thermodynamic analysis of the permeability of biological membranes to non-electrolytes. Biochim Biophys Acta 27:229–246

Kedem O, Katchalsky A (1961) A physical interpretation of the phenomenologic coefficients of membrane permeability. J Gen Physiol 45:143–179

Kedem O, Katchalsky A (1963) Permeability of composite membranes, part 1. Electric current, volume flows and flow of solute through membranes. Trans Farad Soc 59:1918–1930

King-Hele JA, Paulson RW (1977) On the influence of a leaky tight junction on water and solute transport in epithelia. J Theor Biol 67:61–84

Klyce SD, Russel SR (1979) Numerical solution of coupled transport equations applied to corneal hydration dynamics. J Physiol (Lond) 292:107–134

Klyce SD, Russel SR (1980) The viscious flow therory: an adjunct to the standing gradient hypothesis. Fed Proc 39:378

Koefoed-Johnson V, Ussing HH (1953) The contribution of diffusion and flow to the passage of D_2O through living membranes. Effect of neurohypophyseal hormone on isolated anuran skin. Acta Physiol Scand 20:60–76

Kokko JP (1978) Countercurrent exchanger in the small intestine of man: is there evidence for its existence? Gastroenterology 74:791–792

Kokko JP, Burg MB, Orloff J (1971) Characteristics of NaCl and water transport in the renal proximal tubule. J Clin Invest 50:69–76

Kutchai H, Cooper RA, Forster RE (1980) Erythrocyte water permeability. The effects of anesthetic alcohols and alterations in the level of membrane cholesterol. Biochim Biophys Acta 600:542–552

Kyte J (1976) Immunoferritin determination of $(Na^+$-$K^+)$ATPase over the plasma membranes of renal convoluted tubules. II. Proximal segment. J Cell Biol 68:304–318

Lakshminarayanaiah N (1969) Transport phenomena in membranes. Academic, New York

Landis EN (1927) Microinjection studies of capillary permeability. The relation between capillary pressure and the rate at which fluid passes through the walls of single capillaries. Am J Physiol 82:217–238

Lauterbach F (1977) Passive permeabilities of luminal and basolatral membranes in the isolated mucosal epithelium of guinea pig small intestine. Naunyn-Schmiedeberg's Arch Pharmacol 297:201–212

Leaf A (1959) The mechanism of the asymmetrical distribution of endogeneous lactate about the isolated toad bladder. J Cell Comp Physiol 54:103–108

Lee JS (1968) Isoosmotic absorption of fluid from rat jejunum in vitro. Gastroenterology 54:366–374

Lee LS (1969) A micropuncture study of water transport by dog jejunal villi in vitro. Am J Physiol 217:1528–1533

Lee JS (1973) Effects of pressures on water absorption and secretion in rat jejunum. Am J Physiol 224:1338–1344

Lee JS (1974) Glucose concentration and hydrostatic pressure in dog jejunal villus lymph. Am J Physiol 226:675–681

Lee JS (1981) Lymph flow during fluid absorption from rat jejunum. Am J Physiol 240:G312–G316

Lembeck F, Sewing KF, Winne D (1964) Der Einfluß von 5-Hydroxytryptamin auf die Resorption von Tritium-Wasser (HTO) aus dem Dünndarm der Ratte. Naunyn-Schmiedeberg's Arch Pharmacol 247:100–109

Lichtenstein NS, Leaf A (1965) Effect of amphotericin B on the permeability of the toad bladder. J Clin Invest 44:1328–1342

Lichtenstein NS, Leaf A (1966) Evidence for a double series permeability barrier at the mucosal surface of the toad bladder. Ann NY Acad Sci 137:556–565

Lifson N (1979) Fluid secretion and hydrostatic pressure relationships in the small intestine. In: Binder HJ (ed) Mechanisms of intestinal secretion. Riss, New York, pp 249–261

Lindemann B, Solomon AK (1962) Permeability of the luminal surface of intestinal mucosal cells. J Gen Physiol 45:801–810

Lindley BD, Hoshiko T, Leb DE (1964) Effect of D_2O and osmotic gradients on potential and resistance of the isolated frog skin. J Gen Physiol 47:774–793

Lippe C, Bianchi A, Cremaschi D, Capraro V (1965) Different types of asymmetric distribution of hydrosoluble and liposoluble substances at the two sides of a mucosal intestinal preparation. Arch Int Physiol Biochem 73:43–54

Lipschitz-Farber C, Degani H (1980) Kinetics of water diffusion across phospholipid membranes. ^{1}H- and ^{17}O-NMR relaxation studies. Biochim Biophys Acta 600:291–300

Loehry CA, Axon ATR, Hilton PJ, Hider RC, Creamer B (1970) Permeability of the small intestine to substances of different molecular weight. Gut 11:466–470

Loeschke K, Bentzel CJ, Csáky TZ (1970) Asymmetry of osmotic flow in frog intestine: functional and structural correlation. Am J Physiol 218:1723–1731

Love AHG, Mitchell TG, Phillips RA (1968) Water and sodium absorption in the human intestine. J Physiol (Lond) 195:133–140

Lückhoff A, Horster M (1981) Hydraulic permeability coefficient and sodium steady-state luminal concentration of the in vivo perfused rat distal colon. Pflügers Arch 391:301–305

Lundgren O (1974) The circulation of the small bowel mucosa. Gut 15:1005–1013

Lundgren O, Svanvik J (1973) Mucosal hemodynamics in the small intestine of the cat during reduced perfusion pressure. Acta Physiol Scand 88:551–563

Machen TE, Diamond JM (1969) An estimate of the salt concentration in the lateral intercellular spaces of rabbit gallbladder during maximal fluid transport. J Membr Biol 1:194–213

MacRobbie EAC, Ussing HH (1961) Osmotic behaviour of the epithelial cells of frog skin. Acta Physiol Scand 53:348–365

Mailman D (1980) Effects of morphine on canine intestinal absorption and blood flow. Br J Pharmacol 68:617–624

Makhlouf M (1972) Osmotic volume flow in isolated frog gastric mucosa. Fed Proc 31:827

Maude DL, Shehadeh I, Solomon AK (1966) Sodium and water transport in single perfused distal tubules of Necturus kidney. Am J Physiol 211:1043–1049

Mauro A (1957) Nature of solvent transfer in osmosis. Science 126:252–253

McHardy GJR, Parsons DS (1957) The absorption of water and salt from the small intestine of the rat. Q J Exp Physiol 42:33–48

Meschia G, Setnikar I (1958) Experimental study of osmosis through a collodion membrane. J Gen Physiol 42:429–444

Michel CC (1980) Filtration coefficients and osmotic reflexion coefficients of the walls of single frog mesenteric capillaries. J Physiol (Lond) 309:341–355

Miller DL, Hamburger SA, Schedl HP (1979) Effects of osmotic gradients on water and solute transport: in vivo studies in rat duodenum and ileum. Am J Physiol 237:E389–E396

Mills JW, Dibona DR (1978) Distribution of Na^+ pump sites in the frog gallbladder. Nature 271:273–275

Mlekoday HJ, Moore R, Levitt D (1983) Osmotic water permeability of the human red cell. Dependence of direction of water flow and cell volume. J Gen Physiol 81:213–220

Møllgård K, Rostgaard J (1978) Morphological aspects of some sodium transporting epithelia suggesting a transcellular pathway via elements of endoplasmic reticulum. J Membrane Biol 40, special issue: 71–89

Møllgård K, Rostgaard J (1980) The possible role of the endoplasmic reticulum in transepithelial ion transport. J Gen Physiol 76:7a–8a

Møllgård K, Rostgaard J (1981) Morphological aspects of transepithelial transport with special reference to the endoplasmic reticulum. In: Schultz SG (ed) Ion transport by epithelia. Raven Press, New York, pp 209–231

Moody FG, Durbin RP (1969) Water flow induced by osmotic nd hydrostatic pressure in the stomach. Am J Physiol 217:255–261

Moreno JH (1975) Routes of non-electrolyte permeability in gallbladders. Effects of 2,4,6-triaminopyrimidinium (TAP). J Gen Physiol 66:117–128

Mortillaro NA, Taylor AE (1976) Interaction of capillary and tissue forces in the cat small intestine. Circ Res 39:348–358

Munck BG, Rasmussen SN (1977) Paracellular permeability of extracellular space markers across rat jejunum in vitro. Indication of a transepithelial fluid circuit. J Physiol (Lond) 271:473–488

Norman AW, Spielvogel AM, Wong RG (1976) Polyene antibiotic – sterol interaction. Adv Lipid Res 14:127–170

Norman DA, Atkins JM, Seelig LL Jr, Gomez-Sanchez C, Krejs GJ (1980) Water and electrolyte movement and mucosal morphology in the jejunum of patients with portal hypertension. Gastroenterology 79:707–715

Öbrink KJ (1956) Water permeability of the isolated stomach of the mouse. Acta Physiol Scand 36:229–244

Ochsenfahrt H, Winne D (1969) Der Einfluß der Durchblutung auf die Resorption von Arzneimittel aus dem Jejunum der Ratte. Naunyn-Schmiedeberg's Arch Pharmacol 264:55–75

Overton E (1902) Beiträge zur allgemeinen Muskel- und Nervenphysiologie. Pflügers Arch Ges Physiol 92:115–280

Paganelli CV, Solomon AK (1957) The rate of exchange of tritiated water across the human red cell membrane. J Gen Physiol 41:259–277

Pappenheimer JR, Soto-Rivera A (1948) Effective osmotic pressure of the plasma proteins and other quantities associated with the capillary circulation in the hindlimbs of cats and dogs. Am J Physiol 152:471–491

Pappenheimer JR, Renkin EM, Borrero LM (1951) Filtration, diffusion and molecular sieving through peripheral capillary membranes. A contribution to the pore theory of capillary permeability. Am J Physiol 167:13–46

Parisi M, Candia O, Alvarez L (1980) Water permeability of the toad corneal epithelium: The effect of pH and amphotericin B. Pflügers Arch 383:131–136

Parsons DS (1963) Quantitative aspects of pinocytosis in relation to intestinal absorption. Nature 199:1192–1193

Parsons DS (1968) Methods for the investigation of intestinal absorption. In: Handbook of Physiology, Sect 6, vol III. American Physiological Society, Washington DC, chap 64

Parsons DS, Wingate DL (1961) The effect of osmotic gradients on fluid transfer across rat intestine in vitro. Biochim Biophys Acta 46:170–183

Patlak CS, Goldstein DA, Hoffman JF (1963) The flow of solute and solvent across a two-membrane system. J Theor Biol 5:426–442

Pedley TJ, Fischbarg J (1978) The development of osmotic flow through an unstirred layer. J Theor Biol 70:427–447

Pedley TJ, Fischbarg J (1980) Unstirred layer effects on osmotic water flow across gallbladder epithelium. J Membr Biol 54:89–102

Persson E (1970) Water permeability in rat distal tubules. Acta Physiol Scand 78:364–375

Persson E, Ulfendahl HR (1970) Water permeability in rat proximal tubules. Acta Physiol Scand 78:353–363

Persson B-O, Spring KR (1982) Gallbladder epithelial cell hydraulic water permeability and volume regulation. J Gen Physiol 79:481–505

Peters G (1980) Mécanismes de rélage de l'ingestion d'eau. J Physiol (Paris) 76:295–322

Petersen DC (1980) Water permeability through the lipid bilayer membrane. Test of the liquid hydrocarbon model. Biochim Biophys Acta 600:666–677

Phelps CF (1965) The physical properties of inulin solutions. Biochem J 95:41–47

Pietras RJ, Wright EM (1975) The membrane action of antidiuretic hormone (ADH) on toad urinary bladder. J Membr Biol 22:107–123

Polefka TG, Redwood WR, Garrick RA, Chinard FP (1981 a) Permeability of Novikoff hepatoma cells to water and monohydric alcohols. Biochim Biophys Acta 642:67–78

Polefka TG, Garrick RA, Redwood WR (1981 b) Osmotic permeability of Novikoff hepatoma cells. Biochim Biophys Acta 642:79–87
Powell DW, Malawer SJ (1968) Relation between water and solute transport from isoosmotic solutions by rat small intestine in vivo. Am J Physiol 215:49–55
Prescott DH, Zeuthen E (1953) Comparison of water diffusion and water filtration across cell surfaces. Acta Physiol Scand 28:77–94
Rabinovitch J (1927) Factors influencing the absorption of water and chloride from the intestine. Am J Physiol 82:279–289
Rabon E, Takeguchi N, Sachs G (1980) Water and salt permeability of gastric vesicles. J Membr Biol 53:109–117
Redwood WR, Rall E, Perl W (1974) Red cell membrane permeability deduced from bulk diffusion coefficients. J Gen Physiol 64:706–729
Reid EW (1892) Preliminary report on experiments upon intestinal absorption without osmosis. Br Med J i:1133–1134
Reid EW (1900) On the intestinal absorption, especially on the absorption of serum, peptone, and glucose. Philos Trans R Soc Lond [Biol] 102:211–297
Reid EW (1901) Transport of fluid by certain epithelia. J Physiol (Lond) 26:436–444
Reid EW (1902) Intestinal absorption of solutions. J Physiol (Lond) 28:241–256
Renkin EM, Pappenheimer JR (1957) Wasserdurchlässigkeit und Permeabilität der Capillarwände. Ergeb Physiol Biol Chem Exp Pharmakol 49:59–126
Rich GT, Sha'afi RI, Barton TC, Solomon AK (1967) Permeability studies on red cell membranes of dog, cat, and beef. J Gen Physiol 50:2391–2405
Richardson PDI, Granger DN, Mailman D, Kvietys PR (1980) Permeability characteristics of colonic capillaries. Am J Physiol 239:G300–G305
Robbins E, Mauro A (1960) Experimental study of the independence of diffusion and hydrodynamic permeability coefficients in collodion membranes. J Gen Physiol 43:523–532
Rose RC, Nahrwold DL (1976) Electrolyte transport by gallbladders of rabbit and guinea pig: Effect of amphotericin B and evidence of rheogenic Na transport. J Membr Biol 29:1–22
Rusznyak IM, Foldi M, Szabo G (1967) Lymphatics and lymph circulation, 2nd edn. Pergamon, Elmsford, p 971
Sackin H, Boulpaep EL (1975) Models for coupling of salt and water transport. Proximal tubular reabsorption in Necturus kidney. J Gen Physiol 66:671–733
Sato K (1975) Reevaluation of micropuncture techniques: Some of the factors which affect the rate of fluid absorption by proximal tubule. In: Angielski S, Durbach UC (eds) Biochemical aspects of renal function. Curr Probl Clin Biochem 4:175–187
Schafer JA, Andreoli TE (1972) Cellular constraints to diffusion. The effect of antidiuretic hormone on water flows in isolated mammalian collecting tubules. J Clin Invest 51:1264–1278
Schafer JA, Patlak CS, Andreoli TE (1974 a) Osmosis in cortical collecting tubules. A theoretical and experimental analysis of the osmotic transient phenomena. J Gen Physiol 64:201–227
Schafer JA, Troutman SL, Andreoli TE (1974 b) Osmosis in cortical tubules. ADH-independent osmotic flow rectification. J Gen Physiol 64:228–240
Schafer JA, Troutman SL, Andreoli TE (1974 c) Volume reabsorption, transepithelial potential differences, and ionic permeability properties in mammalian superficial proximal straight tubules. J Gen Physiol 64:582–607
Schafer JA, Patlak CS, Andreoli TE (1975) A component of fluid absorption linked to passive ion flows in the superficial pars recta. J Gen Physiol 66:445–471
Schifferdecker E, Frömter E (1978) The AC impedance of *Necturus* gallbladder epithelium. Pfluegers Arch 377:125–133
Schneider M (1964) Einführung in die Physiologie des Menschen, 15. Aufl. Springer, Berlin Göttingen Heidelberg
Schönert H (1980) Anomalous permeation of a reversibly associating substance: hydraulic conductivity and tracer water diffusion. J Membr Biol 52:161–164
Schultz SG (1980) Basic principles of membrane transport. Cambridge University Press, Cambridge

Schultz SG, Frizzell RA, Nellans HN (1974) Ion transport by mammalian small intestine. Ann Rev Physiol 36:51–91
Schultz SG, Frizzel RA, Nellans HN (1977) Active sodium transport and the electrophysiology of the rabbit colon. J Membr Biol 33:351–384
Sharp RR, Sen R (1982) Water permeability of the chromaffin granule membrane. Biophys J 40:17–25
Shepherd AP (1980) Intestinal blood flow autoregulation during foodstuff absorption. Am J Physiol 239:H156–H162
Sidel VW, Solomon AK (1957) Entrance of water into human red cells under an osmotic pressure gradient. J Gen Physiol 41:243–257
Sicgelbauer F (1958) Lehrbuch der normalen Anatomie der Menschen, 8th edn. Urban and Schwarzenberg, München
Siegenbeck van Heukelom J, Van den Ham MD, Albus M, Groot JA (1981) Microscopical determination of the filtration permeability of the mucosal surface of the goldfish intestinal epithelium. J Membr Biol 63:31–39
Simmons NL, Naftalin RJ (1976) Factors affecting the compartmentalization of sodium ion within rabbit ileum in vitro. Biochim Biophys Acta 448:411–425
Simon M, Curci S, Gebler B, Frömter E (1981) Attempts to determine the ion concentrations in the lateral spaces between the cells of Necturus gallbladder epithelium with microelectrodes. In: Ussing HH, Bindslev N, Lassen NA, Sten-Knudsen O (eds) Water transport across epithelia, Alfred Benzon Symposium 15. Munksgaard, Copenhagen, pp 52–63
Singer SJ (1974) The molecular organization of membranes. Annu Rev Biochem 43:805–833
Singer SJ, Nicolson GL (1972) The fluid mosaic model of the structure of cell membranes. Science 175:720–731
Skadhauge E (1967) In vivo perfusion studies on the cloacal water and electrolyte resorption in the fowl (Gallus domesticus). Comp Biochem Physiol 23:483–501
Skadhauge E (1969) The mechanism of salt and water absorption in the intestine of the eel (Anguilla anguilla) adapted to waters of various salinities. J Physiol (Lond) 204:135–158
Skadhauge E (1974) Coupling of transmural flows of NaCl and water in the intestine of the eel (Anguilla anguilla). J Exp Biol 60:535–544
Smulders AP, Wright EM (1971) The magnitude of non-electrolyte selectivity in the gallbladder epithelium. J Membr Biol 5:297–318
Smulders AP, Tormey JMcD, Wright EM (1972) The effect of osmotically induced water flows on the permeability and ultrastructure of the rabbit gallbladder. J Membr Biol 7:164–197
Smyth DH, Taylor CB (1957) Transfer of water and solutes by an in vitro intestinal preparation. J Physiol (Lond) 136:632–648
Smyth DH, Wright EM (1966) Streaming potentials in the rat small intestine. J Physiol (Lond) 182:591–602
Snell FN, Shulman S, Spencer RP, Moos C (1965) Biophysical principles of structure and function. Addison-Wesley, Reading
Soergel KH, Whalen GE, Harris JA (1968) Passive movement of water and sodium across the human small intestinal mucosa. J Appl Physiol 24:40–48
Solomon AK (1968) Characterization of biological membranes by equivalent pores. J Gen Physiol 51:335s–364s
Solomon AK, Gary-Bobo CM (1972) Aqueous pores in lipid bilayers and red cell membranes. Biochim Biophys Acta 255:1019–1021
Spring KR, Hope A (1978) Size and shape of the lateral intercellular space in a living epithelium. Science 200:54–58
Spring KR, Hope A (1979) Fluid transport and the dimensions of cells and interspaces of living Necturus gallbladder. J Gen Physiol 73:287–305
Spring KR, Ericson A-C (1982) Epithelial cell volume modulation and regulation. J Membr Biol 69:167–176
Starling EH (1896) On the absorption of fluid from the connective tissue spaces. J Physiol (Lond) 19:312–326

Staverman AJ (1952) Non-equilibrium thermodynamics of membrane processes. Trans Farad Soc 48:176–185

Stein WD (1967) The movement of molecules across cell membranes. Academic, New York

Stirling ES (1972) Radioautographic localization of sodium pump sites in rabbit intestine. J Cell Biol 53:704–714

Swabb EA, Hynes RA, Donowitz M (1982) Elevated intraluminal pressure alteres rabbit small intestinal transport in vivo. Am J Physiol 242:G58–G64

Tormey JM, Diamond JM (1967) The ultrastructural route of fluid transport in rabbit gall bladder. J Gen Physiol 50:2031–2060

Turnheim K, Lauterbach F (1977) Absorption and secretion of monoquaternary ammonium compounds by the isolated intestinal mucosa. Biochem Pharmacol 26:99–108

Ussing HH (1949) Transport of ions across cellular membranes. Physiol Rev 29:127–155

Ussing HH (1966) Anomalous transport of electrolytes and sucrose through the isolated frog skin induced by hypertonicity of the outside bathing solution. Ann NY Acad Sci 137:543–555

Ussing HH, Erlij D, Lassen U (1974) Transport pathways in biological membranes. Annu Rev Physiol 36:17–49

Van Driessche W, Lindemann B (1979) Concentration dependence of currents through single sodium-selective pores in frog skin. Nature 282:519–520

Van Os CH, Slegers JFG (1973) Path of osmotic water flow through rabbit gallbladder epithelium. Biochim Biophys Acta 291:197–207

Van Os CH, De Jong MD, Slegers JFG (1974) Dimensions of the polar pathways through rabbit gallbladder epithelium. J Membr Biol 15:363–382

Van Os CH, Michels JA, Slegers JFG (1976) Effects of electrical gradients on volume flows across gallbladder epithelium. Biochim Biophys Acta 443:545–555

Van Os CH, Wiedner G, Wright EM (1979) Volume flows across gallbladder epithelium induced by small hydrostatic gradients. J Membr Biol 49:1–20

Vargas FF (1968) Water flux and electrokinetic phenomena in squid axon. J Gen Physiol 51:123s–130s

Vaughan BE (1960) Intestinal electrolyte absorption by parallel determination of unidirectional sodium and water transfers. Am J Physiol 198:1235–1244

Villegas L (1963) Action of histamine on the permeability of frog gastric mucosa to potassium and water. Biochim Biophys Acta 75:377–386

Villegas L (1978) Applied pressures and net water flux across in vitro frog gastric mucosa. Am J Physiol 235:E361–E373

Villegas R, Villegas GM (1960) Characterization of the membranes in the giant nerve fiber of the squid. J Gen Physiol 43 (Suppl 1):73–103

Visscher MB (1957) Transport of water and electrolytes across intestinal epithelia. In: Murphy QE (ed) Metabolic aspects of transport across cell membranes. University of Wisconsin Press, Madison, pp 57–71

Visscher MB, Fetcher ES Jr, Carr CW, Gregor HP, Bushey MS, Barker DE (1944) Isotope tracer studies on the movement of water and ions between intestinal lumen and blood. Am J Physiol 142:550–575

Wade JB, Revel JP, Discala AV (1973) Effect of osmotic gradients on intercellular junctions of the toad bladder. Am J Physiol 224:407–415

Wall BJ, Oschman JL, Schmidt-Nielsen B (1970) Fluid transport: Concentration of the intercellular compartment. Science 167:1497–1498

Wang JH, Robinson CV, Edelman IS (1953) Self-diffusion and structure of liquid water. III. Measurement of the self-diffusion of liquid water with H^2, H^3, and O^{18} as tracers. J Am Chem Soc 75:466–470

Wanitschke R, Nell R, Rummel W (1977) Influence of hydrostatic pressure gradients on net transfer of sodium and water across isolated rat colonic mucosa. Naunyn-Schmiedeberg's Arch Pharmacol 297:191–194

Warren R (1939) Serosal and mucosal dimensions at different levels of the dog's small intestine. Anat Rec 75:427–437

Wedner HJ, Diamond JM (1969) Contributions of unstirred layer effects to apparent electrokinetic phenomena in the gallbladder. J Membr Biol 1:92–108

Weinstein AM, Stephenson JL (1981a) Models of coupled salt and water transport across leaky epithelia. J Membr Biol 60:1–20
Weinstein AM, Stephenson JL (1981b) Coupled water transport in standing gradient models of the lateral intercellular space. Biophys J 35:167–191
Welling DJ, Welling LW (1979) Cell shape as an indicator of volume reabsorption in proximal nephron. Fed Proc 38:121–127
Wells HS (1931) The passage of materials through the intestinal walls. I. The relation between intraintestinal pressure and the rate of absorption of water. Am J Physiol 99:209–220
Wheeler HO (1963) Transport of electrolytes and water across wall of rabbit gallbladder. Am J Physiol 205:427–438
Whitlock RT, Wheeler HO (1964) Coupled transport of solute and water across rabbit gallbladder epithelium. J Clin Invest 43:2249–2265
Whittembury G, Oken DE, Windhager E, Solomon AK (1959) Single proximal tubules of Necturus kidney. IV. Dependence of H_2O movement on osmotic gradients. Am J Physiol 197:1121–1127
Windhager EE, Whittembury G, Oken DE, Schatzmann HJ, Solomon AK (1959) Single proximal tubules of the Necturus kidney. III. Dependence of H_2O movement on NaCl concentrations. Am J Physiol 197:313–318
Windhager E, Bouplpaep E, Giebisch G (1967) Electrophysiological studies in single nephrons. 3rd International congress of nephrology, Washington 1966. Karger, Basel, p 35
Winne D (1966) Der Einfluß einiger Pharmaka auf die Darmdurchblutung und die Resorption tritiummarkierten Wassers aus dem Dünndarm der Ratte. Naunyn-Schmiedeberg's Arch Pharmacol 254:199–224
Winne D (1972) The influence of blood flow and water net flux on the absorption of tritiated water from the jejunum of the rat. Naunyn-Schmiedeberg's Arch Pharmacol 272:417–436
Winne D (1975) The influence of villus countercurrent exchange on intestinal absorption. J Theor Biol 53:145–176
Winne D (1978) Blood flow in intestinal absorption models. J Pharmacokinet Biopharm 6:55–78
Winne D (1979) Influence of blood flow on intestinal absorption of drugs and nutrients. J Pharm Therap 6:333–393
Winne D, Remischovsky J (1971a) Der Einfluß der Durchblutung auf die Resorption von Harnstoff, Methanol und Äthanol aus dem Jejunum der Ratte. Naunyn-Schmiedeberg's Arch Pharmacol 268:392–419
Winne D, Remischovsky J (1971b) Der Einfluß der Durchblutung auf die Resorption von Polyalkoholen aus dem Jejunum der Ratte. Naunyn-Schmiedeberg's Arch Pharmacol 270:22–40
Wood HO (1944) The surface area of the intestinal mucosa in the rat and in the cat. J Anat 78:103–105
Wright EM (1970) The transport across the frog choroid plexus. Brain Res 23:302–304
Wright EM (1977) Passive water transport across epithelia. In: Jungreis AM, Hodges TK, Kleinzeller A, Schultz SG (eds) Water relations in membrane transport in plants and animals. Academic, New York, pp 199–213
Wright EM, Diamond JM (1969) Patterns of non-electrolyte permeability. Proc R Soc Lond [Biol] 172:227–271
Wright EM, Pietras RJ (1974) Routes of nonelectrolyte permeation across epithelial membranes. J Membr Biol 17:293–312
Wright EM, Smulders AP, Tormey JM (1972) The role of the lateral intercellular spaces and solute polarization effects in the passive flow of water across the rabbit gallbladder. J Membr Biol 7:198–219
Yablonski ME, Lifson N (1976) Mechanism of production of intestinal secretion by elevated venous pressure. J Clin Invest 57:904–915

CHAPTER 12

Intestinal Permeability to Calcium and Phosphate

L. R. FORTE

A. Introduction

Calcium and phosphorus are critical elements in the maintenance of living systems. Thus, elegant regulatory mechanisms have evolved by which calcium and phosphorus homeostasis is maintained. In vertebrates, the intestine, kidney, and bone are intimately involved in this process and in fish, the gills appear also to regulate mineral homeostasis. A number of endocrine organs function in the orchestration of mineral homeostasis, including the parathyroid gland, parafollicular cells (C-cells) of the thyroid, and the endocrine kidney. In addition, endocrine factors from the adrenals, gonads, thyroid, and pituitary appear, either directly or indirectly, to influence calcium and phosphorus homeostasis. The purpose of this chapter is to focus primarily on the current views of the mechanisms involved in the intestinal transport of calcium and inorganic phosphate in relation to mineral absorption, with particular emphasis on the physiologic and biochemical mechanisms of calcium and phosphate transport.

In general, land-dwelling vertebrates are exposed to a relatively calcium-poor, phosphate-rich environment. Approximately 99% of the calcium content of the body in humans is found in the skeleton, whereas 85% of phosphorus is localized in bone (PITKIN 1975). Outside of bone mineral reserves of calcium and inorganic phosphate, it may be stated that calcium is primarily an extracellular cation and phosphate is primarily intracellular. It is estimated that ionized calcium levels in the extracellular fluid are in the millimolar range whereas intracellular levels of unbound calcium are in the submicromolar to micromolar range. This suggests that the permeability and transport of calcium across cell membranes is under tight regulation.

B. Calcium Transport

The movement of calcium across the intestinal epithelium may occur by transcellular or paracellular pathways and be in the absorptive (mucosal–serosal) or secretory (serosal–mucosal) direction. Intestinal absorption of calcium is variable according to the physiologic needs of the organism. For many years it has been known that diets low in calcium content cause enhancement of the intestinal absorption of calcium. Balance studies suggested that calcium retention induced by low calcium diets was due to increased intestinal absorption of calcium (FAIRBANKS and MITCHELL 1936; ROTTENSTEN 1938) and the classical studies of NICOLAYSEN (1937 a, b) provided data consistent with an adaptation of intestinal calcium absorption that was dependent upon the administration of vitamin D. Other prominent adaptive features of intestinal calcium absorption are that young growing animals absorb substantially more calcium than mature animals (HENRY and KON 1945; HARRISON and HARRISON 1951; HANSARD et al. 1951; SCHACHTER et al. 1960; AVIOLI et al. 1965; IRELAND and FORDTRAN 1973), and pregnancy and lactation are associated with an increase in the intestinal absorption of calcium (SCHACHTER et al. 1960; KOSTIAL et al. 1969; HEANEY and SKILLMAN 1971; TOVERUD et al. 1976).

The components of calcium transport in the intestine that are thought to be physiologically regulated by 1,25-dihydroxycholecalciferol may be described as an (overall) active transport process in the mucosal–serosal direction. Intestinal absorption and secretion of calcium occurring via the paracellular pathway is a large component of calcium transport, but is not considered to be influenced by the hormone (NELLANS and KIMBERG 1978) whereas cellular transport is regulated by the vitamin D–endocrine system. Using the everted gut sac technique of WILSON and WISEMAN (1954), SCHACHTER et al. (1960) demonstrated that active transport of calcium is more prominent in the proximal small intestine of the rat (i.e., duodenum > jejunum > ileum). This general pattern of intestinal localization of calcium transport has been confirmed by studies using other experimental techniques, notably the ion flux method of Ussing (WALLING 1977) and isolated intestinal loops in vivo (BEHAR and KERSTEIN 1976). Regulation of calcium transport by vitamin D is not limited to the small intestine since it has been shown that 1,25-dihydroxycholecalciferol-stimulated active transport of calcium occurs in the colon (HARRISON and HARRISON 1969; PETITH et al. 1979; LEE et al. 1980; FAVUS et al. 1980, 1981; LEE et al. 1981). Moreover, LEE et al. (1981) found that physiologic doses of 1,25-dihydroxycholecalciferol stimulated calcium transport in duodenum and colon whereas supraphysiologic doses, which caused hypercalcemia, were required to increase calcium transport in the jejunum and ileum. Thus, it is possible that the colon contributes to the vitamin D-regulated portion of intestinal calcium absorption in vivo. In addition, PETITH and SCHEDL (1976) demonstrated that the colon of young growing rats generally exhibited net secretion of calcium when they were fed a 1.2% calcium diet, but generally exhibited net absorption of calcium as an adaptive response to a low calcium (0.02%) diet.

The absorptive transport of calcium is accomplished by the enterocyte through coordinated events at the brush border membrane, intracellular organelles, and the basolateral membrane. Numerous investigations support the general conclusion that the overall calcium transport process is active (e.g., energy dependent and against an electrochemical gradient) and carrier-mediated (SCHACHTER and ROSEN 1959; SCHACHTER et al. 1960). However, it is currently thought that the transport of calcium across the brush border (mucosal) membrane from the lumen into the cell is accomplished by facilitated diffusion down a favorable electrochemical gradient. Therefore, the extrusion of calcium at the serosal (basolateral) membrane by an active, cation-directed transport process appears to be the final pathway for the transcellular transport of calcium. A variety of in vitro techniques have been used to study these transport processes. Undoubtedly, much of the contradictory data obtained in this area relate to the use of so many different methods. Moreover, the viability of the mucosal epithelium has been seriously questioned in those methods where calcium transport across the tissue is evaluated in vitro. Studies have shown that the morphology of the mucosal cells exhibit deterioration within a few minutes after removal of the intestine and incubation of the tissue in vitro (LEVINE et al. 1970). Thus, evaluation of transport data obtained at a time when the epithelium is progressively deteriorating is indeed difficult. Newer techniques may shed light in this area. Notable are the studies with isolated brush border or basolateral membranes, embryonic intestine in organ culture, and isolated epithelial cells.

I. Brush Border Membrane

From studies using the everted gut sac, HARRISON and HARRISON (1960) suggested that the flux of calcium across the mucosal membrane (lumen–cell) was consistent with passive diffusion. Moreover, they concluded that vitamin D regulated the mucosal membrane's permeability specifically to calcium. This effect of vitamin D was noted throughout the small intestine, although in their studies active (concentrative) transport was limited to the duodenum. Studies by other investigators provided additional evidence that vitamin D regulates the permeability of the brush border membrane to calcium (SCHACHTER et al. 1961; WASSERMAN and KALLFELZ 1962; WASSERMAN 1968; WALLING and ROTHMAN 1973; O'DONELL and SMITH 1973; HOLDSWORTH et al. 1975; MELANCON and DELUCA 1970; HAUSSLER et al. 1970; MORIUCHI and DELUCA 1976).

In experiments with chick ileum under short-circuit conditions, ADAMS and NORMAN (1970) found that calcium was actively transported across the epithelium in the mucosal–serosal direction when the tissue was obtained from vitamin D-replete chicks whereas there was no active transport of calcium in vitamin D-deficient intestine. Their data supported the idea that vitamin D regulates the brush border membrane's permeability to calcium. In other studies, it was found that the polyene antibiotic, filipin, when added to the mucosal side of the chick ileum, stimulated calcium flux from mucosa to serosa (ADAMS et al. 1970). Filipin only increased calcium flux in ileum from vitamin D-deficient chicks and only when exposed to the brush border membrane. Thus, filipin in vitro mimicked the effect of administration of vitamin D in vivo by increasing calcium transport across the epithelium. It appears that filipin, perhaps through an interaction with membrane cholesterol, influences the permeability of the mucosal membrane to calcium by altering the lipid milieu of the membrane. These studies (ADAMS and NORMAN 1970; ADAMS et al. 1970) led to the conclusion that calcium transport across the mucosal membrane was accomplished by carrier-mediated passive diffusion. They found evidence of saturation kinetics that supported the existence of a putative carrier (permease) for calcium that was localized in the mucosal membrane.

Confirmation of the existence of a vitamin D-dependent, carrier-mediated diffusion process for the transfer of calcium across the mucosal membrane has been obtained using two experimental techniques: (1) embryonic chick intestine in organ culture; and (2) purified preparations of intestinal brush border membranes. CORRADINO (1978) presented data consistent with the concept that calcium uptake by cultured chick intestine consisted of saturable and nonsaturable components.

The technique used in this study allowed an estimation of the uptake of calcium across the mucosal membrane. Such a procedure appears to be an improvement over the techniques previously used to study intestinal cell uptake which used isolated cell preparations or intestinal slices. With those techniques it was not possible to differentiate readily between uptake of calcium across the mucosal versus the basolateral surface of the mucosal cell or intestinal epithelium. CORRADINO (1978) reported that 1,25-dihydroxycholecalciferol stimulated calcium uptake across the mucosal membrane and that the sterol hormone exerted its effect on a nonsaturable component of calcium transport. The saturable component of calcium transport that appeared not to be affected by 1,25-dihydroxycholecalciferol was saturated at 4–5 m*M* calcium. Mucosal uptake of calcium was relatively independent of metabolic energy and of sodium.

FRANCESCHI and DELUCA (1981 a) extended the investigation of calcium transport using the cultured chick duodenum. They confirmed that calcium uptake was saturable (K_m 0.45 m*M*), but in contrast to the report of CORRADINO (1978) observed that 1,25-dihydroxycholecalciferol specifically stimulated the maximal velocity of calcium transport from 49 to 110 pmol $mg^{-1}min^{-1}$. The nonsaturable component of calcium uptake, measured in the presence of ethyleneglycol-bis(β-aminoethylether)-*N*-tetraacetic acid (EGTA), was not affected by the sterol hormone. A reason for the different results obtained by FRANCESCHI and DELUCA (1981 a) from those of CORRADINO (1978) may be due to the difference in technique in that the former investigation studied calcium uptake by tissue that was immersed in the medium whereas the latter study used a filter paper method for directly examining mucosal uptake of calcium. The report by FRANCESCHI and DELUCA (1981 a) agreed with CORRADINO (1978) in that inhibitors of metabolism which reduced tissue ATP levels by a least 70% did not affect the uptake of calcium. It was concluded that the embryonic chick intestine in organ culture may represent a unique model which allows study of the carrier-mediated, passive diffusion of calcium (which appears to be an important site for regulation by vitamin D) across the mucosal membrane without a substantial influence of the active transport component of calcium transport (basolateral membrane) that is observed in other preparations of intestine (SCHACHTER et al. 1960, 1961; SCHACHTER and ROSEN 1959; PAPWORTH and PATRICK 1970; FREUND and BRONNER 1975 a; KENDRICK et al. 1981).

Currently, the experimental approach that has been most successful in isolating the mucosal component of calcium transport is the technique whereby purified preparations of intestinal brush border membranes are studied in vitro. Reviews of these techniques have appeared recently (MURER and HILDMANN 1981; MURER and KINNE 1980; see also Chap. 7). These methods have provided substantial new information regarding the mechanisms involved in the transport of sugars and amino acids in tissues such as the intestine and kidney. Preparations of brush border membranes from intestine and kidney have been shown to be oriented in the right-side-out configuration (HAASE et al. 1978) so that studies of calcium uptake by the membrane vesicles in vitro provide data analogous to the transport which is postulated to occur across the mucosal membrane in situ.

This technique has been applied to the chick intestine and a preparation of brush border membranes obtained which exhibited a 20-fold purification of the brush border enzyme marker, sucrase (MAX et al. 1978). Treatment of rachitic chicks with 1-hydroxycholecalciferol caused an increase in the phospholipid content of brush border membranes and a concomitant increase in unsaturated fatty acid content of the phosphatidylcholine fraction of the membrane phospholipids. This vitamin D metabolite also enhanced the rate of uptake of calcium by vesicles of brush border membranes when the sterol was administered to rachitic chicks (RASMUSSEN et al. 1979; FONTAINE et al. 1981). These investigators found that calcium uptake by brush border vesicles exhibited two components including a rapid (i.e., 1 min) uptake that was not affected by 1-hydroxycholecalciferol and appeared to be due to calcium binding to the membrane and a sterol hormone-dependent uptake of calcium into an osmotically active space (intravesicular). The latter calcium uptake process reached steady state in about 60 min in vesicles from vitamin D-replete chicks whereas calcium uptake continued progressively for about 5 h in vesicles from vitamin D-deficient intestine. Vitamin D treatment increased the velocity of calcium uptake from 0.25 to 0.68 nmol $mg^{-1}min^{-1}$ and the estimated K_m for calcium was not affected by the hormone (1.4–1.5 mM). Thus, it appears that this technique supports one postulated mechanism for vitamin D regulation of calcium transport in the intestine in that the hormone increased the apparent carrier-mediated, passive diffusion of calcium across the mucosal membrane. Additional support was obtained by these investigators that calcium uptake is related to the regulation of membrane permeability to calcium by experiments with filipin. It was shown that incubation of brush border membranes with filipin (2.5–10 μg/ml) increased the velocity of calcium uptake only in membranes from vitamin D-deficient chicks. This data supports the observation originally made by ADAMS et al. (1970) who reported that filipin specifically enhanced the mucosal–serosal flux of calcium in the intestine from vitamin D-deficient chicks. The calcium ionophore, A23187 was found to stimulate calcium uptake to an equivalent extent in brush border membranes from either vitamin D-replete or D-deficient intestine.

II. Basolateral Membranes

As previously mentioned, the intestinal transport of calcium in the mucosal–serosal direction has been shown to be, at least in part, an active transport process. It has been well documented in studies with the everted gut sac that calcium is transported against its electrochemical gradient, resulting in serosal–mucosal calcium gradients substantially greater than unity (SCHACHTER and ROSEN 1959; HARRISON and HARRISON 1960; SCHACHTER et al. 1960, 1961; KIMBERG et al. 1961; HURWITZ et al. 1967; MARTIN and DELUCA 1969). The original studies from SCHACHTER and co-workers revealed that the active transport process was dependent upon oxidative metabolism since incubation of the tissue under a nitrogen atmosphere or with metabolic inhibitors eliminated the concentrative transport of calcium (SCHACHTER and ROSEN 1959; SCHACHTER et al. 1960). Studies of calcium transport in vivo are consistent with active transport of calcium, thus providing information of the physiologic relevance of the transport processes studied in vitro (WASSERMAN et al. 1961; CRAMER and DUECK 1962; KRAWITT and SCHEDL 1968; WENSEL et al. 1969; BIRGE et al. 1969; URBAN and SCHEDL 1969). In vitro experiments using the isotope flux technique of USSING (1949) provided further support for the existence of an active transport pump for calcium since the flux ratio (mucosa–serosa: serosa–mucosa) under short-circuit conditions exceeded unity in vitamin D-replete chick intestine. For the purpose of the ensuing discussion of calcium transport across the basolateral membrane of the polar enterocyte, it is useful to assume that the active transport pump is localized in that membrane.

Development of the knowledge of relationships between sodium transport and intestinal transport of both sugars and amino acids provided an impetus to examine the effects of sodium on calcium transport. Using the everted sacs of rat duodenum, MARTIN and DELUCA (1969) showed that calcium transport was substantially decreased when sodium was omitted from the buffer medium. It was concluded that sodium did not affect the mucosal membrane's permeability to calcium, thus suggesting that sodium influences the transport of calcium across the basolateral membrane. Such an interpretation was supported by the studies of HOLDSWORTH et al. (1975) using noneverted chick intestine in vitro. They found that low sodium concentrations (25 m*M*), in accord with the investigation of others using chick intestine (HURWITZ et al. 1967), provided optimal conditions for calcium transport and that sodium at physiologic levels was inhibitory to calcium transport. The inhibitor of sodium transport, ethacrynic acid, decreased intestinal calcium transport (HOLDSWORTH et al. 1975). The significance of this finding is unclear, however since ethacrynic acid can inhibit oxidative metabolism, leading to decreased ATP levels (EPSTEIN 1972). Moreover, recent information indicates that ethacrynic acid's pharmacologic mechanism of action in the kidney is associated with the inhibition of active chloride transport with secondary inhibition of sodium transport (BURG and GREEN 1973). Thus, the effect of ethacrynic acid to inhibit an intestinal Na^+, K^+-ATPase, described by BIRGE et al. (1972), is difficult to interpret with respect to its physiologic significance. Moreover, inhibition of the sodium pump with ouabain did not affect intestinal calcium transport (MARTIN and DE LUCA 1969). It is conceivable that the effect of sodium on calcium transport observed by some investigators reflects a sodium–calcium exchange mechanism, perhaps at the basolateral membranes (MURER and HILDMANN 1981). The existence of such a mechanism may be presumed to exist from extrapolation of the occurrence of such a mechanism from other ion-transporting tissues (GMAJ et al. 1979; ULLRICH et al. 1976).

A number of investigations using isolated slices of small intestine, mucosal cells, or other in vitro approaches have studied the process of calcium uptake and found that metabolic inhibitors or a nitrogen atmosphere inhibit calcium uptake (SCHACHTER and ROSEN 1959; HARRISON and HARRISON 1960; SCHACHTER et al. 1961; PAPWORTH and PATRICK 1970; FREUND and BRONNER 1975a). Recently, KENDRICK et al. (1981) prepared intestinal discs from rat duodenum and studied calcium uptake. They found that, in the vitamin D-replete rat, intestinal discs exhibited an O_2-dependent calcium uptake that was saturable (K_m 0.8 m*M*). Treatment of vitamin D-deficient rats with 1,25-dihydroxycholecalciferol enhanced the O_2-dependent uptake three fold. It was found that actinomycin D pretreatment in vivo provided a partial blockade of the stimulation of calcium uptake produced by the sterol hormone. However, actinomycin D was nonspecific in its pharmacologic effects to inhibit calcium uptake since the antibiotic also inhibited calcium uptake into intestinal discs derived from vitamin D-deficient rats. KENDRICK et al. (1981) concluded that the uptake was occurring at the mucosal border since calcium uptake at the serosal side into the muscle layer was a minor component of the uptake process and not affected by lack of oxygen. These studies also demonstrated that food deprivation (7.5–11 h) increased the O_2-dependent uptake of calcium by intestinal discs from both vitamin D-deficient and D-replete animals. The calcium ionophore, A23187, produced no consistent effects on O_2-dependent calcium uptake other than inhibition at some concentrations of the ionophore. These investigators concluded that, if 1,25-dihydroxycholecalciferol acts to increase the passive permeability of the mucosal membrane to calcium, then that process must be tightly coupled to the putative O_2-dependent, active extrusion of calcium from the cell. From this experimental design, which used relatively short incubations, it would be conceivable that the increased "uptake" observed under an oxygen atmosphere is due to extrusion of calcium at the basolateral membrane and the subsequent accumulation of calcium in the extracellular space and other serosal compartments. This is consistent with data from experiments using the everted gut sac and Ussing flux experiments that characteristically require rather long incubations for calcium transport across the entire structure. Calcium absorption in vivo is not reflected by this situation since the calcium extruded at the basolateral membrane is removed by the intestinal capillaries into the circulation of the animal.

Studies of calcium transport processes utilizing basolateral membranes have provided less information than the corresponding studies with brush border membranes. The vesicles of basolateral membranes are a mixture of right-side-out and inside-out orientation. Moreover, their permeability does not reflect the in vivo situation where calcium permeability of the basolateral membrane is low. MURER and HILDMANN (1981) published some preliminary data on calcium transport by vesicles of basolateral membranes. They found that ATP enhanced calcium uptake into the vesicles (inside-out orientation) thus representing calcium extrusion by a calcium pump mechanism in the membrane. This pump may be the Ca^{2+}-ATPase observed by others (BIRGE and GILBERT 1974; GHIJSEN et al. 1979, 1980) and discussed in Sect. D.VI. Inhibitors of ATP-dependent mitochondrial calcium uptake such as oligomycin or ruthenium, according to results from MURER and HILDMANN (1981), did not affect the ATP-dependent uptake of calcium by intestinal basolateral membranes. These investigators related preliminary evidence of a sodium–calcium exchange mechanism existing in intestinal basolateral membranes. After loading of vesicles with calcium, the efflux of calcium was found to be greater with a sodium than a potassium gradient imposed from the extravesicular–intravesicular space. These preliminary observations suggest that this in vitro system may provide additional insight into the mechanism existing for calcium transport at the serosal pole of the enterocyte. It may be speculated that the active transport pump for calcium resides specifically in this membrane whereas the vitamin D-mediated permeability regulation exists at the brush border membrane. A tight coupling between the two membrane events, presumably through other important but intracellular events, could provide and explanation for the overall regulation of calcium absorption produced by 1,25-

dihydroxycholecalciferol in vivo. The existence of a sodium–calcium exchange mechanism at the basolateral membrane may help to explain the effects of sodium on intestinal calcium transport. It is clear that transport in the intestine resembles that for other tissues, notably the kidney where sodium–calcium exchange has been observed at the basolateral (peritubular) membrane (GMAJ et al. 1979; ULLRICH et al. 1976). It will be important to determine the physiologic importance of the putative sodium–calcium exchange system in the gastrointestinal absorption of calcium in vivo.

C. Phosphate Transport

In contrast to the situation for intestinal absorption of calcium previously described, phosphate transport from the intestinal lumen into the mucosal cell is against an electrochemical gradient, suggesting that active transport occurs at the mucosal membrane. Moreover, the transport of phosphate across the basolateral membrane appears to be down a favorable electrochemical gradient which indicates that the process of passive diffusion may be involved in phosphate transport across this membrane barrier. Intestinal phosphate transport has not been as extensively studied as calcium transport and in fact much of the data obtained for phosphate transport have been derived through investigations of the calcium transport mechanisms. Many of the studies of phosphate transport deal with the regulation of that process in the intestine by vitamin D. Therefore, this section will deal primarily with the regulation of phosphate transport by vitamin D and the basic characteristics of the transport mechanism.

It was recognized very early that in the human, vitamin D deficiency was associated with decreased serum phosphorus (HOWLAND and KRAMER 1921). Balance studies in humans (TEFLER 1922) and rats (NICOLAYSEN 1937a) revealed that intestinal phosphate absorption was decreased by vitamin D deficiency and that treatment with vitamin D enhanced both phosphate and calcium absorption. Data from these studies were interpreted to mean that the absorption of phosphate was secondary to that of calcium. Thus, for a substantial period of time it was thought that vitamin D influenced phosphate transport secondarily to its influence on calcium transport, perhaps through vitamin D-mediated stimulation of a cotransport process. More recent studies supported that notion since active calcium transport appeared to require the presence of phosphate (HELBOCK et al. 1966) and the calcium chelator, ethylenediaminetetraacetate (EDTA) inhibited intestinal phosphate transport which was reversed by adding calcium (HARRISON and HARRISON 1961). However, it should be emphasized that the overall body of data strongly suggests that intestinal phosphate transport is independent of calcium transport. CARLSSON (1954) demonstrated that intestinal phosphate absorption was not dependent upon calcium in the intestinal contents and showed that vitamin D stimulated phosphate absorption in rats fed a low calcium diet. COHN and GREENBERG (1939) studied the absorption of phosphate ^{32}P and found that vitamin D decreased fecal phosphate excretion. However, their finding that “the absorption of phosphate by rachitic rats is increased but little by vitamin D” can be explained by their experimental conditions. They studied the effects of vitamin

D on intestinal phosphate absorption 1 h after treatment and found only a slight increase in phosphate absorption. It is now recognized that the lag period following administration of vitamin D before either calcium or phosphate transport is stimulated is due to metabolic activation of the precursor, vitamin D, to form the sterol hormone followed by the induction of RNA and protein synthesis in target cells of the intestine.

Evidence that phosphate transport in the intestine is not coupled to active transport of calcium is derived from the following observations:

1. The vitamin D-stimulated transport of phosphate is greatest in the jejunum whereas calcium transport is greatest in the duodenum (HARRISON and HARRISON 1961; KOWARSKI and SCHACHTER 1969; HURWITZ and BAR 1972; WASSERMAN and TAYLOR 1973; CHEN et al. 1974; WALLING 1977; PETERLIK and WASSERMAN 1978).
2. Vitamin D enhances calcium but not phosphate transport (absorptive) in the colon (LEE et al. 1980, 1981).
3. Intestinal phosphate transport is clearly dependent upon sodium whereas calcium transport appears not to be sodium dependent (HARRISON and HARRISON 1963; TAYLOR 1974b; BERNER et al. 1976; PETERLIK 1978; DANISI and STRAUB 1980).
4. Phosphate transport is not dependent upon the presence of calcium (KOWARSKI and SCHACHTER 1969; WASSERMAN and TAYLOR 1973; TAYLOR 1974b; PETERLIK and WASSERMAN 1978) and calcium transport is not dependent upon the presence of phosphate (WALLING and ROTHMAN 1969; ADAMS and NORMAN 1970).
5. The adaptive increase in phosphate absorption caused by a low phosphate diet is only partly due to enhanced production of 1,25-dihydroxycholecalciferol whereas the correlated increase in calcium transport appears completely dependent upon the parathyroid–renal axis for the observed increase in calcium absorption under these conditions (RIBOVICH and DELUCA 1974; STOLL et al. 1979a, b; CRAMER and MCMILLAN 1980).

Intestinal phosphate transport has been studied in vivo and by a multiplicity of in vitro techniques. The characteristics of the transport process have been revealed through the in vitro techniques of: (1) everted gut sac; (2) ligated intestinal loop in situ; (3) Ussing technique; (4) cultured embryonic intestine; and (5) isolated brush border membrane preparations. Using the everted gut sac, HARRISON and HARRISON (1963) demonstrated that replacement of sodium with choline in the medium markedly reduced the concentrative transport of phosphate as well as the transport of glucose and tyrosine. Absence of sodium did not alter intestinal calcium transport. Studies in the chick intestine confirmed that phosphate transport was dependent upon sodium and extended the information by demonstrating that ouabain inhibited phosphate transfer in everted gut sacs (TAYLOR 1974b). The concentrative transport of phosphate was markedly reduced in gut sacs from vitamin D-deficient relative to D-replete animals and phosphate transport was inhibited by cyanide, anaerobiosis (HARRISON and HARRISON 1961), or omission of an oxidizable substrate such as glucose (CHEN et al. 1974). KOWARSKI and SCHACHTER (1969) used the rat gut sac to demonstrate that vitamin D preferentially enhanced mucosal–serosal phosphate transport whereas serosal–mucosal flux was not affected by vitamin D. They also concluded that phosphate transport was "channelized" in that phosphate ^{32}P did not equilibrate with the intracellular pool of phosphate. Later studies by PETERLIK and WASSERMAN (1978) supported the idea that phosphate transport was coupled or compartmentalized in the mucosal cell of the intestine. They further demonstrated that phosphate transport was a saturable process with a K_m of 0.19–0.2 mM in vitamin D-deficient or D-replete intestine whereas vitamin D enhanced the V_{max} of phosphate transport from 0.13 to 0.32 μmol g^{-1} min^{-1}. Moreover, vitamin D enhanced mucosal–serosal flux by stimulating phosphate influx at the mucosal membrane with no effect on transport from the cell across the basolateral membrane. Calcium had no effect on the flux of phosphate from lumen to cell, but low calcium levels enhanced the movement of phosphate from the cell to lumen. These observations are consistent with the hypothesis that vitamin D regulates phosphate absorption in the intestine by enhancing a sodium-dependent, active transport mechanism in the brush border membrane of mucosal cells, probably by increasing the number of carrier molecules for phosphate.

Using the in situ ligated loop method, WASSERMAN and TAYLOR (1973) studied the phosphate transport system in chick intestine. They observed that phosphate absorption was via a saturable process in duodenum, jejunum, and ileum and was enhanced by treatment of vitamin D-deficient chicks with vitamin D. A lag of about 10 h was found before a dose of 500 IU vitamin D_3 produced an increase in phosphate transport, whereas the maximal response occurred by 48 h. Treatment with EDTA to reduce calcium availability did not affect phosphate transport whereas arsenate, L-phenylalanine, and disodiumethane-1-hydroxy-1,1-diphosphonate (EHDP) inhibited phosphate transport. Arsenate appears to compete with phosphate at the transport (carrier) site, whereas L-phenylalanine inhibits alkaline phosphatase and EHDP inhibits the synthesis of 1,25-dihydroxycholecalciferol. Inhibition of phosphate transport by EHDP appears to be a relatively straightforward phenomenon in that is has been shown that vitamin D metabolites must be 1-hydroxylated by the renal enzyme before they are effective in the stimulation of intestinal phosphate transport (CHEN et al. 1974). The data with L-phenylalanine suggest that phosphate transport may be in some way linked to alkaline phosphatase, an enzyme localized in the brush border and regulated by 1,25-dihydroxycholecalciferol (HOLDSWORTH 1970; NORMAN et al. 1970; BIKLE et al. 1977; MORRISSEY et al. 1978a). A role for alkaline phosphatase in the transport of phosphate is not clear at present, since other studies showed that L-phenylalanine did not inhibit intestinal phosphate transport (TAYLOR 1974b). A potent inhibitor of alkaline phosphatase, L-bromotetramisole, has also been shown not to affect phosphate transport in the proximal tubule of rabbit kidney (BRUNETTE and DENNIS 1982). Recent studies implicate the enzyme, alkaline phosphatase, in a functional role by serving as the phosphatase mechanism which dephosphorylates the tyrosyl phosphate groups of cell protein (SWARUP et al. 1981, 1982). In this manner, alkaline phosphatase would be considered part of the cell machinery associated with the regulation of cell function by growth factors such as epidermal or nerve growth factor which have been shown to react with specific high affinity receptor sites on the surface of target cells with subsequent phosphorylation of the tyrosine moieties of cell protein. If such a role of alkaline phosphatase is further documented, then it would solve a very long-lived puzzle of the physiologic role for this ubiquitous membrane-bound enzyme.

Intestinal phosphate transport has also been studied under short-circuit conditions (Ussing technique). WALLING (1977) demonstrated that phosphate transport was stimulated by 1,25-dihydroxycholecalciferol in all regions of rat small intestine and flux ratios indicated that active transport of absorptive phosphate transport was enhanced by the hormone whereas phosphate secretion was unaffected. The greatest effect of 1,25-dihydroxycholecalciferol was noted in the jejunum in contrast to the duodenum in regard to active calcium transport. They concluded that the data supported the concept that a different distribution of phosphate-absorbing versus calcium-absorbing cells may account for the regional differences in transport that was influenced by 1,25-dihydroxycholecalciferol. Other studies that focused on the effects of vitamin D metabolites on intestinal phosphate transport have demonstrated that the active transport of phosphate is enhanced by biologically active compounds (WALLING and KIMBERG 1975; WALLING et al. 1976, 1977). Administration of 1,25-dihydroxycholecalciferol increased phosphate transport significantly by 3 h and the effects were noted as late as 96 h after administration to vitamin D-deficient rats. In vitamin D-deficient duodenum, net phosphate transport was in the serosal–mucosal (secretory) direction whereas net calcium absorption was found (WALLING and KIMBERG 1975). Administration of 1,25-dihydroxycholecalciferol caused a biphasic increase in both phosphate and calcium transport (mucosa–serosa). It was suggested that the hormone's early effects were on the phosphate transport of existing mucosal cells whereas the late effects (48–96 h) may be explained by effects of the hormone on the transport mechanisms of newly formed enterocytes that migrated to the forefront of the villi. These studies also confirmed that 24,25-dihydroxycholecalciferol was inactive in stimulating intestinal transport in the nephrectomized rat (WALLING et al. 1977). Thus, the 1-hydroxylation of 24,25-dihroxycholecalciferol to the trihydroxy metabolite is necessary for biologic activity in the intestine (BOYLE et al. 1973; HOLICK et al. 1973).

Influx of phosphate was also studied in rabbit duodenum. Both a diffusional process that was not influenced by 1,25-dihydroxycholecalciferol and a sodium-dependent, saturable phosphate influx which was enhanced by the hormone were observed in vitro (DANISI et al. 1980). Inhibition of the renal 1-hydroxylase by treatment with the diphosponate, EHDP, markedly reduced the V_{max} of phosphate influx from 211 to 42 nmol cm^{-2} h^{-1} whereas 1,25-dihydroxycholecalciferol increased the velocity of phosphate uptake to 413 nmol cm^{-2} h^{-1}. The K_m for phosphate influx was relatively constant from 0.21 to 0.37 mM and not considered to be affected by "vitamin D deficiency" or by treatment with 1,25-dihydroxycholecalciferol. Removal of sodium reduced the phosphate influx to that which could be accounted for by passive diffusion into the mucosal cells (DANISI and STRAUB 1980). Arsenate competitively inhibited the active transport of phosphate in rabbit duodenum. Rabbit jejunum and ileum appeared to have only a passive diffusion mechanism for phosphate uptake since influx was a linear function of the phosphate concentration and arsenate or lack of sodium had no effect on phosphate influx. A role for microfilaments and microtubules was proposed in phosphate transport since cytochalasin-B, colchicine, and vinblastine appeared to inhibit mucosal–serosal transfer of phosphate (FUCHS and PETERLIK 1979). The importance of this intracellular system in phosphate transport is unclear at present since these drugs may have other pharmacologic effects on cells. In the chick jejunum, PETERLIK and WASSERMAN (1980) confirmed that inhibition of renal synthesis of 1,25-dihydroxycholecalciferol by pretreatment with strontium markedly reduced phosphate transport. Administration of 1,25-dihydroxycholecalciferol reversed the effects of strontium on phosphate transport, a process that was effectively blocked by the inhibitor of protein synthesis, cycloheximide. This suggests that the hormone regulates phosphate transport in the intestine through induction of de novo protein synthesis although other investigators have demonstrated that inhibitors of RNA and protein synthesis do not block the transport of phosphate that is stimulated by 1,25-dihydroxycholecalciferol (BIKLE et al. 1978). This controversy is discussed in Sect. D.II relative to the cellular mechanism of action of 1,25-dihydroxycholecalciferol.

Phosphate transport has been studied using the cultured embryonic chick intestine technique developed by CORRADINO (1973 a). Vitamin D was shown to increase the uptake of both phosphate and iron in this preparation. PETERLIK (1978) showed that phosphate uptake occurred by a saturable process and that vitamin D in the culture medium increased the V_{max} from 55 to 75 nmol min^{-1} min^{-1} g^{-1} whereas the K_m (0.5 mM) was not affected by the sterol. Protein synthesis inhibitors reduced baseline phosphate uptake and prevented the stimulation of transport by vitamin D. A sodium dependency was noted for the saturable phosphate uptake process, which was inhibited by metabolic poisons. The uptake of phosphate in the absence of sodium or after inhibition of metabolism appeared to be due to passive diffusion and equivalent to that observed in the absence of vitamin D. CORRADINO (1979 b) also reported that vitamin D_3 stimulated phosphate uptake in the embryonic chick intestine cultured in vitro. These observations are generally consistent with those previously discussed although it should be noted that the embryonic chick intestine is unique in that it responds to vitamin D_3 in vitro without apparent conversion to hydroxy metabolites.

Animals fed a phosphate-deficient diet adapt by increasing the intestinal absorption and renal tubular reabsorption of phosphate. Intestinal adaptation of phosphate absorption when animals are phosphate depleted has been well documented (RIZZOLI et al. 1977; FOX and CARE 1978 a, 1978 b; LEE et al. 1979; FOX et al. 1981). Since low phosphorus diets stimulated the production of 1,25-dihydroxycholecalciferol (BAXTER and DELUCA 1976), it was initially considered that the effect of phosphate deficiency on intestinal phosphate absorption was mediated by the sterol hormone in a manner similar to the adaptation that occurs secondary to feeding calcium-deficient diets. However, it has been shown that the adaptation of intestinal phosphate transport occurs, at least in part, by a vitamin D-independent mechanism. Thus, RIBOVICH and DELUCA (1975) found that treatment with 1,25-dihydroxycholecalciferol did not prevent the increase in phosphate transport caused by diets low in phosphorus, whereas the adaptation to a low calcium diet could be mimicked by pretreatment with 1,25-dihydroxycholecalciferol. In a comprehensive study, CRAMER and MCMILLAN (1980) demonstrated that phosphate depletion enhanced the intestinal absorption of phosphate, even when rats were vitamin D deficient. The physiologic mechanism of adaptation was not associated with either the parathyroid or thyroid glands. As discussed in Sect. E, the vitamin D-independent mechanisms of regulating phosphate and calcium transport in the intestine are beginning to be recognized for their potential physiologic significance.

The characteristics of intestinal phosphate transport processes have been further defined recently by use of isolated preparations of brush border membrane vesicles. In experiments with vesicles from rat intestine, BERNER et al. (1976) demonstrated that phosphate uptake was a saturable process that was dependent upon an inward-directed sodium gradient. Arsenate inhibited the uptake of phosphate. K_m for phosphate was estimated to be 0.11 mM whereas K_i for arsenate was 0.34 mM. The electroneutral transport of phosphate with sodium suggested that a cotransport system was operative in vesicles of brush border. Therefore, the active transport of phosphate in vivo would appear to be dependent on the sodium gradient established by the sodium pump mechanism.

The effects of 1,25-dihydroxycholecalciferol on phosphate transport were studied using brush border vesicles from chick duodenum. Vitamin D deficiency reduced and 1,25-dihydroxycholecalciferol treatment stimulated the rate of sodium-dependent phosphate uptake (MATSUMOTO et al. 1980). K_m was unaffected by the vitamin D state (031–0.33 mM) whereas V_{max} of initial phosphate uptake was increased by the hormone from 385 to 750 pmol per milligram protein. Treatment with 1,25-dihydroxycholecalciferol in vivo increased phosphate uptake within 4 h and a maximal increase was noted within 8 h. Cycloheximide pretreatment did not prevent the increased phosphate uptake into vesicles that was caused by pretreatment of vitamin D-deficent chicks with 1,25-dihydroxycholecalciferol. The studies of FUCHS and PETERLIK (1980) also documented that vitamin D stimulates the sodium-dependent uptake of phosphate without affecting the diffusion-mediated entry of phosphate into brush border vesicles. It is apparent that phosphate transport mechanisms in the intestine are similar to those that have been described in the renal tubule (STOLL et al. 1979a, b).

From this discussion, it can be concluded that the absorption of phosphate in the intestine may occur both by passive diffusion and by a cotransport process with sodium which is secondarily active in nature. Thus, dissipation of the sodium gradient by removal of extracellular sodium, inhibition of cellular metabolism, or inhibition of the sodium pump by cardiac glycosides is associated with a reduction in the active transport of phosphate across the mucosal membrane. This membrane barrier appears to be the rate-limiting step for mucosal–serosal transfer of phosphate and is the site which is regulated by vitamin D, although vitamin D-independent regulation of phosphate absorption is thought to be physiologically significant. Vectoral transport of phosphate requires movement through the intracellular compartment followed by transfer across the basolateral membrane. Vitamin D is not thought to exert a major influence on the transfer across the basolateral membrane. It appears that phosphate transport through the enterocyte is somehow coupled or compartmentalized so that the phosphate does not readily mix with intracellular pools of phosphate. It is unlikely that alkaline phosphatase participates in the transport of phosphate per se. Moreover, it is apparent that a great deal of additional exploration is required before a satisfactory understanding of intestinal phosphate transport mechanisms is achieved.

D. Mechanism of Action of 1,25-Dihydroxycholecalciferol

A large body of data suggests that 1,25-dihydroxycholecalciferol regulates calcium absorption through a direct interaction with specific, high affinity receptor sites in the target cell. Because these receptors are soluble cytoplasmic proteins that, after combination with the hormone, are translocated to the chromatin of the nucleus, resulting in the induction of RNA and protein synthesis, we can generally describe the mechanism of action to be of the classical type attributed to steroid and thyroid hormones (for reviews see CHAN and O'MALLEY 1976; GORSKI and GANNON 1976; STERLING 1979). The current state of knowledge is, however, much more unsettled than one may derive from the relatively straightforward

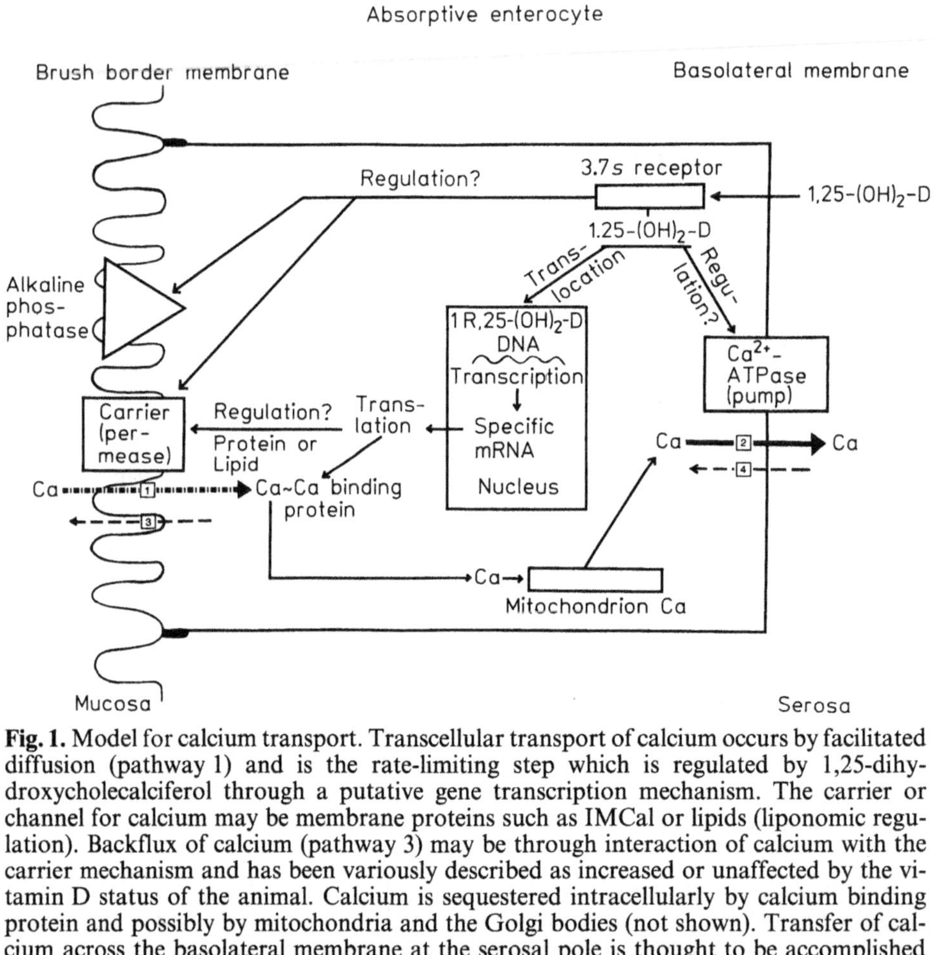

Fig. 1. Model for calcium transport. Transcellular transport of calcium occurs by facilitated diffusion (pathway 1) and is the rate-limiting step which is regulated by 1,25-dihydroxycholecalciferol through a putative gene transcription mechanism. The carrier or channel for calcium may be membrane proteins such as IMCal or lipids (liponomic regulation). Backflux of calcium (pathway 3) may be through interaction of calcium with the carrier mechanism and has been variously described as increased or unaffected by the vitamin D status of the animal. Calcium is sequestered intracellularly by calcium binding protein and possibly by mitochondria and the Golgi bodies (not shown). Transfer of calcium across the basolateral membrane at the serosal pole is thought to be accomplished by an active, energy-dependent transport mechanism (Ca^{2+}-ATPase, pathway 2) against an electrochemical gradient. Pathway 4 probably occurs by passive diffusion. Vitamin D has not been shown conclusively to regulate the Ca^{2+}-ATPase of basolateral membranes. Not shown is a putative sodium–calcium exchange mechanism which may exist and has been proposed largely from its occurrence in other ion-transporting tissues

mechanism already stated in terms of the molecular mechanism by which 1,25-dihydroxycholecalciferol regulates intestinal calcium transport. Figure 1 provides a schematic model for some of the events that appear related to the hormone's action. The following sections will provide a summary of the data that either support or refute the existence of the molecular mechanisms provided in that model.

I. Pharmacology of the Receptors for 1,25-Dihydroxycholecalciferol

The existence of soluble, cytoplasmic binding sites for vitamin D sterols is well established in the small intestine (TSAI and NORMAN 1973b; BRUMBAUGH and HAUSSLER 1974a, b; KREAM et al. 1976) as well as in other tissues that are involved in the specialized transport of calcium such as bone (CHEN et al. 1979; MANOLAGAS et al. 1979; MELLON and DELUCA 1980), placenta (PIKE et al. 1980), mammary gland (COLSTON et al. 1980; FRY et al. 1980), chick embryo chorioallantoic membrane (NARBAITZ et al. 1980; COTY et al. 1981), kidney (CHANDLER et al. 1979; COLSTON and FELDMAN 1979; CHRISTAKOS and NORMAN 1979), and the avian eggshell gland (COTY 1980). Other tissues have been shown to contain the binding proteins, notably skin, pituitary, pancreas, and parathyroid gland (NARBAITZ et al. 1980; SIMPSON and DELUCA 1980; STUMPF et al. 1979; HAUSSLER et al. 1980; PIKE et al. 1980), and furthermore macromolecules have been identified in other portions of the digestive tract such as stomach and large intestine (STUMPF et al. 1979; HIRST and FELDMAN 1981). Therefore, it is reasonable to assume that 1,25-dihydroxycholecalciferol regulates a number of cell types in addition to the generally accepted physiologic effects of the hormone on small intestine and bone. Two macromolecules have been identified that bind vitamin D sterols. The first is a 6.0 *S*, soluble protein which was isolated from the cytosol of cells (HADDAD and BIRGE 1971, 1975; COOKE et al. 1979). Although present in a variety of tissues, more recent evidence from studies with cultured cells (VAN BAELEN et al. 1977; KREAM et al. 1979) suggest that the 6.0 *S* binding protein may not be present in the cytosol, but instead is derived from the plasma vitamin D binding protein (4.1 *S*, 52,000 daltons α_1-globulin). This protein in the plasma appears to play a role in the binding and transport of 25-hydroxy- and 24,25-dihydroxycholecalciferol in the circulation. Thus, we can view this plasma protein in an analogous fashion to other hormone binding (transport) proteins in the plasma which bind steroid and thyroid hormones and describe the protein as an acceptor for those vitamin D metabolites. The binding specificity (HADDAD and WALGATE 1976) and immunoreactivity (KREAM et al. 1979; COOKE et al. 1979) of the 4.1 *S* acceptor relative to the 6.0 *S* cytosolic binding protein are consistent with this view. Whether the acceptor protein is involved in the transfer of 25-hydroxycholecalciferol and/or 24,25-dihydroxycholecalciferol across cell membranes remains an open question. This acceptor protein has been successfully used as the detector for a radioreceptor assay of 25-hydroxy- and 24,25-dihydroxycholecalciferol (BELSEY et al. 1971; HADDAD and CHYU 1971).

The second vitamin D binding protein is also found in cytosol of a number of tissues, is approximately 3.5 *S* (variously described as 3.1–3.7 *S*) when isolated on sucrose gradients, and exhibits high affinity and specificity for 1,25-dihydroxycholecalciferol relative to other vitamin D metabolites (for review see FRANCESCHI et al. 1981). Based on these characteristics and the knowledge that the binding protein when complexed with 1,25-dihydroxycholecalciferol is translocated to nuclear chromatin (TSAI et al. 1972; BRUMBAUGH and HAUSSLER 1974a; STUMPF et al. 1979) with subsequent induction of RNA and protein synthesis (TSAI and NORMAN 1973a; ZERWEKH et al. 1976; TAYLOR and WASSERMAN 1967), it is appropriate to describe the 3.5 *S* protein as a receptor for 1,25-dihydroxycholecalciferol. However, suggesting that this macromolecule is *the* receptor for 1,25-dihydroxycholecalciferol that regulates intestinal calcium transport per se is premature as will become apparent from the state of knowledge summarized in Sect. D.II.

It is worthwhile to consider the pharmacologic characteristics of the cytosolic receptor (affinity, specificity, etc.) in relation to the effects of a series of hydroxy metabolites of vitamin D on intestinal calcium absorption or in some instances the formation of calcium binding protein, which is considered as one gene product induced by 1,25-dihydroxycholecalciferol (TAYLOR and WASSERMAN 1967). In general, the relative potency of vitamin D metabolites in the regulation of calcium transport correlates well with the relative affinities of the metabolites as competing ligands in the radioreceptor assay using the intestinal receptor (cytosol) preparations. Data in Table 1 illustrate the relative specificity of avian and mammalian intestinal receptors for 1,25-dihydroxycholecalciferol in terms of the potency of vitamin D metabolites for competition with radiolabeled 1,25-dihydroxycholecalciferol (IC_{50} molar ratio). It is readily clear that this macromolecule exhibits receptor-like specificity for binding with 1,25-dihydroxycholecalciferol in comparison with its very low affinity for binding the precursor sterols and other metabolites or drugs which have been used as vitamin D-like agents (i.e., dihydrotachysterol). Of interest is the marked increase in potency of dihydrotachysterol when hydroxylated in the C-25 position. Such an increase in apparent affinity provides an explanation for the pharmacologic efficacy of dihydrotachysterol as a structural analog of vitamin D_3. This drug is hydroxylated in vivo at the C-25 position by the hepatic enzyme responsible for hydroxylation of cholecalciferol to 25-hydroxycholecalciferol (LAWSON and BELL 1974; HALLICK and DELUCA 1972). It should be pointed out that the potency of a series of structural analog of cholecalciferol provide information of the structure–activity relationship for binding to this putative receptor, but do not necessarily invoke a correlated potency of the drugs relative to their efficacy as regulators of intestinal calcium absorption. However, the order of potency of these drugs as competitors for receptor binding, in general, correlates with their potency as stimulators of calcium transport. Where differences in this relationship have been found will be discussed in a later section.

The equilibrium dissociation constant K_d of labeled 1,25-dihydroxycholecalciferol binding to the intestinal receptor has been estimated using the Scatchard analysis (SCATCHARD 1949). MELLON and DELUCA (1979), using a high specific activity radioligand (106 Ci/mmol), prepared enzymatically from 25-hydroxycholecalciferol tritium labeled at C-26 and C-27 using the renal 25-hydroxycholecalciferol-1-hydroxylase, demonstrated that chick intestinal receptors had a K_d of 71 p*M* and a concentration of binding sites B_{max} of 0.16 pmol per mil-

Table 1. Specificity of intestinal receptors for 1,25-dihydroxycholecalciferol IC_{50} molar ratio [a]

Analog	
Chick intestinal cytosol – chromatin receptor system [b]	
Unlabeled 1,25-$(OH)_2$-D_3	1
3-Deoxy-1,25-$(OH)_2$-D_3	1
25-OH-D_3	900
1-OH-D_3	900
24R,25-$(OH)_2$-D_3	5,000
24S,25-$(OH)_2$-D_3	5,000
D_3	> 10,000
25-OH-Dihydrotachysterol	90
Dihydrotachysterol	> 10,000
Rat intestinal cytosol receptor system [c]	
1,25-$(OH)_2$-D_3	1
25-OH-D_3	100
1-OH-D_3	333
24R,25-$(OH)_2$-D_3	500
Dihydrotachysterol	> 1,000
D_3	> 1,000

[a] The proportion of unlabeled drug to radioactive ligand required for half-maximal inhibition of binding of tritium-labeled 1,25-$(OH)_2$-D_3

[b] Data taken from PROCSAL et al. (1975); labeled 1,25-$(OH)_2$-D concentration in the radioceptor assay was 20 n*M*

[c] Data taken from FELDMAN et al. (1979); labeled 1,25-$(OH)_2$-D concentration in the radioceptor assay was 1.3 n*M*

ligram protein. They estimated 1,800 binding sites per cell to be present in chick intestine. Other investigators, using lower specific activity radioligand found higher K_d values (lower affinity). For example, BRUMBAUGH and HAUSSLER (1974 a) found a K_d of 2.2 n*M* and TSAI and NORMAN (1973 b) found a K_a of 5.3×10^{10} and binding site density of 5.8 pmol per milligram protein. These absolute values for K_d and B_{max} are difficult to compare between laboratories owing to methodological differences both in the preparation of receptor fractions and the specific activities of radioligands used in vitro. The mammalian intestinal receptor has equivalent high affinity. FELDMAN et al. (1979) reported a K_d of 0.47 n*M* and B_{max} of 445 fmol per milligram protein and WECKSLER et al. (1979) found a K_d of 0.74 n*M* in rat intestinal cytosol preparations. Thus, a generalization can be made that the cytosolic binding sites demonstrate appropriately high affinity, consistent with their putative role as receptors for the hormone, 1,25-dihydroxycholecalciferol. The properties of this receptor have provided the means for assaying plasma and tissue levels of 1,25-dihydroxycholecalciferol using a radioreceptor assay technique (BRUMBAUGH et al. 1974; EISMAN et al. 1976).

Corradino developed a convenient in vitro bioassay for vitamin D sterols using cultured chick embryo duodenum (CORRADINO and WASSERMAN 1971; CORRADINO 1973 a, b, c). This tissue responds appropriately to the hormones by increasing its calcium uptake (CORRADINO 1973a, 1974), probably at the mucosal surface (CORRADINO 1978), and by enhanced mucosal–serosal transport of calcium (CORRADINO et al. 1976). FRANCESCHI and DELUCA (1981a) used this bioassay to demonstrate a saturable calcium uptake response to 1,25-dihydroxycholecalciferol (K*m* for calcium 0.45 m*M*). They studied the pharmacology of cholecalciferol and its hydroxymetabolites using the calcium uptake response in cultured duodenum and related the potency of these compounds to apparent receptor affinity. All of the sterols tested were found to be full agonists with *estimated* effective concentrations for half-maximal increases in calcium uptake (EC_{50}) of: 1,25-dihydroxycholecalciferol $3 \times 10^{-9} M$; 1-hydroxycholecalciferol $2 \times 10^{-8} M$; 25-hydroxycholecalciferol $6 \times 10^{-7} M$; 24R,25-dihydroxycholecalciferol $1.5 \times 10^{-6} M$; and cholecalciferol $3.5 \times 10^{-6} M$. It was of interest that these dose–response relationships did not correlate with the effectiveness of the sterols as competitors with 1,25-dihydroxycholecalciferol in the intestinal radioreceptor assay using cytosol from embryonic duodenum. For example, 1-hydroxy- and 25-hydroxycholecalciferol were equivalently effective in the receptor assay whereas cholecalciferol exhibited no activity, even at a molar ratio of 40,000:1 over the radioligand (1,25-dihydroxycholecalciferol $K_d = 85$ pM, $B_{max} = 86$ fmol per milligram protein). These data demonstrated the considerable difficulty that is encountered when tissue or cell bioassay results are compared with the radioreceptor assay data. An explanation for the surprising effectiveness of cholecalciferol in stimulating calcium uptake may be that intestine hydroxylates cholecalciferol (TUCKER et al. 1973; KUMAR et al. 1978) sufficiently to account for the efficacy of the precursor sterol in this in vitro bioassay, although CORRADINO (1973c) was unable to demonstrate the formation of hydroxy metabolites by this tissue in vitro. The transfer of these drugs across the enterocyte plasma membrane may be different, thus explaining this apparent discrepancy. However, the possibility that alternate cellular mechanisms exist for cholecalciferol-mediated regulation of calcium transport other than that postulated to be mediated via cytosolic receptors should not be discounted. It is possible that alternate receptors for vitamin D compounds may occur in the intestine which exhibit the required affinity for cholecalciferol. Moreover, it is conceivable that such receptor sites may not be cytosolic, but could be membrane-bound receptors. No clear evidence for this type of receptor currently exists.

II. Regulation of Transport Mediated by a Nuclear Action of Vitamin D

Using biochemical techniques, the nuclear localization of 1,25-dihydroxycholecalciferol has been demonstrated. The sterol–receptor complex, like other steroid hormone–cytosolic receptor complexes, appears to be translocated from the cytoplasm to the nucleus by a temperature-dependent process (BRUMBAUGH and HAUSSLER 1974b), with subsequent enhancement of chromatin template activity (ZERWEKH et al. 1976). Thus, association of the 1,25-dihydroxycholecalciferol–receptor complex with nuclear chromatin stimulates RNA polymerase (ZERWEKH et al. 1974), leading to translation of specific messenger RNA which in turn codes for protein synthesis. That both RNA and protein synthesis are induced by 1,25-

dihydroxycholecalciferol in the intestine appears to be well established. Nuclear localization of 1,25-dihydroxycholecalciferol has also been demonstrated in vivo using autoradiography (STUMPF et al. 1979). Not only intestine exhibits nuclear localization when labeled 1,25-dihydroxycholecalciferol is administered in vivo, a number of other tissues including stomach, kidney, skin, pituitary, and parathyroid exhibit preferential nuclear localization of the label (STUMPF et al. 1979, 1980). Presumably, these tissues, notably kidney, are also target tissues for the sterol hormone, although precise physiologic regulatory events have not been clearly established in these tissues.

It would seem that the molecular mechanism of action of 1,25-dihydroxycholecalciferol in regulating intestinal calcium transport is well established according to the classical model for steroid hormones per se. At least one gene product has been demonstrated, i.e., vitamin D-dependent calcium binding protein. However, the evidence for this protein playing a primary role in calcium transport is relatively weak, as discussed in a later section. Moreover, it appears that the primary regulatory event in 1,25-dihydroxycholecalciferol-mediated calcium transport is an increase in the permeability of the brush border membrane to calcium (carrier-mediated passive influx). A great deal of controversy currently exists regarding the mechanism by which this hormone regulates calcium transport. The suggestion has been made that the increased permeability of the brush border membrane to calcium subsequent to exposure of the tissue to 1,25-dihydroxycholecalciferol is *not* dependent on RNA and protein synthesis, whereas the active transport of calcium out of the cell via the basolateral membrane may be dependent on RNA and protein synthesis (for review see BIKLE et al. 1981). Unfortunately, much of the data supporting the notion that the sterol hormone regulates mucosal permeability to calcium independent of RNA and protein synthesis are derived from pharmacologic studies. Inhibitors of RNA or protein synthesis have been shown to inhibit at least in part, the synthesis of RNA and protein (calcium binding protein) in the intestine without blocking the vitamin D-mediated increase in calcium transport in vivo or in vitro (BIKLE et al. 1978; RASMUSSEN et al. 1979). It is also argued that the temporal relationship between the vitamin D-stimulated RNA and protein synthesis and calcium transport are inconsistent with a precursor–product relationship (MORRISSEY et al. 1978a). Increased calcium flux is often observed substantially before the changes in RNA and protein synthesis can be measured. Moreover, calcium influx into mucosal cells occurs rapidly following exposure to 1,25-dihydroxycholecalciferol and accumulation of excess calcium in the cells may occur, even when inhibitors of transcription or translation are concurrently present (MORRISSEY et al. 1977). Thus, it seems plausible that the classical mechanism of action for steroid hormones may be extended to the sequestration (calcium binding protein) and perhaps to the active transport of calcium (Ca^{2+}-ATPase), but not to the regulation of brush border membrane permeability to calcium.

Such a view is, however, inconsistent with all of the available data, since the results of a number of investigations supported the idea that vitamin D- or 1,25-dihydroxycholecalciferol-stimulated calcium uptake or transport by mucosal cells is indeed blocked by inhibitors of RNA or of protein synthesis (NORMAN 1965; ZULL et al. 1965; CORRADINO 1973b; FRANCESCHI and DELUCA 1981b).

Moreover, the use of actinomycin D, cycloheximide, or other drugs of this type in vivo to block intestinal RNA and protein synthesis is fraught with difficulty. The toxicities of such drugs are too great to use at in vivo doses that substantially block RNA or protein synthesis. Therefore, interpreting data showing modest (25%–40%) inhibition of synthesis with no blockade of vitamin D-stimulated calcium transport (BIKLE et al. 1978) must be carried out with more than a little trepidation. Studies by CORRADINO and co-workers and reports from DELUCA's laboratory using the chick embryo duodenal preparation in organ culture provided data which demonstrated that inhibitors of either RNA or protein synthesis blocked the 1,25-dihydroxycholecalciferol-stimulated calcium uptake by the tissue (CORRADINO 1973b, 1974, 1979a; CORRADINO and WASSERMAN 1974; FRANCESCHI and DELUCA 1981b). The reports by CORRADINO of this type have been weakened by the critique that long-term exposure (24–48 h) of the duodenal tissue to actinomycin D or cycloheximide (or similar drugs) would be expected to have toxic effects on the mucosal absorptive cell (FRANCESCHI and DELUCA 1981b; BIKLE et al. 1981). Thus, blockade of the physiologic effects of the sterol hormone on calcium transport might be indirectly related to the primary pharmacologic effects of these inhibitors of transcription and translation and not a direct result of the blockade of cellular RNA and protein synthesis.

FRANCESCHI and DELUCA (1981b) carried out a careful study of the concentration–response and time–response characteristics of embryonic duodenum when exposed to these inhibitors with the objective of selecting doses of the RNA synthesis inhibitors (actinomycin D, α-amanitin) or protein synthesis inhibitors (cycloheximide, anisomycin) that inhibited synthesis of RNA or protein without producing overt toxic effects on the tissue. They found that cycloheximide (5 μM) was capable of inhibiting protein synthesis by about 70% and the effects were reversible, whereas actinomycin D at 5 μM produced approximately 50% inhibition of RNA synthesis. Moreover, actinomycin D was clearly toxic to the tissue in view of the marked decrease in tissue weight and irreversible effects of the antibiotic on calcium uptake. Both drugs effectively blocked the 1,25-dihydroxycholecalciferol-stimulated calcium uptake. Removal of cycloheximide from the medium allowed the effect of the sterol to be quantitatively similar to the effect on tissue that had been exposed only to the hormone and no inhibitor. This was not true for actinomycin D since only about one-half of the control calcium uptake response to 1,25-dihydroxycholecalciferol was found when actinomycin D was removed from the medium. Evidently, actinomycin D produced irreversible effects on cellular function within the conditions of these experiments. The conclusions from this study by FRANCESCHI and DELUCA (1981b), were that RNA and protein synthesis were required for the expression of 1,25-dihydroxycholecalciferol action on calcium uptake by small intestine. Since this uptake is presumed to be due to increased permeability of the brush border membrane to calcium, then the primary regulatory event of this hormone in the absorptive enterocyte may be through the classical gene regulation mechanism.

As previously mentioned, the interpretation of data obtained with inhibitors of RNA or protein synthesis suffers from the lack of specificity of the drugs. A more specific drug, which blocks only the 1,25-dihydroxycholecalciferol-induced RNA and protein synthesis without interfering with other initial metabolic events in the intestine would be a valuable aid in studies of the type described in this section. An example is a competitive antagonist of 1,25-dihydroxycholecalciferol, which would be an excellent pharmacologic tool for studying the hypothesis that this hormone regulates calcium transport by induction of RNA and protein synthesis. Unfortunately, there is no effective antagonist of this sort presently available.

In contrast to these reports, BIKLE et al. (1978) and RASMUSSEN et al. (1979) reported that cycloheximide treatment in vivo in the chick did not block the vitamin D-stimulated level of calcium transport. BIKLE et al. (1978) used the ligated intestinal loop technique for assessing calcium transport, whereas RASMUSSEN et al. (1979) utilized a brush border membrane preparation (vesicles) for measuring calcium uptake which was developed in his laboratory (MAX et al. 1978). Intestinal protein synthesis was stimulated by 1,25-dihydroxycholecalciferol about 2- to 3-fold (BIKLE et al. 1978) and cycloheximide treatment effectively blocked the stimulation of protein synthesis due to the sterol hormone. Of interest were the data obtained on intestinal calcium transport. These investigators found that 1,25-dihydroxycholecalciferol stimulated calcium transport from a control value of 1.52 ± 0.33 (mean $\pm$ standard error) to 3.96 ± 0.26 nmol per milligram protein. The value for calcium transport in the presence of both cycloheximide and 1,25-dihydroxycholecalciferol was 4.31 ± 0.72, which was no different from that due to 1,25-dihydroxycholecalciferol alone. On the other hand, there was an apparent increase in calcium transport by cycloheximide alone (2.88 ± 0.34 nmol/mg). Thus, the increase in calcium transport due to 1,25-dihydroxycholecalciferol was 2.44 nmol/mg whereas that due to the sterol hormone in the presence of cycloheximide was 1.43 nmol/mg (sterol+cycloheximide) minus the cycloheximide control. Based on this rationale, the authors' interpretation that inhibition of protein synthesis by cycloheximide in chick intestine does not result in blockade of calcium transport is not at all clear from these data. BIKLE et al. (1978), also found that actinomycin D did not block the hormone-mediated increase in intestinal calcium transport, but the measured inhibition of RNA synthesis in the absence of 1,25-dihydroxycholecalciferol by this antibiotic was only about 24%. RASMUSSEN et al. (1979) used the same in vivo treatment protocol with cycloheximide as that reported by BIKLE et al. (1978) in an attempt to block the vitamin D-stimulated (in vivo treatment) calcium uptake into brush border vesicles isolated from chick intestine. This study showed that cycloheximide did not block the calcium uptake that was stimulated by the hormone. Since the same cycloheximide treatment protocol was employed in these two studies, this criticism may be applied to the data reported by RASMUSSEN et al. (1979). Thus, from this discussion and the contradictory data reported by FRANCESCHI and DELUCA (1981 b), it is evident that a controversy exists whether or not 1,25-dihydroxycholecalciferol or the parent sterols do indeed regulate intestinal calcium transport (brush border permeability) by the classical gene transcription mechanism. Further experiments will be required to clarify this situation.

III. Regulation of Lipid Metabolism by Vitamin D

An alternate hypothesis for the mechanism of action of 1,25-dihydroxycholecalciferol has recently been proposed (FONTAINE et al. 1981), which stipulates that the regulation of calcium permeability by the hormone at the level of the brush border membrane is accomplished by alteration of specific lipids in the membrane (liponomic control). The observations supporting this hypothesis are: (a) filipin, which interacts with membrane cholesterol, has been shown to enhance calcium uptake in brush border vesicles only in the membranes isolated from vitamin D-deficient chicks (RASMUSSEN et al. 1979); (b) 1,25-dihydroxycholecalciferol stimulates phosphatidylcholine synthesis and alters the fatty acid structure of the phospholipids (MATSUMOTO et al. 1981); and (c) fluidization of brush border membranes by incorporation of *cis*-vaccenic acid in vitro is associated with enhanced calcium uptake into brush border vesicles isolated from vitamin D-deficient, but not D-replete chicks (FONTAINE et al. 1981). Taken as a whole, these studies suggest that the alteration of specific phospholipids by the sterol hormone in vivo may be the mechanism whereby 1,25-dihydroxycholecalciferol exerts its primary regulation of calcium transport through an increase in permeability of the brush border membrane (RASMUSSEN et al. 1982). It was suggested that RNA and protein synthesis was not required for these lipid regulatory and calcium uptake events since cycloheximide treatment in vivo did not block the hormone-mediated changes in either the membrane lipids or calcium uptake (RASMUSSEN et al. 1979). Addition of 1,25-dihydroxycholecalciferol to the brush border membranes in vitro was ineffective, suggesting the sterol did not produce these effects by a direct action on the membrane per se. The criticisms discussed in the previous sections also apply in this experiment regarding the interpretation of cycloheximide effects on this system. However, it should be emphasized that this hypothesis for the molecular mechanism of action of 1,25-dihydroxycholecalciferol is indeed attractive in view of the recent developments in our understanding of how modification of membrane lipids can alter the function of membrane proteins. It is reasonable to consider that the increased fluidity (microviscosity) of critical lipid–protein domains in the brush border membrane could regulate the passive influx of calcium down its electrochemical gradient by a mechanism that may or may not involve the transcription of genetic information and synthesis of protein molecules that could be intimately involved in this process.

IV. Calcium Binding Proteins

As previously discussed, the molecular mechanism of vitamin D action is thought to be through the classical type of regulation exemplified by steroid hormones. Thus, in the intestine, one or more proteins may be induced either by enhanced messenger RNA synthesis or through a modification of the translation of the message at the level of protein synthesis. A number of vitamin D-dependent proteins have been described in the intestinal mucosa and the best characterized is calcium binding protein. This putative gene product, resulting from the expression of hormonal regulation by 1,25-dihydroxycholecalciferol was first described by TAYLOR and WASSERMAN (1966) in chick intestine. They demonstrated that rachitic chicks have nondetectable levels of calcium binding protein and that treatment of the vitamin D-deficient chick with vitamin D_3 markedly increased the intestinal content of this protein (TAYLOR and WASSERMAN 1967).

Intestinal, vitamin D-dependent calcium binding protein may be classified as one of the low molecular weight, soluble (cytoplasmic) proteins in cells that exhibit relatively high affinity for calcium and appear to be involved in calcium-dependent regulation of cellular processes. Examples of other proteins with similar characteristics are calmodulin and troponin (CHEUNG 1980). Intestinal calcium binding protein in the chick is approximately 28,000 daltons (WASSERMAN et al. 1968) whereas the mammalian calcium binding protein is about 10,000 daltons (DRESCHER and DELUCA 1971; FULLMER and WASSERMAN 1973; BRUNS et al. 1977). The affinity of this protein for binding calcium has been reported to be consistent with the intracellular levels of free calcium. Calcium binding protein from chick intestine was shown to have an equilibrium dissociation constant of 0.5 μM and 4 mol calcium were bound for every 1 mol protein (BREDDERMAN and WASSERMAN 1974), whereas the protein from rat intestine has been reported to have a dissociation constant for calcium of 0.3 μM in one report (BRUNS et al. 1977) and 1.4–1.9 μM in another investigation (FREUND and BRONNER 1975a). A binding capacity of about 2 mol calcium for every 1 mol intestinal calcium binding protein was shown in the rat (BRUNS et al. 1977). The protein from bovine intestine has been crystallized and studied by X-ray diffraction (SZEBENYI et al. 1981). They showed that the protein contained four helices and the approximate molecular dimensions were 25 × 30 × 30 Å.

The calcium binding property of this protein has been used successfully as a means of quantifying the content of this protein for bioassay of the physiologic effects of vitamin D. Such an assay is, of course, limited by its lack of specificity and relative insensitivity. The apparent disappearance of intestinal calcium binding protein in the vitamin D-deficient animal has been shown to be due to a decrease in the protein below the limits of detectability by the calcium binding assay technique. More recently, a radioimmunoassay was developed for the calcium binding protein which has higher sensitivity for measurement of calcium binding protein and is also more specific for that molecular entity (TAYLOR and WASSERMAN 1970; CORRADINO and WASSERMAN 1971; TAYLOR and WASSERMAN 1972).

It should be stressed that calcium binding proteins with characteristics similar to those described have been found in a variety of tissues other than intestine. Moreover, as described in Sect. D.I, specific receptors for 1,25-dihydroxycholecalciferol are commonly found in tissues containing calcium binding protein. This suggests that this calcitropic sterol hormone may exert physiologic regulation of calcium and/or phosphate transport in a broad fashion. Examples of tissues where calcium binding protein has been demonstrated are bone (CHRISTAKOS and NORMAN 1978), kidney (TAYLOR and WASSERMAN 1967), parathyroid gland (OLDHAM et al. 1974), brain (TAYLOR 1974a), skin (LAOUARI et al. 1980), avian eggshell gland (CORRADINO et al. 1968; BAR and HURWITZ 1973), and placenta (BRUNS et al. 1978). With the exception of brain, it is readily apparent that these tissues, like intestine, are intimately involved in either the specialized transport of calcium necessary for calcium homeostasis or in the endocrine regulation of calcium homeostasis. However, the dependency of these calcium binding proteins on vitamin D remains controversial. For example, the calcium binding protein of the parathyroid gland was shown to increase in vitamin D-deficient dogs (OLDHAM et al. 1980) and the protein in kidney has been described both as dependent (TAYLOR and WASSERMAN 1967, 1972; HERMSDORF and BRONNER 1975) and independent (RHOTEN and CHRISTAKOS 1981) of the vitamin D status of the animal. A finding of potential relevance to intestinal transport of calcium is that estrogen treatment increases the content of calcium binding protein of the chicken eggshell gland (uterus) presumably in association with enhanced calcium transport during the reproductive cycle (NAVICKIS et al. 1979). Thus, estrogen, as suspected from the high incidence of osteoporosis in the postmenopausal state, may conceivably be an important regulator of intestinal calcium transport in the mammal, although direct evidence is not available to support a putative role for estrogen in this regard. An increase in the intestinal calcium binding protein in avian species is clearly correlated with enhanced calcium absorption during the egg-laying period (BAR and HURWITZ 1972, 1973; BAR et al. 1976). Estrogen may regulate intestinal levels of calcium binding proteins and calcium transport indirectly through a mechanism that involves an increase in the 25-hydroxycholecalciferol-1-hydroxylase of kidney (KENNEY 1976; SPANOS et al. 1978; CASTILLO ET AL. 1977. BAR and HURWITZ 1979). The increased synthesis and elevated circulating levels of 1,25-dihydroxycholecalciferol under the influence of estrogen provides a plausible mechanism of action for the sex steroid's regulation of intestinal calcium transport in the avian species. An alternate view is that the increased calcium demand during reproduction in birds regulates the renal synthesis of 1,25-dihydroxycholecalciferol independent of changes in estrogen levels (BAR et al. 1978a, b).

Although intestinal calcium binding protein formation is regulated by 1,25-dihydroxycholecalciferol, the requirement or role of this protein relative to vitamin D-mediated control of calcium transport is presently controversial. A predominant reason is that the temporal relationship between the appearance of vitamin D-dependent calcium binding protein (i.e., synthesis) and the increase in intestinal calcium transport is inconsistent with the notion that this protein is required for vitamin D stimulation of calcium absorption (HARMEYER and DELUCA 1969). Studies in the chicken (MORIUCHI and DELUCA 1976; SPENCER et al. 1976; MORRISSEY et al. 1978a) and rat (THOMASSET et al. 1979) revealed that 1,25-dihydroxycholecalciferol treatment in vivo in vitamin D-deficient animals caused a marked increase in calcium transport (everted gut sac in vitro, duodenal loops in situ) that preceded a significant increase in calcium binding protein content of the intestinal mucosa. For example, MORRISSEY et al. (1978a) found a significant increase in duodenal calcium transport 2.5 h after an oral dose of 1.0 μg 1,25-dihydroxycholecalciferol in the vitamin D-deficient chick. A measurable increase in calcium binding protein was found 5 h after hormonal treatment. THOMASSET et al. (1979) extended this finding to the rat. A plausible conclusion is that calcium binding protein synthesis is subsequent to vitamin D-stimulated calcium transport and therefore the protein may play a role as a "calcium acceptor" for intracellular calcium. This suggests that calcium binding protein is not a carrier molecule in transmembrane calcium transport, but may be involved in the intracellular regulation of calcium levels in the enterocyte. The equilibrium dissociation constant for calcium binding (approximately 1 μM) is consistent with such a role of calcium binding protein as is the increased level of calcium binding protein observed when extracellular calcium is increased in vitro (CORRADINO 1973 a).

Other investigators have found a better correlation between the formation of calcium binding protein and the increased calcium transport after treatment with 1,25-dihydroxycholecalciferol. WASSERMAN et al. (1977) found an increase in calcium binding protein as early as 2 h after sterol treatment in the chick. Using intestinal cells isolated from the vitamin D-deficient rat duodenum, FREUND and BRONNER (1975 a) demonstrated that $4.7 \times 10^{-8} M$ 1,25-dihydroxycholecalciferol (but not 25-hydroxycholecalciferol) stimulated calcium uptake 2.6-fold after 90 min exposure to the active sterol. They also found an increase in cellular levels of calcium binding protein after 90 min exposure to $4.7 \times 10^{-8} M$ 1,25-dihydroxycholecalciferol. This is one of the earliest responses reported and may reflect the experimental technique of studying the isolated mucosal cell directly in comparison with other studies in vivo or with the everted gut sac technique. It is of interest that a better temporal relationship between the appearance of calcium binding protein and enhanced calcium transport exists in the vitamin D-replete rat than in the vitamin D-deficient animal (BUCKLEY and BRONNER 1980). Thus, in vitamin D-replete animals, 1,25-dihydroxycholecalciferol treatment in vivo increased calcium binding protein two fold by 1 h whereas a maximum response in the vitamin D-deficient rat was not observed until 16–20 h, although the magnitude of change in calcium binding protein content was substantially greater. These investigators speculated that 1,25-dihydroxycholecalciferol may exert its action at either the translational or posttranslational level in addition to stimulating messenger RNA synsthesis. Such an effect may explain the rapid increase in the intestinal content of calcium binding protein since the vitamin D-replete animal would be expected to have the transcribed message readily available for translation. It should be pointed out that the temporal relationship between the decay of both vitamin D-stimulated calcium transport and the levels of calcium binding protein are also inconsistent with the interpretation that this protein is required for calcium transport (MORRISEY et al. 1978 a; THOMASSET et al. 1979).

Additional experimental data that further weakens the case for calcium binding protein was provided by BIKLE et al. (1978). They demonstrated that treatment of rachitic chicks with either actinomycin D or cycloheximide blocked the induction of calcium binding protein synthesis by vitamin D without inhibiting intestinal calcium transport (isolated intestinal loop technique). On the surface, these data support the conclusion that 1,25-dihydroxycholecalciferol does not regulate calcium transport by a specific transcriptional mechanism. However, in other investigations it was shown that inhibition of RNA or protein synthesis in the isolated, embryonic chick intestine in vitro did block the stimulation of calcium transport by 1,25-dihydroxycholecalciferol (CORRADINO 1973 b, 1974, 1979 a; FRANCESCHI and DELUCA 1981 b). CORRADINO (1973 b) reported that actinomycin D, 2 µg/ml, which inhibited RNA synthesis by greater than 90% in vitro, blocked both the calcium binding protein and calcium transport (uptake) responses to 1,25-dihydroxycholecalciferol. Thus, taking the data currently available as whole, it seems that the soluble, cytoplasmic calcium binding protein may not be required for 1,25-dihydroxycholecalciferol to stimulate intestinal calcium transport, yet the protein is clearly the best available candidate for a gene product that is induced by the sterol hormone in vivo. That regulation of intestinal content of calcium binding protein is influenced by other factors such as age and nutritional status (calcium intake) (Freund and Bronner 1975b; Bruns et al. 1977) suggests that this protein may not be controlled only by the vitamin D–endocrine mechanism per se.

Bronner et al. (1982) reviewed the data that support a correlation between intestinal content of calcium binding protein and calcium transport and concluded that a positive correlation was observed. They further demonstrated that rats fed either a high calcium, vitamin D-deficient or a low calcium, vitamin D-replete diet both exhibited a delayed response to 1,25-dihydroxycholecalciferol (i.e., 8 h) whereas rats fed a high calcium, vitamin D-replete diet showed a brisk increase in the content of calcium binding protein by 30 min. It was concluded that vitamin D deficiency retarded this intestinal response to the hormone. Using isolated duodenal cells, Bronner and co-workers demonstrated that the increased calcium binding response to 1,25-dihydroxycholecalciferol could be blocked by cycloheximide but not by actinomycin. They suggested that the increase in calcium binding protein synthesis observed in animals fed a high calcium, vitamin D-replete diet occurred rapidly through an enhancement of translation of existing mRNA and the slower response in other animals required both transcriptional and translational processes. It was of interest that isolated duodenal cells exhibited a temporal relationship in regard to vitamin D-stimulated calcium uptake that correlated reasonably well with the changes in content of calcium binding protein.

The controversy surrounding the role of 1,25-dihydroxycholecalciferol induction of RNA and protein (i.e., calcium binding protein) synthesis as a requirement for the effects of the hormone on intestinal calcium transport has been addressed in an attempt to clarify the situation. Walling and Kimberg (1975) demonstrated, using the Ussing technique, that mucosal–serosal calcium flux increased in a biphasic manner to a single dose of 270 ng 1,25-dihydroxycholecalciferol administered to vitamin D-deficient rats. The first peak in calcium transport occurred at 6 h, followed by a decrease at 12 h and then a gradual prolonged increase in transport from 12 to 96 h. They suggested that the initial response to the hormone was due to enhanced transport in existing cells of the villus whereas the prolonged response was due to an action of 1,25-dihydroxycholecalciferol in new cells forming at the base of the villus and subsequently migrating to the villus tip. This biphasic response has been confirmed using the everted gut sac by Halloran and DeLuca (1981b). It was concluded that the increased synthesis of calcium binding protein correlated with the second, prolonged peak of increased calcium transport which may explain some of the discordant opinions regarding either the correlation or lack of correlation between the stimulation of calcium transport and appearance of calcium binding protein found in the literature (DeLuca et al. 1982). Such an interpretation is supported by the studies that demonstrated the appearance of calcium binding protein in cells at the base of the villus 6–8 h after treatment with 1,25-dihydroxycholecalciferol. By 18 h, the protein was detectable throughout the villus length (Morrissey et al. 1978b). It is conceivable that this biphasic calcium transport to vitamin D may also contribute to the discrepancies previously discussed in regard to the effects of inhibitors of RNA and or protein synthesis on this action of the hormone.

V. Membrane-Bound Calcium Binding Protein

A vitamin D-dependent calcium binding protein has also been described as an integral membrane protein of mucosal cells (KOWARSKI and SCHACHTER 1975, 1980; SCHACHTER and KOWARSKI 1982). The earliest studies reported that a high molecular weight component of mucosal cell membranes, termed "calcium binding complex," was of physiologic significance because this intestinal activity was greater in the duodenum than jejunum, decreased by vitamin D deficiency, enhanced by treatment of vitamin D-deficient rats with vitamin D, increased by a calcium-deficient diet, and decreased in the aged animal relative to young rats. All are consistent with the direction of changes previously observed for intestinal calcium transport under those conditions. In addition, cycloheximide pretreatment prevented the vitamin D stimulation of calcium binding activity and this complex was shown to occur in brush border membranes. In a subsequent study, KOWARSKI and SCHACHTER (1980) demonstrated that the calcium binding complex also contained calcium-dependent ATPase and *p*-nitrophenylphosphatase activities. However, the enzymatic activities were resolved from the calcium binding complex by DEAE-cellulose and hydroxylapatite chromatography when solubilized from the membranes using either *n*-butanol or Triton X-100. The apparent molecular weight was about 200,000 and SDS electrophoresis revealed that the complex could be dissociated to monomers of molecular weight 20,500. In contrast, the cytosolic calcium binding protein exhibited a different electrophoretic mobility (11,500 daltons) and the relative affinities (for calcium) of the two proteins were different. Of interest was the finding that the membrane protein had a K_d for calcium of 0.37 μM whereas the soluble calcium binding protein had a K_d of 2.25 μM. Clearly, the affinity of the membrane calcium binding protein is within the range to be considered physiologically significant. KOWARSKI and SCHACHTER (1980) termed the protein IMCal for intestinal membrane calcium binding protein.

MORIUCHI and DELUCA (1976) have also described a high molecular weight membrane protein (i.e., 230,000 daltons) which appears in the brush border membranes following treatment with 1,25-dihydroxycholecalciferol. This protein had both calcium binding and alkaline phosphatase activities and could be solubilized with *n*-butanol. The protein in membranes from vitamin D-deficient chick intestine did not have calcium binding activity and appeared to be smaller (i.e., 200,000 daltons). MILLER et al. (1979) described a calcium binding protein that was associated with brush border membranes but was not an intrinsic membrane protein. Its molecular weight was 18,500 and enhancement of its activity by vitamin D was quite variable. FEHER and WASSERMAN (1978) found the cytosolic calcium binding protein of chick intestine was associated with membranes and released from membranes by Triton X-100. The physiologic significance of this finding remains unclear. The protein (IMCal) described by KOWARSKI and SCHACHTER (1980) was shown not to be the cytosolic calcium binding protein by its electrophoretic mobility, affinity for binding calcium, and by differences in amino acid composition between IMCal and cytosolic calcium binding protein. SCHACHTER and KOWARSKI (1982) concluded that IMCal may conceivably be a component of the brush border membrane that serves as the calcium channel (carrier, permease) that is regulated by vitamin D, resulting in the enhancement of facilitated diffusion of calcium across the brush border membranes. This protein appears to vary in activity in proportion to the quantitative level of calcium transport, thus providing impetus for further studies in this area. The relationship of IMCal to the "liponomic regulation" of calcium transport by vitamin D proposed by RASMUSSEN et al. (1982) should be a fruitful area for additional research. In addition, FREEDMAN et al. (1977) reported that Golgi membranes exhibit vitamin D-dependent uptake of calcium and WERINGER et al. (1978) found that intracellular calcium was localized in both Golgi and mitochondrial compartments. This suggests that the Golgi apparatus may play a role in the translocation of calcium during calcium absorption in vivo.

VI. Calcium-Dependent Adenosine Triphosphatase

Knowledge of the pivotal role played by the sodium–potassium-dependent adenosine triphosphatase (Na^+,K^+-ATPase) in the active transport of sodium and potassium by cells has stimulated the search for a similar transport enzyme (pump) that would be responsible for the active transport of calcium in the intestine. According to the biochemical mechanism of action suggested for regulation of intestinal calcium transport by 1,25-dihydrocholecalciferol, it appeared plausible that a Ca^{2+}-ATPase may be induced or in some fashion regulated by the sterol hormone. Such an enzyme activity has been demonstrated to exist in the enterocyte and its activity is well correlated with the relative quantitative differences in calcium absorption along the small intestine (WALLING 1977; MIRCHEFF et al. 1977). The Ca^{2+}-ATPase of intestine has been shown to be increased in activity by vitamin D (MARTIN et al. 1969; HAUSSLER et al. 1970). However, a great deal of confusion exists regarding the nature of this enzymatic activity since a number of investigations supported the notion that the intestinal Ca^{2+}-ATPase activity may be attributed largely to the fact that alkaline phosphatase (EC 3.1.3.1) also is found, at very high levels, in the intestinal mucosa brush border and also has been shown to occur in basolateral membranes (MARTIN et al. 1969; BIRGE and GILBERT 1974; HAUSSLER et al. 1970; HANNA et al. 1978). This enzyme is activated by divalent cations, notably magnesium, zinc, cobalt, and calcium (HARKNESS 1968; HIWADA and WACHSMUTH 1974). However, the K_m for calcium activation of this zinc-containing enzyme is in the millimolar range and has relatively poor specificity for the hydrolysis of ATP relative to other phosphate ester compounds (GHIJSEN et al. 1980). Thus, the physiologic significance of alkaline phosphatase relative to its involvement in the cellular mechanism of calcium transport is questionable, although a role in phosphate transport has been proposed (see Sect. C). Additional complicating factors are that the velocity of ATP hydrolysis by alkaline phosphatase is much greater than that attributed to the Ca^{2+}-ATPase in brush border preparations and the two enzyme activities appear to copurify, suggesting that both activities may be attributed to alkaline phosphatase per se (OKU and WASSERMAN 1978; HANNA et al. 1978).

A physiologic role for the intestinal alkaline phosphatase has been suggested by recent studies (SWARUP et al. 1981, 1982). Using alkaline phosphatase from bovine intestine and liver or from *Escherichia coli,* they demonstrated that the enzyme exhibited a high degree of specificity for hydrolysis of the tyrosyl phosphate moiety of either histones or cell membrane proteins that had been phosphorylated exclusively on the tyrosine residues in vitro. These investigators reasoned that *p*-nitrophenylphosphate is structurally similar to tyrosine phosphate. Thus, the substrate that has been used in the classical studies of alkaline phosphatase activity was inadvertently measuring an enzyme that may be involved in the dephosphorylation of cell protein, apparently including membrane proteins. SWARUP et al. (1982) found a particulate phosphatyrosylprotein phosphatase that also hydrolyzed *p*-nitrophenylphosphate in cell membranes from TCRC-12 cells. They also found that alkaline phosphatase exhibited a very high specificity for hydrolysis of the phosphate–ester bond of tyrosine phosphate in comparison with serine or threonine phosphate residues of protein. The pH optimum was between 7 and 8 which also supports the idea that alkaline phosphatase may exert a physiologically relevant effect on the dephosphorylation of cell protein. This putative role of alkaline phosphatase should be evaluated further in view of the marked enhancement of the intestinal activity of this enzyme by vitamin D. In addition, the reported stimulation by 1,25-dihydroxycholecalciferol of the in vitro phosphorylation of an 84,000 daltons protein in the intestinal brush border membrane may have significance in this regard (WILSON and LAWSON 1981). However, these investigators reported that this protein appeared to be phosphorylated on serine and threonine residues since the phosphate ester was acid resistant and labile to hydrolysis with 1 *M* NaOH, suggesting that the phosphorylated product was not phosphotyrosine. It may be speculated that vitamin D may be involved in the regulation of protein phosphorylation–dephosphorylation in vivo in concert with the effects of the hormone on maturation of the intestinal villi.

The existence of a Ca^{2+}-ATPase which has the kinetic characteristics consistent with those required of a calcium transport pump has recently been demonstrated in the rat intestine (GHIJSEN and VAN OS 1979; GHIJSEN et al. 1980). These investigators separated the mucosal cell membranes into brush border and basolateral fractions. From a large body of data, it is reasonable to suggest that the intestinal calcium transport mechanism under regulation by 1,25-dihydroxycholecalciferol is by facilitated diffusion across the brush border membrane and an active, energy-dependent process across the basolateral membrane (see Sect. B). Therefore, a Ca^{2+}-ATPase (pump) should be found in the basolateral membrane of the enterocyte. GHIJSEN and VAN OS 1979, reported that both membrane preparations exhibited putative Ca^{2+}-ATPase activity, but the enzyme activity at physiologically relevant calcium concentrations (0.5 μ*M*) was highest in the basolateral membranes. Both membrane fractions exhibited high (K_m 0.5–1.0 μ*M*) and low affinity (K_m 50–70 μ*M*) sites for calcium. The low affinity site (50–70 μ*M* calcium) for calcium-stimulated ATPase activity presumably was due to the presence of alkaline phosphatase.

In a subsequent report GHIJSEN et al. (1980) provided evidence that the physiologically significant Ca^{2+}-ATPase activity was preferentially localized to the basolateral membrane of intestinal cells, whereas alkaline phosphatase was found in both brush border and basolateral fractions. These investigators used the criteria of substrate specificity and differential inhibition of Ca^{2+}-ATPase versus alkaline phosphatase with specific inhibitors under physiologic conditions of intracellular calcium concentration, i.e., micromolar levels of calcium. At calcium concentrations below 25 μM, the hydrolysis of phosphate esters showed a high specificity for ATP relative to ADP, AMP, and *p*-nitrophenylphosphate with the basolateral membranes. High calcium (0.2 m*M*) levels provided the expression of alkaline phosphatase activity which did not reveal the physiologically required difference in substrate specificity between ATP, ADP, AMP, and *p*-nitrophenylphosphate. Brush border membranes showed no preference for ATP as substrate at physiologically relevant levels of calcium whereas 0.2 m*M* calcium increased the hydrolysis of ADP and AMP preferentially to that observed with ATP and *p*-nitrophenylphosphate. Inhibitors of oxidative metabolism (oligomycin, azide) did not inhibit either enzyme activity. However, GHIJSEN et al. (1980), demonstrated that chlorpromazine effectively inhibited the Ca^{2+}-ATPase of basolateral membranes whereas theophylline and L-phenylalanine inhibited the alkaline phosphatase of both membrane fractions even at physiologic concentrations of calcium. Chlorpromazine has been shown to inhibit the Ca^{2+}-ATPase (pump) of erythrocytes and sarcoplasmic reticulum (SCHATZMANN 1975; BALZER et al. 1968). This pharmacologic data with chloropromazine implicates a calmodulin-like mechanism since the phenothiozines are effective inhibitors of calmodulin-regulated processes. From the pharmacologic effects of these drugs on the enzyme activities it can be summarized that a chlorpromazin-sensitive, calcium-stimulated ATPase exists only on the basolateral membrane and that both membrane fractions exhibit theophylline- and L-phenylalanine-sensitive alkaline phosphate. The brush border membranes had about tenfold higher alkaline phosphatase activity than did the basolateral membranes, which agrees with the investigation of HANNA et al. (1980).

1,25-dihydroxycholecalciferol or vitamin D treatment of rachitic animals clearly enhances alkaline phosphatase activity of the intestine (HOLDSWORTH 1970; NORMAN et al. 1970; BIKLE et al. 1977) although it has been described as a Ca^{2+}-ATPase (MELANCON and DELUCA 1970). However, from the previous discussion it is clear that this enzymatic activity is probably not directly involved in intestinal calcium transport. Moreover, it has been shown that the increase in alkaline phosphatase activity by 1,25-dihydroxycholecalciferol, like calcium binding protein, lags behind the sterol-mediated increase in calcium transport (MORRISSEY et al. 1978a). The results of GHIJSEN et al. (1980) already discussed, provide an impetus for future experiments designed to investigate the temporal relationship between 1,25-dihydroxycholecalciferol-mediated changes in calcium transport with the specific, high affinity Ca^{2+}-ATPase that appears to be localized in the basolateral membrane of the enterocyte. It is conceivable that vitamin D regulation of the Ca^{2+}-ATPase could be an early event which is due to the transcription and translation of genetic information resulting from the sterol induction of RNA and protein synthesis in the intestine. Alternatively, the calcium pump may increase its activity subsequent to a vitamin D-mediated increase in permeability of the brush border membrane to calcium as appears to be true for the increased intestinal content of vitamin D-dependent calcium binding protein.

VII. Adenylate Cyclase

Increased levels of cyclic AMP in the intestine and stimulation of adenylate cyclase activity by treatment with vitamin D have been demonstrated (NEVILLE and HOLDSWORTH 1969; CORRADINO 1974). These changes appear to correlate with the increased synthesis of RNA and protein, which has led to the suggestion of a role for cyclic AMP as a second messenger involved in this metabolic process (WASSERMAN and CORRADINO 1973). Analogs of cyclic AMP such as the dibutyryl derivative appear to increase intestinal calcium transport (HARRISON and HARRISON 1970; CORRADINO 1974). Whether this is due to a direct effect of dibutyryl cyclic AMP enhancing the activity of cyclic AMP-dependent protein kinase activity is questionable since this analog has very low affinity for the regulatory subunit of that enzyme and has equally low efficacy as an activator of cyclic AMP-dependent protein kinase of other tissues (FORTE et al. 1975). Perhaps the dibutyryl derivative is converted to N^6-monobutyryl cyclic AMP by the enterocyte. This analog is a potent activator of cyclic AMP-dependent protein kinase (FORTE et al. 1975). Alternatively, dibutyryl cyclic AMP, like the methylxanthines, may affect intestinal transport through inhibition of phosphodiesterase, thus increasing cyclic AMP levels. It is of related interest that 1,25-dihydroxycholecalciferol treatment in vivo enhances the phosphorylation of an 84,000 daltons brush border membrane protein by a cyclic AMP-*independent* protein kinase (WILSON and LAWSON 1981). This 84,000 daltons protein's synthesis appears also to be regulated by 1,25-dihydroxycholecalciferol (WILSON and LAWSON 1981; MAX et al. 1978). The relationship of this protein substrate for phosphorylation with that of the intestinal mucosal cell cyclic AMP system is presently unknown, if a relationship indeed exists.

The data currently available do not provide compelling evidence that the cyclic AMP system of the absorptive enterocyte is involved in the cellular mechanism of action of vitamin D. Changes in cyclic AMP content and adenylate cyclase activity may be secondary to distant morphological and functional alterations in the intestine due to vitamin D. Moreover, the demonstration that dibutyryl cyclic AMP increases calcium uptake could be unrelated to the vitamin D–endocrine system since it is well recognized that agonists which increase cyclic AMP levels also increase calcium flux. A better pharmacologic tool for stuying cyclic AMP-dependent mechanisms is the recently discovered activator of adenylate cyclase, forskolin (SEAMON et al. 1981). This diterpene, isolated from *Coleus forskohlii,* has potent cardiovascular activity (LINDNER et al. 1978) and reversibly activates the adenylate cyclase in both whole cells and isolated plasma membranes (SEAMON et al. 1981). Forskolin reportedly activates adenylate cyclase by a direct effect on the catalytic unit (SEAMON et al. 1981) although FORTE et al. (1982) have demonstrated that the bare catalytic unit of mammalian sperm adenylate cyclase is not activated by forskolin. The drug does not appear to activate this enzyme through either the hormone receptor-dependent or guanyl nucleotide-dependent mechanisms. Since forskolin is a potent agonist which markedly increases tissue cyclic AMP levels, is reversible, and exhibits no appreciable lag period (unlike cholera toxin), it is reasonable to speculate that this drug would be an effective tool by which to examine the question of whether 1,25-dihydroxycholecalciferol regulates calcium transport in the intestine via the second messenger, cyclic AMP. Studies could be carried out in both vitamin D-deficient and D-replete tissue in order to evaluate the effects of forskolin on intestinal cyclic AMP in correlation with putative changes in calcium uptake. Forskolin could also be used to evaluate in more detail the role of cyclic AMP in the regulation of intestinal water transport in view of the marked changes in this parameter resulting from the action of cholera toxin on the intestine.

E. Vitamin D-Independent Regulation of Intestinal Calcium Absorption

The 1970s provided a virtual explosion of new information concerning both the mechanisms which regulate the metabolism of vitamin D and the subsequent physiologic effects of the hydroxy metabolites on intestinal calcium and phosphorus absorption. Before these physiologic mechanisms involving the hormone, 1,25-dihydroxycholecalciferol, were known it was generally appreciated that other hormones, notably parathyroid hormone, were involved in the regulation of intestinal calcium transport. Moreover, direct effects of parathyroid hormone and of 1,25-dihydroxycholecalciferol on the intestine have recently been demonstrated in regard to enhanced release of lysosomal enzymes and increased calcium uptake (NEMERE and SZEGO 1981 a, b). Thus, the intestine may indeed be a target tissue for this peptide hormone. However, the contemporary view is that parathyroid hormone does indeed regulate calcium absorption, but accomplishes this primarily through regulation of the renal hydroxylation of 25-hydroxycholecalciferol (FRASER and KODICEK 1973; GARABEDIEN et al. 1972, 1974; HENRY et al. 1974). Such a mechanism was thought to account for the important adaptive response of the intestine that had been described in a number of animals during periods of increased need for calcium by the organism. Excellent examples are provided by animals placed on a calcium-restricted diet (NICOLAYSEN 1943; RIBOVICH and DELUCA 1975; OMDAHL and DELUCA 1977) or the female during the reproductive cycle (HEANEY and SKILLMAN 1971; KOSTIAL et al. 1969; TOVERUD 1976; HURWITZ and GRIMINGER 1960). In mammalian and avian species, physiologic adaptation occurs in both instances such that the transport of calcium (absorption) is markedly enhanced. The adaptation of the intestine due to calcium deprivation by dietary means appears to be due to the stimulation of parathyroid hormone secretion which in turn increases the synthesis of 1,25-dihydroxycholecalciferol by the kidney. The resulting increased circulating levels of the sterol hormone (PIKE et al. 1979; HALLORAN et al. 1979; BOASS et al. 1977; KUMAR et al. 1979; STEICHEN et al. 1980) would then produce enhanced calcium absorption by the intestine. Such a mechanism is a plausible explanation of the results of experiments in the young animal. However, intestinal adaptation to calcium-restricted diets is markedly attenuated in the aged rat (ARMBRECHT et al. 1980 a, 1981), presumably due to a reduction in the response of the renal 1-hydroxylase to calcium deficiency (ARMBRECHT et al. 1980 b).

Adaptation of intestinal calcium absorption during reproduction in birds and mammals is a well-recognized phenomenon that appears related to the increased need for calcium for eggshell production and to provide the calcium for fetal mineralization of bone, respectively. From the foregoing discussion, it is believed that reproduction in these animals is associated with stimulation of the renal 1-hydroxylase, leading to increased circulating levels of 1,25-dihydroxycholecalciferol. Although preliminary experiments suggest that estrogen does not directly regulate the renal 1-hydroxylase system (HENRY 1981), estrogen appears to be implicated as a regulator of this hydroxylation mechanism in the kidney (KENNY 1976; CASTILLO et al. 1977). Thus, a reasonable rationale could be developed by which the process of intestinal calcium absorption adapts to the enhanced need for calcium during reproduction involving the vitamin D–endocrine system. However, a series of recent studies clearly demonstrated that physiologic regulation of intestinal calcium transport is not solely dependent upon this vitamin D–endocrine mechanism. The remainder of this section will review the evidence supporting such a notion.

Because of the hypothesis that the vitamin D–endocrine system played a central role in the regulation of intestinal calcium transport, it was somewhat surprising that investigators were able to raise female rats on a diet devoid of vitamin D from the weanling stage to sexual maturity, successfully breed the females, have them carry out a relatively normal pregnancy, and deliver offspring that were viable (HALLORAN and DELUCA 1979; THOMAS and FORTE 1982). This was noteworthy even though WARKANY (1943) had previously carried out a similar study, feeding rats a vitamin D-deficient diet that was supplemented with 2% dessicated pig liver. However, since the liver would be expected to contain vitamin D, it is probable that WARKANY's animals were not truly vitamin D deficient. The female animals raised on a vitamin D-deficient diet by HALLORAN and DELUCA (1979) exhibited classic signs of vitamin D deficiency, including profound hypocalcemia and nondetectable levels of both 25-hydroxy- and 1,25-dihydroxycholecalciferol. THOMAS and FORTE (1981) demonstrated the same degree of hypocalcemia in vitamin D-deficient rats and also found that circulating levels of immunoreactive parathyroid hormone were markedly increased in female rats to the same general extent as age-matched male animals. It was of considerable interest that calcium transport increased during pregnancy in these animals (HALLORAN and DELUCA 1980a). The surprising fact that female rats can reproduce in the absence (or marked deficiency) of 1,25-dihydroxycholecalciferol suggests that prominent physiologic mechanisms exist which promote intestinal calcium absorption via vitamin D-independent mechanisms. Thus, the adaptation of the intestine to increase calcium absorption during pregnancy is not explained adequately by the previously stated vitamin D–endocrine mechanism. This was further substantiated by the investigation of THOMAS and FORTE (1982) who demonstrated that the serum calcium levels of vitamin D-deficient rats increased substantially during the first 17 days of pregnancy and then decreased just prior to parturition. The decrease in serum calcium at the end of gestation was probably due to enhanced transfer of calcium from the maternal circulation to satisfy the fetal demands for calcium required for mineralization of the fetal skeleton and is known to occur in the vitamin D-replete rat. It is reasonable to suggest that the increased serum calcium elicited by pregnancy in the vitamin D-deficient rat may be derived from increased intestinal calcium absorption, although enhanced mineral mobilization from bone cannot be ruled out. Therefore, an endocrine factor during pregnancy may contribute an important component to the regulation of intestinal calcium absorption during pregnancy per se; sex steroids and/or prolactin may be candidates. It has been shown in a preliminary fashion that prolactin treatment of vitamin D-deficient *male* rats increased serum calcium and stimulated intestinal calcium transport (PAHUJA and DELUCA 1981). These data, however, cannot be readily extrapolated to the female vitamin D-deficient rat as a mechanism explaining the vitamin D-independent increase in serum calcium observed during pregnancy by THOMAS and FORTE(1982).

Related studies that provide data which underscore the vitamin D-independent mechanisms regulating intestinal calcium transport have been obtained during lactation in the rat. Lactation is a greater stress to the calcium homeostasis mechanism than pregnancy per se in this species. Thus, the intestine and bone must provide large quantities of calcium for secretion of calcium into milk, resulting in a substantial increase in intestinal transfer of calcium (KOSTIAL et al. 1969; TOVERUD et al. 1976) and a very significant mobilization of bone mineral. This causes substantial demineralization of bone in the vitamin D-replete animal (KOMARKOVA et al. 1967; RASMUSSEN 1977; HALLORAN and DELUCA 1980b). BOASS et al. (1981) demonstrated that the intestine adapts to the increased calcium requirements imposed during lactation in the vitamin D-deficient rat. Moreover, the results of HALLORAN and DELUCA (1980b) showed a similar vitamin D-independent mobilization of bone mineral during lactation in this animal model. Indeed, the extent of demineralization that occurred during lactation was similar in vitamin D-deficient and D-replete animals. A study by THOMAS and FORTE (1982) revealed that the enhanced transfer of calcium from intestine and/or bone during lactation was associated with a significant "overshoot" in maternal serum calcium when pups were removed from the mother after 21 days of lactation. The extent of this physiologic calcemic response was similar between vitamin D-replete and D-deficient animals. In the vitamin D-replace rat, it has been shown that the lactating rat characteristically becomes hypercalcemic when pups are removed from the mother (PIKE et al. 1979). The reason for this was thought to be related to the marked increase in circulating levels of 1,25-dihydroxycholecalciferol observed during lactation (PIKE et al. 1979). The experiments of THOMAS and FORTE (1982), however, indicate that the overshoot or rebound calcemia following lactation is associated with a vitamin D-independent stimulation of calcium transport by the intestine and/or bone. It is reasonable to speculate that prolactin could play a role in this vitamin D-independent mechanism of regulating calcium transport (PAHUJA and DELUCA 1981).

A third body of data providing evidence for vitamin D-independent regulation of intestinal calcium absorption has been derived from studies in the developmental period. Thus, HALLORAN and DELUCA (1980c) found that during the first 2 weeks of life, the absorption of calcium by the intestine was similar in magnitude whether the pups were from vitamin D-replete or D-deficient mothers. The pups at this time did not respond to 1,25-dihydroxycholecalciferol with enhanced calcium transport, but did respond later during lactation after solid food was being ingested. Appearance of responsiveness to the sterol was subsequently shown to be related to the appearance of specific receptors for 1,25-dihydroxycholecalciferol in the intestine (HALLORAN and DELUCA 1981a). A correlated increase in the calcium binding protein content of intestine late in the period of lactation has also been demonstrated (DELORME et al. 1979). Thus, maturation of the intestine in the neonatal rat appears to proceed functionally from a vitamin D-independent mode during the first 2 weeks of life, when intestinal absorption of milk appears to be primarily accomplished by pinocytosis of food particles (WISSIG and GRANEY 1968), to the more selective type of transport which is regulated by the vitamin D–endocrine system and other mechanisms both at the end of lactation and in adult life. Such developmental changes would explain the relative normocalcemia and normal growth of rat pups from vitamin D-deficient mothers during the period of lactation when pups only consume milk. Moreover, these findings are consistent with data from our laboratory (M. L. THOMAS and L. R. FORTE 1981, unpublished work) which revealed that fetal and newborn animals from vitamin D-deficient mothers are relatively normocalcemic and euparathyroid, even though the mothers are markedly hypocalcemic and hyperparathyroid.

In summary, physiologic regulation of intestinal calcium transport is quite clearly more complex than previously recognized and is not solely dependent upon the vitamin D–endocrine system. A number of factors may be involved, but it is reasonable to suspect that other endocrine factors such as prolactin or sex steroids may play important roles in the regulation of intestinal calcium absorption. Further studies of perinatal calcium metabolism using the vitamin D-deficient rat as the experimental model may provide further insights into the mechanisms involved in this area of intestinal function.

F. Summary

Intestinal calcium permeability is regulated by vitamin D at the level of the brush border membrane. Transport at this site appears to be accomplished by a process of facilitated diffusion and is thought to be the rate-limiting step for calcium transport through the mucosal cell. Vitamin D regulates both lipid and protein synthesis of brush border components which may constitute a molecular mechanism for the control of this transport site. The sterol hormone may accomplish this through a gene transcription mechanism although evidence to the contrary is available. Intracellular organelles appear to be responsible for the intracellular sequestration of calcium, including mitochondria, Golgi apparatus and the cytosolic, vitamin D-dependent calcium binding protein. A calcium-dependent ATPase exists in the basolateral membrane and may be responsible for the active, energy-dependent transport of calcium against an electrochemical gradient. At this pole of the enterocyte, a sodium–calcium exchange process may account for part of the calcium transport, although data supporting such a mechanism are sparse. Much of intestinal calcium transport in the absorptive and secretory directions is accomplished via a paracellular pathway which is not affected by vitamin D. This process may be regulated during pregnancy and lactation as a component of the vitamin D-independent regulation of transport that may be physiologically significant, especially during pregnancy and lactation.

Phosphate transport across the brush border is thought to occur by cotransport with sodium utilizing the sodium gradient established by the sodium–potassium pump mechanism. Therefore, phosphate transport is secondarily active in nature. Vitamin D appears to regulate the transport of phosphate across this membrane by a gene transcription mechanism, although the molecular mechanism is unknown. Phosphate transport across the enterocyte is coupled since the radiolabeled phosphate does not readily equilibrate with intracellular phosphate pools. Transport of phosphate across the basolateral membrane is by passive diffusion down a favorable electrochemical gradient. The distribution of vitamin D-dependent phosphate transport in the intestine is greatest in the jejunum whereas calcium transport is greatest in the duodenum. Moreover, the large intestine exhibits vitamin D-stimulated transport of calcium, but not phosphate. Intestinal phosphate transport is not dependent upon calcium transport as was originally proposed.

References

Adams TH, Norman AW (1970) Studies on the mechanism of action of calciferol. I. Basic parameters of vitamin D-mediated calcium transport. J Biol Chem 245:4421–4431

Adams TH, Wong RG, Norman AW (1970) Studies on the mechanism of action calciferol. II. Effects of the polyene antibiotic, filipin, on vitamin D-mediated calcium transport. J Biol Chem 245:4432–4442

Armbrecht HJ, Zenser TV, Davis BB (1980a) Effect of age on the conversion of 25-hydroxy-vitamin D_3 to 1,25-dihydroxyvitamin D_3 by kidney of rat. J Clin Invest 66:1118–1123

Armbrecht HJ, Zenser TV, Gross CJ, Davis BB (1980b) Adaption to dietary calcium and phosphorus restriction changes with age in the rat. Am J Physiol 239:E322–E327

Armbrecht HJ, Gross CJ, Zenser TV (1981) Effect of dietary calcium and phosphorus restriction on calcium and phosphorus balance in young and old rats. Arch Biochem Biophys 210:179–185

Avioli LV, McDonald JE, Lee SW (1965) The influence of age on the intestinal absorption of ^{47}Ca in women and its relation to ^{47}Ca absorption in postmenopausal osteoporosis. J Clin Invest 44:1960–1967

Balzer H, Makinose M, Hasselbach W (1968) The inhibition of the sarcoplasmic calcium pump by prenylamine, reserpine, chlorpromazine, and imipramine. Naunyn Schmiedeberg's Arch Pharmacol 260:444–455

Bar A, Hurwitz S (1972) Relationship of duodenal calcium-binding protein to calcium absorption in the laying fowl. Comp Biochem Physiol 41B:735–744

Bar A, Hurwitz S (1973) Uterine calcium-binding protein in the laying fowl. Comp Biochem Physiol 45:579–486

Bar A, Hurwitz J (1979) The interaction between dietary calcium and gonadal hormones in their effect on plasma calcium, bone 25-hydroxycholecalciferol-1-hydroxylase and duodenal calcium-binding protein, measured by a radioimmunoassay in chicks. Endocrinology 104:1455–1460

Bar A, Norman AW (1981) Studies on the mode of action of calciferol. XXXIV. Relationship of the distribution of 25-hydroxyvitamin D_3 metabolites to gonadal activity and egg shell formation in the quail. Endocrinology 109:950–955

Bar A, Dubrov D, Eisner U, Hurwitz S (1976) Calcium-binding protein and calcium absorption in the laying quail (*Coturnix Coturnix Japonica*). Poult Sci 55:622–628

Bar A, Cohen A, Edelstein S, Shemesh M, Montecuccoli G, Hurwitz S (1978a) Involvement of cholecalciferol metabolism in birds in the adaptation of calcium absorption to the needs during reproduction. Comp Biochem Physiol 59B:245–249

Bar A, Cohen A, Eisner U, Risenfeld G, Hurwitz S (1978b) Differential response of calcium transport system in laying hens to exogenous and endogenous changes in vitamin D status. J Nutr 108:1322–1328

Baxter LA, DeLuca HF (1976) Stimulation of 25-hydroxyvitamin D_3-1α-hydroxylase by phosphate depletion. J biol Chem 251:3158–3161

Behar J, Kerstein MD (1976) Intestinal calcium absorption: Differences in transport between duodenum and ileum. Am J Physiol 230:1255–1260
Belsey RE, DeLuca HF, Potts JT Jr (1971) Competitive binding assay for vitamin D and 25-OH vitamin D. J Clin Endocrinol Metab 33:554–557
Berner W, Kinne R, Murer H (1976) Phosphate transport into brush-border membrane vesicles isolated from rat small intestine. Biochem J 160:467–474
Bikle DD, Empson RN Jr, Herman RH, Morrissey RL, Zolock DR (1977) The effect of 1,25-dihydroxyvitamin D_3 in the distribution of alkaline phosphatase activity along the chick intestinal villus. Biochem Biophys Acta 499:61–66
Bikle DD, Zolock DT, Morrissey RL, Herman RH (1978) Independence of 1,25-dihydroxyvitamin D_3-mediated calcium transport from de novo RNA and protein synthesis. J Biol Chem 253:484–488
Bikle DD, Morrissey RL, Zolock DT, Rasmussen H (1981) The intestinal response to vitamin D. Rev Physiol Biochem Pharmacol 89:63–142
Birge SJ, Gilbert HR (1974) Identification of an intestinal sodium and calcium-dependent phosphatase stimulated by parathyroid hormone. J Clin Invest 54:710–717
Birge SJ, Peck WA, Berman M, Whedon GD (1969) Study of calcium absorption in man: A kinetic analysis and physiologic model. J Clin Invest 48:1705–1713
Birge SJ Jr, Gilbert HR, Avioli LV (1972) Intestinal calcium transport: The role of sodium. Science 176:168–170
Boass AI, Toverud SU, McCain TA, Pike JW, Haussler MR (1977) Elevated serum levels of 1α,25-dihydroxycholecalciferol in lactating rats. Nature 267:630–632
Boass A, Toverud SU, Pike JW, Haussler MR (1981) Calcium metabolism during lactation: Enhanced intestinal calcium absorption in vitamin D-deprived hypocalcemic rats. Endocrinology 109:900–907
Boyle IT, Omdahl JL, Gray RW, DeLuca HF (1973) The biological activity and metabolism of 24,25-dihydroxyvitamin D_3. J Biol Chem 248:4174–4180
Bredderman PL, Wasserman RH (1974) Chemical composition, affinity for calcium and some related properties of the vitamin D-dependent calcium-binding protein. Biochemistry 13:1687–1694
Bronner F, Lipton J, Pansa D, Buckley M, Singh R, Miller A (1982) Molecular and transport effects of 1,25-dihydroxyvitamin D_3 in rat duodenum. Fed Proc 41:61–65
Brumbaugh PF, Haussler MR (1974a) 1α,25-dihydroxycalciferol receptors in intestine: I. Association of 1α,25-dihydroxycholecalciferol with intestinal mucosa chromatin. J Biol Chem 249:1251–1257
Brumbaugh PF, Haussler MF (1974b) 1α,25-dihydroxycholecalciferol receptors in intestine. II. Temperature-dependent transfer of the hormone to chromatin via a specific cytosol receptor. J Biol Chem 249:1258–1262
Brumbaugh PF, Haussler DH, Bursac KM, Haussler MR (1974) Filter assay for 1α,25-dihydroxyvitamin D_3. Utilization of the hormone's target tissue chromatin receptor. Biochemistry 13:4091–4097
Brunette MG, Dennis VW (1982) Effects of L-bromotetramisole on phosphate transport by the proximal renal tubule: Failure to demonstrate a direct involvement of alkaline phosphatase. Can J Physiol Pharmacol 60:276–281
Bruns MEH, Fliesher EB, Avioli LV (1977) Control of vitamin D-dependent calcium-binding protein in rat intestine by growth and fasting. J Biol Chem 252:4145–4150
Bruns EH, Fausto A, Aviolo LV (1978) Placental calcium binding protein in rats. Apparent identity with vitamin D-dependent calcium binding protein from rat intestine. J Biol Chem 253:3186–3190
Buckley M, Bronner F (1980) Calcium-binding protein biosynthesis in the rat: Regulation by calcium and 1,25-dihydroxyvitamin D_3. Arch Biochem Biophys 202:235–241
Burg M, Green N (1973) Effect of ethacrynic acid on the thick ascending limb of Henle's loop. Kidney Int 4:301–308
Carlsson A (1954) The effect of vitamin D on the absorption of inorganic phosphate. Acta Physiol Scand 31:301–307
Castillo L, Tanaka Y, DeLuca HF, Sunde ML (1977) The stimulation of 25-hydroxyvitamin D_3-1α hydroxylase by estrogen. Arch Biochem Biophys 179:211–217

Chan L, O'Malley BW (1976) Mechanism of action of sex hormones. N Engl J Med 294:1322–1328, 1372–1381, 1430–1437

Chandler JS, Pike JW, Haussler MR (1979) 1,25-dihydroxyvitamin D_3 receptors in rat kidney cytosol. Biochem Biophys Res Commun 90:1057–1063

Chen TC, Castillo L, Korycka-Dahl M, DeLuca HF (1974) Role of vitamin D metabolites in phosphate transport of rat intestine. J Nutr 104:1056–1060

Chen TL, Hirst MA, Feldman D (1979) A receptor-like binding macromolecule for 1α,25-dihydroxycholecalciferol in cultured mouse bone cells. J Biol Chem 254:7491–7494

Cheung WY (1980) Calmodulin plays a pivotal role in cellular regulation. Science 207:12–27

Christakos S, Norman AW (1978) Vitamin D_3-induced calcium binding protein in bone tissue. Science 202:70–71

Christakos S, Norman AW (1979) Studies on the mode of action of calciferol. XVIII. Evidence for a specific high affinity binding protein for 1,25-dihydroxyvitamin D_3 in chick kidney and pancreas. Biochem Biophys Res Comm 89:56–63

Cohn WE, Greenberg DM (1939) Studies in mineral metabolism with the aid of artificial radioactive isotopes. III. The influence of vitamin D on the phosphorus metabolism of rachitic rats. J Biol Chem 130:625–634

Colston KW, Feldman D (1979) Demonstration of a 1,25-dihydroxycholecalciferol cytoplasmic receptor-like binder in mouse kidney. J Clin Endocrinol Metab 49:798–800

Colston K, Hirst M, Feldman D (1980) Organ distribution of the cytoplasmic 1,25-dihydroxycholecalciferol receptor in various mouse tissues. Endocrinology 107:1916–1922

Cooke NE, Walgate J, Haddad JG Jr (1979) Human serum binding protein for vitamin D and its metabolites. I. Physicochemical and immunological identification in human tissues. J Biol Chem 254:5958–5964

Corradino RA (1973a) Embryonic chick intestine in organ culture: A unique system for the study of the intestinal calcium absorptive mechanism. J Cell Biol 58:64–78

Corradino RA (1973b) 1,25-Dihydroxycholecalciferol: Inhibition of action in organ-cultured intestine by actinomycin D and α amanitin. Nature 243:41–43

Corradino RA (1973c) Embryonic chick intestine in organ culture: Response to vitamin D_3 and its metabolites. Science 179:402–405

Corradino RA (1974) Embryonic chick intestine in organ culture: Interaction of adenylate cyclase system and vitamin D_3-mediated calcium absorptive mechanism. Endocrinology 94:1607–1614

Corradino RA (1978) A simple technique for the measurement of unidirectional calcium influx at the mucosal surface of organ-cultured embryonic chick duodenum. Anal Biochem 91:60–69

Corradino RA (1979a) Embryonic chick intestine in organ culture: Hydrocortisone and vitamin D-mediated processes. Arch Biochem Biophys 192:302–310

Corradino RA (1979b) Hydrocortisone and vitamin D_3 stimulation of ^{32}Pi-phosphate accumulation by organ-cultured chick embryo duodenum. Horm Metab Res 11:519–523

Corradino RA, Wasserman RH (1971) Vitamin D_3: Induction of calcium-binding protein in embryonic chick intestine in vitro. Science 172:731–733

Corradino RA, Wasserman RH (1974) 1,25-dihydroxycholecalciferol-like activity of solanum malacoxylon extract on calcium transport. Nature 252:716–718

Corradino RA, Wasserman RH, Pubols MH, Chang SI (1968) Vitamin D_3 induction of a calcium-binding protein in the uterus of laying hen. Arch Biochem Biophys 125:378–380

Corradino RA, Fullmer CS, Wasserman RH (1976) Embryonic chick intestine in organ culture: Stimulation of calcium transport by exogenous vitamin D-induced calcium binding protein. Arch Biochem Biophys 174:738–743

Coty WA (1980) A specific, high affinity binding protein for 1α,25-dihydroxy vitamin D in the chick oviduct shell gland. Biochem Biophys Res Commun 93:285–292

Coty WA, McConkey CL Jr, Brown TA (1981) A specific binding protein for 1α,25-dihydroxyvitamin D in the chick embryo chorioallantoic membrane. J Biol Chem 256:5545–5549

Cramer CF, Dueck J (1962) In vivo transport of calcium from healed thiry-Vella fistulas in dogs. Am J Physiol 202:161–164

Cramer CF, McMillan J (1980) Phosphorus adaptation in rats in absence of vitamin D or parathyroid glands. Am J Physiol 239:G261–G265

Danisi G, Straub RW (1980) Unidirectional influx of phosphate across the mucosal membrane of rabbit small intestine. Pflügers Arch 385:117–122

Danisi G, Bonjour JP, Straub RW (1980) Regulation of Na-dependent phosphate influx across the mucosal border of duodenum by 1,25-dihydroxycholecalciferol. Pflügers Arch 388:227–232

Delorme AC, Marche P, Garel JM (1979) Vitamin D-dependent calcium-binding protein. Changes during gestation, prenatal and postnatal development in rats. J Dev Physiol 1:181–194

DeLuca HF, Franceschi RT, Halloran BP, Massaro ER (1982) Molecular events involved in 1,25-dihydroxyvitamin D_3 stimulation of intestinal calcium transport. Fed Proc 41:66–71

Drescher D, DeLuca HF (1971) Possible precursor of the vitamin D-stimulated calcium-binding protein in rats. Biochemistry 10:2308–2312

Eisman JA, Hamstra AJ, Kream BE, DeLuca HF (1976) A sensitive, precise and convenient method for determination of 1,25-dihydroxyvitamin D in human plasma. Arch Biochem Biophys 176:235–243

Epstein RW (1972) The effects of ethacrynic acid on active transport of sugars and ions and on other metabolic processes in rabbit kidney cortex. Biochim Biophys Acta 274:128–139

Fairbanks BW, Mitchell HH (1936) The relation between calcium retention and the store of calcium in the body, with particular reference to the determination of calcium requirements. J Nutr 11:551–572

Favus MJ, Kathpalia SC, Coe FL, Mond AE (1980) Effects of diet calcium and 1,25-dihydroxyvitamin D_3 on colon calcium active transport. Am J Physiol 238:G75–G78

Favus MJ, Kathpalia SC, Coe FL (1981) Kinetic characteristics of calcium absorption and secretion by rat colon. Am J Physiol 240:G350–G354

Feher JJ, Wasserman RH (1978) Evidence for a membrane-bound fraction of chick intestinal calcium-binding protein. Biochim Biophys Acta 540:134–143

Feldman D, McCain TA, Hirst MA, Chen TL, Colston KW (1979) Characterization of a cytoplasmic receptor-like binder for 1α,25-dihydroxycholecalciferol in rat intestinal mucosa. J Biol Chem 254:10378–10384

Fontaine O, Matsumoto T, Goodman DBP, Rasmussen H (1981) Liponomic control of Ca^{2+} transport: Relationship to mechanism of action of 1,25-dihydroxyvitamin D_3. Proc Natl Acad Sci USA 78:1751–1754

Forte LR, Chao WTH, Walkenbach RJ, Byington KH (1975) Studies of kidney plasma membrane adenosine-3′,5′-monophosphate-dependent protein kinase. Biochim biophys Acta 389:84–96

Forte LR, Bylund DB, Zahler WL (1982) Forskolin: Mechanism of activation of adenylate cyclase. Fed Proc 41:1471

Fox J, Care AD (1978a) Effect of low calcium and low phosphorus diets on the intestinal absorption of phosphate in intact and parathyroidectomized pigs. J Endocrinol 77:225–231

Fox J, Care AD (1978b) Stimulation of duodenal and ileal absorption of phosphate in the chick by low-calcium and low-phosphorus diets. Calcif Tissue Res 26:243–245

Fox J, Bunnett NW, Farrar AR, Care AD (1981) Stimulation by low phosphorus and low calcium diets of duodenal absorption of phosphate in betamethasone-treated chicks. J Endocrinol 88:147–153

Franceschi RT, DeLuca HF (1981a) Characterization of 1,25-dihydroxyvitamin D_3-dependent calcium uptake in cultured embryonic chick duodenum. J Biol Chem 256:3840–3847

Franceschi RT, DeLuca HF (1981b) The effect of inhibitors of protein and RNA synthesis on 1α,25-dihydroxyvitamin D_3-dependent calcium uptake in cultured embryonic chick duodenum. J Biol Chem 256:3848–3852

Franceschi RT, Simpson RU, DeLuca HF (1981) Binding proteins for vitamin D metabolites: Serum carriers and intracellular receptors. Arch Biochem Biophys 210:1–13
Fraser DR, Kodicek E (1973) Regulation of 25-hydroxycholecalciferol-1-hydroxylase activity in kidney by parathyroid hormone. Nature 241:163–166
Freedman RA, Weiser MM, Isselbacher KJ (1977) Calcium translocation by Golgi and lateral-basal membrane vesicles from rat intestine: Decrease in vitamin D-deficient rats. Proc Natl Acad Sci USA 74:3612–3616
Freund T, Bronner F (1975a) Stimulation in vitro by 1,25-dihydroxyvitamin D_3 of intestinal cell calcium uptake and calcium-binding protein. Science 190:1300–1302
Freund T, Bronner F (1975b) Regulation of intestinal calcium-binding protein by calcium intake in the rat. Am J Physiol 228:861–869
Fry JM, Curnow DH, Gutteridge DH, Retallack RW (1980) Vitamin D in lactation. I. The localization, specific binding and biological effect of 1,25-dihydroxyvitamin D_3 in mammary tissue of lactating rats. Life Sci 27:1255–1263
Fuchs R, Peterlik M (1979) Vitamin D-induced transepithelial phosphate and calcium transport by chick jejunum. Effect of microfilamentous and microtubular inhibitors. FEBS Lett 100:357–359
Fuchs R, Peterlik M (1980) Vitamin D-induced phosphate transport in intestinal brush border membrane vesicles. Biochem Biophys Res Commun 93:87–92
Fullmer CS, Wasserman RH (1973) Bovine intestinal calcium-binding proteins. Purification and some properties. Biochim Biophys Acta 317:172–186
Garabedian M, Holick MF, DeLuca HF, Boyle IT (1972) Control of 25-hydroxycholecalciferol metabolism by parathyroid glands. Proc Natl Acad Sci USA 69:1673–1676
Garabedian M, Tanaka Y, Holick MF, DeLuca HF (1974) Response of intestinal calcium transport and bone calcium mobilization of 1,25-dihydroxyvitamin D_3 in thyroparathyroidectomized rats. Endocrinology 94:1022–1027
Ghijsen WEJM, Van Os CH (1979) Ca-stimulated ATPase in brush border and basolateroal membranes of rat duodenum with high affinity sites for Ca ions. Nature 279:802–803
Ghijsen WEJM, DeLong MD, Van Os CH (1980) Dissociation between Ca^{2+}-ATPase and alkaline phosphatase activities in plasma membranes of rat duodenum. Biochim Biophys Acta 599:538–551
Gmaj P, Murer H, Kinne R (1979) Calcium ion transport across plasma membranes isolated from rat kidney cortex. Biochem J 178:549–557
Gorski J, Gannon F (1976) Current models of steroid hormone action: A critique. Annu Rev Physiol 38:425–450
Haase W, Schafer A, Murer H, Kinne R (1978) Studies on the orientation of brush-border membrane vesicles. Biochem J 172:57–62
Haddad JG Jr, Birge SJ (1971) 25-Hydroxycholecalciferol: Specific binding by rachitic tissue extracts. Biochem Biophys Res Commun 45:829–834
Haddad JG, Birge SJ (1975) Widespread, specific binding of 25-hydroxycholecalciferol in rat tissues. J Biol Chem 250:299–303
Haddad JG, Chyu KJ (1971) Competitive protein-binding radioassay for 25-hydroxycholecalciferol. J Clin Endocrinol Metab 33:992–998
Haddad JG Jr, Walgate J (1976) 25-Hydroxyvitamin D transport in human plasma. J Biol Chem 251:4803–4809
Hallick RB, DeLuca HF (1972) Metabolites of dihydrotachysterol$_3$ in target tissues. J Biol Chem 247:91–97
Halloran BP, DeLuca HF (1979) Vitamin D deficiency and reproduction in rats. Science 204:73–74
Halloran BP, DeLuca HF (1980a) Calcium transport in small intestine during pregnancy and lactation. Am J Physiol 239:E64–E68
Halloran BP, DeLuca HF (1980b) Skeletal changes during pregnancy and lactation: The role of vitamin D. Endocrinology 107:1923–1929
Halloran BP, DeLuca HF (1980c) Calcium transport in small intestine during early development: Role of vitamin D. Am J Physiol 239:G473–G479

Halloran BP, DeLuca HF (1981 a) Appearance of the intestinal cytosolic receptor for 1,25-dihydroxyvitamin D_3 during neonatal development in the rat. J Biol Chem 256:7338–7342

Halloran BP, DeLuca HF (1981 b) Intestinal calcium transport: Evidence for two distinct mechanisms of action of 1,25-dihydroxyvitamin D_3. Arch Biochem Biophys 208:477–486

Halloran BP, Barthell EN, DeLuca HF (1979) Vitamin D metabolism during pregnancy and lactation in the rat. Proc Natl Acad Sci USA 76:5549–5553

Hanna S, Mircheff A, Wright E (1978) Purification of alkaline phosphatase and Ca^{++}-ATPase from basal lateral membranes of rat duodenum. Biophys J 21:203 a

Hansard SL, Comar CL, Plumlee MP (1951) Effect of calcium status, mass of calcium administered and age in Ca^{45} metabolism in the rat. Proc Soc Exp Biol Med 78:455–460

Harkness DR (1968) Studies on human placental alkaline phosphatase. II. Kinetic properties and studies on the apoenzyme. Arch Biochem Biophys 126:513–523

Harmeyer J, DeLuca HF (1969) Calcium-binding protein and calcium absorption after vitamin D administration. Arch Biochem Biophys 133:247–254

Harrison HC, Harrison HE (1969) Calcium transport by rat colon in vitro. Am J Physiol 217:121–125

Harrison HE, Harrison HC (1951) Studies with radiocalcium: The intestinal absorption of calcium. J Biol Chem 188:83–90

Harrison HE, Harrison HC (1960) Transfer of Ca^{45} across intestinal wall in vitro in relation to action of vitamin D and cortisol. Am J Physiol 199:265–271

Harrison HE, Harrison HC (1961) Intestinal transport of phosphate: Action of vitamin D, calcium and potassium. Am J Physiol 201:1007–1012

Harrison HE, Harrison HC (1963) Sodium, potassium and intestinal transport of glucose, l-tyrosine, phosphate and calcium. Am J Physiol 205:107–111

Harrison HC, Harrison HE (1970) Dibutyryl cyclic AMP, vitamin D and intestinal permeability to calcium. Endocrinology 86:756–760

Haussler MR, Nagode LA, Rasmussen H (1970) Induction of intestinal brush border alkaline phosphatase by vitamin D and identify with Ca-ATPase. Nature 228:1199–1201

Haussler MR, Manolagas SC, Deftos LJ (1980) Evidence for a 1,25-dihydroxyvitamin D_3 receptor-like macromolecule in rat pituitary. J Biol Chem 255:5007–5010

Heaney RP, Skillman TG (1971) Calcium metabolism in normal human pregnancy. J Clin Endocrinol Metab 33:661–670

Helbock JH, Forte JG, Saltman P (1966) The mechanism of calcium transport by rat intestine. Biochim Biophys Acta 126:81–93

Henry HL (1981) 25(OH)D_3 metabolism in kidney cell culture: Lack of a direct effect of estradiol. Am J Physiol 240:E119–E124

Henry HL, Midgett RJ, Norman AW (1974) Regulation of 25-hydroxyvitamin D_3-1-hydroxylase in vivo. J Biol Chem 249:7584–7592

Henry KM, Kon SK (1945) Effect of advancing age on the assimilations of calcium by the rat. Biochem J 39:xxi

Hermsdorf CL, Bronner F (1975) Vitamin D-dependent calcium-binding protein from rat kidney. Biochim Biophys Acta 379:553–561

Hirst MA, Feldman D (1981) 1,25-dihydroxyvitamin D_3 receptors in mouse colon. J Steroid Biochem 14:315–319

Hiwada K, Wachsmuth ED (1974) Catalytic properties of akaline phosphatase from pig kidney. Biochem J 141:283–291

Holdsworth ES (1970) The effect of vitamin D on enzyme activities in the mucosal cells of the chick small intestine. J Membr Biol 3:43–53

Holdsworth ES, Jordan JE, Keenan E (1975) Effects of cholecalciferol on the translocation of calcium by non-everted chick ileum in vitro. Biochem J 152:181–190

Holick MF, Kleiner-Bossaller A, Schnoes HK, Kasten PM, Boyle IT, DeLuca HF (1973) 1,24,25-trihydroxyvitamin D_3: A metabolite of vitamin D_3 effective on intestine. J biol Chem 248:6691–6696

Howland J, Kramer B (1921) Calcium and phosphorus in the serum in relation to rickets. Am J Dis Child 22:105–119

Hurwitz S, Bar A, (1972) Site of vitamin D action in chick intestine. Am J Physiol 222:761–767
Hurwitz S, Griminger P (1960) Observations on the calcium balance of laying hens. J Agric Sci 54:373–377
Hurwitz S, Harrison HC, Harrison HE (1967) Effect of vitamin D_3 on the in vitro transport of calcium by the chick intestine. J Nut 91:319–323
Hurwitz S, Bar A, Cohen I (1973) Regulation of calcium absorption by fowl intestine. Am J Physiol 225:150–154
Ireland P, Fordtran JS (1973) Effect of dietary calcium and age on jejunal calcium absorption in humans studied by intestinal perfusion. J Clin Invest 52:2672–2681
Kendrick NC, Kabakoff B, DeLuca HF (1981) Oxygen-dependent 1,25-dihydroxycholecalciferol-induced calcium ion transport in rat intestine. Biochem J 194:178–186
Kenney AD (1976) Vitamin D metabolism: Physiological regulation in the egg-laying Japanese Quail. Am J Physiol 230:1609–1615
Kimberg DV, Schachter D, Schenker H (1961) Active transport by intestine: Effects of dietary calcium. Am J Physiol 200:1256–1262
Komarkova A, Zahor Z, Czabanova V (1967) The effect of lactation on the composition of long bones in rats. J Lab Clin Med 69:102–109
Kostial K, Gruden N, Durakovic A (1969) Intestinal absorption of calcium-47 and strontium-85 in lactating rats. Calcif Tissue Res 4:13–19
Kowarski S, Schachter D (1969) Effects of vitamin D on phosphate transport and incorporation into mucosal constituents of rat intestinal mucosa. J Biol Chem 244:211–217
Kowarski S, Schachter D (1975) Vitamin D-dependent, particulate calcium-binding activity and intestinal calcium transport. Am J Physiol 229:1198–1204
Kowarski S, Schachter D (1980) Intestinal membrane calcium-binding protein. Vitamin D-dependent membrane component of the intestinal calcium transport mechanism. J Biol Chem 255:10834–10840
Krawitt EL, Schedl HP (1968) In vivo calcium transport by rat small intestine. Am J Physiol 214:232–236
Kream BE, Reynolds RD, Knutson JC, Eisman JA, DeLuca HF (1976). Intestinal cytosol binders of 1,25-dihydroxyvitamin D_3 and 25-hydroxyvitamin D_3. Arch Biochem Biophys 176:779–787
Kream BE, DeLuca HF, Moriarity DM, Kendrick NC, Ghazarian JG (1979) Origin of 25-hydroxyvitamin D_3 binding protein from tissue cytosal preparations. Arch Biochem Biophys 192:318–323
Kumar R, Schnoes HK, DeLuca HF (1978) Rat intestinal 25-hydroxyvitamin D_3- and 1α,25-dihydroxyvitamin D_3-24-hydroxylase. J Biol Chem 253:3804–3809
Kumar R, Cohen WR, Silva P, Epstein FH (1979) Elevated 1,25-dihydroxyvitamin D plasma levels in normal human pregnancy and lactation. J Clin Invest 63:342–344
Laouari D, Pavlovitch H, Deceneux G, Balsan S (1980) A vitamin D-dependent calcium-binding protein in rat skin. FEBS Lett 3:285–289
Lawson DEM, Bell PA (1974) Metabolism of dihydrotachysterol and 5,6-transcholecalciferol in the chick and rat. Biochem J 142:37–46
Lee DBN, Brautbar N, Walling MW, Silis V, Coburn JW, Kleeman CR (1979) Effect of phosphorus depletion on intestinal calcium and phosphorus absorption. Am J Physiol 236:E451–E457
Lee DBN, Walling MW, Gafter U, Silis V, Coburn JW (1980) Calcium and inorganic phosphate transport in rat colon. Dissociated response to 1,25-dihydroxyvitamin D_3. J Clin Invest 65:1326–1331
Lee DBN, Walling MW, Levine BS, Gafter U, Silis V, Hodsman A, Coburn JW (1981) Intestinal and metabolic effect of 1,25-dihydroxyvitamin D_3 in normal adult rat. Am J Physiol 240:G90–G96
Levine RR, McNary WF, Kornguth PJ, LeBlanc R (1970) Histological reevaluation of everted gut technique for studying intestinal absorption. Eur J Pharmacol 9:211–219
Lindner E, Wohadwalla AN, Bhattacharya BK (1978) Positive inotropic and blood pressure lowering activity of a diterpene derivative isolated from Coleus forskohli: Forskolin. Arzneimittelforsch 28:284–289

Manolagas SC, Taylor CM, Anderson DC (1979) Highly specific binding of 1,25-dihydroxycholecalciferol in bone cytosol. J Endocrinol 80:35–39

Martin DL, DeLuca HF (1969) Influence of sodium on calcium transport by the rat small intestine. Am J Physiol 216:1351–1359

Martin TFJ, Ronning SA (1981) Multiple mechanisms of growth inhibition by cyclic AMP derivatives in rat GH pituitary cells: Isolation of an adenylate cyclase-deficient variant. J Cell Physiol 190:289–297

Martin DL, Melancon MJ Jr, DeLuca HF (1969) Vitamin D stimulated, calcium-dependent adenosine triphosphatase from brush borders of rat small intestine. Biochem Biophys Res Commun 35:819–823

Matsumoto T, Fontaine O, Rasmussen H (1980) Effect of 1,25-dihydroxyvitamin D-3 on phosphate uptake into chick intestinal brush border membrane vesicles. Biochim Biophys Acta 599:13–23

Matsumoto T, Fontaine O, Rasmussen H (1981) Effect of 1,25-dihydroxyvitamin D_3 on phospholipid metabolism in chick duodenal mucosal cell. J Biol Chem 256:3354–3360

Max EE, Goodman DBP, Rasmussen H (1978) Purification and characterization of chick intestine brush border membrane. Effects of 1α(OH) vitamin D_3 treatment. Biochim Biophys Acta 511:224–239

Melancon MJ Jr, DeLuca HF (1970) Vitamin D stimulation of calcium-dependent adenosine triphosphatase in chick intestinal brush borders. Biochemistry 9:1658–1664

Mellon WS, DeLuca HF (1979) An equilibrium and kinetic study of 1,25-dihydroxyvitamin D_3 binding to chicken intestinal cytosol employing high specific activity 1,25-dihydroxy[^{3}H-26,27]vitamin D_3. Arch Biochem Biophys 197:90–95

Mellon WS, DeLuca HF (1980) A specific 1,25-dihydroxyvitamin D_3 binding macromolecule in chicken bone. J biol Chem 255:4081–4086

Miller A III, Ueng TH, Bronner F (1979) Isolation of a vitamin D-dependent calcium-binding protein from brush borders of rat duodenal mucosa. FEBS Lett 103:319–322

Mircheff AK, Walling MW, Van Os CH, Wright EM (1977) Distribution of alkaline phosphatase and Ca-ATPase in intestinal epithelial cell plasma membranes: Differential response to 1,25-$(OH)_2$-D_3. In: Norman AW, Schaefer K, Coburn JW, DeLuca HF, Fraser D, Grigoleit, Herrath DV (eds) Vitamin D: Biochemical, chemical and clinical aspects related to calcium metabolism. De Gruyter, Berlin, pp 281–283

Moriuchi S, DeLuca HF (1976) The effect of vitamin D_3 metabolites on membrane proteins of chick duodenal brush borders. Arch Biochem Biophys 174:367–372

Morrissey RL, Zolock DT, Bikle DD, Mellick PW (1977) Role of vitamin D-dependent calcium-binding protein in intestinal calcium absorption. Fed Proc 36:1097

Morrissey RL, Zolock DT, Bikle DD, Empson RN Jr, Bucci TJ (1978 a) Intestinal response to 1α,25-dihydroxycholecalciferol: I. RNA polymerase, alkaline phosphatase, calcium and phosphorus uptake in vitro and in vivo calcium transport and accumulation. Biochim Biophys Acta 538:23–33

Morrissey RL, Empson RN Jr, Zolock DT, Bikle DD, Bucci TJ (1978 b) Intestinal response to 1α,25-dihydroxycholecalciferol: II. A timed study of the intracellular localization of calcium binding protein. Biochim Biophys Acta 538:34–41

Murer H, Hildmann B (1981) Transcellular transport of calcium and inorganic phosphate in the small intestinal epithelium. Am J Physiol 240:G409–G416

Murer H, Kinee R (1980) The use of isolated membrane vesicles to study epithelial transport processes. J Membr Biol 55:81–95

Narbaitz R, Stumpf W, Sar M, DeLuca HF, Tanaka Y (1980) Autoradiographic demonstration of target cells for 1,25-dihydroxycholecalciferol in the chick embryo chorioallantoic membrane, duodenum and parathyroid glands. Gen Comp Endocrinol 42:283–289

Navickis RJ, Katzenellenbogen BS, Nalbandov AV (1979) Effects of the sex steroid hormones and vitamin D_3 on calcium-binding proteins in the chick shell gland. Biol Reprod 21:1153–1162

Nellans HN, Kimberg DV (1978) Cellular and paracellular calcium transport in rat ileum: Effects of dietary calcium. Am J Physiol 235:E726–E737

Nellans HN, Kimberg DV (1979) Anomalous calcium secretion in rat ileum: Role of paracellular pathway. Am J Physiol 236:E473–E481

Nemere I, Szego CM (1981 a) Early actions of parathyroid hormone and 1,25-dihydroxycholecalciferol on isolated epithelial cells from rat intestine: I. Limited lysosomalenzyme release and calcium uptake. Endocrinology 108:1450–1462

Nemere I, Szego CM (1981 b) Early actions of parathyroid hormone and 1,25-dihydroxycholecalciferol on isolated epithelial cells from rat intestine: II. Analyses of additivity, contribution of calcium, and modulatory influence of indomethacin. Endocrinology 109:2180–2187

Neville E, Holdsworth ES (1969) A "second messenger" for vitamin D. FEBS Lett 2:313–316

Nicolaysen R (1937 a) Studies upon the mode of action of vitamin D. III. The influence of vitamin D on the absorption of calcium and phosphorus in the rat. Biochem J 31:122–129

Nicolaysen R (1937 b) Studies upon the mode of action of vitamin D. IV. The absorption of calcium chloride, xylose and sodium sulphate from isolated loops of the small intestine and of calcium chloride from the abdominal cavity in the rat. Biochem J 31:323–328

Nicolaysen R (1943) The absorption of calcium as a function of body maturation with calcium. Acta Physiol Scand 6:201–209

Norman AW (1965) Actinomycin D and the response to vitamin D. Science 149:184–186

Norman AW, Mircheff AK, Adams TH, Spieluogel A (1970) Studies on the mechanism of action of calciferol: III. Vitamin D-mediated increase of intestinal brush border alkaline phosphatase activity. Biochim Biophys Acta 215:348–359

O'Donnell JM, Smith MW (1973) Influence of cholecalciferol (vitamin D_3) on the initial kinetics of the uptake of calcium by rat small intestinal mucosa. Biochem J 134:667–669

Oku T, Wasserman RH (1978) Properties of vitamin D-stimulated calcium-dependent adenosinetriphosphatase (CaATPase) and alkaline phosphatase in chick intestinal brush borders. Fed Proc 37:408

Oldham SB, Fischer JA, Shen LH, Arnaud CD (1974) Isolation and properties of a calcium-binding protein from porcine parathyroid glands. Biochemistry 13:4790–4796

Oldham SB, Mitnick SA, Coburn JW (1980) Intestinal and parathyroid calcium-binding proteins in the dog. J Biol Chem 225:5789–5794

Omdahl JL, DeLuca HF (1977) Mediation of calcium adaptation by 1,25-dihydroxycholecalciferol. J Nutr 107:1975–1980

Pahuja DN, DeLuca HF (1981) Stimulation of intestinal calcium transport and bone calcium mobilization by prolactin in vitamin D-deficient rats. Science 214:1038–1039

Papworth DG, Patrick G (1970) The kinetics of influx of calcium and strontium into rat intestine in vitro. J Physiol 210:999–1020

Peterlik M (1978) Phosphate transport by embryonic chick duodenum. Stimulation by vitamin D_3. Biochim Biophys Acta 514:164–171

Peterlik M, Wasserman RH (1978) Effect of vitamin D on transepithelial phosphate transport in chick intestine. Am J Physiol 234:E379–E388

Peterlik M, Wasserman RH (1980) Regulation by vitamin D of intestinal phosphate absorption. Horm Metab Res 12:216–219

Petith MM, Schedl HP (1976) Intestinal adaptation to dietary calcium restriction: In vivo cecal and colonic calcium transport in the rat. Gastroenterology 71:1039–1042

Petith MM, Wilson HD, Schedl HP (1979) Vitamin D dependence of in vivo calcium transport and mucosal calcium binding protein in rat large intestine. Gastroenterology 76:99–104

Pike JW, Parker JB, Haussler MR, Boass A, Toverud SU (1979) Dynamic changes in circulating 1,25-dihydroxyvitamin D during reproduction in rats. Science 204:1427–1429

Pike JW, Gooze LL, Haussler MR (1980) Biochemical evidence for 1,25-dihydroxyvitamin D receptor macromolecules in parathyroid, pancreatic, pituitary and placental tissues. Life Sci 26:407–414

Pitkin RM (1975) Calcium metabolism in pregnancy: A review. Am J Obstet Gynecol 121:724–737

Procsal DA, Okamura WH, Norman AW (1975) Structural requirements for the interaction of 1α,25-$(OH)_2$-vitamin D_3 with its chick intestinal receptor system. J Biol Chem 250:8382–8388

Rasmussen P (1977) Calcium deficiency, pregnancy and lactation in rats. Calcif Tissue Res 23:87–94

Rasmussen H, Fontaine O, Max EE, Goodman DBP (1979) The effect of 1α-hydroxyvitamin D_3 administration on calcium transport in chick intestine brush border membrane vesicles. J Biol Chem 264:2993–2999

Rasmussen H, Matsumoto T, Fontaine O, Goodman DBP (1982) Role of changes in membrane lipid structure in the action of 1,25-dihydroxyvitamin D_3. Fed Proc 41:72–77

Rhoten WB, Christakos S (1981) Immunocytochemical localization of vitamin D-dependent calcium binding protein in mammalian nephron. Endocrinology 109:981–983

Ribovich ML, DeLuca HF (1975) The influence of dietary calcium and phosphorus on intestinal calcium transport in rats given vitamin D metabolites. Arch Biochem Biophys 170:529–535

Rizzoli R, Fleisch H, Bonjour JP (1977) Role of 1,25-dihydroxyvitamin D_3 on intestinal phosphate absorption in rats with a normal vitamin D supply. J Clin Invest 60:639–647

Rottensten KV (1938) The effect of body stores on the efficiency of calcium utilization. Biochem J 32:1285–1292

Scatchard G (1949) The attractions of protein for small molecules and ions. Ann NY Acad Sci 51:660–672

Schachter D, Kowarski S (1982) Isolation of the protein IMCal, a vitamin D-dependent membrane component of the intestinal transport mechanism for calcium. Fed Proc 41:84–87

Schachter D, Rosen SM (1959) Active transport of Ca^{45} by the small intestine and its dependence on vitamin D. Am J Physiol 196:357–362

Schachter D, Dowdle EB, Schenker H (1960) Active transport of calcium by the small intestine of the rat. Am J Physiol 198:263–268

Schachter D, Kimberg DV, Schenker H (1961) Active transport of calcium by intestine; action and bioassay of vitamin D. Am J Physiol 200:1263–1271

Schatzmann HJ (1975) In: Bronner F, Kleinzeller A (eds) Current topics in membrane transport. Academic, New York, pp 125–168

Seamon KB, Padgett W, Daly JW (1981) Forskolin: Unique diterpene activator of adenylate cyclase in membranes and intact cells. Proc Natl Acad Sci USA 78:3363–3367

Simpson RU, DeLuca HF (1980) Characterization of a receptor-like protein for 1,25-dihydroxyvitamin D_3 in rat skin. Proc Natl Acad Sci USA 77:5822–5826

Spanos E, Colston KW, Evans IMS, Galante LS, McCauley SJ, MacIntyre I (1976) Effects of prolactin on vitamin D metabolism. Mol Cell Endocrinol 5:163–167

Spanos E, Barret DI, Chong KT, MacIntyre I (1978) Effect of oestrogen and 1,25-dihydroxycholecalciferol on 25-hydroxycholecalciferol metabolism in primary chick kidney cell cultures. Biochem J 174:231–236

Spencer R, Charman M, Wilson P, Lawson E (1976) Vitamin D-stimulated intestinal calcium absorption may not involve calcium-binding protein directly. Nature 263:161–163

Steichen JJ, Tsang RC, Gratton TL, Hamstra A, DeLuca HF (1980) Vitamin D homeostasis in the perinatal period: 1,25-dihydroxyvitamin D in maternal, cord and neonatal blood. N Engl J Med 302:315–319

Sterling K (1979) Thyroid hormone action at the cell level. N Engl J Med 300:117–123, 173–177

Stoll R, Kinne R, Murer H (1979a) Effect of dietary phosphate intake on phosphate transport by isolated rat renal brush border vesicles. Biochem J 180:465–470

Stoll R, Kinne R, Murer H, Fleisch H, Bonjour JP (1979b) Phosphate transport by rat renal brush border membrane vesicles: Influence of dietary phosphate, thyroparathyroidectoma and 1,25-dihydroxyvitamin D_3. Pflügers Arch 380:47–52

Stumpf WE, Sar M, Reid FA, Tanaka Y, DeLuca HF (1979) Target cells for 1,25-dihydroxyvitamin D_3 in intestinal tract, stomach, kidney, skin, pituitary, and parathyroid. Science 206:1188–1190

Stumpf WE, Sar M, Narbaitz R, Reid FA, DeLuca HF, Tanaka Y (1980) Cellular and subcellular localization of 1,25-$(OH)_2$-vitamin D_3 in rat kidney. Comparison with localization of parathyroid hormone and estradiol. Proc Natl Acad Sci USA 77:1149–1153

Swarup G, Cohen S, Garbers DL (1981) Selective dephosphorylation of proteins containing phosphotyrosine by alkaline phosphatase. J Biol Chem 256:8197–8201

Swarup G, Speeg KV Jr, Cohen S, Garbers DL (1982) Phosphatyrosylprotein phosphatase of TCRC-2 cells. J Biol Chem 257:7298–7301

Szebenyi DME, Obendorf SK, Moffat K (1981) Structure of vitamin D-dependent calcium-binding protein from bovine intestine. Nature 294:327–332

Taylor AN (1974a) Chick brain calcium-binding protein: Comparison with intestinal vitamin D-induced calcium-binding protein. Arch Biochem Biophys 161:100–108

Taylor AN (1974b) In vitro phosphate transport in chick ileum: Effect of cholecalciferol, calcium, sodium and metabolic inhibitors. J Nutr 104:489–494

Taylor AN, Wasserman RH (1966) Vitamin D D_3-induced calcium-binding protein in chick intestinal mucosa. Science 152:791–793

Taylor AN, Wasserman RH (1967) Vitamin D_3-induced calcium-binding protein: Partial purification, electrophoretic visualization and tissue distribution. Arch Biochem Biophys 119:536–540

Taylor AN, Wasserman RH (1970) Immunofluorescent localization of vitamin D-dependent calcium-binding protein. J Histochem Cytochem 18:107–115

Taylor AN, Wasserman RH (1972) Vitamin D-induced calcium-binding protein: Comparative aspects in kidney and intestine. Am J Physiol 223:110–114

Tefler SV (1922) Studies on calcium and phosphorus metabolism. Partetabolism of calcium and phosphorus in rickets. Q J Med 16:63–72

Thomas ML, Forte LR (1981) Sex differences during the development of vitamin D deficiency in the rat: Serum parathyroid hormone, calcitonin, calcium and phosphorus. Endocrinology 109:1528–1532

Thomas ML, Forte LR (1982) Serum calcium and parathyroid hormone during the reproductive cycle in normal and vitamin D-deficient rats. Endocrinology 110:703–707

Thomasset M, Cuisinier-Gleizes P, Mathieu H (1979) 1,25-Dihydroxycholecalciferol: Dynamic of the stimulation of duodenal calcium-binding protein, calcium transport and bone calcium mobilization in vitamin D and calcium-deficient rats. FEBS Lett 107:91–94

Toverud SU, Harper C, Munson PL (1976) Calcium metabolism during lactation: Enhanced effects of thyrocalcitonin. Endocrinology 99:371–378

Tsai HC, Norman AW (1973a) Studies on the mode of action of calciferol: VI. Effect of 1,25-dihydroxy-vitamin D_3 on RNA synthesis in the intestinal mucosa. Biochem Biophys Res Commun 54:622–627

Tsai HC, Norman AW (1973b) Studies on calciferol metabolism: VIII. Evidence for a cytoplasmic receptor for 1,25-dihydroxy-vitamin D_3 in the intestinal mucosa. J Biol Chem 248:5967–5975

Tsai HC, Wong RG, Norman AW (1972) Studies on calciferol metabolism. IV. Subcellular localization of 1,25-dihydroxy-vitamin D_3 in intestinal mucosa and correlation with increased calcium transport. J Biol Chem 247:5510–5519

Tucker G III, Gagnon RE, Haussler MR (1973) Vitamin D_3-25-hydroxylase: Tissue occurrence and apparent lack of regulation. Arch Biochem Biophys 155:47–57

Ullrich KJ, Rumrich G, Klöss S (1976) Active Ca^{2+} reabsorption in the proximal tubule of the rat kidney. Dependence on sodium and buffer transport. Pflügers Arch 364:223–228

Urban E, Schedl HP (1969) Comparison of in vivo and in vitro effects of vitamin D on calcium transport in the rat. Am J Physiol 217:126–130

Ussing HH (1949) The distinction by means of tracers between active transport and diffusion. The transfer of iodide across the isolated frog skin. Acta Physiol Scand 19:43–56

Van Baelen H, Bouillon R, DeMoor P (1977) Binding of 25-hydroxycholecalciferol in tissues. J Biol Chem 252:2515–1518

Walling MW (1977) Intestinal Ca and phosphate transport: Differential responses to vitamin D_3 metabolites. Am J Physiol 223:E488–E494

Walling MW, Rothman SS (1969) Phosphate-independent, carrier-mediated active transport of calcium by rat intestine. Am J Physiol 217:1144–1148
Walling MW, Rothman SS (1973) Adaptive uptake of calcium at the duodenal brush border. Am J Physiol 225:618–623
Walling MW, Kimberg DV (1975) Effects of 1α,25-dihydroxyvitamin D_3 and *Solanum glaucophyllum* on intestinal calcium and phosphate transport and on plasma Ca, Mg, and P levels in the rat. Endocrinology 97:1567–1576
Walling MW, Kimberg DV, Wasserman RH, Feinberg RR (1976) Duodenal active transport of calcium and phosphate in vitamin D-deficient rats: Effects of nephrectomy, Cestrum diurnum and 1α,25-dihydroxyvitamin D_3. Endocrinology 98:1130–1134
Walling MW, Hartenbower DL, Coburn JW, Norman AW (1977) Effects of 1α,25-24R,25- and 1α,24R,25-hydroxylated metabolites of vitamin D_3 on calcium and phosphate absorption by duodenum from intact and nephrectomized rats. Arch Biochem Biophys 182:251–257
Warkany J (1943) Effect of maternal rachitogenic diet on skeletal development of young rat. Am J Dis Child 66:511–516
Wasserman RH (1968) Calcium transport by the intestine: A model and comment on vitamin D action. Calcif Tissue Res 2:301–313
Wasserman RH, Corradino RA (1973) Vitamin D, calcium and protein synthesis. Vitam Horm 31:43–103
Wasserman RH, Kallfelz FA (1962) Vitamin D_3 and unidirectional calcium fluxes across the rachitic chick duodenum. Am J Physiol 203:221–224
Wasserman RH, Taylor AN (1973) Intestinal absorption of phosphate in the chick: Effect of vitamin D_3 and other parameters. J Nutr 103:586–599
Wasserman RH, Kallfelz FA, Comar CL (1961) Active transport of calcium by rat duodenum in vivo. Science 133:883–884
Wasserman RH, Corradino RA, Feher J, Armbrecht HJ (1977) Temporal patterns of response of the intestinal absorptive system and related parameters to 1,25-dihydroxycholecalciferol. In: Norman AW, Schaefer K, Coburn JW, DeLuca HF, Fraser D, Grigoleit HG, Herrath D (eds) Vitamin D, biochemical, chemical, and clinical aspects related to calcium metabolism. DeGruyter, New York, p 331
Weckslér WR, Ross FP, Norman AW (1979) Characterization of the 1α,25-dihydroxyvitamin D_3 receptor from rat intestinal cytosol. J Biol Chem 254:9488–9491
Wensel RH, Rich C, Brown AC, Volwiler W (1969) Absorption of calcium measured by intubation and perfusion of the intact human small intestine. J Clin Invest 48:1768–1775
Weringer EJ, Oldham SB, Bethune JE (1978) A proposed cellular mechanism for calcium transport in the intestinal epithelial cell. Calcif Tissue Res 26:71–79
Wilson PW, Lawson DEM (1981) Vitamin D-dependent phosphorylation of an intestinal protein. Nature 289:600–602
Wilson TH, Wiseman G (1954) The use of sacs of everted small intestine for the study of the transferase of substances from the mucosal to the serosal surface. J Physiol 123:116–125
Wissig SL, Graney DO (1968) Membrane modification in the apical endocytic complex of ileal epithelial cells. J Cell Biol 39:564–579
Zerwekh JE, Haussler MR, Lindell TJ (1974) Rapid enhancement of chick intestinal DNA-dependent RNA polymerase II activity by 1α,25-dihydroxyvitamin D_3, in vivo. Proc Natl Acad Sci USA 71:2337–2341
Zerwekh JE, Lindell TJ, Haussler MR (1976) Increased intestinal chromatin template activity. J Biol Chem 251:2388–2394
Zull JE, Czarnowska-Misztal E, DeLuca HF (1965) Actinomycin D inhibition of vitamin D action. Sience 149:182–184

CHAPTER 13

Protein-Mediated Epithelial Iron Transfer *

H. HUEBERS and W. RUMMEL

A. Introduction

Iron, the fourth most abundant element of the Earth's crust, is unsurpassed in its versatility as a biologic catalyst (AISEN 1977). The adult human being contains 3–4 g total body iron of which the majority is present in circulating hemoglobin (HUGHES 1980). The second largest fraction of iron within the body is storage iron in the form of ferritin and hemosiderin. Essential tissue iron is present in myoglobin and in the cell enzymes. Only 4 mg iron is bound to plasma transferrin whose important function is iron transport and exchange between body tissues.

All proteins which affect oxygen transport, iron transfer, and iron storage have extremely high affinities for iron (association constants higher than 10^{20}). The concentration of free ionic iron, therefore, both in extracellular and intracellular fluids of organisms is kept extremely low. This condition is most desirable since the availability of iron is a prerequisite for bacterial growth (SCHADE and CAROLINE 1946) and since free ionic iron is highly toxic. The toxicity relates in part to the high affinity of free iron for enzyme proteins whose structure can consequently be irreversibly altered (HUGHES 1980). Another physiologic advantage of the high stability of protein–iron complexes is the effective restriction of iron losses from organisms. For example, the half-life of hemoglobin iron in adult humans was found to be about 8 years (FINCH and LODEN 1959). The excretion of iron by the kidneys is extremely low. Therefore, in contrast to the homeostasis of alkali and alkaline earth metals, that of iron is not regulated by renal excretion. The iron balance is maintained by adjustment of the intestinal absorption of iron in accordance with body needs. To solve this problem, nature had to develop ingenious mechansims for the transport of iron across the membranes of the intestinal mucosa. The problem is quite similar in the placenta, where the syncytiotrophoblasts have to perform the iron transfer from the mother to the fetus (LARKIN et al. 1970; FAULK and GALBRAITH 1979). The aim of this chapter is to summarize our present views of the mechanism of iron absorption and regulation and to discuss the evidence which forms the basis for the current understanding of iron absorption as a protein-mediated process.

B. Mucosal Uptake, Storage, and Transfer of Iron

The translocation of iron from the luminal to the contraluminal side of the intestinal epithelium is conventionally subdivided into two distinct steps, namely, the entry of iron into the enterocytes, "mucosal uptake," and its release from the cells

* Dedicated to Dr. ARTHUR L. SCHADE on the occasion of his 70th birthday

into the bloodstream, "transfer" (MANIS and SCHACHTER 1962a). Iron uptake into the mucosa is more rapid than its release on the serosal side by in vitro measurements. Thus, the transfer is the rate-limiting step. Mucosal uptake increases in response to the concentration of luminal iron, even in the range where the release to the serosal side remains constant and maximal. Furthermore, mucosal uptake of a given iron concentration in segments from various regions of the small intestine does not differ significantly, but transfer is notably higher in the upper part of the small intestine (MANIS and SCHACHTER 1962a). In addition, the two steps can be discriminated with certain tools. Cobalt, for example, inhibits the transfer, but not the uptake of iron (BECKER et al. 1979a).

With the advent of techniques for isolation and identification of proteins, the assumption that ferritin is the protein which is responsible for epithelial iron transfer was shown to be untenable (BRITTIN and RAVAL 1970; HUEBERS et al. 1971b, 1976). BOTHWELL and FINCH (1957) had already shown that "the intestinal ferritin is not in any clear way connected with the mechanism of absorption." In spite of these facts, there are still textbooks which do not acknowledge current information. Ferritin also functions in the intestinal mucosa as an iron

Table 1. Characteristics of the intestinal iron transfer system

Properties	References [a]
Dependence on metabolic energy	JACOBI et al. (1956); BROWN and JUSTUS (1958); DOWDLE et al. (1960); MANIS and SCHACHTER (1962a, b); PEARSON and REICH (1965); HELBOCK and SALTMAN (1967); RUMMEL and FORTH (1968)
Limited capacity	HAHN et al. (1951); MANIS and SCHACHTER (1962a, b); WHEBY et al. (1964); FORTH and RUMMEL (1965, 1966); BECKER et al. (1979a)
Adaptation to demand	WACK and WYATT (1959); BANNERMAN et al. (1962); MANIS and SCHACHTER (1962b); RULIFFSON and HOPPING (1963); CONRAD et al. (1964); CHARLTON et al. (1965); FORTH et al. (1965); FORTH and RUMMEL (1965, 1966); PEARSON and REICH (1965); CHIRASIRI and IZAK (1966); HELBOCK and SALTMAN (1967); PEARSON et al. (1967); EL-SHOBAKI and RUMMEL (1978)
Anisotropy: mucosa → serosa	MANIS and SCHACHTER (1962a); FORTH et al. (1966, 1968a); FORTH (1970); FORTH and RUMMEL (1971)
Genetically controlled adaptation to demand	PINKERTON and BANNERMAN (1967); PINKERTON (1968); BANIS et al. (1969); MANIS (1970, 1971); PINKERTON et al. (1970); HUEBERS et al. (1973); EDWARDS and HOKE (1978)
Dependence on protein synthesis	GREENBERGER and RUPPERT (1966a, b); YEH and SHILS (1966); GREENBERGER et al. (1967)

[a] For further references see FORTH and RUMMEL (1971, 1973, 1975)

storage protein. Because of ferritin's particular location in the intestinal mucosa at the entrance into the body, it can inhibit absorption by trapping iron until the absorptive cells are exfoliated (CROSBY 1963).

The characteristics of the mucosal iron transfer system can be summarized as follows: (1) dependence on metabolic energy, (2) limited capacity; (3) adaptation to demand; (4) preference of mucosal to serosal transport; (5) specificity for iron; (6) genetic control; and (7) dependence on protein synthesis (Table 1).

I. Experimental Models

Various experimental models have been used for elucidating the mechanism of iron absorption in humans and in small animals (particularly the rat). In addition, gut segments, perfused in vitro and in vivo, suspensions of isolated mucosal cells, and purified fractions of the mucosal tissue have been investigated (FINCH and LODEN 1959; HEINRICH 1970; FORTH and RUMMEL 1973; KIMBER et al. 1973; CALLENDER 1974; TURNBULL 1974; BOTHWELL et al. 1979; MARX 1979). While in vitro preparations permit a more direct study of interaction between iron and the mucosal epithelium, the small amount of iron transferred by such preparations, approximately 1% of in vivo transfer (BOTHWELL et al. 1979), raises questions of their physiologic validity. Only one publication is known to us which reports on iron and cobalt transfer in isolated vascularly perfused intestinal segments (FORTH 1967).

In the majority of animal studies reported, iron was administered in tied-off jejunal loops in situ with intact blood supply. This technique permits standardization of the luminal conditions employed and differentiation between mucosal iron uptake and transfer with a precision not usually achieved when iron is administered orally via a stomach tube. The latter technique, however, has been used to evaluate the role of the stomach and of pancreatic secretion in mucosal iron uptake and transfer (JACOBS et al. 1968).

II. Choice of the Experimental Conditions and Iron Test Doses

The amount of iron absorbed from a test dose depends on the status of iron metabolism, on the concentration of luminal iron, on the chemical form of iron, and on the possible interaction of iron with food components and gut secretions (FORTH and RUMMEL 1973; TURNBULL 1974; MARX 1979). In food there are two types of absorbable iron. One is heme iron (organic iron) which is taken up as such (CALLENDER et al. 1957; TURNBULL et al. 1962; CORNRAD et al. 1966) and catabolized inside the mucosal cell; the second is nonheme iron (inorganic iron) which is taken up as free iron and/or in a protein-bound form.

The absorbability of inorganic iron is greatly influenced by dietary composition and the pH of the luminal fluid. The availability of heme iron can be greater than that of inorganic iron because its mucosal uptake is unaffected by the composition of the diet and the pH of the luminal fluid. The absorption of heme iron is increased in iron deficiency, but much less than that of nonheme iron. The interaction with binding sites at the surface of the luminal membrane is different for organic and inorganic iron (KIMBER et al. 1973). After disintegration of heme by heme oxygenase within the mucosal cell (RAFFIN et al. 1974), the iron appears to enter the same pool as nonheme iron and is released to the blood side by the same transfer mechanism. Therefore, the study of nonheme iron absorption furnishes information relevant to the mucosal transfer of both types of iron available in food (HALLBERG and BJÖRN-RASMUSSEN 1972). The experimental animal widely preferred to study the process of iron absorption is the rat. Experiments with guinea pigs, mice, and other animals have also been reported (FORTH and RUMMEL 1973). Heme iron is less well absorbed in the rat (COOK et al. 1973) making this animal more suitable as a model for absorption studies of inorganic iron.

The most active parts of the small intestine for the absorption of inorganic iron are the duodenum and the upper jejunum (FORTH and RUMMEL 1973). Iron is absorbed through the mucosa in two phases, a rapid phase of 30–60 min at the most, and a slow phase of about 24 h (HALLBERG and SÖLVELL 1960; BROWN 1963; WHEBY and CROSBY 1963). This temporal course has been observed in both laboratory animals and humans. Not all the iron, however, which enters the mucosa from the lumen is transferred to the plasma. A variable proportion is retained within rat epithelial cells and is eventually discarded after about 2–3 days when these cells exfoliate (CONRAD and CROSBY 1963).

The absorption of inorganic iron salts rather than nonheme food iron has usually been studied. The valency of the iron used was either ferric or ferrous (FORTH and RUMMEL 1973). A summary of the dose ranges used in experimental studies in different species is given in Table 2. The relation to the therapeutic dose range can be estimated by taking into account that usually about 1.5 mg/kg are given as a single dose in humans. This is about 2.5×10^{-5} mol/kg.

Table 2. Dose range of iron in publications dealing with dependence of the absorption on the dose

Species	Oral iron dose (mol/kg)	Reference
Human	4.60×10^{-7} –3.07×10^{-5}	HAHN et al. (1951)
Human	2.56×10^{-10}–2.56×10^{-5}	SMITH and PANNACCIULLI (1958)
Rat	4.48×10^{-7} –8.95×10^{-5}	BANNERMAN et al. (1962)
Mouse	7.67×10^{-7} –3.84×10^{-3}	GITLIN and CRUCHAUD (1962)
Human	1.43×10^{-7} –1.28×10^{-5}	HEINRICH (1970)
Rat	2.00×10^{-8} –2.00×10^{-4}	SCHADE et al. (1970)
Rat	2.10×10^{-6} –5.70×10^{-4}	BECKER et al. (1979 b)
Experiments on tied-off duodenal segments		
N rat [a]	2.71×10^{-7} –2.71×10^{-6}	WHEBY et al. (1964)
N rat	2.50×10^{-8} –5.00×10^{-6}	BECKER et al. (1979 b)
N rat	5.00×10^{-8} –5.00×10^{-6}	BECKER et al. (1979 a)
D rat [b]	2.71×10^{-7} –2.71×10^{-5}	WHEBY et al. (1964)
D rat	2.50×10^{-8} –5.00×10^{-6}	BECKER et al. (1979 b)
D rat	5.00×10^{-8} –5.00×10^{-6}	BECKER et al. (1979 a)

[a] N normal rat
[b] D iron-deficient rat

Although the proportion of iron absorbed drops with increasing dosage in human, rat, and mouse, there is a progressive rise in the absolute amount absorbed, indicating that there is no defined upper limit to absorption (SMITH and PANNACCIULLI 1958; BOTHWELL and FINCH 1962; FLANAGAN et al. 1980). It has been suggested that the transfer of iron at low dosage levels is carrier mediated (SMITH and PANNACCIULLI 1958; GITLIN and CRUCHAUD 1962; FORTH and RUMMEL 1973), whereas elevated absorption values after high iron dosage are predominantly due to diffusion (GITLIN and CRUCHAUD 1962; FLANAGAN et al. 1980). The latter interpretation is not completely satisfactory since it has been shown that far less iron is absorbed from high doses injected distally into the small intestine, although diffusion is comparable at all small intestinal levels (PERMEZEL and WEBLING 1971). In contradistinction to the availability of organic iron as heme iron, inorganic iron depends on the low pH value of the intestinal content for absorption. This is particularly true for ferric iron. The absorptive utilization of a test dose administered in solution at pH 2 is ten times higher than that from a solution of pH 6 (FORTH and RUMMEL 1973).

The pH dependence of iron availability is particularly relevant for physiologic iron absorption. Iron bound to food constituents is liberated by gastric acid and dissolved in gastric fluid as ionized iron. After emptying from the stomach it remains available for the iron transfer system of the duodenal epithelium as long as the pH is low enough. Chelating agents (peptides, amino acids, ascorbic or citric acid) prevent its transformation into very stable nonabsorbable complexes of ferrioxide–polyhydrates (Fig. 1). When higher doses (20–50 μg iron) are given to normal rats, the absorption of ferric salts is considerably lower than that of ferrous salts (FORTH and RUMMEL 1973; HUEBERS et al. 1983). Similar observations have been reported for humans (MOORE et al. 1944; HEINRICH 1970). In iron-deficient rats, the difference related to the valency of iron is less striking. This obser-

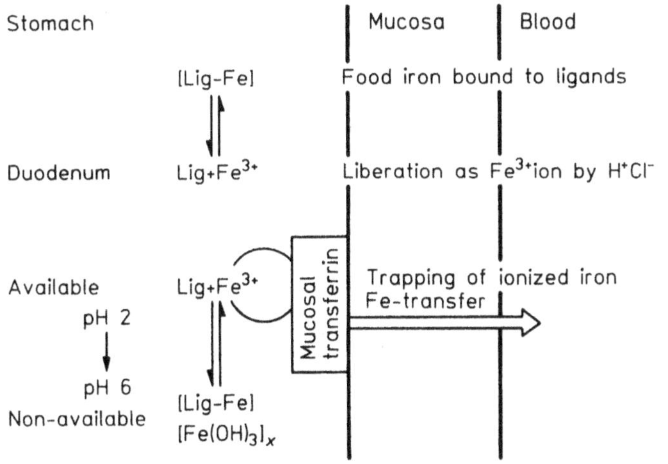

Fig. 1. Absorption of food iron. The availability of iron for absorption at the epithelial surface as a function of the intraluminal pH. After HUEBERS and RUMMEL (1977)

vation indicates that factors other than mere solubility of ferric iron must be important (HUEBERS unpublished).

By adding ligands which form soluble complexes with iron, an attempt has been made to promote the absorption of ferric salts by preventing the precipitation of ferric iron as ferric hydroxide and/or its polymers. These ligands include citric acid, ascorbic acid, amino acids, and others. A high molar excess of the chelating agent generally has to be present to guarantee the stability of a soluble iron chelate at pH values around 7 (FORTH and RUMMEL 1973). By use of the gut loop technique, it has been shown that the amount of iron absorbed from these iron complexes is much less than the same amount of iron introduced in the ionized form at pH 2 (FORTH and RUMMEL 1973; TURNBULL 1974). However, there are other disadvantages in using iron chelating agents. When present in millimolar concentrations, these chelates have been shown to mediate iron exchange between a number of high molecular weight iron binding substances, particularly transferrin and ferritin (AISEN and BROWN 1977). It is also possible that this exchange may alter the original distribution of iron within the mucosal tissue or in the subsequent mucosal cell homogenate. In addition, some of these ligands may prevent the detection of less stable endogenous low molecular weight iron components of the mucosal cell. To avoid such interference by exogenous chelates, simple iron salts have ben used in search for iron binding intermediates during intestinal absorption of iron. The disadvantage when using inorganic iron salts at pH 2 is the short time of iron availability which makes absorption nonlinear. This can be overcome by adding albumin. In spite of the fact that the pH of the albumin solution is above 7, absorption remains linear for 60 min and is three times higher than without albumin (HUEBERS et al. 1983).

III. Molecular Aspects of Iron Absorption: Search for Mucosal Iron Carriers

While the capability of organisms to regulate iron absorption is well recognized, the molecular nature of the absorptive mechanism and the manner in which it is regulated is not yet completely clear. Indications that proteins might be involved in iron absorption are given by the observations that iron absorption is increased after activation of protein synthesis by phenobarbital (see Table 1) or by polychlorinated hydrocarbons (e.g., 2,3,7,8-tetrachlorobenzo-*p*-dioxin; MANIS and KIM 1979). Conversely, pretreatment with inhibitors of protein synthesis decreases activity of the iron transport system (GREENBERGER and RUPPERT 1966 a, b; YEH and SHILS 1966; GREENBERGER et al. 1967).

The aim of the studies to be reviewed is to identify the essential components of the epithelial iron transfer system and to analyze the changes which are significant for low and high absorptive states. The capacity of rat small intestine to absorb iron is greatly increased in experimental iron deficiency, whether it is produced by bleeding or a low iron diet (FORTH and RUMMEL 1973). Most of our present knowledge about the mechanisms of iron absorption is derived from fractionation studies or morphological analyses of duodenal and jejunal tissue from normal and iron-deficient rats.

1. Subcellular Distribution

Information about the subcellular distribution of iron during absorption is a prerequisite in the search for iron binding components possibly involved in duodenal and jejunal absorptive transfer of iron. Special methods to fractionate the constituents of intestinal mucosal epithelium have been described (HUEBERS et al. 1971 c; WORWOOD and JACOBS 1971; HUEBERS 1972; HALLIDAY et al. 1975; BATEY and GALLAGHER 1977). They include differential centrifugation, as well as density gradient systems. With these methods the amount of ^{59}Fe which appeared in particulate and nonparticulate fractions of the mucosal tissue was followed as a function of time after injection of a ^{59}Fe test dose into the intestinal lumen of a tied-off duodenal or jejunal loop (HUEBERS et al. 1971 b, c; HUEBERS 1972; POLLACK and LASKY 1975).

a) Nonparticulate Fraction

In rats, after the administration of a ^{59}Fe-labeled test dose, 60% or more of the radioiron in the mucosal tissue was present in the nonparticulate fraction and only 5% of this amount was dialyzable. By means of electrophoresis and column chromatography it was determined that the radioiron was bound to two proteins. These two proteins have been isolated and characterized as mucosal transferrin and mucosal ferritin (HUEBERS et al. 1971 b, c, 1976; HALLIDAY et al. 1976; EL-SHOBAKI and RUMMEL 1977). Rat mucosal transferrin has the same molecular weight as serum transferrin and binds two atoms of iron, but differs in amino acid composition and isoelectric point from plasma transferrin (HUEBERS et al. 1976). Differences between mucosal and plasma transferrin were found by in vitro tagging with radioiron (POLLACK et al. 1972; HUEBERS 1975).

The second iron binding protein in the gut mucosa, mucosal ferritin, was compared with the ferritins of rat spleen and liver as to its molecular weight, isoelectric point, amino acid composition, and tryptic peptide pattern (HUEBERS et al. 1974, 1976). All three ferritins were distinctly different in their electrophoretic behavior (HUEBERS 1975; HUEBERS et al. 1976). In addition, the iron content of mucosal ferritin was found to be much lower than that of liver and spleen ferritins. In the iron-replete animal, most of the iron taken up by intestinal mucosa is deposited as ferritin and ultimately is lost from the body as the body's cells are exfoliated into the gut (CONRAD and CROSBY 1963). In iron deficiency, virtually no mucosal ferritin can be demonstrated, but the amounts of mucosal transferrin and the activity of the iron transport system within the mucosa is manyfold increased (HUEBERS et al. 1971 b; SAVIN and COOK 1977, 1980; EL-SHOBAKI and RUMMEL 1978; OSTERLOH 1979).

In Fig. 2, the time course of the appearance and disappearance of absorbed ^{59}Fe in the mucosal transferrin and ferritin fraction is illustrated. It is evident in iron-deficient rats that the rapid uptake of iron into the mucosa and its subsequent release into the body is accelerated by mucosal transferrin (HUEBERS 1972). In normal rats, however, mucosal transferrin plays an insignificant role in the time course of the ^{59}Fe content in the cytosol fraction. In this case, the time dependence of the ^{59}Fe content in the cytosol correlates with that of mucosal ferritin.

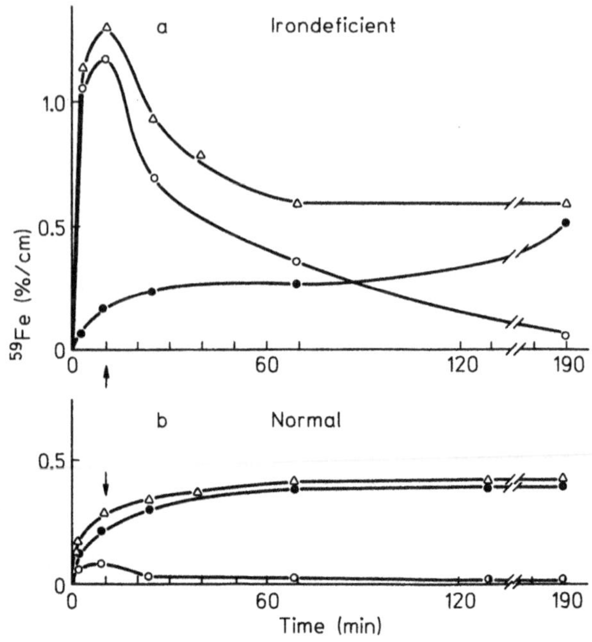

Fig. 2a, b. Content of absorbed iron in the particle-free fraction of homogenized jejunal mucosa and its distribution between mucosal transferrin and ferritin as a function of time in iron-deficient (**a**) and normal rats (**b**). Ordinate: ^{59}Fe content per centimeter length of the jejunal segment as a percentage of the dose (10 nmol $^{59}FeCl_3$) administered in 2 ml 0.9% NaCl solution (pH 2.0) into a tied-off segment of 12–17 cm length). Abscissa: time in minutes. The *arrows* indicate the end of the exposure time (10 min) and the removal of the iron-containing solution by perfusion with 25 ml 0.9% NaCl solution (pH 7.4). Hemoglobin content per 100 ml blood: normal rats 14 g, iron-deficient rats 8 g. *Full circles*, ^{59}Fe in mucosal ferritin; *open circles*, ^{59}Fe in mucosal transferrin; *triangles*, ^{59}Fe in the total particle-free fraction. $N=5$; s, $\leqq 0.04$. After HUEBERS et al. (1971 b)

The correlation in time between the disappearance of ^{59}Fe from the mucosal transferrin fraction and its appearance in the animal (HUEBERS 1972) suggests strongly that mucosal transferrin plays a dominant role among the factors which are involved in the translocation of iron across the epithelium (HUEBERS et al. 1971 b). Further evidence for this important functional role of mucosal transferrin was obtained when measuring the amount of mucosal transferrin by a two-site immunoradiometric assay. In the intestinal mucosa of rats of varying iron status, a good correlation was found between iron absorption and the mucosal content of transferrin (SAVIN and COOK 1977, 1980).

The ability to adapt the absorptive utilization of a given dose to higher demand is genetically determined. Unlike normal mice, mice with sex-liked congenital anemia (SLA mice) are unable to increase the absorptive utilization when the body's need for iron is enhanced. Subcellular fractionation studies showed that the characteristic increase of absorbed iron which appears in the fraction of mucosal transferrin does not occur in mice with sex-linked anemia (HUEBERS et al. 1973; EDWARDS and HOKE 1978).

Low molecular weight iron binding components, e.g., citrate, ascorbate, and "free iron" present in the nonparticulate fraction, have been reported (SHEEHAN and FRENKEL 1972; LINDER and MUNRO 1975; HALLIDAY et al. 1975, 1976; EL-SHOBAKI and RUMMEL 1977, 1979; BATEY and GALLAGHER 1977). Without additional studies, however, it might be cautioned that these findings are due to the addition of chelates to the iron test dose or from the degradation of proteins leading to the formation of low molecular weight iron complexes. In addition, certain buffers used (e.g., phosphate) are likely to release iron from mucosal transferrin during column chromatography, even at neutral pH (HUEBERS et al. 1981).

b) Particulate Fraction

After in vivo tagging with ^{59}Fe, the particulate fraction of mucosal homogenates was separated into microsomal, mitochondrial, brush border, and nuclear fractions (HUEBERS et al. 1971c; HUEBERS 1972). Studies on the subcellular distribution of radioiron as a function of time did not provide evidence of direct involvement of mitochondrial and microsomal fractions in the process of iron absorption (HUEBERS 1972). Possibly, the original cellular distribution of iron was disturbed by homogenization. Earlier suggestions of the involvement of mitochondria in the iron transport system (WORWOOD and JACOBS 1971) have meanwhile been revised (HUMPHRYS et al. 1977). Attempts have been made to identify the nature of the radioiron bound to the various particulate fractions of mucosal cell homogenates by using membrane solubilizing detergents. From these studies, it appears likely that the major part of the radioiron on the particulate fraction is in the form of membrane-bound ferritin and transferrin and that no other membrane protein could be isolated which binds iron (YOSHINO and MANIS 1973; KAUFMAN et al. 1976, 1977; EL-SHOBAKI and RUMMEL 1977). These findings emphasize the fundamental roles of the two iron binding mucosal proteins in intestinal iron absorption.

IV. Studies in Purified Fractions of Mucosal Epithelium and Mucosal Cell Suspension

There have been many attempts to elucidate the process of iron absorption by studying iron uptake by purified mucosal cell fractions and by the use of mucosal cell suspension (GREENBERGER et al. 1969; HALLIDAY et al. 1976; SAVIN and COOK 1978; BOTHWELL et al. 1979). While these studies do not permit conclusions to be made relative to iron transfer, they do provide observations on the binding of iron to membranes or cells under well-defined conditions.

1. Binding of Iron by Brush Borders

The binding of iron to the luminal membrane of enterocytes has been studied with preparations of isolated brush borders (GREENBERGER et al. 1969; HUEBERS et al. 1971a; HUEBERS 1972; KIMBER et al. 1973; COX and O'DONNELL 1980, 1981; O'DONNELL and COX 1981). Brush borders from the cells of the proximal small intestine bind iron in preference to other biometals such as cobalt, copper, zinc, and manganese. Furthermore, the membrane-bound iron, in contradistinction to cobalt, cannot be removed by repeated washings. Neither of these features is seen with brush borders from the distal ileal mucosa (HUEBERS et al. 1971 a, HUEBERS 1972). These observations suggest that the more efficient uptake of iron in the proximal small bowell is associated with the presence of more specific receptors for iron on the luminal cell membranes. In addition, preparations of brush borders isolated from the distal ileum of iron-deficient animals bind more iron than those from animals with normal iron stores, while proximal iron binding is inhibited in iron-loaded animals (KIMBER et al. 1973).

The role of the surface glycoproteins in iron absorption was studied in isolated brush borders by incubating them with ferric citrate at various pH and temperature ranges (MUKHERJEE 1972). Iron was bound mainly to the glycocalyx and this binding was maximal at pH 7.4 at 37 °C. Furthermore, a spotty uptake of iron among adjacent isolated brush borders was observed. This uneven distribution is paralleled by the localization of transferrin in some enterocytes and hepatocytes and not in others, as demonstrated by the immunoperoxidase staining method (MASON and TAYLOR 1978) and by the fluorescent antibody technique (LANE 1967). Both methods revealed transferrin-positive cells in close proximity to negative cells. Similar observations have also been made through use of the Prussian blue technique (PARMLEY et al. 1978).

It seems probable that certain glycoproteins on the luminal surface play a significant role for the absorptive utilization of iron, particularly in iron deficiency. Since it is known that the glycoproteins of the surface coat are continuously produced by the enterocytes (ITO and REVEL 1964; ITO 1969; BENNETT 1970; BENNETT and LEBLOND 1970), it is not unreasonable to assume that transferrin, which is also a glycoprotein (AISEN and BROWN 1977), can be "secreted" by enterocytes (HUEBERS et al. 1974).

2. Uptake of Iron by Duodenal Biopsy Specimens

The ability of a range of homologous transferrin-like proteins to donate iron to pieces of human duodenal mucosa was examined after incubation in vitro (COX and PETERS 1978; COX et al. 1979). Lactoferrin was able to yield its iron to intestinal tissue, but not to reticulocytes; in contrast, serum transferrin and ovotransferrin were able to donate their iron to reticulocytes, but not to intestinal tissue (COX and PETERS 1978). Doubly tagged lactoferrin preparations (^{59}Fe and ^{125}I) indicated that the intact protein was unable to enter into enterocytes. The authors concluded that specific cell surface receptors for lactoferrin at the brush border membrane are involved. These in vitro results do not agree with results in vivo in humans and animals, showing that lactoferrin inhibits rather than enhances iron absorption (DE LAEY et al. 1968; DE VET and VAN GOOL 1974; MCMILLAN et al. 1977). In iron-overloaded patients with primary hemochromatosis, the uptake of iron by the biopsy specimens was exceptionally high (COX and PETERS 1978). Kinetic analysis suggested that this was the result of affinity for iron being increased in a carrier protein in the enterocyte (COX et al. 1979).

3. Release of Iron from the Mucosal Cell to the Plasma

The final step in the epithelial transfer of iron is the release of iron from the mucosal cell to the plasma. In vitro experiments using isolated intestinal epithelial cells from rats previously tagged with ^{59}Fe have shown that the release of ^{59}Fe induced by iron-deficient serum is greater than by normal serum and that isolated serum transferrin is able to liberate the same amount of ^{59}Fe as serum (LEVINE et al. 1972). Further, it has been found that the released ^{59}Fe had the same electrophoretic mobility as serum transferrin (SAVIN and COOK 1978). This result and the demonstration that ^{125}I-labeled plasma apotransferrin is able to bind to intestinal epithelial cells led to the conclusion that plasma apotransferrin binds to receptors on the contraluminal side of intestinal epithelial cells, removes iron from the cell, and returns to the plasma once it is saturated with iron (LEVINE et al. 1972). However, experiments using isolated enterocytes do not permit a decision to be made whether iron release occurs at the luminal or contraluminal side of the cells. Furthermore, the conclusions of these authors are not supported by the work of others (WHEBY and JONES 1963; SCHADE et al. 1969). In addition, recent studies have shown that rat serum causes a complement-dependent cytolysis of isolated intestinal epithelial cells (SULLIVAN and WEINTRAUB 1979). Such cytolysis makes the results of all experiments using isolated intestinal cells in presence of serum questionable.

It has been further shown that iron absorption continues after the iron binding capacity of the plasma transferrin has been saturated (WHEBY and JONES 1963). In addition, a preparation of isolated duodenum with an artificial circulation transfers iron rapidly to the blood side, even when there is no transferrin in the vascular perfusate (JACOBS et al. 1966), and increasing the amount of transferrin in the plasma does not affect absorption (POLLACK et al. 1963). It is therefore clear that the release of iron from the contraluminal pole of the mucosal cell is at least not predominantly dependent on the availability of free iron binding sites on plasma transferrin. Finally, the total rate of transcapillary exchange of serum transferrin and the rate of passage of plasma transferrin into the extravascular compartment of the intestinal mucosa are quantitatively insufficient to explain the amount of iron actually transferred from the mucosa to the blood (MORGAN 1980).

V. Morphological Studies

For the morphological demonstration in rats of the pathway which iron takes during the translocation from the luminal to the serosal side of the mucosa, doses between 0.3 and 7.0 μmol/kg were used (CONRAD and CROSBY 1963; BÉDARD et al. 1971, 1973; HUMPHRYS et al. 1977; PARMLEY et al. 1978). Under pharmacotherapeutic conditions, about 25 μmol/kg are usually given (see Table 2).

1. Radioautography

Radioautography has been employed to visualize the passage of radioiron through the mucosal cell of the duodenum in mice and rats (BÉDARD et al. 1971, 1973; HUMPHRYS et al. 1977). It is found that, 5 min after the administration of ^{55}Fe-labeled $FeSO_4$ (7 μmol/kg, for comparison see Table 2) into the stomach of normal mice (BÉDARD et al. 1971), activity spots appear in the duodenal wall over the brush border, the terminal web, in the cytoplasm, allegedly over the rough endoplasmic reticulum, and already over the lamina propria near capillary walls.

The authors felt that spots were never seen over pinocytotic vacuoles near the terminal web and that therefore there was no evidence for the participation of micropinocytosis in iron uptake into the mucosa. Using radioautography it is difficult to draw conclusions about precise localization over small structures such as pinocytotic vesicles and rough endoplasmic reticulum. A spot count reached a peak at 30 min over the brush border and then decreased steeply to very low values from 90 min onwards. A sharp peak was seen within the cytoplasm at 60 min. Up to 1 h, very few spots were seen over or near lysosomes and their maximal labeling was achieved at 3 h, when the number of lysosomes was increased. The authors believe that the frequency of spots in relation to clumps of ferritin granules was increased. Epithelial cells other than the absorptive cells, i.e., undifferentiated, goblet, Paneth, and argentaffin cells, show only very scanty spots and therefore do not appear to participate in mucosal iron transfer (BÉDARD et al. 1971). The time course of the appearance and disappearance of the ^{55}Fe activity spots is accelerated in iron deficiency and retarded in iron-overloaded and sex-linked anemic mice (BÉDARD et al. 1973). Thus, these radioautographic observations confirm the results obtained in kinetic studies.

2. Prussian Blue Reaction

Ferrocyanide and ferricyanide staining technique (Prussian blue reaction) permits an ultrastructural cytochemical visualization of iron and its subcellular distribution in the mucosal tissue of the rat (PARMLEY et al. 1978). In addition, the ionic state of absorbed inorganic iron can be morphologically discerned. The dose used was about 10 µmol/kg. These studies suggest that ferrous iron is converted to ferric iron at the microvillus membrane and appears subsequently epithelially as small nonmembrane-bound stain deposits which are concentrated in the apical cytoplasm. The staining of cells varied widely. It was greatest among differentiated cells at the tips of the intestinal villi. Single epithelial cells exhibit abundant staining often not seen in adjacent cells. Extracellular spaces and endothelial cells are also generally stained. No staining was observed in lymphatic channels of the lamina propria. The appearance of larger stained deposits in the lateral and in the basal extracellular spaces, along the intraluminal and extraluminal outer plasmalemma of adjacent endothelial cells in the lamina propria, suggests passage of iron from epithelial cells through the lamina propria to blood vessels. These findings are in agreement with the previously described radioautographic observations (BÉDARD et al. 1971, 1973). The fact that stain deposits in epithelial cells were not observed in microendocytotic caveolae and that the majority of iron in epithelial cells was not membrane bound suggested that iron is not absorbed by endocytotic processes. As with radioautography, this technique provides no information about iron binding to particular proteins which may play a role in iron transfer across the cell. They do, however, complement the biochemically oriented cell fractionation studies.

3. Immunoperoxidase Technique

An immunohistologic method which makes possible the identification and localization of iron binding proteins in the intestinal mucosa during iron absorption was used by MASON and TAYLOR (1978). In their studies, an immunoperoxidase staining technique was used for detecting the three major iron binding proteins (transferrin, ferritin, and lactoferrin) in routine histologic paraffin sections of human tissue. In epithelial cells of the duodenum, strong granular staining was noted for transferrin, both at the tips of villi and in cells lying along the sides of the villi. The reaction was most intense just beneath the brush border of the cells. For ferritin, positive reactions were noted within epithelial cells at the tips of villi, similar in distribution to that of transferrin. Lactoferrin was detected in some intestinal epithelial cells of the absorptive type. Unlike transferrin, it was usually confined to the tips of villi. Lactoferrin-positive cells tended to be in groups clearly demarcated from adjacent negative ones.

An important stimulus for studies on the assessment of the postulated role of the mucosal iron binding proteins for the process of iron absorption came from the work of ISOBE et al. (1978). In their communications they described the localization of ferritin, lactoferrin, and transferrin in the small intestine as observed microscopically using a direct immunoperoxidase technique. The material was derived from pieces of normal duodenum which were taken from moderately anemic patients during abdominal operations such as gastrectomy for gastric ulcer. In some of these patients, ferrous sulfate (105 mg Fe^{2+}) was administered orally 3 h before operation. The results clearly showed that all the three iron binding proteins: ferritin, lactoferrin, and transferrin, occur in the epithelium with distinct localization. Under moderately anemic conditions, these proteins were present in the intestinal epithelium, but in small amounts. After iron administration, however, the levels of these proteins in the mucus of goblet cells increased appreciably. The authors concluded that the administration of iron stimulated the secretion of these proteins from goblet cells. Severe reservations about immunolocalization of transferrin and ferritin must be voiced because this tissue was frozen, sectioned, and thawed prior to application of labeled antibodies; under these circumstances proteins can migrate from their original locations in vivo (TAYLOR 1981). It is conceivable that the secreted iron binding proteins were in the apo form, since these proteins failed to stain with Prussian blue (ISOBE et al. 1978).

C. Regulation of Iron Absorption

The homeostasis of iron metabolism is maintained by the regulation of iron absorption, with no recognizable control of its excretion (MCCANCE and WIDDOWSON 1937; BOTHWELL and FINCH 1962). The regulation is performed directly by the epithelium of the upper small intestine (FORTH and RUMMEL 1973). This has been substantiated by numerous studies since 1973 (HUEBERS et al. 1973, 1974, 1975; KIMBER et al. 1973; POLLACK and LASKY 1975; HALLIDAY et al. 1975, 1976; FURUGOURI and KAWABATA 1976; BATEY and GALLAGHER 1977; HUMPHRYS et al. 1977; SAVIN and COOK 1977, 1980; EDWARDS and HOKE 1978; COX and PETERS 1980).

I. The Significance of Mucosal Iron Binding Proteins

The determining role of mucosal transferrin and ferritin in the epithelial regulation of iron absorption was clearly demonstrated in experiments in which iron deficiency and iron overload in rats was produced by a changeover from the normal state to that of iron deficiency and back again (EL-SHOBAKI and RUMMEL 1977). During the development of iron deficiency, the content of absorbed iron in the mucosal transferrin fraction increased simultaneously with the transfer of absorbed iron from the epithelium to the body. The content of absorbed iron in the mucosal ferritin fraction, however, diminished with the degree of iron deficiency (Fig. 3). These results in the rat model resemble those obtained in growing piglets (FURUGOURI 1977), indicating some interspecies validity. This association of an increased absorption of iron with a decrease in absorbed iron bound to mucosal ferritin was also described in pregnant rats (BATEY and GALLAGHER 1977). In mice with sex-linked anemia, however, in which mucosal iron uptake was intact but transfer impaired (MANIS 1970, 1971; HUEBERS et al. 1973), the mucosal amount of iron (PINKERTON 1968; BÉDARD et al. 1973) and ferritin (EDWARDS et al. 1977; EDWARDS and HOKE 1978) was increased despite the existing iron deficiency anemia. In iron-deficient rats during the recompensation by iron repletion, the decrease of absorption was associated with a sharp rise in ferritin-bound iron (EL-SHOBAKI and RUMMEL 1977). Early during iron repletion, the mucosal ferritin level increases (BRITTIN and RAVAL 1970; LINDER et al. 1975; KAUFMAN et al. 1976, 1977; EL-SHOBAKI and RUMMEL 1977). Therefore, the conclusion has been drawn that the two mucosal iron binding proteins are involved in a reciprocal manner in the regulation of the epithelial transfer of absorbed iron to the body. This conclusion is suported by results which SAVIN and COOK (1980) obtained by determining the amount of mucosal transferrin and ferritin with a highly sensitive two-site immunoradiometric assay in isolated mucosal cells from normal and iron-deficient rats. With increasing iron absorption, the amount of mucosal transferrin increased and the amount of mucosal ferritin decreased inversely. The decrease of mucosal ferritin during the development of iron deficiency was also described by others (LINDER et al. 1975; SETSUDA et al. 1980). The ratio of mucosal

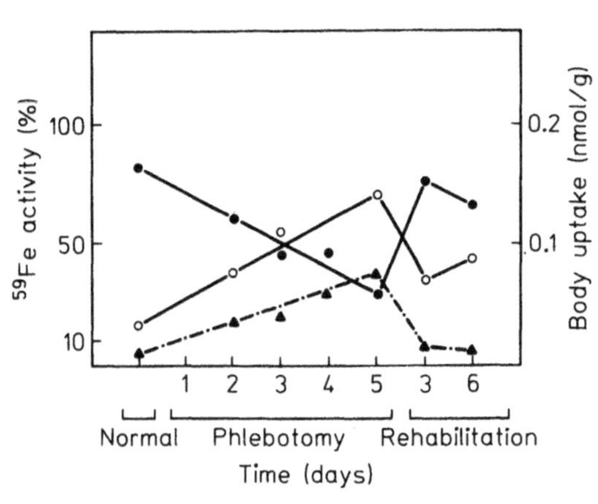

Fig. 3. Distribution of ^{59}Fe activity between mucosal ferritin and transferrin in the "cytosol" fraction correlated with ^{59}Fe absorption (body uptake) after different times of phlebotomies and rehabilitation (*full circles*, ferritin fraction; *open circles*, transferrin fraction; *triangles*, body uptake). EL-SHOBAKI and RUMMEL (1977)

transferrin to mucosal ferritin showed a very high correlation ($r = 0.95$; SAVIN and COOK 1980) with the degree of absorptive utilization of a given iron dose.

From these studies, the shape of the curves of Fig. 3 can be interpreted as follows: (1) the increase in the slope of the transferrin curve reflects an increase of newly synthesized mucosal apotransferrin induced by a decreased iron content within a certain iron pool of the epithelium; (2) the increase in newly synthesized mucosal ferritin is caused by an increase in the intraepithelial iron pool. If this interpretation is correct, it can be stated that the reciprocal dependence of the synthesis of mucosal transferrin and ferritin on the iron status resembles that of hepatic transferrin and ferritin under similar conditions. Results obtained in isolated perfused rat livers taken from iron-deficient and iron-refed animals showed that in iron deficiency the synthesis of transferrin was increased while, after refeeding with iron, an increase in hepatic ferritin concentration was associated with a reduction in transferrin synthesis (MORTON and TAVILL 1977). The latter result was previously obtained by LANE (1968) by use of the fluorescent antibody technique to visualize the transferrin synthesis in rats.

The determining role of mucosal transferrin and ferritin in the epithelial regulation of iron absorption has been convincingly demonstrated by the results of a crucial experiment. When hemoglobin synthesis in rats has been reduced by dietary protein deficiency, the iron stores in the liver increased. Thus, despite the fact that the diet was also lacking in iron, the epithelial transfer of iron did not increase, probably due to a defective transferrin synthesis. This is a degree of iron deficiency in the diet which, in the absence of a protein deficiency, would have increased the epithelial iron transfer to the body fivefold (Fig. 4; EL-SHOBAKI and RUMMEL 1978). The distribution ratio of the iron taken up into the epithelium be-

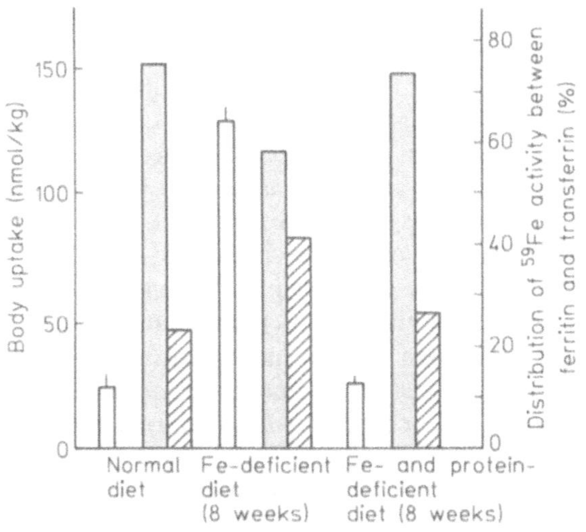

Fig. 4. Interdependence of iron absorption (*white columns*) and incorporation of absorbed ^{59}Fe into the mucosal ferritin (*dark columns*) and transferrin fraction (*striped columns*) of rats on normal, iron-deficient, and iron-deficient plus protein-deficient diet. After EL-SHOBAKI and RUMMEL (1978)

tween mucosal transferrin and ferritin was 0.36 : 1 after feeding an iron-deficient and protein-deficient diet, i.e., it was approximately the same as under normal conditions (0.3 : 1). For comparison, the distribution ratio was 0.7 : 1 when feeding a diet with the same iron deficiency, but with a normal protein content. Under comparable conditions, using endotoxin treatment of rats as a model for infection anemia, it could be shown that the inhibition of iron absorption is also associated with a decrease of the transferrin to ferritin ratio (RUMMEL et al. 1984).

II. Luminal Factors

The question whether gastric or pancreatic juice might have a regulating function in iron absorption has been repeatedly discussed (for references, see FORTH and RUMMEL 1973). The name "gastroferrin" was created for a protein which was presumed to activate iron absorption. However, this protein has never been isolated or identified. Meanwhile, interest has become focused on duodenal and jejunal secretions and also on bile.

1. Gastric Juice

In contrast to the earlier assumption, there exists to date no conclusive evidence that the amount of iron binding and absorption activating factors in gastric juice vary in relation to the body's demand for iron (MIGNON et al. 1965; FORTH and RUMMEL 1968; JACOBS and MILES 1968; SMITH et al. 1969; POWELL and WILSON 1970). The same holds true for pancreatic secretions, although in certain diseases the reduction in the bicarbonate content of pancreatic juice might affect iron absorption because of a change in luminal pH values.

2. Bile

The role of bile in iron absorption is not yet clear. In normal rats, ligation of the bile duct reduced absorption of ferric and ferrous iron, but in iron-deficient animals only that of ferric iron (CONRAD and SCHADE 1968; JACOBS and MILES 1970). It was suggested that ascorbic acid in bile promoted iron absorption by making soluble iron complexes. This proposal cannot provide the full explanation because inorganic iron also forms soluble absorbable complexes with bile salts (JACOBS and MILES 1970). The iron complexes in the bile are soluble at neutral pH and would act to maintain iron in solution in the lumen of the intestine. H. HUEBERS and W. RUMMEL (1980, unpublished work) observed that, after intravenous injection of ^{59}Fe-tagged transferrin into normal and iron-deficient rats, the ^{59}Fe activity found in the bile after a 1-h collection period was exclusively transferrin bound. Also in humans, the occurrence of transferrin in bile has been described (DE VET 1971). Whether the transferrin secreted with the bile is a participant in the regulation of iron absorption is an open question.

3. Duodenal and Jejunal Secretions

Duodenal and jejunal secretions have been investigated, particularly in relation to the absorption of hemoglobin (WHEBY et al. 1962), but there also exist reports

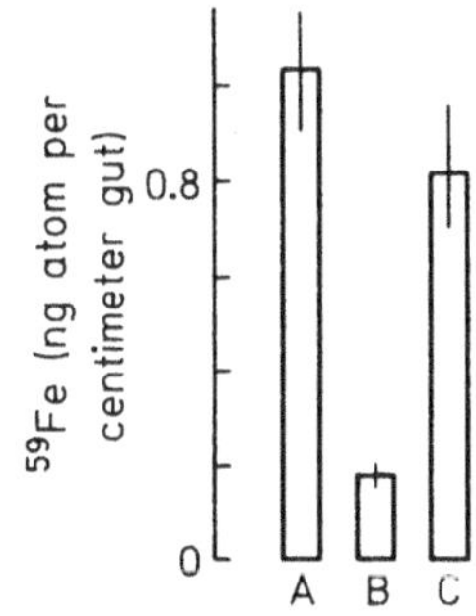

Fig. 5. Effect on iron absorption of an elutable component obtained from jejunal segments of iron-deficient rats. Dose: 165 nmol $^{59}FeCl_3$ in 1 ml isotonic saline at pH 2.0; (*A, B*); and 165 nmol $^{59}FeCl_3$ in 1 ml solution (pH 4.8) obtained as residue of a $^{59}FeCl_3$ solution (540 nmol, pH 2.0) after 2 min of exposure to jejunal segments of iron-deficient donor rats (*C*). In *B* and *C*, the rats have been perfused for 10 min with isotonic saline (pH 7.4 buffered with 0.3 m*M* phosphate) at a flow rate of 4.5 ml/min. Exposure time 10 min. Mean ± standard deviation, $N=6$. After HUEBERS et al. (1974, 1975)

about the influence of duodenal and jejunal secretions in the absorption of nonheme iron in rats. A high molecular weight iron binding factor has been found on the surface of jejunal mucosa in iron-deficient animals, which is called "elutable factor" because it can be washed away (HUEBERS et al. 1974, 1975; HUEBERS and RUMMEL 1977). The absorptive utilization of an iron test dose is remarkably decreased after the elution of this factor (Fig. 5). It can be restored nearly to the original high degree of absorptive utilization in iron deficiency by transferring the elutable factor from other iron-deficient animals.

From these observations it can be concluded that the "elutable factor" is an essential component for the first step of absorption and that it is at least partially responsible for the increased absorptive utilization of an iron test dose in iron deficiency. Mucosal transferrin is probably one constituent of the elutable iron binding factor. In experiments designed to answer the question whether transferrin-bound iron itself is available for intestinal iron absorption, it was shown that rat plasma transferrin-bound iron can actually enter the mucosal epithelium of the small intestine in rats (HUEBERS 1979; HUEBERS et al. 1979 a). In duodenal segments of iron-deficient rats, a 4 µg transferrin-bound iron dose was completely absorbed within 1 h and more than two-thirds of the amount taken up into the mucosa was transferred to the body. Jejunal segments were less active and the transferrin-bound iron taken up in the ileum was not transferred at all. Normal rats absorbed less than one-tenth of the amount of transferrin iron compared with the iron-deficient group. Subcellular fractionation studies in the mucosal homogenates of the respective groups revealed that most of the radioiron in normal rats was found in ferritin, whereas in iron-deficient rats more radioiron was bound to transferrin.

The origin of mucosal transferrin on or in the mucosa under physiologic conditions is not yet clear. The suggestion by ISOBE et al. (1978) that it may be stored or secreted by goblet cells may or may not be artifactual (ISOBE K and ISOBE Y,

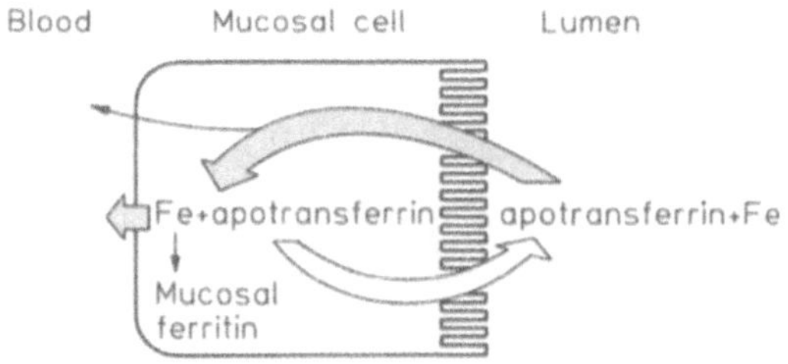

Fig. 6. Model for uptake and release of transferrin by the mucosal cell. Apotransferrin present in the secretions of the duodenal and jejunal mucosa reacts with food iron to form transferrin. Subsequently, the transferrin-bound iron is taken up into the mucosal cell without appreciable degradation, probably by an endocytotic process. Within the cell, the iron released from the transferrin can either enter the blood or be deposited in the mucosal ferritin. In iron deficiency, release to the blood is predominant whereas in iron overload, deposition as ferritin iron is prevalent. Small amounts of transferrin iron (about 5%–10% of the dose) can enter the circulation in a physiologically intact form. This transfer system does not exist in the ileal epithelium. After HUEBERS et al. (1983)

1983). Another possibility is that the protein is synthesized and secreted by mucosal cells (HUEBERS et al. 1974, 1975; see also Sect. B.V.3). At any rate, mucosal transferrin may serve as a carrier in a shuttle mechanism to move iron from the intestinal lumen into the mucosal cell, in a fashion similar to that assumed for reticulocytes (AISEN and BROWN 1977; for references see MORGAN 1981). Supportive of this theory is the observation that plasma transferrin saturated with iron is not subject to enzymatic degradation in the gut lumen. If the same holds true for mucosal transferrin, this would be in favor of its iron carrying role (HUEBERS 1979). Possibly, there are specific binding sites at the brush border membrane comparable to the transferrin binding sites demonstrated on the reticulocyte membrane (for references see MORGAN 1981).

In rats, absorption experiments using doubly tagged (^{125}I and ^{59}Fe) plasma transferrin injected into the lumen showed transferrin within the mucosa in intact form (HUEBERS 1979). A measurable amount of the dose administered, 5%–10%, was transferred without disintegration to the blood (Fig. 6). One is tempted to assume that, as in reticulocytes, a part is recycled as apotransferrin into the intestinal lumen. In any case, these experiments demonstrated at least that luminal transferrin-bound iron was transported into the mucosa of the upper part of the small intestine (HUEBERS et al. 1979a, 1983). Chromium III bound to transferrin, which is poorly absorbed when given as free aquocomplex, is easily taken up by the duodenal mucosa, but only in 100 times smaller amounts by the ileal mucosa. This also indicates a receptor-mediated transferrin uptake across the luminal membrane (WOLLENBERG et al. 1982).

Iron loading of the apotransferrin present in the lumen or within the mucosal cell might be enzymatically controlled. An enzyme capable of accomplishing this function has been identified in rabbit intestinal mucosa (TOPHAM 1973; TOPHAM et al. 1981). Differential centrifugation indicated that the enzyme is contained primarily in the particle-free supernatant of mucosal homogenates. The mucosal enzyme, which is not ceruloplasmin, is not inhibited by azide, has a pH optimum of 7.4, and a single K_m for Fe^{2+} of 43 μM. This enzyme may function similarly in iron absorption as ceruloplasmin does in mobilizing iron from liver stores. Furthermore, variations in the amount or activity of this enzyme in the mucosa could regulate the fraction of the total mucosal iron that becomes incorporated into transferrin and eventually enters the body.

D. Heavy Metal Interaction with the Iron Transfer System: Sites of Interaction

In iron deficiency, the absorption of chromium, manganese, cobalt, nickel, and zinc is also increased (POLLACK et al. 1965; FORTH et al. 1966; FORTH and RUMMEL 1971; for additional references see FORTH and RUMMEL 1973, 1975), suggesting that these heavy metals utilize the epithelial iron transfer system to some degree. It was also pointed out that this phenomenon is analogous to the increased uptake of manganese, cobalt, and zinc by reticulocytes as compared with erythrocytes (FORTH and RUMMEL 1971). Moreover, a mutual inhibition of iron and cobalt with respect to the uptake into reticulocytes has been described (FORTH et al. 1968 b). Such a mutual inhibition was also shown in the intestinal absorption for iron, manganese, cobalt, and zinc (SCHADE et al. 1970; FORTH and RUMMEL 1971, 1973; FLANAGAN et al. 1980) and for iron, cadmium, and lead. These latter interactions are of particular interest with respect to their toxicologic consequences since iron deficiency resulting from small amounts of dietary cadmium and lead can be explained by the competition of these metals with iron providing sites on transferrin or other possible transport proteins. Increased toxicity of cadmium and lead in iron deficiency may be caused by the increased absorption of both metals. A protective effect of additional dietary iron against cadmium and lead toxicity has also been observed and is fairly well explained by competition for binding sites (cadmium: PINDBORG et al. 1946; BERLIN and FRIBERG 1960; HILL et al. 1963; BUNN and MATRONE 1966; BANIS et al. 1969; FOX and FRY 1970; FOX et al. 1971; POND and WALKER 1972; FREELAND and COUSINS 1973; MAJI and YOSHIDA 1974; HAMILTON and VALBERG 1974; VALBERG et al. 1976; SUZUKI and YOSHIDA 1977, 1978; FLANAGAN et al. 1978; RADI and POND 1979; lead: WATSON et al. 1958; SIX and GOYER 1972; RAGAN 1977; BARTON et al. 1978; CONRAD and BARTON 1978; HAMILTON 1978; FLANAGAN et al. 1979; CERKLEWSKI 1980; BARTON et al. 1981).

The search for sites in the intestinal epithelium where the interactions between iron and these heavy metals occur has yielded new instructive information. To localize the sites it is useful to discriminate between three steps of the absorption process: (1) the binding at the luminal surface by the "elutable factor" (HUEBERS et al. 1974, 1975) and the brush border membrane (GREENBERGER et al. 1969; HUEBERS et al. 1971 a; KIMBER et al. 1973; COX and O'DONNELL 1981); (2) the uptake through the luminal membrane into the epithelial cell; and (3) the delivery across the contraluminal membrane to the portal blood. With respect to cobalt absorption in iron deficiency, it has been shown that the first step, in contradistinction to iron, is not dependent on the "elutable factor" and is not responsible for the higher absorptive utilization (HUEBERS et al. 1974, 1975). By studying the kinetics of iron uptake and release in the epithelium during iron absorption in iron deficiency, it was observed that the interaction between cobalt and iron occurs at the contraluminal side of the epithelium. The resulting inhibition of the iron transfer causes a stagnation of absorbed iron in the epithelium (BECKER et al. 1979a). The further elucidation of the interactions between iron and other heavy metals in absorption was approached at the molecular level by questioning whether mucosal transferrin was one of the sites at which this interaction takes place. This seemed to be reasonable with respect to the functional significance of the mucosal transferrin (HUEBERS and RUMMEL 1977) and since interactions between iron and other heavy metals had already been described for plasma and ovotransferrin (SCHADE et al. 1949; FRAENKEL-CONRAT and FEENEY 1950; WARNER and WEBER 1953; AASA et al. 1963; WOODWORTH 1966; AISEN 1975; TAN and WOODWORTH 1976).

Copper proved a good tool and yielded the first success. It belongs to those multivalent heavy metal cations which are bound to plasma transferrin with the same stoichiometry as iron (SCHADE et al. 1949; SCHADE and REINHART 1966; WOODWORTH 1966; AISEN 1975). It was known that a decrease of iron stores in the liver (CASSIDY and EVA 1958; BUNCH et al. 1963; RITCHIE et al. 1963) and anemia (WALLACE et al. 1960; BUNCH et al. 1961) can be induced by adding copper to the diet in pigs. Supplementary iron afforded protection against copper-induced anemia (SUTTLE and MILLS 1966a, b; HEDGES and KORNEGAY 1973). Therefore, the conclusion can be drawn that copper inhibits iron absorption. Actually, when copper is administered together with iron in a ratio of 10:1 (Cu:Fe), iron absorption in iron-deficient rats is inhibited by more than 90%. Simultaneously, the amount of iron bound to mucosal transferrin is also remarkably decreased. In other experiments, it was demonstrated that copper is bound by mucosal transferrin and can be displaced by iron (EL-SHOBAKI and RUMMEL 1979).

This displacement has already been shown to occur with ovotransferrin and plasma transferrin (WOODWORTH 1966; TAN and WOODWORTH 1976). In contradistinction to copper, no binding of cobalt to mucosal transferrin could be demonstrated, at least by chromatographic elution on Sepharose 6B (EL-SHOBAKI and RUMMEL, unpublished). This negative result might indicate that the affinity of cobalt for the binding sites of the mucosal transferrin is lower than that of iron.

Cadmium also binds to mucosal transferrin (HUEBERS et al. 1979b). Iron delivery from the mucosal epithelium to the blood decreases with an increasing ratio of Cd:Fe, whereas the fraction of iron taken up into the mucosa measured in the cytosol rises (HUEBERS et al. 1979b). Therefore, the conclusion can be drawn that iron deficiency anemia produced by dietary cadmium results from inhibition of iron absorption caused by cadmium competing for iron binding sites on luminal and mucosal transferrin. Consequently, the development of cadmium anemia can be prevented by the addition of higher iron doses to the diet (for references see earlier in this section).

In conclusion, it can be stated that iron transfer through the intestinal epithelium is inhibited by several multivalent heavy metals. Apart from causing massive lesions of the epithelium in high doses with consequent loss of all its absorptive functions, some heavy metals compete with iron for its binding sites on mucosal transferrin and thereby cause a specific inhibition of the epithelial iron transfer and secondary iron deficiency anemia.

E. Conclusions

Iron absorption is a complex process by which the translocation of iron, primarily in the upper small intestine from the luminal side of the mucosal epithelium to the blood, occurs. Several membranes have to be crossed in this passage. During this process, the iron taken up from the luminal fluid interacts with at least two iron binding proteins, the mucosal transferrin and the mucosal ferritin. Mucosal ferritin functions, as in other tissues, as an intracellular store for iron. At least a part of the iron remains trapped there until the epithelial cells are exfoliated. Thus, mucosal ferritin prevents all iron taken up into the mucosa from being transferred to the body. In iron deficiency, the content of ferritin in the mucosal cells is very low and mucosal transferrin determines the fate of the absorbed iron. The disappearance of the absorbed iron from the mucosal transferrin pool and the appearance of iron in the body are reciprocally correlated. Obviously, mucosal transferrin is involved in the epithelial regulation of iron absorption and enhances the transfer of iron in iron deficiency, at least during the initial rapid phase. Recent observations point to the possibility that apotransferrin secreted by the liver in bile, by goblet cells, and/or by mucosal cells chelates the ionized iron in the acid bolus emptied into the duodenum. Then transferrin interacts with receptors at the luminal membranes preferentially localized in the upper part of the small intestine and absorption starts.

The capability of the epithelial iron transfer system to adapt to the body's demand for iron is of great importance to preserve homeostasis of iron metabolism because regulation through iron excretion is not possible. Full details of the regulatory process are still unknown. Present information supports the assumption that the synthesis of either mucosal iron binding protein, mucosal transferrin, or ferritin is inhibited or enhanced, respectively, in response to the size of a certain intracellular iron pool in a manner demonstrated in bacterial iron chelating and transfer systems.

Iron can circumvent its physiologic transfer system, probably by diffusion when the system's capacity is overwhelmed by high iron dosages or when iron is offered in the form of a very stable absorbable chelate which, in contradistinction to heme, cannot be degraded within the mucosal cells. The interference of some heavy metals with iron at its binding sites within the epithelial transfer system is of toxicologic relevance because it provides an explanation on a molecular basis for the development of iron deficiency anemias caused by those heavy metals.

Acknowledgments. The authors were supported in part by grants from the Sonderforschungsbereich 38, Membrane Research, DFG, Federal Republic of Germany and Research Grant HL 06242 from the National Institute of Heart, Lung and Blood, U.S. National Institutes of Health.

References

Aasa R, Malmström BG, Saltman P, Vänngard T (1963) The specific binding of iron (III) and copper (II) to transferrin and conalbumin. Acta Biochim Biophys 75:203–222

Aisen P (1975) The transferrins. In: Eichhorn GL (ed) Inorganic biochemistry. Elsevier, Amsterdam, p 280

Aisen P (1977) Some physicochemical aspects of iron metabolism. In: Porter R, Fitzsimons DW (eds) Iron metabolism. Elsevier, Amsterdam, pp 1–17

Aisen P, Brown EB (1977) The iron-binding function of transferrin in iron metabolism. Semin Hemat 14:31–53
Banis RJ, Pond WG, Walker EF Jr, O'Connor JR (1969) Dietary cadmium, iron and zinc interactions in the growing rat. (33659) Proc Soc Exp Biol Med 130:802–806
Bannerman RM, O'Brien JRP, Witts LJ (1962) Studies in iron metabolism. IV. Iron absorption in experimental iron-deficiency. Blood 20:532–546
Barton JC, Conrad ME, Nuby S, Harrison L (1978) Effects of iron on the absorption and retention of lead. J Lab Clin Med 92:536–547
Barton JC, Conrad ME, Holland R (1981) Iron, lead, and cobalt absorption: similarities and dissimilarities. Proc Soc Exp Biol Med 166:64–69
Batey RG, Gallagher ND (1977) Study of the subcellular localization of ^{59}Fe and iron-binding proteins in the duodenal mucosa of pregnant and nonpregnant rats. Gastroenterology 73:267–272
Becker G, Hübers H, Rummel W (1979a) Intestinal absorption of cobalt and iron: mode of interaction and subcellular distribution. Blut 38:397–406
Becker G, Korpilla-Schäfer S, Osterloh K, Forth W (1979b) Capacity of the mucosal transfer system and absorption of iron after administration in rats. Blut 38:127–134
Bédard YC, Pinkerton PH, Simon GT (1971) Radioautographic observations on iron absorption by the normal mouse duodenum. Blood 38:232–245
Bédard YC, Pinkerton PH, Simon GT (1973) Radioautographic observations on iron absorption by the duodenum of mice with iron overload, iron deficiency, and x-linked anemia. Blood 42:131–140
Bennett C (1970) Migration of glycoprotein from Golgi apparatus to cell coat in the columnar cells of the duodenal epithelium. J Cell Biol 45:668–673
Bennett G, Leblond CP (1970) Formation of cell coat material for the whole surface of columnar cells in the rat small intestine as visualized by radioautography with L-fucose-3H. J Cell Biol 46:409–416
Berlin M, Friberg L (1960) Bone-marrow activity and erythrocyte destruction in chronic cadmium poisoning. Arch Environ Health 1:478
Bothwell TH, Finch CA (1957) The intestine in iron metabolism. Its role in normal and abnormal states. Am J Dig Dis NS 2:145
Bothwell TH, Finch CA (1962) Iron absorption. In: Bothwell TH, Finch CA (eds) Iron metabolism. Little Brown, Boston, pp 92–120
Bothwell TH, Charlton RW, Cook JD, Finch CA (1979) Iron metabolism in man. Blackwell Scientific, Oxford
Brittin GM, Raval D (1970) Duodenal ferritin synthesis during iron absorption in the iron-deficient rat. J Lab Clin Med 75:811–817
Brown EB (1963) The absorption of iron. Am J Clin Nutr 12:205–213
Brown EB; Justus BW (1958) In vitro absorption of radioiron by everted pouches of rat intestine. Am J Physiol 194:319–326
Bunch RJ, Speer VC, Hays VW, Hawbaker JH, Catron DV (1961) Effects of copper sulfate, copper oxide and chlortetracycline on baby pig performance. J Anim Sci 20:723–726
Bunch RJ, Speer VC, Hays VW, McCall JT (1963) Effects of high levels of copper and chlortetracycline on performance of pigs. J Anim Sci 22:56–60
Bunn CR, Matrone G (1966) In vivo interactions of cadmium, copper, zinc, and iron in the mouse and rat. J Nutr 90:395–399
Callender ST (1974) Iron absorption. In: Smyth DH (ed) Biomembranes, vol 4B, Intestinal absorption. Plenum, New York, pp 761–791
Callender ST, Mallet BJ, Smith MD (1957) Absorption of haemoglobin iron. Br J Haematol 3:186–192
Cassidy J, Eva JK (1958) Relationship between the copper and iron concentrations in pigs' livers. Proc Nutr Soc 17:Abstract XXXI
Cerklewski FL (1980) Reduction in neonatal lead exposure by supplemental dietary iron during gestation and lactation in the rat. J Nutr 110:1398–1408
Charlton RW, Jacobs P, Torrance JD, Bothwell TH (1965) The role of the intestinal mucosa in iron absorption. J Clin Invest 44:543–554

Chirasiri L, Izak G (1966) The effect of acute haemorrhage and acute haemolysis on intestinal iron absorption in the rat. Br J Haematol 12:611–622
Conrad ME, Barton JC (1978) Factors affecting the absorption and excretion of lead in the rat. Gastroenterology 74:731–740
Conrad ME, Crosby WH (1963) Intestinal mucosal mechanisms controlling from absorption. Blood 22:406–415
Conrad ME, Schade SG (1968) Ascorbic and chelate in iron absorption: A role for hydrochloric acid and bile. Gastroenterology 55:35–45
Conrad ME, Weintraub LR, Crosby WH (1964) The role of the intestine in iron kinetics. J Clin Invest 43:963–974
Conrad ME, Weintraub LR; Sears DA, Crosby WH (1966) Absorption of hemoglobin iron. Am J Physiol 211:1123–1130
Cook JD, Hershko C, Finch CA (1973) Storage iron kinetics. V. Iron exchange in the rat. Br J Haematol 25:695–706
Cox TM, O'Donnell WW (1980) Iron uptake by purified intestinal microvillus membranes. Gut 21:A908, T54
Cox TM, O'Donnell MW (1981) Studies on the binding of iron by rabbit intestinal microvillus membranes. Biochem J 194:753–759
Cox TM, Peters TM (1978) Uptake of iron by duodenal biopsy specimens from patients with iron-deficiency anaemia and primary hemachromatosis. Lancet I:123–124
Cox TM, Peters TJ (1980) Cellular mechanisms in the regulation of iron absorption by the human intestine: studies in patients with iron deficiency before and after treatment. Br J Haematol 44:75–86
Cox TM, Mazurier J, Spike G, Montreuil J, Peters TJ (1979) Iron binding proteins and influx of iron across the duodenal brush border, evidence for specific lactotransferrin receptors in the human intestine. Biochem Biophys Acta 588:120–128
Crosby WH (1963) The control of iron balance by the intestinal mucosa. Blood 22:441–449
De Laey P, Masson PL, Heremans JF (1968) The role of lactoferrin in iron absorption. Protides Biol Fluids Proc Colloq 16:627–632
De Vet BHC (1971) Iron metabolism and iron-binding proteins in human bile. Folia Med Neerl 14:123
De Vet BHCM, Van Gool J (1974) Lactoferrin and iron absorption in the small intestine. Acta Med Scand 196:393–402
Dowdle EB, Schachter D, Schenker H (1960) Active transport of ^{59}Fe by everted segments of rat duodenum. Am J Physiol 198:609–613
Edwards JA, Hoke JE (1978) Mucosal iron binding proteins in sex-linked anemia and microcytic anemia of the mouse. J Med 9:353–364
Edwards JA, Hoke JE, Mattiolo M, Reichlin M (1977) Ferritin distribution and synthesis in sex-linked anemia. J Lab Clin Med 90:68–76
El-Shobaki FA, Rummel W (1977) Mucosal transferrin and ferritin factors in the regulation of iron absorption. Res Exp Med 171:243–253
El-Shobaki FA, Rummel W (1978) The role of mucosal iron binding proteins in adaptation of iron absorption during protein deficiency and rehabilitation. Res Exp Med 173:119–129
El-Shobaki FA, Rummel W (1979) Binding of copper to mucosal transferrin and inhibition of intestinal iron absorption in rats. Res Exp Med 174:187–195
Faulk WP, Galbraith GMP (1979) Transferrin and transferrin-receptors of human trophoblst. In: Hemmings WA (ed) Protein transmission through living membranes. Elsevier, Amsterdam, pp 55–61
Finch CA, Loden B (1959) Body iron exchange in man. J Clin Invest 38:392–396
Flanagan PR, McLellan JS, Haist J, Cherian MG, Chamberlain MJ, Valberg LS (1978) Increased dietary cadmium absorption in mice and human subjects with iron deficiency. Gastroenterology 74:841–846
Flanagan PR, Hamilton DL, Haist J, Valberg LS (1979) Interrelationships between iron and lead absorption in iron-deficient mice. Gastroenterology 77:1074–1081

Flanagan PR, Haist J, Valberg LS (1980) Comparative effects of iron deficiency induced by bleeding and a low-iron diet on the intestinal absorptive interactions of iron, cobalt, manganese, zinc, lead, and cadmium. J Nutr 110:1754–1763

Forth W (1967) Eisen- und Kobalt-Resorption am perfundierten Dünndarmsegment. 3. Konferenz der Gesellschaft für Biologische Chemie, 27–29 April 1967; Oestrich/ Rheingau. Springer, Berlin Heidelberg New York

Forth W (1970) Absorption of iron and chemically related metals in vitro and in vivo; the specificity of an iron binding system in the intestinal mucosa of the rat. In: Mills CF (ed) Trace element metabolism in animals. Livingstone, London, p 298

Forth W, Rummel W (1965) Eisen-Resorption an isolierten Dünndarmpräparaten von normalen und anämischen Ratten. Arch Exp Pathol Pharmakol 252:205–223

Forth W, Rummel W (1966) Beziehungen zwischen Eisen-Konzentration und -Resorption am isolierten Dünndarm normaler und anämischer Ratten. Med Pharmacol Exp 14:289–296

Forth W, Rummel W (1968) Zur Frage der Regulation der Eisenresorption durch Gastroferrin, ein eisenbindendes Protein des Magensaftes. Klin Wochenschr 46:1003–1005

Forth W, Rummel W (1971) Absorption of iron and chemically related metals in vitro and in vivo: specificity of the iron binding system in the mucosa of the jejunum. In: Skoryna SC, Waldron-Edward D (eds) Intestinal absorption of metal ions, trace elements and radionuclides. Pergamon, Oxford, pp 173–191

Forth W, Rummel W (1973) Iron absorption. Physiol Rev 53:724–792

Forth W, Rummel W (1975) Gastrointestinal absorption of heavy metals. In: Peters G (executive ed), Forth W, Rummel W (section eds) IEPT – Pharmacology of intestinal absorption: gastrointestinal absorption of drugs, sect 39B, vol II. Pergamon, Oxford, pp 599–746

Forth W, Pfleger K, Rummel W, Seifen E, Richmond SJ (1965) Der Einfluß verschiedener Liganden auf Resorption, Verteilung und Ausscheidung von Eisen nach oraler Verabfolgung. Arch Exp Pathol Pharmakol 252:242–257

Forth W, Rummel W, Becker PJ (1966) Die vergleichende Prüfung von Bindung und Durchtritt von Eisen Kobalt und Kupfer durch isolierte Jejunum-Segmente normaler und anämischer Ratten. Med Pharmacol Exp 15:179–186

Forth W, Leopold G, Rummel W (1968 a) Eisendurchtritt von der Mucosa- zur Serosaseite und umgekehrt an isolierten eisenarmen und normalen Segmenten von Jejunum und Ileum. Naunyn Schmiedebergs Arch Pharmacol 261:434–440

Forth W, Rummel W, Crüsemann D, Simon J (1968 b) Die Bindung von Eisen und verwandten Schwermetallen in der Membran und ihre Aufnahme in Reticulozyten. In: Deutsch E, Gerlach E, Moser K (eds) Stoffwechsel und Membranpermeabilität von Erythrocyten und Thrombocyten. Thieme, Stuttgart, pp 444–446

Fox MRS, Fry BE Jr (1970) Cadmium toxicity decreased by dietary ascorbic acid. Science 169:989–991

Fox MRS, Fry BE Jr, Harland BF, Schertel ME, Weeks CE (1971) Effect of ascorbic acid on cadmium toxicity in the young coturnix. J Nutr 101:1295–1306

Fraenkel-Conrat H, Feeney RE (1950) The metal-binding activity of conalbumin. Arch Biochem 29:101–113

Freeland JH, Cousins RJ (1973) Effect of dietary cadmium on anemia, iron absorption, and cadmium binding protein in the chick. Nutr Rep Int 8:337–347

Friberg L (1950) Health hazards in the manufacture of alkaline accumulators with special reference to chronic cadmium poisoning. Acad Med Scand 138 (Suppl):240

Furugouri K (1977) Iron binding substances in the intestinal mucosa of neonatal piglets. J Nutr 107:487–494

Furugouri K, Kawabata A (1976) Iron absorption by neonatal pig intestine in vivo. J Anim Sci 42:1460–1464

Gitlin D, Cruchaud A (1962) On the kinetics of iron absorption in mice. J Clin Invest 41:344–350

Greenberger NJ, Ruppert RD (1966 a) Inhibition of protein synthesis: a mechanism for the production of impaired iron absorption. Clin Res 14:298

Greenberger NJ, Ruppert RD (1966 b) Tetracycline induced inhibition of iron absorption. Clin Res 14:432

Greenberger NJ, Ruppert RD, Cuppage FE (1967) Inhibition of intestinal iron transport induced by tetracycline. Gastroenterology 53:590–599

Greenberger NJ, Balcerzak SP, Ackerman GA (1969) Iron uptake by isolated intestinal brush borders: changes induced by alterations in iron stores. J Lab Clin Med 73:711–721

Hahn PF, Carothers EL, Darby WJ, Martin M, Sheppard CW, Cannon RO, Beam AS, Deusen PM, Petterson JS, McClellan CS (1951) Iron metabolism in human pregnancy as studied with the radioactive isotope Fe^{59}. Am J Obstet Gynecol 61:477–486

Hallberg L, Björn-Rasmussen E (1972) Determination of iron absorption from whole diet. A new two-pool model using two radioiron isotopes given as haem and non-haem iron. Scand J Haematol 9:193–197

Hallberg L, Sölvell L (1960) Absorption of a single dose of iron in man. Acta Med Scand 358 (Suppl):19–42

Halliday JW, Powell LW, Mack U (1975) Intestinal iron-binding-complex in iron absorption. In: Crichton RR (ed) Proteins of iron storage and transport in biochemistry and medicine. Elsevier, Amsterdam, pp 405–410

Halliday JW, Powell LW, Mack U (1976) Iron absorption in the rat: The search for possible intestinal mucosal carriers. Br J Haematol 34:237–250

Hamilton DL (1978) Lead retention in iron deficient mice. Proc Can Fed Biol Soc 21:88

Hamilton DL, Valberg LS (1974) Relationship between cadmium and iron absorption. Am J Physiol 227:1033–1037

Hedges JD, Kornegay ET (1973) Interrelationship of dietary copper and iron as measured by blood parameters, tissue stores and feedlot performance of swine. J Animal Sci 37:1147–1154

Heinrich HC (1970) Intestinal iron absorption in man – methods of measurements, dose relationship, diagnostic and therapeutic applications. In: Hallberg L, Harwerth HG, Vannotti A (eds) Iron deficiency. Academic, London, pp 213–294

Helbock HI, Saltman P (1967) The transport of iron by rat intestine. Biochim Biophys Acta 135:979–990

Hill CH, Matrone G, Payne WL, Barber CW (1963) In vivo interactions of cadmium with copper, zinc, and iron. J Nutr 80:227–235

Huebers H (1972) Eine Methode zur Herstellung stabiler Dichtegradienten und ihre Anwendung beim Studium der Eisenresorption. Dissertation; Mathematisch-Naturwissenschaftliche Fakultät der Universität des Saarlandes

Huebers H (1975) Identification of iron binding intermediates in intestinal mucosa tissue of rats during absorption. In: Crichton RR (ed) Proteins of iron storage and transport. North-Holland, Amsterdam, pp 281–288

Huebers H (1979) Die enterale Resorption von Transferrin-Eisen: Bedeutung für die Eisenresorption. Dissertation; Medizinische Fakultät der Universität des Saarlandes

Huebers H, Huebers E, Forth W, Leopold G, Rummel W (1971 a) Binding of iron and other metals in brush borders of jejunum and ileum of the rat in vitro. Acta Pharmacol Toxicol 29 (Suppl 4):22

Huebers H, Huebers E, Forth W, Rummel W (1971 b) Binding of iron to a non-ferritin protein in the mucosal cells of normal and iron-deficient rats during absorption. Life Sci 10:1141–1148

Huebers H, Huebers E, Simon J, Forth W (1971 c) A method for preparing stable density gradients and their application for fractionation of intestinal mucosal cells. Life Sci 10:377–384

Huebers H, Huebers E, Forth W, Rummel W (1973) Iron absorption and iron-binding proteins in intestinal mucosa of mice with sex linked anaemia. Hoppe Seyler's Z Physiol Chem 354:1156–1158

Huebers H, Huebers E, Rummel W (1974) Dependence of increased iron absorption by iron-deficient rats on an elutable component of jejunal mucosa. Hoppe Seylers Z Physiol Chem 355:1159–1161

Huebers H, Huebers E, Rummel W (1975) Mechanisms of iron absorption: iron-binding proteins and dependence of iron absorption on an elutable factor. In: Kief H (ed) Iron metabolism and its disorders. Excerpta Medica, Amsterdam, pp 13–21

Huebers H, Huebers E, Rummel W, Crichton RR (1976) Isolation and characterization of iron-binding proteins from rat intestinal mucosa. Eur J Biochem 66:447–455

Huebers H, Huebers E, Csiba E, Rummel W, Finch CA (1979a) The intestinal absorption of transferrin bound iron. Blood 54 (Suppl 53):40a

Huebers H, Huebers E, Rummel W (1979b) Iron absorption as influenced by cadmium: studies on a molecular level. Blood 54 (Suppl 54)

Huebers H, Csiba E, Josephson B, Huebers E, Finch CA (1981) Interaction of human diferric transferrin with reticulocytes. Proc Natl Acad Sci USA 86(1):621–625

Huebers H, Rummel W (1977) Iron binding proteins: mediators in iron absorption. In: Kramer M, Lauterbach F (eds) Intestinal permeation. Excerpta Medica, Amsterdam, pp 377–380

Huebers H, Huebers E, Csiba E, Rummel W, Finch CA (1983) The significance of transferrin for intestinal iron absorption. Blood 61:283–290

Hughes ER (1980) Human iron metabolism, chap 9. In: Siegel H (ed) Metal ions in biological systems, vol 7. Iron in model and natural compounds. Dekker, New York, pp 351–376

Humphrys J, Walpole B, Worwood M (1977) Intracellular iron transport in rat intestinal epithelium: Biochemical and ultrastructural observations. Br J Haematol 36:209–217

Isobe K, Isobe Y (1983) Localization of transferrin in rat duodenal mucosa by immunoperoxidase technique. Acta Haematol. Jap 46: 9–19

Isobe K, Sakurami T, Isobe Y (1978) Studies on iron transport in human intestine by immunoperoxidase technique. I. The localization of ferritin, lactoferrin, and transferrin in human duodenal mucosa. Acta Haematol Jap 41:294–299

Ito S (1969) Structure and function of the glycocalyx. Fed Proc 28:12–25

Ito S, Revel JP (1964) Incorporation of radioactive sulfate and glocuse on the surface coat of enteric microvilli. J Cell Biol 23:44A

Jacobi H, Pfleger K, Rummel W (1956) Komplexbildner und aktiver Eisentransport durch die Darmwand. Arch Exp Pathol Pharmakol 229:198–206

Jacobs A, Miles PM (1968) The iron-binding properties of gastric juice. Clin Chim Acta 24:87–92

Jacobs A, Miles PM (1970) The formation of iron complexes with bile and bile constituents. Gut 11:732–734

Jacobs P, Bothwell TH, Charlton RW (1966) Intestinal iron transport: studies using a loop of gut with an artificial circulation. Am J Physiol 210:694–700

Jacobs P, Charlton RW, Bothwell TH (1968) The influence of gastric factors on the absorption of iron salts. S Afr J Med Sci 33:53–57

Kaufman N, Newkirk M, Wyllie JC (1976) Effect of iron absorption on plasma membrane proteins of small intestinal mucosal cells from iron-deficient rats. Biochem Biophys Res Commun 73:1036–1041

Kaufman N, Wyllie JC, Newkirk M (1977) Two microsomal-associated iron-binding proteins observed in rat small intestinal cells during iron absorption. Biochim Biophys Acta 497:719–727

Kimber CL, Mukherjee T, Deller DJ (1973) In vitro iron attachment to the intestinal brush border; effect of iron stores and other environmental factors. Dig Dis Sci 18:781–791

Lane RS (1967) Localization of transferrin in human and rat liver by fluorescent antibody technique. Nature 215:161–162

Lane RS (1968) Transferrin synthesis in the rat: A study using the fluorescent antibody technique. Br J Haematol 15:355–364

Larkin EC, Weintraub LR, Crosby WH (1970) Iron transport across rabbit allantoic placenta. Am J Physiol 218:7–11

Levine PH, Levine AJ, Weintraub LR (1972) The role of transferrin in the control of iron absorption: studies on a cellular level. J Lab Clin Med 80:333–341

Linder MC, Munro HN (1975) Ferritin and free iron in iron absorption. In: Crichton RR (ed) Proteins of iron storage and transport in biochemistry and medicine. North-Holland, Amsterdam, pp 395–400
Linder MC, Dunn V, Isaacs E, Jones D, Lim S, Van Volkom M, Munro HN (1975) Ferritin and intestinal iron absorption: Pancreatic enzymes and free iron. Am J Physiol 228:196–204
Maji T, Yoshida A (1974) Therapeutic effect of dietary iron and ascorbic acid on cadmium toxicity of rats. Nutr Rep Int 10:139–149
Manis JG (1970) Active transport iron by intestine: selective genetic defection mouse. Nature 227:385–386
Manis JG (1971) Intestinal iron-transport defect in the mouse with sex-linked anemia. Am J Physiol 220:135–139
Manis J, Kim G (1979) Stimulation of iron absorption by polychlorinated aromatic hydrocarbons. Am J Physiol 236:e763–e768
Manis JG, Schachter D (1962a) Active transport of iron by intestine: features of the two-step mechanism. Am J Physiol 203:73–80
Manis JG, Schachter D (1962b) Active transport of iron by intestine: effects of oral iron and pregnancy. Am J Physiol 203:81–86
Marx JJM (1979) Iron absorption and its regulation. A review. Haematologica 64:479–493
Mason DY, Taylor CR (1978) Distribution of transferrin, ferritin, and lactoferrin in human tissues. J Clin Pathol 31:316–327
McCance RA, Widdowson EM (1937) Absorption and excretion of iron. Lancet 1:680–684
McMillan JA, Oski FA, Lourie G, Tomarelli RM, Landaw SA (1977) Iron absorption from human milk, simulated human milk, and proprietary formulas. Pediatrics 60:896–900
Mignon M, Semb LS, Finch CA, Nyhus LM (1965) Effect of gastric juice on the absorption of iron. Surg Forum 16:319–321
Moore CA, Dubach R, Minnich V, Roberts HK (1944) Absorption of ferrous and ferric radioactive iron by human subjects and by dogs. J Clin Invest 23:755–767
Morgan EH (1980) The role of plasma transferrin in iron absorption in the rat. Q J Exp Physiol 65:239–252
Morgan EH (1981) Transferrin, biochemistry, physiology, and clinical significance. Mol Aspects Med 4:1–123
Morton AG, Tavill AS (1977) The role of iron in the regulation of hepatic transferrin synthesis. Br J Haematol 36:383–394
Mukherjee T (1972) Factors affecting iron attachment to microvilli. Med J Aust 2:378–381
O'Donnell MW, Cox TM (1981) Iron-binding glycoconjugates from intestinal microvilli. FEBS Meeting Edinburgh. Biochem Soc Trans 9:Tue-S10–13
Osterloh KS (1979) Die Bestimmung von mucosalem Transferrin im Mucosahomogenat von Duodenum, Jejunum und Ileum normaler und eisenarmer Ratten. Phd Dissertation, Ruhr-Universität Bochum
Parmley RT, Barton JC, Conrad ME, Austin RL (1978) Ultrastructural cytochemistry of iron absorption. Am J Pathol 93:707–728
Pearson WN, Reich M (1965) In vitro studies of Fe^{59}-absorption by everted intestinal sacs of rat. J Nutr 87:117–124
Pearson WN, Reich M, Frank H, Salamat L (1967) Effects of dietary iron level on gut iron levels and iron absorption in the rat. J Nutr 92:53–65
Permezel NC, Webling DDA (1971) The length and mucosal surface area of the small and large gut in young rats. J Anat 108:295–296
Pindborg EV, Pindborg JJ, Plum CM (1946) The relation beetween cadmium poisoning and iron metabolism. Acta Pharmacol Toxicol 2:302–306
Pinkerton PH (1968) Histological evidence of disordered iron transport in the x-linked hypochromic anemia of mice. J Pathol Bacteriol 95:155–165
Pinkerton PH, Bannerman RM (1967) Hereditary defect in iron absorption in mice. Nature 216:482–483
Pinkerton PH, Bannerman RM, Doeblin TD, Benisch BM, Edwards JA (1970) Iron metabolism and absorption studies in x-linked anemia of mice. Br J Haematol 18:211–228

Pollack S, Lasky FD (1975) A new iron binding protein in intestinal mucosa. In: Crichton RR (ed) Proteins of iron storage and transport in biochemistry and medicine. North-Holland, Amsterdam, pp 389–393

Pollack S, Balcerzak SP, Crosby WH (1963) Transferrin and the absorption of iron. Blood 21:33–38

Pollack S, George JN, Reba RC, Kaufman R, Crosby WH (1965) The absorption of non-ferrous metals in iron deficiency. J Clin Invest 44:1470–1473

Pollack S, Campana T, Arcario A (1972) A search for a mucosal iron carrier. Identification of mucosal fractions with rapid turnover of Fe^{59}. J Lab Clin Med 80:322–332

Pond WG, Walker EF Jr (1972) Cadmium-induced anemia in growing rats: Prevention by oral or parenteral iron. Nutr Rep Int 5:365–370

Powell LW, Wilson E (1970) In vivo intestinal mucosal uptake of iron, body iron absorption and gastric juice iron-binding in idopathic haemochromatosis. Aust Ann Med 19:226–231

Radi SA, Pond WC (1979) Effect of dietary cadmium on fate of parenterally administered ^{59}Fe in the weanling pig. Nutr Rep Int 19:695–701

Raffin SB, Woo CH, Roost KT, Price DC, Schmid R (1974) Intestinal absorption of hemoglobin iron-heme cleavage by mucosal heme oxygenase. J Clin Invest 54:1344–1352

Ragan HA (1977) Effects of iron deficiency on the absorption and distribution of lead and cadmium in rats. J Lab Clin Med 90:700–706

Ritchie HD, Luecke RW, Baltzer BV, Miller ER, Ullrey DE, Hoefer JA (1963) Copper and zinc interrelationships in the pig. J Nutr 79:117–123

Ruliffson WS, Hopping JM (1963) Maturation, iron deficiency and ligands in enteric radioiron transport in vitro. Am J Physiol 204:171–175

Rummel W, Forth W (1968) Zur Frage der metabolischen Abhängigkeit von Eisenbildung und -durchtritt durch den isolierten Dünndarm. Naunyn Schmiedebergs Arch Pharmacol 260:50–57

Rummel W, El-Shobaki FA, Wollenberg P (1984) Mucosal iron binding proteins and inhibition of iron absorption by endotoxin. In: Urushizaki I (ed) Proteins of iron storage and transport. Elsevier North-Holland, Amsterdam (in press)

Savin MA, Cook JD (1977) Interrelationship between mucosal cell transferrin and iron absorption. Clin Res 25:573A

Savin MA, Cook JD (1978) Iron transport by isolated rat intestinal mucosal cells. Gastroenterology 75:688–694

Savin MA, Cook JD (1980) Mucosal iron transport by rat intestine. Blood 56:1029–1035

Schade AL, Caroline L (1946) An iron-binding component in human blood plasma. Science 104:340–341

Schade AL, Reinhart RW (1966) Carbon dioxide in the iron and copper siderophilin complexes (sect A, metal-binding proteins). In: Peeters H (ed) Protides of the biological fluids, vol 14. Pergamon, Oxford, pp 75–81

Schade AL, Reinhart RW, Levy H (1949) Carbon dioxide and oxygen in complex formation with iron and siderophilin, the iron binding component of human plasma. Arch Biochem 20:170–172

Schade SG, Bernier GM, Conrad ME (1969) Normal iron absorption in hypertransferrinanemic rats. Br J Haematol 17:187–190

Schade SG, Felsher BF, Glader BE, Conrad ME (1970) Effect of cobalt upon iron absorption. Proc Soc Exp Biol Med 134:741–743

Setsuda T, Yamamoto Y, Shimoura Y (1980) Absorption, distribution and metabolism of iron in rats with nutritional anemia, particularly viewed from the ferritin levels of the organs. Acta Haematol (Jpn) 43:115–123

Sheehan RG, Frenkel EP (1977) The control of iron absorption by the gastrointestinal mucosa cell. J Clin Invest 51:224–231

Six KM, Goyer RA (1972) The influence of iron deficiency on tissue content and toxicity of ingested lead in the rat. J Lab Clin Med 79:128–136

Smith MD, Pannacciulli IM (1958) Absorption of inorganic iron from graded doses. Its significance in relation to iron absorption tests and the mucosal block theory. Br J Haematol 4:428–434

Smith PM, Studley F, Williams R (1969) Postulated gastric factor enhancing iron absorption in haemochromatosis. Br J Haematol 16:443–449

Sullivan AL, Weintraub LR (1979) In vivo studies on transferrin binding by rat intestinal epithelial cells. Blood 54 (5):Abstr no 70

Suttle NF, Mills CF (1966 a) Studies of the toxicity of copper to pigs. 1. Effects of oral supplements of zinc and iron salts on the development of copper toxicosis. Br J Nutr 20:135–148

Suttle NF, Mills CF (1966 b) Studies of the toxicity of copper to pigs. 2. Effect of protein source and other dietary components on the response to high and moderate intakes of copper. Br J Nutr 20:149–161

Suzuki T, Yoshida A (1977) Effect of dietary iron and ascorbic acid on the recovery from cadmium toxicity in rats. Nutr Rep Int 16:769–778

Suzuki T, Yoshida A (1978) Long-term effectiveness of dietary iron and ascorbic acid in the prevention and cure of cadmium toxicity in rats. Am J Clin Nutr 31:1491–1498

Tan AT, Woodworth RC (1976) Ultraviolet difference spectral studies of conalbumin complexes with transitional metal ions. Biochemistry 8:3711–3716

Taylor AN (1981) Immunocytochemical localization of the vitamin D-induced calcium-binding protein: relocation of antigen during frozen section processing. J Histochem Cytochem 29(1):65–73

Topham RW (1978) Isolation of an intestinal promotor of Fe^{3B}-transferrin formation. Biochem Biophys Res Commun 85:1339–1345

Topham RW, Woodruff JH, Walker MC (1981) Purification and characterization of the intestinal promoter of iron(3+)-transferrin formation. Biochemistry 20:319–324

Turnbull A (1974) Iron absorption. In: Jacobs A, Worwood M (eds) Iron in biochemistry and medicine. Academic, London, pp 369–403

Turnbull A, Cleton F, Finch CA (1962) Iron absorption. IV. The absorption of hemoglobin iron. J Clin Invest 41:1897–1907

Valberg LS, Sorbie J, Hamilton DL (1976) Gastrointestinal metabolism of cadmium in experimental iron deficiency. Am J Physiol 231:462–467

Wack JP, Wyatt JP (1959) Studies on ferrodynamics. I. Gastrointestinal absorption of 59-Fe in the rat under differing dietary states. Pathology 67:237–247

Wallace HD, McCall JT, Bass B, Combs GE (1960) High level copper for growing-finishing swine. J Anim Sci 19:1153–1163

Warner RC, Weber I (1953) The metal combining properties of conalbumin. J Am Chem Soc 75:5094–5101

Watson RJ, Decker E, Lichtman HC (1958) Hematologic studies of children with lead poisoning. Pediatrics 21:40–46

Wheby MS, Crosby WH (1963) The gastrointestinal tract and iron absorption. Blood 22:410–428

Wheby MS, Jones LG (1963) Role of transferrin in iron absorption. J Clin Invest 42:1007–1016

Wheby MS, Conrad ME, Hedberg SE, Crosby WH (1962) The role of bile in the control of iron absorption. Gastroenterology 42:319–324

Wheby MS, Jones LG, Crosby WH (1964) Studies on iron absorption. Intestinal regulatory mechanism. J Clin Invest 43:1433–1442

Wollenberg P, Huebers H, Rummel W (1982) Intestinal absorption and binding of chromium and iron. In: Saltman P, Hegenauer J (eds) The biochemistry and physiology of iron. Elsevier North-Holland, New York, pp 287–289

Woodworth RC (1966) The mechanism of metal binding to conalbumin and siderophilin (sect A, metal-binding proteins). In: Peeters H (ed) Protides of the biological fluids, vol 14. Pergamon, Oxford, pp 37–44

Worwood M, Jacobs A (1971) Absorption of ^{59}Fe in the rat: Iron binding substances in the soluble fraction of intestinal mucosa. Life Sci 10:1363–1373

Yeh SD, Shils ME (1966) Effect of tetracycline on intestinal absorption of various nutrients by the rat. Proc Soc Exp Biol Med 123:367–370

Yoshino Y, Manis J (1973) Iron-binding substance isolated from particulate fraction of rat intestine. Am J Physiol 225:1276–1281

CHAPTER 14

Intestinal Absorption of Heavy Metals

E. C. FOULKES

A. Introduction

Heavy metals have always been present in the natural environment; in addition, throughout history, anthropogenic sources have also contributed to metal accumulation in the human body. For nonsmokers outside of occupational environments, it is the ingestion of metal compounds which constitutes the major source of the body burden. Introduction of metals into the human food chain or water supplies thus poses potentially serious problems. A tragic example of this fact is Itai-Itai disease in Japan, attributed to Cd contamination of irrigation waters used in rice cultivation (FRIBERG et al. 1975). Minamata disease represents another intance of excessive oral metal exposure, caused by consumption of fish contaminated with methylmercury. Metal contamination of the environment generally tends to increase with industrial and agricultural activities, owing to the presence of these elements in fossil fuels, agricultural fertilizers, by-products of mining or metallurgical industry, etc. There is some urgency, therefore, in the search for ways for explaining and controlling intestinal metal absorption.

In spite of extensive work in this area, no accepted model of the absorption processes for heavy metals has yet emerged. The present chapter, therefore, discusses first general problems and characteristics of intestinal metal uptake; it will then review in more detail what is known about absorption of specific heavy metals. Of course, the term heavy metal in the biologic context seldom stands for an element as such, or even for its free ionic form; rather the term refers to salts and other compounds. The metals primarily considered here are Cd, Zn, Pb, Cu, and Hg. While some of these possess biologic functions, others are of purely toxicologic concern. In each case, however, similar processes seem to be involved in intestinal absorption. The handling of Fe, Ca, and Mg is described elsewhere in this volume.

B. Experimental Problems

As in the study of other solutes, a great variety of techniques has been brought to bear on intestinal absorption of heavy metals. They range from feeding studies in humans or intact animals to analysis of metal uptake by small rings of intestine in vitro. Each of these approaches can yield useful information, but no one technique can provide a complete picture of the total process. This section deals with specific limitations of different techniques in the study of metal absorption.

A prime factor underlying these limitations arises from the ease with which metals form coordination complexes with proteins and other biologic molecules.

No significant fraction of heavy metal is therefore likely to be present in free, ionized form when dissolved in biologic fluids or mixed with food digests. Binding by various ligands may render the metals more or less absorbable, as further discussed in Sect. C.IV. The complexing of metals in the intestinal lumen implies that study of metal absorption under physiologic conditions may often resolve itself into analysis of transport of metal complexes. It follows that study of metal uptake from ligand-free saline solutions may possess only limited quantitative relevance to the problem of absorption under physiologic conditions.

Another consequence of the high reactivity of metals with biologic macromolecules is in many cases their avid retention in the intestinal mucosa (see Sect. C.II). This is of particular importance in the study of the toxic metals Cd, Hg, and Pb (NEATHERY and MILLER 1975). When studying transmural movement of metals in the everted sac, in the absence of vascular perfusion, their reaction with tissue constituents would interfere with their ability to move from mucosa to the serosal fluid, even if the mucosa did not retain them in the first place. Sacs have, of course, been applied to great advantage to the study of absorption of such diffusible solutes as sugars and amino acids. Unlike the metals, these compounds can move across the thick intestinal wall without significant binding to the tissue.

The extent to which transmural absorption rates of metals into sacs are depressed by tissue binding varies from metal to metal, as does trapping in or on mucosal cells in the first place (Sect. C.II). The everted sac is therefore likely to provide more useful information on absorption of some metals than of others. The major disadvantage of the everted sac for the study of metal absorption can be avoided by use of intestinal segments doubly perfused in vitro, through the lumen and the vascular system (SMITH and COUSINS 1980). In such a preparation, both removal of Zn from the lumen, and its appearance in vascular perfusate, can be readily demonstrated.

The problem of the physiologic relevance of metal absorption from ligand-free perfusates has already been raised and is further discussed in Sect. C.IV. Another difference between luminally perfused but isolated intestinal segments, in vitro or in vivo, and the intestine of the intact animal, may be the absence from the lumen of endogenous modulators of metal absorption. For example, certain bile salts have been observed to inhibit Cd absorption in the rat jejunum (FOULKES and VONER 1981). This phenomenon is further discussed in Sect. D.I and appears to be related to micelle formation. Transport of some other metals is also influenced by bile or bile salts (CIKRT and TICHY 1975; GOLLAN et al. 1971; HOLDSWORTH and WEBLING 1971; ANTONSON et al. 1979). Another endogenous factor which could conceivably affect metal transport is calcium in intestinal secretions. Addition of Ca to the lumen interferes with absorption of several metals, as for instance Cd (e.g., FOULKES 1980). Absence of normal constituents of luminal fluid such as bile salts, Ca, or other factors, thus complicates the extrapolation from an isolated segment to the intact gut. Little is known of the mechanism whereby humoral factors may influence metal absorption. However, the pronounced response of the absorption of certain metals to a variety of physiologic stimuli, such as Zn deficiency or stress in the case of Zn (Sect. D.II), or vitamin D in the case of Cd KOO et al. 1978) and other metals, makes it likely that endogenous factors are important in the control of metal transport.

Interpretation of results obtained with intact animals also raises certain questions. For instance, enterohepatic circulation of a metal, or its intestinal secretion or mucosal retention may interfere with calculation of unidirectional absorptive flux. In summary, some of the gaps in our understanding of mechanisms mediating intestinal metal transport may be attributed to experimental difficulties. Nevertheless, considerable information has accumulated in this field and will be further analyzed in this chapter.

C. General Characteristics of Heavy Metal Absorption

I. Kinetics

There is some disagreement about the basic nature of metal transport out of the intestinal lumen. First-order kinetics have occasionally been reported to describe this process adequately (e.g., KOJIMA and KIYOZUMI 1974). These reports, however, are mostly based on the results of in vitro studies with relatively high metal concentrations. The vascularly perfused sac in vitro, as pointed out in Sect. B, avoids some of the difficulties associated with other in vitro procedures, and permitted the demonstration that transmural Zn absorption is a saturable process (SMITH and COUSINS 1980). Similarly, with an intact segment of intestine in vivo, disappearance of Cd from a low concentration in the lumen is clearly subject to saturation and inhibition phenomena (see Sect. D.I). The weight of evidence therefore suggests that simple diffusion cannot explain metal absorption under physiologic conditions of concentration and vascular perfusion; in all likelihood cellular transport phenomena are involved. This conclusion cannot, of course, imply active transport of these heavy metals as long as their electrochemical activities in lumen, cells, and blood are not known. Evidence adduced to support the involvement of active transport in, for instance, Zn absorption (PEARSON et al. 1966) is not compelling. Inhibitory effects of cyanide or anoxia, or high tissue levels of Zn, cannot per se prove uphill transport.

At an initial concentration of 20 μM in the lumen, jejunal uptake of ^{109}Cd follows first-order kinetics (Sect. D.I). On the other hand, uptake of ^{65}Zn under the same conditions represents a multicompartment process (see Sect. D.II). In any case, uptake from lumen into mucosa may be regarded as the first step in a two-step series process, in which the second step describes translocation of the metal from mucosa into the body. This model is schematically illustrated in Fig. 1. The model does not specify any particular molecular mechanism of metal transport; it simply states the self-evident fact that the first step in absorption of a solute must be its transfer from lumen to intestinal mucosa (step I). The model does, however, exclude parallel and independent pathways for: (1) cellular accumulation of metals; and (2) their transmural movement, perhaps through tight junctions in the mucosal epithelium. Possible existence of such pathways has repeatedly been suggested, but usually at excessively high and possibly acutely toxic concentrations of the metals. Thus, KOO et al. (1978) concluded that Cd uptake out of the chicken intestine could not be saturated by Cd concentrations as high as 1 mM; inspection of their results provides some indication, however, for a process of Cd absorption approaching saturation in the range of 0.01–0.10 mM. At

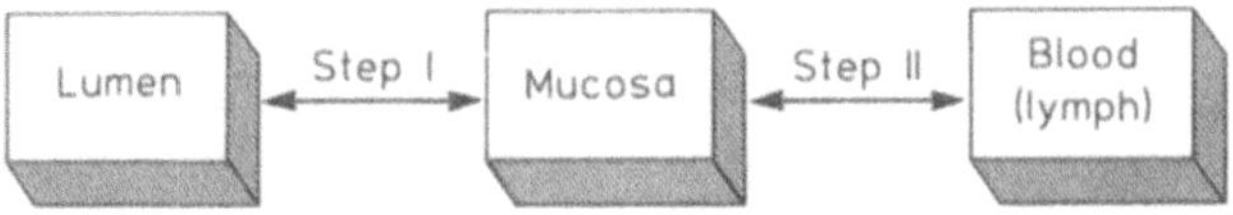

Fig. 1. Schematic representation of intestinal metal absorption

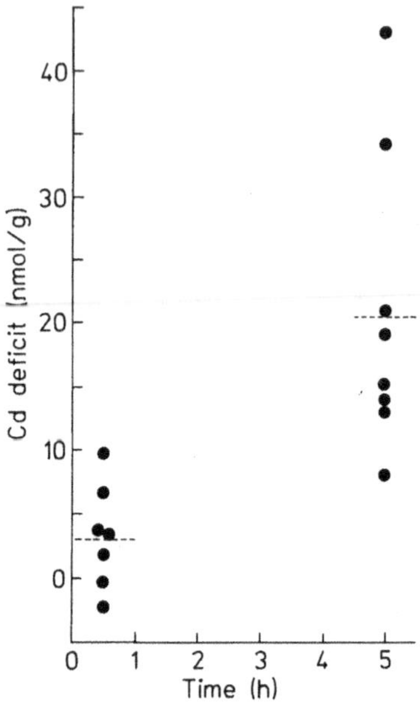

Fig. 2. Determination of step II of Cd absorption; for details, see Table 2. Step II is equated to the deficit in Cd recovery from the tissue, i.e., Cd removed from lumen minus Cd accumulated in tissue. KELLO et al. (1979)

lower concentrations, occurrence of parallel pathways of metal transport, in which appearance of metal in serosal fluid is claimed to be independent of mucosal uptake, has also been proposed (BLAIR et al. 1979; MEREDITH et al. 1977): BLAIR et al. (1979) measured the amount of Pb accumulated in or on the tissue of everted sacs of rat intestine, as well as the amount appearing in serosal fluid; recalculation of their results, however, shows that over a 500-fold concentration range of Pb in mucosal fluid, the ratio of serosal to serosal plus tissue Pb changed very little. Such a finding is fully compatible with the series model of Fig. 1.

Direct evidence against independent function of parallel pathways is seen in the work of KELLO et al. (1979). The critical experiment is shown in Fig. 2. Here essentially all Cd removed from the perfusate, i.e., all Cd transported by step I, was recovered in the intestinal wall at the end of the perfusion; Table 2, Sect. D.I further illustrates the fact that all this tissue Cd is actually accumulated in the mucosa. The conclusion states that step I leads to mucosal accumulation of Cd. By 5 h later, part of this accumulation has been dissipated into the body (step II). Step II is here simply equated to the difference between net Cd transport by step I, and recovery of Cd in the intestinal wall.

Table 1. Steps in Zn absorption at different Zn concentrations (E. C. FOULKES and C. VONER 1981, unpublished work)

Zn concentration in perfusate (μM)	Zn absorption (nmol g^{-1} min^{-1})[a]	
	2 (N=7)	200 (N=7)
Step I[b]	0.14 ± 0.05	10.8 ± 1.6
Step II[b]	0.05 ± 0.02	3.2 ± 1.0
Step II/I (%)[c]	32 ± 4	30 ± 6

[a] Mean ± standard deviation
[b] Steps I and II were measured as in the work of KELLO et al. (1979)
[c] Mean of ratios from individual animals

Another experimental finding, this time referring to Zn absorption, also supports the proposed model. The rate of step II of Zn transport closely varies with that of step I. This is illustrated in Table 1, where the ratio of step II to step I is seen to have remained constant over a 100-fold concentration range of Zn in the lumen. Such a result would be highly coincidental if steps I and II represented independent processes. In summary, therefore, the scheme of Fig. 1 adequately predicts absorption characteristics of various metals at low concentrations.

Another point to be noted in the proposed scheme is that it specifically states the possibility of reverse fluxes, from blood into lumen. Such secretion was described for instance by EVANS et al. (1979) for Zn. KOJIMA et al. (1976) and FOULKES (1980) reported a small return flux of Cd back into the lumen in the presence of various chelating compounds. The possibility of backflux must, therefore, be taken into account in experimental studies of metal absorption, as otherwise its occurrence could lead to faulty estimates of the absolute size of steps I and II. This problem may become especially significant in isotope studies, where the possibility of isotope dilution must not be neglected (EVANS et al. 1979).

No implications about mechanisms are made in Fig. 1. Nor does the scheme distinguish between various possible metal compartments in the mucosa. That such compartmentation occurs has been reported by several investigators. Thus, for instance, Cd is distributed in the mucosa between cytosol and particulate fractions; cytosolic Cd, in turn, is bound to a series of ligands of different molecular weights (KELLO et al. 1979). Each ligand may possess a characteristic affinity for the metal. The role, if any, of these cytosolic ligands in controlling transmural Cd movement remains unclear (see Sect. D.I).

II. Role of Mucosal Metal Retention

Step II in Fig. 1 provides the major fraction of total body burden of various metals. It is interesting to note, therefore, that the ratio of step II to step I, both expressed in amounts of metal transported per unit time by a given segment of jejunum, amounts only to about 0.01 : 1 for Cd. In contrast, the equivalent ratio

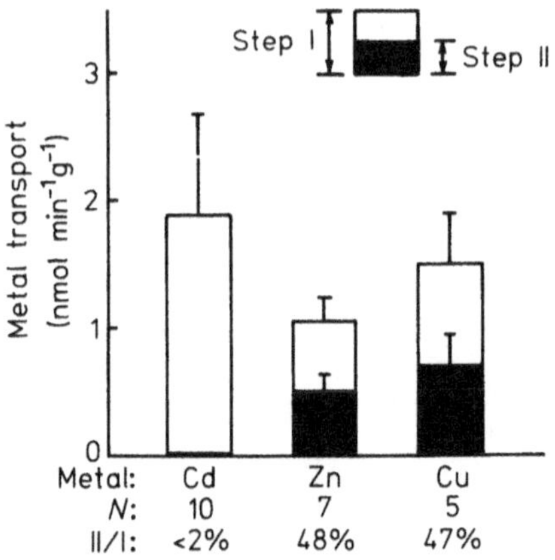

Fig. 3. Steps I and II in jejunal transport of ^{109}Cd, ^{65}Zn, and ^{64}Cu. In each case, the rat jejunum was perfused in situ with 5 m*M* glucose in saline containing 0.02 m*M* metal. After 25 min, the jejunal segment was washed and its isotope content determined. Step II was equated to the difference between step I and the recovery in the tissue. *Height of bars* represents mean $\pm$ standard error. BONEWITZ et al. (1982)

for the essential metals Cu and Zn is much higher and may reach 0.5 : 1. This fact, which is illustrated in Fig. 3, is implicit in earlier work which showed, for instance, that appearance of Zn in the vascular compartment is very much faster than that of Cd (SMITH et al. (1978).

Figure 3 illustrates that the mucosa represents the major barrier to absorption of the toxic metal Cd. This same mechanism also reduces absorption of Pb (CONRAD and BARTON 1978); mucosal retention of this metal was further found to be independent of total body burden, i.e., there is no evidence for any homeostatic mechanism controlling Pb absorption.

The concept of homeostasis is, of course, inappropriate for toxic metals. In general, absorption of such metals as Hg, Cd, and Pb is slow and independent of body burden (NEATHERY and MILLER 1975). On the other hand, a homeostatic role of mucosal Zn retention has been proposed by RICHARDS and COUSINS (1975), who suggested that accumulation of Zn-metallothionein (see Sect. D.II) provides the means of controlling Zn absorption according to bodily requirements; metal taken up into the mucosa, but not further transferred to the body (step II) would be excreted following desquamation of the epithelial cells. A similar role has been attributed to mucosal binding of iron.

III. Specificity of Absorption Mechanisms

A major question relates to the similarities and differences between mechanisms mediating absorption of different metals. Metal–metal antagonism in nutrition and metabolism is very common, and includes mutual interference at the level of intestinal absorption. For instance, BREMNER (1978) reviewed interactions of Cd in vivo with Ca, Fe, Zn, and Cu; in each case effects on absorption appear to be involved. HAMILTON and VALBERG (1974) reported a positive correlation between rates of intestinal Fe and Cd uptake. Mutual effects of several heavy metals on metal absorption were explored in vitro by SAHAGIAN et al. (1967). Perhaps because the results were derived from studies with nonvascularly perfused intestinal segments, they are not in full agreement with those from in vivo studies. In any case, occurrence of metal–metal interaction at the level of intestinal absorption is well documented.

Cadmium and zinc mutually depress each other's transport out of the lumen of the rat jejunum, possibly in a competitive manner (N. SUGAWARA and E. C. FOULKES 1980, unpublished work); if this interpretation were correct it would suggest involvement of a common site in absorption of the two metals. On the other hand, Zn absorption is increased in Zn-deficient rats (BECKER and HOEKSTRA 1971), while that of Cd is independent of the Zn status of the animals (FOULKES and VONER 1981). It follows that not all aspects of the mechanisms responsible for Cd and Zn absorption can be identical in spite of their interaction, i.e., interaction is not necessarily synonymous with identity of the absorption processes.

Further evidence against the concept of a common carrier nonspecifically mediating absorption of different metals is the variation observed in certain cases between the pattern of their absorption along the gastrointestinal tract. Thus Cd but not Zn is absorbed from the stomach (VAN CAMPEN and MITCHELL 1965). It must be emphasized, however, that such distinctive absorption patterns could reflect the presence of specific endogenous modulators of metal transport in various segments; reference in this regard has already been made to the bile salts (Sect. B). A more clear-cut argument for the involvement of specific transport systems in intestinal absorption of heavy metals is provided by Menkes' disease (DANKS et al. 1972), a condition associated with a hereditary defect in Cu absorption; the patients show no sign of abnormal Zn metabolism. Similarly, patients suffering from acrodermatitis enteropathica present with impaired intestinal absorption of Zn (LOMBECK et al. 1975).

While some specific transport mechanisms may thus exist, it seems unlikely a priori that separate mechanisms should exist for each metal, and especially so for nonessential toxic elements like Cd and Pb. Presumably the small fractional absorption of these metals reflects, at least in part, the less than complete specificity of mechanisms for absorption of essential metals.

IV. Chemical Form of Absorbed Metals

Binding of metals to nonabsorbed macromolecular ligands obviously will interfere with their absorption. This has already been referred to in Sect. B and leads, as corollary, to the conclusion that ligands which form diffusible metal complexes may increase intestinal transport of different metals. For instance, presence of a low molecular weight Zn binding ligand in human milk, tentatively identified as citric acid by HURLEY et al. (1979), may explain under certain conditions the greater bioavailability of Zn from that source than from bovine milk. The latter contains more of its Zn bound to high molecular weight constituents than does human milk (ECKHERT et al. 1977). The low molecular weight compounds, in this and similar cases, may be visualized as competing with larger ligands to render the metal more absorbable. Such an explanation also accounts for the observation that ethylenediaminetetraacetate (EDTA) increases Zn absorption in the presence of phytic acid, a high molecular weight nonabsorbable metal ligand (OBERLEAS et al. 1966). Reference may be made in this regard also to the parallel role of filterable metal complexes in determining reabsorption of heavy metals by renal tubular epithelium (FOULKES 1974). Some chelators, on the other hand, may also be found to depress luminal uptake of metal by preventing its reaction with appropriate receptor sites on cell membranes. Finally, and independently of competition with nonabsorbable complexes, binding of a metal into a lipophilic chelate, e.g., diiodohydroxyquin (DELVES et al. 1975) could directly enhance metal absorption. Such an effect may explain the therapeutic effect of Diodoquin in the treatment of acrodermatitis enteropathica, attributed by DELVES et al. (1975) to the formation of readily absorbed Zn complex.

Numerous further examples may be cited to illustrate these points. KOJIMA and KIYOZUMI (1974) found that Cd transport across intestinal sacs in vitro is greatly enhanced by addition of EDTA and other chelators. EVANS and coworkers (EVANS 1980; EVANS and JOHNSON 1980) proposed that picolinic acid plays an essential role as endogenous ligand in mediating Zn absorption. Even somewhat larger molecules may contribute to transport of metals: Thus, CHERIAN (1979) reported that Cd-metallothionein, a cysteine-rich protein of molecular weight around 6,000 can cross the intestinal barrier and be recovered as such from the kidney.

In spite of the strong evidence for a permissive role of various exogenous or endogenous ligands in metal absorption, there is evidence against the view that this role is obligatory. Thus, the studies of FOULKES and collaborators (FOULKES 1980; KELLO et al. 1979; BONEWITZ et al. 1982) on Cd and Zn transport out of the lumen of a segment of rat jejunum in vivo utilized a perfusate free of exogenous ligands. Both metals were rapidly absorbed from such a solution. To test further whether an endogenous mediator of metal absorption might be secreted into the perfusate, rates of metal removal were compared from a recirculating solution, and one that passed through the lumen only once. The single-pass perfusion should diminish accumulation of a putative ligand secreted into the perfusate, and therefore permit only slower absorption than occurs from a recirculated solution. No such difference was observed. It is unnecessary, therefore, to postulate that soluble metal ligands of the type envisioned by EVANS (1980) in the lumen are essential for Cd or Zn absorption. Presumably, the metals react directly with cell membranes; it is unlikely, however, that their further movement involves free metal ions. Absence of unbound metal from mucosal homogenates has repeatedly been demonstrated (e.g., KELLO et al. 1979), although metals may of course be redistributed during homogenization. Some of the metal complexes observed in such homogenates may represent storage compounds, or may even be directly involved in transmural metal movement. In summary, it is not known in what chemical form absorbed metals finally reach blood or lymph.

In the case of metallic elements which can exist under physiologic conditions in more than one valence state, the degree of oxidation of the metal may also greatly affect its intestinal absorption. This has been observed, for instance, in the case of chromium (MERTZ 1969): Compounds of trivalent Cr are in general much less soluble and more poorly absorbed than are those of hexavalent Cr; in addition, it is possible that anions like chromate or dichromate, containing the element in its hexavalent state, might cross cell membranes through anion channels. Another element whose valence state may well determine the degree of its absorption is copper. The preferential absorption of iron in the ferrous state is well documented.

V. Effects of Age

The efficiency of its absorption is a characteristic of each metal. In general, essential metals are absorbed to a greater extent than are toxic metals (NEATHERY and MILLER 1975). Certain factors, however, can be identified which strongly influence metal absorption in general. One of these, the presence of fibers or other nonabsorbed macromolecular metal ligands in the diet, has repeatedly been referred to. Another important variable is the age of the animal, and its stage of development.

In the developing rat, the time of weaning corresponds to the stage at which fractional absorption of several metals declines from relatively high neonatal to much lower adult values (BALLOU and THOMPSON 1961; KELLO and KOSTIAL 1977; FORBES and REINA 1972; KOSTIAL et al. 1971). Presumably, both changes in diet and maturational factors are responsible for this decline. The neonatal intestine is indeed well known to differ extensively in function from the mature tissue. Because of their relatively efficient absorption mechanisms, neonatal animals (and humans) are a class at special risk of intoxication with heavy metals.

D. Absorption of Some Individual Metals

Previous sections dealt with general characteristics of heavy metal absorption. Here we proceed to consider in greater detail the intestinal handling of specific metals. In no case, however, has the process of metal absorption been clarified to the point where an adequate model can yet be proposed.

I. Cadmium

Cadmium is one of those toxic metals for which no biologic function is known, and whose fractional net absorption into the body from the intestinal lumen of adult human or animal amounts to only a few percent of the oral load (NEATHERY and MILLER 1975; MOORE et al. 1973). This value is independent of the body burden (COTZIAS et al. 1961), in further support of the conclusion that Cd is not an essential element in mammalian nutrition. Toxicity of the metal, and its metabolism, are however related to the fact that its chemical properties closely resemble those of the essential metal Zn, and it has indeed repeatedly been suggested that Cd primarily acts by interfering with Zn metabolism. The evidence previously discussed in Sect. C.III, however, points to differences between the processes of Cd and Zn absorption from the jejunum. While common reaction sites may be involved, the processes are not identical.

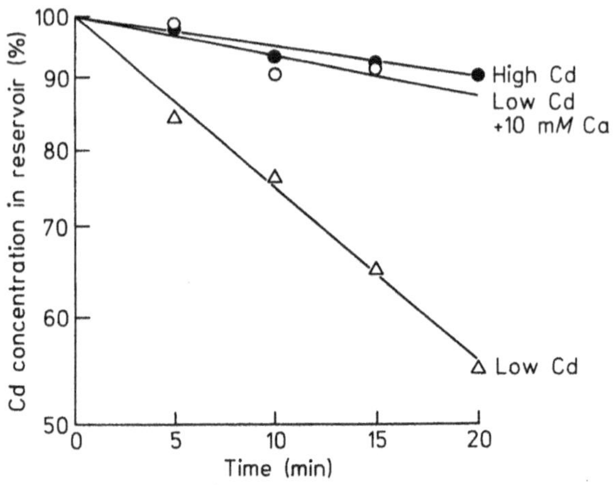

Fig. 4. Kinetics of jejunal Cd transport. Low Cd (20 μ*M*) and high Cd (200 μ*M*) in glucose saline was recirculated through the lumen of the rat jejunum in situ. Note saturation at high Cd concentration, and inhibition by Ca. Foulkes (1980)

In an isolated segment of the rat jejunum perfused in situ with 20 μ*M* $CdCl_2$ in glucose–saline, the metal is removed from the lumen by a process which follows first-order kinetics, but can be saturated at higher concentrations; this is illustrated in Fig. 4. Further, the process is subject to inhibition, for instance by Ca (Foulkes 1980). Cytotoxicity cannot explain the depression of fractional absorption seen at the higher Cd concentration, as sugar and volume absorption both continue at normal rates. In addition, the depression is largely reversible by dilution, although this does not lead to significant washout of Cd from the tissue. In other words, it is the concentration of Cd at the cell membrane rather than that in the cells which governs the rate of step I of Cd uptake (Foulkes 1980). These observations suggest that a membrane mechanism controls the rate of Cd uptake. Little is known of this proposed membrane mechanism. Kinetic analysis yields an affinity constant of the order of 0.1 m*M* (Foulkes 1980). Bovine serum albumin added to the perfusate in a concentration of 30 mg/ml greatly reduces Cd transport, presumably by competing for the metal with mucosal binding sites involved in absorption (Foulkes and Voner 1981).

At the end of a 25-min perfusion period with 0.02 m*M* Cd as is depicted in Fig. 4, essentially all Cd lost from the perfusate can be recovered in the jejunal mucosa (Table 2). As pointed out in Sect. C.II, mucosal retention of Cd is very strong, and further movement of the metal into the body (step II) is quite slow. Reasons for this retention are not clearly defined. As can be seen in Table 2, the freshly absorbed Cd is distributed among a wide spectrum of cell constituents, including the metal binding protein metallothionein in the cytosol. This low molecular weight protein possesses a very high affinity for Cd and was therefore believed to trap the metal in the mucosa (Squibb et al. 1976; Valberg et al. 1976). A direct test of this hypothesis, in which transmural Cd movement was compared in animals with low and with high metallothionein levels in the mucosa, failed to establish any correlation between metallothionein concentration and mucosal Cd

Table 2. Uptake and distribution of Cd in rat jejunum[a] (after KELLO et al. 1979)

I Cd removed from lumen in 25 min	II Cd in mucosal homogenate at 25 min		III Deficit at 25 min (I–II)	IV Cd in intestinal wall at 5 h	V Deficit at 5 h (I–IV)
25.1 (step I)	*Supernatant*		0.6	20.9	4.2
	Molecular weight				
	> 10,000	7.3			
	6,000–10,000	3.3[b]			
	< 6,000	1.3			
	Subtotal	11.9			
	Residue	12.6			
	Total	24.5			

[a] Results are expressed as nmol Cd, and are mean values obtained with segments of jejunum (average weight 1.4 g) perfused in situ with 0.02 mM $CdCl_2$ for 25 min. The lumen was then rinsed and the intestine assayed, either immediately or after having been returned to the animal for the balance of 5 h

[b] This fraction contains metallothionein

retention (KELLO et al. 1979). Other workers have attributed the prolonged Cd retention to extracellular adsorption (SASSER and JARBOE 1977; SAHAGIAN et al. 1967). Since relatively little Cd has been reported to bind to nuclei, mitochondria, and endoplasmic reticulum (BHATTACHARJEE et al. 1979), a large portion of the Cd recovered in the insoluble portion of mucosal homogenates by KELLO et al. (1979) (see also Table 2) may well have been bound to cell membranes, as was found by TAGUCHI and SUZUKI (1978).

Cadmium absorption in other isolated sections of the small intestine has not been studied in as much detail as in jejunum. The physiologic significance of comparing activity in specific isolated portions of the intestine is muted by the fact that they may not contain the same concentrations of endogenous modulators of Cd absorption as may be present in the intact intestine. One class of such endogenous compounds is the bile salts (FOULKES and VONER 1981; see also Sect. B).

The action of selected bile salts in depressing jejunal Cd absorption in the rat is fully reversible, and under specified conditions affects only Cd, not Zn (FOULKES and VONER 1981). A dose–effect relationship for glycocholate is shown in Fig. 5 and indicates that the critical inhibitory concentration falls near the concentration at which this bile salt tends to form micelles. Similar results have been obtained with taurocholate; in contrast, the nonmicelle-forming taurodehydrocholate exerted no inhibition. While details of the mechanism responsible for inhibition of step I of jejunal Cd absorption by bile salts remain to be elucidated, the occurrence of the effect indicates the strong likelihood that endogenous compounds can modulate metal absorption in various segments of the intestine. Absorption of Cd, like that of several other metals, is depressed in presence of Ca in the lumen (FOULKES 1980, KOO et al. 1978), and by systemic calciferol and the calcium status of the animal (KOO et al. 1978). As discussed in Sect. D.III for Pb, there is no direct evidence involving the mucosal Ca binding protein in this effect.

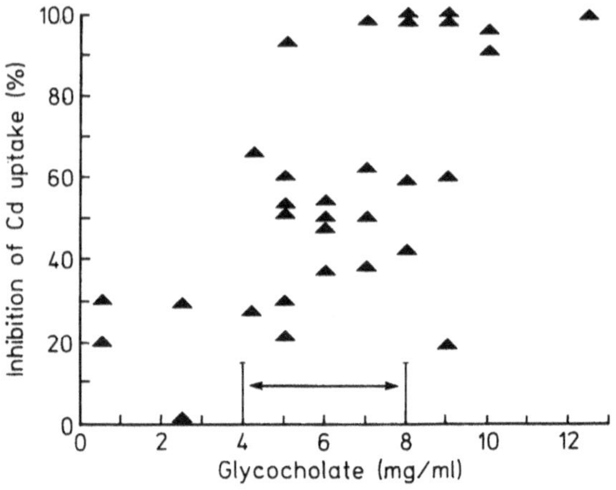

Fig. 5. Effect of glycocholate on jejunal Cd absorption. Each point represents the result from one rat. The *arrow* indicates the critical micellar range of glycocholate. FOULKES and VONER (1981)

II. Zinc

Zinc is an essential metal, and its absorption from the intestine is generally much more complete than that of Cd. The site of maximal absorption in the rat is claimed to be the ileum (ANTONSON et al. 1979; EMES and ARTHUR 1975); other investigators found faster uptake in duodenal segments, followed by ileum and jejunum (VAN CAMPEN and MITCHELL 1965). Values for fractional absorption have been quoted as ranging from 5% (FEASTER et al. 1955) to as high as 98% (HETH et al. 1966). This wide range undoubtedly reflects the fact that Zn absorption is sensitive to a variety of physiologic variables such as age, stress, state of nutrition, and, of course, the composition of the diet. As is true of other metals, Zn may become nutritionally unavailable owing to reaction with nonabsorbed ligands such as phytic acid, fibers, etc. (PECOUD et al. 1975). Thus, Zn deficiency has actually been observed in children practicing pica with clay-containing soils (OBERLEAS et al. 1966). On the other hand, various low molecular weight ligands may accelerate absorption, as discussed in Sect. C.IV, presumably by competing with nonabsorbable macromolecular ligands and thus rendering luminal Zn more available.

To the extent discussed so far, uptake of Zn from the intestinal lumen resembles that of Cd. The similarities extend further: Zn and Cd inhibit each other's uptake in rat jejunum (N. SUGAWARA and E.C. FOULKES 1980, unpublished work), and both processes are depressed by Ca. Nevertheless, important differences between the handling of the two metals in the intestine have also been reported. A major characteristic of the absorption of Zn, as contrasted with that of Cd, is its dependence on body burden of the metal. Indeed, homeostatic control of Zn uptake may be a major mechanism determining the steady state level of Zn in the body. The ability of the intestine thus to respond to the Zn requirements of the body is probably related to the influence of a variety of hormonal and other

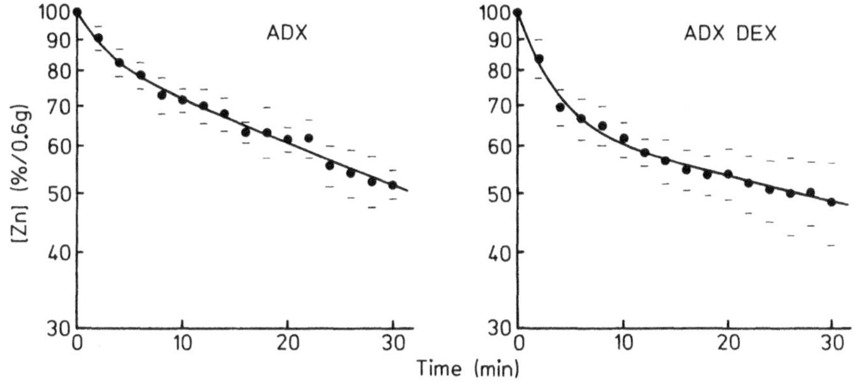

Fig. 6. Dexamethasone and jejunal Zn transport in the rat. The plot shows the mean Zn concentration with 1 standard deviation in a perfusate initially containing 20 μ*M* Zn and recirculated through the jejunum of adrenalectomized (ADX) rats in situ. Results were normalized for an average jejunal weight of 0.6 g. DEX indicates 2 mg dexamethasone per kilogram body weight, injected 7 h previously. After BONEWITZ et al. (1983)

endogenous factors on Zn absorption (e.g., PEKAREK and EVANS 1975; SAS and BREMNER 1979).

In general, stress, as mediated presumably by steroid hormones, increases Zn uptake. It is interesting, therefore, that the kinetics of Zn absorption are affected by dexamethasone, as shown by BONEWITZ et al. (1983). This work involved a compartmental analysis of the removal of Zn from the rat jejunum perfused in vivo. The process, as in the case of Cd, shows saturation kinetics. However, whereas Cd uptake may be described by a single exponential (see Fig. 4), that of Zn reflects at least two components, as illustrated in Fig. 6 (BONEWITZ et al. 1983). Dexamethasone (2 mg/kg, injected 7 h previously) increases the relative contribution of the fast component to total Zn uptake. The nature of the two components, and of the action of the hormone, have not been fully elucidated. One explanation considered was that the steroid induces metallothionein synthesis in jejunal mucosa, as it does in liver; it was further hypothesized that this metallothionein could then trap a certain amount of Zn, and by preventing its backflux into the lumen, transiently increase the net rate of Zn uptake from the lumen. This explanation had to be abandoned when dexamethasone was found not to stimulate metallothionein synthesis in jejunal mucosa (BONEWITZ et al. 1983).

Animals receiving adequate amounts of Zn in their diets absorb the metal more slowly than do Zn-deficient animals (BECKER and HOEKSTRA 1971). At the same time, a high Zn diet also increases the concentration of metallothionein in the intestinal mucosa; this inverse correlation between metallothionein levels in the mucosa and the rate of Zn absorption led RICHARDS and COUSINS (1975) to propose the following scheme for homeostatic control of Zn absorption. The high concentration of metallothionein in the mucosa of Zn-fed animals would trap Zn and prevent its further translocation into the body; mucosal Zn-metallothionein would then be excreted after desquamation of epithelial cells. The hypothesis

Table 3. Jejunal Zn absorption after Cd pretreatment[a] (after SUGAWARA 1982)

N	Control 11	Cd-treated 10
Removed from lumen (step I)	40.9±9.5	44.9±8.0
Retained in mucosa	13.8±1.9	20.0±3.9
Transferred into body (step II)	26.6±9.1	24.8±6.6

[a] Pretreated rats had received 50 ppm Cd in their drinking water for 9 days, sufficient to increase mucosal metallothionein by a factor of about 4 (KELLO et al. 1979; see Sect. D.I). Isolated jejunal segments were perfused in situ for 20 min with 50 μ*M* Zn in glucose–saline. Each value represents men ± standard deviation from *N* animals, and is expressed in nmol per gram tissue 20 min

therefore predicts that step II of Zn absorption will be decreased in Zn-loaded animals; step I should not be affected. Experimental test of these predictions by measurement of tracer fluxes is complicated by the likelihood of greater isotope dilution in Zn-replete than in Zn-deficient animals.

An accelerating action of metallothionein on Zn absorption was claimed by STARCHER et al. (1980). Interpretation of these results is somewhat uncertain, however, since Zn absorption was evaluated only indirectly, by recovery of ^{65}Zn from the liver. Increased hepatic accumulation of Zn in these experiments could have resulted simply from the induction of hepatic metallothionein synthesis, and need not be related to raised metallothionein levels in the intestinal mucosa. A role of metallothionein in determining Zn absorption was further questioned by SUGAWARA (1982). Induction of metallothionein synthesis in the mucosa by exposure of rats to Cd in their drinking water was indeed accompanied by increased Zn retention in that tissue, but the total transfer of the metal into the body (step II) was not significantly reduced. These findings are described in Table 3; use of Cd instead of Zn to increase mucosal metallothionein levels diminishes the potential difficulty posed by isotopic dilution of tracer Zn during the uptake studies. In summary, a role of metallothionein in the control of intestinal Zn absorption has not been established, any more so than in the case of Cd (Sect. D.I).

In addition to metallothionein, other factors may well be involved in the homeostatic control of Zn absorption. COTZIAS et al. (1962) had previously concluded that Zn homeostasis is based both on absorption of the metal and on its intestinal excretion. EVANS et al. (1979) proposed that Zn secretion into the lumen is the major factor in the dependence of net Zn absorption on the level of Zn in the body.

III. Lead

Intestinal absorption of Pb in the adult organism is generally slow, like that of the other nonessential toxic metals Hg and Cd (NEATHERY and MILLER 1975).

Little is known of the mechanism responsible for the small fraction of oral Pb which is absorbed into the body. Because of its great industrial significance, and the consequently large number of people exposed, extensive work has been carried out on uptake of lead by humans, especially through the gastrointestinal tract. Some of the investigations were balance studies (KEHOE 1961) and can therefore give information only on net retention of Pb, not on the rate of its absorption. More recently tracer methodology has been applied to humans (RABINOWITZ et al. 1980). The stable isotope ^{204}Pb was ingested with meals by two adult males. On the basis of fecal excretion of the isotope and its specific activity, net fractional absorption was determined as 6.5% and 8.5% for the two subjects. CHAMBERLAIN et al. (1978) utilized ^{203}Pb and calculated a fractional absorption of 7.1%.

Considerable information has been collected also on lead absorption in the experimental animal. Thus, several investigators studied the effects of Ca on Pb absorption or retention. Low dietary Ca has been shown to increase symptoms of lead intoxication (MAHAFFEY et al. 1973). The antagonistic action of Ca on Pb intoxication is probably related at least in part to events at the level of intestinal absorption (QUARTERMAN and MORRISON 1975). BARTON et al. (1978) suggested that Ca in the intestinal lumen interferes with Pb absorption, while dietary Ca deprivation may influence Pb retention. The interaction between Ca and Pb at the level of intestinal absorption is correlated with a competition between the two metals for the two main soluble Pb binding proteins, the low molecular weight, heat-stable calcium binding protein (CaBP) induced by vitamin D, and a protein in the high molecular weight fraction (BARTON et al. 1978). It is interesting that altering the mucosal CaBP content by changing the Ca content of the diet exerts no effect on Pb absorption. This recalls the similar lack of influence of the Cd binding protein metallothionein on Cd absorption (Sect. D.I), and does not support the concept that CaBP plays any part in the control of Pb absorption. Vitamin D itself does not appear to exert a direct effect on Pb absorption (BARTON et al. 1980).

In spite of its high Ca centent, milk has been reported to increase Pb absorption (KOSTIAL et al. 1978), although the distinction between unidirectional absorption and retention in this case is difficult, especially in light of a significant biliary Pb excretion (CIKRT and TICHY 1975). On the assumption that the increased retention of Pb on a milk diet may be equated with increased absorption, the low iron content of milk has been invoked as the critical factor determining absorption (HAMILTON 1978). Fe deficiency is indeed known to increase retention of ingested Pb (SIX and GOYER 1972). Another interesting suggestion for how milk may facilitate Pb absorption arises from the observation that lactose accelerates Pb absorption in segments of the small intestine of the rat (BUSHNELL and DELUCA 1981). Thus sugar affects metabolism of several metals, including Ca, Fe, and Zn. The effect is specific for lactose as compared with other sugars (Table 4), and may contribute greatly to the high susceptibility of the newborn to Pb.

No action of lactose on Ca metabolism is seen after parenteral lactose administration (LENGEMANN 1959); sugar and Ca must be present simultaneously in the same segment of intestine. Presumably the sugar acts directly at the level of the

Table 4. Effect of sugars on Pb absorption in rats[a] (after BUSHNELL and DE LUCA 1981)

Sugar	Pb absorbed (step II) (μmol) (mean ± standard error)
None	0.39 ± 0.05
Glucose	0.46 ± 0.05
Galactose	0.49 ± 0.06
Maltose	0.41 ± 0.10
Lactose	0.71 ± 0.05

[a] Fasted weanling rats were given by gavage 1 ml 1 m*M* Pb acetate labeled with ^{110}Pb and 3 mg sugar per gram body weight, and tissues were collected about 20 h later for analysis

intestine. Unlike the role of ligands in accelerating, for example, Cd absorption (KOJIMA and KIYOZUMI 1974), the action of lactose may involve a nonselective increase of tissue permeability to cations by alteration of the transmural electrical potential (MARTIN and DELUCA 1969). The result would be to permit greater passive diffusion of Pb and other cations across the intestinal barrier. A significant contribution of passive diffusion to uptake of metals at low concentrations in vivo has, however, not been unequivocally established. BLAIR et al. (1979) interpreted their results on Pb absorption in terms of a first-order, nonsaturable process, but, as pointed out in Sect. C.I, an alternative interpretation is possible.

IV. Copper

Copper, although toxic in high concentrations, is an essential metal. Unlike the nonessential metals Cd, Pb, and Hg, it is trapped only to a relatively small extent in the intestinal mucosa (see Sect. C.II). A useful review on some of the older work on Cu absorption was published by EVANS (1973). Absorption has been described in stomach and duodenum of the rat (VAN CAMPEN and MITCHELL 1965) and of humans (VAN BERGE HENEGOUWEN et al. 1977). The characteristic distribution of absorptive activity, as well as the existence of a specific Cu malabsorption syndrome (DANKS et al. 1972; CARTWRIGHT and WINTROBE 1964) suggest that a specific mechanism mediates Cu absorption (see Sect. C.III).

Few details are known of this mechanism. GITLIN et al. (1960) fed mice 0.2 ml solution containing various amounts of Cu and concluded that the metal is absorbed by two processes. One of these reaches saturation when the dose of Cu amounts to 25 μg (i.e., 2 m*M* solution), whereas no saturation was evident for the second component at much higher concentrations. The biologic significance of these findings is difficult to evaluate because of the excessively high Cu concentrations employed. CRAMPTON et al. (1965) used everted sacs of hamster intestine to study both uptake from mucosal fluid into the tissue, and appearance of Cu on the serosal side. Unlike tissue accumulation, the transmural movement of Cu could be saturated and inhibited by dinitrophenol and anoxia. These findings do not necessarily imply that Cu is actively transported across the tissue, and the overall quantitative evaluation of the results, as pointed out in Sect. B, is rendered uncertain by the absence of vascular perfusion of the tissue.

MARCEAU et al. (1970) calculated the initial rate of appearance of ^{64}Cu from plasma activity curves, and observed that the rate increased linearly with dose up to 12 µg in 300 g rats. Beyond this dose level, the response became nonlinear, perhaps owing to saturation of transport mechanisms. The fact, however, that the metal was administered in presence of a twofold molar excess of histidine may have significantly influenced the results observed. Amino acids indeed greatly facilitate absorption of Cu (KIRCHGESSNER and GRASSMAN 1970). On that basis, EVANS (1973) suggested a model in which Cu absorption results from active transport of a Cu–amino acid complex across the basolateral membrane of mucosal epithelium. There is no evidence, however, that amino acid carriers can transport Cu–amino acid complexes, nor that transfer of amino acids across epithelial cells involves basolateral amino acid carriers.

During absorption of ^{64}Cu out of the chicken duodenum (STARCHER 1969), the metal is found associated with a metallothionein-like protein. This finding was extended by EVANS et al. (1970a), who concluded that competition between Zn, Cd, and Cu for metallothionein could explain the interaction between these metals. The assignment to metallothionein of a major role in the regulation of metal uptake is not supported however by the experiments discussed in Sects. D.I and D.II on Cd and Zn absorption; this, of course, does not exclude the possibility of metallothionein being involved in control of Cu absorption.

When ascorbic acid is placed together with Cu into a ligated segment of the rat intestine, it interferes with Cu absorption (VAN CAMPEN and GROSS 1968). A reduction of cupric to cuprous ion does not readily explain this effect as the acid also influences movement of Zn and Cd (see also SAHAGIAN et al. 1967). EVANS et al. (1970b) correlated the ascorbate inhibition with a direct effect on metallothionein. Again, in light of the negative evidence on the role of metallothionein in absorption of Cd and Zn, the significance of the correlation remains uncertain.

V. Mercury

Although exposure to mercury, in its elemental form, is primarily a pulmonary problem, ingested mercury compounds represent the major source of body mercury under nonoccupational conditions. The process of mercury absorption has been studied in some detail, expecially in vitro (SAHAGIAN et al. 1967; AARONSON and SPIRO 1973; CIKRT 1970). Interpretation of in vitro results, as discussed in Sect. B, is difficult, and especially so in this case because of the high affinity of tissue proteins for mercury. Ligated segments of the rat intestine were used in situ by CIKRT (1970); uptake of Hg by the intestinal wall (step I in absorption) was much faster than its further transfer from intestinal wall into the body (step II). Intestinal handling of Hg thus resembles that of Cd and Pb, as opposed to the much smaller trapping of nutritionally essential metals (NEATHERY and MILLER 1975). The absorption of Hg was ascribed to passive movement, but no specific evidence was offered to support this view. It seems likely, however, that disappearance of Hg from the lumen is to a significant extent the result of more or less specific protein binding, not always relevant to the process of Hg absorption into the body.

Binding to constituents of the intestinal mucosa presumably also explains the observation of SASSER et al. (1978) that over 90% of a tracer dose of $^{203}HgCl_2$, instilled into ligated segments of the rat gastrointestinal tract in vivo, was retained in these segments even after 4 h; step II of absorption during that period in, for example, the jejunum amounted to only 2% of the administered dose, an amount even smaller than that observed with Cd (KELLO et al. 1979).

In contrast to inorganic mercury, organic mercurials are in many cases absorbed relatively readily. Of particular interest in this regard is methylmercury (monomethylmercuric chloride), the source of several episodes of severe poisoning in human populations. The compound is readily absorbed from the intestine (ABERG et al. 1969); SASSER et al. (1978) found its absorption in the rat to proceed at a rate 15–35 times faster than that of inorganic mercury, depending on the site of measurement. This ready uptake into the body is certainly related to the high lipid solubility of methylmercury which also accounts for its ability to cross the blood–brain barrier. At the same time, lipid solubility is not the only factor involved in facilitating methylmercury absorption. Thus, cysteine greatly accelerates movement of methylmercury into the body, although the cysteine complex is less lipid-soluble than is the free compound (HIRAYAMA 1975). Possibly cysteine acts be reducing the trapping of methylmercury in the mucosa. The fact that acetylcysteine cannot be substituted for cysteine could arise from the need for a free amino group in the reaction with mercury; alternatively one might invoke a transport system for methylmercury complexes specific for the unsubstituted amino acid.

As with other metals, presence of nonabsorbable ligands reduces uptake of Hg from the lumen. Advantage has been taken of this fact not only to prevent absorption, but even to reverse it (TAKAHASHI and HIRAYAMA 1971; CLARKSON et al. 1973). Keratin, in the form of reduced hair powder, and a synthetic polythiol resin both decreased the level of residual methylmercury in mice poisoned with this compound, presumably by inhibiting reabsorption of methylmercury excreted in the bile. The synthetic resin reduced by 50% the rate of absorption of methylmercury from food.

VI. Other Metals

There are several other heavy metals of toxicologic and/or nutritional interest whose intestinal absorption has not been specifically reviewed in this chapter. In general, similar factors govern their transport as do that of other metals (Sect. C). Little further detail is known of the mechanisms involved in their intestinal absorption.

E. Summary and Conclusions

Absorption of heavy metals from the intestine, following their ingestion in food and water, constitutes the major source of these metals in the body under normal conditions. Detailed analysis of the absorption process is complicated by questions about the applicability of some commonly used experimental techniques. In all probability, only intestine with normal blood supply in situ, or with at least some vascular perfusion in vitro, can provide an adequate model for the study of metal absorption. Step I in this process, the transfer of metal from lumen into the mucosa, can, or course, be followed in simpler systems. It is the measurement of step II, the further movement of the metals from mucosa into the body, which cannot be readily studied in vitro. Perhaps because of these experimental difficulties no generally accepted scheme for the mechanism of intestinal metal absorption has yet emerged.

In general, the extent of absorption of metals is determined by a variety of factors (humoral, dietary, etc.). Uptake of the essential metals (Zn, Cu) is subject to homeostatic control, and is distinguished further from that of the nonessential toxic metals by a variable and smaller retention in the mucosa. These facts, together with the ability to saturate or to inhibit uptake, suggest that simple physical diffusion cannot explain intestinal absorption of essential heavy metals. Further, the occurrence of specific malabsorption syndromes, and the different absorptive patterns for Zn and Cu along the gastrointestinal tract point to the existence of relatively specific absorption mechanisms.

Absorption of toxic, nonessential metals is independent of their body burden, and is generally depressed by their avid retention in the mucosa. At the same time, saturable membrane sites may be involved in step I of the absorption process. The strong interaction between nonessential toxic and essential metals, such as between Pb and Ca, Cd and Zn, etc. suggests the possibility that the toxic metals share at least in part step I of the absorption mechanism of chemically similar essential metals. On this view, the absorption of the toxic metals reflects the less than complete specificity of the transport systems responsible primarily for absorption of essential metals. It would indeed be illogical to postulate that special mechanisms should be present for absorption of such metals as Pb, Cd, and Hg. On the other hand, the evidence is not compelling that interaction between, for instance, Cd and Zn results from competition for common binding sites.

The fact that step I for metals, at least in the case of Cd, seems to involve membrane mechanisms provides a means for selectively altering metal uptake by addition of transport inhibitors. In addition to such exogenous modulators of metal transport, endogenous compounds also may help determine the extent of absorption of the metals. No details are known of the mechanism of step II in the absorption of the various metals. Here again the possibility must be considered that transfer of the toxic metals utilizes the mechanisms available to the essential metals. Alternatively, step II of all the metals may depend primarily on their relative affinity for binding sites on nondiffusible cell constituents and on various diffusible ligands. There is no need to assume that such diffusible ligands are obligatory components of step I of the absorption process. The form in which absorbed metals finally reach blood or lymph remains uncertain.

Acknowledgments. The preparation of this chapter, and unpublished work quoted, were supported by grant ES 02416 from the U.S. National Institutes of Health, and grant R 805840 from the U.S. Environmental Protection Agency.

References

Aaronson RM, Spiro HM (1973) Mercury and the gut. Am J Digest Dis 18:583–594

Aberg B, Ekman L, Falk R, Greitz U, Persson G, Snihs JO (1969) Metabolism of methyl mercury compounds (^{203}Hg) in man. Arch Environ Health 19:478–484

Antonson DL, Barak AJ, Vanderhoof JA (1979) Determination of the site of zinc absorption in rat small intestine. J Nutr 109:142–147
Ballou JE, Thompson RE (1961) Metabolism of Zinc^{65} in the rat. Consideration of permissible exposure limits. Health Phys 6:6–18
Barton JC, Conrad ME, Harrison L, Nuby S (1978) Effects of calcium on absorption and retention of lead. J Lab Clin Med 91:366–376
Barton JC, Conrad ME, Harrison L, Nuby S (1980) Effects of vitamin D on the absorption and retention of lead. Am J Physiol 238:G124–G130
Becker WM, Hoekstra WG (1971) The intestinal absorption of Zn. In: Skoryna SC, Waldron-Edward D (eds) Intestinal absorption of metal ions, trace elements and radionuclides. Pergamon, Oxford, pp 229–256
Bhattacharjee D, Shetty TK, Sundaram K (1979) Studies on the distribution of cadmium-115m in mice tissues. Indian J Exp Biol 17:74–76
Blair JA, Coleman IPL, Hilburn ME (1979) The transport of the lead cation across the intestinal membrane. J Physiol 286:343–350
Bonewitz RF, Voner C, Foulkes EC (1982) Uptake and absorption of zinc in perfused rat jejunum: The role of endogenous factors in the lumen. Nutr Res 2:301–307
Bonewitz RF, Foulkes EC, O'Flaherty EJ, Hertzberg V (1983) Kinetics of zinc absorption by the rat jejunum: Effects of adrenalectomy and dexamethasone. Am J Physiol 244:G314–G320
Bremner I (1978) Cadmium toxicity. World Rev Nutr Diet 32:165–197
Bushnell PJ, DeLuca HF (1981) Lactose facilitates the intestinal absorption of lead in weanling rats. Science 211:61–63
Cartwright GE, Wintrobe MM (1964) The question of copper deficiency in man. Am J Clin Nutr 15:94–110
Chamberlain AC, Heard MJ, Little P, Newton D, Wells AC, Wiffen RD (1978) Atomic energy research establishment report R9198. HMSO, London
Cherian MG (1979) Metabolism or orally administered Cadmium-metallothionein in mice. Environ Health Perspect 28:127–130
Cikrt M (1970) The uptake of Hg^{203}, Cu^{64}, Mn^{52}, and Pb^{212} by the intestinal wall of the duodenal and ileal segment in vitro. Int Z Klin Pharmacol Ther Toxicol 4:351–357
Cikrt M (1971) Absorption of $Hg^{203}Cl_2$ from ligated intestinal segment in the rat in vivo. Int Arch Arbeitsmed 28:12–25
Cikrt M, Tichy M (1975) Role of bile in intestinal absorption of lead-203 in rats. Experientia 31:1320–1321
Clarkson TW, Small H, Norseth T (1973) Excretion and absorption of methyl mercury after polythiol resin treatment. Arch Environ Health 26:173–176
Conrad ME, Barton JC (1978) Factors affecting the absorption and excretion of lead in the rat. Gastroenterology 74:731–740
Cotzias GC, Borg DC, Selleck B (1961) Virtual absence of turnover in cadmium metabolism: Cd^{109} studies in the mouse. Am J Physiol 201:927–930
Cotzias GC, Borg DC, Selleck B (1962) Specificity of zinc pathway through the body: Turnover of Zn^{65} in the mouse. Am J Physiol 202:359–363
Crampton RF, Matthews DM, Poisner R (1965) Observations on the mechanism of absorption of copper by the small intestine. J Physiol 178:111–126
Danks DM, Campbell PE, Stevens BJ, Mayne V, Cartwright E (1972) Menkes's kinky hair syndrome. An inherited defect in copper absorption with widespread effects. Pediatrics 50:188–201
Delves HT, Harries JT, Lawson MS, Mitchell JD (1975) Zinc and diodoquin in Acrodermatitis Enteropathica. Lancet 2:929
Eckhert CD, Sloan MV, Duncan JR, Hurley LS (1977) Zinc binding a difference between human and bovine milk. Science 195:789–790
Emes JH, Arthur D (1975) The site of Zinc absorption in the rat small intestine (38481). Proc Soc Exp Biol Med 148:86–88
Evans GW (1973) Copper homeostasis in the mammalian system. Physiol Rev 53:535–570
Evans GW (1980) Normal and abnormal Zinc absorption in man and animals: The tryptophan connection. Nutr Rev 38:137–141

Evans GW, Johnson EC (1980) Zinc absorption in rats fed a low-protein diet and a low-protein diet supplemented with tryptophan or picolinic acid. J Nutr 110:1076–1080
Evans GW, Majors PF, Cornatzer WE (1970a) Mechanism for cadmium and zinc antagonism of copper metabolism. Biochem Biophys Res Commun 40:1142–1148
Evans GW, Majors PF, Cornatzer WE (1970b) Ascorbic acid interaction with metallothionein. Biochem Biophys Res Commun 41:1244–1247
Evans GW, Johnson EC, Johnson PE (1979) Zinc absorption in the rat determined by radioisotope dilution. J Nutr 109:1258–1264
Feaster JP, Hansard SL, McCall JT, Davis GK (1955) Absorption, deposition and placental transfer of $Zinc^{65}$ in the rat. Am J Physiol 181:287–290
Forbes GB, Reina JC (1972) Effect of age on gastrointestinal absorption (Fe, Sr, Pb) in the rat. J Nutr 102:647–652
Foulkes EC (1974) Excretion and retention of cadmium, zinc, and mercury by rabbit kidney. Am J Physiol 227:1356–1360
Foulkes EC (1980) Some determinants of intestinal cadmium transport in the rat. J Environ Pathol Toxicol 3:471–481
Foulkes EC, Voner C (1981) Effects of Zn status, bile and other endogenous factors on jejunal Cd absorption. Toxicology 22:115–122
Friberg L, Kjellstrom T, Nordberg G, Piscator M (1975) Cadmium in the environment – a toxicological and epidemiological appraisal. Rpt 650/2-75/049. US Environmental Protection Agency, Washington DC
Gitlin D, Hughes WL, Janeway CA (1960) Absorption and excretion of copper in mice. Nature 188:150–151
Gollan JL, Davis PS, Deller DJ (1971) Effects of human alimentary secretions on ^{64}Cu diffusion in an in vitro system. Aust J Biol Sci 24:605–608
Hamilton DL (1978) Interrelationships of lead and iron retention in iron-deficient mice. Toxicol Appl Pharmacol 46:651–661
Hamilton DL, Valberg LS (1974) Relationship between cadmium and iron absorption. Am J Physiol 227:1033–1037
Heth DA, Becker WM, Hoekstra WG (1966) Effect of calcium, phosphorus and zinc on Zinc-^{65} absorption and turnover in rats fed semipurified diets. J Nutr 88:331–337
Hirayama K (1975) Transport mechanism of methyl mercury intestinal absorption, biliary excretion and distribution of methyl mercury. Kumamoto Med J 28:151–163
Holdsworth ES, Webling DDA (1971) The effect of bile, bile salts and detergents on the absorption of calcium and other cations. In: Skoryna SC, Waldron-Edward D (eds) Intestinal absorption of metal ions, trace elements and radionuclides. Pergamon, Oxford, pp 339–357
Hurley LS, Lonnerdal B, Stanislowski AG (1979) Zinc citrate, human milk, and acrodermatitis enteropathica. Lancet 1:677–678
Kehoe RA (1961) The metabolism of lead in man in health and disease. J R Inst Pub Health Hyg 24:101–120
Kello D, Kostial K (1977) Influence of age and milk diet on cadmium absorption from the gut. Tox Appl Pharmacol 40:277–282
Kello D, Sugawara N, Voner C, Foulkes EC (1979) On the role of metallothionein in cadmium absorption by rat jejunum in situ. Toxicology 14:199–208
Kirchgessner M, Grassmann E (1970) The dynamics of copper absorption. In: Mills CF (ed) Trace element metabolism in animals. Livingstone, Edinburgh, pp 277–287
Kojima S, Kiyozumi M (1974) Studies on poisonous metals. I. Transfer of cadmium chloride across rat small intestines in vitro and effects of chelating agents on its transfer. Yakugaku Zasski 94:695–701
Kojima S, Kiyozumi M, Saito K (1976) Studies on poisonous metals: II. Effect of chelating agents on excretion of cadmium through bile and gastrointestinal mucosa in rats. Chem Pharm Bull (Tokyo) 24:16–21
Koo SI, Fullmer CS, Wasserman RH (1978) Intestinal absorption and retention of ^{109}Cd: Effects of cholecalciferol, calcium status and other variables. J Nutr 108:1812–1822
Kostial K, Simonovic I, Pisonic M (1971) Lead absorption from the intestine in newborn rats. Nature 233:564

Kostial K, Kello D, Jugo S, Rabar I, Maljkovic T (1978) Influence of age on metal metabolism and toxicity. Environ Health Perspect 25:81–86

Lengemann FW (1959) The site of action of lactose in the enhancement of calcium utilization. J Nutr 69:23–27

Lombeck I, Schnippering HG, Ritzl F, Feinendegen IE, Bremer HJ (1975) Letter: Absorption of zinc in Acrodermatitis Enteropathica. Lancet 1:855

Mahaffey KR, Goyer R, Haseman JK (1973) Dose-response to lead ingestion in rats fed low dietary calcium. J Lab Clin Med 82:92–100

Marceau N, Aspin N, Sass-Kortsak A (1970) Absorption of copper-64 from gastrointestinal tract of the rat. Am J Physiol 218:377–383

Martin DL, DeLuca HF (1969) Influence of sodium on calcium transport by the rat small intestine. Am J Physiol 216:1351–1359

Meredith PA, Moore MR, Goldberg A (1977) The effect of calcium on lead absorption in rats. Biochem J 166:531–537

Mertz W (1969) Chromium occurrence and function in biological systems. Physiol Rev 49:163–239

Moore W Jr, Stara JF, Crocker WC (1973) Gastrointestinal absorption of different compounds of ^{115}cadmium and the effect of different concentrations in the rat. Environ Res 6:159–164

Neathery MW, Miller WJ (1975) Metabolism and toxicity of cadmium, mercury and lead in animals: A review. J Dairy Sci 58:1767–1781

Oberleas D, Muhrer ME, O'Dell BL (1966) Dietary metal-complexing agents and zinc availability in the rat. J Nutr 90:56–62

Pearson WN, Schwink T, Reich M (1966) In vitro studies of Zn absorption in the rat. In: Prasad AS (ed) Zinc metabolism. Thomas, Springfield, p 239

Pecoud A, Donzel P, Schelling JL (1975) Effect of foodstuffs on the absorption of zinc sulfate. Clin Pharmacol Ther 17:469–474

Pekarek RS, Evans GW (1975) Effect of acute infection and endotoxemia on zinc absorption in the rat. Proc Soc Exp Biol Med 150:755–758

Prasad AS, Schulert AR, Miale A Jr, Farid Z, Sandstead HH (1963) Zinc and iron deficiencies in male subjects with dwarfism and hypogonadism but without ancylostomiasis, schistosomiasis or severe anemia. Am J Clin Nutr 12:437–444

Quarterman J, Morrison JN (1975) The effect of dietary calcium and phosphorus on the retention and excretion of lead in rats. Br J Nutr 34:351–362

Rabinowitz MB, Kopple JD, Wetherill GW (1980) Effect of food intake and fasting on gastrointestinal lead absorption in humans. Am J Clin Nutr 33:1784–1788

Richards MP, Cousins RJ (1975) Mammalian zinc homeostasis: Requirement for RNA and metallothionein synthesis. Biochem Biophys Res Commun 64:1215–1223

Sahagian BM, Harding-Barlow I, Perry HM (1967) Transmural movements of zinc, manganese, cadmium and mercury by rat small intestine. J Nutr 93:291–300

Sas B, Bremner I (1979) Effect of acute stress on the absorption and distribution of zinc and on Zn-metallothionein production in the liver of the chick. J Inorg Biochem 11:67–76

Sasser LB, Jarboe GE (1977) Intestinal absorption and retention of cadmium in neonatal rat. Toxicol Appl Pharmacol 41:423–431

Sasser LB, Jarboe GE, Walter BK, Kelman BJ (1978) Absorption of mercury from ligated segments of the rat gastrointestinal tract. Proc Soc Exp Biol Med 157:57–60

Six KM, Goyer RA (1972) The influence of iron deficiency on tissue content and toxicity of ingested lead in the rat. J Lab Clin Med 79:128–136

Smith KT, Cousins RJ (1980) Quantitative aspects of zinc absorption by isolated, vascularly perfused rat intestine. J Nutr 110:316–323

Smith KT, Cousins RJ, Silbon BL, Failla ML (1978) Zinc absorption and metabolism by isolated, vascularly perfused rat intestine. J Nutr 108:1849–1857

Squibb KS, Cousins RJ, Silbon BL, Levin S (1976) Liver and intestinal metallothionein: Function in acute cadmium toxicity. Exp Mol Pathol 25:136–171

Starcher BC (1969) Studies on the mechanism of copper absorption in the chick. J Nutr 97:321–326

Starcher BC, Glauber JG, Madaras JG (1980) Zinc absorption and its relationship to intestinal metallothionein. J Nutr 110:1391–1397
Sugawara N (1982) Role of metallothionein in Zn uptake from rat jejunum. In: Foulkes EC (ed) Biological roles of metallothionein. Elsevier-North Holland, Amsterdam, pp 155–162
Taguchi T, Suzuki S (1978) Cadmium binding components in the supernatant fraction of the small intestinal mucosa of rats administered cadmium. Jpn J Hyg 33:467–473
Takahashi H, Hirayama K (1971) Accelerated elimination of methyl mercury from animals. Nature 232:201–202
Valberg LS, Sorbie J, Hamilton DL (1976) Gastrointestinal metabolism of cadmium in experimental iron deficiency. Am J Physiol 231:462–467
Van Berge Hennegouwen GP, Tangedahl TN, Hofmann AF, Northfield TC, LaRusso NF, McCall JT (1977) Biliary secretion of copper in healthy man. Gastroenterology 72:1228–1231
Van Campen D, Gross E (1968) Influence of ascorbic acid on the absorption of copper by rats. J Nutr 95:617–622
Van Campen DR, Mitchell EA (1965) Absorption of Cu^{64}, Zn^{65}, Mo^{99}, and Fe^{59} from ligated segments of the rat gastrointestinal tract. J Nutr 86:120–124

CHAPTER 15

Intestinal Permeability of Water-Soluble Nonelectrolytes: Sugars, Amino Acids, Peptides

G. ESPOSITO

A. General Functions of the Enterocyte

The epithelial barrier is a layer of cells separating the lumen (the external environment) from the internal milieu of the organism. Most of these cells are columnar absorbing cells, also named enterocytes. Their main function is to absorb and/or secrete solutes and water selectively. Many of these solutes are water-soluble nonelectrolyte molecules such as nutrients, e.g., sugars and amino acids. In order to be transported from the lumen to the subepithelial spaces and then to the bloodstream or the lymph, these molecules must cross two in-series plasma membranes: the brush border and the basolateral membrane. However, these substances have dimensions that hinder their movement through water pores of plasma membranes or even through junctional complexes between cells; therefore, specific transport mechanisms have developed to allow the transepithelial movement of these solutes. In order to achieve a net transport, these mechanisms must be asymmetrically distributed in the two opposite plasma membranes: the luminal and the contraluminal (Fig. 1).

There is experimental evidence that these mechanisms involve in some way a carrier molecule. First of all, the kinetics of transport of these solutes is a typical

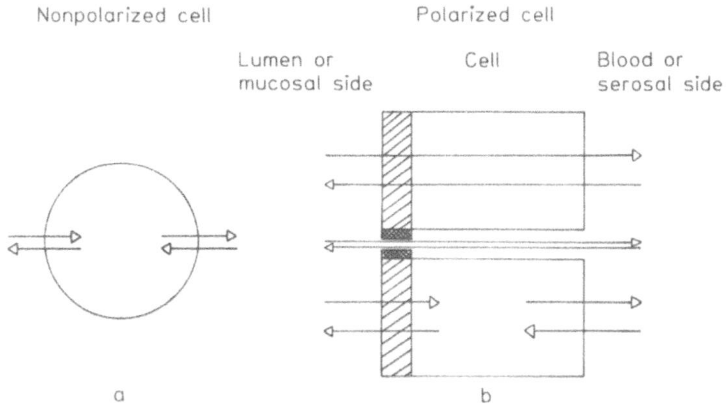

Fig. 1 a, b. Schematic representation of a functionally nonpolarized (**a**) and polarized cell (**b**). Two polarized cells are shown in **b**, connected by a tight junction and separated by a lateral intercellular space. Transmembrane, transmucosal, and transjunctional unidirectional fluxes are also illustrated

saturation kinetics; this fact seems to suggest the presence of a carrier molecule. Second, during their transport, substances of the same group display a mutual competition; in other words, if present, the carrier molecule shows a substrate specificity so that when, for instance, two or more monosaccharides are present, a competition for transport results. Third, there are inhibitors that specifically block intestinal transport. Finally, if a carrier-mediated transport is driven by metabolic energy, any substance blocking cellular energy-making mechanisms stops the transport.

Many enzymes are specifically located in the apical and/or the basolateral membrane of the enterocyte. For that reason these cells participate also in the digestive function of the gastrointestinal tract while some enzymes are involved in transport activities. The functionality of the enterocyte may vary according to its location along the intestinal tract (small, or large intestine) and even along the villus. It is known, for instance, that the cells of the villus tip have the highest transport activity together with the highest content of the Na^+, K^+-ATPase and other enzymes (Kinter 1961; Nordstrom and Dahlqvist 1973; Charney et al. 1974). On the contrary, the cells of the crypts or of the villus base are involved in secretory processes (Serebro et al. 1969; Hendrix and Bayless 1970). In conclusion, the epithelium of the intestine acts as a selective barrier as far as the movement of electrolytes, nonelectrolytes, and water is concerned. This selectivity resides mainly in the chemical (chemical composition), biochemical (enzyme content), and physiologic (transport mechanisms) characteristics of the plasma membrane and the junctional complexes of the enterocytes.

B. Intestinal Permeability to Sugars

The major component of carbohydrate in a normal diet is represented by starch which is a polymer of glucose. Also glycogen is introduced with food, but in a far less amount. In addition, the diet can contain disaccharides (sucrose, lactose, maltose); however, we know that carbohydrates can be absorbed only as monosaccharides. The mechanisms utilized by these molecules during their movement across the intestinal barrier are different and they will be discussed here in some detail. In addition, since most data available on this topic have been obtained in the small intestine, we will limit our discussion mainly to this intestinal tract.

I. Simple Diffusion

The simple or thermal diffusion of a water-soluble nonelectrolyte molecule across a biologic membrane is the amount of material crossing unit area in unit time along the chemical potential gradient. The law describing this flux is Fick's first law. It is known that, even in the absence of structured pores (water-filled channels), there is always a certain number of dynamic pores due to the random movement of the hydrophobic chains of polar lipids present in the lipid bilayer of the plasma membrane. Through these pores a water-soluble nonelectrolyte, such as mannose or other monosaccharides with rather high molecular weight (around 180) can nevertheless move, even with difficulty; therefore, a small flux of these substances due to simple diffusion is always present. In other words, even if a substance is transported via a carrier, there is always a small fraction (depending on the molecular weight and dimension) that passively moves for simple diffusion. Even glucose, which is known to be actively transported by the intestine, shows some simple diffusion. This has been demonstrated in patients with glucose–galactose malabsorption syndrome: in this case with an intestinal lumen initially empty of glucose, the gut lumen finally contained the same concentration of glucose as the blood. In addition, by using an "exorption" technique (i.e., by studying the movement of glucose from the blood to the lumen) it has been demonstrated that some simple diffusion of this sugar occurs (LOEHRY et al. 1970; AXON 1971). The kinetics of jejunal glucose absorption in vivo shows a curve in which, superimposed on the curve of active transport, there is a passive transport component (DEBNAM and LEVIN 1975).

At the very beginning of studies on intestinal absorption of sugars it was found that the absorption rate of some monosaccharides was directly proportional to their conentration in the lumen, the concentration in the blood being practically zero. A sugar behaving in this way was sorbose (VERZÁR 1935). Other sugars showing similar behavior are mannose (VERZÁR 1935), fructose (WILSON and VINCENT 1955; RIKLIS and QUASTEL 1958), and xylose (VERZÁR 1935). However, a linear relationship between absorption and concentration does not necessarily mean a simple diffusion; as a matter of fact a straight line-correlation is also compatible with a carrier-mediated transport mechanism with a high apparent K_m value. As we will see later, these sugars seem to utilize a carrier-mediated transport. In any case, it is reasonable to conclude that many naturally occurring nonelectrolyte solutes are polar molecules; therefore, except in a very small fraction, they do not permeate by simple diffusion, but enter the intestinal epithelium via a carrier-mediated mechanism.

II. Facilitated Diffusion and Active Transport

In general, a mobile carrier is probably a molecule with a specific binding site that recognizes the molecule to be transported, therefore it probably contains a protein part. In additon, it should also be a molecule that rapidly and easily permeates the lipid layer of plasma membranes and consequently it probably contains a lipid matrix.

There is an increasing interest in studies concerning the structure of the carrier involved in transmembrane movement. The investigations regard mostly the Na^+/D-glucose cotransporter system. A 160,000-MW protein has been extracted from brush border membrane and inserted into liposomes (MALATHI et al. 1980); this protein seems to be involved in D-glucose transport. Further studies of the Semenza's group seem to show an asymmetric insertion of the Na^+/D-glucose cotransporter in the membrane. Its mode of operation resembles that of a gated channel with multiple conformational states (KLIP et al. 1980).

From kinetic approaches, the existence has been suggested of a gated pore mechanism operating the translocation of transported solutes across the membrane barrier (HOPFER and GROSECLOSE 1980). Such transport system is probably achieved by a rocker-type conformational change of the transporter molecule.

One could assume the existence of two kinds of carriers: an equilibrating carrier performing a nonactive, facilitated diffusion and an accumulating carrier involved in active transport. The former operates a net transport that ceases when the concentration of the solute to be transported has reached the same value in the two compartments separated by the biologic barrier; in other words, the "facilitated diffusion" refers to a carrier-mediated transport mechanism which accelerates the rate of attainment of diffusion equilibrium, but no energy supply is involved. This mechanism possesses, however, some characteristics similar to those of active transport such as saturation kinetics, competitive inhibition by analogous substances and a high temperature coefficient. On the other hand, the latter also performs a net transport when the concentration in the two opposite compartments separated by the biologic barrier is the same or even when this transport takes place against a chemical potential difference, thus utilizing metabolic energy supplied by the cell.

1. The Role of Na^+ in Sugar Transport

It has been known for many years that Na^+ is involved in transport of many nonelectrolyte molecules across the intestine, including sugars (MCHARDY and PARSONS 1957; RIKLIS and QUASTEL 1958; CSÁKY and THALE 1960), but the precise role of this cation is still a subject of debate. It seems that the presence of Na^+ is essential on the luminal side, but not on the serosal one (CSÁKY and THALE 1960) although some authors claim that partial replacement of Na^+ in the serosal bathing medium inhibits active glucose absorption in hamster small intestine (SMULDERS and WRIGHT 1971). Anyway, the absence of Na^+ prevents active transport of hexoses as well as their tissue accumulation. The lack of Na^+, however, does not irreversibly damage the enterocyte since the active transport can be gradually restored after reintroducing Na^+ into the medium bathing the mucosal surface (CSÁKY and ZOLLICOFFER 1960). Whatever the mechanism of the Na^+ effect on nonelectrolyte transport, the relationship is a reciprocal one, that is to say, the presence of actively transported sugars in the mucosal solution causes an increase in the rate of net transintestinal Na^+ transport both in vitro (SCHULTZ and ZALUSKY 1964; ESPOSITO et al. 1964a, b; FRIZZELL et al. 1973) and in vivo (SLADEN and DAWSON 1969; ADIBI 1970; MODIGLIÀNI and BERNIER 1972). The relationship between Na^+ and sugar transport has been amply reviewed (SCHULTZ and CURRAN 1970; HEINZ 1972). The effect of Na^+ on transport of nonelectrolytes could be at the level of the brush border membrane and/or the basolateral membrane or even on the supply of energy needed for active transport. However, many recent studies seem to prove that the Na^+ effect is mainly at the level of the brush border membrane.

a) Influence of Na^+ on Sugar Transport at the Level of Brush Border Membrane

It was suggested years ago (CRANE 1965) that the chemical potential gradient of Na^+ between the mucosal solution and the cytosol of the enterocyte is essential for accumulation of sugars within the cell. The cation dependence of this process led to the suggestion of the Na^+ gradient hypothesis for intestinal transport of nonelectrolytes. In other words, the Na^+ concentration gradient across the apical membrane is the driving force required for accumulation of sugars. In the apical membrane there would be a carrier molecule with two binding sites, one for Na^+ and the other for the sugar; a ternary complex would thus be formed. This cotransport system is driven by the Na^+ concentration gradient between the outside and the inside of the cell. This gradient is maintained by the activity of the Na^+-pump which continuously extrudes the Na^+ across the basolateral membrane. Therefore, a direct input of metabolic energy for sugar accumulation is not needed. In other words, the apparent active accumulation of sugars within the cell is driven by coupling to Na^+ entry, not by direct coupling to the metabolism. It must also be remembered that Na^+ movement from the luminal side to the cell interior is also favored by the electrical potential gradient between these two regions; therefore, the total driving force for sugar entry and accumulation is the electrochemical potential gradient of Na^+. It seems that extracellular Na^+ concentration is essential for the coupled mechanism of sugar transport (and that of many other nonelectrolytes). As a matter of fact if, in an in vitro preparation, the chemical potential gradient of Na^+ is artificially reversed, i.e., cellular Na^+ concentration is higher than outside, the sugar within the cell can move outwards, even against its chemical potential gradient (CRANE 1964). Moreover, recent observations on brush border vesicles prepared from rat and human intestine (MURER and HOPFER 1974; LÜCKE et al. 1978) have shown that rendering the interior of the vesicle more and more electronegative increases sugar accumulation inside the vesicles. In contrast, when agents are used which dissipate the Na^+ gradient (e.g., *p*-chloromercurobenzene sulfonate), the overshoot of D-glucose found in brush border membrane vesicles disappears (WILL and HOPFER 1979). It seems reasonable to conclude that electrochemical gradients can provide energy for the apparent active accumulation of sugars within the cell (RANDLES and KIMMICH 1978; KIMMICH 1981). It is interesting to note that the presence of actively transported sugars in the mucosal bathing solution results in a rapid depolarization of the electrical potential difference across the brush border membrane (WHITE and ARMSTRONG 1971; ROSE and SCHULTZ 1971). This means that the cotransport of sugars and Na^+ from the mucosal side to the cell interior involves charge movement. In other words, the entry of Na^+ along with D-glucose is electrogenic; this cation enters on the carrier without an attached counterion.

Thermodynamically, the maximum free energy required for sugar accumulation is given by the steady state electrochemical potential difference of Na^+

$$\Delta\bar{\mu}_{Na} = \Delta\mu_{Na} + F\Delta E\,,$$

where $\Delta\bar{\mu}_{Na}$ and $\Delta\mu_{Na}$ represent the electrochemical and the chemical potential difference of Na^+ and ΔE the electrical potential difference between the outside and the inside of the cell, whereas F is the faraday ($\sim$96,500 C/mol). This kind of approach has been experimentally studied in the bullfrog intestine; the conclusion is that the energy available from $\Delta\bar{\mu}_{Na}$ is sufficient to account for apparent active sugar accumulation (ARMSTRONG et al. 1973; ARMSTRONG 1975). There are, however, data which do not fit the hypothesis that ion gradients provide the major source of energy for uphill transport (BAKER et al. 1974). It has recently been suggested that membrane potential is more important in the modifications of transport kinetics than the Na^+ chemical gradient (CARTER-SU and KIMMICH 1980).

What is, however, the precise role of Na^+ in the formation and function of the complex movement across the brush border membrane? Looking through the literature, it seems that there are animal species differences. For instance, in the case of rat and hamster intestines it seems that Na^+ modifies the K_m value, but not the maximum influx J_{max} of actively transported sugars. The reverse seems to happen in human and rabbit intestine. In the former case, Na^+ influences the K_m value of sugar–carrier complex formation. At high Na^+ concentration, as present in the lumen, the carrier molecule reacts with Na^+ thus achieving more affinity for the sugar which in turn binds to the carrier. Therefore, the first step of the ternary complex formation is necessarily the binding of Na^+ to the carrier; sugar could not bind to the carrier first. The ternary complex diffuses across the apical membrane and reaches the cytoplasmic side where the Na^+ concentration is kept lower by the activity of the Na^+-pump located in the contraluminal membrane. Consequently, Na^+ leaves the complex; the carrier molecule loses its affinity for the sugar which in turn is released within the cytoplasm. This model is based on the variation of K_m (the affinity factor) which is regulated by Na^+ concentration. The K_m is low on the outside and high in the inside of the apical membrane, therefore, the lumen–cytoplasm flux is higher than the cytoplasm–lumen flux. They become identical only when the cell glucose concentration becomes very high.

In the case of rabbit and human, the presence of Na^+ positively affects the maximum influx J_{max} of the sugar without modifying the K_m value. Therefore, in this case, it is immaterial if Na^+ or sugar binds first to the carrier; now it is the ternary complex which permeates the membrane more easily than the binary complex. Since the cell Na^+ concentration is lower than outside, less ternary complex will be formed on the cytoplasmic side of the apical membrane than on the luminal side of the same membrane; consequently the outflux of sugar is much lower than its lumen–cytoplasm flux with a consequent cell sugar accumulation.

A last point concerns the stoichiometry between sodium and sugar transport. Several authors have reported a 1:1 stoichiometry in the intestine (GOLDNER et al. 1969; OKADA 1979; HOPFER and GROSECLOSE 1980; SEMENZA 1982). However, KESSLER and SEMENZA (1983) have recently pointed out that also a Na^+/D-glucose flux ratio of 2 must be considered a real possibility. Other authors, on the basis of the fact that Na^+ entry into the intestinal cell is, in part, a potential-dependent event, suggest a Na^+/glucose stoichiometry of 2:1 (KIMMICH and RANDLES 1980; KIMMICH 1981). In fact, in the presence of an actively transported sugar the membrane potential undergoes a partial depolarization due to rheogenic Na^+ entry, with a consequent decrease in Na^+ entry via other routes, and this event must be considered when calculating the coupling stoichiometry.

In conclusion, the difference in Na^+ concentration between the lumen and the cytoplasm regulates the K_m or the J_{max} of sugar transport, thus facilitating the influx and reducing the outflux. In this way the energy released by Na^+ entering the cell along its favorable electrochemical potential gradient is utilized by sugar molecules to move against their chemical potential gradient.

Therefore, it seems reasonable to say that, in the case of actively transported sugars, we are dealing with a typical secondary active transport. Some authors have, however, stressed that there is a Na^+-independent transport system together with a Na^+-dependent one, or even that Na^+ is not essential for active transport of sugars. These conclusions have been reached by in vitro studies with isolated intestinal cells (KIMMICH 1970, 1973; KIMMICH and RANDLES 1977) as well as in vivo (OLSEN and INGELFINGER 1968; FÖRSTER and HOOS 1972; SALTZMAN et al. 1972).

With regard to in vivo studies it has been observed that, in human jejunum and ileum, Na^+ replacement has no effect on glucose absorption, provided that luminal glucose concentration exceeds 6 mM (OLSEN and INGELFINGER 1968). Replacement of Na^+ with xylitol results in an insignificant reduction of glucose absorption in rat small intestine perfused in vivo (FÖRSTER and HOOS 1972) nor did replacement of Na^+ with mannitol or K^+ significantly influence glucose absorption in human, dog, and rat ileum in vivo (SALTZMAN et al. 1972). However, it must be kept in mind that, especially in in vivo experiments, a conspicuous unstirred water layer close to the brush border membrane could exist; if this is the case, Na^+ concentration in the bulk luminal solution when the intestine is perfused with an initial Na^+-free solution is not the same as that close to the brush border where the Na^+ concentration can reach considerable values, owing to the Na^+ backflux from plasma to lumen. The existence of these unstirred water layers can be indirectly demonstrated by using an increased perfusion rate; in this case the glucose absorption increase (MODIGLIANI and BERNIER 1971). This fact could also explain the observation that apparent K_m values for sugar and amino acid absorption determined in vivo are greater than those found in vitro (WINNE 1973). The effect of luminal Na^+ removal on sugar absorption has also been recently discussed (FORDTRAN 1975). In conclusion, some complicating results are still observed; together with results demonstrating that removal of Na^+ in the in vivo luminal perfusing solution greatly reduces sugar absorption (CSÁKY and ZOLLICOFFER 1960; CSÁKY 1963), other results lead to opposite conclusions, as already mentioned. Also, the active absorption of sugars depending on the presence of Na^+ in the mucosal and/or the serosal solution, is still controversial (CSÁKY and THALE 1960; SMULDERS and WRIGHT 1971; BOYD et al. 1975; RINALDO et al. 1975; NAFTALIN and HOLMAN 1976).

b) Influence of Na^+ on the Basolateral Membrane

It has been repeatedly stressed that the vectorial transport operated by the enterocyte can be accomplished if two different mechanisms are asymmetrically distributed in the two opposite in-series plasma membranes. We have just seen that the mechanism of sugar entry from the lumen is Na^+ dependent; we therefore presume that the mechanism of sugar exit from the cell to the subepithelial spaces should be Na^+ independent. For a long time it has been assumed that sugars, actively accumulated within the cell, diffuse out of it by simple diffusion (MCDOUGAL et al. 1960). However, owing to the impermeability characteristics of the basolateral membrane it is improbable that sugar molecules can simply diffuse; in order to exit from the cell, another carrier mechanism is needed. We have, however, very little information concerning the properties of this membrane because access to it is more difficult than to the brush border membrane. However, it seems that sugars probably cross the contraluminal membrane by a facilitated transport mechanism. Experimental evidence demonstrates that this mechanism is entirely independent of Na^+ (BIHLER and CYBULSKY 1973; NAFTALIN and CURRAN 1974). These results have been obtained with different techniques and in no instance has Na^+ dependence been detected at the basolateral membrane. Contrary to the brush border membrane, sugar transport is not inhibited by phlorhizin, but it is sensitive to its aglycone, phloretin (KIMMICH and RANDLES 1975; RANDLES and KIMMICH 1978). Many experiments indicate that the Na^+-independent, phloretin-sensitive system is mainly localized in the basolateral membrane of the enterocyte (MURER et al. 1974; HOPFER et al. 1975, 1976). Similar conclusions have been obtained by other authors by using basolateral membrane vesicles from rat duodenum, jejunum, and ileum (WRIGHT et al. 1980). Furthermore, it seems that there is a stereospecificity, since D-glucose equilibration is 25 times faster than that of L-glucose and this uptake displays saturation kinetics and phloretin inhibition. Moreover, the rate of transport is independent from Na^+.

In addition, this transport system shows a specificity for different sugars transported that is quite different from the specificity of the brush border transport system (BIHLER and CYBULSKY 1973). For instance, 2-deoxy-D-glucose is a substrate transported specifically by the basolateral membrane system (KIMMICH and RANDLES 1976). Also, the competitive inhibition is different in the two opposite aspects of the enterocyte plasma membrane. In fact, 2-deoxy-D-glucose, D-fructose, and D-mannose, which are not actively transported by the Na^+-dependent system for glucose at the brush border membrane, are sugar transport inhibitors at the basolateral membrane. On the contrary, α-methyl-D-glucoside, which is actively transported at the brush border membrane, does not act as an inhibitor in the basolateral membrane (BIHLER and CYBULSKY 1973). Finally, as to the competition during sugar transport, it was observed that while a free OH group on C-2 in the D-glucose configuration is essential for Na^+ cotransport in brush border membrane (see below), this configuration is not required for the transport system across the basolateral membrane.

2. Specificity, Competition, and Inhibition Phenomena in Sugar Transport

It has been mentioned that there exists a specificity for monosaccharide transport. It also appears that there exist two separate ways for sugar entry into the epithelial cell: a Na^+-dependent and a Na^+-independent one. From the analysis of the kind of transported sugars utilizing the former way and from their transport rate it is possible to deduce which functional groups of the monosaccharide molecule are important in order for it to be transported. The minimum structural requirement for intestinal transport of sugars is the pyranose ring with the OH group at C-2 oriented as in D-glucose (Fig. 2; WILSON et al. 1960; CRANE 1960). In fact D-mannose, which differs from D-glucose because its OH group at C-2 is oriented in the opposite way is still Na^+ cotransported, but its rate of transport is very low (Fig. 2; CSÁKY and HO 1966). As a matter of fact, 2-deoxy-D-glucose is not Na^+ cotransported. The OH group in C-2 can, however, be substituted by a methoxy (OCH_3) group; in this case the cotransport is much lower, but still present. The possibility of a covalent bond formation with the oxygen of the OH group at C-2 of glucose being connected with an active transport mechanism has been ruled out (SWAMINATHAN and EICHHOLZ 1973).

The OH groups at C-1, C-5, and C-6 are much less important. However, if they are substituted by methoxy groups, the transport which results is 30%–40%

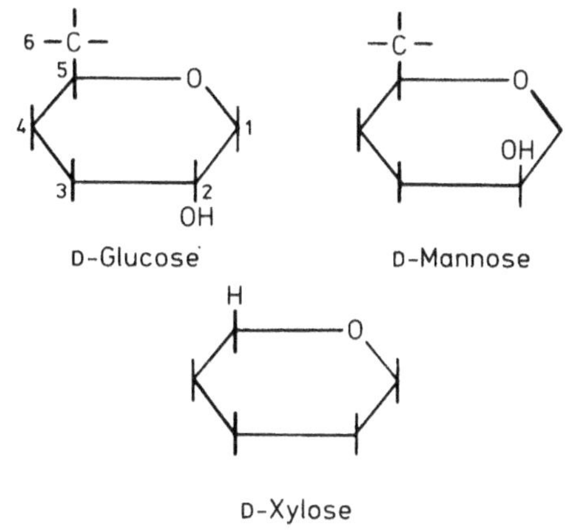

Fig. 2. Some molecular configurations, showing the structural requirements for intestinal transport of sugars

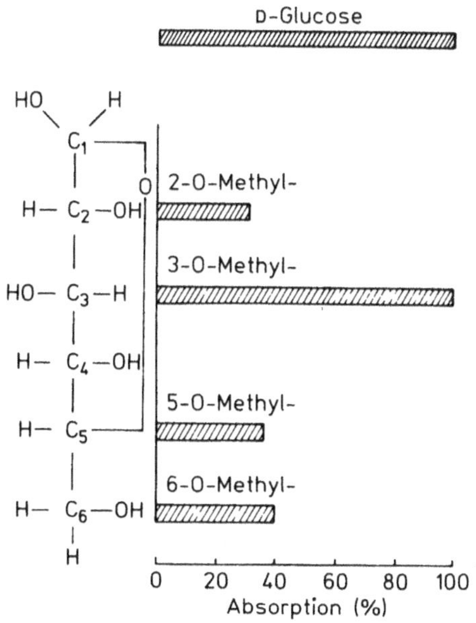

Fig. 3. Absorption of different *O*-methyl derivates of glucose, referred to the D-glucose absorption set equal to 100%. After CSÁKY (1942)

of that of D-glucose. On the contrary, the OH group at C-3 does not seem to be of great importance since 3-*O*-methyl-D-glucose is very well transported (Fig. 3; CSÁKY 1942), but since it has been shown that also D-xylose, which has a ring conformation different from D-glucose, is actively Na^+ cotransported, the specific requirements for the pyranose ring do not seem to be so strict (CSÁKY and LASSEN 1964). It also seems that there is no kinetic preference for α-D-glucose and β-D-glucose by the sugar carrier (SEMENZA 1969).

It has also been demonstrated that L-glucose, at low concentration, is actively transported by the small intestine (CASPARY and CRANE 1968; NEALE and WISEMAN 1968; BIHLER et al. 1969). Its transport is Na^+ dependent, inhibited by phlorhizin, and competes with other sugars for transport. However, its apparent K_m is only slightly influenced by the presence of Na^+, i.e., it is 8 times less in the presence than in the absence of this ion (in the case of D-galactose, the K_m is 130 times lower in the presence of Na^+). This fact could explain why its active transport is very low and can be observed at low concentrations only.

With regard to the Na^+-independent sugar entry mechanism it seems to be accepted that it does not lead to uphill accumulation. Fructose, 2-deoxy-D-glucose, and sorbitol seem to be transported by this system which differs from the Na^+-dependent one. A nonspecific entry for 2-deoxy-D-glucose and D-arabinose has been shown (GOLDNER et al. 1969a; SCHULTZ and YU-TU 1970). Particularly, D-arabinose influx across the brush border of rabbit ileum seems to be predominantly the result of simple diffusion.

Concerning fructose transport, a relatively specific mechanism has been demonstrated, different from the Na^+-dependent one (SCHULTZ and STRECHTER 1970). However, in rat intestine, a Na^+-dependent active transport has been demonstrated (GRACEY et al. 1972). This transport mechanism does not seem to share the glucose transport system. By in vivo studies it has been suspected that fructose transport utilizes a specific mechanism. Its absorption is not inhibited by glucose (HOLDSWORTH and DAWSON 1964), but the rate of absorption, as compared with that of other monosaccharides such as sorbose, is much higher (HOLDSWORTH and DAWSON 1965) even if the size and the characteristics of the molecule are similar to those of passively diffusing monosaccharides. Therefore, also by in vivo experiments, it is presumed that fructose absorption is not due to simple diffusion.

Many experiments seem to prove that the specificity, competition, and inhibition of sugar movement across the two opposite plasma membranes are different. This has been achieved by methods in which one of the two membranes has been blocked or, even better, by using vesicles made of either the microvillus plasma membrane or basolateral membrane (BIHLER and CYBULSKY 1973; HOPFER et al. 1973; MURER et al. 1974; LÜCKE et al. 1978; MURER and KINNE 1980). As already described, it seems that there is some overlap in specificities between transport systems located in the two opposite plasma membranes of the enterocyte. Both membranes transport D-glucose and D-galactose; the differences are: 2-deoxy-D-glucose, D-fructose, and D-mannose which do not utilize the Na^+-dependent system for D-glucose at the apical plasma membrane are effective inhibitors of 3-*O*-methyl-D-glucose (which uses the Na^+-dependent transport system) at the basolateral membrane, while α-methyl-D-glucoside (which is Na^+ cotransported at the apical pole) is not. The three sugars mentioned are not inhibited by D-glucose and D-galactose. Several sugars, apart from galactose, show appreciable Na^+-independent entry into the enterocyte. Some of them, such as 3-*O*-methyl-D-glucose, α-methyl-D-glucoside, and D-xylose, share also the Na^+-dependent entry across the brush border. Three others, L-rhamnose, L-arabinose, and L-fucose do not, nevertheless, they enter more rapidly across the basolateral membrane. In addition the uptake of D-glucose by brush border vesicles is much faster than that of L-glucose in either plasma membrane. However, in the presence of a Na^+-gradient,

D-glucose is taken up five times faster than L-glucose. On the other hand, Na^+ stimulates D-glucose transport by the apical membrane, but not by the basolateral membrane. Moreover, D-glucose uptake, but not that of L-glucose, is inhibited by D-galactose at the microvillus membrane.

The apical membrane possesses a transport system for D-fructose that is different from that of D-glucose (SIGRIST-NELSON and HOPFER 1974). Also in the kidney two sugar transport systems, one Na^+-dependent and one Na^+-independent, have been found to display different specificity characteristics (KLEINZELLER 1970; ARONSON and SACKTOR 1975; ULLRICH et al. 1974). Concerning inhibition, it seems that sugar transport across the apical membrane is preferentially inhibited by phlorhizin while phloretin specifically acts on the basolateral membrane system (KIMMICH and RANDLES 1975; HOPFER et al. 1976; BIHLER 1977; MURER and HOPFER 1977).

Uranyl nitrate inhibits glucose and galactose transport, but not that of fructose and arabinose in vivo (PONZ and LLUCH 1958). In in vitro experiments (NEWEY et al. 1966) uranyl nitrate at low concentration prevents glucose entry from the mucosal side into the cell, while at higher concentration it inhibits glucose metabolism and reduces glucose, galactose, and 3-*O*-methylglucose transport. Other inhibitors, such as atebrine, atractyloside, and selenite cause strong inhibitory effects on active hexose transport in vivo (NADAL and PONZ 1965). Phenolphthalein can inhibit the Na^+-dependent active transport of 3-*O*-methyl-D-glucose in vitro, especially its entry step, probably by competitively inhibiting the hexose carrier (ADAMIČ and BIHLER 1967). Theophylline, cytochalasin B, and various flavonoids selectively inhibit the facilitated diffusion pathway of D-glucose without interfering with Na^+-dependent transport (KIMMICH 1981).

3. Factors Affecting Sugar Absorption

There are substances affecting sugar absorption: for instance DMSO (dimethylsulfoxide) strongly and reversibly increases D-glucose (CSÁKY and HO 1966), but not 3-*O*-methyl-D-glucose absorption. This stimulation seems based on the formation of an apolar glucose–DMSO complex which is easily membrane soluble thus bypassing the glucose carrier system.

Ethanol at a concentration between 3% and 5% (v/v) depresses D-glucose and 3-*O*-methyl-D-glucose absorption, both in vitro and in vivo (FOX et al. 1978; KUO and SHANBOUR 1978). This phenomenon does not seem to be due to an osmotic effect. It probably involves interference of ethanol with the carrier-mediated coupled entrance of Na^+ and glucose or a depressive action on cell metabolism (DINDA et al. 1975). Cytochalasin-B, a fungal metabolite, depresses the basolateral sugar transport of the enterocyte which utilizes a Na^+-independent transport system (BIHLER 1977; KIMMICH and RANDLES 1979).

Also, unconjugated bile salts inhibit fluid, electrolyte, and actively transported sugars (FAUST and WU 1965; FORTH et al. 1966; ROY et al. 1970; GRACEY et al. 1971) in the small intestine. Some unconjugated bile salts cause shedding of absorbing cells from the jejunum and ileum villi. It seems, however, that the histologic damage is reversible so that intestinal absorption recovers with tissue recovery (HARRIES and SLADEN 1972; TEEM and PHILLIPS 1972). It has also been shown that deoxycholate, unlike cholate and taurocholate, can enter the cell and affect the Na^+,K^+-ATPase thus inhibiting Na^+-coupled transport (Guiraldes et al. 1975).

Many humoral factors can influence sugar absorption. Epinephrine or norepinephrine increase the transport of glucose and Na^+ in rat small intestine in vitro (Auselbrook 1965c). It seems that their action displays some specificity since dopamine or glucagone are ineffective. It also seems that cyclic AMP is in some way involved in these catecholamine effects on glucose and Na^+ absorption. The administration of thyroid hormones to thyroidectomized rats increases the capacity of the enterocytes to accumulate galactose (Bronk and Parsons 1965), Anyway, a review on the effects of hormones on the absorptive capacity of the small intestine has been reported by Levin (1969). Cyclic AMP, too, besides increasing membrane permeability to small nonelectrolytes, strongly stimulates net glucose transport in rat small intestine (Esposito et al. 1972).

There are many drugs influencing sugar absorption; reserpine, for instance, enhances intestinal transport of glucose and Na^+ (Auselbrook 1965b). This drug acts both in vivo and in vitro. Although it releases many humoral substances such as catecholamines, the adrenal medulla is not involved; the most plausible action of reserpine in vitro is a direct one on the intestine, probably by releasing catecholamines from intestinal storage sites. Harmaline inhibits Na^+ and Na^+-dependent transport mechanisms (sugar and amino acids) in intestinal brush border membrane preparation without affecting the Na^+-independent component. Phenolphthalein at a lower concentration inhibits Na^+-coupled D-glucose transport without influencing Na^+-coupled L-alanine transport. At the level of basolateral membrane, both drugs inhibit (Na^+,K^+)-ATPase activity but do not affect the Na^+-independent, phloretin-sensitive D-glucose movement (Im et al. 1980).

Cardiac glycosides, besides impairing Na^+ transport, inhibit active sugar transport indirectly. In fact, since they depress the Na^+-pump, the cellular concentration of this cation increases and the Na^+-coupled mechanism of sugar entry across the brush border is thus altered. This has been found by using many cardiac glycosides (Bolufer et al. 1973). Nicotine decreases the Na^+-dependent glucose uptake in brush border membrane vesicles, probably by a direct effect upon the D-glucose transport system (Ling and Faust 1982).

As far as anesthetic agents are concerned, it has been observed that in general they do not affect monosaccharide absorption, at least in rats (Fullerton and Parsons 1956).

Among diuretics, hydrochlorothiazide and chlorothiazide, while inhibiting Na^+ and water absorption, do not affect glucose absorption in the intestine (Rummel and Stupp 1962; Binder et al. 1966; Esposito et al. 1978). Unlike ouabain, chlorothiazide does not affect cellular Na^+ concentration so that sugar entry across the luminal membrane of the enterocyte takes place under a normal Na^+ concentration gradient.

Biguanides are substances inhibiting intestinal absorption of hexoses in animals and humans (Love 1969; Caspary and Creutzfeld 1971; Arvanitakis et al. 1972; Luisier and Robinson 1973) and thus are used as hypoglycemic agents. Also, these compounds seem to act by abolishing the Na^+ concentration gradient across the brush border membrane on which sugar transport depends and/or by interfering with the cellular energy-making systems responsible for the function of transport activities.

During pregnancy, an increased intestinal transport of glucose has been observed; this seems an important factor in maintenance of homeostasis during this physiologic condition (LARRALDE et al. 1966). Several chemical and physical factors affect sugar absorption. It is known that pH strongly influences the transport of weak electrolytes; however, pH variations can also affect intestinal sugar transport. For instance, in the everted sacs of hamster small intestine, it has been observed that the pH value corresponding to maximum glucose transport was 5.9. Below and above this value glucose transport gradually decreases (IIDA et al. 1968). However, studies performed with rat intestinal loops perfused in vivo showed that the optimum pH for glucose absorption was around 7.0. Even a slight decrease of pH inhibits sugar absorption while a considerable pH increase is necessary in order to reduce sugar absorption. The effect, however, is fully reversible (CSÁKY 1971; CSÁKY and AUTENRIETH 1975). It seems that not only the Na^+-pump can be affected by variations of H^+ concentration, but that such variations can modify the leakage of tight junctions. Also, the motility of the intestine modifies the rate of sugar absorption. The serosal transfer of glucose is almost tripled during peristalsis in comparison with the quiescent condition (GWEE and YEOH 1969). Other authors have confirmed these results, provided that luminal fluid did not contain bile salts (SCHNEIDER et al. 1969).

A factor that strongly influences sugar absorption in vivo is the rate of blood flow. At normal blood flow, the rate of solute appearance in blood draining the intestine has a higher value than in the case where the blood flow is reduced or artificially stopped (BOYD and PARSONS 1978; for a complete review of this topic see WINNE 1979). It had already been found that a sustained reduction of blood supply decreases the ATP content of the mucosa which in turn affects glucose absorption negatively (VARRÓ et al. 1965).

There are physical factors that strongly inhibit intestinal sugar absorption; irradiation of the intestine with X-rays depresses oxygen consumption and alters the cell respiratory systems of strips of rat jenunum (JORDANA and PONZ 1969) as well as active transport of sugars in everted sacs (NADAL and PONZ 1966) and in vivo (PONZ and LLUCH 1967). It is interesting to note that the presence of cysteamine in the solutions bathing the intestine during the irradiation, prevents the deleterious effects on glucose absorption (LLUCH and PONZ 1966). Changing the osmolality of the mucosal solution results in variation of sugar transport. Hypotonicity of the mucosal fluid causes a statistical increase of glucose absorption, but a moderate hypertonicity does not affect glucose absorption while fluid transport is statistically reduced. These results have been obtained in hamster small intestine (DINDA et al. 1972; ESPOSITO et al. 1976); similar results have been found in rat small intestine (MAINOYA 1975).

III. Enzymes Related to Sugar Transport

It has been known for many years that the intestinal absorption of hexoses could be advantageous if they are offered to the brush border in the form of disaccharides (CHAIN et al. 1960). Both hydrolysis and absorption of sucrose are very efficient in human jejunum; in addition it has been found that considerable amounts of glucose and fructose released from sucrose hydrolysis move into the lumen where they are absorbed subsequently; the hydrolyzing enzymes are mucosa-bound enzymes (GRAY and INGELFINGER 1965). Further experiments by these authors revealed a saturation kinetics nearly identical for sucrose hydrolysis and glucose product absorption, suggesting an interdependence of these two processes (GRAY and INGELFINGER 1966).

Work by PARSON's group has suggested, by using a preparation of perfused amphibian intestine, a very close relationship between brush border disaccharidases and the glucose transport system (PARSONS and PRICHARD 1965, 1968, 1971). It seems that there is a "kinetic advantage" for the transport of hexoses derived from the brush border disaccharidases. More precisely, there would be a spatial organization between sucrase and the glucose transport carriers, both placed in the superficial region of the brush border (CRANE 1966). Experiments by other authors support the view that the disaccharide hydrolysis and the consequent hexose transport are sequential and separate events (DAVIDSON and LEESE 1977).

Besides the well-known Na^+-dependent glucose transport system, there is also a membrane transport system for glucose requiring that this sugar be presented to it in the form of a disaccharide. This system is Na^+ independent and the glucose released does not mix with the pool of luminal glucose before crossing the apical membrane of the enterocyte. These brush border enzymes seem to act as vectorial enzymes in order to transport their products directly across the apical membrane in a way independent of glucose or fructose transport carriers. Most probably, the disaccharidases acting as vectorial enzymes "could impart an inward vectorial component to some of the hexoses liberated from glycosidic linkage at the membrane interface and thus directly subserve a transport function" (CRANE 1975).

The experiments of SEMENZA's group seem to be in agreement with this view. If a purified sucrase–isomaltase complex is incorporated into an artificial lipid membrane, it has been observed that this black lipid membrane is more permeable to glucose and fructose when they are present in the form of sucrose than when they are in the form of free monosaccharides (STORELLI et al. 1972). However, it seems that this system which seems to bypass the Na^+-dependent glucose transport system is not a significant route for the entry of glucose into the cell (CRANE et al. 1977), i.e., only 5%–10% of the sugars released by disaccharidases use the disaccharidase-dependent transport system in the natural membrane (RAMASWAMY et al. 1974). Anyway, besides sucrose, other glycosides act as substrates for this hydrolase-dependent transport system: maltose, trehalose, lactose, and phlorhizin (DIEDRICH et al. 1975).

SEMENZA's view concerning the role of sucrase–isomaltase as a direct translocator of glucose coming from sucrose is that 90%–95% of this enzyme is present in the natural membrane with its active sites located outside and far from the acidic region of the lipid bilayer; this region has an excess of negative charge. In such orientation the disaccharidase is deprotonated and its enzymic activity is inhibited by $Tris^+$(Hydroxymethyl)aminomethane. On the other hand, 5%–10% of the sucrase–isomaltase molecules have their active sites located within the lipid bilayer. Only these enzyme molecules would act both as sugar translocators and hydrolytic enzymes since they are in an acidic microenvironment owing to the excess negative charge of the lipid bilayer. Consequently, both their activities would be very slightly sensitive to inhibition by $Tris^+$.

This view explains why $Tris^+$ inhibits the hydrolytic activity much more than the disaccharidase-dependent transport system. Therefore, in natural membranes, most of the monosaccharides released by the action of membrane-bound disaccharidases on glucosides would be efficiently picked up by the carriers for free monosaccharides. The particular structure of the brush border region covered by its fuzzy coat constitutes a barrier to the backdiffusion of released monosaccharides into the lumen, thus favoring their absorption locally. Only a small fraction would enter the cell as translocated by the enzyme molecules. This view is described by SEMENZA (1976). It has been reported that a sucrase–isomaltase complex, a dimeric glycoprotein with a molecular weight of approximately 220,000, is anchored in the intestinal brush border membrane via a hydrophobic segment which represents less than 10% of the total protein mass; the catalytic centers of this complex are readily accessible from the lumen and the major part of the enzyme seems to protrude from the external luminal surface of the membrane (FRANK et al. 1978; BRUNNER et al. 1979).

At the level of the basolateral membrane, there is a sugar transport system which is Na^+ independent, phlorhizin insensitive, and inhibited by phloretin. It seems that 2-deoxyglucose shares this system; the sugar undergoes intracellular phosphorylation by the action of hexokinase. The phosphorylated sugar is then unavailable for a backflux through the carrier-mediated transport system so that a lack of cellular accumulation of free sugar against a concentration gradient does not occur (KIMMICH and RANDLES 1976). It seems improbable that hexokinase is present in the basolateral membrane (HÜLSMANN 1977). Its presence in basolateral membranes from rat kidney proximal tubules has been recently ruled out (KELJO et al. 1978). Hexokinase activity is mainly accounted for in terms of cytosolic and mitochondrial enzyme contributions. The absorbed sugars could be phosphorylated and then dephosphorylated at the level of the plasma membrane during their transport, but the amount of glucose-6-phosphatase present in the plasma membrane of the enterocytes seems to be very low (NORDLIE and JORGENSON 1976) together with the observation, already mentioned, that hexokinase activity is not present in the plasma membrane. Anyway, the involvement of sugar phosphorylation during its transport has been disregarded for many years (see WILSON 1962 for the pros and cons of phosphorylation).

IV. Sugar Binding Sites

It has been reported that the brush border region, including the microvillus core, possesses the capacity to bind D-glucose in preference to D-mannose and L-glucose and that this binding activity is Na^+ dependent (FAUST 1975). It seems that this binding of sugar (and amino acids as well) takes place in a protein macromolecule in the brush border core. Then the movement of sugars and amino acids from the core to the intracellular compartment may be operated by the contraction of active filaments that have been demonstrated in the brush border (TINLEY and MOOSEKER 1971).

Other authors by using brush border of rat intestine came to a similar conclusion (OLSEN and ROGERS 1971), i.e., that there is a specific uptake of D-glucose by brush borders and that this phenomenon is at least part of the overall process of glucose absorption. Previous reports have shown that hamster intestinal brush borders and their subfractions show a binding specificity towards several sugars; this specificity, however, differs from that of intestinal active transport and does not require Na^+. Finally, this binding activity is highest in the distal portion of the small intestine (EICHHOLZ et al. 1969). By using vesicles derived from brush borders of rabbit intestinal mucosal cells, a close parallelism between the high affinity phlorihizin binding and D-glucose transport has been demonstrated. It seems, therefore, that this substance is a fully competitive inhibitor of Na^+-dependent monosaccharide transport across small intestinal brush border membranes (TOGGENBURGER et al. 1978).

The Na^+–sugar cotransport model, based on a mobile carrier hypothesis, predicts that the transmembrane electrical potential difference may influence this model, depending on whether the Na^+ binding site of the carrier is charged either in the unloaded or loaded state. It has been found that the influence of the electrochemical potential difference of Na^+ across the apical membrane on phlorhizin binding shows a close similarity to that on D-glucose transport, so that phlorhizin seems indeed bound to the D-glucose transporting protein (TOGGENBURGER et al. 1978, 1982). It has also been shown previously that the high affinity of phlorhizin binding is due to its contemporaneous binding to the sugar binding site and to an adjacent aglycone binding site (DIEDRICH 1966; ALVARADO 1967). Finally, it seems that the transmembrane electrical potential difference (PD) can modulate this binding activity.

V. The Role of Brush Border and Basolateral Membranes in Sugar Transport

As previously seen, the brush border membrane differs widely from the basolateral membrane as far as sugar transport systems are concerned. It is commonly accepted that, in the brush border membrane, a cotransport system operates, favoring sugar entry which is driven by the electrochemical potential gradient of Na^+. This entry follows a Michaelis–Menten kinetics and is independent of metabolic energy (CRANE 1964, 1965; for a complete review see SCHULTZ and CURRAN 1970; MURER et al. 1974; WRIGHT et al. 1981). The cotransported sugar is then released intracellularly where it accumulates; this accumulation is different for the different monosaccharides actively transported. The degree of accumulation depends on the sugar concentration in the mucosal fluid and on the characteristics of the transport system as well as on the type of tissue preparation used in in vitro experiments (BRONK and LEESE 1974). On the contrary, the sugars not actively transported by the enterocyte, but utilizing a carrier-mediated mechanism, do not accumulate inside the cell.

The influence between sugar and Na^+ entry is reciprocal, i.e., not only is Na^+ essential for the transport of sugars, but the transport of the latter compounds enhances the rate of Na^+ transport. All this series of events explains the effect of glucose in the lumen and the increase of short-circuit current (SCHULTZ and ZALUSKY 1964; ROSE and SCHULTZ 1971). This sugar entry is specifically inhibited by phlorhizin which displays a very high affinity for the carrier-mediated system. Once the sugar has accumulated within the cell it moves downhill towards the subepithelial spaces across the basolateral membrane. This movement also requires a carrier-mediated transport system, but in this case neither Na^+ nor energy seem to be involved; in addition, this system shows a different chemical specificity from that of the brush border and a much lower sensitivity to phlorhizin. Even a very low concentration of phloretin displays a great inhibitory effect on this Na^+-independent transport system. This substance significantly increases the steady state sugar level within the enterocyte because this inhibitor preferentially affects the sugar exit across the basolateral membrane (KIMMICH and RANDLES 1975; BIHLER 1977). Phloretin inhibition at the level of the contraluminal membrane has also been observed in experiments with basolateral membrane vesicles (MURER et al. 1974; HOPFER et al. 1976). The use of theophylline, a phosphodiesterase inhibitor, increases the intracellular sugar level because it seems to inhibit basolateral fluxes (HOLMAN and NAFTALIN 1975, 1976). This substance induces a cellular sugar accumulation much higher than that obtained with phloretin, probably because the latter compound exerts a possible inhibitory effect, even if small, on the Na^+-dependent influx, probably due to an elevated cellular Na^+ concentration (RANDLES and KIMMICH 1978).

Now the question could be raised: are intracellularly accumulated sugars in an osmotically free form or bound, completely or partially, to intracellular components? Experimental evidence seems to suggest that sugars are within the cell in an unbound osmotically active form (SCHULTZ et al. 1966; CSÁKY and ESPOSITO 1969; ARMSTRONG 1970). As a matter of fact, when sugar accumulates intracellularly it draws water from the outside and, as a consequence, the cell undergoes a corresponding swelling (Table 1). In the presence of an actively transported sugar or amino acid, cell water increases which in turn dilutes cell Na^+ and K^+, whereas the total cell content of these cations remains unaltered. If this is the case, the accumulated sugars can move, whatever the mechanism, toward the subepithelial spaces. It is very highly improbable that sugars accumulated within the cell can simply diffuse toward the subepithelial spaces because of the impermeability of the basolateral plasma membrane to sugars.

It has been shown (and reported repeatedly) by in vitro experiments, that sugar movement (as well as that of some amino acids) occurs via a carrier-mediated diffusion from the cell to the serosal compartment across the basolateral membrane (HAJJAR et al. 1972; BIHLER and CYBULSKY 1973; MURER et al. 1974). In agreement with the notion that the enterocyte performs a net transport is the fact that two transport systems, namely a Na^+-dependent entry from the lumen and a Na^+-independent exit towards the subepithelial spaces, are asymmetrically distributed in the two opposite plasma membranes of the absorbing epithelial cells. However, the possibility of an active sugar extrusion mechanism at the level of the basolateral membrane has also been postulated (ESPOSITO et al. 1973, 1977). This conclusion comes mainly from in vivo experiments. It has been found that the intracellular concentration of D-glucose, as well as of the nonmetabolizable

Table 1. Water and solute content and concentrations in the enterocyte

Experimental conditions	Animal	Cell content [c]			Cell concentration [d]		
		Water (ml per gram dry weight)	Na^+ (μmol per gram dry weight)	K^+ (μmol per gram dry weight)	Na^+ (mM)	K^+ (mM)	Solute (mM)
Controls (11)	Bullfrog [a]	2.49±0.12	135±11	261±11	55±6	106±3	
3-O-methyl-D-glucose, 10 mM (7)		3.19±0.13	136±15	259±12	42±4	78±3	33±2
Controls (10)	Rabbit [b]	3.33±0.09	209±15	483±24	62±4	143±6	
L-alanine, 5 mM) (19)		3.78±0.06	204±12	465±17	54±3	123±4	51±1

[a] CSÁKY and ESPOSITO (1969)
[b] SCHULTZ et al. (1966)
[c] Cell water is given in ml per gram dry tissue weight of scraped mucosa; cell Na^+ and K^+ content are expressed in μmol per gram dry tissue weight of scraped mucosa
[d] Cell concentrations are given in mmol per liter cell water. Mean values ± standard error are reported; number of experiments in parentheses

sugar 3-*O*-methyl-D-glucose, is lower than the concentration in the lumen and in the blood. In spite of that, net transepithelial sugar transport is higher in vivo than in vitro even if, in the latter condition, a cellular sugar accumulation occurs. The low intracellular sugar concentration in vivo has ben found in rat small intestine (ESPOSITO et al. 1973; SMIRNOVA and UGOLEV 1974). The main criticism of this explanation is that the cellular sugar concentration is an average one; therefore, the actual intracellular sugar concentration could be higher than that in the external media. However, from many experimental tests and from accurate determinations of intestinal extracellular spaces, it seems that such criticism can be ruled out (ESPOSITO et al. 1976, 1977, 1979). Therefore, it seems that a basolateral mechanism extruding sugars towards subepithelial spaces could exist.

This mechanism could be partially dissociated from the activity of the Na^+-pump. In fact, ouabain at low concentration (0.5×10^{-3} M) has a stimulating effect on net Na^+ transport in hamster small intestine in vitro, without affecting net glucose transport. At higher concentration (10^{-2} M) it blocks net Na^+ transport, but not that of glucose which is still present even if reduced to 25% of control values. By using chlorothiazide (2–4 mM) which is another Na^+ transport inhibitor, it is possible to reduce net Na^+ transport strongly with only a slight reduction of net glucose transport (ESPOSITO et al. 1978). These results agree with those reported by others (BINDER et al. 1966).

Generalizing, it seems that sugars enter the cell across the apical plasma membrane coupled with Na^+ along its gradient; this happens both in vitro and in vivo. When sugar transport is conspicuous (in vivo), it does not increase intracellularly because, as soon as it enters, it is extruded towards the subepithelial spaces. When transport activity is lower (in vitro) more sugar enters the cell than is extruded until a new steady state condition is reached where the same amount of sugar en-

Table 2. Cell electrolyte concentrations and cell water[a] in rat jejunum in vitro and in vivo

Incubating or perfusing fluid	Cell Na^+ (m*M*)	Cell K^+ (m*M*)	Cell water (ml/g)
Rat jejunum in vitro (5)	60 ± 5	89 ± 6	5.8 ± 0.3
Rat jejunum in vivo (11)	21 ± 1	139 ± 3	3.7 ± 0.1

[a] Cell water is given in ml per gram dry tissue weight of scraped mucosa; cell Na^+ and K^+ concentrations are expressed in mmol per liter cell water. Mean values $\pm$ standard error are reported; number of experiments in parentheses

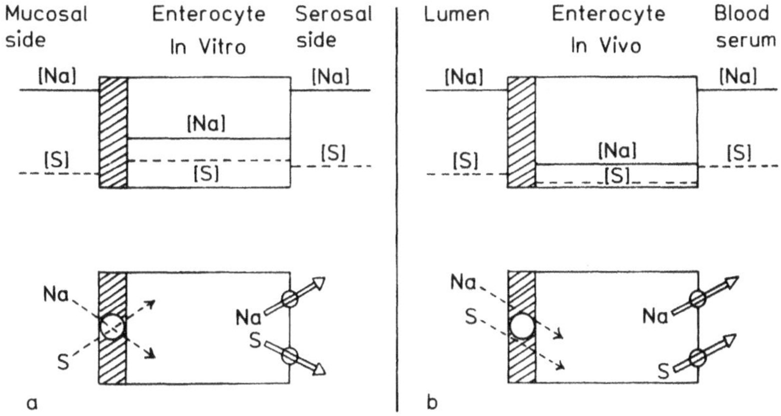

Fig. 4 a, b. Solute concentration profiles and transport models in the two opposite plasma membranes of the enterocyte, in vitro (**a**) and in vivo (**b**). Note that cell Na^+ concentration is lower in vivo and that sugar (S) accumulation takes place only in vitro. In both conditions, there is a net transmural active transport of sugar. In vitro, there is a Na^+–sugar cotransport in the brush border membrane with an uphill movement of the sugar. The Na^+ is then actively extruded across the basolateral membrane; the sugar extrusion (active?) occurs downhill. In vivo, there is still a Na^+–sugar cotransport in the brush border membrane with both solutes moving downhill. Na^+ and sugar extrusion occur uphill across the basolateral membrane

ters and leaves the cell. Obviously, the in vivo intestine possesses a better transport activity than in vitro. As a matter of fact, in the latter condition there is a cell electrolyte imbalance, namely cellular Na^+ concentration increases while cellular K^+ concentration decreases (Table 2). In addition, the in vivo small intestine transports more Na^+ and glucose than in vitro (Love et al. 1965; Esposito et al. 1973). Finally, by artificially increasing blood glucose concentration, cellular sugar concentration increases and concomitantly net sugar transport decreases (Esposito et al. 1977).

Figure 4 describes the concentration profiles in the three main compartments for Na^+ and sugar as well as transport mechanisms, asymmetrically distributed in the luminal and contraluminal plasma membranes, both in vitro and in vivo.

All these data indicate, but do not necessarily prove, that an active sugar extrusion mechanism operates in the basolateral membrane of the enterocyte.

It is known that experimentally induced diabetes increases sugar absorption in vitro as well as in vivo (Laszt and Vogel 1946; Crane 1961; Auselbrook 1965 a; Flores and Shedl 1968; Dubois and Roy 1969; Axelrad et al. 1970). Moreover, it has been found that a prolonged sustained hyperglycemia per se is able to stimulate net transintestinal sugar transport in vitro (Csáky and Fischer 1977; Esposito et al. 1981). This stimulation has been ascribed to an increased synthesis of transport carriers, mainly at the level of the basolateral membrane of the enterocyte. These conclusions are supported by the observation that cycloheximide completely inhibits the increased sugar transport and that phloretin, but not phlorhizin, eliminates this transport activity. As a matter of fact, phloretin inhibits the Na^+-independent carrier-mediated sugar transport in the basolateral membrane of the absorbing cell.

VI. Energetics of Sugar Transport

A detailed description of sugar transport energetics is beyond the purpose of this chapter. However, a few comments on this topic will be given here. An important question is: where does the energy necessary for sugar transport come from? This topic has been faced for many years and excellent reviews of this problem are reported by Smyth (1971) and Parsons (1975). There are sugars which are transported (like glucose, galactose, fructose), sugars which are metabolized (like mannose), and those which are both transported and metabolized (like glucose). It has been suggested that there is an intracellular pool of energy derived from sugars coming from the serosal side (mannose, glucose) and from the mucosal one (glucose); this fuel is used by transport mechanisms requiring energy. If total supply of energy exceeds utilization, there is no interference between different energy-requiring transport systems (e.g., sugars, and amino acids); if it does not, then competition for energy occurs among actively transported solutes.

Within the cell, the ultimate source of energy is ATP hydrolysis. The intestinal epithelium needs energy either for a basal performance (ion pumping for maintenance of cell volume, cell growth, and differentiation) or for a work performance (active transport of solutes). It is known that transport activity of in vivo intestine is higher than in vitro. As a matter of fact the energy charge of the in vitro enterocyte is lower than that of the corresponding in vivo enterocyte and decreases with time (Laners and Hülsmann 1973; Bronk and Leese 1973; Faelli et al. 1976, 1979; Watford et al. 1979). If ATP is the major source of energy, the addition of this nucleotide to an in vitro preparation should stimulate intestinal transport activity. As a matter of fact, exogenous ATP stimulates electrical activity and Na^+ transport in the small intestine (Kohn et al. 1970; Gerencser and Armstrong 1972). However, ATP added to the incubating media of the everted sac of rat small intestine has an inhibitory effect on amino acid and sugar absorption (Hardcastle 1974). This negative effect has been ascribed to an increase of passive permeability of the luminal aspect of mucosal cells so that the efflux of accumulated sugar is increased.

Many substances, other than sugars, can supply energy for transport activities. It is interesting to observe that some potential energy suppliers cannot readily cross the lipid bilayer of plasma membrane. Acetate, for instance, does not stimulate water transport, at least in rat jejunum (PARSONS 1967). However, if offered to the cell as ethylacetate it can easily permeate the lipid barrier; the latter compound, split into acetate by cell esterase, stimulates water, sodium, and glucose transport (CSÁKY et al. 1971; ESPOSITO et al. 1976).

C. Intestinal Permeability to Amino Acids and Peptides

It is known that proteins introduced with the diet are absorbed mostly as free amino acids and, to some extent, as dipeptides or oligopeptides, though in general only free amino acids enter the portal blood. The latter compounds are mostly transported unchanged to the blood although some of them may be metabolized, such as glutamic and aspartic acids, asparagine, and ornithine. The dipeptides, as we shall see later, are mostly hydrolyzed to their constituent amino acids, partly at the level of the brush border membrane, partly intracellularly; finally, they enter the blood as free amino acids and only in small amounts as small peptides.

The mechanism by which the amino acids are transported has been extensively studied and partly elucidated thanks to many in vitro and in vivo techniques introduced in the early 1950s and to the biochemical methods introduced in order to determine specifically α-NH_2 groups and L- and D-stereoisomers. We will briefly review the most important results obtained in studies concerning the mechanisms of intestinal amino acid and peptide absorption.

I. Specific Transport Systems of L- and D-Amino Acids

It must be pointed out first that amino acids are absorbed faster than polyhydric alcohols of similar molecular volume and that at high concentration their absorption shows a saturation kinetics (HÖBER and HÖBER 1937). However, the mechanism of amino acid absorption was still a subject of debate since some authors felt that these solutes were absorbed passively and that the two stereoisomers did not show a substantial difference in absorption rate. The method often used in the first studies of amino acids movement across the intestine was that of CORI (1925) and consists in introducing, by a stomach tube, an amino acid solution and then analyzing the collected material for unabsorbed amino acids. The first convincing evidence that special mechanisms exist for the absorption of L-amino acids comes from the experiments of WISEMAN's group (GIBSON and WISEMAN 1951; WISEMAN 1951). The interesting experimental approach was that of the specific enzymic determination of the two enantiomorphs of the amino acids. From a loop of rat small intestine in vivo it was thus demonstrated that from a racemic mixture of amino acids the L-isomer was absorbed more rapidly than the D-enantiomorph. Some L-amino acids, like histidine, were absorbed six times as fast as the D-isomer. Similar results were obtained in other animal species. Subsequently, by using an in vitro technique it was also possible to demonstrate that L-amino acids are actively transported by the intestine (that is to say they move against a chemical potential difference), while D-isomers did not (WILSON and WISEMAN 1954). Experiments performed with tissue segments of intestine incubated in a solution containing amino acids have shown a tissue accumulation of L-, but not of D-amino acids (Agar et al. 1954). The movement of some amino acids is passive, thus the amount absorbed displays a linear relationship with luminal concentration. However, high concentrations of some amino acids, actively or passively transported, may be damaging for the intestinal tissue so that at these concentrations the rate of absorption decreases (Matthews and Laster 1965). The active transport of some L-amino acids cannot be detected unless the initial concentration in the incubating fluid is very low so that caution should be used when deciding if an L-amino acid is actively transported or not; see, for instance, the case of L-tryptophan transport (Spencer and Samiy 1960). The active transport of L-amino acids has also been demonstrated in vivo (Christensen et al. 1963).

1. Specificity of Amino Acid Transport

As just seen, amino acids, like sugars, can be actively transported against a concentration gradient. The different amino acids, although Na^+ cotransported (see Sect. C.I.2) do not display the same transport mechanism. At least four transport systems have been found: (a) one for neutral amino acids, including histidine; (b) one for basic amino acids which is also used by L-cystine (in addition to mechanism a); (c) one for dicarboxylic amino acids; (d) one for *N*-substituted amino acids (proline, hydroxyproline, sarcosine, betaine, *N,N*-dimethylglycine). Proline and hydroxyproline also use mechanism (a) efficiently. With regard to the first system, it is worth pointing out that a number of neutral amino acids compete with each other for transport; some of them behave as better inhibitors than others (Wiseman 1955). In order to be actively transported, the neutral amino acids must have the carboxylic and amino groups free as well as the hydrogen bound to the asymmetric carbon atom placed in the α position. Also, the side chain is important because it is involved in the degree of lipid solubility of the amino acid which in turn affects the accessibility of the active site of the carrier and the ease of penetration. As to the second group (basic amino acids), it has been shown that they are actively transported (Hagihira et al. 1961), albeit at a rate 10–20 times lower than the neutral amino acids. For some of them, however, like L-lysine, the influx across the brush border is similar to that of neutral amino acids; the outflux across the basolateral membrane is, however, much reduced (Munck and Schultz 1969). It should be mentioned that basic amino acids placed in the presence of neutral ones partially compete for the transport of the latter amino acids even if to a small extent. On the contrary, neutral amino acids strongly reduce the transport of basic amino acids.

As to the third group, it has been found that they cross the intestinal barrier following a saturation kinetics, can be competitively inhibited, and their absorption is influenced by the Na^+ concentration in the medium. A detailed study of their movement across the brush border has shown a carrier-mediated process and a Na^+ dependence (Schultz et al. 1970). This study has also shown the effect that the amino acid charge displays on the binding affinity for Na^+. The dicarboxylic amino acids are not actively transported, but undergo transamination during their transport (Neame and Wiseman 1957). In fact, after introducing glutamic acid into the luminal solution, a high concentration of alanine was found in the blood coming from the same intestinal tract. It has been found recently that

L-glutamic acid exit across the basolateral membrane is low compared to that of L-alanine; on the other hand, the influx of this amino acid across the contraluminal membrane is faster than that of L-alanine, suggesting that the rate of transamination of glutamic acid to alanine is regulated by the basolateral membrane transport of these amino acids (BOYD and PERRING 1980).

As to the fourth group, by using sacs of hamster intestine it has been shown that substances belonging to this group are actively transported (HAGIHIRA et al. 1961). These solutes compete with one another, but they have no effect on the transport of neutral amino acids; most of the latter compounds have relatively little effect on betaine transport.

In subsequent studies, it has been shown that some D-amino acids can be actively transported only when the corresponding L-forms are not present (JERVIS and SMYTH 1959); in addition many D-amino acids show some affinity for the transporting system of their group (neutral, basic); however, such affinity is so low that active transport under normal conditions is practically negligible, owing to the competing exogenous and endogenous L-amino acids. Further details concerning the specificity of amino acid transport mechanisms are reported by WILSON (1962) and WISEMAN (1974).

2. Effect of Na^+ on Amino Acid Transport

Na^+-dependent amino acid transport in the small intestine has been demonstrated by many authors (CSÁKY 1961; ROSENBERG et al. 1965; REISER and CHRISTIANSEN 1967). In general, together with a net transintestinal transport of an actively transported amino acid, one observes an intracellular accumulation which in turn depends on the Na^+ concentration difference between the lumen and the cell (SCHULTZ et al. 1966). If the cell is artificially loaded with Na^+ so that the concentration gradient is now reversed, one observes an uphill movement of the amino acid from the cell to the lumen. Finally, as Na^+ activates the amino acid transport, so the amino acid activates the Na^+ transport. As in the case of sugars, the influx and the accumulation of an amino acid is the result of a Na^+ cotransport process. By blocking ATP production (with metabolic inhibitors) which drives the Na^+-pump or by inhibiting the pump directly with ouabain, the cell concentration of Na^+ increases and the Na^+ gradient disappears while amino acid accumulation and net transepithelial transport are concomitantly abolished.

It has to be mentioned here that, unlike sugars, the amino acid influx is not entirely dependent on Na^+ cotransport processes; in other words, in Na^+-free media the influx of sugars is negligible while that of amino acids is still present, even if reduced. For instance, lysine transport by isolated rabbit ileum is partly a Na^+-dependent fraction and partly a Na^+-independent one (MUNCK and SCHULTZ 1969; REISER and CHRISTIANSEN 1973a); the latter system is able to perform an uphill accumulation but, in the case of lysine which is a cationic amino acid, the electrical potential difference across the plasma membrane of the enterocyte might account for its accumulation. It is also possible that an exchange transport mechanism between an intracellular amino acid moving outwards and Na^+-independent lysine uptake, could occur (REISER and CHRISTIANSEN 1973b). It has been found that aliphatic neutral amino acids possess a transstimulatory effect on lysine influx across the brush border of rat small intestine. This effect is probably $Na^+\Delta$ dependent, induced by an electrical hyperpolarization of the apical membrane owing to the Na^+-coupled efflux across this membrane of the preloaded neutral amino acid (MUNCK 1980).

In order to understand as comprehensively as possible the mechanism of transepithelial transport of a solute, information deriving only from net transepithelial movements, bidirectional transepithelial fluxes, or cell accumulations is incomplete. What is needed is a knowledge of bidirectional movements of a solute across the apical and basolateral membranes of the enterocyte as well as diffusional movements through the paracellular shunt pathways.

The effect of Na^+ on amino acid influx across the brush border has been extensively studied (CURRAN et al. 1967; SCHULTZ et al. 1967; HAJJAR et al. 1970; CURRAN et al. 1970). It has been shown that amino acid influx, at a constant mucosal Na^+ concentration, increases by increasing the concentration of mucosal amino acid and shows, however, a tendency to saturation, as does the active amino acid transport across the whole epithelium. The lack of Na^+ in the mucosal fluid causes a great decrease of amino acid influx at any given concentration of amino acid in the mucosal compartment; however, the maximum rate of amino acid influx V_{max} can be reached, but in this case the amino acid concentration in the mucosal fluid has to be raised much more than in the presence of Na^+. This seems to indicate that the absence of Na^+ does not influence the V_{max} but increases the apparent Michaelis constant K_m. This result is opposite to that found, also in rabbit ileum, in the case of an actively transported sugar, 3-*O*-methyl-D-glucose (GOLDNER et al. 1969 b) in which the mucosal Na^+ concentration affects the V_{max} but not the K_m of the process. The rabbit jejunum behaves like the ileum, but in this case the amino acid influx is twice as much as that present in the ileum (ALVAREZ et al. 1969).

It is interesting to observe that amino acid influx seems to be independent of cellular Na^+ concentration; as a matter of fact, by depleting the cell of Na^+, the amino acid influx is identical to that found in normal Na^+ conditions (SCHULTZ et al. 1967). These conclusions seem to indicate that the extracellular, rather than the intracellular Na^+ concentration is important in regulating amino acid influx. On the contrary, the importance of the cellular Na^+ concentration has been stressed by NEWEY et al. (1970). As to the amino acid efflux across the brush border, it has been shown that it is a saturating process which depends on cell Na^+ concentration. If this concentration is artificially increased, the amino acid efflux increases as well; this seems to indicate that the K_m value of this process has decreased (HAJJAR et al. 1970).

Finally, the increase in amino acid influx is associated with the increase of Na^+ influx and the coupling coefficient of these two influxes depends on mucosal Na^+ concentration. In other words, this coefficient is zero when the amino acid influx occurs in the absence of Na^+ and approaches unity at normal mucosal Na^+ concentration. All these observations are consistent with a kinetic model in which the amino acid interacts with a membrane carrier to form a binary complex (amino acid–carrier) which can either move across the apical membrane and liberate the amino acid inside the cell, or combine with Na^+ to form a ternary complex (amino acid–carrier–Na^+) which then crosses the membrane and liberates

Na^+ and amino acid inside the cell. The formation of the binary complex would allow for the transport of amino acid in the absence of external Na^+. If the permeability coefficients of the carrier, the binary, and the ternary complexes are identical and are assumed to be small so that the movement across the membrane is the rate-limiting step, the association–dissociation reactions at the membrane boundaries could be considered at equilibrium.

Recent reports (SMITH and SEPULVEDA 1979; PATERSON et al. 1979, 1980) have described in more detail the mechanism of amino acid entry and Na^+ dependence across the brush border membrane of rabbit ileum. Alanine, for instance, utilizes two mediated entry systems, one fully dependent on Na^+ in the mucosal medium with high affinity and low transport capacity, and the other Na^+ independent, with low affinity and high transport capacity. As to the first transport system, a stoichiometry of two Na^+ ions per alanine molecule has been shown. Anyway, both mechanisms can operate in the presence of Na^+ and each of the two systems has a higher affinity for larger hydrophobic amino acids which are mostly essential amino acids. An interesting observation is that the presence of an amino acid in the mucosal compartment causes an increase in transmural electrical potential difference PD_{ms} (SCHULTZ and ZALUSKY 1965). This is due to the increase of Na^+ movement caused by the presence of the amino acid, as demonstrated also by the increase in short-circuit current. The increase of potential (the serosal side becomes more positive) is very rapid (within a few seconds), thus excluding the involvement of a metabolic effect. That this phenomenon is linked to a Na^+ influx is demonstrated by the fact that the stimulation of the PD_{ms} does not occur in the absence of Na^+, when the amino acid is placed only in the serosal side, or when ouabain is used. Such PD_{ms} increase due to the presence of amino acids has also been demonstrated in other animal species, like the Greek tortoise (BALLIEN and SCHOFFENIELS 1962) and fish (MEPHAM and SMITH 1966). The increase in PD_{ms} due to the presence of an actively transported sugar is further increased by the addition of an actively transported amino acid.

Before drawing conclusions on the effects of amino acids on the transmural PD_{ms} it is important to know the PD profile across the two in-series membranes of the enterocyte and the modifications they undergo by the presence of amino acids. Under control conditions the PD across the apical membrane PD_{mc} is negative across the cytoplasm-facing membrane and the PD across the basolateral membrane PD_{cs} is higher than PD_{mc} (negative across the cytoplasm-facing membrane). The transmural electrical potential difference is thus the result of the algebraic difference between these two membrane PDs (GILLES-BALLIEN and SCHOFFENIELS 1965; ROSE and SCHULTZ 1971).

The presence of an amino acid in the mucosal solution causes a depolarization of the brush border membrane in the sense that it stimulates Na^+ influx (ROSE and SCHULTZ 1971). In this respect, this influx is a rheogenic one, i.e., it is a current-generating process. This fact has been recently confirmed by studies with brush border membrane vesicles (SIGRIST-NELSON et al. 1975; LÜCKE et al. 1977). The resulting increased PD_{ms} is thus mainly due to the higher depolarization of the brush border in comparison with the basolateral membrane (Fig. 5). Similar results have also been obtained by other authors (WHITE and ARMSTRONG 1971). However, opposite conclusions have been reached by others (GILLES-BALLIEN and

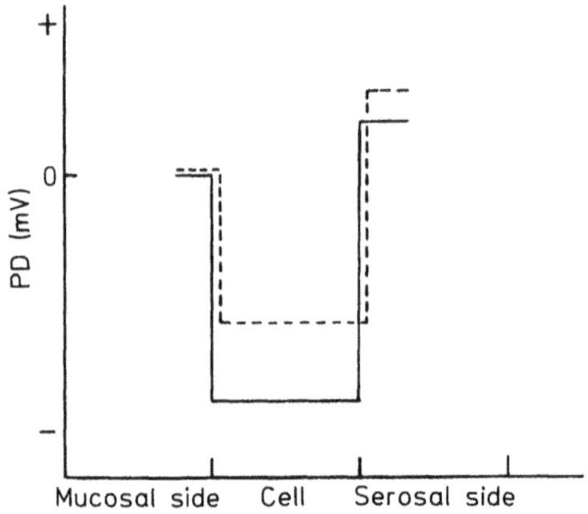

Fig. 5. Electrical potential differences (PD) across the brush border and the basolateral membranes of the enterocyte. *Full line* represents PD in the absence of an actively transported solute; *broken line* represents PD in the presence of an actively transported solute. After ROSE and SCHULTZ (1971)

SCHOFFENIELS 1965) in the sense that they found that addition of an amino acid causes an increase of PD_{cs} without modifying the PD_{mc}. The final result is always an increase in PD_{ms}.

It is worth knowing how an amino acid accumulated intracellularly can now move across the basolateral membrane towards the subepithelial space via a downhill process. It is difficult to believe, however, that the exit process is a simple diffusion because most biologic membranes are impermeable to hexoses and many amino acids. A carrier-mediated amino acid movement across the basolateral membrane is the most likely process. In the case of a cationic amino acid, like lysine, it seems that there is a carrier-mediated exit (MUNCK and SCHULTZ 1969) since this movement is a saturable function of cellular lysine concentration. Further experiments (HAJJAR et al. 1972) have shown that amino acid movement across the contraluminal membrane is due to a Na^+-independent carrier-mediated process with symmetric properties.

In order to achieve a net transintestinal movement of a solute it is important, as mentioned elsewhere, that two asymmetric mechanisms be located in the opposite plasma membranes of the enterocyte, namely the apical and the basolateral membrane. In fact, it has been reported that the entry mechanism across the brush border is Na^+ dependent, while the exit across the opposite membrane is Na^+ independent. At a steady state condition, the higher or lower accumulation of a solute intracellularly, and the higher or lower rate of transmural transport, would be the result of the rate of the net entry into the cell from the lumen and of the net exit towards the subepithelial space.

By using a vascularly perfused preparation, it has been found that, in addition to the importance of Na^+ role in brush border solute transport, there is an important role of this cation in expanding extracellular spaces within the intestinal mucosa (especially intercellular spaces) with consequent effect on the clearance of transported solutes from these spaces (BOYD et al. 1975). Further support for this interpretation has been subsequently reported for amino acids (CHEESEMAN 1979).

Recent results obtained with purified basolateral plasma membranes present evidence of the presence of different amino acid transport systems, partly Na^+ dependent and partly Na^+ independent (MIRCHEFF et al. 1980; WRIGHT et al. 1981). The former systems seem to operate in providing the enterocytes with amino acids in the absence of dietary protein; the latter ones would represent the normal movement of the amino acid from the cell towards the subepithelial spaces. It is worth pointing out that some authors have also put forward the suggestion that the movement of the amino acid across the basolateral membrane from the cell to the serosal side is a metabolically dependent process (NEWEY and SMYTH 1962; ESPOSITO et al. 1964b; GILLES-BALLIEN and SCHOFFENIELS 1966). Other authors in in vitro and in vivo experiments have suggested the existence of two transport systems: one responsible for solute uptake into the intestinal cell, the other allowing movement from the cell to the serosal compartment. The latter system is inhibited by anoxia and metabolic inhibitors (JACOBS and TARNASKY 1963; NEWEY and SMYTH 1964). Another possible explanation for the uphill exit of an amino acid across the basolateral membrane could be that of a coupled movement of K^+ or protons.

II. Interactions Between Amino Acid and Sugar Transport

If a Na^+ cotransported sugar (like glucose or galactose) is present together with amino acids, a mutual and partial competitive inhibition is observed, i.e., net transport of sugar and amino acid is lowered. It has been found in dog intestine that, in the presence of glucose or galactose, the rate of the absorption of some amino acids is decreased. This fact has not been observed with fructose (ANNEGERS 1966). In order to explain this interaction, several suggestions have been proposed.

The first suggestion is that of an allosteric interaction, i.e., competition for a common carrier. The latter should act as a polyfunctional carrier present in the microvillus membrane where an interaction between the two substrates should take place (ALVARADO 1966). This hypothesis has been amply discussed by ROBINSON and ALVARADO (1977). A comparative analysis in different animal species has supported this hypothesis. It seems also that there is a countertransport effect between sugars and amino acids across the brush border membrane (ROBINSON and ALVARADO 1971). The partial competitive inhibition would be due to the binding of the competitor to a carrier site which is not the same but very close to the site where the substrate binds. The latter binding site is thus allosterically modified with a consequent increase of the K_m value, but without modification of J_{max}. This interpretation has been criticized by some authors (SCHULTZ and CURRAN 1970) especially on the grounds that the alanine influx across the brush border is not inhibited by the sugars, at least in rabbit ileum, but the alanine efflux across the brush border is even enhanced by sugars (CHEZ et al. 1966).

The latter observation leads to the second suggestion, accelerated efflux, i.e., the decreased influx of a solute could simply result from an accelerated efflux from the cell, the latter being induced by a concomitant influx of another solute which in turn increases the cellular Na^+ concentration as a result of the concomitant movement of the competitive solute together with its own Na^+. This fact could change the Na^+ gradient, thus favoring the efflux of the entering solute (Read 1967). The hyperconcentration of Na^+ built up by one solute could display an inhibitory trans effect on the other solute (Semenza 1971). A competition of the sugar and amino acid transport systems for Na^+ has been found in experiments with brush border vesicles (Murer et al. 1975). D-Glucose influx is inhibited by the simultaneous influx of L-alanine only when Na^+ is present, not in its absence. Most probably, in the presence of a Na^+ gradient, these two substances compete for the electrochemical potential gradient between the medium and the interior of the brush border membrane vesicle.

It has been found that cellular alanine has a transstimulating effect on influx of galactose across the brush border membrane. This fact seems due to an electrical hyperpolarization of the luminal membrane of the enterocyte as a consequence of a Na^+-coupled alanine efflux (Munck 1980). The third suggestion concerns a competition for a source of energy available for transport. The energy is divided among the different substances actively transported; consequently each of these substances could become competitive in relation to the others because the cell does not possess enough energy to allow each transport process to work at maximum capacity (Newey and Smyth 1964; Bingham et al. 1966; Reiser and Christiansen 1969). However, glucose, a metabolizable sugar, being able to increase the availability of ATP, stimulates amino acid transport (Newey and Smyth 1964). If one artificially increases the supply of energy to the intestine, the reciprocal inhibition of sugar and amino acid transport can be partially counteracted (Bihler and Sawh 1973). Studies concerning net transmural transport of Na^+ in the presence of glucose and amino acids in an everted rat jejunum preparation have shown the existence of a positive linear relationship between net Na^+ transport and net glucose transport as well as net amino acid transport. However, at a given amount of Na^+ transported, the amount of glucose transported is lower when the amino acid is transported at the same time than when glucose is the only solute transported (Esposito et al. 1964a, b). This correlation may simply be due to the fact that, in all instances, net transport of Na^+ is a linear function of the energy at the disposal of the epithelial cells, but the coefficient of proportionality is different according to the number of substances available for transport. In other words, the proportion of the total energy available for the Na^+ transport seems to be smaller the more the number of transported solutes increases.

Another suggestion concerns the mutual inhibition due to the formation of toxic sugar metabolites of one of the transported solutes which antagonize the movement of the other solute (Saunders and Isselbacher 1965a, b). Finally, by using the vascularly perfused anuran small intestine, it has been found that some amino acids are able to inhibit the exit of a monosaccharide (α-methyl-D-glucopyranoside) from the cell to the vascular bed across the basolateral membrane of the enterocyte (Boyd 1979), while they stimulate, to a lesser extent, the backflux of this sugar from the cell towards the lumen.

III. Absorption and Transport of Peptides

It has been known for many years that the digestion products of protein could be absorbed as amino acids, but also as dipeptides and small oligopeptides. At the end of the last century it was thought that proteins could be partially hydrolyzed and then absorbed into the blood as peptones (SHORE 1890; REID 1900; BOTTAZZI 1901). When techniques for revealing amino acids became more accurate, the studies and the interest in dipeptides diminished. During the first years of this century was found that after a protein meal the concentration of free amino acids in the blood increased (VAN SLYKE and MEYER 1912), but the distinction between the uptake of substrate by the enterocyte and the movement towards the subepithelial spaces was not taken into account.

With in vitro techniques, it was shown that a small amount of dipeptide was absorbed by the intestine (AGAR et al 1953). The conclusion was that amino acids, appearing in the serosal compartment during peptide absorption, were due to two processes: a hydrolysis of peptide on the mucosal side with a consequent transepithelial transport of liberated amino acids, and an absorption of intact peptides followed by an intracellular hydrolysis. It has also been demonstrated that some dipeptides can be taken up unmodified by the cell and that they do not derive from a synthesis from intracellular amino acids (PETERS and MACMAHON 1970; ADIBI 1971; BOULLIN et al. 1973). Intact peptide absorption has also been found in vivo (HELLIER et al. 1972). In rat small intestine it was shown that almost one-third of the nitrogen appearing in the serosal compartment is in the form of peptides (GARDNER 1975).

SMYTH's group did a lot of work in order to elucidate the mechanism of absorption and hydrolysis of peptides (NEWEY and SMYTH 1959, 1960, 1962). It was first concluded that these compounds could either enter the absorbing cell and then undergo hydrolysis or be hydrolyzed at the mucosal surface with a subsequent uptake of derived free amino acids. It was then observed that the amount of amino acids liberated by hydrolysis and appearing in the mucosal compartment was too low to explain the amount of amino acids transported towards the serosal compartment. Therefore, it was concluded that peptides were mostly hydrolyzed within the enterocytes, although some hydrolysis could also take place at the brush border level.

For some time it was believed that a peptide molecule could not enter the cell; consequently its hydrolysis should have taken place at the mucosal surface of the absorbing cell. This interpretation was probably due to the fact that disaccharides are hydrolyzed at the brush border level where disaccharidases have been found. It seemed that hydrolysis of disaccharides and peptides were phenomena that could take place in the same region, namely the brush border (UGOLEV et al. 1964; UGOLEV and KUSHAK 1966). It has been shown that two hydrolases (aminopeptidase and maltase) have a portion facing the outside of the brush border membrane and possessing an enzymatic activity. One portion is inserted in the membrane and another short portion penetrates into the cytoplasm (MAROUX et al. 1979). This enzyme could represent a kinetic advantage for the transport of liberated amino acids. However, some confusion has arisen over the definition of "superficial" and "intracellular" hydrolysis. Some classifications of different types of hydrolysis have been given (PARSONS 1972; SMYTH 1972; MATTHEWS 1975 a). For instance, superficial hydrolysis is used to designate the process in which amino acids are released by membrane hydrolases; these amino acids then behave as if released in free solution from where they are taken up as from an amino acid mixture. Intracellular hydrolysis (SMYTH 1972) means a process apparently occurring within the enterocyte, namely in the inner region of the plasma membrane of the brush border, or in the cytosol, or associated with an intracelluar organelle. In this case the amino acids liberated behave differently from the same amount of free amino acids present in the external mucosal fluid. In this respect, the process of membrane digestion (UGOLEV 1974) could partly be included as intracellular hydrolysis.

1. Mechanisms of Peptide Absorption

It is now known that amino acids can be absorbed more rapidly if derived from small peptides than from an equivalent mixture of free amino acids (ADIBI and PHILLIPS 1968; MATTHEWS et al. 1968; SILK et al. 1973). This phenomenon appears more evident when the luminal peptide concentration increases. In addition, it seems that there is no competition between peptides and constituent amino acids during their absorption, while di- and tripeptides compete with each other; in fact during their absorption they display a competition among themselves while single amino acids do not interfere, or very little, with peptide absorption (see for instance RUBINO et al. 1971). This seems to mean that two different mechanisms of uptake, one for peptides and the other for free amino acids, are present in the brush border membrane. Two separate transport systems, one for glycine and the other for glycylglycine have also been reported in guinea pig small intestine (HIMUKAI et al. 1978). In this respect it has been shown that semistarvation and starvation reduce the mediated peptide influx more severely than that of the amino acid (SCHEDL et al. 1979). Also, the kinetics of peptide uptake and that of uptake of constituent amino acids are different. The presence of two separate mechanisms of uptake is proved also by the existence of congenital diseases involving defects in absorbing certain groups of free amino acids. However, these patients are able to absorb the same amino acids completely when they are offered as dipeptides (MILNE and ASATOOR 1975).

The kinetics of absorption resembles a typical Michaelis–Menten kinetics, characterized by a V_{max} higher than that of amino acids. A saturable process during peptide absorption has been reported by many authors (CHEESEMAN and SMYTH 1973; MATTHEWS et al. 1974). It is rather difficult to demonstrate the active uptake of peptides since most of them are rapidly hydrolyzed; this demonstration can, however, be performed when using peptides resistent to hydrolysis, like glycylsarcosine (ADDISON et al. 1972), glycylsarcosylsarcosine, β-alanylhistidine, etc. In this case the peptide concentration ratio between cell water and the medium reaches a value of 3:1 or even more. The energy dependence of this process is demonstrated by the fact that, in the presence of metabolic inhibitors, this accumulation is strongly reduced, while the Na^+ dependence is proved by substituting Na^+ with other monovalent cations which reduce the peptide accumulation. By using an everted sac preparation, it has also been shown that some peptides appear as intact molecules in the serosal side together, of course, with the free constituent amino acids. As mentioned before and also reported by MATTHEWS and BURSTON (1977), the absorption of amino acids from a peptide is more rapid than in the free form. By assuming that a dipeptide, such as glycylglycine, and glycine alone are taken up at the same rate, mole per mole, two results are worth mentioning. First, the absorption of amino acids derived from an equimolar solution of peptide will be double than that of amino acids present alone initially. Second, the absorption of amino acids from an equivalent solution of the peptide (such that the complete hydrolysis liberates the same amount of amino acid as that of the amino acid present alone) and of amino acid present alone initially, has been found more rapid in the case of the peptide.

Interestingly enough, it seems that there is a stereospecificity during peptide absorption. D-Peptides containing D-amino acids are poorly absorbed and hydrolyzed. Their uptake seems due to a carrier-mediated process. This transport system is a very poor one. Peptides with D-amino acids can also utilize the transport system of peptides with L-amino acids, but the latter are potent inhibitors of the former (as seen previously for free amino acid transport systems).

As seen before, the enterocyte is able to absorb di- and tripeptides by an active and Na^+-dependent mechanism. This absorption has also been recently demonstrated by using isolated brush border vesicles where peptides can be taken up inside the vesicle (SIGRIST-NELSON 1975). This uptake system is specific for peptides and different from that utilized by free amino acids. Also in this preparation there is no competition for transport between peptides and free amino acids while competition among peptides has been demonstrated as well as stereospecificity between D- and L-forms of peptides. An interesting observation found with this preparation concerns the presence of a countertransport phenomenon. More precisely, the amino acids inside the vesicle, liberated from peptide hydrolysis, can stimulate the external amino acids to enter the vesicle.

Very recently, it has been confirmed in brush border membrane vesicles from mouse intestine that peptide transport is the result of two complementary processes, namely uptake of free amino acids liberated by the hydrolysis of membrane-bound oligopeptides and intact peptide transport. The latter, however, seems to take place down a concentration gradient by a non-Na^+ dependent transport system (both passive and facilitated diffusion). These results have been obtained in normal and papain-treated brush border membrane vesicles; the enzyme treatment suggests that both γ-glutamyltransferase and oligopeptidases are not involved in intact peptide translocation (BERTELOOT et al. 1981, 1982). For a review see GANAPATHY and LEIBACH 1982.

Is the intestine able to absorb tetra- or higher peptides? Evidence has been presented on the existence of a simple common carrier for the uptake of di- and tripeptides by hamster small intestine (SLEISENGER et al. 1976). A tetrapeptide does not utilize this peptide carrier system nor does it affect the di- and tripeptide uptake. Further evidence supporting this view has been presented by others (SMITHSON and GRAY 1977): these authors have shown that, for tetrapeptide disappearance from rat small intestinal lumen, a brush border aminopeptidase plays an important role in this process, suggesting that the first step in the uptake of the tetrapeptide does not implicate a transport process, but rather a hydrolytic process.

Other experiments have demonstrated that intestinal disappearance of tetraglycine is mainly due to a hydrolytic process by brush border activity of an oligopeptidase, rather than to its uptake by a peptide carrier system (ADIBI and MORSE 1977). Evidence that tetrapeptides do not enter the intestinal tissue intact has been presented (BURSTON et al. 1979). However, it has also been found (CHUNG et al. 1979 a) that a tetrapeptide seems to be transported intact by the rat small intestine in vivo by means of a transport system different from that of di- and tripeptides. All these results seem to indicate an excellent coordination between peptide transport activity and hydrolytic processes in order to achieve a better intestinal absorption of oligopeptides. In other words, for di- and tripeptides that undergo intracellular hydrolysis, the transport by the peptide carrier system represents their major route of luminal disappearance; for tetrapeptides that undergo brush border hydrolysis this process represents their major route of disappearance from the luminal compartment. Finally, it has been demonstrated that the presence of dipeptides in the lumen stimulates water and electrolyte absorption in human jejunum (SILK et al. 1975). The same results were obtained by others (HELLIER et al. 1973).

2. Importance of Peptide Absorption

Experimental evidence now available suggests that peptide absorption plays an important role in protein absorption and therefore in nutritional problems. Under certain conditions, this way of absorption may account for the most important part of the absorption of protein digestive products. Many congenital defects of amino acid absorption are efficiently overcome by peptide absorption so that no malnutrition symptoms are observed.

By feeding three types of protein meal, it was observed that the absorption was so rapid in relation to the rate of in vitro hydrolysis that it seemed unlikely that a complete intraluminal hydrolysis to free amino acids had occurred (NIXON and MAWER 1970). This fact implies probably that quantitative digestion and absorption of a protein is complete after an ingested meal has passed along the total small intestinal length (CHUNG et al. 1979 b).

Peptide absorption seems to present further advantages. If their intracellular hydrolysis is efficient enough, in order to maintain a low cellular peptide concentration, they can easily enter the cell along their concentration gradient without expenditure of energy. In this respect, peptide hydrolysis acts as a modulating process while working according to the needs of the cell. In addition, the peptide transport requires no more energy than the transport of a single amino acid; moreover, the energy derived from hydrolysis can probably be utilized for other transport processes (PARSONS 1972). Peptide absorption may also overcome the differences existing among different amino acids (offered as free amino acid mixtures) as far as their preferential rate of absorption is concerned, thus avoiding amino acid imbalance. This would probably explain why young animals fed on diets made by partial hydrolysates of protein grow better than if fed on mixtures of free amino acids, even if these mixtures simulate the composition of diet proteins.

Finally, it is worth mentioning that some biologically active peptides can be absorbed intact by the small intestine. The mechanisms of their absorption are still obscure. These oligopeptides could utilize the mechanism for protein absorption or could move across plasma membranes, thanks to their lipid solubility. This topic has been reviewed by MATTHEWS (1975 b).

D. Concluding Remarks

The different mechanisms used by some important nutrients during their intestinal absorption have been mentioned in some detail. In this respect, it should be kept in mind that the intestine (together with the kidney) is of the utmost importance in maintaining the energy as well as the water and electrolyte homeostasis of the entire organism. In fact, the intestinal epithelium can be considered a biologic barrier separating the outside from the internal milieu of the organism. This barrier selectively allows the movement of many solutes thanks to its peculiar structure and the ensemble of transport mechanisms present in it; the cells of this barrier can thus modulate the processes required for the homeostasis of the organism.

References

Adamič Š, Bihler I (1967) Inhibition of intestinal sugar transport by phenolphthalein. Mol Pharmacol 3:188–194

Addison JM, Burston D, Matthews DM (1972) Evidence for active transport of the dipeptide glycylsarcosine by hamster jejunum in vitro. Clin Sci 43:907–911

Adibi SA (1970) Leucine absorption rate and net movements of sodium and water in human jejunum. J Apl Physiol 28:753–757

Adibi SA (1971) Intestinal transport of dipeptides in man: relative importance of hydrolysis and intact absorption. J Clin Invest 50:2266–2275

Adibi SA, Morse EL (1977) The number of glycine residues which limits intact absorption of glycine oligopeptides in human jejunum. J Clin Invest 60:1008–1016

Adibi SA, Phillips E (1968) Evidence for greater absorption of amino acid from peptides than from free form by human intestine. Clin Res 16:446

Agar WT, Hird FJR, Sidhu GS (1953) The active absorption of amino acids by the intestine. J Physiol (Lond) 121:255–263

Agar WT, Hird FJR, Sidhu GS (1954) The uptake of amino acids by the intestine. Biochim Biophys Acta 14:80–84

Alvarado F (1966) Transport of sugars and amino acids in the intestine: evidence for a common carrier. Science 151:1010–1013

Alvarado F (1967) Hypothesis for the interaction of phlorizin and phloretin with membrane carriers for sugars. Biochim Biophys Acta 135:483–495

Alvarez O, Goldner AM, Curran PF (1969) Alanine transport in rabbit jejunum. Am J Physiol 217:946–950

Annegers JH (1966) Some effects of hexoses on the absorption of amino acids. Am J Physiol 210:701–704

Armstrong WMcD (1975) Electrophysiology of sodium transport by epithelial cells of the small intestine. In: Csáky TZ (ed) Intestinal absorption and malabsorption. Raven, New York, pp 45–65

Armstrong WMcD, Musselman DL, Reitzug HC (1970) Sodium, potassium, and water content of isolated bullfrog small intestinal epithelia. Am J Physiol 219:1023–1026

Armstrong WMcD, Byrd BJ, Hamang PM (1973) The Na^+ gradient and D-galactose accumulation in epithelial cells of bullfrog small intestine. Biochim Biophys Acta 330:237–241

Aronson PS, Sacktor B (1975) The Na^+-gradient dependent transport of D-glucose in renal brush border membranes. J Biol Chem 250:6032–6039

Arvanitakis C, Lorenzsonn V, Olson W (1972) Effect of phenformin on glucose and water absorption in man. Gastroenterology 62:837

Auselbrook KA (1965a) Intestinal transport of glucose and sodium: changes in alloxan diabetes and effects of insulin. Experientia 21:346–347

Auselbrook KA (1965b) Intestinal transport of glucose and sodium: stimulation by reserpine and the humoral mechanism involved. Proc Soc Exp Biol Med 119:387–389

Auselbrook KA (1965c) Intestinal absorption of glucose and sodium: effects of epinephrine and norepinephrine. Biochem Biophys Res Commun 18:165–169

Axelrad AD, Lawrence AL, Hazelwood RL (1970) Fasting and alloxan diabetes effects on intestinal transport of monosaccharides. Am J Physiol 219:860–864

Axon ATR (1971) Sugar absorption studied by an exorption technique. Gut 12:856

Baker RD, Lo CS, Nunn AS (1974) Galactose fluxes across brush border of hamster jejunal epithelium: effects of mucosal anaerobiosis. J Membr Biol 19:55–78

Ballien M, Schoffeniels E (1962) Action des acid aminée sur la différence de potential électrique et sur la courrant de court-circuitage au niveau de l'épithélium isolé de l'intestin grêle de la tortue grecque. Arch Int Physiol Biochim 70:140–142

Berteloot A, Khan AH, Ramaswany K (1981) Characteristics of dipeptide transport in normal and papain-treated brush border membrane vesicles from mouse intestine. I. Uptake of glycylphenylalanine. Biochim Biophys Acta 649:179–188

Berteloot A, Khan AH, Ramaswamy K (1982) Characteristics of dipeptide transport in normal and papain-treated brush border membrane vesicles from mouse intestine. II. Uptake of glycyl-L-leucine. Biochim Biophys Acta 686:47–54

Bihler I (1977) Sugar transport at the basolateral membrane of the mucosal cell. In: Kramer M, Lauterbach F (eds) Intestinal permeation. Excerpta Medica, Amsterdam, pp 85–92

Bihler I, Cybulsky R (1973) Sugar transport of the basal and lateral aspects of the small intestinal cell. Biochim Biophys Acta 298:429–437

Bihler I, Sawh PC (1973) The role of energy metabolism in the interaction between amino acid and sugar transport in the small intestine. Can J Physiol Pharmacol 51:378–382

Bihler I, Kim ND, Sawh PC (1969) Active transport of L-glucose and D-xylose in hamster intestine, in vitro. Can J Physiol Pharmacol 47:525–532

Binder HJ, Katz LA, Spencer RP, Spiro HM (1966) The effect of inhibitors of renal transport on the small intestine. J Clin Invest 45:1854–1858

Bingham JK, Newey H, Smyth DH (1966) Interaction of sugars and amino acids in intestinal transfer. Biochim Biophys Acta 130:281–284

Bolufer J, Anselmi E, Larralde J (1973) Efecto de algunos glucósidos cardiotonicos sobre el transporte activo de azúcares por intestino de hamster. Rev Esp Fisiol 29:267–272

Bottazzi F (1901) Chimica Fisiologica. Soc Ed Libraria, Milano, vol 1

Boullin DJ, Crampton RF, Heading CE, Pelling D (1973) Intestinal absorption of dipeptides containing glycine, phenylalanine, proline, β-alanine or histidine in the rat. Clin Sci 45:849–858

Boyd CAR (1979) Studies on amino acid inhibition of monosaccharide exit from anuran small intestinal epithelium. J Physiol (Lond) 294:195–210

Boyd CAR, Parsons DS (1978) Effects of vascular perfusion on the accumulation, distribution and transfer of 3-*O*-methyl-D-glucose within and across the small intestine. J Physiol (Lond) 274:17–36

Boyd CAR, Perring VS (1980) Interactions between amino acids during exit from small intestinal epithelium. In: Proc XXVIII Congress Physiol Sciences, Budapest, p 335

Boyd CAR, Cheeseman CI, Parsons DS (1975) Effects of sodium on solute transport between compartments in intestinal mucosal epithelium. Nature 256:747–749

Bronk JR, Leese HJ (1973) Changes in adenine nucleotide content of preparations of the rat small intestine in vitro. J Physiol (Lond) 235:183–196

Bronk JR, Leese HJ (1974) Accumulation of amino acids and glucose by the mammalian small intestine. In: Sleigh MA, Jennings DH (eds) Transport at the cellular level. Symp Soc Exp Biol 28:283–304

Bronk JR, Parsons DS (1965) Influence of the thyroid gland on the accumulation of sugars in rat intestinal mucosa during absorption. J Physiol (Lond) 179:323–332

Brunner J, Hauser H, Braun H, Wilson KJ, Wacker H, O'Neill B, Semenza G (1979) The mode of association of the enzyme complex sucrase-isomaltase with the intestinal brush border membrane. J Biol Chem 254:1821–1828

Burston D, Taylor E, Matthews DM (1979) Intestinal handling of two tetrapeptides by rodent small intestine in vitro. Biochim Biophys Acta 553:175–178

Carter-Su C, Kimmich GA (1980) Effect of membrane potential on Na^+-dependent sugar transport by ATP-depleted intestinal cells. Am J Physiol 238:C37–C80

Caspary WF, Crane RK (1968) Inclusion of L-glucose within the specificity limits of the active sugar transport system of hamster small intestine. Biochim Biophys Acta 163:395–400

Caspary WF, Creutzfeldt W (1971) Analysis of the inhibitory effect of biguanides on glucose absorption: inhibition of active sugar transport. Diabetologia 7:379–385

Chain EB, Mansford KRL, Pocchiari F (1960) The absorption of sucrose, maltose and higher oligosaccharides from the isolated rat small intestine. J Physiol (Lond) 154:39–51

Charney AN, Gots RE, Giannella RA (1974) (Na^+-K^+)-stimulated adenosine triphosphatase in isolated intestinal villus tip and crypt cells. Biochim Biophys Acta 367:265–270

Cheeseman CI (1979) Factors affecting the movement of amino acids and small peptides across the vascularly perfused anuran small intestine. J Physiol (Lond) 293:457–468

Cheeseman CI, Smyth DH (1973) Specific transfer process for intestinal absorption of peptides. J Physiol (Lond) 229:45P–46P

Chez RA, Schultz SG, Curran PF (1966) Effect of sugars on transport of alanine in intestine. Science 153:1012–1013

Christensen HN, Feldman BH, Hastings AB (1963) Concentrative and reversible character of intestinal amino acid transport. Am J Physiol 205:255–260

Chung YC, Silk DBA, Kim YS (1979a) Intestinal transport of a tetrapeptide, L-leucylglycylglycylglycine, in rat small intestine in vivo. Clin Sci 57:1–11

Chung YC, Kim YS, Shadchehr A, Garrido A, Macgregor IL, Sleisenger MH (1979b) Protein digestion and absorption in human small intestine. Gastroenterology 76:1415–1421

Cori CF (1925) The fate of sugar in the animal body. I. The rate of absorption of hexoses and pentoses from the intestinal tract. J Biol Chem 66:691–715

Crane RK (1960) Intestinal absorption of sugars. Physiol Rev 40:789–825

Crane RK (1961) The effect of alloxan diabetes on the active transport of sugars by rat small intestine in vitro. Biochem Biophys Res Commun 4:436–440

Crane RK (1964) Uphill outflow of sugar from intestinal cells induced by reversal of the Na^+ gradient: its significance for the mechanism of Na^+-dependent active transport. Biochem Biophys Res Commun 17:481–485

Crane RK (1965) Na^+-dependent transport in the intestine and other animal tissues. Fed Proc 24:1000–1005

Crane RK (1966) Structural and functional organization of an epithelial cell brush border. In: Warren KB (ed) Symp Int Soc Cell Biol 5:71–102

Crane RK (1975) 15 years of struggle with the brush border. In: Csáky TZ (ed) Intestinal absorption and malabsorption. Raven, New York, pp 127–141

Crane RK, Malathi P, Preiser H (1977) Reconstitution of Na^+ gradient-coupled carrier functions of brush border membranes of intestine and kidney in sonicated liposomes. In: Semenza G, Carafoli E (eds) Biochemistry of membrane transport, FEBS-Symposium no 42. Springer, Berlin Heidelberg New York, pp 261–268

Csáky TZ (1942) Über die Rolle der Struktur des Glucosemoleküls bei der Resorption aus dem Dünndarm. Hoppe-Seyler's Z Physiol Chem 277:47–57

Csáky TZ (1961) Significance of sodium ion in active intestinal transport of nonelectrolytes. Am J Physiol 201:999–1001

Csáky TZ (1963) A possible link between active transport of electrolytes and nonelectrolytes. Fed Proc 22:3–7

Csáky TZ (1971) Physiological considerations of the relationship between intestinal absorption of electrolytes and nonelectrolytes. In: Armstrong WMcD, Nunn AS Jr (eds) Intestinal transport of electrolytes, amino acids and sugars. Charles C Thomas, Springfield Illinois, pp 188–207

Csáky TZ, Autenrieth B (1975) Transcellular and intercellular intestinal transport. In: Csáky TZ (ed) Intestinal absorption and malabsorption. Raven, New York, pp 177–185

Csáky TZ, Esposito G (1969) Osmotic swelling of intestinal epithelia cells during active sugar transport. Am J Physiol 217:753–755

Csáky TZ, Fischer E (1977) Induction of an intestinal epithelial sugar transport system by high blood sugar. Experientia 33:223–224

Csáky TZ, Ho PM (1966) Active transport of D-mannose in the small intestine. Life Sci 5:1025–1030

Csáky TZ, Lassen UV (1964) Active intestinal transport of D-xylose. Biochim Biophys Acta 82:215–217

Csáky TZ, Thale M (1960) Effect of ionic environment on intestinal sugar transport. J Physiol (Lond) 151:59–65

Csáky TZ, Zollicoffer L (1960) Ionic effect on intestinal transport of glucose in the rat. Am J Physiol 198:1056–1058

Csáky TZ, Esposito G, Faelli A, Capraro V (1971) Stimulation of the water transport in the jejunum of the rat by ethyl acetate. Proc Soc Exp Biol Med 136:242–244

Curran PF, Schultz SG, Chez RA, Fuisz RE (1967) Kinetic relations of the Na-amino acid interaction at the mucosal border of the intestine. J Gen Physiol 50:1261–1286

Curran PF, Hajjar JJ, Glynn IM (1970) The sodium-alanine interaction in rabbit ileum. Effect of alanine on sodium Fluxes. J Gen Physiol 55:297–308

Davidson RE, Leese HJ (1977) Sucrose absorption by the rat small intestine in vivo and in vitro. J Physiol (Lond) 267:237–248

Debnam ES, Levin RJ (1975) An experimental method of identifying and quantifying the active transfer electrogenic component from the diffusive component during sugar absorption measured in vivo. J Physiol (Lond) 246:181–196

Diedrich DF (1966) Competitive inhibition of intestinal glucose transport by phlorizin analogs. Arch Biochem Biophys 117:248–256

Diedrich DF, Hanke DW, Evans JO (1975) Relationship between glycosidase activity and sugar transport in the intestine. In: Csáky TZ (ed) Intestinal absorption and malabsorption. Raven, New York, pp 143–153

Dinda PK, Beck M, Beck IT (1972) Effect of changes in the osmolality of the luminal fluid on water and glucose transport acorss the hamster jejunum. Can J Physiol Pharmacol 50:83–86

Dinda PK, Beck IT, Beck M, McElligott TF (1975) Effect of ethanol on sodium-dependent glucose transport in the small intestine of the hamster. Gastroenterology 68:1517–1526

Dubois RS, Roy CC (1969) Insulin stimulated transport of 3-*O*-methyl glucose across the rat jejunum. Proc Soc Exp Biol Med 130:931–934

Eichholz A, Howell K, Crane RK (1969) Studies on the organization of the brush border in intestinal epithelial cells. VI. Glucose binding to isolated intestinal brush borders and their subfractions. Biochim Biophys Acta 193:179–192

Esposito G, Faelli A, Capraro V (1964a) Influence of the transport of amino acids on glucose and sodium transport across the small intestine of the albino rat incubated in vitro. Experientia 20:122–124

Esposito G, Faelli A, Capraro V (1964b) Sul meccanismo del trasporto transepiteliale di amino acidi e suoi rapporti col trasporto contemporaneo di sodio e di glicoso in un preparato intestinale in vitro. Arch Sci Biol (Bologna) 48:341–356

Esposito G, Faelli A, Garotta G, Parotelli R, Capraro V (1972) Relationship between permeability and active transport activity of the isolated rat intestine. Possible involved mechanisms. In: Bolis L, Keynes RD, Wilbrandt W (eds) Role of membranes in secretory processes. North-Holland, Amsterdam, pp 332–337

Esposito G, Faelli A, Capraro V (1973) Sugar and electrolyte absorption in the rat intestinal perfused in vivo. Pflügers Arch 340:335–348

Esposito G, Faelli A, Capraro V (1976) Effect of ethyl acetate on the transport of sodium and glucose in the hamster small intestine in vitro. Biochim Biophys Acta 426:489–498

Esposito G, Faelli A, Caprano V (1977) A critical evaluation of the existence of an outward sugar pump in the basolateral membrane of the enterocyte. In: Kramer M, Lauterbach F (eds) Intestinal permeation. Excerpta Medica, Amsterdam, pp 107–113

Esposito G, Faelli A, Capraro V (1978) Intestinal sugar transport at the basolateral membrane of the enterocyte. In: Varró V, Balint GA (eds) Current views in gastroenterology. 10th International congress of gastroenterology, Budapest 1976, Hungarian Society of Gastroenterology Edition, Budapest, pp 105–114

Esposito G, Faelli A, Tosco M, Burlini N, Capraro V (1979) Extracellular space determination in rat small intestine by using markers of different molecular weights. Pflügers Arch 382:67–71

Esposito G, Faelli A, Tosco M, Capraro V (1981) Hyperglycemia and net transintestinal glucose and sodium transport in the rat. Pflügers Arch 390:202–206

Faelli A, Esposito G, Capraro V (1976) Energy-rich phosphates and transintestinal transport in rat intestine incubated in vitro at different temperatures. Biochim Biophys Acta 455:759–766

Faelli A, Esposito G, Burlini N, Tosco M, Capraro V (1979) The rat and hamster jejunum during transintestinal transport in vitro. Arch Int Physiol Biochim 87:73–86

Faust RG (1975) The intestinal brush border as an organelle. In Csáky TZ (ed) Intestinal absorption and malabsorption. Raven, New York, p 155

Faust RG, Wu SML (1965) The action of bile salts on fluid and glucose movement by rat and hamster jejunum in vitro. J Cell Physiol 65:435–448

Flores P, Schedl HP (1968) Intestinal transport of 3-*O*-methyl-D-glucose in the normal and alloxan-diabetic rat. Am J Physiol 214:725–729

Fordtran JS (1975) Intestinal absorption of sugars in the human in vivo. In: Csáky TZ (ed) Intestinal absorption and malabsorption. Raven, New York, pp 229–234

Förster H, Hoos I (1972) The excretion of sodium during the active absorption of glucose from the perfused small intestine of rats. Hoppe-Seyler's Z Physiol Chem 353:88–94

Forth W, Rummel W, Glasner H, Andres H (1966) Resorption-inhibiting action of bile acids. Arch Exp Pathol Pharmakol 254:364–380

Fox JE, McElligott TF, Beck IT (1978) The correlation of ethanol-induced depression of glucose and water transport with morphological changes in the hamster jejunum in vivo. Can J Physiol Pharmacol 56:123–131

Frank G, Brunner J, Hauser H, Wacker H, Semenza G, Zuber H (1978) The hydrophobic anchor of small intestinal sucrase-isomaltase. N-terminal sequence of the isomaltase subunit. FEBS Lett 96:183–188

Frizzell RA, Nellans HN, Schultz SG (1973) Effects of sugars and amino acids on sodium and potassium influx in rabbit ileum. J Clin Invest 52:215–217

Fullerton PM, Parsons DS (1956) The absorption of sugars and water from rat intestine in vivo. Q J Exp Physiol 41:387–397

Ganapathy V, Leibach FH (1982) Peptide transport in intestinal and renal brush border membrane vesicles. Life Sci 30:2137–2146

Gardner MLG (1975) Absorption of amino acids and peptides from a complex mixture in the isolated small intestine of the rat. J Physiol (Lond) 253:233–256

Gerencser GA, Armstrong WMcD (1972) Sodium transport in bullfrog small intestine. Stimulation by exogenous ATP. Biochim Biophys Acta 255:663–674

Gibson QH, Wiseman G (1951) Selective absorption of stereo-isomers of amino acids from loops of the small intestine of the rat. Biochem J 48:426–429

Gilles-Ballien M, Schoffeniels E (1965) Site of action of L-alanine and D-glucose on the potential difference across the intestine. Arch Int Physiol Biochim 73:355–357

Gilles-Ballien M, Schoffeniels E (1966) Metabolic fate of L-alanine actively transported across the tortoise intestine. Life Sci 5:2253–2255

Goldner AM, Hajjar JJ, Curran PF (1969a) 2-Deoxyglucose transfer in rabbit intestine. Biochim Biophys Acta 173:572–574

Goldner AM, Schultz SG, Curran PF (1969b) Sodium and sugar fluxes across the mucosal border of rabbit ileum. J Gen Physiol 53:362–383

Gracey M, Burke V, Oshin A (1971) Reversible inhibition of intestinal active sugar transport by deconjugated bile salt in vitro. Biochim Biophys Acta 225:308–314

Gracey M, Burke V, Oshin A (1972) Intestinal transport of fructose. Biochim Biophys Acta 266:397–406

Gray GM, Ingelfinger FJ (1965) Intestinal absorption of sucrose in man: the site of hydrolysis and absorption. J Clin Invest 44:390–398

Gray GM, Ingelfinger FJ (1966) Intestinal absorption of sucrose in man: Interrelation of hydrolysis and monosaccharide product absorption. J Clin Invest 45:388–398

Guiraldes E, Lamabadusuriya SP, Oyesiku JEJ, Whitfield AE, Harries JT (1975) A comparative study on the effects of different bile salts on mucosal ATPase and transport in the rat jejunum in vivo. Biochim Biophys Acta 389:495–505

Gwee MCE, Yeoh TS (1969) Serosal transfer of glucose during peristalsis. J Pharm Pharmacol 21:131

Hagihira H, Lin ECC, Wilson TH (1961) Active transport of lysine, ornithine, arginine, and cystine by the intestine. Biochem Biophys Res Commun 4:478–481

Hajjar JJ, Lamont AS, Curran PF (1970) The sodium-alanine interaction in rabbit ileum. Effect of sodium on alanine fluxes. J Gen Physiol 55:277–296

Hajjar JJ, Khuri RN, Curran PF (1972) Alanine efflux across the serosal border of turtle intestine. J Gen Physiol 60:720–734

Hardcastle PT (1974) The effect of ATP on the transport of hexoses and amino acids in everted sacs of rat small intestine. Biochim Biophys Acta 332:114–121

Harries JT, Sladen GE (1972) The effect of different bile salts on the absorption of fluid, electrolytes and monosaccharides in the small intestine of the rat in vivo. Gut 13:596–603

Hellier MD, Holdsworth CD, McColl I, Perrett D (1972) Dipeptide absorption in man. Gut 13:965–969

Hellier MD, Thirumalai C, Holdsworth CD (1973) The effect of amino acids and dipeptides on sodium and water absorption in man. Gut 14:41–45

Hendrix TR, Bayless TM (1970) Digestion: Intestinal secretion. Ann Rev Physiol 32:139–164

Himukai M, Suzuki Y, Hoshi T (1978) Differences in characteristics between glycine and glcylglycine transport in guinea pig small intestine. Jpn J Physiol 28:499–510

Höber R, Höber J (1937) Experiments on the absorption of organic solutes in the small intestine of rats. J Cell Physiol 10:401–422

Holdsworth CD, Dawson AM (1964) The absorption of monosaccharides in man. Clin Sci 27:371–379

Holdsworth CD, Dawson AM (1965) Absorption of fructose in man. Proc Soc Exp Biol Med 118:142–145

Holman GD, Naftalin RJ (1976) Transport of 3-*O*-methylglucose and β-methyl-D-glucoside by rabbit ileum. Biochim Biophys Acta 433:597–614

Hopfer U, Groseclose R (1980) The mechanism of Na^+-dependent D-glucose transport. J Biol Chem 255:4453–4462

Hopfer U, Nelson K, Perrotto J, Isselbacher KJ (1973) Glucose transport in isolated brush border membrane from rat small intestine. J Biol Chem 248:25–32

Hopfer U, Sigrist-Nelson K, Murer H (1975) Intestinal sugar transport: studies with isolated plasma membranes. Ann NY Acad Sci 264:414–427

Hopfer U, Sigrist-Nelson K, Amman E, Murer H (1976) Differences in neutral amino acid and glucose transport between brush border and basolateral plasma membrane of intestinal epithelial cells. J Cell Physiol 89:805–810

Hülsmann WC (1977) Energy metabolism in different preparations of rat small intestinal epithelium. In: Kramer M, Lauterbach F (eds) Intestinal permeation. Excerpta Medica, Amsterdam, pp 229–238

Iida H, Moore EW, Broitman SA, Zamcheck N (1968) Effect of pH on active transport of D-glucose in the small intestine of hamsters. Proc Soc Exp Biol Med 127:730–732

Im WB, Misch DW, Powell DW, Faust RG (1980) Phenolphtalein- and harmaline-induced disturbances in the transport functions of isolated brush border and basolateral membrane vesicles from rat jejunum and kidney cortex. Biochem Pharmacol 29:2307–2317

Jacobs FA, Tarnasky WG (1963) Primary and secondary transport systems for amino acids in the intact intestine. J Am Med Assoc 183:765–768

Jervis EL, Smyth DH (1959) Competition between enantiomorphs of amino acids during intestinal absorption. J Physiol (Lond) 145:57–65

Jordana R, Ponz F (1969) Effects of the X-irradiation in vitro on the O_2 uptake and on the utilization of glucose by the intestine. Rev Esp Fisiol 25:129–136

Keljo DJ, Kleinzeller A, Murer H, Kinne R (1978) Is hexokinase present in the basal lateral membranes of rat kidney proximal tubular epithelial cells? Biochim Biophys Acta 508:500–512

Kessler M, Semenza G (1983) The small-intestinal Na^+, D-glucose cotransporter: an asymmetric gateal channel (or pore) responsive to $\Delta\psi$. J Membr Biol 76:27–56

Kimmich GA (1970) Active sugar accumulation by isolated intestinal epithelial cells, a new model for sodium dependent metabolite transport. Biochemistry 9:3669–3677

Kimmich GA (1973) Coupling between Na^+ and sugar transport in small intestine. Biochim Biophys Acta 300:31–78

Kimmich GA (1981) Gradient coupling in isolated intestinal cells. Fed Proc 40:2474–2479

Kimmich GA, Randles J (1975) A Na^+-independent, phloretin-sensitive monosaccharide transport system in isolated intestinal epithelial cells. J Membr Biol 23:57–76

Kimmich GA, Randles J (1976) 2-deoxyglucose transport by intestinal epithelial cells isolated from chick. J Membr Biol 27:363–379

Kimmich GA, Randles J (1977) A Na^+-independent transport system for sugars in intestinal epithelial cells: specificity, kinetics and interaction with inhibitors. In: Kramer M, Lauterbach F (eds) Intestinal permeation. Excerpta Medica, Amsterdam, pp 94–106

Kimmich GA, Randles J (1979) Energetics of sugar transport by isolated intestinal epithelial cells: Effects of cytochalasin B. Am J Physiol 237:C56–C63

Kimmich GA, Randles J (1980) Evidence for an intestinal Na^+:sugar transport coupling stoichiometry of 2.0. Biochim Biophys Acta 596:439–444

Kinter WB (1961) Autoradiographic study of intestinal transport. In: Metcoff J (ed) Proceedings of the 12th annual conference of the nephrotic syndrome. National Kidney Disease Foundation, New York, pp 59–68

Kleinzeller A (1970) The specificity of the active sugar transport in kidney cortex cells. Biochim Biophys Acta 211:264–276

Klip A, Grinstein S, Semenza G (1980) The small-intestinal sodium, D-glucose cotransporter is inserted in the brush border membrane asymmetrically. Ann NY Acad Sci 358:374–377

Kohn PG, Newey H, Smyth DH (1970) The effect of adenosine triphosphate on the transmural potential in rat small intestine. J Physiol (Lond) 208:203–220

Kuo YJ, Shanbour LL (1978) Effects of ethanol on sodium, 3-*O*-methyl-glucose, and L-alanine transport in the jejunum. Am J Dig Dis 23:51–56

Lamers JMJ, Hülsmann WC (1973) The effect of fructose on the stores of energy-rich phosphate in rat jejunum in vivo. Biochim Biophys Acta 313:1–8

Larralde J, Fernandez-Otero P, Gonzales M (1966) Increased active transport of glucose through the intestine during pregnancy. Nature 209:1356–1357

Laszt L, Vogel H (1946) Resorption of glucose from the small intestine of alloxan-diabetic rats. Nature 157:551–552

Levin RJ (1969) The effects of hormones on the absorptive, metabolic and digestive functions of the small intestine. J Endocrinol 45:315–348

Ling KY, Faust RG (1982) Effect of caffeine, theophylline and nicotine on D-glucose and folate transport in rat jejunal brush border membrane vesicles. Int J Biochem 14:1047–1050

Lluch M, Ponz F (1966) Immediate effects of X irradiation on the intestinal absorption of glucose and radioprotection by cysteamine. Rev Esp Fisiol 22:109–114

Loehry CA, Axon ATR, Hilton PJ, Hider RC, Creamer B (1970) Permeability of the small intestine to substances of different molecular weight. Gut 11:466–470

Love AH, Mitchell TG, Neptune EM Jr (1965) Transport of sodium and water by rabbit ileum in vitro and in vivo. Nature 206:1158

Love AHG (1969) The effect of biguanides on intestinal absorption. Diabetologia 5:422

Lücke H, Haase W, Murer H (1977) Amino acid transport in brush-border-membrane vesicles isolated from human small intestine. Biochem J 168:529–532

Lücke H, Berner W, Menge H, Murer H (1978) Sugar transport by brush border membrane vesicles isolated from human small intestine. Pflügers Arch 373:243–248

Luisier AL, Robinson JWL (1973) Inhibition of intestinal sugar and amino acid transport by N-butyl-biguanide. In: Bolis L, Schmidt-Nielsen K, Maddrell Shp (eds) Comparative physiology. North Holland, Amsterdam, pp 465–475

Mainoya JR (1975) Effect of prolactin on sugar and amino acid transport by the rat jejunum. J Exp Zool 192:149–154

Malathi P, Preiser H, Crane RK (1980) Protease-resistent integral brush border membrane proteins and their relationship to sodium-dependent transport of D-glucose and L-alanine. Ann NY Acad Sci 358:253–266

Maroux S, Louvard D, Semeriva M, Desnuelle P (1979) Hydrolases bound to the intestinal brush border: an example of transmembrane protein. Ann Biol Anim Biochim Biophys 19:787–790

Matthews DM (1975a) Intestinal absorption of peptides. Physiol Rev 55:537–608

Matthews DM (1975b) Absorption of peptides by mammalian intestine. In: Matthews DM, Payne JW (eds) Peptide transport in protein nutrition. North Holland, Amsterdam, pp 61–146

Matthews DM, Burston D (1977) Intestinal transport of peptides. In: Martin K, Lauterbach F (eds) Intestinal permeation. Excerpta Medica, Amsterdam, pp 136–143

Matthews DM, Laster L (1965) The kinetics of intestinal active transport of five neutral amino acids. Am J Physiol 208:593–600

Matthews DM, Craft IL, Geddes DM, Wise IJ, Hyde CW (1968) Absorption of glycine and glycine peptides from the small intestine of the rat. Clin Sci 35:415–424

Matthews DM, Addison JM, Burston D (1974) Evidence for active transport of the dipeptide carnosine (β-alanyl-L-hystidine) by hamster jejunum in vitro. Clin Sci 46:693–705

McDougal DB Jr, Little KD, Crane RK (1960) Studies on the mechanism of intestinal absorption of sugars. IV. Localization of galactose concentrations within the intestinal wall during active transport in vitro. Biochim Biophys Acta 45:483–489

McHardy GJR, Parsons DS (1957) The absorption of water and salt from the small intestine of the rat. Q J Exp Physiol 42:33–48

Mepham TB, Smith MW (1966) Amino acid transport in the goldfish intestine. J Physiol (Lond) 184:673–684

Milne MD, Asatoor AM (1975) Peptide absorption in disorders of amino acid transport. In: Matthews DM, Payne JW (eds) Peptide transport in protein nutrition. North Holland, Amsterdam, pp 167–182

Mircheff AK, Van Os CH, Wright EM (1980) Pathways for alanine transport in intestinal basal lateral membrane vesicles. J Membr Biol 52:83–92

Modigliani R, Bernier JJ (1971) Absorption of glucose, sodium, and water by the human jejunum studied by intestinal perfusion with a proximal occluding balloon and at variable flow rates. Gut 12:184–193

Modigliani R, Bernier JJ (1972) Effects of glucose on net and unidirectional movements of water and electrolytes in the human small intestine. Biol Gastro-Enterol 5:165–174

Munck BG (1980) Lysine transport across isolated rabbit ileum. J Gen Physiol 53:157–182

Munck BG, Schultz SG (1969) Lysine across the small intestine. Stimulating and inhibitory effects of neutral amino acids. J Membr Biol 53:45–53

Murer H, Hopfer U (1974) Demonstration of electrogenic Na^+-dependent D-glucose transport in intestinal brush border membranes. Proc Natl Acad Sci USA 71:484–488

Murer H, Hopfer U (1977) The functional polarity of the intestinal epithelial cell: studies with isolated plasma membrane vesicles. In: Kramer M, Lauterbach F (eds) Intestinal permeation. Excerpta Medica, Amsterdam, pp 294–311

Murer H, Kinne R (1980) The use of isolated membrane vesicles to study epithelial transport processes. J Membr Biol 55:81–95

Murer H, Hopfer U, Kinne-Saffran E, Kinne R (1974) Glucose transport in isolated brush-border and lateral-basal plasma membrane vesicles from intestinal epithelial cells. Biochim Biophys Acta 345:170–179

Murer H, Sigrist-Nelson K, Hopfer U (1975) On the mechanism of sugar and amino acid interaction in intestinal transport. J Biol Chem 250:7392–7396

Nadal J, Ponz F (1965) Inhibición del transporte activo de azucares por el intestino de rata in vitro. II. Accion de la atebrina, atractiloside y selenito. Rev Esp Fisiol 21:81–84

Nadal J, Ponz F (1966) Inhibition of the active transport of sugars by X irradiation in vitro of intestinal sacs. Rev Esp Fisiol 22:105–108

Naftalin RJ, Curran PF (1974) Galactose transport in rabbit ileum. J Membr Biol 16:257–278

Naftalin RJ, Holman GD (1976) The effects of removal of sodium ions from the mucosal solution on sugar absorption by rabbit ileum. Biochim Biophys Acta 419:385–390

Neale RJ, Wiseman G (1968) Active intestinal absorption of L-glucose. Nature 218:473–474

Neame KD, Wiseman G (1957) The transamination of glutamic and aspartic acids during absorption by the small intestine of the dog, in vivo. J Physiol (Lond) 135:442–450

Newey H, Smyth DH (1959) The intestinal absorption of some dipeptides. J Physiol (Lond) 145:48–56

Newey H, Smyth DH (1960) Intracellular hydrolysis of dipeptides during intestinal absorption. J Physiol (Lond) 152:367–380

Newey H, Smyth DH (1962) Cellular mechanisms in intestinal transfer of amino acids. J Physiol (Lond) 164:527–551

Newey H, Smyth DH (1964) The transfer system for neutral amino acids in the rat small intestine. J Physiol (Lond) 170:328–343

Newey H, Rampone AJ, Smyth DH (1964) The relation between L-methionine uptake and sodium in rat small intestine in vitro. J Physiol (Lond) 211:539–549

Newey H, Sanford PA, Smyth DH (1966) The effect of uranyl nitrate on intestinal transfer of hexoses. J Physiol (Lond) 186:403–502

Newey H, Rampone AJ, Smyth DH (1970) The relation between L-methionine uptake and sodium in rat small intestine in vitro. J Physiol (Lond) 211:539–549

Nixon SE, Mawer GE (1970) The digestion and absorption of protein in man. 2. The form in which digested protein is absorbed. Br J Nutr 24:241–258

Nordlie RC, Jorgenson RA (1976) Glucose-6-phosphatase. In: Martonosi A (ed) The enzymes of biological membranes, vol 2. Biosynthesis of cell components. Wiley, New York, pp 465–491

Nordstrom C, Dahlqvist A (1973) Quantitative distribution of some enzymes along the villi and crypts of human small intestine. Scand J Gastroenterol 8:407–413

Olsen WA, Ingelfinger FJ (1968) The role of sodium in intestinal absorption in man. J Clin Invest 47:1133–1142

Olsen WA, Rogers L (1971) Glucose binding by intestinal brush borders of rats. Comp Biochem Physiol 39B:617–625

Okada Y (1979) Solute transport process in intestinal epithelial cells. Membr Biochem 2:339–365

Parsons DS (1967) Salt and water absorption by the intestinal tract. Br Med Bull 23:252–257

Parsons DS (1972) Summary. In: Burland WL, Samuel PD (eds) Transport across the intestine. Livingstone, Edinburgh, pp 253–275

Parsons DS (1975) Energetics of intestinal transport. In: Csáky TZ (ed) Intestinal absorption and malabsorption. Raven, New York, pp 9–36

Parsons DS, Prichard JS (1965) Hydrolysis of disaccharides during absorption by the perfused small intestine of amphibia. Nature 208:1097–1098

Parsons DS, Prichard JS (1968) A preparation of perfused small intestine for the study of absorption in amphibia. J Physiol (Lond) 198:405–434

Parsons DS, Prichard JS (1971) Relationships between disaccharide hydrolysis and sugar transport in amphibia small intestine. J Physiol (Lond) 212:299–319

Paterson JYF, Sepulveda FV, Smith MW (1979) Two-carrier influx of neutral amino acids into rabbit ileal mucosa. J Physiol (Lond) 292:339–350

Paterson JYF, Sepulveda FV, Smith MW (1980) A sodium-independent low affinity transport system for neutral amino acids in rabbit ileal mucosa. J Physiol (Lond) 298:333–346

Peters TJ, MacMahon MT (1970) the absorption of glycine and glycine dipeptides by the rat. ClinSci 39:811–821

Ponz F, Lluch M (1958) The effect of cytochrome c and uranyl on the active trnsport of sugars by the intestine. Rev Esp Fisiol 14:217–224

Ponz F, Lluch M (1967) Effect of X irradiation on the active transport of glucose through the intestine of the rat in vivo. Rev Esp Fisiol 23:117–126

Ramaswamy K, Malathi P, Caspary WF, Crane RK (1974) Studies on the transport of glucose from disaccharides by hamster small intestine. II. Characteristics of the disaccharidase-related transport system. Biochim Biophys Acta 345:39–48

Randles J, Kimmich GA (1978) Effects of phloretin and theophylline on 3-*O*-methylglucose transport by intestinal epithelial cells. Am J Physiol 234:C64–C72

Read CP (1967) Studies on membrane transport. I. A common transport system for sugars and amino acids. Biol Bull 133:630–642

Reid EW (1900) On intestinal absorption, especially on the absorption of serum, peptone and glucose. Philos Trans R Soc Lond [Biol] 192:211–297

Reiser S, Christiansen PA (1967) Intestinal transport of valine as affected by ionic environment. Am J Physiol 212:1297–1302

Reiser S, Christiansen PA (1969) Intestinal transport of amino acids as affected by sugars. Am J Physiol 216:915–924

Reiser S, Christiansen PA (1973a) The properties of Na^+-dependent and Na^+-independent lysine uptake by isolated intestinal epithelial cells. Biochim Biophys Acta 307:212–222

Reiser S, Christiansen PA (1973b) Exchange transport and amino acid charge as the basis for Na^+-independent lysine uptake by isolated intestinal epithelial cells. Biochim Biophys Acta 307:223–233

Riklis E, Quastel JH (1958) Effects of cations on sugar absorption by isolated surviving guinea pig intestine. Can J Biochem Physiol 36:347–362

Rinaldo JE, Jennings BL, Frizzell RA, Schultz SG (1975) Effects of unilateral sodium replacement on sugar transport across in vitro rabbit ileum. Am J Physiol 228:854–860

Robinson JWL, Alvarado F (1971) Interaction between the sugar and amino-acid transport at the small intestinal brush border: A comparative study. Pflügers Arch 326:48–75

Robinson JWL, Alvarado F (1977) Comparative aspects of the interactions between sugar and amino acid transport systems. In: Kramer M, Lauterbach F (eds) Intestinal permeation. Excerpta Medica, Amsterdam, pp 145–162

Rose RC, Schultz SG (1971) Studies on the electrical potential profile across rabbit ileum. Effect of sugars and amino acids on transmural and transmucosal electrical potential differences. J Gen Physiol 57:639–663

Rosenberg IA, Coleman A, Rosenberg L (1965) The role of sodium ion in the transport of amino acids by the intestine. Biochim Biophys Acta 102:161–171

Roy CC, Dubois RS, Philippon F (1970) Inhibition by bile salts of the jejunal transport of 3-*O*-methylglucose. Nature 225:1055–1056

Rubino A, Field M, Shwachman H (1971) Intestinal transport of amino acid residues of dipeptides. 1. Influx of the glycine residue of glycyl-L-proline across mucosal border. J Biol Chem 246:3542–3548

Rummel W, Stupp HF (1962) The influence of diuretics on the absorption of salt, glucose and water from the isolated small intestine of the rat. Experientia 18:303–309

Saltzman DA, Rector FC Jr, Fordtran JS (1972) The role of intraluminal sodium in glucose absorption in vivo. J Clin Invest 51:876–885

Saunders SJ, Isselbacher KJ (1965 a) Inhibition of intestinal amino acid transport by hexoses. Biochim Biophys Acta 102:397–409

Saunders SJ, Isselbacher KJ (1965 b) Inhibition of intestinal amino acid transport by sugars. Nature 205:700–701

Schedl HP, Burston D, Taylor E, Matthews DM (1979) Kinetics of uptake of an amino acid and a dipeptide into hamster jejunum and ileum: the effect of semistarvation and starvation. Clin Sci 56:487–492

Schneider R, Burdett K, Pover WFR (1969) Intestinal motility and the absorption of glucose and fatty acid. Life Sci 8:123–130

Schultz SG, Curran PF (1970) Coupled transport of sodium and organic solutes. Physiol Rev 50:637–718

Schultz SG, Strechter CK (1970) Fructose influx across the brush border of rabbit ileum. Biochim Biophys Acta 211:586–588

Schultz SG, Yu-Tu L (1970) D-Arabinose influx across the brush border of rabbit ileum. Biochim Biophys Acta 196:351–353

Schultz SG, Zalusky R (1964) Ion transport in isolated rabbit ileum. II. The interaction between active sodium and active sugar transport. J Gen Physiol 47:1043–1059

Schultz SG, Zalusky R (1965) Interactions between active sodium transport and active amino-acid transport in isolated rabbit ileum. Nature 204:292–294

Schultz SG, Fuisz RE, Curran PF (1966) Amino acid and sugar transport in rabbit ileum. J Gen Physiol 49:849–866

Schultz SG, Curran PF, Chez RA, Fuisz RE (1967) Alanine and sodium fluxes across mucosal border of rabbit ileum. J Gen Physiol 50:1241–1260

Schultz SG, YU-TU L, Alvarez OO, Curran PF (1970) Dicarboxylic amino acid influx across brush border of rabbit ileum. Effects of amino acid charge on the sodium-amino acid interaction. J Gen Physiol 56:621–639

Semenza G (1969) Studies on intestinal sucrase and sugar transport. VII. A method for measuring intestinal uptake. The absorption of the anomeric forms of some monosaccharides. Biochim Biophys Acta 173:104–112

Semenza G (1971) On the mechanism of mutual inhibition among sodium-dependent transport systems in the small intestine. A hypothesis. Biochim Biophys Acta 241:637–649

Semenza G (1976) Small intestinal disaccharidases: their properties and role as sugar translocators across natural and artificial membranes. In: Martonosi A (ed) The enzymes of biological membranes. Plenum, New York, pp 349–382

Semenza G (1982) Asymmetric and kinetic properties of the small intestinal Na$^+$-D-glucose cotransporter. A plausible model. In: Gilles-Baillen M (ed) Intestinal transport. Fundamental and comparative aspects. Fourth conference, Bielefeld, FRG. ESCPB, Liège, p 72

Serebro HA, Iber FL, Yardley JH, Hendrix TR (1969) The inhibition of cholera toxin action in the rabbit by cycloheximide. Gastroenterology 56:506–511

Shore LE (1890) On the fate of peptone in the lymphatic system. J Physiol (Lond) 11:528–565

Sigrist-Nelson K (1975) Dipeptide transport in isolated intestinal brush border membrane. Biochim Biophys Acta 394:220–226

Sigrist-Nelson K, Hopfer U (1974) A distinct D-fructose transport system in isolated brush border membrane. Biochim Biophys Acta 367:247–254

Sigrist-Nelson K, Murer H, Hopfer U (1975) Active alanine transport in isolated brush border membrane. J Biol Chem 250:5674–5680

Silk DBA, Perrett D, Clark ML (1973) Intestinal transport of two dipeptides containing the same two neutral amino acids in man. Clin Sci 45:291–299

Silk DBA, Fairclough PD, Park NJ, Lane AE, Webb JPW, Clark ML, Dawson AM (1975) A study of relations between the absorption of amino acids, dipeptides, water and electrolytes in the normal human jejunum. Clin Sci 49:401–408

Sladen GE, Dawson AM (1969) Interrelationship between the absorptions of glucose, sodium and water by the normal human jejunum. Clin Sci 36:119–132

Sleisenger MH, Burston D, Dalrymple JA, Wilkinson S, Matthews DM (1976) Evidence for a single common carrier for uptake of a dipeptide and a tripeptide by hamster jejunum in vitro. Gastroenterology 71:76–81

Smirnova LF, Ugolev AM (1974) Transport and accumulation of glucose in the mucosa of the small intestine. Dokl Akad Nauk SSSR 215:230–233

Smulders AP, Wright EM (1971) Galactose transport across the hamster small intestine. The effect of sodium electrochemical potential gradients. J Physiol (Lond) 212:277–286

Smith MW, Sepulveda FV (1979) Sodium dependence of neutral amino acid uptake into rabbit ileum. Biochim Biophys Acta 555:374–378

Smithson KW, Gray GM (1977) Intestinal assimilation of a tetrapeptide in the rat. Obligate function of brush border aminopeptidase. J Clin Invest 60:665–674

Smyth DH (1971) Energetics of intestinal transfer. In: Armstrong WMcD, Nunn AS Jr (eds) Intestinal transport of electrolytes, amino acids and sugars. Charles C Thomas, Springfield, Illinois, pp 52–75

Smyth DH (1972) Peptide transport by mammalian gut. In: Elliott K, O'Connor M (eds) Peptide transport in bacteria and mammalian gut. Ciba Found Symp 37:59–66

Spencer RP, Samiy AH (1960) Intestinal transport of L-triptophan in vitro. Inhibition by high concentrations. Am J Physiol 199:1033–1036

Storelli C, Vögeli H, Semenza G (1972) Reconstitution of a sucrase-mediated sugar transport system in lipid membranes. FEBS Lett 24:287–292

Swaminathan N, Eichholz A (1973) Studies on the mechanism of active intestinal transport of glucose. Biochim Biophys Acta 298:724–731

Teem MV, Phillips SF (1972) Perfusion of the hamster jejunum with conjugated and unconjugated bile acids: Inhibition of water absorption and effects on morphology. Gastroenterology 62:261–267

Tilney LG, Mooseker M (1971) Actin in the brush border of epithelial cells of the chicken intestine. Proc Natl Acad Sci USA 68:2611–2615

Toggenburger G, Kessler M, Rothstein A, Semenza G, Tannenbaum C (1978) Similarly in effects of Na$^+$ gradients and membrane potentials on D-glucose transport by, and phlorizin binding to, vesicles derived from brush border of rabbit intestinal mucosal cells. J Membr Biol 40:269–290

Toggenburger G, Kessler M, Semenza G (1982) Phlorizin as a probe of the small intestinal Na$^+$, D-glucose cotransporter. A model. Biochim Biophys Acta 688:557–571

Ugolev AM (1974) Membrane (contact) digestion. In: Smyth DH (ed) Biomembranes. Intestinal absorption, vol 4A. Plenum, London, pp 285–362

Ugolev AM, Kushak RI (1966) Hydrolysis of dipeptides in cells of the small intestine. Nature 212:859–860

Ugolev AM, Iesuitova NN, Timofeeva NM, Fediushina IN (1964) Location of hydrolysis of certain disaccharides and peptides in the small intestine. Nature 202:807–809

Ullrich KJ, Rumrich G, Klöss S (1974) Specificity and sodium dependence of the active sugar transport in the proximal convolution of the rat kidney. Pflügers Arch 351:35–48

Van Slike DD, Meyer GM (1912) The amino-acid nitrogen of the blood. Preliminary experiments on protein assimilation. J Biol Chem 12:399–410

Varró V, Jung I, Szarvas F, Csernay L (1965) Glucose absorption in relation to ATP content of the small-intestine mucosa in the dog. Am J Dig Dis 10:178–182

Verzar F (1935) Die Rolle von Diffusion und Schleimhautaktivität bei der Resorption von verschiedenen Zuckern aus dem Darm. Biochem Z 276:17–27

Watford M, Lund P, Krebs HA (1979) Isolation and metabolic characteristics of rat and chicken enterocytes. Biochem J 178:589–596

White JF, Armstrong WMcD (1971) Effect of transported solutes on membrane potentials in bullfrog small intestine. Am J Physiol 221:194–201

Will PC, Hopfer U (1979) Apparent inhibition of active non-electrolyte transport by an increased sodium permeability of the plasma membrane. J Biol Chem 254:3806–3811

Wilson TH (1962) Intestinal absorption. Saunders, Philadelphia

Wilson TH, Vincent TN (1955) Absorption of sugars in vitro by the intestine of golden hamster. J Biol Chem 216:851–866

Wilson TH, Wiseman G (1954) The use of sacs of everted small intestine for the study of the transference of substances from the mucosal to the serosal surface. J Physiol (Lond) 123:116–125

Wilson TH, Lin ECC, Landau BR, Jorgensen CR (1960) Intestinal transport of sugars and amino acids. Fed Proc 19:870–875

Winne D (1973) Unstirred layers, source of biased Michaelis constant in membrane transport. Biochim Biophys Acta 298:27–31

Winne D (1979) Influence of blood flow on intestinal absorption of drugs and nutrients. Farmac Ther, vol 6. Pergamon, Oxford, pp 333–393

Wiseman G (1951) Active stereochemically selective absorption of amino-acids from rat small intestine. J Physiol (Lond) 114:7P–8P

Wiseman G (1955) Preferential transference of amino-acids from amino-acid mixtures by sacs of everted small intestine of the golden hamster (Mesocricetus auratus). J Physiol (Lond) 127:414–422

Wiseman G (1974) Absorption of protein digestion products. In: Smyth DH (ed) Intestinal absorption. Biomembranes 4A:363–481

Wrights EM, Van Os CH, Mircheff AK (1980) Sugar uptake by intestinal basolateral membrane vesicles. Biochim Biophys Acta 597:112–124

Wright EM, Harms V, Mircheff AK, Van Os CH (1981) Transport properties of intestinal basolateral membranes. Ann NY Acad Sci 372:626–635

CHAPTER 16

Pharmacologic Aspects of Intestinal Permeability to Lipids (Except Steroids and Fat-Soluble Vitamins)

A. GANGL

A. Introduction

Lipids are important constituents of human food. Their physical and chemical properties have been well defined (SMALL 1968, 1970; CAREY and SMALL 1970) and the mechanisms of absorption of dietary lipids by intestinal mucosa have been explored in great detail during the past century. In addition to dietary or exogenous lipids, intestinal mucosa is continuously exposed to endogenous lipids from two opposite sides: the intestinal lumen and the plasma pool. This duality of endogenous lipid supply, particularly of fatty acids to the intestinal mucosa has attracted attention more recently (GANGL and OCKNER 1974a, b, 1975a; GANGL and RENNER 1978; GANGL et al. 1980).

While the physiology and pathophysiology of fat absorption have been the subject of many extensive reviews in the past (GAGE and FISH 1924; FRAZER 1952; SENIOR 1964; JOHNSTON 1968; GANGL and OCKNER 1975b; ROMMEL et al. 1976; SHIAU 1981), pharmacologic aspects of the intestinal permeability to lipids have not been studied that extensively. Therefore, it is the aim of this chapter to outline only briefly the physiology of intestinal permeability to lipids and to pay attention mainly to mechanisms by which drugs may affect the intestinal permeability to lipids and to focus on some specific agents such as ethanol, hormones, cytostatic agents, and dietary fiber and their modes of action upon the intestinal permeability to lipids.

B. Brief Outline of the Physiology of Intestinal Permeability to Lipids

I. Permeation from the Intestinal Lumen (Fat Absorption)

Dietary fat consists mainly of triglycerides, up to about 10% phospholipids, and contains only minute amounts of steroids, fat-soluble vitamins, fatty acids, and other lipids. In addition to exogenous dietary lipids, endogenous lipids (KARMEN et al. 1963), mainly biliary phospholipids and lipids from shed epithelial cells (SHRIVASTAVA et al. 1967; OCKNER et al. 1969), enter the intestinal lumen. They are admixed to the dietary lipids and subjected to the very same digestive and absorptive processes as exogenous lipids (Fig. 1). During the luminal phase of fat absorption, long-chain triglycerides are hydrolyzed to a small extent in the stomach by pharyngeal lipase (HAMOSH and SCOW 1973; HAMOSH et al. 1975) and

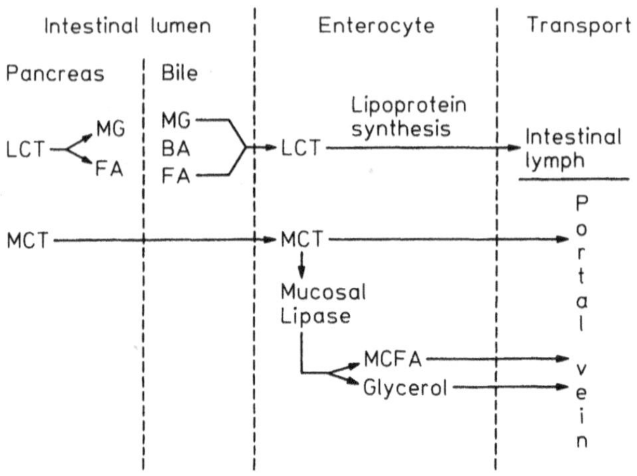

Fig. 1. Schematic representation of differences in the intestinal absorption of long-chain and medium-chain triglycerides (*LCT*, long-chain triglyceride; *MCT*, medium-chain triglyceride; *MG*, monoglyceride; *FA*, fatty acids; *BA*, bile acids; *MCFA*, medium-chain fatty acids)

mainly in the intestinal lumen by pancreatic lipase and colipase in the presence of conjugated bile acids to free fatty acids and β-monoglycerides (for review see ROMMEL et al. 1976; SHIAU 1981). Phospholipids are hydrolyzed partially by pancreatic (for review see DE HAAS et al. 1978) and intestinal (MANSBACH et al. 1982) phospholipases, and cholesterol esters are split by cholesterolesterase into free cholesterol and free fatty acids. The products of fat hydrolysis are solubilized in the intestinal watery contents mainly in mixed bile salt–lipid micelles and to some extent by other mechanisms, most likely involving proteins (MEYER et al. 1976). The delivery of gastric contents, bile, and pancreatic enzymes into the duodenum is guarded by cholecystokinin, secretin, and possibly other hormonal and neural stimuli (MEYER 1975; JOHNSON 1977).

The first step in the permeation of the intestinal mucosa by the products of intraluminal lipid hydrolysis, the uptake, requires the direct contact of these products with the absorptive surface of the intestinal epithelium. This takes place only after a mixed bile acid–lipid micelle of the bulk phase within the intestinal lumen has penetrated the layer of watery phase immediately adjacent to the microvillous membrane of the absorptive intestinal epithelial cell. This layer has been termed the unstirred layer (WILSON et al. 1971; WILSON and DIETSCHY 1972) and is not equilibrated with the bulk phase of intestinal contents. In some way it acts like a "hydrophilic membrane" interposed between the bulk phase and the hydrophobic brush border membrane. Therefore, it has been claimed that this unstirred layer may be rate limiting for the uptake of lipids from the intestinal lumen into intestinal mucosa (WILSON et al. 1971; WILSON and DIETSCHY 1972). Mixed bile salt–lipid micelles are not incorporated in toto into the epithelial cell, but dissociate before uptake and only the products of intraluminal lipid hydrolysis carried in the mixed micelle are taken up into the brush border membrane by passive diffusion (for recent review see SHIAU 1981), while the bile salt micelle remains extracellularly in the intestinal lumen. Conjugated bile acids are absorbed later on, mainly in the ileum (WILSON and DIETSCHY 1972).

While the uptake of luminal lipids into the microvillous membrane occurs by passive diffusion, the transport of long-chain fatty acids from the plasma membrane to the endoplasmic reticulum and presumably to other intracellular sites of long-chain fatty acid metabolism is facilitated by a protein with low molecular weight, termed fatty acid binding protein (OCKNER et al. 1972a; OCKNER and MANNING 1974, 1976). Absorbed long-chain fatty acids are then reesterified, mainly with monoglycerides to di- and triglycerides and in part also to phospholipids and cholesterol esters. The site of this reesterification is the smooth endoplasmic reticulum which is known to contain all requisite enzymes (RAO and JOHNSTON 1966). The smooth endoplasmic reticulum, the rough endoplasmic reticulum, and the Golgi apparatus represent an intricate tubular system which is thought to channel the reesterified lipids through the absorptive epithelial cell for secretion, while it imposes all the biochemical transformations leading to the formation of chylomicrons. Among others, this process involves the attachement of a number of apoproteins to the lipid core (for review see GANGL and OCKNER 1975b). This sequence of events finally leads to the exocytosis of a bulk of complete chylomicrons by fusion of the prechylomicron-containing Golgi vacuoles with the basolateral plasmalemma (FRIEDMANN and CARDELL 1972a; SABESIN and FRASE 1977).

Evidence has been presented that the movement of chylomicron-filled Golgi vesicles may be guided by the microtubular system (GLICKMAN et al. 1976; ARREAZA-PLAZA et al. 1976; GANGL et al. 1979), which is present also in the absorptive epithelial cells. And it is speculated that recognition sites for Golgi vesicles may exist and be located on specific areas of the plasmalemma (BERGERON et al. 1973) and that microtubules would be able to direct the Golgi vesicles to such specific recognition sites. The definite proof of this speculation is still pending, however.

Chylomicrons secreted into the intercellular space pass into the lamina propria and then enter intestinal lymphatics which finally gain access to the systemic blood circulation. Contrary to long-chain triglycerides, medium-chain triglycerides (see Fig. 1) may enter the intestinal mucosa, even unhydrolyzed, and are split after their uptake within the intestinal mucosa by virtue of a mucosal lipase into medium-chain fatty acids and glycerol. Medium-chain fatty acids are not reesterified and not absorbed into lymphatics, but enter the portal bloodstream. These differences have been reviewed in detail previously (GREENBERGER et al. 1966; GREENBERGER and SKILLMAN 1969).

II. Permeation from the Plasma Pool (Uptake and Metabolism of Plasma Free Fatty Acids)

More recently it has been shown that, in addition to luminal fatty acids, the intestinal mucosa of rats and of humans takes up and utilizes fatty acids from the plasma pool as well (GANGL and OCKNER 1974a, b, 1975a; GANGL and RENNER 1978). Quantitatively, the fractional uptake of long-chain plasma free fatty acids by intestinal mucosa has been estimated as about 1%. In the plasma, fatty acids are carried bound to serum albumin, they traverse the wall of the capillaries, and enter the enterocyte at its basal pole, opposite to the brush border.

Within the enterocyte, long-chain fatty acids derived from the intestinal lumen and fatty acids derived from the plasma pool are compartmentalized (GANGL and OCKNER 1975a). While luminal long-chain fatty acids are mainly esterified to triglycerides and only a minute fraction is oxidized by intestinal mucosa, plasma long-chain fatty acids are mainly oxidized and incorporated into phospholipids. Unsaturated long-chain fatty acids are esterified at a higher rate by intestinal mucosa than saturated long-chain fatty acids regardless of whether the long-chain fatty acids are derived from the intestinal lumen (OCKNER et al. 1972b) or from the plasma pool (GANGL et al. 1980). This difference in the esterification rate between fatty acids with different degrees of saturation most likely is related to the fatty acid binding protein, which exerts a higher binding affinity to unsaturated than to saturated long-chain fatty acids and which in addition to its role in intracellular fatty acid transport has been shown to enhance fatty acid esterification.

C. Mechanisms by which Drugs May Affect the Intestinal Permeability to Lipids

Theoretically, one can imagine many ways by which drugs might affect the permeation of the intestinal wall by lipids from both the intestinal lumen and the plasma pool. Thus, drugs may interfere with intraluminal events of fat absorption, e.g., by affecting the motility of the stomach and of the intestine, the lipolysis, or the formation of mixed bile acid–lipid micelles, e.g., by changes in the secretion, intraluminal binding, or precipitation of conjugated bile acids (Table 1). Drugs may also disturb the integrity of the intestinal mucosa or interfere with in-

Table 1. Pharmacologic interactions with premucosal events of lipid absorption

I. Gastrointestinal motility
   1. Gastric emptying
      a) Delayed by: morphine, ethanol, dietary fiber
      b) Accelerated by: motilin, ethanol
   2. Intestinal transit
      a) Delayed by: morphine, atropine
      b) Accelerated by: sorbitol, dietary fiber, motilin

II. Lipolysis
   1. Inhibited by: simple and mixed bile salt micelles, chlortetracycline, neomycin, cyclophosphamide, 5-fluorouracil, ethanol, fenfluramine, hyperacidity; somatostatin(?)
   2. Stimulated by: cholecystokinin, secretin

III. Micellar solubilization inhibited by:
   1. Bile salt binding: cholestyramine, cholestipol, polydexide, lignin; pectin(?)
   2. Bile salt precipitation: hyperacidity, neomycin

IV. Displacement of fatty acids from fatty acid–albumin complex of plasma: e.g., by chlorophenoxyisobutyrate

Table 2. Pharmacologic interactions with mucosal events of intestinal permeation by lipids

I. Disturbance of intestinal mucosal integrity and reduction of absorptive surface area
   1. Surfactants, ethanol, neomycin
   2. Inhibition of cell renewal: aminopterin, 5-fluorouracil, Cyclophosphamide, etc.
   3. Somatostatin(?)

II. Effects on intracellular events of intestinal lipid and lipoprotein metabolism
   1. Inhibition of fatty acid transport by FABP inhibitors: flavaspidic acid, α-bromopalmitate
   2. Modification of lipid reesterification
      a) Stimulation by: ethanol, corticosteroids
      b) Inhibition by: aminopterin
   3. Modification of fatty acid oxidation
      a) Stimulation by: glucagon
      b) Inhibition by: ethanol
   4. Inhibition of lipoprotein synthesis and secretion by:
      a) Protein synthesis inhibitors: acetoxycycloheximide, puromycin, DL-ethionine
      b) Antimicrotubular agents: colchicine, vinblastine

III. Alteration of intestinal lymph flow: increase by neostigmine, intraduodenal saline infusion, or ethanol causes enhanced transmucosal fat transport

tracellular events of intestinal lipid and lipoprotein metabolism (Table 2). On the other hand, drugs causing changes of intestinal lymph and blood flow are also likely to affect the permeability of the intestine to lipids from either side, the lumen and the plasma.

I. Interference with Intraluminal Events of Fat Absorption

1. Gastrointestinal Motility

The jejunum is the main site of fat absorption and therefore gastric emptying and intestinal transit time can be expected to affect the absorption of lipids from the intestinal lumen. Morphine has long been known as an inhibitor of intestinal propulsion by increasing the general tone of the small intestine (INGELFINGER 1943). In the rat, a single dose of morphine, 32 mg/kg, was shown to depress the absorption of saponifiable fat (coconut oil emulsion) from the intestinal lumen by 44% for 2 h. This effect was due to regurgitation of fat into the stomach by intestinal spasm, thus reducing the rate at which fat was presented to the small intestine for absorption, while the permeability of the intestinal mucosa to lipids was not affected (BENNET et al. 1962). Crystalline atropine sulfate, a drug which depresses all phases of intestinal motility, given in the same experiment at a constant rate of 1 mg kg^{-1} h^{-1}, did not interfere with the intestinal absorption and lymphatic transport of a coconut oil emulsion infused constantly into the duodenum. The only effect of the interference of atropine with intestinal propulsion was a transfer of the location of fat absorption to a more proximal site of the small intestine (BENNET et al. 1962).

While morphine and atropine slow passage through the proximal small intestine, motilin has been shown to accelerate gastric emptying (CHRISTOFIDES et al. 1979) and intestinal transit time (RUPPIN et al. 1976) in humans. However, gastric emptying of fat is not stimulated by low-dose exogenous motilin (CHRISTOFIDES et al. 1981). Studies of the effect of motilin on the absorption of lipids from the intestinal lumen have not been published, so far.

Small bowel transit time, which has been estimated in humans as ranging from 72 min using lactulose and breath hydrogen analysis (BOND and LEVITT 1975) to 130 min using barium (LEVANT et al. 1974), not only affects fat absorption via the time available for presentation of lipids to the absorptive surface for absorption, but may also act on fat absorption indirectly, as it has been shown that acute alterations in small bowel transit time significantly affect the biliary excretion rate of bile acids (HARDISON et al. 1979). Thus, sorbitol shortens transit time by 38% and increases the hourly bile acid excretion rate by 31%, while atropine increases transit time by 38% and decreases hourly bile acid excretion rate by 38%. As conjugated bile acids are intimately involved in intraluminal lipid emulsification, hydrolysis (MORGAN and HOFFMAN 1971; BORGSTRÖM and ERLANSON 1973), and micellar solubilization (CAREY and SMALL 1972), changes in bile acid excretion are likely to affect intestinal lipid absorption.

2. Intestinal Lipolysis

Hydrolysis of long-chain triglycerides by pancreatic lipase is an obligatory step before their subsequent intestinal absorption. Lipase is secreted by the pancreas in an active form, has a pH optimum of 8.0 (BORGSTRÖM 1954) and is inactivated irreversibly by low pH (GO et al. 1970).

The possibility of interfering pharmacologically at this step of intestinal lipid absorption was evidenced by ROKOS et al. (1958), who observed an inhibition of the lipase activity of acetone extracts of dried pancreas of hog and of pancreatic juice of rat by chlortetracycline. In vivo studies in rats showed no effect of chlortetracycline on the rate of gastric emptying and confirmed the inhibitory action of this antibiotic upon pancreatic lipase (KRONDL et al. 1962). A similar inhibitory effect of chlortetracycline upon the lipolytic activity of digestive juice was shown in humans (KRONDL et al. 1959). Neomycin administered orally has also been shown in vitro (MEHTA et al. 1967) and in vivo (ROGERS et al. 1966) to inhibit intraluminal intestinal lipolysis. Additional intraluminal and mucosal effects of neomycin upon intestinal lipid absorption will be discussed later.

Taurodeoxycholate at a concentration of 0.8 m*M* inhibits pancreatic lipase activity by preventing the adsorption of enzyme at the oil–water interface, resulting in the physical separation of enzyme and substrate (MOMSEN and BROCKMAN 1976a). Colipase, a protein cofactor, reverses these inhibitory effects of bile salt by providing a high affinity binding site for the lipase at this interface (MOMSEN and BROCKMAN 1976b). The human pancreatic lipase–colipase activity is not only inhibited by simple bile salt micelles, but by mixed dihydroxy bile salt–phosphatidylcholine micelles as well (PATTON and CAREY 1981).

Lipid digestion and absorption from rat intestine is impaired in vitro and in vivo by fenfluramine, an anorectic drug (BIZZI et al. 1973; DANNENBURG et al. 1973; COMAI et al. 1978). This observation was ascribed to an inhibitory action of fenfluramine to pancreatic lipase activity (DANNENBURG and WARD 1971; COMAI et al. 1978). More recently it was shown, however, that in vitro lipase alone is inhibited only insignificantly by fenfluramine and rather that this drug is a potent inhibitor of the complex pancreatic lipase–colipase–bile salt system (BORSTRÖM and WOLLESEN 1981).

3. Micellar Solubilization

The mechanism whereby bile acid micelles increase the rate of fatty acid and cholesterol uptake into the intestinal mucosal cell has been reevaluated by WESTERGAARD and DIETSCHY (1976). Their experimental results indicate that the principal role of the micelle in facilitating lipid absorption is to overcome unstirred layer resistance, while the actual process of fatty acid and cholesterol absorption occurs through a monomer phase in equilibrium with the micelle (WESTERGAARD and DIETSCHY 1976).

Conjugated bile acids form micelles only at a concentration equal to or higher than the critical micellar concentration, which varies with pH, temperature, presence of other lipids, and of counterions between 2 and 5 m*M* (CAREY and SMALL 1972). Any decrease of the amount of conjugated bile acids in the bowel lumen to below this critical micellar concentration will interfere with the formation of mixed bile acid–lipid micelles. Under these conditions, the solubilization of the products of intraluminal lipid hydrolysis may be insufficient to permit satisfactory transport to the absorptive epithelium.

Such a decreased concentration of bile acid in the jejunal lumen may be due either to the interruption of the flow of bile from the liver into the intestinal lumen by obstruction of the bile duct, by bile diversion (experimental or postoperative states), or by the interruption of the enterohepatic circulation of bile acids following ileal disease (MANSBACH et al. 1972) or resection (HARDISON and ROSENBERG 1967; VAN DEEST et al. 1968; MCLEOD and WIGGINS 1968) and, less commonly, intraluminal bile acid precipitation (GO et al. 1970), dilution (MCLEOD and WIGGINS 1968; DI MAGNO 1972) or bacterial deconjugation (SWITZ et al. 1970). Furthermore, liver cell failure may also be associated with a decrease in the rate of hepatic bile acid synthesis and secretion (THEODOR et al. 1968; VLAHCEVIC et al. 1971, 1972). Pharmacologically, the intrajejunal bile acid concentration can be altered by the peroral (intraluminal) application of bile acid sequestering agents, such as cholestyramine, cholestipol, and polydexide, and furthermore by bile acid precipitating factors such as changes of intraluminal pH or by neomycin.

a) Binding of Bile Acids

Cholestyramine, a quaternary ammonium anion exchange resin (TENNENT et al. 1960), which is not absorbed from the intestine, binds bile salts tightly (GALLO et al. 1965) within the intestinal lumen, thus interfering with enterohepatic circulation and thereby causing increased loss of bile acids in feces. Within limits, the fecal loss of luminal bile acids is compensated by an increase of hepatic bile acid synthesis. With daily doses of cholestyramine below 15 g, the associated fecal loss of triglyceride is negligible (DANHOF 1966; HASHIM et al. 1961), and only after a daily dose of about 30 g cholestyramine the absorption of triolein is impaired, while that of oleic acid (HASHIM et al. 1961) or of medium-chain triglyceride (ZURIER et al. 1965) is not. The effects of cholestyramine on lipid metabolism have been the subject of recent reviews (LEVY et al. 1972; HAVEL and KANE 1973).

Cholestipol, a high molecular weight basic anion exchange resin, is also a very potent bile acid sequestrant polymer, which, like cholestyramine, is not absorbed from the gastrointestinal tract (PARKINSON et al. 1970). Its oral administration in a daily dose of three times 5 g for periods up to 36 months does not cause impaired intestinal fat absorption, however (SACHS and WOLFMAN 1974; HARVENGT and DESAGER 1976). A third bile sequestering agent, polydexide, which has the skeleton of dextran, is also effective in decreasing elevated serum cholesterol, but does not alter fecal fat excretion or serum levels of fat-soluble vitamins and triglycerides (RITLAND et al. 1975).

b) Altering the Intraluminal pH

Another mechanism whereby the intrajejunal concentration of conjugated bile acids may be reduced involves the pH of the small intestinal contents, as only dissociated conjugated bile acids form micelles. At a pH lower than their pK_a, bile salts do not dissociate (CAREY and SMALL 1972), but are precipitated and rapidly absorbed by passive diffusion (DIETSCHY 1968).

Thus, hyperacidity within the intestinal lumen as it occurs in the Zollinger–Ellison syndrome due to overproduction of the gastrointestinal hormone gastrin, may also result in intestinal fat malabsorption (SHIMODA et al. 1968). Bile acid precipitation by low pH is reversible however (GO et al. 1970) and with increasing intraluminal pH in the lower small intestine, bile acids return into solution. Pharmacologically, the duodenal pH can be increased by cimetidine, which was found effectively to correct fat maldigestion in pancreatic insufficiency (REGAN et al. 1979).

c) Bile Salt Precipitation by Neomycin

Precipitation of bile acids can be achieved in vitro also by neomycin, a polybasic member of the aminoglucoside series of antibiotics (DE SOMER et al. 1964; VAN DEN BOSCH and CLAES 1967; FALOON et al. 1966). The mechanisms which are operative during neomycin-induced steatorrhea in vivo (RODGERS et al. 1966) are more complex, however. For the purpose of a systematic discussion, the effects of neomycin and its derivatives on intestinal lipid absorption can be divided according to their site of action into intraluminal and mucosal effects.

With regard to the intraluminal phase of lipid absorption, conflicting results have been published concerning the effect of neomycin upon pancreatic lipase activity: while RODGERS et al. (1966), who studied two adult male volunteers, presented evidence for an inhibitory effect of neomycin (4 and 8 g/day) upon intraluminal fat hydrolysis, THOMPSON et al. (1971) studying five healthy physicians, found no effect of a single 1-g dose of neomycin sulfate on the pancreatic lipase concentration in aspirated intestinal contents.

Furthermore, neomycin does not alter the pH of intestinal contents (THOMPSON et al. 1971). Earlier studies in rats on the influence of neomycin on digestion and absorption of fat in vivo had also shown no influence upon the rate of lipolysis (KRONDL et al. 1962). More recently, further evidence has been presented that the addition of neomycin sulfate to simple micellar solutions of bile salts in vitro induces precipitation of the taurine conjugates of dihydroxy bile acids, but not of trihydroxy bile acids. When mixed bile salt–lipid micelles are used as substrate, neomycin causes precipitation of most of the fatty acids, monoglycerides, and cholesterol, however, only a small proportion of bile salt is precipitated (THOMPSON et al. 1970). In vivo, the uptake of oleic acid ^{14}C and labeled cholesterol from mixed micelles, given to rats intraduodenally, is markedly decreased by the simultaneous administration of 10–50 mg neomycin sulfate (THOMPSON et al. 1970). As in rats with cannulated intestinal lymphatics and bile ducts the lymphatic transport of labeled fatty acids and cholesterol is also inhibited by neomycin sulfate (and its basic derivatives), although the intestinal absorption and biliary reexcretion of taurocholate and taurodeoxycholate is not, one can assume that neomycin and its basic derivatives precipitate mixed micellar solutions primarily by their ionic interaction with fatty acids, thus interfering with fat absorption (THOMPSON et al. 1970). This concept was confirmed also by in vivo studies in healthy humans and provides an explanation for the intraluminal mode of action of neomycin on the process of fat absorption (THOMPSON et al. 1971). Failure to find a consistent increase in fecal acidic steroids following daily administration of two times 1 g neomycin in four patients for at least 5 weeks was advocated more recently against the concept of neomycin being a bile acid sequestrant in vivo (SEDAGHAT et al. 1975).

In addition to the intraluminal action of neomycin, morphological (JACOBSON et al. 1960) and functional alterations (KESSLER et al. 1978) of intestinal mucosa caused by neomycin have been described which may affect intestinal mucosal permeability to lipids more directly. These effects of neomycin will be discussed later.

II. Disturbance of Intestinal Mucosal Integrity

1. Physiology of the Interface Between Luminal Contents and Absorptive Surface

A prerequisite for the permeation of the intestinal mucosa by any substance to be absorbed from the small bowel lumen is the direct contact of this substance with the absorptive surface. According to present concepts of fat absorption, a lipid molecule has to traverse an unstirred layer of the watery phase which is directly adjacent to the brush border membrane of the absorptive epithelial cell. The thickness of this unstirred layer has been estimated in vitro to be 150–207 μm (SALLEE and DIETSCHY 1973; LUKIE et al. 1974; WILSON and DIETSCHY 1974) and in vivo 416–530 μm (DEBNAM and LEVIN 1975; WINNE 1976) in the rat, and 487–634 μm (READ et al. 1976) in humans.

For some lipids, e.g., medium-chain fatty acids, which are water soluble, this unstirred layer represents only little diffusion resistance. The majority of dietary lipids, however, require solubilization after lipolysis. The absorption of these lipids is facilitated by the formation of mixed bile acid–lipid micelles, which increase the net diffusive flux, e.g., of long-chain fatty acids through the unstirred layer by a factor of 100–200 (HOFMANN 1976). The actual process of fatty acid absorption, however, occurs through a monomer phase in equilibrium with the micelle (WESTERGAARD and DIETSCHY 1976). While WESTERGAARD and DIETSCHY (1976) suggested that the absorption of fatty acid from the unstirred layer leads to further release of fatty acid from the mixed bile acid–lipid micelles, because free fatty acids of the unstirred layer are in equilibrium with micellar fatty acids, more recently, other explanations for micellar dissociation have been proposed, involving a pH gradient between the bulk phase and the area adjacent to the epithelial cell (SHIAU and LEVINE 1980). This area directly adjacent to the epithelial cell was termed the "acidic microclimate" and its formation attributed to intestinal hydrogen secretion. The existence of such a unique acidic microclimate was shown in rat proximal jejunum (LUCAS et al. 1975) by direct measurement by pH microelectrode. These newer concepts of fat digestion and absorption have been reviewed by SHIAU (1981).

The luminal side of the microvillous membrane is covered by a structure, known as the glycocalyx, surface coat, fuzzy coat, or fuzz (ITO 1965, 1974; TRIER 1968; SWIFT and MUKHERJEE 1976). The function of this structure, which represents the interface between the unstirred layer and the luminal surface of the microvillous membrane and which contains an appreciable amount of glycoproteins and negatively charged sulfated mucopolysaccharides is not fully elucidated yet (ALPERS and SEETHARAM 1977).

2. Effect of Surfactants

While conjugated trihydroxy bile salts at physiologic concentrations do not induce ultrastructural or biochemical alterations of the brush border membrane, other, more potent surfactants are able to do so. These effects of surfactants upon structure and function of the intestinal brush border membrane have attracted considerable interest. Thus, deoxycholate at concentrations of 5 and 10 mM causes net water secretion, alteration in permeability to inulin, dextran, and albumin, release of DNA and sucrase, and ultrastructural changes of epithelial cells and cell exfoliation, particularly at the villus tips of small intestine of hamster (GULLIKSON et al. 1977) and of ileal mucosa of rabbit (GAGINELLA et al. 1977). Several other anionic, cationic, and nonionic surfactants were shown to accelerate the release of protein and phospholipid from the mucosal surface of rat jejunum and, with increasing concentrations, begin to cause membrane damage (WHITMORE et al. 1979; BRYAN et al. 1980).

Studies of lipid absorption under these conditions have not been reported; they are likely to show a decrease in intestinal lipid absorption rather than an increase. This view can be supported by recent findings that neomycin and its *N*-methylated derivative, which retains the polycationic properties of the original molecule, but is devoid of antibiotic activity, affect the permeability of the intestinal absorptive membrane of rats in a manner similar to surfactants, without causing an increase in the secretion of very low density lipoproteins (KESSLER et al. 1978) by intestinal mucosa.

III. Interference with Intracellular Events of Intestinal Lipid and Lipoprotein Metabolism

Following the uptake of lypolytic products by absorptive intestinal epithelial cells, a series of biochemical reactions takes place, starting with the activation of long-chain fatty acids, which is a prerequisite step for the subsequent reesterification of absorbed lipids.

1. Physiology of Lipid Reesterification

The translocation of long-chain fatty acids from the inner surface of the brush border membrane to the site of activation at the smooth endoplasmic reticulum (SER) is facilitated by a fatty acid binding protein (FABP) (OCKNER et al. 1972a; OCKNER and MANNING 1974) which, in addition to this carrier function, increases the activity of both microsomal and mitochondrial acyl-CoA synthetase (OCKNER and MANNING 1976; BURNETT et al. 1979). Experimentally in vitro, this carrier function can be inhibited by flavaspidic acid and α-bromopalmitate which exert an inhibitory effect on the binding of long-chain fatty acids to FABP without affecting uptake of fatty acids by everted jejunal sacs or transacylation (OCKNER and MANNING 1976).

The activation of long-chain fatty acids with CoA requires the presence of ATP and fatty acid CoA ligase (acyl-CoA synthetase, thiokinase) and results in the formation of acyl-CoA, which then serves as acyl donor for both the monoglyceride and the phosphatidic acid pathways of triglyceride synthesis (for review see GANGL and OCKNER 1975b). In the monoglyceride pathway, acyl-CoA is esterified by acyl-CoA monoglyceride acyltransferase with absorbed monoglyceride to diglyceride, which then is esterified to triglyceride by acyl-CoA diglyceride acyltransferase. These lipid reesterifying enzymes are located at the SER in close proximity to each other and the entire complex of enzymes is also referred to as triglyceride synthetase (RAO and JOHNSTON 1966). During absorption of the usual dietary fat, which consists mainly of triglycerides, the monoglyceride pathway is the major esterification mechanism and contributes more than 70% of total intestinal triglyceride synthesis (KAYDEN et al. 1967). In the phosphatidic acid pathways α-glycerophosphate, derived mainly from glucose metabolism, is the acyl receptor and this pathway is involved both in triglyceride and in phospholipid synthesis. The fatty acid esterification activity exists along a proximal–distal gradient (DAWSON and ISSELBACHER 1960; CLARK et al. 1973; SHIAU et al. 1979), and along the villus crypt unit fatty acid esterification capacity is concentrated more apically (SHIAU et al. 1980).

The lipid reesterification process can be modified by the presence of the lipid substrate in the intestinal lumen, as indicated by an increase of ileal lipid reesterifying enzyme activities of rats following jejunal removal (RODGERS and BOCHENEK 1970) and a decrease of the lipid reesterifying capacity of the rat small bowel following the reduction of lipid absorption due to complete bile diversion (TANDON et al. 1972) or to parenteral nutrition (KOTLER et al. 1980). Furthermore, in jejunoileal bypass patients, jejunum in continuity possesses higher esterification activity than bypassed jejunum (GOLDBERG et al. 1981).

2. Pharmacologic Modification of Lipid Reesterification

The reesterification of absorbed lipids is susceptible to pharmacologic stimuli as well, however. Thus, it has been shown that the acute intraduodenal administration of ethanol at a dose of 5 g/kg exerts a specific stimulating effect on lipid reesterifying enzymes of the rat small bowel (CARTER et al. 1971; RODGERS and O'BRIEN 1975). On the other hand, the folic acid antagonist, aminopterin, given intramuscularly to rats as a single dose of 250 μg/100 g causes a significant decrease of the specific and total activities of intestinal mucosal fatty acid CoA ligase and monoglyceride acyltransferase. This decrease is most pronounced 3 days after application of aminopterin (FROMM and RODGERS 1971), and results in malabsorption of lipid.

3. Formation and Secretion of Chylomicrons

The next step after uptake of digested lipid from the intestinal lumen and reesterification of absorbed lipid, the formation of chylomicrons and their subsequent transport into lymph, can also be influenced pharmacologically. In this regard, particularly the effects of protein synthesis inhibition and of agents interfering with the assembly of microtubules upon the formation and the secretion of chylomicrons have been studied.

a) Effect of Protein Synthesis Inhibition

The first evidence that protein synthesis in some way could be related to the production and secretion of chylomicrons was derived from observations made in patients with the rare inborn error of lipid metabolism called abetalipoproteinemia. Among other features, this disorder is characterized by undetectable levels of normal apolipoprotein B, absence of low density lipoprotein (LDL) from plasma and extremely low levels of plasma cholesterol (SALT et al. 1960; ISSELBACHER et al. 1964; GOTTO et al. 1971; HERBERT et al. 1978). Patients with this disease are unable to form chylomicrons after a fatty meal and triglyceride accumulates in the absorptive epithelial cells. As apolipoprotein B is the main apoprotein of LDL but is also found in chylomicrons and very low density lipoprotein (VLDL), it was speculated that apolipoprotein B somehow was required for the exit of chylomicrons and VLDL from the absorptive epithelial cell. Reasoning, therefore, that a similar condition could be created experimentally if intestinal synthesis of protein, including apolipoprotein B, were inhibited pharmacologically, rats were injected intraperitoneally with puromycin or with acetoxycycloheximide, which are potent inhibitors of protein synthesis and indeed, after the administration of corn oil by intubation, triglyceride accumulated within the absorptive intestinal cell and rats pretreated in this manner failed to develop the normal postprandial hyperlipemia (SABESIN and ISSELBACHER 1965).

A similarly marked impairment of the intestinal absorption of long-chain fatty acids and triglycerides was observed after the administration of another inhibitor of protein synthesis, DL-ethionine (HYAMS et al. 1966; KARVINEN and MIETTINEN 1966; KESSLER et al. 1969). It was argued by others (REDGRAVE and ZILVERSMIT 1969), however, that protein synthesis inhibitors may have delayed gastric emptying, thus complicating the interpretation of the lipid absorption data. Furthermore, chylomicron release from the small bowel into lymph was observed, despite significant impairment of protein synthesis by the small bowel (REDGRAVE 1969; GLICKMAN et al. 1970). On the other hand, studies have been reported indicating increased portal vein transport of lipid in the form of nonesterified fatty acid after administration of puromycin (KAYDEN and MEDICK 1969) and subsequent experiments (GLICKMAN et al. 1972; GLICKMAN and KIRSCH 1973) clearly demonstrated a diminished recovery of labeled fatty acid from intestinal lymph after intraduodenal administration of micellar lipid under conditions of protein synthesis inhibition by acetoxycycloheximide in the rat. During this protein synthesis inhibition, mesenteric lymph chylomicrons exhibit a dramatic increase in size, which is associated with a decrease of the protein: triglyceride ratio (GLICKMAN et al. 1972) and with significant changes in their apoprotein content (GLICKMAN and KIRSCH 1973). Teleologically, this phenomenon can be regarded as an adaptive mechanism which permits the transport of more triglyceride in fewer but larger particles, thereby conserving surface apoproteins when their supply is limited.

The exact site and mechanism of the interaction of protein synthesis inhibitors with chylomicron formation and secretion is not definitely clear. In view of the many intracellular events required for the conversion of absorbed lipid into completed lipoprotein particles which are ready for secretion into mesenteric lymph, it is likely that impaired protein synthesis may affect the transepithelial lipid and lipoprotein transport in several ways. This view is supported by the experimental demonstration of specific phospholipid biosynthesis inhibition in isolated rat jejunal mucosal cells (O'DOHERTY et al. 1972) and by the finding of a significant impairment of glucosamine ^{14}C incorporation into chylomicrons (YOUSEF and KUKSIS 1972) by puromycin. Furthermore, significant ultrastructural alterations of the rat intestine following puromycin treatment have been described, the most striking being the appearance of large lipid droplets within the absorptive epithelial cell, which apparently fail to enter Golgi vesicles (FRIEDMAN and CARDELL 1972 b). In the rat liver, puromycin also causes ultrastructural changes of the Golgi complex and inhibits glycoprotein synthesis in the Golgi apparatus (STURGESS et al. 1975). These dramatic effects of protein synthesis inhibition upon ultrastructure and specific functions of the Golgi apparatus, associated with significant changes of structure and composition of lymph chylomicrons, are consistent with the current concept that the Golgi apparatus is the site of final assembly of prechylomicrons (KESSLER et al. 1975; SABESIN 1976).

b) Effect of Interference with Microtubules

The final process of lipoprotein completion and secretion from the intestinal epithelial cell can be affected pharmacologically not only by inhibitors of protein synthesis, but also by colchicine, a known inhibitor of microtubular function (WILDON et al. 1974). Microtubules are a system of filaments found in the cytoplasm of eukaryotic cells throughout the animal and plant kingdoms. This organelle participates in a variety of cellular functions, including cell motility, cytoskeletal functions, and mitosis (PORTER 1966; TILNEY 1968; MOHRI 1976; SAKAI 1980). More recent evidence suggests that microtubules may be important also in the directed movement of secretory vesicles and somehow are involved in the transport of a variety of newly synthesized products out of cells (LE MARCHAND et al. 1974; EHRLICH et al. 1974; CHAJEK et al. 1975; NICKERSON et al. 1980), including the hepatocellular transport and release of hepatic lipoproteins (LE MARCHAND et al. 1973; STEIN and STEIN 1973; STEIN et al. 1974; REAVEN and REAVEN 1980) and biliary lipids in the rat (GREGORY et al. 1978).

In the absorptive intestinal epithelial cell, microtubules are localized predominantly in the apical cytoplasm and in the Golgi area (REAVEN and REAVEN 1977;

PAVELKA and GANGL 1978; GANGL et al. 1979), regions known to be associated with lipid transport, and the microtubule content within the apical and Golgi regions is significantly reduced during the absorption of a fat-containing meal (REAVEN and REAVEN 1977). In rats, the administration of colchicine (0.05–5 mg/kg) or of vinblastine sulfate (40 mg/kg) also reduces the microtubule content of enterocytes greatly, thereby causing an accumulation of lipid in apical regions of enterocytes (REAVEN and REAVEN 1977; GLICKMAN et al. 1976). Colchicine-treated rats with indwelling mesenteric lymph cannulas show a marked delay as well as a decrease in the lymphatic absorption of oleic acid ^{14}C (GLICKMAN et al. 1976). During micellar lipid absorption (GLICKMAN et al. 1976), during absorption of ingested margarine emulsion (ARREAZA-PLAZA et al. 1976), and even in the fasting state (GANGL et al. 1979), colchicine causes a severalfold increase of intestinal mucosal triglyceride, indicating that the impairment of lipid transport induced by colchicine takes place at a site distal to triglyceride resynthesis. Contrary to the effect of protein synthesis inhibitors (GLICKMAN and KIRSCH 1973), colchicine does not induce alterations in the apolipoprotein content of lymph chylomicrons (GLICKMAN et al. 1976). Taking these observations together and considering the delay in the lymphatic absorption of oleic acid ^{14}C (GLICKMAN et al. 1976) and the absence of a rise in plasma triglyceride concentration after a fatty meal in rats treated with 5 mg/kg colchicine (ARREAZA-PLAZA et al. 1976), the impairment in lipid transport induced by colchicine and vinblastine sulfate is envisioned as an "exit block" (GLICKMAN et al. 1976).

IV. Interactions with Intestinal Metabolism of Plasma Free Fatty Acids

The fractional uptake of plasma free fatty acids (FFA) by small bowel mucosa in the fasting state was estimated in rats as 1% (GANGL and OCKNER 1975a) and in humans as 0.7% (GANGL and RENNER 1978). It is well established that serum albumin is the major carrier of the FFA in the plasma and the characteristics of the binding of fatty acid to plasma albumin have been explored in great detail (SPECTOR 1975; WOSILAIT et al. 1976).

As it has been suggested that the unbound fraction of a fatty acid is an obligatory intermediate in the translocation of a fatty acid from the albumin to a cell surface (SPECTOR et al. 1965; SPECTOR 1968) and this fraction is very small (0.009–0.4 μmol/l) (WOSILAIT et al. 1976), it appears that the rate of dissociation of palmitate from albumin may be of great importance and might be affected pharmacologically. Indeed, chlorophenoxyisobutyrate, a hypolipidemic drug, was shown in vitro effectively to displace palmitate from a palmitate–bovine ^{14}C serum albumin complex (MEISNER 1975). However, no studies have been published so far, regarding this consideration with respect to intestinal uptake and metabolism of plasma FFA in vivo.

It was shown that, compared with fasting rats, the intraduodenal infusion of glucose is associated with a slight decrease in the concentration of plasma FFA and of mucosal FFA concentration, but does not affect mucosal metabolism of intravenous palmitate ^{14}C, while an intraduodenal ethanol infusion inhibits mucosal oxidation of plasma FFA by 60% and increases their incorporation into triglycerides about twofold (GANGL and OCKNER 1975a).

The intraduodenal infusion of sodium taurocholate at concentrations of 10 and 30 m*M* does not affect the intestinal mucosal uptake and metabolism of plasma FFA (GANGL 1975). The intravenous injection of 3 μg/kg glucagon is followed by a slight decrease of intravenous palmitate ^{14}C uptake by intestinal mucosa and by an increase of mucosal oxidation of plasma palmitate (GANGL 1975). The contribution of plasma FFA to intestinal mucosal and lymph triglycerides is minimal in the fasting state, but increases during fat absorption (GANGL and OCKNER 1975a). It is conceivable that this contribution of plasma FFA to intestinal mucosal and mesenteric lymph triglycerides may be affected by certain drugs as well, yet detailed studies have not been published.

D. Agents which Affect the Intestinal Permeability to Lipids in a More Complex Manner

I. Ethanol

Ethanol has long been known as a drug and is widely used (and abused) as a nutrient. The well-known hepatic and gastrointestinal manifestations of chronic alcoholism include alcoholic liver disease (which may be complicated by portal hypertension, associated with ascites and esophageal varices), pancreatitis, gastritis, gastrointestinal motor dysfunction, diarrhea, and several malabsorption syndromes (for review see BODE 1980; VAN THIEL et al. 1981). Furthermore, marked effects of acute exposure of the small intestine to ethanol on intestinal transport of sugar, amino acids, water, minerals, and electrolytes have been described (for review see WILSON and HOYUMPA 1979; BECK and DINDA 1981). As steatorrhea is a well-known finding in alcoholics with (BARAONA et al. 1962; LINSCHEER et al. 1966; SUN et al. 1967) or without (ROGGIN et al. 1969; MEZEY et al. 1970) liver cirrhosis and the effect of ethanol upon the transport of dietary lipids across the intestinal mucosal epithelium has not been studied directly, it seems justified to discuss at least briefly several effects of ethanol which may contribute to alterations in the intestinal absorption and metabolism of lipids.

Larger doses of ethanol (3 g/kg or more) administered acutely into the stomach of rats simultaneously with corn oil, delay the absorption of the oil markedly (BARBORIAK and MEADE 1969; BOQUILLON 1976), probably owing to the retention of lipids in the stomach (BARBORIAK and MEADE 1970; BOQUILLON 1976). However, inconsistent results have been reported with respect to the effect of ethanol on gastric emptying (FRANKEN 1928; BARLOW et al. 1936; BREWSTER et al. 1966; BARBORIAK and MEADE 1970; KAUFMAN and KAYE 1979; MOORE et al. 1981) ranging from delaying effects, via no effect at all, to enhancing effects. A major causative factor for fat malabsorption in chronic alcoholics most likely is a reduction in pancreatic lipase activity (pancreatic insufficiency) due to chronic pancreatitis (FAST 1959; GOEBELL et al. 1970; FILIPPINI and LÖFFLER 1972; ROGGIN et al. 1972; SARLES 1974; SARLES et al. 1977).

Contrary to the studies referred to thus far, studies of the effect of exposure of the small intestine to ethanol provide information which is more directly relevant to intestinal permeability. After acute ethanol intake, controversial morphological effects have been reported, however. While HAYTON (1975) found no structural changes of the rat jejunal epithelium after in vivo perfusion with ethanol at low concentration (0.05%) and the duodenal mucosa of dogs showed no histologic abnormality after exposure to a solution of 20% ethanol (HIMAL and GREENBERG 1977), GILLESPIE and LUCAS (1961) described intestinal hemorrhage in 15% of malnourished rats after the intragastric administration of ethanol at a concentration ranging from 12%to 76%. Following intragastric administration of ethanol in concentrations ranging from 5% to 49%, BARAONA et al. (1974) observed epithelial damage, which was most pronounced at the villus tips and appears to be dose related. Similar morphological alterations of the intestinal mucosa owing to exposure to ethanol were reported more recently (HOYUMPA et al. 1975; DINDA et al. 1975; BROITMAN et al. 1976; FOX et al. 1978; MILLAN et al. 1980). The influence of these morphological changes of the absorptive epithelium on the permeability to lipids has not been studied directly; however, the findings of MENDENHALL et al. (1974) that, in rats, ethanol enhanced the appearance of orally administered labeled tripalmitin in the chyle and stimulated lipid uptake by isolated mucosal cells, and the observations of BARAONA and LIEBER (1975) of an increased output of dietary lipids into the lymph during acute administration of ethanol suggest an increased permeability of the intestinal mucosa during acute ethanol administration.

The enhanced transport of dietary fat from the intestinal lumen into mesenteric lymph during the acute administration of ethanol-containing diets is associated with a marked increase in intestinal lymph flow (BARAONA and LIEBER 1975). As the intraduodenal injection of neostigmine (0.05 mg/kg) or the intraduodenal infusion of large amounts of saline, which also cause an increased lymph flow, are associated with an enhanced output of intraduodenally administered labeled fatty acids into mesenteric lymph as well (BARAONA and LIEBER 1975), it is likely, that an increase in the mesenteric lymph flow per se enhances the transmucosal fat transport by an as yet unknown mechanism.

Chronic administration of ethanol is also followed by ultrastructural changes of the intestinal mucosal epithelium. In jejunal and ileal villi of rats, degenerative alterations of microvilli and mitochondria and dilation of the SER and of the Golgi cisternae were observed (RUBIN et al. 1972; KRAWITT et al. 1975; WORTHINGTON et al. 1978). But, contrary to the acute administration of ethanol, chronic ethanol ingestion was shown to result in a moderate decrease of intestinal fat absorption (BARAONA and LIEBER 1975).

In addition to structural alterations of the intestinal mucosa, important functional effects of ethanol on the intestinal lipid metabolism have been described, which also may affect the intestinal permeability to lipids. In rats, the constant intraduodenal infusion of ethanol (5 g/kg) over a period of 8 h is associated with a fourfold increase of intestinal mucosal triglyceride levels and a significant increase of intestinal lymph output of endogenous triglyceride and phospholipid (MISTILIS and OCKNER 1972). Furthermore, ethanol was shown to decrease oxidation of endogenous fatty acids by intestinal mucosa (GANGL and OCKNER 1974, 1975a) and to enhance the activities of intestinal enzymes (acyl-CoA synthetase, acyl-CoA monoglyceride acyltransferase) involved in lipid absorption (CARTER et al. 1971; RODGERS and O'BRIEN 1975).

Thus, the effect of ethanol on the intestinal permeability to lipids is complex indeed, including effects on the permeability of the plasma membrane, effects on intracellular metabolic processes, particularly fatty acid activation, esterification, and oxidation, and effects on the mesenteric lymph flow. Detailed studies are required, however, to determine more directly the effect of ethanol on the intestinal mucosal membrane permeability, and on the various intracellular steps of the transepithelial lipid transport.

II. Hormones

1. Cholecystokinin and Secretin

The gastrointestinal hormones cholecystokinin and secretin (for review see RAYFORD et al. 1976; JOHNSON 1977) are thought to play an important role in the physiology of fat absorption. Cholecystokinin, an effective stimulant of pancreatic enzyme secretion (STENING and GROSSMAN 1969), gallbladder contraction (AMER 1969), and bile flow (JONES and GROSSMAN 1970) is released from cholecystokinin-secreting cells of intestinal mucosa (POLAK et al. 1975) by amino acids (ERTAN et al. 1971; JOHNSON 1974), fatty acids, and other nutrients (MEYER 1975) when they enter the duodenal and small intestinal lumen from the stomach. The cholecystokinin-induced secretion of pancreatic enzymes is further stimulated by secretin (for review see JOHNSON 1977). Pharmacologic interactions with these "regulatory chemical messengers" (GROSSMAN 1979) are conceivable, the effect of such interactions upon the intestinal permeability to lipids in a broader sense has not yet been explored.

2. Somatostatin

Somatostatin, a known suppressor of pancreatic exocrine secretion (BODEN 1975; BLOOM et al. 1975) predictably should interfere with intestinal triglyceride hydrolysis. Indeed an intravenous bolus of 1 mg somatostatin and the subsequent intravenous infusion of 1 mg/h somatostatin over a period of 3 h in ten healthy volunteers prevented the expected increase in serum triglyceride after a test meal containing 100 g neutral fat (POINTNER et al. 1977). However, pancreatic lipase activity or intestinal mucosal functions were not studied in this investigation. Nevertheless, by steady state perfusion experiments with either glucose- and amino acid-containing test solutions or a plasma-like electrolyte solution in the jejunum of healthy subjects, it was demonstrated by others (KREJS et al. 1980), however, that during intravenous somatostatin infusion, 8 $\mu g\ kg^{-1}\ h^{-1}$, glucose and amino acid absorption were inhibited by a direct effect on the intestinal mucosa, possibly by a selective reduction of functional mucosal surface area of the intestine.

3. Corticosteroids

Studies performed by RODGERS et al. (1967) in adrenalectomized rats in vivo suggest that adrenal corticosteroids are required for the maintenance of normal intestinal absorption of fatty acids and triglycerides. As adrenalectomized rats exhibited malabsorption not only of triglycerides, but of free fatty acids as well, it seemed likely that adrenalectomy interferes with intestinal mucosal function rather than with the intraluminal process of triglyceride hydrolysis. In vitro experiments in intestinal slices of adrenalectomized rats indeed demonstrated an abnormal mucosal cell function and showed that the lack of adrenal corticosteroids was associated with decreased activities of intestinal thiokinase, monoglyceride acylase, and diglyceride acylase. When adrenalectomized rats received hydrocortisone, the activities of the lipid esterifying enzymes not only returned to the normal range, but became even greater than normal (RODGERS et al. 1967).

4. Insulin

More recently the effect of insulin on in vitro intestinal fatty acid esterification was studied by SHIAU and HOLTZAPPLE (1980) in the rat. Although glucose metabolism plays an important role in modifying intestinal fatty acid esterification (SHIAU et al. 1978), insulin itself has no effect on intestinal fatty acid esterification (SHIAU and HOLTZAPPLE 1980).

5. Glucagon

Contrary to insulin, glucagon administered intravenously as a bolus of 3 μg/kg in the rat is followed by a slight, but statistically significant decrease of the intestinal uptake of plasma FFA and by an increase of their intestinal oxidation at the expense of their esterification (GANGL 1975).

6. Sex Hormones

Profound sex differences in the utilization of long-chain fatty acids at concentrations within and below the physiologic range have been shown in rat hepatocyte suspensions and attributed to corresponding differences in cytosolic FABP concentration (OCKNER et al. 1979). Whether similar differences exist in enterocytes, where FABP also serves important functions in the cellular utilization of long-chain fatty acids (OCKNER et al. 1972a, b; OCKNER and MANNING 1964, 1976; O'DOHERTY and KUKSIS 1975) has not been explored and one could only speculate about possible pharmacologic implications.

These few examples of hormonal interactions with intestinal lipid absorption and metabolism provide only scanty hints for a possible endocrine regulation of the intestinal permeability to lipids and demonstrate that much more work is needed to explore this area more precisely.

III. Cytostatic Agents

Cytostatic chemotherapy aims at the suppression of tumor cell proliferation. The suppressive effect of cytostatic agents is not confined to tumor cells, however, but is seen in normal cells as well, particularly in those with a high rate of turnover. Many side effects of cytostatic therapy can be explained on this account (e.g., leuko- and thrombocytopenia, due to suppression of the hematopoietic system). As small bowel mucosa is characterized by a rapid turnover of its epithelial cells, resulting in complete renewal of the mucosal lining every 4–6 days (for review see

WEINSTEIN 1974; EASTWOOD 1977), it is not surprising that mitotic inhibition, loss and damage of intestinal cells, accompanied by mucosal dysfunction have been demonstrated repeatedly after the administration of a variety of cytostatic agents (for review see ECKNAUER and ROMMEL 1978). The effect of cytostatic chemotherapy upon lipid absorption or intestinal permeability to lipids has received only little attention, however.

1. Cyclophosphamide

Studies in rats pretreated with cyclophosphamide (FLEISCHER and FIEDLER 1973) demonstrated a depression of the pancreatic exocrine secretion of protein and enzymes, including lipase. In patients on cytotoxic treatment for malignancy, a single dose of 30–40 mg/kg cyclophosphamide did not reduce pancreatic lipase output; however, following combination treatment with procarbazine, vincristine, and cyclophosphamide, a significant reduction of pancreatic lipase secretion was observed (FLEISCHER and MECKEL 1975). Intestinal fat absorption was not studied in this investigation. Whether the observed depression of pancreatic enzyme secretion is due to a nonspecific pancreatic lesion resulting from cytotoxic drug administration, to protein synthesis inhibition, or both, remains to be clarified.

2. Aminopterin

The folic acid antagonist, aminopterin does not affect lipase activity of the biliary–pancreatic secretions of rats after intramuscular application at a dose of 250 μg per 100 g body weight, and the marked reduction in the absorption of octanoic acid and trioctanoate observed under these conditions was attributed to a reduction of the absorptive surface area (VALDIVIESO and SCHWABE 1965).

More detailed studies in humans showed, that the intravenous injection of 2–5 mg/kg aminopterin is followed by a dramatic mitotic inhibition of jejunal epithelium for at least 48 h (TRIER 1962a), and by marked ultrastructural changes of villous absorptive and other intestinal mucosal cells (TRIER 1962b). These alterations resolve spontaneously by 96 h after aminopterin administration (TRIER 1962a, b). An inhibitory effect of aminopterin on the absorption of fat into the lymph was demonstrated in unanesthetized rats, by a technique of steady duodenal perfusion (REDGRAVE and SIMMONDS 1967). This inhibitory effect on fat absorption can be related to the age of the intestinal mucosal cells: after inhibition of mitosis with 250 μg intramuscular aminopterin, the absorption of olive oil emulsions remains normal for 32 h and is then severely impaired for a period of 2 days. On the fifth day after aminopterin administration, which is about 24 h after the recommencement of mitosis in the crypts, fat absorption begins to recover (REDGRAVE and SIMMONDS 1967). Although aminopterin exerts its toxic effects mainly by directly inhibiting DNA synthesis (MARGOLIS et al. 1971), the effect of aminopterin on the mucosal phase of fat absorption is not confined to the inhibition of cell renewal, causing a reduction of the absorptive surface area, but includes also an inhibitory effect on the specific activities of intestinal lipid reesterifying enzymes (FROMM and RODGERS 1971) and possibly interferes with the process of lipoprotein production and secretion as well. The profound effects of protein synthesis inhibition by acetoxycycloheximide (SABESIN and ISSELBACHER 1965; GLICKMAN et al. 1972; GLICKMAN and KIRSCH 1973), puromycine (SABESIN and ISSELBACHER 1965; KAYDEN and MEDICK 1969; YOUSEF and KUKSIS 1972; O'DOHERTY et al. 1972; FRIEDMAN and CARDELL 1972b) and DL-ethionine (HYAMS et al. 1966; KARVINEN and MIETTINEN 1966; KESSLER et al. 1969) and the effects of colchicine, an inhibitor of microtubular function (GLICKMAN et al. 1976; ARREAZA-PLAZA et al. 1976; REAVEN and REAVEN 1977; GANGL et al. 1979) upon intestinal lipoprotein production and secretion have been discussed earlier in this chapter.

3. 5-Fluorouracil

An other metabolite, 5-fluorouracil, which is widely used in the treatment of advanced gastrointestinal cancer, appears to inhibit both pancreatic zymogen production and lipase secretion (KUGLER et al. 1967) and causes morphological and functional changes of intestinal mucosa (LEVIN 1968; HARTWICH et al. 1974). Everted sac preparations of rats pretreated by daily intramuscular injections of 5-fluorouracil (12.5 mg/kg) for 5 days exhibited a significant reduction in the uptake of palmitic acid ^{14}C (CAPEL et al. 1979), however, more detailed studies of the effect of 5-fluorouracil on the intestinal lipid absorption have not been published.

In the light of the extensive use of cytotoxic chemotherapy in the treatment of many, mostly malignant, diseases, which often feature malnutrition, the further exploration of the interactions of cytotoxic drugs with intestinal fat absorption has important clinical implications and represents an intriguing and promising area for future research.

IV. Dietary Fiber

Dietary fibers are the various constituents of plant foods that cannot be digested and absorbed by the human gastrointestinal tract. They represent a heterogeneous mixture of water-insoluble (cellulose, lignin, many hemicelluloses) and water-soluble substances (Pectins, some hemicelluloses, mucilages, gums, polysaccharides, etc.), which are mostly carbohydrates. The decreasing intake of these natural components of human food has been linked to the development of disease in civilized societies (for review see KELSAY 1978; MATZKIES and BERG 1978) and therefore more recently the enrichment of human food or diets with dietary fiber has been proposed for treatment of a variety of health disorders, including spastic colon, constipation, and diverticular disease of the colon, and as a therapeutic or prophylactic adjuvant in various disorders of glucose, lipid, and lipoprotein metabolism (for review see KELSAY 1978; ANDERSON and CHEN 1979).

Although conflicting results have been reported with regard to the effect of dietary fiber upon plasma lipid levels of experimental animals and humans, varying from virtually no effect on plasma cholesterol and triglyceride (ANTONIS and

BERSOHN 1962 b; PRATHER 1964; EASTWOOD et al. 1973; BREMNER et al. 1975; CONNELL et al. 1975; DURRINGTON et al. 1975; HUTH and FETTEL 1975; JENKINS et al. 1975 a; TRUSWELL 1975; WALTERS et al. 1975; HEATON et al. 1976), to significant reduction of plasma cholesterol (KEYS et al. 1960, 1961; DE GROOT et al. 1963; GRANDE et al. 1965; PALMER and DIXON 1966; MATHUR et al. 1968; SHURPALEKAR et al. 1971; MENON and KURUP 1974; JENKINS et al. 1975 b; PERSSON et al. 1976; DURRINGTON et al. 1976; KIRBY et al. 1981), plasma triglyceride (EASTWOOD 1969; HEATON and POMARE 1974), or both (CHEN et al. 1981), these results warrant a brief consideration of mechanisms by which dietary fiber might affect intestinal permeability to lipids.

Changes in gastrointestinal motility are likely to affect intestinal fat absorption, and indeed profound effects of dietary fiber on gastrointestinal motility have been observed: the rate of gastric emptying is decreased by dietary fiber (JENKINS et al. 1978; HOLT et al. 1979; MALAGELADA et al. 1980) and gastrointestinal transit has been described as accelerated (MCCANCE et al. 1953; PAYLER 1973, PAYLER et al. 1975; WALKER 1975). Contradictory observations have been reported however (EASTWOOD et al. 1973; HARVEY et al. 1973) and studies of the effects of fiber-induced motility alterations on intestinal fat absorption have not been published.

Intraluminal binding of absorbable lipid or of bile salts by dietary fiber would be another possibility of interference with intestinal fat absorption. Particularly lignin, a predominantly aromatic and water-insoluble, major component of vegetable fiber was shown to adsorb bile salts by hydrophobic bonding (EASTWOOD and HAMILTON 1968). Furthermore, evidence has been presented that pectin lowers plasma and liver cholesterol levels in cholesterol-fed rats by inhibiting bile acid absorption and also by reducing cholesterol absorption (LEVEILLE and SAUBERLICH 1966). Intraluminal binding of bile acids and cholesterol by certain fractions of dietary fiber and the acceleration of the gastrointestinal transit presumably are causally related to the finding of increased amounts of bile acids and sterols (ANTONIS and BERSOHN 1962; SHURPALEKAR et al. 1971; MENON and KURUP 1974; WALTERS et al. 1975; KIRBY et al. 1981), fatty acids (ANTONIS and BERSOHN 1962 a), and lipids (SOUTHGATE and DURNIN 1970; WALKER 1975; BRODRIBB and HUMPHREYS 1976; SOUTHGATE et al. 1976) in stools during increased fiber intake.

Pectins, gums, mucilages, and storage polysaccharides may form gels in the small bowel lumen (MCCONNELL et al. 1974) which may interact with the unstirred layer or acidic microclimate at the interface between luminal contents and absorptive surface, however, these aspects have not been investigated with regard to intestinal permeability to lipids. Removal of fiber from the diet of weanling rats was found to delay villus development into broad ridges in the jejunum of maturing rats, while feeding a diet containing 10% pectin induced villus evolution (TASMAN-JONES et al. 1978), but again the effect of such morphological consequences of dietary fiber on the intestinal permeability to lipids has not been studied. Thus it appears that, despite the existence of a large body of evidence for a profound effect of dietary fiber upon the intestinal absorption of lipids, our present knowledge of the mechanisms of such interactions of dietary fiber and intestinal permeability to lipids is scanty and further studies are needed to unravel those mechanisms.

E. Concluding Remarks

The permeation of the intestinal mucosa by dietary or endogenous lipids from the intestinal lumen or by lipids derived from the plasma pool involves a series of physical and biochemical processes, which has been explored in many details. Virtually every step in this sequence of reactions can be modified by drugs. As a matter of fact, pharmacologic interference with distinct steps of fat absorption and of intestinal metabolism of lipids offered to the mucosa from the lumen or from the plasma pool is a valuable experimental tool both in vitro and in vivo.

From a clinical point of view, it is remarkable that the intestinal permeability to lipids is susceptible to influences exhibited by substances commonly used in health and disease, for instance, ethanol, dietary fiber, and possibly sex hormones (contraceptives). And although the physiology and pathophysiology of intestinal lipid absorption are well explored, present knowledge of the interactions of these substances with the intestinal permeability to lipids is very limited and needs to be improved. Furthermore, cytostatic and immunosuppressive chemotherapy appears to exert profound effects upon the structure and function of intestinal mucosa which in part are intimately related to the intestinal permeability to lipids; as such drugs are frequently used repeatedly for long periods in diseases featuring malnutrition, the further exploration of the interactions of cytotoxic drugs with intestinal fat absorption also has important clinical implications.

References

Alpers DH, Seetharam B (1977) Pathophysiology of diseases involving intestinal brush-border proteins. N Engl J Med 296:1047–1050

Amer MS (1969) Studies with cholecystokinin. II. Cholecystokinetic potency of porcine gastrins I and II and related peptides in three systems. Endocrinology 84:1277–1281

Anderson JW, Chen WJL (1979) Plant fiber. Carbohydrate and lipid metabolism. Am J Clin Nutr 32:346–363

Antonis A, Bersohn I (1962a) The influence of diet on fecal lipids in South African white and Bantu prisoners. Am J Clin Nutr 11:142–155

Antonis A, Bersohn I (1962b) The influence of diet on serum lipids in South African white and Bantu prisoners. Am J Clin Nutr 10:484–499

Arreaza-Plaza CA, Bosch V, Otayek MA (1976) Lipid transport across the intestinal epithelial cell. Effect of colchicine. Biochim Biophys Acta 431:297–302

Baraona E, Lieber CS (1975) Intestinal lymph formation and fat absorption: Stimulation by acute ethanol administration and inhibition by chronic ethanol feeding. Gastroenterology 68:495–502

Baraona E, Orrego H, Fernandez O, Amenabar E, Maldonado E, Tag F, Salinas A (1962) Absorptive function of the small intestine in liver cirrhosis. Am J Dig Dis 7:318–330

Baraona E, Pirola RC, Lieber CS (1974) Small intestinal damage and changes in cell population produced by ethanol ingestion in the rat. Gastroenterology 66:226–234

Barboriak JJ, Meade RC (1969) Impairment of gastrointestinal processing of fat and protein by ethanol in rats. J Nutr 98:373–377

Barboriak JJ, Meade RC (1970) Effect of alcohol on gastric emptying in man. Am J Clin Nutr 62:1151–1153

Barlow OW, Beams AJ, Goldblatt H (1936) Studies on the pharmacology of ethyl alcohol. I. A comprehensive study of pharmacologic effects of grain and synthetic alcohols. J Pharmacol 56:117–146

Beck IT, Dinda PK (1981) Acute exposure of small intestine to ethanol. Effects on morphology and function. Dig Dis Sci New Series 26:817–838

Bennett S, Shepherd P, Simmonds WJ (1962) The effect of alterations in intestinal motility induced by morphine and atropine on fat absorption in the rat. Aust J Exp Biol Med Sci 40:225–232
Bergeron JJM, Ehrenreich JH, Siekevitz P, Palade GE (1973) Golgi functions prepared from rat liver homogenates. II. Biochemical characterization. J Cell Biol 59:73–88
Bizzi A, Veneroni E, Garattini S (1973) Effect of fenfluramine on the intestinal absorption of triglycerides. Eur J Pharmacol 23:131–136
Bloom SR, Joffe SN, Polak JM (1975) Effect of somatostatin on pancreatic and biliary function. Gut 16:836–837
Bode JC (1980) Alcohol and the gastrointestinal tract. In: Frick P, Von Harnack GA, Martini GA, Prader A (eds) Advances in internal medicine and pediatrics, vol 45. Springer, Berlin Heidelberg New York, pp 1–75
Boden G (1975) Somatostatin suppresses secretin and pancreatic exocrine secretion. Science 190:163–165
Bond JH Jr, Levitt MD (1975) Investigation of small bowel transit time in man utilizing pulmonary hydrogen (H_2) measurements. J Lab Clin Med 85:546–555
Boquillon M (1976) Effect of acute ethanol ingestion on fat absorption. Lipids 11:848–852
Borgström B (1954) On the mechanism of pancreatic lipolysis of glycerides. Biochim Biophys Acta 13:491–504
Borgström B, Erlanson C (1973) Pancreatic lipase and Co-lipase. Interactions and effects of bile salts and other detergents. Eur J Biochem 37:60–68
Borgström B, Wollesen C (1981) Effect of fenfluramine and related compounds on the pancreatic colipase/lipase system. FEBS Lett 126:25–28
Bremner WF, Brooks PM, Third JLHC, Lawrie TDV (1975) Bran in triglyceridemia. A failure of response. Br Med J 3:574
Brewster AC, Lankford HG, Schwartz MG, Sullivan JF (1966) Ethanol and alimentary lipemia. Am J Clin Nutr 19:255–259
Brodribb AJM, Humphreys DM (1976) Diverticular disease: three studies. Br Med J 1:424–430
Broitman SA, Gottlieb LS, Vitale JJ (1976) Augmentation of ethanol absorption by mono- and disaccharides. Gastroenterology 70:1101–1107
Bryan AJ, Kaur R, Robinson G, Thomas NW, Wilson CG (1980) Changes in rat intestine exposed to polyethylene glycol 2000 and polyoxyethylene (40) stearate. Br J Pharmacol 72:557P–558P
Burnett DA, Lysenko N, Manning JA, Ockner RK (1979) Utilization of long chain fatty acids by rat liver: studies of the role of fatty acid binding protein. Gastroenterology 77:241–249
Capel ID, Pinnock MH, Williams DC (1979) An in vitro assessment of the effect of cytotoxic drugs upon the intestinal absorption of nutrients in rats. Eur J Cancer 15:127–131
Carey MC, Small DM (1970) the characteristics of mixed micellar solutions with particular reference to bile. Am J Med 49:590–608
Carey MC, Small DM (1972) Micelle formation by bile salts. Physical-chemical and thermodynamic considerations. Arch Intern Med 130:506–527
Carter EA, Drummey GD, Isselbacher KJ (1971) Ethanol stimulates triglyceride synthesis by the intestine. Science 174:1245–1247
Chajek T, Stein O, Stein Y (1975) Interference with the transport of heparin-releasable lipoprotein lipase in the perfused rat heart by colchicine and vinblastine. Biochim Biophys Acta 388:260–267
Chen WJL, Anderson JW, Gould MR (1981) Effects of oat bran, oat gum and pectin on lipid metabolism of cholesterol-fed rats. Nutr Rep Int 24:1093–1098
Christofides ND, Modlin IM, Fitzpatrick ML, Bloom SR (1979) Effect of motilin on the rate of gastric emptying and gut hormone release during breakfast. Gastroenterology 76:903–907
Christofides ND, Long RG, Fitzpatrick ML, McGregor GP, Bloom SR (1981) Effect of motilin on the gastric emptying of glucose and fat in humans. Gastroenterology 80:456–460

Clark SB, Lawergran B, Martin JV (1973) Regional intestinal absorptive capacities for triolein: an alternative to markers. Am J Physiol 225:574–585

Comai K, Triscari J, Sullivan AC (1978) Comparative effects of amphetamine and fenfluramine on lipid biosynthesis and absorption in the rat. Biochem Pharmacol 27:1987–1994

Connell AM, Smith CL, Somsel M (1975) Absence of effect of bran on blood lipids. Lancet 1:496–497

Danhof IE (1966) the effct of cholestyramine on fecal excretion of ingested radioiodinated lipids. Am J Clin Nutr 18:343–349

Dannenburg WN, Ward JW (1971) The inhibitory effect of fenfluramine on pancreatic lipase activity. Arch Int Pharmacodyn Ther 191:58–65

Dannenburg WN, Kardian BC, Norell LY (1973) Fenfluramine and triglyceride synthesis by microsomes of the intestinal mucosa in the rat. Arch Int Pharmacodyn Ther 201:115–124

Dawson AM, Isselbacher KJ (1960) The esterification of palmitate-1-C by homogenates of intestinal mucosa. J Clin Invest 39:150–160

Debnam ES, Levin RJ (1975) Effects of fasting and semi-starvation on the kinetics of active and passive sugar absorption across small intestine in vivo. J Physiol (Lond) 252:681–700

De Groot AP, Luyken R, Pikaar NA (1963) Cholesterol-lowering effect of rolled oats. Lancet 2:303–304

De Haas GHA, Slotboom AJ, Verheij HM, Jansen EH, De Aroujo JM, Vidal JC (1978) Interaction of phospholipase A_2 with lipid-water interfaces. Adv Prostaglandin Tromboxane Res 3:11–21

De Somer P, Vanderhaeghe H, Eyssen H (1964) Influence of basic antibiotics on serum and liver cholesterol concentration in chicks. Nature 204:1306

Dietschy JM (1968) Mechanisms for the intestinal absorption of bile acids. J Lipid Res 9:297–309

Di Magno EP, Go VLW, Summerskill WHJ (1972) Impaired cholecystokinin-pancreozymin secretion, intraluminal dilution and maldigestion of fat in sprue. Gastroenterology 63:25–32

Dinda PK, Beck IT, Beck M, McElligot TF (1975) Effect of ethanol on sodium-dependent glucose transport in the small intestine of the hamster. Gastroenterology 68:1517–1526

Durrington P, Wicks ACB, Heaton KH (1975) Effect of bran on blood lipids. Lancet 2:133

Durrington PN, Manning AP, Bolton CH, Hartog M (1976) Effect of pectin on serum lipids and lipoproteins, wholegut transit time and stool weight. Lancet 2:394–396

Eastwood GL (1977) Gastrointestinal epithelial renewal. Gastroenterology 72:962–975

Eastwood M (1969) Dietary fiber and serum-lipids. Lancet 2:1222–1224

Eastwood MA, Hamilton D (1968) Studies on the adsorption of bile salts to nonabsorbed components of diet. Biochim Biophys Acta 152:165–173

Eastwood MA, Kirkpatrick JR, Mitchell WD, Bone A, Hamilton T (1973) Effects of dietary supplements of wheat bran and cellulose on faeces and bowel function. Br Med J 4:392–394

Ecknauer R, Rommel K (1978) Zytostatica und Dünndarm. Klin Wochenschr 56:579–592

Ehrlich HP, Ross R, Bornstein P (1974) Effects of anti-microtubular agents on the secretion of collagen. A Biochemical and morphological study. J Cell Biol 62:390–405

Ertan A, Brooks FP, Ostrow JD, Arvan DA, Williams CN, Cerda JJ (1971) Effect of jejunal amino acid perfusion and exogenous cholecystokinin on the exocrine pancreatic and biliary secretions in man. Gastroenterology 61:686–692

Falloon WW, Paes IC, Woolfolk D, Nankin H, Wallace K, Haro EN (1966) Effect of neomycin and kanamycin upon intestinal absorption. Ann NY Acad Sci 132:879–887

Fast BB, Wolfe SJ, Stormont JM, Davidson CS (1959) Fat absorption in alcoholics with cirrhosis. Gastroenterology 37:321–324

Filippini L, Löffler A (1972) Exokrine Pankreasfunktion bei chronischem Alkoholkonsum. Dtsch Med Wochenschr 97:596–600

Fleischer K, Fiedler R (1973) die Wirkung von Cyclophosphamid auf die exkretorische Funktion des Rattenpankreas. Arch Pharmacol 277:R17

Fleischer K, Meckel H (1975) Exocrine pancreatic function in man after cytotoxic treatment. Acta Hepato-Gastroenterol 22:392–398

Fox JE, McElligot TF, Beck IT (1978) Effect of ethanol on the morphology of hamster jejunum. Am J Dig Dis 23:201–209

Franken G (1928) Untersuchungen über Alkohol. VII. Mitteilung: Alkoholwirkungen auf die Magenverdauung. Arch Exp Pathol Pharmakol 134:129–141

Frazer AC (1952) Fat metabolism. Annu Rev Biochem 21:245–272

Friedman HI, Cardell RR Jr (1972 a) Morphological evidence for the release of chylomicra from intestinal absorptive cells. Exp Cell Res 75:57–62

Friedman HI, Cardell RR Jr (1972 b) Effects of puromycin on the structure of rat intestinal epithelial cells during fat absorption. J Cell Biol 52:15–40

Fromm H, Rodgers JB Jr (1971) Effect of aminopterin on lipid absorption: depression of lipid reesterifying enzymes. Am J Physiol 221 (4):998–1003

Gage SH, Fish PA (1924) Fat digestion, absorption, and assimilation in man and animals as determined by the darkfield microscope, and a fat-soluble dye. Am J Anat 34:1–85

Gaginella TS, Lewis JC, Phillips SF (1977) Rabbit ileal mucosa exposed to fatty acids, bile acids, and other secretagogues. Scanning electron microscopic appearances. Am J Digest Dis, New Series 22:781–790

Gallo DG, Bailey KR, Shaffner AL (1965) The interaction between cholestyramine and drugs. Proc Soc Exp Biol Med 120:60–65

Gangl A (1975) Der Fettstoffwechsel des Dünndarms und seine Beziehung zum Lipid- und Lipoproteinstoffwechsel des Gesamt-Organismus. Acta Med Austriaca 2 (Suppl 2) 1–49

Gangl A, Ockner R (1974 a) Intestinal metabolism of plasma free fatty acids. Clin Res 22:358A

Gangl A, Ockner R (1974 b) Intestinal metabolism of plasma free fatty acids. Gastroenterology 66:187A

Gangl A, Ockner RK (1975 a) Intestinal metabolism of plasma free fatty acids. Intracellular compartmentation and mechanisms of control. J Clin Invest 55:803–813

Gangl A, Ockner RK (1975 b) Intestinal metabolism of lipids and lipoproteins. Gastroenterology 68:167–186

Gangl A, Renner F (1978) In vivo metabolism of plasma free fatty acids by intestinal mucosa of man. Gastroenterology 74:847–850

Gangl A, Pavelka M, Klose B (1979) Evidence for functional significance of microtubuli in intestinal transepithelial lipid transport. In: Peeters H (ed) Protides of the biological fluids. Pergamon, Oxford, pp 527–530

Gangl A, Kornauth W, Mlczoch J, Sulm O, Klose B (1980) Different metabolism of saturated and unsaturated long chain plasma free fatty acids by intestinal mucosa of rats. Lipids 15:75–79

Gillespie RJG, Lucas CC (1961) Effect of single intoxicating doses of ethanol on the gastric and intestinal mucosa of rats. Can J Biochem Physiol 39:237–241

Glickman RM, Kirsch K (1973) Lymph chylomicron formation during the inhibition of protein synthesis. J Clin Invest 52:2910–2920

Glickman RM, Alpers DH, Drummey GD, Isselbacher KJ (1970) Increased lymph alkaline phosphatase after fat feeding: effects of medium chain triglycerides and inhibition of protein synthesis. Biochim Biophys Acta 201:226–235

Glickman RM, Kirsch K, Isselbacher KJ (1972) Fat absorption during the inhibition of protein synthesis: studies of lymph chylomicrons. J Clin Invest 51:356–363

Glickman RM, Perotto JL, Kirsch K (1976) Intestinal lipoprotein formation: effect of colchicine. Gastroenterology 70:347–352

Go VLW, Poley JR, Hofmann AF, Summerskill WHJ (1970) Disturbances in fat digestion induced by acidic jejunal pH due to gastric hypersecretion in man. Gastroenterology 58:638–646

Goebell H, Bode C, Bastian H, Strohmeyer G (1970) Klinisch asymptomatische Funktionsstörungen des exokrinen Pankreas bei chronischen Alkoholikern. Dtsch Med Wochenschr 95:808–814

Goldberg PB, Shiau YF, Levine GM, Rosato EF (1981) Intestinal fatty acid esterification activity in jejunoileal bypass patients. Am J Clin Nutr 34:2742–2747

Gotto AM, Levy RI, John K, Fredrickson DS (1971) On the protein defect in abetalipoproteinemia. N Engl J Med 284:813–818

Grande F, Anderson JT, Keys A (1965) Effect of carbohydrates of leguminous seeds, wheat and potatoes on serum cholesterol concentration in man. J Nutr 86:313–317

Greenberger NJ, Skillman TG (1969) Medium-chain triglycerides. Physiologic considerations and clinical implications. N Engl J Med 280:1045–1058

Greenberger NJ, Rodgers JB, Isselbacher KJ (1966) Absorption of medium and long chain triglycerides. Factors influencing their hydrolysis and transport. J Clin Invest 45:217–227

Gregory DH, Vlahcevic ZR, Prugh MF, Swell L (1978) Mechanism of secretion of biliary lipids: role of a microtubular system in hepatocellular transport of biliary lipids in the rat. Gastroenterology 74:93–100

Grossman MI (1979) Chemical messenger: a view from the gut. What shall we call them? Fed Proc 38:2341–2343

Gullikson GW, Cline WS, Lorenzsonn V, Benz L, Olsen WA, Bass P (1977) Effects of anionic surfactants on hamster small intestinal membrane structure and function: Relationship to surface activity. Gastroenterology 73:501–511

Hamosh M, Scow RO (1973) Lingual lipase and its role in the digestion of dietary fat. J Clin Invest 52:88–95

Hamosh M, Klaeveman HL, Wolf RO, Scow RO (1975) Pharyngeal lipase and digestion of dietary triglyceride in man. J Clin Invest 55:908–913

Hardison WGM, Rosenberg IH (1967) Bile salt deficiency in the steatorrhoea following resection of the ileum and proximal colon. N Engl J Med 277:337–342

Hardison WGM, Tomaszewski N, Grundy SM (1979) Effect of acute alterations in small bowel transit time upon the biliary excretion rate of bile acids. Gastroenterology 76:568–574

Hartwich G, Domschke W, Matzkies F, Pesch HJ, Prestele H (1974) Disaccharidasen der Dünndarmschleimhaut der Ratte unter einer cytostatischen Behandlung mit 5-Fluorouracil. Klin Wochenschr 52:930–938

Harvengt C, Desager JP (1976) Colestipol in familial type II hyperlipoproteinemia: a three-year trial. Clin Pharmacol Ther 20:310–314

Harvey RF, Pomare EW, Heaton KW (1973) Effects of increased dietary fibre on intestinal transit. Lancet 1:1278–1280

Hashim SA, Bergen SS Jr, Van Itallie TB (1961) Experimental steatorrhea induced in man by bile acid sequestrant. Proc Soc Exp Biol Med 106:173–175

Havel RJ, Kane JP (1973) Drugs and lipid metabolism. Annu Rev Pharmacol Toxicol 13:287–308

Hayton WL (1975) Effects of normal alcohols on intestinal absorption of salicylic acid, sulfapyridine, and prednisolone in rats. J Pharm Sci 64:1450–1456

Heaton KW, Pomare EW (1974) Effect of bran on blood lipids. Lancet 1:49–50

Heaton KW, Manning AP, Hartog M (1976) Lack of effect on blood lipid and calcium concentrations of young men on changing from white to wholemeal bread. Br J Nutr 35:55–60

Herbert PN, Gotto AM Jr, Fredrickson DS (1978) Familial lipoprotein deficiency (Abetalipoproteinemia, Hypolipoproteinemia and Tangier disease). In: Stanbury JB, Wyngaarden JB, Fredrickson DS (eds) The metabolic basis of inherited disease, 3rd edn. McGraw-Hill Book, New York, pp 544–588

Himal HS, Greenberg L (1977) The effect of ethanol and bile on electrolyte movement across canine proximal duodenal mucosa. Am J Gastroenterology 68:45–50

Hofmann AF (1976) Fat digestion: the interaction of lipid digestion products with micellar bile acid solutions. In: Rommel K, Goebell H, Boehmer R (eds) Lipid absorption: biochemical and clinical aspects. MTP Press, Lancaster, pp 3–18

Holt S, Heading RC, Carter DC, Prescott LF, Tothill P (1979) Effect of gel fibre on gastric emptying and absorption of glucose and paracetamol. Lancet 1:636–639

Hoyumpa AM, Breen KJ, Schenker S, Wilson FA (1975) Thiamine transport across the rat intestine. II. Effect of ethanol. J Lab Clin Med 86:803–816

Huth K, Fettel M (1975) Bran and blood lipids. Lancet 2:456

Hyams DE, Sabesin SM, Greenberger NJ, Isselbacher KJ (1966) Inhibition of intestinal protein synthesis and lipid transport by ethionine. Biochim Biophys Acta 125:166–173

Ingelfinger FJ (1943) The modification of intestinal motility by drugs. N Engl J Med 229:114–122

Isselbacher KJ, Scheig R, Plotkin GR, Caulfield JB (1964) Congenital β-lipoprotein deficiency: an hereditary disorder involving a defect in the absorption and transport of lipids. Medicine 43:347–361

Ito S (1965) The enteric coat on cat intestinal microvilli. J Cell Biol 27:475–491

Ito S (1974) Form and function of the glycocalyx on free cell surfaces. Philos Trans R Soc Lond [Biol] 268:55–66

Jacobson ED, Prior JT, Faloon WW (1960) Malabsorptive syndrome induced by neomycin: morphological alterations in the jejunal mucosa. J Lab Clin Med 56:245–250

Jenkins DJA, Hill MS, Cummings JH (1975 a) Effect of wheat fiber on blood lipids, fecal steroid excretion and serum iron. Am J Clin Nutr 28:1408–1411

Jenkins DJA, Leeds AR, Newton C, Cummings JH (1975 b) Effect of pectin, guar guin, and wheat fibre on serum cholesterol. Lancet 1:1116–1117

Jenkins DJA, Wolever TMS, Leeds AR, Gassull MA, Haisman P, Dilawari J, Goff D, Metz GL, Alberti KGMM (1978) Dietary fibres, fibre analogues, and glucose tolerance: importance of viscosity. Br Med J 1:1392–1394

Johnson LR (1974) Gastrointestinal hormones, gastrointestinal physiology. In: Jacobson ED, Shanbour LL (eds) MTP International review of Science, Physiology Series One, vol 4. University Park Press, Baltimore, pp 1–43

Johnson LR (1977) Gastrointestinal hormones and their functions. Annu Rev Physiol Toxicol 39:135–158

Johnston JM (1968) Mechanism of fat absorption. American Physiological Society, Washington, DC, pp 1353–1375 (Handbook of physiology, vol 3, sect 6)

Jones RS, Grossman MI (1970) Choleretic effects of cholecystokinin, gastrin II and caerulein in the dog. Am J Physiol 219:1014–1018

Karmen A, Whyte M, Goodman DS (1963) Fatty acid esterification and chylomicron formation during fat absorption. I. Triglycerides and cholesterol esters. J Lipid Res 4:312–321

Karvinen E, Miettinen M (1966) Effect of ethionine on the absorption of palmitic acid-1-^{14}C in the rat. Acta Physiol Scand 68:228–230

Kaufman SE, Kaye MD (1979) Effect of ethanol upon gastric emptying. Gut 20:688–692

Kayden HJ, Medick M (1969) The absorption and metabolism of short and long chain fatty acids in puromycin treated rats. Biochim Biophys Acta 176:37–43

Kayden HJ, Senior JR, Mattson FH (1967) the monoglyceride pathway of fat absorption in man. J Clin Invest 46:1695–1703

Kelsay JL (1978) A review of research on effects of fiber intake on man. Am J Clin Nutr 31:142–159

Kessler JI, Mishkin S, Stein J (1969) Effect of DL-ethionine on the intestinal absorption and transport of palmitic acid-1-^{14}C and tripalmitin-^{14}C. Role of intramucosal factors in the uptake of luminal lipids. J Clin Invest 48:1397–1407

Kessler JI, Narcessian P, Mauldin DP (1975) Biosynthesis of lipoproteins by intestinal epithelium. Site of synthesis and sequence of association of lipid, sugar and protein moieties. Gastroenterology 68:1058/A-201

Kessler JI, Sehgal AK, Turcotte R (1978) Effect of neomycin on amine acid uptake and on synthesis and release of lipoproteins by rat intestine. Can J Physiol Pharmacol 56:420–427

Keys A, Anderson JT, Grande F (1960) Diet-type (fats constant) and blood lipids in man. J Nutr 70:257–266

Keys A, Grande F, Anderson JT (1961) Fiber and Pectin in the diet and serum cholesterol concentration in man. Proc Soc Exp Biol Med 106:555–558

Kirby RW, Anderson JW, Sieling B, Rees ED, Chen WJL, Miller RE, Kay RM (1981) Oat-bran intake selectively lowers serum low-density lipoprotein cholesterol concentrations of hypercholesterolemic men. Am J Clin Nutr 34:824–829

Kotler DP, Shiau YF, Levine GM (1980) Effects of luminal contents on jejunal fatty acid esterification in the rat. Am J Physiol 238:H414–G418

Krawitt EL, Sampson HW, Katagiri CA (1975) Effect of 1,25-dihydroxycholecalciferol on ethanol mediated suppression of calcium absorption. Calcif Tissue Res 18:119–124

Krejs GJ, Browne R, Raskin P (1980) Effect of intravenous somatostatin on jejunal absorption of glucose, amino acids, water, and electrolytes. Gastroenterology 78:26–31

Krondl A, Vavrinkova H, Michalec C, Placer Z (1959) Beitrag zur Emulgation und Spaltung der Fette in vitro. Dtsch Z Verdau Stoffwechselkr 19:283–292

Krondl A, Vokáč V, Vavřínková H (1962) Influence of chlortetracycline and neomycin on digestion and absorption of fat in rats. Am J Physiol 202 (3):437–439

Kugler JH, Levin RJ, Martin BF, Sneddon V (1967) The effects of 5-fluorouracil on the storage and secretion of pancreatic lipase and zymogen granules. J Physiol 190:42P–44P

Le Marchand Y, Singh A, Assimacopoulos-Jeannet F, Orci L, Rouiller C, Jeanrenaud B (1973) A role for the microtubular system in the release of very low density lipoproteins by perfused mouse livers. J Biol Chem 248:6862–6870

Le Marchand Y, Patzelt C, Assimacopoulos-Jeannet F, Loten E, Jeanrenaud B (1974) Evidence for a role of the microtubular system in the secretion of newly synthesized albumin and other proteins by the liver. J Clin Invest 53:1512–1517

Levant JA, Kun TL, Jachna J, Richard A, Sturdevant L, Isenberg JI (1974) The effects of graded doses of C-terminal octapeptide of cholecystokinin on small intestinal transit time in man. Am J Dig Dis 19:207–209

Leveille GA, Sauberlich HE (1966) Mechanism of the cholesterol-depressing effect of pectin in the cholesterol-fed rat. J Nutr 88:209–214

Levin RJ (1968) Anatomical and functional changes of the small intestine induced by 5-fluorouracil. J Physiol 197:73P–74P

Levy RI, Fredrickson DS, Shulman R, Bilheimer DW, Breslow JL, Stone NJ, Lux SE, Sloan HR, Krauss RM, Herbert PN (1972) Dietary and drug treatment of primary hyperlipoproteinemia. Ann Intern Med 77:267–294

Linscheer WG, Patterson JF, Moore EW, Clermont RJ, Robins SJ, Chalmers TC (1966) Medium and long chain fat absorption patients with cirrhosis. J Clin Invest 45:1317–1325

Lucas ML, Schneider W, Haberich FJ, Blair JA (1975) Direct measurement by pH microelectrode of the pH microclimate in rat proximal jejunum. Proc R Soc Lond [Biol] 192:39–48

Lukie BE, Westergaard H, Dietschy JM (1974) Validation of a chamber that allows measurement of both tissue uptake rates and unstirred layer thicknesses in the intestine under conditions of controlled stirring. Gastroenterology 67:562–661

Malagelada JR, Carter SE, Brown ML, Carlson GL (1980) Radiolabeled fiber. A physiologic marker for gastric emptying and intestinal transit of solids. Dig Dis Sci (New Series) 25:81–87

Mansbach CM, Garbutt JT, Tyor MP (1972) Bile salt and lipid metabolism in patients with ileal disease with and without steatorrhoea. Am J Dig Dis 17:1089–1099

Mansbach CM, Pieroni G, Verger R (1982) Intestinal phospholipase, a novel enzyme. J Clin Invest 69:368–376

Margolis S, Philips FS, Sternberg SS (1971) The cytotoxicity of methotrexate in mouse small intestine in relation to inhibition of folic acid reductase and of DNA synthesis. Cancer Res 31:2037–2046

Mathur KS, Kahn MA, Sharma RD (1968) Hypocholesterolaemic effect of Bengal gram: a long term study in man. Br Med J 1:30–31

Matzkies F, Berg G (1978) Dietary fiber syndrome as the cause of disease in civilised societies. Acta Hepato-Gastroenterol 25:402–407

McCance RA, Prior KM, Widdowson EM (1953) A radiological study of the rate of passage of brown and white bread through the digestive tract of man. Br J Nutr 7:98–104

McConnell AA, Eastwood MA, Mitchell WD (1974) Physical characteristics of vegetable foodstuffs that could influence bowel function. J Sc Food Agric 25:1457–1464
McLeod GM, Wiggins HS (1968) Bile salts in small intestinal contents after ileal resection and in other malabsorption syndromes. Lancet 1:873–876
Mehta SK, Weser E, Sleisenger MH (1967) Neomycin inhibition of lipolysis in vitro. Proc Soc Exp Biol Med 125:905–907
Meisner H (1975) Displacement of palmitate from albumin by chlorophenoxyisobutyrate. Biochem Biophys Res Commun 66:1134–1140
Mendenhall CL, Greenberger PA, Greenberger JC, Julian DJ (1974) Dietary lipid assimilation after acute ethanol ingestion in the rat. Am J Physiol 227:377–382
Menon PVG, Kurup PA (1974) Hypolipidaemic action of the polysaccharide from Phaseolus mungo (blackgram). Effect on glycosaminoglycans, lipids and lipoprotein lipase activity in normal rats. Atherosclerosis 19:315–326
Meyer JH (1975) Release of secretin and cholecystokinin. In: Thompson JC (ed) Gastrointestinal hormones. University of Texas Press, Austin, pp 475–489
Meyer JH, Stevenson EA, Watts HD (1976) The potential role of protein in the absorption of fat. Gastroenterology 70:232–239
Mezey E, Jow E, Slavin RE, Tobon F (1970) Pancreatic function and intestinal absorption in chronic alcoholism. Gastroenterology 59:657–664
Millan MS, Morris GP, Beck IT, Henson JT (1980) Villous damage induced by suction biopsy and by acute ethanol intake in the normal human small intestine. Dig Dis Sci 25:513–525
Mistilis SP, Ockner RK (1972) Effects of ethanol on endogenous lipid and lipoprotein metabolism in small intestine. J Lab Clin Med 80:34–46
Mohri H (1976) The function of tubulin in motile systems. Biochim Biophys Acta 456:85–127
Momsen WE, Brockman HL (1976a) Effects of colipase and taurodeoxycholate on the catalytic and physical properties of pancreatic lipase B at an oil-water interface. J Biol Chem 251:378–383
Momsen WE, Brockman HL (1976b) Inhibition of pancreatic lipase B activity by taurodeoxycholate and its reversal by colipase. Mechanism of action. J Biol Chem 251:384–388
Moore JG, Christian PE, Datz FL, Coleman RE (1981) Effect of wine on gastric emptying in humans. Gastroenterology 81:1072–1075
Morgan RGH, Hoffman NE (1971) The interaction of lipase, lipase cofactor and bile salts in triglyceride hydrolysis. Biochim Biophys Acta 248:143–148
Nickerson SC, Smith JJ, Keenan TW (1980) Role of microtubules in milk secretion – Action of colchicine on microtubules and exocytosis of secretory vesicles in rat mammary epithelial cells. Cell Tissue Res 207:361–376
Ockner RK, Manning JA (1974) Fatty acid-binding protein in small intestine. Identification, isolation, and evidence for its role in cellular fatty acid transport. J Clin Invest 54:326–338
Ockner RK, Manning JA (1976) Fatty acid binding protein. Role in esterification of absorbed long chain fatty acid in rat intestine. J Clin Invest 58:632–641
Ockner RK, Hughes FB, Isselbacher KJ (1969) Very low density lipoproteins in intestinal lymph: origin, composition and role in lipid transport in the fasting state. J Clin Invest 48:2079–2088
Ockner RK, Manning JA, Poppenhausen RB, Ho WKL (1972a) A binding protein for fatty acids in cytosol of intestinal mucosa, liver, myocardium and other tissues. Science 177:56–58
Ockner RK, Pittman JP, Yager JL (1972b) Differences in the intestinal absorption of saturated and unsaturated long chain fatty acids. Gastroenterology 62:981–992
Ockner RK, Burnett DA, Lysenko N, Manning JA (1979) Sex differences in long chain fatty acid utilization and fatty acid binding protein concentration in rat liver. J Clin Invest 64:172–181
O'Doherty PJA, Kuksis A (1975) Stimulation of triacylglycerol synthesis by a protein in rat liver and intestinal mucosa. FEBS Lett 60:256–258

O'Doherty PJA, Yousef IM, Kuksis A (1972) Differential effect of puromycin on triglyceride and phospholipid biosynthesis in isolated mucosal cells. Fed Proc 31:701 (Abstr)
Palmer GH, Dixon DG (1966) Effect of pectin dose on serum cholesterol levels. Am J Clin Nutr 18:437–442
Parkinson TM, Gunderson K, Nelson NA (1970) Effects of colestipol (U26597-A), a new bile acid sequestrant on serum lipids in experimental animals and man. Atherosclerosis 11:531–537
Patton JS, Carey MC (1981) Inhibition of human pancreatic lipase-colipase activity by mixed bile salt-phospholipid micelles. Am J Physiol 241:G328–G336
Pavelka M, Gangl A (1978) Die Ultrastruktur der Dünndarmepithelzelle nach Colchizinverabreichung – Untersuchungen im Nüchternzustand und während Fettresorption. Verh Anat Ges 72:687–689
Payler DK (1973) Food fibre and bowel behavior. Lancet 1:1394
Payler DK, Pomare EW, Heaton KW, Harvey RF (1975) The effect of wheat bran on intestinal transit. Gut 16:209–213
Persson I, Raby K, Fønss-Bech P, Jensen E (1976) Effect of prolonged bran administration on serum levels of cholesterol, ionized calcium and iron in the elderly. J Am Geriatr Soc 24:334–335
Pointner H, Hengl G, Bayer PM, Flegel U (1977) Hemmung des postprandialen Triglyzeridanstiegs im Serum durch Somatostatin beim Menschen. Wien Klin Wochenschr 89:224–227
Polak JM, Pearse AGE, Bloom SR, Buchan AMJ, Rayford PL, Thompson JC (1975) Identification of cholecytokinin-secreting cells. Lancet 2:1016–1018
Porter KR (1966) Cytoplasmic microtubules and their functions. In: Wolstenholm GEW, O'Connor M (eds) Principles of biomolecular organization. Little Brown, Boston, pp 308–345 (CIBA Found Symp)
Prather ES (1964) Effect of cellulose on serum lipids in young women. J Am Diet Assoc 45:230–233
Rao GA, Johnston JM (1966) Purification and properties of triglyceride synthetase from the intestinal mucosa. Biochim Biophys Acta 125:465–473
Rayford PL, Miller TA, Thompson JC (1976) Secretin, cholecystokinin and newer gastrointestinal hormones. Medical Progress. N Engl J Med 294:1093–1101
Read NW, Holdsworth CD, Levin RJ (1976) The role of jejunal unstirred layer thickness in interpretation of changes in electrogenic glucose absorption in coeliac disease (Abstr). Eur J Clin Invest 6:314
Reaven EP, Reaven GM (1977) Distribution and content of microtubules in relation to the transport of lipid. An ultrastructural quantitative study of the absorptive cell of the small intestine. J Cell Biol 75:559–572
Reaven EP, Reaven GM (1980) Evidence that microtubules play a permissive role in hepatocyte very low density lipoprotein secretion. J Cell Biol 84:28–39
Redgrave TG (1969) Inhibition of protein synthesis and absorption of lipid into thoracic duct lymph in rats. Proc Soc Exp Biol Med 130:776–780
Redgrave TG, Simmonds WJ (1967) Effect of aminopterin on the absorption of fat into the lymph of unanaesthetized rats. Gastroenterology 52:54–66
Redgrave TG, Zilversmit DB (1969) Does puromycin block release of chylomicrons from the intestine? Am J Physiol 217:336–340
Regan PT, Malagelada JR, Dimagno EP, Go VLW (1979) Reduced intraluminal bile acid concentrations and fat maldigestion in pancreatic insufficiency: correction by treatment. Gastroenterology 77:285–289
Ritland S, Fausa O, Gjone E, Blomhoff JP, Skrede S, Lanner A (1975) Effect of treatment with a bile-sequestring agent (Secholex®) on intestinal absorption, duodenal bile acids, and plasma lipids. Scand J Gastroenterol 10:791–800
Rodgers JB, Bochenek W (1970) Localization of lipid esterifying enzymes of the rat small intestine. Effects of jejunal removal on ileal enzyme activities. Biochim Biophys Acta 202:426–435
Rodgers JB, O'Brien RJ (1975) The effect of acute ethanol treatment on lipid-reesterifying enzymes of the rat small bowel. Am J Dig Dis 20:354–358

Rodgers JB, Riley EM, Drummey JD, Isselbacher KJ (1967) Lipid absorption in adrenalectomized rats: the role of altered enzyme activity in the intestinal mucosa. Gastroenterology 53:547–556

Rodgers AI, Vloedman DA, Bloom EC, Kalser MH (1966) Neomycin-induced steatorrhea. A preliminary report on the in vivo hydrolysis of a long-chain unsaturated fat. JAMA 197:185–190

Roggin GM, Iber FL, Kater RMH, et al. (1969) Malabsorption in the chronic alcoholic. Johns Hopkins Med J 125:321–330

Roggin GM, Iber FL, Linscheer WG (1972) Intraluminal fat digestion in the chronic alcoholic. Gut 13:107–111

Rokos J, Burger M, Prochazka P (1958) Effect of calcium ions on the inhibition of hydrolases by chlortetracycline. Nature 181:1201

Rommel K, Goebell H, Böhmer R (eds) (1976) Lipid absorption: biochemical and clinical aspects. MTP Press, Lancaster

Rubin E, Rybak BJ, Lindenbaum J, Gerson CD, Walker G, Lieber CS (1972) Ultrastructural changes in the small intestine, induced by ethanol. Gastroenterology 63:801–814

Ruppin H, Sturm G, Westhoff D, Domschke S, Domschke W, Wünsch E, Demling L (1976) Effect of 13-Nlemotilin on small intestinal transit time in healthy subjects. Scand J Gastroenterol 11 (Suppl 39):85–88

Sabesin SM (1976) Ultrastructural aspects of the intracellular assembly, transport and exocytosis of chylomicrons by rat intestinal absorptive cells. In: Rommel K, Goebell H, Böhmer R (eds) Lipid absorption: biochemical and clinical aspects. MTP Press, Lancaster, pp 113–148

Sabesin SM, Frase S (1977) Electron microscopic studies of the assembly, intracellular transport, and secretion of chylomicrons by rat intestine. J Lipid Res 18:496–511

Sabesin SM, Isselbacher KJ (1965) Protein synthesis inhibition: mechanism for the production of impaired fat absorption. Science 147:1149–1151

Sachs BA, Wolfman L (1974) Colestipol therapy of hyperlipidemia in man (38419). Proc Soc Exp Biol Med 147:694–697

Sakai H (1980) Regulation of microtubule assembly in vitro. Biomed Res 1:359–375

Sallee VL, Dietschy JM (1973) Determinants of intestinal mucosal uptake of short- and medium-chain fatty acids and alcohols. J Lipid Res 14:475–484

Salt HB, Wolff OH, Lloyd JK, Fosbrokke AS, Cameron AH, Hubble DV (1960) On having no beta-lipoprotein. A syndrome comprising beta-lipoproteinemia, acanthocytosis, and steatorrhea. Lancet 2:325–329

Sarles H (1974) Chronic calcifying pancreatitis – chronic alcoholic pancreatitis. Gastroenterology 66:604–616

Sarles H, Discornia D, Talasciano G (1977) Chronic alcoholism and canine exocrine pancreas secretion: a long-term follow up study. Gastroenterology 72:238–243

Sedaghat A, Samuel P, Crouse JR, Ahrens EH Jr (1975) Effects of neomycin on absorption, synthesis and/or flux of cholesterol in man. J Clin Invest 55:12–21

Senior JR (1964) Intestinal absorption of fats. J Lipid Res 5:495–521

Shiau YF (1981) Mechanisms of intestinal fat absorption. Editorial Review. Am J Physiol 240:G1–G9

Shiau YF, Holtzapple PG (1980) Effect of insulin on in vitro intestinal fatty acid esterification in the rat. Am J Physiol 238:E364–E370

Shiau YF, Levine GM (1980) pH dependence of micellar diffusion and dissociation. Am J Physiol 239:G177–G182

Shiau YF, Long WB, Weiss JB (1978) Effect of sugar and monoolein on intestinal fatty acid esterification in rat. Am J Physiol 234:E236–E242

Shiau YF, Umstetter C, Kendall K, Koldovsky O (1979) Development of fatty acid esterification mechanisms in rat small intestines. Am J Physiol 237:E399–E403

Shiau YF, Boyle JT, Umstetter C, Koldovsky O (1980) Apical distribution of fatty acid esterification capacity along the villus-crypt unit of rat jejunum. Gastroenterology 79:47–53

Shimoda SS, Saunders DR, Rubin CE (1968) The Zollinger-Ellison syndrome with steatorrhea. II. The mechanisms of fat and vitamin B_{12} malabsorption. Gastroenterology 55:705–723

Shrivastava BK, Redgrave TG, Simmonds WJ (1967) The source of endogenous lipid in the thoracic duct lymph of fasting rats. Q J Exp Physiol 52:305–312

Shurpalekar KS, Doraiswamy TR, Sundaravalli OE, Rao MN (1971) Effect of inclusion of cellulose in an "atherogenic" diet on the blood lipids of children. Nature 232:554–555

Small DM (1968) A classification of biologic lipids based upon their interaction in aqueous systems. J Am Oil Chem Soc 45:108–119

Small DM (1970) Surface and bulk interactions of lipids and water with a classification of biologically active lipids based on these interactions. Fed Proc 29:1320–1326

Southgate DAT, Durnin JVGA (1970) Caloric conversion factors. An experimental reassessment of the factors used in the calculation of the energy value of human diets. Br J Nutr 24:517–535

Southgate DAT, Branch WJ, Hill MJ, Drasar BS, Walters RL, Davies PS, Baird IM (1976) Metabolic responses to dietary supplements of bran. Metabolism 25:1129–1135

Spector AA (1968) Lipids, hormones, and atherogenesis. The transport and utilization of free fatty acid. Ann NY Acad Sci 149:768–783

Spector AA (1975) Fatty acid binding to plasma albumin. K Lipid Res 16:165–179

Spector AA, Steinberg D, Tanaka A (1965) Uptake of free fatty acids by Ehrlich Ascites Tumor Cells. J Biol Chem 240:1032–1041

Stein O, Stein Y (1973) Colchicine-induced inhibition of very low density lipoprotein release by rat liver in vivo. Biochim Biophys Acta 306:142–147

Stein O, Sanger L, Stein Y (1974) Colchicine-induced inhibition of lipoprotein and protein secretion into the serum and lack of interference with secretion of biliary phospholipids and cholesterol by rat liver in vivo. J Cell Biol 62:90–103

Stening GF, Grossman MI (1969) Gastrin-related peptides as stimulants of pancreatic and gastric secretion. Am J Physiol 217:262–266

Sturgess JM, Mitranic MM, Moscarello MA (1975) The Golgi complex. III. The effects of puromycin on ultrastructure and glycoprotein synthesis. Chem Biol Interact 11:207–224

Sun DCH, Albacete RA, Chen JK (1967) Malabsorption studies in cirrhosis of the liver. Arch Intern Med 119:567–572

Swift JG, Mukherjee TM (1976) Demonstration of the fuzzy surface coat of rat intestinal microvilli by freeze etching. J Cell Biol 69:491–494

Switz DM, Hislop IG, Hofmann AF (1970) Factors influencing the absorption of bile acids by the human jejunum. Gastroenterology 59:999 (Abstr)

Tandon R, Edwards RH, Rodgers JB (1972) Effects of bile diversion on the lipid-reesterifying capacity of the rat small bowel. Gastroenterology 63:990–1003

Tasman-Jones C, Jones AL, Owen RL (1978) Jejunal morphological consequences of dietary fiber in rats. Gastroenterology 74:1102A

Tennent DM, Siegel H, Zanetti ME, Kuron GW, Ott WH, Wolf FJ (1960) Plasma cholesterol lowering action of bile acid binding polymers in experimental animals. J Lipid Res 1:469–473

Theodor E, Spritz N, Sleisenger MH (1968) Metabolism of intravenously injected isotopic cholic acid in viral hepatitis. Gastroenterology 55:183–190

Thompson GR, Mac Mahon M, Claes P (1970) Precipitation by neomycin compounds of fatty acid and cholesterol from mixed micellar solutions. Eur J Clin Invest 1:40–47

Thompson GR, Barrowman J, Gutierrez L, Dowling RH (1971) Action of neomycin on the intraluminal phase of lipid absorption. J Clin Invest 50:319–323

Tilney LG (1968) The assembly of microtubules and their role in the development of cell form. Dev Biol (Suppl) 2:63–102

Trier J (1962 a) Morphologic alterations induced by methotrexate in the mucosa of human proximal intestine. I. Serial observations by light microscopy. Gastroenterology 42:295–305

Trier JS (1962b) Morphologic alterations induced by methotrexate in the mucosa of human proximal intestine. II. Electron microscopic observations. Gastroenterology 42:407–424

Trier JS (1968) Morphology of the epithelium of the small intestine. American Physiological Society, Washington, DC, pp 1125–1175 (Handbook of physiology, vol 3, sect 6)

Truswell AS, Kay RM (1975) Absence of effect of bran on blood lipids. Lancet 1:922–923

Valdivieso VD, Schwabe AD (1965) Alteration of intestinal epithelial function and medium chain fat absorption. Clin Res 13:98

Van-Deest BW, Fordtran JS, Morawski SG, Wilson JD (1968) Bile salt and micellar fat concentration in proximal small bowel contents of ileectomy patients. J Clin Invest 47:1314–1324

Van den Bosch JF, Claes PJ (1967) Correlation between the bile salt precipitating capacity of derivatives of basic antibiotics and their plasma cholesterol lowering effect in vivo. Prog Biochem Pharmacol 2:97–104

Van Thiel DH, Lipsitz HD, Porter LE, Schade RR, Gottlieb GP, Graham TO (1981) Gastrointestinal and hepatic manifestations of chronic alcoholism. Clinical conference. Gastroenterology 81:594–615

Vlahcevic ZR, Buhac I, Farrar JT, Bell CC, Swell L (1971) Bile acid metabolism in patients with cirrhosis. I. Kinetic aspects of cholic acid metabolism. Gastroenterology 60:491–498

Vlahcevic ZR, Juttijudata P, Bell CC Jr, Swell L (1972) Bile acid metabolism in patients with cirrhosis. II. Cholic and chenodeoxycholic acid metabolism. Gastroenterology 62:1174–1181

Walker ARP (1975) Effect of high crude fiber intake on transit time and the absorption of nutrients in South African Negro school children. Am J Clin Nutr 28:1161–1169

Walters RL, Baird IM, Davies PS, Hill MJ, Drasar BS, Southgate DAT, Green J, Morgan B (1975) Effects of two types of dietary fibre on fecal steroid and lipid excretion. Br Med J 2:536–538

Weinstein WM (1974) Epithelial cell renewal of the small intestinal mucosa. Med Clin North Am 58:1375–1386

Westergaard H, Dietschy JM (1976) The mechanism whereby bile acid micelles increase the rate of fatty acid and cholesterol uptake into the intestinal mucosal cell. J Clin Invest 58:97–108

Whitmore DA, Brookes LG, Wheeler KP (1979) Relative effects of different surfactants on intestinal absorption and the release of proteins and phospholipids from the tissue. J Pharm Pharmacol 31:277–283

Wilson FA, Dietschy JM (1972) Characterization of bile acid absorption across the unstirred water layer and brush border of the rat jejunum. J Clin Invest 51:3015–3025

Wilson FA, Dietschy JM (1974) The intestinal unstirred layer: its surface area and effect on active transport kinetics. Biochim Biophys Acta 363:112–126

Wilson FA, Hoyumpa AM Jr (1979) Ethanol and small intestinal transport. Gastroenterology 76:388–403

Wilson FA, Sallee VL, Dietschy JM (1971) Unstirred water layers in intestine: rate determinant of fatty acid absorption from micellar solutions. Science 174:1031–1033

Wilson L, Bamburg JR, Mizel SB, Grisham L, Creswell KM (1974) Interaction of drugs with microtubule proteins. Fed Proc 33:158–166

Winne D (1976) Unstirred layer thickness in perfused rat jejunum in vivo. Experientia 32:1278–1279

Worthington BS, Meserole L, Syrotuck JA (1978) Effect of daily ethanol ingestion on intestinal permeability to macromolecules. Am J Dig Dis 23:23–32

Wosilait WD, Soler-Argilaga C, Nagy P (1976) A theoretical analysis of the binding of palmitate by human serum albumin. Biochem Biophys Res Commun 71:419–426

Yousef IM, Kuksis A (1972) Release of chylomicrons by isolated cells of rat intestinal mucosa. Lipids 7:380–386

Zurier RB, Hashim SA, Van Itallie TB (1965) Effect of medium chain triglyceride on cholestyramine-induced steatorrhea in man. Gastroenterology 49:490–495

CHAPTER 17

Intestinal Absorption of the Fat-Soluble Vitamins: Physiology and Pharmacology

J. A. BARROWMAN

A. Introduction

By definition, the fat-soluble vitamins comprise a group of lipophilic essential micronutrients. Their lipid solubility is their only common feature and their chemical structures are as diverse as their metabolic and biochemical functions. Nevertheless, their common physicochemical property results in shared mechanisms in the stages of intestinal absorption, notably their solubilisation in intestinal content and the participation of bile salts in this process, and in the route of transport of the compounds from the intestine after the absorption step. It is particularly at the intestinal mucosal cell level that the handling of these vitamins has to be considered individually. Before considering the absorption of the fat-soluble vitamins it is worthwhile to review in a general way the currently understood scheme of lipid digestion and absorption in the mammalian intestine as this is essential for an appreciation of the events in fat-soluble vitamin absorption.

B. Lipid Digestion and Absorption

The following brief synopsis describes the current concepts of fat digestion and absorption with particular attention to the major lipid species, long-chain triglyceride. It is generally accepted that there is no substantial absorption of intact triglyceride in the small intestine, but that lipolysis is a necessary step in triglyceride assimilation. Endogenous and exogenous lipases are responsible for this. A lipase of pharyngeal and lingual origin is present in several species including humans (HAMOSH et al. 1975). This enzyme, with a pH optimum of about 5, initiates lipolysis in the pharynx and stomach. In the stomach there is lipase activity which is principally active against triglycerides containing medium- and short-chain fatty acids, but relatively inefficient against long-chain triglycerides (COHEN et al. 1971; LEVY et al. 1981). It is probable that this enzymic activity is mainly of physiological importance in the newborn.

Until food enters the small intestine the hydrolysis of dietary triglyceride is only of limited extent. In the duodenum and jejunum, as a result of neurohumoral mechanisms, the gastric chyme mixes with bile, pancreatic juice and intestinal secretions. Lipolysis proceeds rapidly at this stage as a result of the action of pancreatic lipase. In the newborn, the activity of pancreatic lipase is rather low and lipolytic activity in the intestine is augmented by a bile salt-stimulated lipase present in milk, a form of physiological oral enzyme supplementation (HERNELL and OLIVECRONA 1974). Triglycerides of gastric chyme exist as a coarse emulsion of oil droplets covered by a variety of substances such as the hydrophobic proteins albumin and β-lactoglobulin, and amphiphilic lipids such as phospholipids. In the small intestine, bile salts clear the interface of such proteins (BORGSTRÖM and ERLANSON 1978), and phospholipase A_2 digests the phospholipids (BORGSTRÖM 1980). The result is a bile salt- and fatty acid-stabilised oil–water emulsion. This bile salt-covered interface repels pancreatic lipase which tends to bind to oil–water interfaces, undergoing irreversible inactivation probably as a result of conformational changes. Colipase, the polypeptide cofactor of pancreatic lipase, is secreted in pancreatic juice. It binds to lipase in the presence of bile salts and also anchors lipase to the triglyceride–water interface overcoming the repulsion of lipase by bile salts (BORGSTRÖM et al. 1979). Lipolysis can then proceed efficiently and the split products, fatty acids and monoglycerides, are cleared from the interface by forming mixed micelles with bile salts thus facilitating the progress of the lipolytic reaction.

Pancreatic lipase is responsible for hydrolysis of the ester bonds in the 1 and 3 positions of triglyceride yielding two fatty acid molecules and a 2-monoglyceride which are subsequently absorbed by the enterocyte. Although isomerisation of 2-monoglyceride can occur yielding a 1- or 3-monoglyceride which could be split by lipase, this is too slow to be of quantitative importance. The result of triglyceride lipolysis is the generation of a micellar phase in the small intestine comprising mixed bile salt: fatty acid: monoglyceride micelles. This micellar phase is further complicated by the presence of biliary and dietary phospholipid, principally lecithin, and its hydrolysis product, lysolecithin, produced by the action of pancreatic phospholipase A_2. Other lipid solutes in the micelles include cholesterol, the fat-soluble vitamins and small amounts of the plant sterols. These micelles are also presumably a medium for solubilisation of foreign lipophilic substances.

Until recently it was considered that intraluminal fat digestion involved only the two phases described above, viz. the oil phase and a mixed bile salt micellar phase. This appears however to be an oversimplification. In recent studies by PATTON and CAREY (1979) lipolysis has been followed by light microscopy and two other visible lipid phases which appear in sequence have been detected. These are a lamellar liquid crystalline phase containing calcium and ionised fatty acids and subsequently a viscous isotropic phase composed mostly of monoglycerides and fatty acids. Lipophilic solutes such as the fat-soluble vitamins presumably dissolve in these phases. While it is generally accepted that lipid absorption by the enterocyte involves transfer of solutes from mixed bile salt micelles to the cell, the role of these newly described phases in intestinal fat absorption is presently unknown.

Before leaving lipolysis in the small intestine it is important to recognise the presence of lipases other than pancreatic lipase and its cofactor. As already mentioned there is a potent phospholipase A_2 which is secreted by the pancreas as a zymogen, prophospholipase, which is activated by tryptic digestion. This enzyme splits the ester bond at the 2 position of lecithin yielding lysolecithin, a water-soluble "lipid" with strong detergent properties (DE HAAS et al. 1968). An enzyme active against a wide range of substances such as sterol esters, monoglycerides and retinol esters in bile salt micellar solution and a variety of synthetic water-soluble esters of short-chain fatty acids, is also secreted in pancreatic juice (MORGAN et al. 1968). These enzymes are not greatly involved in long-chain triglyceride digestion, but their action on their own substrates will affect the overall physicochemical state of the lipid mixture in the small intestine during digestion and absorption.

Dietary and endogenous lipids in the small intestinal lumen exist in three main physicochemical states in equilibrium with each other, viz. the oil phase, the micellar phase, and the monomeric form. A fourth phase can be envisaged under circumstances where unabsorbable substances are present in the diet, such as lignins which offer the possibility of hydrophobic bonding with some lipids; this phase could be designated the precipitate. Despite the very low aqueous solubility of lipids such as long-chain fatty acids and monoglycerides, it is from the monomeric phase that these lipids are thought to be absorbed by the apical membrane of the enterocyte. Between the stirred bulk aqueous phase of the lumen and the "brush border" or apical microvillous membrane of the enterocyte is the "unstirred" aqueous layer, variously estimated to be 100–500 μm in thickness, depending on experimental conditions. This unstirred layer creates a resistance to diffusion of mixed micelles and lipid monomers towards the lipid phase of the cell membrane (WILSON et al. 1971). As the uptake by the cell of fatty acids and monoglycerides is considered to be a passive process depending on chemical diffusion gradients, bile salt micelles in the aqueous phase have an important role in creating a high chemical potential for diffusion across the unstirred layer and by their own diffusion into this layer can enhance the local concentration of monomer at the lipid–water interface of the cell membrane.

From the enterocyte membrane, the transport of the split products of lipolysis to the smooth endoplasmic reticulum is probably mediated by carrier proteins such as the fatty acid binding protein of the intestinal mucosal cell (OCKNER and MANNING 1974). Through the enzyme complex "triglyceride resynthetase" the absorbed 2-monoglycerides are acylated by a stepwise stereospecific mechanism to triglycerides. This is achieved following the activation of the absorbed fatty acids to their acyl-CoA derivatives. This is the preferred resynthetic process for triglyceride in the enterocyte. The alternative pathway for triglyceride resynthesis via the glycerol-3-phosphate pathway is inhibited by monoglycerides and this inhibition may be viewed as a means by which the energetically more conservative monoglyceride pathway is facilitated while excess monoglyceride is available during active lipid absorption (JOHNSTON 1976). A third mechanism for triglyceride biosynthesis, the dihydroxyacetone phosphate pathway, has also been shown to exist in intestinal mucosa (RAO et al. 1970).

The resynthesized triglycerides are subsequently given a polar coat in the form of phospholipid and apoproteins within the endoplasmic reticulum, becoming chylomicrons. The apoproteins of chylomicrons receive added carbohydrate moieties during their subsequent passage through the Golgi complex. In order for transfer of nascent chylomicrons from the endoplasmic reticulum to the Golgi complex to occur, apoproteins must be added to their surface and this transport step is inhibited by conditions which interfere with lipoprotein synthesis. Chylomicrons are the major form of lipoprotein particle elaborated and secreted by the enterocyte during fat absorption. Very low density lipoproteins are also synthesised by intestinal epithelium and this seems to be chiefly during fasting. The lipids secreted under these conditions will be of endogenous origin. Chylomicrons have the following approximate composition: 81%–97% triglyceride, 2%–9% phospholipid, 0.9%–3% cholesterol, 1%–4% cholesterol ester, and 0.5%–2% protein.

The exit of mature chylomicrons from the enterocyte is by the process of exocytosis or reverse pinocytosis involving fusion of Golgi vesicle membranes with the lateral plasmalemma. The chylomicrons subsequently pass between the lateral walls of adjacent enterocytes to cross the basement membrane of these cells and make their way through the lamina propria of the intestinal villi to enter the central lacteal via gaps between endothelial cells of these initial lymph vessels. Thence this particulate fat is transported via mesenteric lymph vessels to the cisterna chyli, thoracic duct and jugular vein.

It has long been known that absorbed lipid partitions between intestinal venous blood and lymph. The general principles of this partition are that medium- and short-chain fatty acids are principally transported in portal venous blood in the unesterified form bound to proteins, mainly albumin. The changeover point is at 12 carbon atoms chain length; that is, above 14 carbon atoms chain length the bulk of the fatty acid is esterified as triglyceride and transported in intestinal lymph. Nevertheless, a proportion of long-chain fatty acid appears to be carried in portal venous blood and this amount is increased in bile salt deficiency in the intestinal lumen and in conditions of defective reesterification of fatty acid in the enterocyte (SAUNDERS and DAWSON 1963). The partition is not only governed by chain length; the degree of saturation of the fatty acid is also important and the polyunsaturated fatty acids of the diet are carried to a larger extent in the portal vein than their saturated counterparts (MCDONALD and WEIDMAN 1978). The key to the partition seems to be the facility with which the fatty acids are esterified in the enterocyte. Where lymphatic drainage is defective it is probable that some increase in portal venous transport of long-chain fatty acids can occur. As minor dietary lipids, the fat-soluble vitamins can be seen as interacting with this overall process of lipid absorption at every stage.

C. The Fat-Soluble Vitamins

I. Vitamins A

The principal dietary forms of vitamin A are retinol (Fig. 1) and its long-chain fatty acid esters which are derived from animal sources, and the carotenoid, β-carotene, of plant origin which undergoes conversion to retinal (Fig. 2) with subsequent reduction to retinol, during passage through the enterocyte.

II. Vitamins D

Although vitamin D is traditionally included in the category of fat-soluble vitamins it is unique in that it is the precursor of a substance which fulfils the criteria of a hormone. Furthermore, since cholecalciferol (vitamin D_3) can be formed from its precursor, 7-dehydrocholesterol in the skin by ultraviolet light in the wavelength region of 300 nm, it is only a vitamin for individuals whose environ-

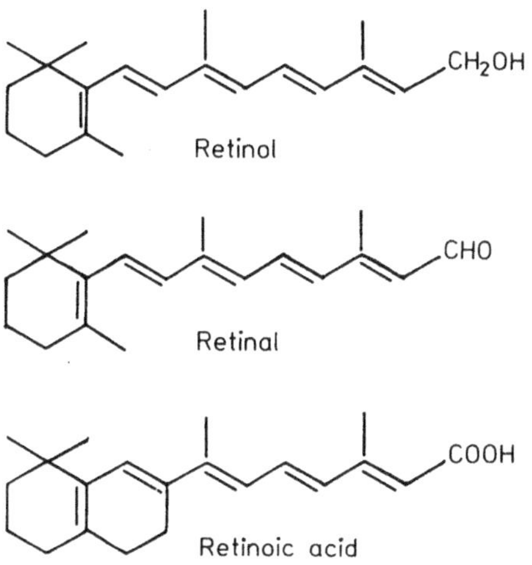

Fig. 1. Forms of vitamin A

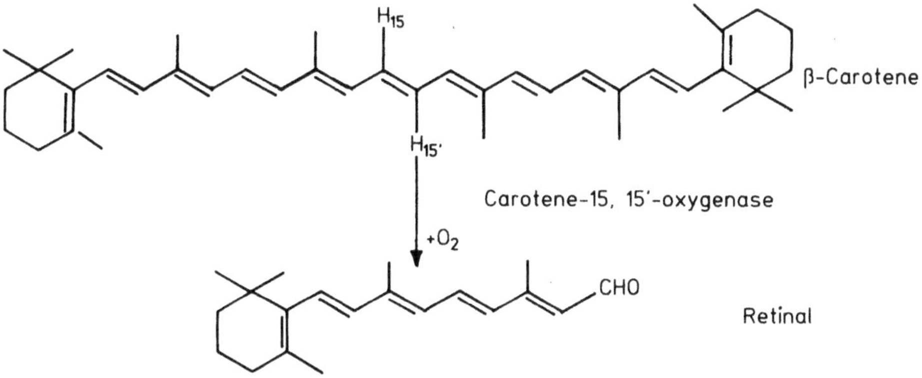

Fig. 2. Cleavage of β-carotene

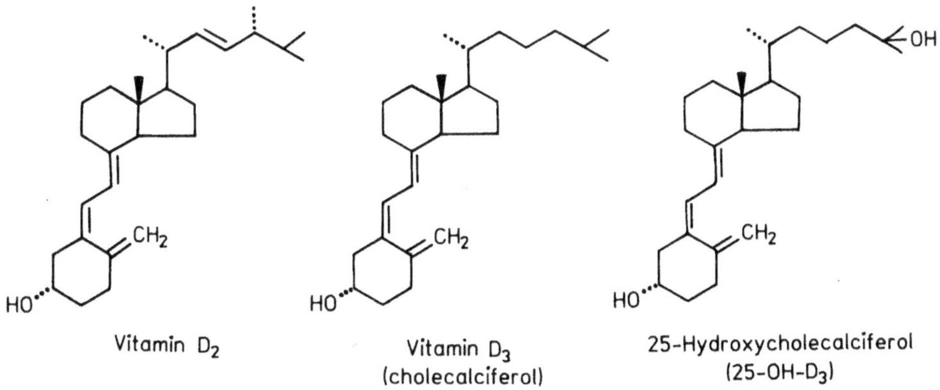

Fig. 3. The vitamins D

ments allow limited exposure to ultraviolet light. Vitamin D is not widely distributed in nature. Fish liver oils are rich sources, but fortification of foods such as dairy products and cereals offers a palatable and consistent means of delivering an adequate daily supply. Hydroxylation of cholecalciferol at the 25 position (Fig. 3) in the liver produces an active hormone and a more potent derivative, 1,25-dihydroxycholecalciferol, results from further hydroxylation in the kidney.

III. Vitamins E

This term refers to a group of tocols and tocotrienols of which α-tocopherol (Fig. 4) is the most potent. These compounds are found in seed oils and lipids of green plants. The tocopheramines, which are referred to in Sect. H.III, do not occur naturally. The status of vitamin E has been the subject of uncertainty, partly on account of the difficulty in defining nutritional requirements. This difficulty arises because the requirements for vitamin E are dependent on the concurrent dietary intake of pro- and antioxidant agents.

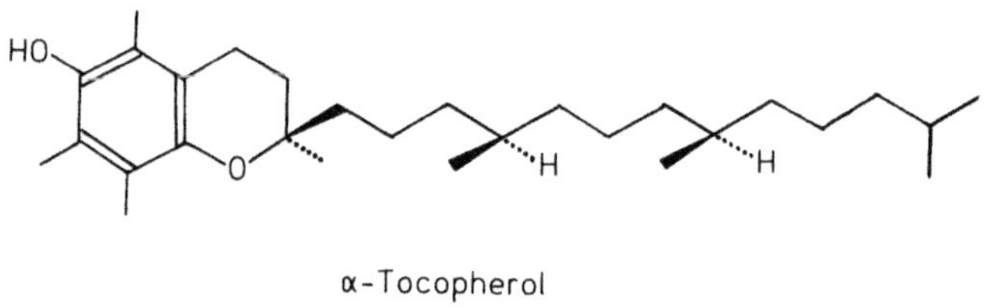

Fig. 4. α-Tocopherol

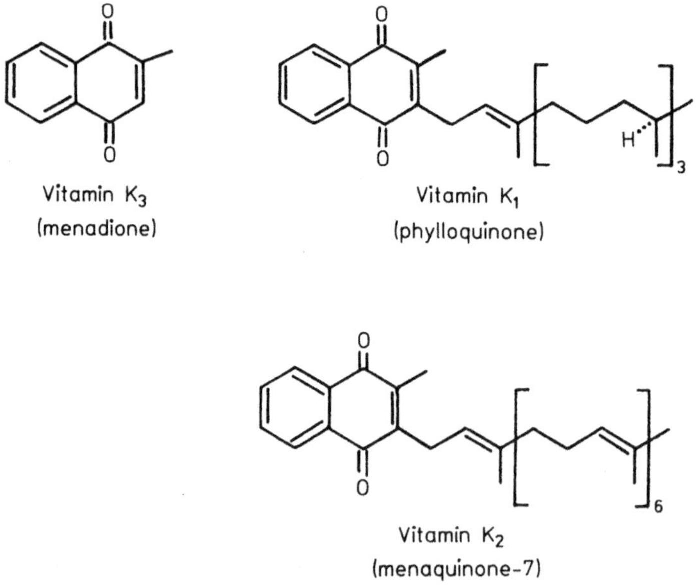

Fig. 5. The vitamins K

Table 1. Nomenclature of the vitamins K

Vitamin	IUPAC name	Chemical name
K_3	Menadione	2-methyl-1, 4-naphthoquinone
K_1	Phylloquinone	2-methyl-3-phythyl-1, 4-naphthoquinone
$K_{2(35)}$	Menaquinone-7 (MK-7)	2-methyl-3-farnesylgeranyl geranyl-1, 4-naphthoquinone
$K_{2(n)}$	Menaquinone-*n* (MK-*n*)	2-methyl-3-multiprenyl-1, 4-naphthoquinone

[a] IUPAC International Union of Pure and Applied Chemistry

IV. Vitamins K

The structures of vitamins K_1, K_2, and K_3 are shown in Fig. 5. All the vitamins K are derivatives of 2-methyl-1,4-napththoquinone (vitamin K_3), a synthetic compound. Vitamin K_1, which has a phytyl side chain, occurs in the photosynthetic portion of many plants. Vitamin K_2 is a bacterial product with an unsaturated side chain of variable length. The nomenclature for the K vitamins which is used in this chapter is shown in Table 1.

D. Hydrolysis of Esters of the Fat-Soluble Vitamins

I. Intraluminal Digestion

Most of the available information indicates that hydrolysis is a necessary step converting fatty acid esters of the vitamins A, D, and E into the free alcohols prior to absorption, but there is surprisingly little information about this aspect of their assimilation. Studies by GANGULY and his colleagues have indicated this to be the case for vitamin A (GANGULY 1969) and dietary protein restriction impairs the assimilation of vitamin A from its esterified form in chickens by reducing the hydrolytic enzyme content of pancreas and intestine (NIR et al. 1967). GALLO-TORRES (1970 a, b) has obtained evidence which suggests that intraluminal hydrolysis of tocopherol esters is of great importance for the absorption of the free vitamin though it is not an absolute prerequisite since tocopheryl pivalate which strongly resists hydrolysis by pancreatic juice enzymes is absorbed intact into rat thoracic duct lymph (NAKAMURA et al. 1975). It is probable that vitamin D esters need to be hydrolysed prior to intestinal absorption. In these respects the fat-soluble vitamin esters seem to be similar to cholesterol esters which have been more extensively studied and where it is known that intraluminal hydrolysis is an absolute requirement for the absorption of the sterol (VAHOUNY and TREADWELL 1964).

As far as sources of hydrolytic activity in the intestinal lumen are concerned, the likely origins are the pancreas and/or the intestinal mucosa. For vitamin A esters a retinyl ester hydrolase activity has been recognised in many species in pancreatic extracts and in pancreatic juice. Its activity however has never been fully characterised though studies by GANGULY and his co-workers suggested that the enzyme activity was distinct from cholesterol esterase activity and from pancreatic lipase (GANGULY 1969). However, ERLANSON and BORGSTRÖM (1968) demonstrated that gel filtration of rat pancreatic juice yielded fractions containing activity against emulsified triglyceride, that is, pancreatic lipase, which were also active in hydrolysing emulsified vitamin A palmitate. Similarly, fractions containing esterolytic activity against a variety of water-soluble esters also attacked bile salt micellar solutions of vitamin A palmitate. This latter enzyme is a carboxyl ester hydrolase of broad specificity which encompasses the activity of "cholesterol esterase". It is probably best termed "nonspecific lipase".

A fascinating aspect of lipolysis has been investigated by FREDRIKZON et al. (1978) who have demonstrated the presence of a bile salt-dependent lipase in human milk whose activity is probably of considerable importance in lipid absorption in the newborn at time when the infant's endogenous pancreatic enzyme activities are often at a very low level. This enzyme has been shown to hydrolyse retinyl esters which are present in the milk and though the concentration of vitamin A in milk is low, this is the only source of this vitamin in the newborn. The vitamin is essential for normal growth and development and the role of the bile salt-stimulated lipase in making retinol available from retinyl esters, which incidentally comprise more than 80% of the vitamin A in human milk, is evident. This enzyme appears to be the same as pancreatic non specific lipase.

Little is known about the other hydrolytic activities in the gut lumen as regards the esters of vitamin D or vitamin E. MULLER et al. (1976) however, have demonstrated that in human duodenal content fractionated by gel filtration, the major activity against tocopheryl acetate appears to correspond to nonspecific lipase. A recent study by this same group has shown in the rat that while the bulk of tocopheryl esters are hydrolysed in the intestinal lumen by pancreatic esterase prior to absorption some α-tocopheryl acetate appears to pass intact into the enterocyte to be hydrolysed by a mucosal esterase associated with the endoplasmic reticulum (MATHIAS et al. 1981). This enzyme when liberated from shed enterocytes also probably contributes to the total intraluminal hydrolytic activity towards tocopheryl esters. As far as esters of vitamin D are concerned it appears that vitamin D_3 oleate is not as readily assimilated as the free vitamin in rats (BELL and BRYAN 1969). Rat pancreatic juice and porcine pancreatic extract can hydrolyse the ester and can esterify cholecalciferol with oleic acid. The activity of these crude enzyme preparations towards vitamin D_3 and its ester is considerably less than that towards cholesterol and cholesterol oleate.

In humans it seems from a recent study that the broad specificity enzyme, nonspecific lipase of pancreatic juice hydrolyses esters of vitamin A, tocopherol and vitamin D_3 in the presence of bile salts. In addition to solubilising the substrates, the trihydroxy bile salts activate this enzyme (LOMBARDO and GUY 1980). This enzyme under acid conditions can also catalyse the synthesis of esters of vitamins A, D, and E though it is doubful if this phenomenon is of any physiological significance (LOMBARDO et al. 1980). Thus, at present, there is no evidence for specific retinyl ester, cholecalciferol ester or tocopherol ester hydrolases in pancreatic juice. Rather, the activity against these esters resides in enzymes of broader specificity such as nonspecific lipase and possibly pancreatic lipase. The activity of these enzymes against fat-soluble vitamin esters is determined by the physicochemical state of the substrate rather than its specific chemical structure.

II. Membrane Digestion of Fat-Soluble Vitamin Esters

Although pancreatic hydrolases are probably responsible for splitting most of the fatty acid esters of retinol, MAHADEVAN et al. (1963) identified hydrolytic enzyme activity associated with the luminal membrane of the enterocyte. Whether contact digestion of retinyl esters at the brush border has any quantitative importance in dietary retinol assimilation is not known.

E. Role of Bile Salts in Fat-Soluble Vitamin Absorption

In the absence of bile salts, cholesterol absorption is effectively abolished and it seems from several studies that the fat-soluble vitamins have a similar requirement for their absorption. In a series of human studies, FORSGREN (1969) demonstrated severe impairment of absorption of labelled vitamins A, D, E, and K_1 as judged by recoveries from thoracic duct lymph in the presence of complete biliary obstruction. The impairment of vitamin D absorption which occurs in patients with primary biliary cirrhosis has also been ascribed to bile salt deficiency in the intestine (DANIELSSON et al. 1982). It has been noted in patients with biliary obstruction and coincidental pancreatic exocrine insufficiency that vitamin K_1 absorption is even more markedly impaired than in the presence of normal pancreatic function (FORSGREN 1969). This is in keeping with animal observations which suggest that both bile and pancreatic juice are necessary for optimum vitamin K_1 absorption. Vitamin K_3, however, does not seem to depend on bile salts for absorption (JACQUES et al. 1954). Vitamin E absorption in rats requires bile salts in the intestine (GALLO-TORRES 1970a; PEARSON andLEGGE 1972; MACMAHON and THOMPSON 1970). The latter authors showed that while a polar lipid, oleic acid, was absorbed nearly as well from an emulsion as a bile salt micellar solution, α-tocopherol uptake from the emulsion into intestinal mucosa was less than from the micellar solution, indicating the greater importance of micellar solubilisation for the absorption of less polar lipids. Bile salts are also required for optimal vitamin D absorption in the rat (SCHACHTER et al. 1964). The means by which bile salts enhance fat-soluble vitamin absorption is not clear, but since these vitamins are very hydrophobic lipids they may simply depend on bile salt micellar solubilisation to achieve sufficiently high monomeric concentrations in aqueous solution close to the enterocyte brush border to promote uptake by the cell membrane.

In an in vitro study in 1968, BORGSTRÖM examined the partition of lipids between emulsified oil and micellar phases of glyceride–fatty acid–bile salt dispersions. Nonglyceride lipids in such a system partition between oil and micellar phases, the distribution seemingly governed to a large extent by their polarity. Thus, cholesteryl oleate partitioned much more in favour of the oil phase than cholesterol. Nevertheless the highly nonpolar hydrocarbon octadecane partitioned more in favour of the micellar phase than cholesteryl oleate and many of the cholesteryl ethers, suggesting that stereochemical fit into the micellar core may also be important. This might also explain the interesting observation that the degree of saturation of the fatty acid in the micellar phase is important as it was shown that cholesterol partitions more in favour of the micellar phase when the fatty acid species is oleic acid rather than linoleic acid.

Relatively few studies have examined the solubility behaviour of fat-soluble vitamins in intestinal content though DAVID and GANGULY (1967) found that when rats were given retinyl acetate in groundnut oil, analysis of intestinal content showed retinyl esters favouring the oil phase and free retinol distributing towards the micellar phase. In humans, vitamin D_3 fed in a liquid test meal is subsequently solubilised in mixed fatty acid–bile salt micelles in the jejunum prior to absorption (RAUTUREAU and RAMBAUD 1981).

Similar in vitro studies to those of BORGSTRÖM have been carried out where the interaction of certain fat-soluble vitamins with bile salts, fatty acids, triglycerides and partial glycerides has been examined. EL-GORAB and UNDERWOOD (1973) have shown that β-carotene and retinol are solubilised by mixed bile salt–lipid micelles. Retinol is almost ten times more readily dissolved in these micelles than is β-carotene. There is no competition between these two solutes for micellar solubilisation. The proportion of glycine to taurine conjugates does not influence solubility of the two forms of vitamin A but with increasing proportion of trihydroxy versus dihydroxy bile salts lesser amounts of the vitamins are solubilised. This is explicable by a higher critical micellar concentration and lowered saturation ratio (moles solute: moles bile salt) with an increasing ratio of trihydroxy to dihydroxy bile salt.

Since retinol is more polar than β-carotene, it may be incorporated into a more polar region of the bile salt micelle and may compete with polar lipids such as fatty acid for micellar inclusion. β-Carotene, on the other hand, is probably solubilised in the hydrophobic core of the micelle and its solubility would be enhanced by expansion of the micelle with polar lipids. Other physicochemical factors which may vary in the small intestimal lumen and affect micellar solubilisation of such substances as β-carotene and retinol include sodium ion concentration and pH. In the case of sodium concentration it appears that micellar solubilisation, particularly of β-carotene is enhanced by increasing sodium concentration and this is due to a fall in the critical micellar concentration and an increase in micellar size as estimated by the saturation ratio. In the pH range 4.5–7.0 no effects on micellar solubility of retinol or β-carotene are seen, but below pH 4.5 the solubility of both falls mainly due to precipitation of the weaker species of bile acids since in the nonionised form these acids are rather insoluble.

In an in vitro study of the behaviour of α-tocopherol in a model two-phase oil–bile salt micellar system the vitamin is found to partition strongly in favour of the oil phase, whether long-chain or medium-chain triglyceride (TAKAHASHI and UNDERWOOD 1974). Addition of monoglyceride and lecithin of long-chain fatty acids to the system greatly enhances micellar solubilisation of α-tocopherol though the medium-chain derivatives have much less of this effect. Probably this is because the long-chain monoglyceride and lecithin, having larger hydrophobic regions than the medium-chain derivatives, expand more effectively that part of the micelle which accommodates the tocopherol.

These sophisticated models of intestinal content give some indication of how a micellar solute such as a fat-soluble vitamin will behave in the mixture of lipids and bile salts in the intestinal lumen, but still fall far short of describing the in vivo situation which is a dynamic process. Lipolysis progressively alters the oil phase volume while uptake by the enterocyte of micellar lipids promotes the completion of the digestive process. Furthermore, hydrolysis of lecithin to lysolecithin by phospholipase A_2 will alter micellar characteristics. Thus, the conditions are constantly changing and the vitamins will partition between the phases according to physicochemical principles. The mixture is immensely complex and other interactions between solutes such as those already described are undoubtedly occurring. It is clear that the micellar solubility characteristics of each lipid must be considered separately and these are governed by polarity and stereochemical "fit". Their interactions in the micelle with other dietary lipid species can probably be explained on these grounds.

Many studies have demonstrated interactions of different lipids fed concurrently on the absorption of a fat-soluble vitamin. For example, polyunsaturated fatty acids appear to depress the absorption of retinol (HOLLANDER and MURALIDHARA 1977), phylloquinone (HOLLANDER et al. 1977a), α-tocopherol (MURALIDHARA and HOLLANDER 1977; GALLO-TORRES et al. 1971) and vitamin D_3 (HOLLANDER et al. 1978a). In these experiments displacement of the vitamin from bile salt micelles by the fatty acids is probably not responsible since with the addition of the fatty acid the micellar content of the fat-soluble vitamin, in the case of retinol and phylloquinone at least, did not drop. Thus the effect must be exerted at a later stage in the absorptive process, such as micellar diffusion into the unstirred water layer governed by micellar size, uptake at the enterocyte membrane, metabolism in the cell or even at the exit step from the cell. On the other hand, the observation by GALLO-TORRES et al. (1978) that medium-chain triglyceride feeding enhances tocopherol absorption may have its explanation in an effect at any of these steps, but it also could be earlier, that is at the micellar solubilisation stage. Bile salts are also involved in providing a suitable substrate, that is a micellar solution of the fat-soluble vitamin esters for the hydrolytic activity of the carboxyl ester hydrolase of pancreatic juice and the activity of this enzyme towards these esters is specifically enhanced by the trihydroxy bile acids (LOMBARDO and GUY 1980).

To what extent do bile salts influence stages of absorption beyond micellar solubilisation and ester digestion? There is relatively little known about this, but the finding that the absence of bile salts in the gut lumen may alter the route of transport of absorbed vitamin A from a lymphatic to portal venous route (GAGNON and DAWSON 1968) is in keeping with intracellular effects of bile salts on the handling of the vitamin. A study by EL-GORAB et al. (1975) has tackled this problem. Using bile salts and the synthetic detergents Tween 20 and hexadecyltrimethylammonium bromide, they showed that bile salt micellar solutions at about their critical micellar concentration enhance retinol and β-carotene uptake by everted small intestinal sacs when compared with emulsions of the vitamins. With β-carotene, higher concentrations of bile salts depressed uptake while retinol absorption did not decline. Their results suggest that bile salts function only as micellar solubilisers in retinol uptake, but in the case of β-carotene bile salts may play a role in the interaction of this compound with the cell membrane or promote its uptake by an effect on its intracellular handling. Cleavage of absorbed β-carotene by the oxygenase enzyme of the cell to yield retinal which was subsequently reduced to retinol and esterified with long-chain fatty acids occurred only in the presence of bile salts in the medium and was abolished by the synthetic detergents while retinol absorption and esterification occurred with all the detergents which were tested. The higher the proportion of tri- to dihydroxy bile acids the more readily the carotene and retinol were converted to retinyl esters. Vitamin D absorption also involves interactions with bile salts the nature of which are unclear. The important studies of SCHACHTER et al. (1964) indicate that taurocholate enhances vitamin D absorption to a greater degree than either taurodeoxycholate or taurochenodeoxycholate, suggesting some specific interaction between the bile salt and vitamin.

Bile salts therefore, are very important in several aspects of fat-soluble vitamin assimilation. Their most obvious roles involve their ability to dissove the vitamins in micellar solution. This is particularly favourable for achieving high concentrations of the vitamins close to the brush border of the enterocyte, but it should also be remembered that micellar solutions of the esters form good substrates for pancreatic nonspecific lipase. There is good evidence that bile salts also exert an influence on metabolic events involving absorbed lipids within the enterocyte such as the cleavage of β-carotene. The observation that concurrent feeding enhances the absorption of certain fat-soluble vitamin preparations such as α-tocopheryl nicotinate (HASEGAWA et al. 1981) might be explained by stimulation of biliary and pancreatic secretion resulting in improved micellar solubilisation of the vitamin.

F. Route of Transport of Fat-Soluble Vitamins from the Intestine

I. Lymphatic Route

Like other nonpolar dietary lipids such as sterols and their esters, the fat-soluble vitamins are extensively transported in intestinal lymph as components of chylomicrons. Many in vivo studies have used animals with small intestinal lymph fistulae to estimate absorption of the fat-soluble vitamins. These are subject to certain limitations: first, the lymph collection may not be complete; second, lymphaticovenous anastomoses may divert some material from lymph to blood and third, there is good evidence that lymph is not the exclusive route for fat-soluble vitamin transport.

The early observations by DRUMMOND et al. (1935) established the importance of lymphatic uptake of vitamin A and carotene in a patient with a chylothorax and this was confirmed and extended to vitamin D by FORBES (1944) in a similar study. POPPER and VOLK (1944), using fluorescence microscopy demonstrated the presence of vitamin A in rat intestinal lymph vessels after feeding the vitamin and studies by THOMPSON et al. (1950) confirmed the importance of the lymphatic route for vitamin A absorption in the rat. In a number of other species, bullocks and sheep (EDEN and SELLERS 1949), pigs (COATES et al. 1950) and guinea-pigs

(WOYTKIV and ESSELBAUGH 1951) the importance of this route has been further established. In rat lymph most absorbed vitamin A is present in chylomicrons, principally as retinyl palmitate, even though the free vitamin, retinol, or its precursor β-carotene was fed (HUANG and GOODMAN 1965). Similar observations have been made in humans (GOODMAN et al. 1966; BLOMSTRAND and WERNER 1967).

In the case of vitamin D, SCHACHTER et al. (1963) demonstrated rapid absorption of radiolabelled vitamin D_2 in the rat, the vitamin being incorporated into chylomicrons in the unesterified form. Similar data were obtained for vitamin D_3 by the same authors in 1964. Unlike retinol, relatively little mucosal esterification of vitamin D occurs (FRASER and KODICEK 1968; SCHACHTER et al. 1964). Some absorbed 25-hydroxy-vitamin D_3 undergoes esterification prior to appearing in intestinal lymph (MAISLOS et al. 1981). While lymph may be the most important route of transport of vitamin D given in large doses, a study in rats suggests that a major proportion of both vitamin D_3 and 25-hydroxycholecalciferol, when given in physiological doses, is transported in portal venous blood rather than intestinal lymph (SITRIN et al. 1982). This study also showed that approximately half of the absorbed vitamin D_3 transported in lymph is associated with chylomicrons, the remainder being associated with the plasma protein fraction of lymph. Only 13% of lymph 25-hydroxycholecalciferol was found in chylomicrons. These figures contrast with those for retinol since more than 80% of absorbed retinol in lymph is found in the chylomicron fraction. It should be recognised that vitamin D in lymph can probably be readily transferred from chylomicrons to plasma proteins, most likely vitamin D binding protein (DUELAND et al. 1982).

In rats the tocopherols are mainly carried in lymph (JOHNSON and POVER 1962; PEAKE et al. 1972) and this is also the case in humans (BLOMSTRAND and FORSGREN 1968 a). Tocopherols are found in the lymph in the unesterified form. Chronic thoracic duct fistulae in rats lead to hypoprothrombinaemia, indicating the importance of lymph in vitamin K transport. Phylloquinone (vitamin K_1) appears to be mainly transported by lymph in these animals (JACQUES et al. et al. 1954) and menadione (vitamin K_3) is, at least partly, transported by intestinal lymph. In humans too, lymph is a major route for transport of absorbed vitamin K_1 which appears mainly as the unaltered vitamin in chylomicrons (BLOMSTRAND and FORSGREN 1968 b).

II. Portal Venous Route

As with long-chain fatty acids, the lymph–portal venous blood partition for fat-soluble vitamins favours the lymphatic route, but there is evidence for portal venous transport of some of the more polar subspecies of these vitamins. Thus in a study of rats and dogs, MEZICK et al. (1968) concluded that menadione (vitamin K_3) is probably transported from the intestine by both portal venous and lymphatic routes as judged by ratios of the compound in portal and aortic blood. Similarly, retinoic acid which can be produced by retinol oxidation in the intestinal mucosa appears to be substantially transported in portal venous blood (FIDGE et al. 1968). Under these conditions it probably is bound to serum albumin and not to retinol binding protein (SMITH et al. 1973). After an intraduodenal injection of retinal ^{14}C, CRAIN et al. (1967) found that about 40% of the radioactivity appeared in the portal venous blood in rats as various retinol metabolites, which included a substantial proportion of retinoic acid, giving further support to the notion of portal venous transport of some forms of vitamin A. 25-Hydroxy-vitamin D_3, a metabolite of vitamin D_3 which is excreted in bile is transported from the intestine both by lymph and portal venous blood (HOLLANDER et al. 1979; MAISLOS et al. 1981), while 1,25-dihydroxy-vitamin D_3 is transported mainly via portal blood (SITRIN et al. 1981; MAISLOS et al. 1981).

In birds, the transport of absorbed fat differs from that in mammals. Lipid particles similar in size and composition to chylomicrons are transported in portal venous blood (BENSADOUN and ROTHFELD 1972). In chickens, GALLO-TORRES (1970 b) has shown that α-tocopheryl nicotinate is absorbed intact since this ester appears in plasma and liver. Presumably it has been transported by portal venous blood.

There are some indications that not all absorbed vitamin A is transported by the lymphatic route. For example, LAWRENCE et al. (1966) showed considerable liver uptake of vitamin A in rats with thoracic duct fistulae fed vitamin A palmitate. Similarly there appears to be a minor transport of α-tocopherol in portal venous blood in the rat since feeding radiolabelled α-tocopherol to rats with mesenteric lymphatic and bile fistulae results in a significant biliary excretion of radioactivity and the finding of a higher concentration of radioactivity in portal venous blood than aortic blood supports this notion (MACMAHON et al. 1971). In a group of children with abetalipoproteinaemia, serum tocopherol levels were undetectable, but rose with very large oral doses of vitamin E (MULLER et al. 1974). These patients who are unable to form chylomicrons lack the major vehicle for transport of absorbed tocopherol, but by feeding massive doses of the vitamin a significant absorption occurs, possibly via the portal venous route.

Certain physiological circumstances may also favour portal venous transport of the fat-soluble vitamins. PIHL et al. (1970) have suggested that feeding vitamin D_3 in medium-chain triglyceride as compared with long-chain triglyceride might divert the vitamin to the portal venous route, but there is comparatively little information on the effect of concomitant medium-chain triglyceride feeding on the extent and route of absorption of very hydrophobic substances. The concurrent absorption of polyunsaturated long-chain fatty acids appears to divert some absorbed retinol from the lymphatic to the portal venous route (HOLLANDER 1980). Finally, intraluminal bile salt deficiency in the small intestine which seems to favour portal venous transport of long-chain fatty acids may also augment the amount of vitamin A carried in the portal vein (GAGNON and DAWSON 1968). Such an effect has also been suggested in humans (FORSGREN 1969).

In summary, lymph provides a major but not exclusive route for transport of absorbed fat-soluble vitamins. The more polar a compound is, however, the greater will be the proportion carried in portal venous blood. Bile salt deficiency probably diverts the vitamins towards the portal venous route. The extent of lymphatic transport of a fat-soluble vitamin after an oral dose reflects its absorption but for the reasons already outlined, it cannot be used as a quantitative measure of the absorption of that vitamin.

G. Enterohepatic Circulation of the Fat-Soluble Vitamins

There is evidence that fat-soluble vitamins or their metabolites appear in bile and thus may be available for reabsorption. A pool of endogenous and exogenous vitamin can be envisaged in the intestine from which absorption occurs. The extent and importance of the endogenous contribution to this pool is unknown. Since the lymphatic route is of major importance in the absorption of these vitamins, the enterohepatic circulation of these substances involves a circuitous route including the thoracic duct and the systemic circulation.

Following intraperitoneal injection of labelled vitamins K_1, K_2, and K_3 in rats, substantial biliary excretion was found, especially for vitamins K_2 and K_3 and over 12 h about 75% of the dose of vitamin K_2 was recovered by this route and 35% of vitamin K_3 (KONISHI et al. 1973). In the isolated perfused rat liver, menadione (2-methyl-1,4-naphthoquinone) added to the perfusate is conjugated with glucuronic acid and excreted in the bile. Other unidentified metabolites are also present in this bile (LOSITO et al. 1967). The handling of phylloquinone in this preparation differs in that the liver retains much more of this vitamin. In rats with bile fistulae significant biliary excretion occured after feeding 2-(methyl ^{14}C)-vitamin K_1 and K_3 (JACQUES et al. 1954). Following intravenous injection of vitamin K_1 ^3H in humans, radioactivity is found in the duodenum within 20–40 min. This is mainly as water-soluble metabolites, probably conjugates, which may subsequently undergo deconjugation in the gut becoming lipid soluble (SHEARER et al. 1972). Of an oral dose of tritiated vitamin K_1, 5%–25% is recovered in T-tube bile in humans (FORSGREN 1969). Similar results with phylloquinone have been obtained in humans by BLOMSTRAND and GÜRTLER (1971) and these authors also showed a considerable biliary excretion of glucuronide metabolites of phytylubiquinone (a model compound related to coenzyme Q) after oral dosage of this substance.

Tocopherols are also present in bile. KLATSKIN and MOLANDER (1952) found that biliary tocopherol levels in humans are similar to those in plasma and no increase in biliary concentrations was found after oral administration of a large dose of tocopherol. In rats, MELLORS and BARNES (1966) found negligible amounts of radioactivity in the bile after oral administration of α-tocopherol ^{14}C though somewhat higher recoveries in bile were found by SCHMANDKE and PROLL (1964) when the tocopherol was given by intravenous injections. By contrast, an oral dose of labelled α-tocopherol given to rats with bile fistulae produced a well-defined "tolerance curve" pattern of excretion of radioactivity in the bile (CHERNENKO and BARROWMAN 1979, unpublished work). Metabolites of tocopherol including water-soluble species are to be found in bile; the extent of biliary excretion of vitamin E metabolites requires further study (BIERI and FARRELL 1976).

Vitamin D secretion in the bile of humans (AVIOLI et al. 1967) and animals (BELL and KODICEK 1969) is well recognised, but an interesting situation exists in that 25-hydroxycholecalciferol is excreted in bile. This compound which is a metabolite of cholecalciferol (vitamin D_3) is formed in the liver (PONCHON et al. 1969) being the major circulating form of the vitamin (LAWSON et al. 1969). It has greater biological potency than cholecalciferol (BLUNT et al. 1968). In rats, this compound is excreted in the bile largely as a water-soluble glucuronide conjugate

(SITRIN et al. 1978). Using a single-pass small intestinal perfusion technique in the unanaesthetised rat, HOLLANDER et al. (1979) demonstrated that 25-hydroxy-vitamin D_3 is absorbed by a passive diffusion mechanism and in a group of animals with biliary and lymphatic fistulae 16.3% and 18.5% of infused radiolabelled 25-hydroxy-vitamin D_3 were recovered from bile and lymph respectively. Thus an enterohepatic circulation of 25-hydroxy-vitamin D_3, also demonstrated by GASCON-BARRE (1982), appears to exist in the rat. By comparison with cholecalciferol, 25-hydroxycholecalciferol appears to be approximately three times more readily absorbed and the hydroxylation of cholecalciferol could be interpreted as a mechanism favouring the conservation of vitamin D_3 during its enterohepatic circulation.

In humans too, an enterohepatic circulation of 25-hydroxycholecalciferol exists. In subjects with an intraduodenal catheter it was shown that following an intravenous injection of isotopic 25-hydroxycholecalciferol, one-third of the radiolabel was excreted into the doudenum within 24 h, probably in bile. Subsequently, over 85% of this secreted radioactivity was reabsorbed as judged by faecal excretion of the isotope, indicating an extensive enterohepatic circulation (ARNAUD et al. 1975). In patients with malabsorption due to small intestinal resection or bypass given an intravenous dose of 25-hydroxycholecalciferol, increased faecal excretion of the vitamin reflects an interruption in its enterohepatic circulation (COMPSTON et al. 1982).

Other vitamin D metabolites are present in bile; following an intravenous injection of 1,25-dihydroxycholecalciferol, a complex mixture of water-soluble metabolites is excreted in rat bile (ONISKO et al. 1980). Although some of these products have been identified, it is not known whether they have any biological activity or are purely degradation products. Some of these compounds can be subsequently reabsorbed by the small intestine (KUMAR et al. 1980a). A similar enterohepatic circulation of 1,25-dihydroxycholecalciferol and its more polar metabolites also occurs in humans (WIESNER et al. 1980). Another metabolite of vitamin D, 24,25-dihydroxy-vitamin D_3 also undergoes enterohepatic circulation (KUMAR et al. 1980b).

In the case of vitamin A, DUNAGIN et al. (1965) showed that retinoic acid is excreted in bile as a glucuronide conjugate. A recent study indicates that retinoyl β-glucuronide is only one of several retinoic acid metabolic in bile (ZILE et al. 1980). In summary, all the fat-soluble vitamins undergo some degree of enterohepatic circulation and the biliary excretion products are frequently more polar than the parent compound. The magnitude of these enterohepatic circulations is not known. The presence of an enterohepatic circulation makes it difficult to asses the extent of absorption of a fat-soluble vitamin by conventional balance techniques.

H. Intestinal Uptake of the Fat-Soluble Vitamins

It is generally accepted that the absorption of the fat-soluble vitamins is incomplete, but attempts to measure the proportion of a dose absorbed are hampered by difficulties in quantitative collection of absorbed vitamin since lymph is not the exclusive route of fat-soluble vitamin transport. Estimates of absorption are available from conventional balance techniques: vitamin D, 62%–91% (THOMPSON et al. 1966), vitamin K, 40%–80% (BLOMSTRAND and FORSGREN 1968b; SHEARER et al. 1970) and vitamin E, 55%–78% (MACMAHON andNEALE 1970). These figures only indicate net absorption and may give erroneously low estimates because of enterohepatic cycling of the compounds.

I. Vitamin A

Early studies of small intestinal absorption of very large doses of vitamin A palmitate in rat and humans by in vitro techniques suggested that an active, energy-dependent process is involved (LORAN and ALTHAUSEN 1959; LORAN et al. 1961). However, HOLLANDER and MURALIDHARA (1977) reexamined in the rat the intestinal uptake of retinol in perfused isolated small intestinal segments with intact vascular and lymphatic channels. In the physiological range of dosage, apparent saturation kinetics were found for the uptake (Fig. 6). This effect is obscured when pharmacological doses are given where a linear relationship exists between concentration and absorption rate (Fig. 7). Further analysis of the uptake in the

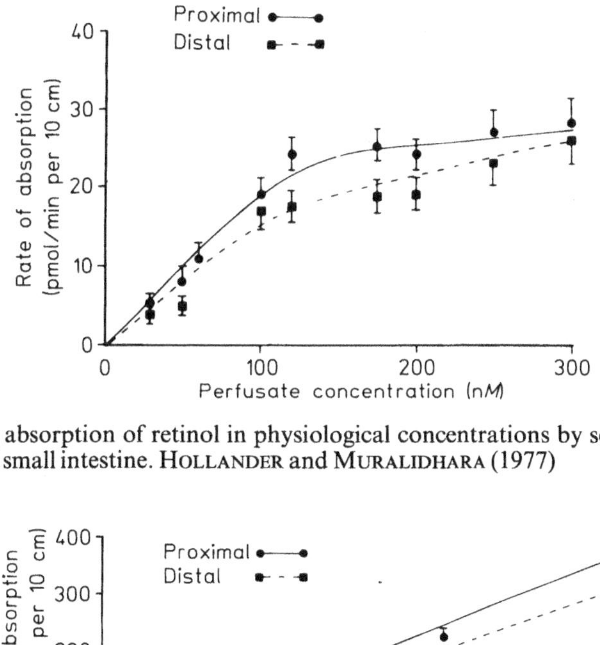

Fig. 6. In vivo absorption of retinol in physiological concentrations by segments of proximal and distal small intestine. HOLLANDER and MURALIDHARA (1977)

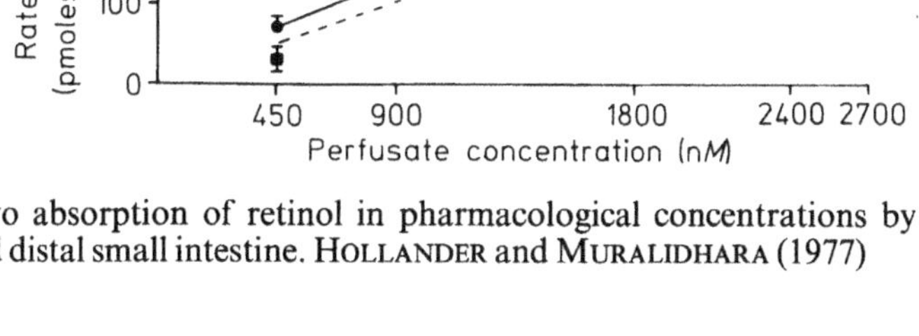

Fig. 7. In vivo absorption of retinol in pharmacological concentrations by segments of proximal and distal small intestine. HOLLANDER and MURALIDHARA (1977)

physiological range was carried out in everted gut sacs where it was shown that uptake was not affected by anoxia or by uncouplers or inhibitors of oxidative phosphorylation. Cytochrome oxidase inhibition with potassium cyanide similarly did not affect uptake. These observations suggest a carrier-mediated passive absorptive process such as a carrier protein in the enterocyte.

A retinol binding macromolecule in cytosols from various rat tissues including intestinal mucosa has been identified as a protein of approximate molecular weight 16,000 (BASHOR et al. 1973). A subsequent study by HOLLANDER et al. (1978b) has confirmed that rat intestinal mucosa contains a binding component for retinol and fatty acids in the molecular weight range 12,000–17,000. Retinol ^{3}H was shown to be displaced from this substance by retinol, retinyl acetate, octanoic, linoleic and linolenic acids, but not by butyric acid. These competitive binding studies are of particular interest since HOLLANDER and MURALIDHARA (1977) had shown that linoleic (C 18:2) and linolenic (C 18:3) acids decrease retinol absorption when added to the perfusate during their in vivo studies of retinol absorption. If the retinol binding protein of the enterocyte acts as a carrier facilitating retinol uptake by promoting its intracellular transport through the cytosol to intracellular organelles, the inhibition of uptake of retinol by polyunsaturated fatty acids might result from competition for the binding agent. The fact that this macromolecule binds a wide variety of structurally dissimilar substances suggests that it may be responsible for intracellular transport of many different lipid species. It is therefore interesting that HOLLANDER's group has shown that polyunsaturated fatty acids inhibit absorption of other fat-soluble vitamins. The binding protein may be related to the intestinal mucosal fatty acid binding protein described by OCKNER and MANNING (1974).

Small intestinal absorption of retinol in the rat is affected by the age of the animal. In a study using perfused segments of small bowel a linear rise in absorption with age was demonstrated such that at 39 months retinol uptake was 50% higher than at 1.5 months (HOLLANDER and MORGAN 1979). The mechanism of this effect is not presently known.

1. β-Carotene Absorption and Intracellular Metabolism

After crossing the cell membrane by a passive process (HOLLANDER and RUBLE 1978), this compound undergoes cleavage by carotene-15,15′-oxygenase, an enzyme associated with the soluble protein fraction of homogenates of intestinal mucosa (GOODMAN and HUANG 1965). The uptake by the cell of β-carotene is promoted by bile salts (EL-GORAB et al. 1975), but it is not clear at which stage in uptake the bile salts exert their effect. It is known, however, that there is an absolute requirement for bile salts for the cleavage of β-carotene by the oxygenase (GOODMAN and HUANG 1965) and also that this reaction is stimulated by fatty acids (GOODMAN et al. 1967). The product, retinal, is readily reduced by another soluble enzyme in the mucosal epithelium which requires a reduced pyridine nucleotide (FIDGE and GOODMAN 1968). The resulting retinol probably enters a pool together with absorbed retinol to be esterified mainly with palmitic acid and to a lesser extent stearic acid. Only minor amounts of retinyl oleate and linoleate are formed (WHYTE et al. 1965).

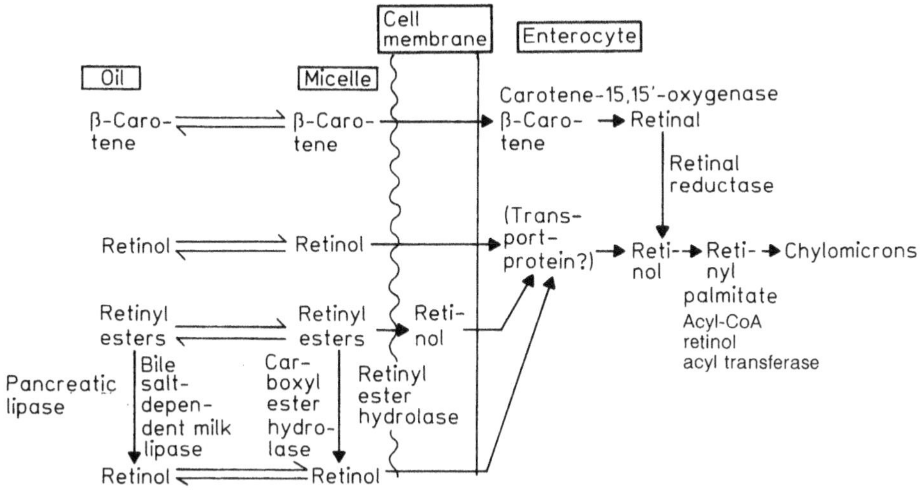

Fig. 8. Vitamin A and *β*-carotene absorption and metabolism in the enterocyte. This scheme does not include the pathway in which a small proportion of retinal formed by *β*-carotene cleavage is oxidised in the intestine to retinoic acid which is subsequently transported, protein-bound, in portal venous blood to the liver

The conversion of *β*-carotene to retinol in humans is less complete than in the rat since significant amounts of labelled *β*-carotene appear in thoracic duct lymph in patients with thoracic duct fistulae fed this compound (BLOMSTRAND and WERNER 1967); virtually no dietary *β*-carotene is absorbed intact into rat lymph (WAGNER et al. 1960; HUANG and GOODMAN 1965; OLSON 1961). A scheme for the processes of digestion, absorption and intracellular handling of the major dietary forms of vitamin A is presented in Fig. 8.

II. Vitamin D

Like the other fat-soluble vitamins, the vitamins D are strongly dependent on the presence of bile salts for their absorption (GREAVES and SCHMIDT 1933; TAYLOR et al. 1935; HEYMAN 1937). However, the interaction of bile salts with the various stages of vitamin D absorption by the enterocyte and its intracellular handling have not been explored. From balance studies in humans it seems that the major part of a physiological oral dose of vitamin D is absorbed. For example, THOMPSON et al. (1966) estimated that 62%–91% of a 0.5–1.0 mg dose of vitamin D_3 is absorbed and HOLLANDER et al. (1971) obtained figures in the same range after intraduodenal or intrajejunal infusion of the vitamin. These estimates are probably low in view of the enterohepatic circulation of vitamin D and its metabolites. Approximately 50% of a fed dose of labelled vitamin D was recovered in thoracic duct lymph in human subjects (BLOMSTRAND and FORSGREN 1967).

The vitamins D are chiefly absorbed in the upper small intestine. In rats, SCHACHTER et al. (1964) have shown that the midjejunum is the site of maximal absorption of vitamin D_2 and vitamin D_3. In humans, HOLLANDER et al. (1971) using faecal excretion measurements, found that comparable amounts of vitamin D are absorbed after the vitamin is infused into duodenum or jejunum thus demonstrating that the duodenum does not have a unique role in vitamin D absorption and in vitro studies of intestinal uptake of pharmacological doses in the rat showed that the proximal and middle portions of the intestine are more efficient than the distal small bowel in this respect. Since the uptake appears to be a passive process these observations may be simply explained by the greater absorptive surface area of the proximal intestine.

Intestinal absorption of vitamin D_3 appears to be a passive diffusion process requiring no energy or carrier as tested in vitro with everted intestinal sacs or in vivo with intestinal loop perfusion (HOLLANDER 1976; HOLLANDER et al. 1978a). In the in vivo studies, the addition of medium-chain fatty acid and unsaturated long-chain fatty acid to the bile salt micelles containing the vitamin diminished its absorption; the site of this interaction is not clear. A possible cause is reduced diffusibility of expanded mixed micelles through the unstirred water layer. This layer is important in vitamin D_3 absorption since reduction in its size by stirring results in enhanced vitamin uptake.

In contrast to HOLLANDER's results, THOMPSON et al. (1969) found enhancement of vitamin D transport in rat lymph by inclusion of long-chain fatty acids in bile salt micellar solutions of vitamin D_3 and the increase in lymphatic transport of the vitamin correlated with increase in lymph triglyceride transport. Initial intestinal mucosal uptake of vitamin D_3 was not affected by inclusion of the fatty acid in the micelles and these authors concluded that the fatty acid affected the exit of the vitamin from the enterocyte to the lymph, the slower of these two stages of vitamin D absorption (SCHACHTER et al. 1964). This important conflict of data regarding the effects of fatty acids on vitamin D absorption needs to be resolved. Little is known about the transport of vitamin D through the enterocyte. It appears from several studies that only very minor amounts of the vitamin are esterified prior to inclusion in chylomicrons. As rats age, triglyceride and vitamin D_3 absorption decrease. The impairment appears to be due either to defective lipoprotein assembly or lipid discharge from the enterocyte (HOLT and DOMINGUEZ 1981). The recent demonstration of impaired intestinal absorption of vitamin D_3 in uraemic rats (VAZIRI et al. 1983) is of great interest. The stage of absorption affected is unknown but the observation adds an extra mechanism to the derangements of vitamin D metabolism and bone disease in patients with chronic renal failure.

1. 25-Hydroxyvitamin D_3

This important metabolite of vitamin D_3 undergoes enterohepatic circulation. Single-pass small intestinal perfusion in rats with bile salt micellar solutions of the compound show that absorption is by a passive diffusion mechanism uninfluenced by the presence of fatty acids in the solution. Reduction of the thickness of the unstirred water layer enhances absorption. 25-Hydroxy-vitamin D_3 is more readily absorbed than its parent compound and seems to be transported by the portal vein to a significant degree as judged by biliary excretion in animals with lymph fistulae (HOLLANDER et al. 1979). A binding substance for 25-hydroxycholecalciferol, presumably a protein, is found in the cytosol of many different tissues including the small intestinal mucosa (HADDAD and BIRGE 1975). Whether this substance plays any part in the absorption of the vitamin is not known. In patients with malabsorption and steatorrhoea, or with intestinal resection there is significant impairment of 25-hydroxycholecalciferol absorption (COMPSTON and CREAMER 1977; DAVIES et al. 1980). The absorption of vitamin D_3, however, is more seriously impaired with steatorrhoea than is the absorption of 25-hydroxycholecalciferol.

2. 1,25-Dihydroxyvitamin D_3

This metabolite, the most potent form of vitamin D, is excreted in bile. It is available as a therapeutic agent for the treatment of metabolic bone disease. In rats, 86% of a dose of 1,25-dihydroxy-vitamin D_3 in a bile salt micellar solution is absorbed from a loop of small intestine in 6 h with approximately 7% appearing in lymph and 12% in bile, indicating that the portal venous route is more important than lymph in uptake of the compound; bile salts appear to promote its transport into lymph. Absorbed 1,25-dihydroxy-vitamin D_3 appears in the unchanged form in lymph, but only a small proportion is associated with chylomicrons. When compared with vitamin D_3 absorption under similar conditions, 1,25-dihydroxy-vitamin D_3 is approximately twice as efficiently absorbed. A major proportion of absorbed vitamin D_3 in lymph is associated with chylomicrons and its intestinal absorption is linked with normal chylomicron formation. The absorption of 1,25-dihydroxy-vitamin D_3 on the other hand appears to be independent of chylomicron formation (SITRIN et al. 1981). Compared with the parent compound, the absorption of the hydroxylated derivatives of vitamin D_3 into portal venous blood and lymph is considerably more rapid (MAISLOS et al. 1981); the explanation for this is not clear at present. In general the hydroxylated derivatives of vitamin D_3 are more rapidly absorbed than the parent compound. This applies to 24,25-dihydroxycholecalciferol in addition to 25-hydroxycholecalciferol and 1,25-dihydroxycholecalciferol (NECHAMA et al. 1977).

III. Vitamin E

Like other fat-soluble vitamins, α-tocopherol is incompletely absorbed, though most estimates in humans suggest that 50%–90% of a dose is absorbed (SCHMANDKE et al. 1969; MACMAHON and NEALE 1970). In patients with thoracic duct fistulae, BLOMSTRAND and FORSGREN (1968a) examined the proportion of radiolabel recovered in lymph lipids after feeding various radioactive tocopherol derivatives. The greatest recovery was found after administration of *N*-(methyl)-DL-tocopheramine followed in order by DL-α-tocopheramine, DL-α-tocopheryl acetate and DL-α-tocopherol. The bulk of the labelled material recovered in lymph was found in chylomicrons, mainly between 2 and 8 h after feeding. Tocopherol and tocopheramine were recovered as such, but after feeding tocopheryl acetate the main compound in lymph was free tocopherol. In patients with biliary obstruction only minimal amounts of radioactivity were recovered in lymph.

In rats, α-tocopherol appears to be absorbed by a passive mechanism. Everted small intestinal sacs incubated in a bile salt micellar solution of oleic acid, monoolein and α-tocopherol showed uptake of the vitamin increasing linearly with increasing concentration of tocopherol and unaffected by 2,4-dinitrophenol, sodium azide or potassium cyanide; a passive diffusion would explain these results. Interestingly, more of the tocopherol was taken up by sacs from the mid-small bowel than from the proximal or distal parts (Hollander et al. 1975). No transmural transport of the tocopherol took place and autoradiography demonstrated that the vitamin had accumulated in submucosal lymphatics.

The passive nature of α-tocopherol absorption in the rat small intestine was confirmed by Muralidhara and Hollander (1977) in perfusion studies in unanaesthetised animals. As with other fat-soluble vitamins the presence of polyunsaturated fatty acids depressed uptake of the vitamin. A series of C_{18} fatty acids all depressed α-tocopherol absorption. Linolenic (C 18:3) was more effective in this respect than stearic (C 18:0), oleic (C 18:1) or linoleic acid (C 18:2). In rats with lymphatic fistulae, Gallo-Torres et al. (1971) have also demonstrated that linoleic acid depresses absorption of α-tocopherol. Whether the effect of these fatty acids in depressing α-tocopherol uptake is intraluminal or intracellular needs to be established.

The relative absorption in vivo of α, β, γ, and δ-tocopherols has been examined by Pearson and Barnes (1970) by measuring the disappearance of these compounds following the injection of the vitamins in glyceryl trioleate solution into small intestinal loops in the rat. Over the 6-h test period 32% of the α-, 30% of the γ-, 18% of the β-, and 1.8% of the δ-tocopherol disappeared. No further analysis of this interesting selectivity is reported.

The concomitant digestion and absorption of other lipid species influences tocopherol absorption in rats. Medium-chain triglycerides as compared with long-chain triglycerides appear to enhance tocopherol absorption (Davies et al. 1972; Gallo-Torres et al. 1978). This is surprising since one might expect a large flux of lipid via the normal route for tocopherol transport, that is, the lymphatics, to promote tocopherol uptake. Perhaps medium-chain triglyceride absorption, involving as it does the portal venous route, in some way channels absorbed tocopherol in this direction also. It is known that minor amounts of tocopherol are transported by the portal venous route (MacMahon et al. 1971). Nevertheless, effects of medium-chain triglyceride digestion on micellar solubilisation of tocopherol and its presentation to the brush border of the enterocyte cannot be ignored. This possibility could be examined with various in vitro models.

Finally, mention should be made of a possible interference with tocopherol absorption by vitamin A in the chick as demonstrated by Combs and Scott (1974). A recent study has shown that vitamin A in the diet impairs α-tocopherol absorption as judged by lymphatic transport of the absorbed tocopherol. Retinoic acid was found to be much more potent than retinol in this respect (Bieri et al. 1981). The mechanism of this inhibition, which is reversed by the addition of 0.2% taurocholate to the diet (Bieri and Tolliver 1982) is presently unknown, but an interesting parallel exists in terms of vitamin A effects on the vitamin K status of rats in that retinoic acid is much more effective in producing hypoprothrombinaemia than retinol (Matschiner andDoisy (1962). The possibility of interference among the fat-soluble vitamins at the intestinal uptake step needs further study.

IV. Vitamin K

Following an oral dose of labelled phylloquinone in humans, radioactivity appears in plasma at 30 min and reaches a peak between 2 and 4 h after feeding. Most of this radioactivity is associated with unchanged vitamin K_1 and is probably present in chylomicrons. Faecal excretion data suggest that at least 50% of the dose is absorbed (SHEARER et al. 1970). This figure is in agreement with the results of BLOMSTRAND and FORSGREN (1968 b).

While the small intestine is an important site for absorption of the K vitamins there are interesting differences in the handling of the three major forms of the vitamin by the rat small bowel. Using everted small intestinal sacs, HOLLANDER (1973) showed that the proximal small intestine absorbs vitamin K_1 to a greater extent than the distal small intestine. When sacs are incubated under an atmosphere of nitrogen or in the presence of 2,4-dinitrophenol, a marked reduction in uptake is found only in the proximal intestinal preparation. These results point to an active energy-dependent uptake of phylloquinone by the upper small intestine. Similar studies with labelled vitamin K_2 (menaquinone-9, MK-9) showed a linear relationship between concentration and rate of uptake to a concentration of 900 n*M* unaffected by metabolic uncouplers and inhibitors, indicating that this form of vitamin K is absorbed by a passive noncarrier-mediated diffusion process (HOLLANDER and RIM 1976). This bacterial product may be available in sufficient amounts in the distal small intestine to contribute to the animal's requirements by absorption in the lower ileum and colon. Finally, vitamin K_3 transport appears to be a passive process in the small intestine and occurs most rapidly in the distal small intestine (HOLLANDER and TRUSCOTT 1974 a).

The active nature of the absorptive process in the small intestine for vitamin K_1 was confirmed by in vivo perfusion studies by HOLLANDER et al. (1977 a). The site of this active process in the cell is not yet identified. It might involve a coupling of phylloquinone with a carrier protein or might possibly operate at a later stage in the transcellular transport of the vitamin. Addition of the polyunsaturated fatty acid, linoleic acid, depressed absorption. A similar interaction has been noted between linoleic acid and other fat-soluble vitamins and competition for an intracellular binding protein could explain these observations. Perhaps the interference of vitamin K absorption by vitamin A (DOISY and MATSCHINER 1970) might be explained by a similar mechanism.

Using animals with lymphatic and biliary fistulae, HOLLANDER and RIM (1978) demonstrated again that polyunsaturated fatty acids in the intestinal infusion mixture depress total vitamin K_1 absorption as estimated by combined lymphatic and biliary recoveries. The addition of short- and medium-chain fatty acids to the infusate greatly enhanced the biliary recovery of radioactivity though the lymphatic transport fell. This again raises the interesting possibility that concomitant absorption of a lipid which partitions in favour of the portal vein might in some way direct more of the vitamin towards this route. As with all the other fat-soluble vitamins there is need for further analysis of their interaction with other dietary lipids at each step in the assimilation process.

1. Colonic Absorption of Vitamin K

Of the fat-soluble vitamins, vitamin K is unique in that in humans and other animals there is a potential endogenous source. Vitamin K_2 is synthesised by bacteria of the distal ileum and colon. This compound, first isolated from putrefied fish meal is one of a series of multiprenylmenaquinones (vitamin $K_{2(n)}$), see Table 1. It is of some interest that faecal microorganisms are capable of splitting off the side chain of phylloquinone (vitamin K_1) and thereafter converting the free methylnaphthoquinone into forms of vitamin K_2 (MARTIUS 1967).

The importance of an endogenous source of vitamin K is underscored by the difficulty of producing experimental vitamin K deficiency in humans. Only by rigorous purgation and the addition of broad-spectrum antibiotics to a vitamin K-deficient diet is it possible to achieve this (DOISY 1971; FRICK et al. 1967). In humans, therefore, ileal or colonic absorption of K vitamins seems possibly to be of physiological importance. As already discussed, dietary vitamin K_1 is probably absorbed in the jejunum by active transport. Rats, being coprophagous, may derive some of their supplies of vitamin K by this means though colonic absorption of vitamin K probably also occurs. Vitamin K can be absorbed from the colon in birds since rectal instillation of phylloquinone and menadione in vitamin K-deficient chicks lowers prothrombin times (BERDANIER and GRIMINGER 1968).

There has been conflicting data in humans about the ability of the colon to absorb vitamin K. Instillation of vitamin K_3 into the rectum of newborn infants has been shown to correct vitamin K-deficiency coagulation defects (ABALLI et al. 1966), but UDALL (1965) was unable to correct the prothrombin time in anticoagulated patients by caecal infusions of vitamin K_1. The explanation for the discrepancy, however, might be in the chemical and physical differences of the two forms of the vitamin used in these studies.

Colonic absorption of vitamin K_3 (2-methyl-1,4-naphthoquinone) the parent compound of the vitamin K series has been investigated by HOLLANDER and TRUSCOTT (1947b). The colon is capable of absorbing several classes of nutrient including sugars, amino acids and medium-chain fatty acids; nonionised lipid-soluble compounds are fairly well absorbed by the colonic mucosa. In everted rat colonic segments, vitamin K_3 is readily absorbed by a nonsaturable process up to a mucosal concentration of 900 μM. Anoxic conditions or the presence of dinitrophenol, an uncoupler of oxidative phosphorylation, do not interfere with the process and the absence of a concentration gradient across the mucosa abolishes the process. Thus there is every indication that the colon can take up vitamin K_3 by a passive process. This differs from the energy-dependent process responsible for vitamin K_1 absorption in the upper small intestine of the rat. On the other hand, in vitro studies of chick intestine suggest that vitamins K_1 and K_2 can be accumulated in the mucosa of the large intestine against a concentration gradient (BERDANIER and GRIMINGER 1968).

To examine colonic absorption of the most physiological form of vitamin K (vitamin K_2) in the large intestine, HOLLANDER et al. (1976) studied the uptake by everted rat colonic sacs in vitro of a tritiated bacterially synthesised vitamin K_2 (MK-9). The mean rate of absorption under these conditions was 20 p/mol/min per 100 g tissue at 300 nM mucosal concentration of the vitamin. Again, as with vitamin K_3, metabolic inhibitors such as 2,4-dinitrophenol, KCN and sodium azide did not interfere with absorption. Absorption was linear up to 900 n*M*. The compound was not transported transmurally which might reflect the absence of a drainage route, the lymphatics, in this preparation. Radioautography demonstrated accumulation of the vitamin in mucosal and submucosal layers of the bowel wall. Thus vitamin K_2 in rat colon, like vitamin K_3, appears to be taken up by a passive nonsaturable process independent of energy or the participation of a carrier.

These studies all indicate the ability of colonic mucosa in vitro to take up various forms of vitamin K by a passive process. However, the conditions employed, including the form of presentation of the vitamin, as emulsion or micellar solution with the nonionic detergent pluronic F-68, are far removed from the physiological situation obtaining in the intact colon. In the conscious rat, HOLLANDER et al. (1977b) have examined the ability of the ileum and colon to take up MK-9 under more physiological circumstances, demonstrating a linear relationship between perfusate concentration and absorption. These results are in keeping with the previous demonstration of passive uptake of the vitamin by in vitro preparations of rat colon. In this study the vitamin was presented as a bile salt micellar solution using sodium taurocholate. In these regions of the gut, bile salt concentration may not reach critical micellar levels; thus these studies may overestimate ileocolic uptake of MK-9. Increased perfusion of the ileum but not the colon enhanced absorption, possibly indicating that the unstirred water layer of the colon is less of a barrier to absorption than that of the ileum. As in other parts of the small intestine the inclusion of unsaturated long-chain fatty acids in the micelles diminished vitamin K_2 absorption in the ileum and colon. It is difficult to determine whether this inhibition of absorption from mixed fatty acid–bile salt micelles is of clinical importance in malabsorption states where increased amounts of fatty acids reach the ileocolic area since such a micellar phase probably does not exist in this region of the gut.

V. Absorption of the Ubiquinones

This class of compounds which are involved in mitochondrial electron transport chains is related to both vitamins E and K. Little is known about their absorption, but they seem to be transported from the intestine mainly in intestinal lymph. Thus, after oral administration, although only about 1% of an oral dose of tritiated coenzyme Q_{10} was recovered from thoracic duct lymph in rats in 48 h, less than half this amount could be recovered from urine and the liver (KATAYAMA and FUJITA 1972). In humans, BLOMSTRAND and GÜRTLER (1971) recovered large proportions of an oral dose of phytylubiquinone (hexahydroubiquinone-4) in thoracic duct lymph. The handling of such compounds by intestinal epithelial cells is not known.

J. Summary of Intestinal Absorption of Fat-Soluble Vitamins

The need for bile salts is a common feature of the absorption of all these vitamins. Their principal function is solubilisation of these lipophilic substances, achieving high local concentrations of the vitamins close to the apical membrane of the enterocyte. Their influence on the absorption is more complex however. Micellar solutions are a preferred substrate for the broad-spectrum enzyme, nonspecific lipase which hydrolyses the esters of vitamins A, D, and E. This hydrolysis appears to be a necessary step for efficient absorption of these vitamins. Bile salts appear to influence the intracellular handling of the absorbed fat-soluble vitamins, the best established effect being that on the cleavage of β-carotene. It is possible that bile salts also influence reesterification processes within the enterocyte and indirectly determine the ultimate route of transport of the vitamins from the intestinal mucosa.

The lymphatics are undoubtedly a major route of transport of absorbed fat-soluble vitamins, but the more polar derivatives of these compounds are extensively transported by the portal vein. It is possible that under conditions where lymphatic transport of the vitamins is compromised, the portal venous route may play a more important part in this step of the assimilation process. The mucosal uptake of the vitamins is largely a passive process, but from the studies of HOLLANDER and his colleagues in the rat, there is evidence that a carrier-mediated step is involved in retinol absorption and phylloquinone absorption is an active process in this species (Table 2). From the foregoing account of the physiological aspects of fat-soluble vitamin absorption the natural dietary substances which appear to influence this are the polyunsaturated fatty acids. As a general rule the absorption of all the fat-soluble vitamins is impaired by concomitant absorption of polyunsaturated fatty acids whether this is studied in vitro or in vivo. Whether the effect of these polyunsaturated fatty acids on absorption is exerted at the same step in each case is not known. In the case of vitamin A, at least, there is some evidence that the competition between these fatty acids and retinol for a binding protein in the cytosol of the enterocyte may be the important event. The remainder of this chapter considers those nonnutrient substances which may influence fat-soluble vitamin absorption.

Table 2. Summary of characteristics of fat-soluble vitamin absorption in the rat. Data collected from papers of HOLLANDER and colleagues. For details, see text

Vitamin	Site of absorption	Nature of absorptive process
Retinol	Small intestine	Passive, carrier-mediated, saturable
Cholecalciferol	Proximal and mid-small intestine	Passive
25-Hydroxycholecalciferol	Small intestine	Passive
α-Tocopherol	Mid-small intestine	Passive
Phylloquinone	Proximal small intestine	Active, saturable
Menaquinone-9 (MK-9)	Small intestine	Passive
	Colon	Passive
Menadione	Distal small intestine	Passive
	Colon	Passive

K. Nonnutrient Substances which Interfere with Fat-Soluble Vitamin Absorption

I. Bile Salt Sequestrants

The need for therapeutic measures to reduce hypercholesterolaemia and consequently to lower the morbidity and mortality from arteriosclerotic disease has led to the development of a number of drugs which bind bile acids in the intestinal lumen. If sufficient amounts of bile acids are precipitated, the micellar phase in the intestine will be reduced and cholesterol absorption will decrease since its absorption depends on micellar solubilisation. In addition, the binding of bile acids by such substances will increase their faecal excretion and since bile acids are the major metabolic end product of cholesterol metabolism this will result in a drain on liver cholesterol towards the excretory route with a consequent reduction in serum cholesterol. Since fat-soluble vitamins, like cholesterol, require a bile acid micellar phase for their absorption and as the management of hypercholesterolaemia is a lifelong problem the possibility of deficiency of these vitamins developing insidiously during treatment must be considered.

Most bile salt sequestrants are nonabsorbable polymers with functional ionic groups and they bind bile salts and other anions by an ion exchange effect though hydrophobic bonding forces also operate. The ion exchange group includes cholestyramine, diethylaminoethyl- (DEAE)-dextran derivatives and colestipol. Certain aminoglycoside antibiotics, notably neomycin, which is very poorly absorbed by the intestine, seem to bind and precipitate bile salts by ionic interaction. Lignins, derived from dietary vegetables, bind bile salts probably by a hydrophobic interaction.

In addition to reducing serum cholesterol, bile salt sequestrants such as cholestyramine have been found useful in the management of conditions in which bile salt physiology is deranged. These include cholerrhoeic enteropathy due to ileal resection or bypass in which diarrhoea results from the secretagogue action of unabsorbed bile acids on the colonic mucosa. In states of impaired bile salt secretion such as primary biliary cirrhosis, congenital biliary atresia and certain forms of acquired extrahepatic biliary obstruction cholestyramine has been effective in relieving pruritus.

1. Cholestyramine

This is the most frequently used bile salt sequestrant in clinical practice. It is a styrene–divinyl benzene copolymer containing quaternary ammonium functional groups and acts as a strongly basic anion exchanger. Electrostatic binding of bile salts is therefore the main mechanism of action of cholestyramine, but hydrophobic bonding of lipid substances to its hydrocarbon chain also occurs. Studies in vitro show that it binds bile salts and fatty acids (JOHNS and BATES 1970) and that its affinity for bile salts increases as the number of hydroxyl groups on the bile salt falls; thus it would bind chenodeoxycholate and deoxycholate more readily than cholate. Its affinity for fatty acids increases with chain length, but falls with increasing degree of unsaturation of the hydrocarbon chain.

In large doses, cholestyramine causes steatorrhoea in both rats (HARKINS et al. 1965) and humans (HASHIM et al. 1961). Experimental animal studies show that fat-soluble vitamin absorption can be impaired by the addition of this drug to the diet. In weanling rats, the addition of 2% cholestyramine to a diet rich in fat but containing vitamin A in growth-limiting amounts caused a reduced body weight gain compared with animals receiving the same diet but no cholestyramine (WHITESIDE et al. 1965); this dose of cholestyramine is comparable to human doses. The effect on growth could be offset by adding more vitamin A to the diet, but liver stores of vitamin A were still reduced compared with control values. If the vitamin was present in the diet as retinyl palmitate rather than retinol the effects of cholestyramine on liver stores of vitamin A were more marked. This could indicate that the depletion of free intraluminal bile salt interfered with retinyl ester hydrolysis by nonspecific lipase, possibly by reducing the concentration of the ester in the micellar solubilised form and by sequestering some of the trihydroxy bile acids which activate the enzyme. Vitamin D malabsorption can be induced in rats by the addition of 4% cholestyramine to their diet (THOMPSON and THOMPSON 1969) and α-tocopherol absorption is also impaired by cholestyramine. This effect is more marked in the presence of a long-chain than a medium-chain triglyceride diet (DAVIES et al. 1972). The explanation for this is not apparent though it is known that tocopherol absorption is greater in the presence of medium-chain as compared with long-chain triglycerides (DAVIES et al. 1972; GALLO-TORRES et al. 1978). Chickens on a marginally low vitamin K intake develop prolonged prothrombin times on a 2% cholestyramine diet, but the effect does not seem to occur in dogs (ROBINSON et al. 1964).

Some studies in humans indicate impaired vitamin A uptake from test meals when it is given with cholestyramine. A dose of 8 g cholestyramine fed with a meal containing 250,000 USP units vitamin A reduced plasma vitamin A levels, but 4 g did not have any significant effect (LONGENECKER and BASU 1965) while BARNARD and HEATON (1973) observed a 60% reduction in the anticipated rise in serum vitamin A which follows a dose of 5,000 IU/kg when 12 g cholestyramine was added to the test meal. Whether these effects of cholestyramine on the tolerance curves following pharmacological doses of vitamin A are relevant to long-term problems of fat-soluble vitamin absorption is debatable.

In patients with hyperlipidaemia on long-term cholestyramine treatment, CASDORPH (1970) has reported moderate increases in prothrombin time in 6 of 12 cases, but no prolonged prothrombin times were found in 9 hypercholesterolaemic subjects treated with 13.3 g cholestyramine daily for periods of 1 month to 4 years (HASHIM and VAN ITALLIE 1965). Similarly in a group of patients suffering from hypercholesterolaemia and hypertriglyceridaemia BRESSLER et al. (1966) found no disturbance of vitamin A or K metabolism after several months of therapy with cholestyramine at doses ranging between 12 and 36 g daily.

A number of single case reports document fat-soluble vitamin depletion in patients on cholestyramine treatment. For example, VISINTINE et al. (1961) found a marked alteration in prothrombin time in a patient with xanthomatous biliary cirrhosis receiving 15 g cholestyramine daily for 4 months and ROE (1968) reported a similar effect in a patient with xanthomatosis treated with 20 g/day.

In some patients there may already be disturbed bile salt metabolism, such as extensive terminal ileal disease, resection or bypass with malabsorption of bile salts and a reduced bile salt pool; this could be aggravated by cholestyramine. Thus, osteomalacia occurred in a patient with a terminal ileal bypass whose diarrhoea was treated for more than 2 years with the drug (HEATON et al. 1972) while GROSS and BROTMAN (1970) reported hypoprothrombinaemia and haemorrhage after only 3 weeks of treatment of postirradiation enterocolitis with cholestyramine. The treatment of cholerrhoeic enteropathy with cholestyramine always carries the risk of further reduction in bile salt concentrations in the proximal small intestine. Similarly, cholestyramine treatment of the pruritus of primary biliary cirrhosis might reduce intraluminal bile salt concentrations to a critical level. These patients, however, usually receive supplements of the fat-soluble vitamins as a routine, in view of the precarious state of their absorption of these vitamins.

In children where fat-soluble vitamin deficiencies would be very important, WEST and LLOYD (1975) found a significant decrease in serum levels of vitamins A and E in patients with hypercholesterolaemia treated for a 2-year period, but a study by GLUECK et al. (1974) showed no such change in a 10-month period of treatment with 12 g cholestyramine daily. In adults with the same condition, 20 g cholestyramine given daily for 18 weeks produced no evidence of malabsorption of any of the fat-soluble vitamins (SCHADE et al. 1976). The general clinical experience suggests that fat-soluble vitamin deficiency with cholestyramine treatment is rather uncommon. However, patients with impaired bile salt metabolism and those on high-dose, long-term treatment for hyperlipidaemia, particularly children, are at risk and should receive supplements of the vitamins.

2. DEAE-Sephadex

This substance belongs to a group of anion exchangers based on cellulose or dextran which are widely used in analytical chemistry. These include DEAE-cellulose, DEAE-Sephadex, and guanidoethyl-cellulose. They all sequester bile acids and all of them have been shown to lower serum cholesterol in cockerels with experimental hypercholesterolaemia (PARKINSON 1967). In dogs with normal or raised serum cholesterol, DEAE-Sephadex lowers the serum concentration and faecal bile acid output increases. CECIL et al. (1973) found a depletion of hepatic vitamin A stores in pregnant, newborn and weanling rats treated with this compound.

A study by BORGSTRÖM (1970) has shown that DEAE-Sephadex alters the enzyme-catalysed equilibrium of triglyceride digestion by pancreatic lipase in vitro, increasing the proportion of monoglyceride in the mixture. This presumably results from sequestration of fatty acids produced during the reaction. Thus this anion exchanger, and probably others, would tend to alter the composition of the micellar phase in the small intestinal lumen.

A number of studies have shown that DEAE-Sephadex (Secholex), poly-[2-(diethylamino)ethyl]polyglycerylenedextran hydrochloride reduces serum cholesterol in hypercholesterolaemia (HOWARD and HYAMS 1971; COURTENAY EVANS and LANNER 1974; RITLAND et al. 1975). In none of these studies was there any direct evidence of interference with fat-soluble vitamin absorption though GUSTAFSON and LANNER (1974) noted a rise in serum alkaline phosphatase in some patients. It is interesting that RITLAND et al. (1975) found a significant increase in the concentration of bile acids in duodenal aspirates of patients taking the drug, suggesting some form of compensation. At the time of writing, this drug is not available for clinical use.

3. Colestipol

A newer addition to the bile salt sequestrant group, colestipol is a high molecular weight copolymer of tetraethylene pentamine and epichlorhydrin with one of the five amino nitrogens as the chloride salt. Compared with cholestyramine, colestipol has approximately two-thirds the affinity for bile salts when tested in vitro. KO and ROYER (1974) have demonstrated that when sodium taurocholate micellar solutions of vitamins A, D, and K are exposed to colestipol, major amounts of the vitamins are removed from solution either bound to the copolymer or thrown out of micellar solution as a precipitate.

However, studies with experimental animals do not suggest that fat-soluble vitamin deficiency occurs with colestipol treatment. Dogs receiving the drug in doses equivalent to ten times the human therapeutic doses did not develop any physical signs or biochemical abnormalities indicating fat-soluble vitamin deficiency (PARKINSON et al. 1973) nor did weanling rats given colestipol 2,000 mg kg^{-1} day^{-1} for 18 months (WEBSTER, cited by PARKINSON et al. 1973).

In humans too, fat-soluble vitamin deficiencies with colestipol treatment are rare. MILLER et al. (1973) found small but significant changes in serum calcium and alkaline phosphatase possibly related to vitamin D deficiency and, in one patient, a prolonged prothrombin time in a study of eight patients with hypercholesterolaemia treated with the drug for 4–6 months. On the other hand, GUNDERSEN (cited by PARKINSON et al. 1973) found no evidence of fat-soluble vitamin deficiency in healthy male subjects taking 12–15 g colestipol daily for more than 3 years and GLUECK et al. (1972) reported normal prothrombin times in 25 patients with type II hyperlipidaemia given 20 g colestipol daily for 4 months. In a study of 23 children with heterozygous familial hypercholesterolaemia treated with long-term colestipol, serum vitamin A and E levels fell significantly during 24 months of treatment, but these levels still remained within normal limits (SCHWARTZ et al. 1980). Serum 25-hydroxycholecalciferol concentrations and prothrombin times were not affected. It is difficult to interpret the falls in serum vitamin A and E since they may have reflected alterations in serum lipoprotein concentrations rather than a direct effect of colestipol on intestinal absorption of the vitamins.

4. Neomycin

This polybasic aminoglycoside antibiotic is very poorly absorbed by the gastrointestinal tract. A major therapeutic use of the drug is to suppress bacterial growth in the large intestine in the management of hepatic encephalopathy. It binds fatty acids and to a lesser extent bile acids in the intestine, disrupting the micellar phase (THOMPSON et al. 1970).

Neomycin produces a reversible malabsorption syndrome by complex effects on the gut. At 12 g/day in human subjects steatorrhoea occurs, but at lower doses such as 2 g/day it has a hypocholesterolaemic effect without steatorrhoea. LEVINE (1967) has documented reduced serum carotene and vitamin A levels with neomycin treatment while UDALL (1965) found prolonged prothrombin times. This latter effect is difficult to interpret since the antibiotic action might reduce endogenous bacterial vitamin K contributions. In patients with chronic liver disease on long-term neomycin treatment, failure of hepatic synthesis of prothrombin will contribute further to hypoprothrombinaemia. A single dose of neomycin given with a test meal containing vitamin A depresses the subsequent rise in plasma retinol (BARROWMAN et al. 1973).

How neomycin causes hypocholesterolaemia and interferes with fat-soluble vitamin absorption is not clear. Cholesterol absorption decreases and faecal neutral steroid excretion rises with neomycin treatment (SEDAGHAT et al. 1975).

Micellar disruption due to bile acid and fatty acid precipitation (THOMPSON et al. 1971) is an attractive hypothesis but SEDAGHAT et al. (1975) found no sustained rise in faecal acidic steroid excretion, when 2 g neomycin were given daily, despite significant reduction in plasma cholesterol. At that dose, therefore, neomycin does not seem to be an effective bile acid sequestrant though transient sequestration in the upper small intestine with subsequent dissociation of neomycin–bile acid complexes in the distal ileum and reabsorption of the bile acids is a possibility. The extent to which the toxic action of neomycin on the intestinal mucosa (see Sect. K.III) contributes to cholesterol and fat-soluble vitamin malabsorption is not established. The related aminoglycoside, kanamycin also causes mild steatorrhoea, but has a weaker affinity for bile acids than neomycin (FALOON et al. 1966).

5. Lignins and Dietary Fibre

These compounds which have been used in the treatment of type II hyperlipidaemia and postileectomy diarrhoea are present in plant foodstuffs; they consist of amorphous phenylpropane polymers. They may form hydrophobic bonds with bile acids, particularly the less polar species, precipitating them from solution. An increasing degree of methylation of the phenolic hydroxyl groups enhances this binding capacity. Lignins are much less effective than cholestyramine in binding bile acids in vivo (HEATON et al. 1971) and it would be unlikely that any impairment of fat-soluble vitamin absorption could result from the use of lignin. BARNARD and HEATON (1973) found that large doses of lignin had no effect on the rise of serum vitamin A which follows a large oral load of the vitamin. Dietary fibre from various sources, wheat bran, cellulose, apple pectin, guar flour, carob bean flour or carrageenan fed with a similar large dose of vitamin A was found to enhance its absorption (KASPER et al. 1979). The explanation for this effect is not clear.

6. Aluminium-Based Antacids

The observation that aluminium antacids interfere with vitamin A absorption (HOFFMAN and DYNIEWICZ 1945) might be worth reinvestigating in the light of recent studies by CLAIN et al. (1977) which have demonstrated that aluminium hydroxide is an effective precipitant of bile acids. It is possible, however, that there is no great disturbance of bile acids in the small intestine since aluminium is probably precipitated there largely as the phosphate which has little affinity for bile acids.

II. Nonabsorbable Lipids

1. Mineral Oil

Mineral oils have long been used as stool softeners and lubricants sometimes in combination with osmotic laxatives such as magnesium salts. A number of early publications suggested that mineral oils impair fat-soluble vitamin absorption (CURTIS and KLINE 1939; CURTIS and BALLMER 1939; JAVERT and MACRI 1941; MORGAN 1941) and occasional case reports such as that of SINCLAIR (1967) record deficiencies of individual fat-soluble vitamins where excessive amounts of mineral oil are ingested. When rats are given a diet containing 20% by weight mineral oil hypoprothrombinaemia develops, correctable by injection of vitamin K (ELLIOTT et al. 1940). Presumably the effect results from the solution of the vitamins in a nonassimilable lipid phase in the intestine which carries them out in the faeces. The dangers of fat-soluble vitamin deficiency are probably exaggerated, but in older patients who are the main consumers of these laxatives a relative dietary deficiency could be amplified by mineral oil. For the maximum effect the oil would need to be fed with the meal in large amounts. In a study by MAHLE and PATTON (1947) 30 ml mineral oil fed to human subjects daily at bedtime for 51 days failed to cause any abnormal decrease in plasma retinol concentrations. Squalene, another indigestible hydrocarbon, when added to rat diets interrupts vitamin K absorption (MATSCHINER et al. 1967). The mechanism for this effect is unknown, but is probably similar to that of mineral oil.

2. Sucrose Polyester

The search for hypocholesterolaemic agents has produced sucrose polyester, (SPE) a mixture of hexa-, hepta-, and octa-esters of sucrose with long-chain fatty acids. This substance is physically similar to triglycerides, but cannot be digested by enzymes within the intestinal lumen (MATTSON and VOLPENHEIN 1972a) and consequently cannot be absorbed (MATTSON and NOLEN 1972; MATTSON and VOLPENHEIN 1972b). Cholesterol absorption is impaired by SPE and since cholesterol partitions similarly between bile salt micelles and either triglyceride or SPE oil the decrease in absorption is attributed to the presence of an undigested oil phase of SPE dissolving dietary and endogenous cholesterol and carrying these through the gastrointestinal tract (MATTSON et al. 1976). A similar mechanism presumably accounts for reductions of 10% and 21% respectively in plasma concentrations of vitamin A and E in human subjects treated with SPE as a hypocholesterolaemic agent (FALLAT et al. 1976). In rats, MATTSON et al. (1979) measuring vitamin A levels in the liver, demonstrated that when SPE replaces cottonseed oil in the diet, a very substantial decrease in hepatic vitamin A storage results. If SPE is to be considered as a possible long-term means of regulating serum cholesterol, attention to fat-soluble vitamin status will be important.

III. Drugs Affecting Small Intestinal Mucosal Morphology and Metabolism

Neomycin, in addition to producing steatorrhoea by intraluminal biochemical effects, causes malabsorption of glucose, xylose, vitamin B_{12}, and iron. A reversible reduction of mucosal disaccharidases occurs (PAES et al. 1967). Histological changes in human small intestinal mucosa include clubbing of the villi and infiltration of the lamina propria with inflammatory cells and pigment-containing macrophages. Crypt mitotic counts rise and electron microscopy shows ballooning of microvilli and evidence of injury to mitochondria and endoplasmic reticulum of crypt cells (DOBBINS et al. 1968).

Colchicine by mouth in doses between 1.9 and 3.9 mg/day produces a malabsorption syndrome in humans which includes a mild steatorrhoea with reduced serum carotene levels (RACE et al. 1970). Intestinal disaccharidase concentrations also fall and mild histological abnormalities including mucosal oedema and infiltration with chronic inflammatory cells are observed. These changes are all reversible on discontinuing the drug.

IV. Other Drugs Which Cause Steatorrhoea

Table 3 lists a group of miscellaneous drugs which have been reported to cause steatorrhoea in humans or experimental animals by a variety of mechanisms. These could presumably interfere with fat-soluble vitamin absorption. Chronic alcoholism is often associated with a moderate degree of steatorrhoea.

Table 3. Miscellaneous agents which produce steatorrhoea in humans or animals

Drug	Reference
Calcium carbonate	KRAMER (1967)
p-Aminosalicylic acid	LEVINE (1968)
Phenindione	JUEL-JENSEN (1959)
Phenolphthalein	FRENCH et al. (1956)
Mefenamic acid	MARKS and GLEESON (1975)
Polymixin–bacitracin mixture	POWELL et al. (1962)
Tetracycline	YEH and SHILS (1966)

L. Other Effects of Drugs on Fat-Soluble Vitamin Absorption

As discussed in Sect. H.IV.1, vitamin K supplies are partly derived from endogenous sources, that is bacterial metabolism in the lower intestine, in many species including humans. Purgation and broad-spectrum antibiotics will eventually produce a vitamin K deficit in humans (FRICK et al. 1967). VESSELL (1972) has reported that phenothiazines which can induce cholestasis can aggravate the hypoprothrombinaemia produced by the coumarin group of anticoagulants.

It has long been recognised that excess vitamin A can cause hypoprothrombinaemia in rats (LIGHT et al. 1944). This does not seem to occur in humans. Possible explanations in addition to systemic interaction include inhibition of bacterial synthesis of vitamin K (QUICK and STEFANINI 1948), formation of an unabsorbable complex between retinoic acid and vitamin K (see DOISY and MATSCHINER

1970) or antagonism at some stage in the absorptive process. This question is not fully resolved, but the finding of an interaction between vitamins A and K in germ-free rats (WOSTMANN and KNIGHT 1965) argues against an effect on bacterial production of vitamin K.

As fat-soluble vitamin deficiency can be anticipated in malabsorption syndromes with steatorrhoea resulting from pancreatic or small intestinal disease, ablation or bypass, correction of these conditions when possible will improve the absorption of these vitamins. Dietary or parenteral supplementation with fat-soluble vitamins may be necessary. Deficiency of the fat-soluble vitamins has been documented in patients with chronic alcoholic pancreatitis receiving treatment with pancreatic enzyme preparations (DUTTA et al. 1979). The enzyme treatment, however, was only partially successful as these patients still had significant steatorrhoea. Fat-soluble vitamin supplements should be given to such patients.

Attempts have been made to overcome the failure of lipid emulsification and micelle formation of bile salt deficiency with artificial detergents. Tween 80, polyoxyethylene sorbitan monooleate, has been reported to prevent cholestyramine-induced fat malabsorption in rats (DU BOIS et al. 1964) and JONES et al. (1948) first reported improved fat and vitamin A absorption with this substance in a variety of malabsorption problems in humans. A more recent study by KING et al. (1979) has shown that Tween 80 reduces steatorrhoea in patients with bile salt deficiency, increasing the concentration of fatty acid and phospholipid in the micellar phase of intestinal content, and might improve fat-soluble vitamin absorption in these patients.

M. Summary of Drug Effects on Fat-Soluble Vitamin Absorption

Although absorption of fat-soluble vitamins is often impaired in diseases of the pancreas and small intestine, drugs and nonnutrient substances in the diet seldom interfere with this process. Since bile acids play an important part in their absorption, bile acid sequestering agents, often given as long-term treatment, could lead to deficiencies of the fat-soluble vitamins. Nonabsorbable lipid substances might also produce this effect if given in substantial amounts over long periods.

References

Aballi AJ, Howard CE, Triplett RF (1966) Absorption of vitamin K from the colon in the new born infant. J Pediatr 68:305–308

Arnaud SB, Goldsmith RS, Lambert PW, Go VLW (1975) 25-hydroxy-vitamin D_3: evidence of an enterohepatic circulation in man. Proc Soc Exp Biol Med 149:570–572

Avioli LV, Lee SW, McDonald JE, Lund J, De Luca HF (1967) Metabolism of vitamin D_3 – ^3H in human subjects: distribution in blood, bile, faeces, and urine. J Clin Invest 46:983–992

Barnard DL, Heaton KW (1973) Bile acids and vitamin A absorption in man: the effects of two bile acid binding agents, cholestyramine and lignin. Gut 14:316–318

Barrowman J, D'Mello A, Herxheimer A (1973) A single dose of neomycin impairs absorption of vitamin A (retinol) in man. Eur J Clin Pharmacol 5:199–202

Bashor MM, Toft DO, Chytil F (1973) In vitro binding of retinol to rat-tissue components. Proc Natl Acad Sci USA 70:3483–3487

Bell NH, Bryan P (1969) Absorption of vitamin D_3 oleate in the rat. Am J Clin Nutr 22:425–430

Bell PA, Kodicek E (1969) Investigations on metabolites of vitamin D in rat bile. Separation and partial identification of a major metabolite. Biochem J 115:663–669

Bensadoun A, Rothfeld A (1972) The form of absorption of lipids in the chicken, Gallus domesticus. Proc Soc Exp Biol Med 141:814–817

Berdanier DC, Griminger P (1968) In vitro and in vivo absorption of three vitamin K analogs by chick intestine. Int Z Vitamin Ernährungsforsch [Beih] 38:376–382

Bieri JG, Farrell PM (1976) Vitamin E. Vitam Horm 34:31–75

Bieri JG, Tolliver TJ (1982) Reversal by bile acid on the inhibition of α-tocopherol absorption by retinoic acid. J Nutr 112:401–403

Bieri JG, Wu AL, Tolliver TJ (1981) Reduced intestinal absorption of vitamin E by the low dietary levels of retinoic acid in rats. J Nutr 111:458–467

Blomstrand R, Forsgren L (1967) Intestinal absorption and esterification of vitamin D_3-1,2-^{3}H in man. Acta Chem Scand 21:1652–1663

Blomstrand R, Forsgren L (1968 a) Labelled tocopherols in man. Intestinal absorption and thoracic duct lymph transport of DL-alpha-tocopheryl-3,4-$^{14}C_2$ acetate, DL-alpha-tocopheramine-3,4-$^{14}C_2$, DL-alphatocopherol-(5-methyl-^{3}H) and N-(methyl-^{3}H)-DL-gamma tocopheramine. Int Z Vitamin Ernährungsforsch [Beih] 38:328–344

Blomstrand R, Forsgren L (1968 b) Vitamin K_1-^{3}H in man. Its intestinal absorption and transport in the thoracic duct lymph. Int Z Vitamin Ernährungsforsch [Beih] 38:45–64

Blomstrand R, Gurtler J (1971) Studies on the intestinal absorption and metabolism of phytylubiquinone-(1′,2′-^{3}H) (hexahydroubiquinone-4) in man. Int J Vitam Nutr Res 41:189–203

Blomstrand R, Werner B (1967) Studies on the intestinal absorption of radioactive β-carotene and vitamin A in man. Scand J Clin Lab Invest 19:339–345

Blunt JW, Deluca HF, Schnoes HK (1968) 25-Hydroxycholecalciferol. A biologically active metabolite of vitamin D_3. Biochemistry 7:3317–3322

Borgström B (1968) Partition of lipids between emulsified oil and micellar phases of glyceride-bile salt dispersions. J Lipid Res 8:598–608

Borgström B (1970) Effect of ion-exchange substances on the lipolysis catalysed by pancreatic lipase. Scand J Gastroenterol 5:549–553

Borgström B (1980) Importance of phospholipids, pancreatic phospholipase A_2 and fatty acid for the digestion of dietary fat. Gastroenterology 78:954–962

Borgström B, Erlanson C (1978) Interaction of serum albumin and other proteins with porcine pancreatic lipase. Gastroenterology 75:382–386

Borgström B, Erlanson-Albertsson C, Wieloch T (1979) Pancreatic colipase: chemistry and physiology. J Lipid Res 20:805–816

Bressler R, Nowlin J, Bogdonoff MD (1966) Treatment of hypercholesterolemia and hypertriglyceridemia by anion exchange resin. South Med J 59:1097–1103

Casdorph HR (1970) Safe uses of cholestyramine. Ann Intern Med 72:759

Cecil HC, Harris SJ, Bitman J Dryden LP (1973) Effect of DEAE-Sephadex on liver vitamin A of lactating rats and their offspring. J Nutr 103:43–48

Clain JE, Malagelada JR, Chadwick VS, Hoffman AF (1977) Binding properties in vitro of antacids for conjugated bile acids. Gastroenterology 73:556–559

Coates ME, Thompson SY, Kon SK (1950) Conversion of carotene to vitamin A in the intestine of the pig and of the rat: transport of vitamin A by the lymph. Biochem J 46:30P–31P

Cohen M, Morgan RGH, Hofmann AF (1971) Lipolytic activity of human gastric and duodenal juice against medium and long chain triglycerides. Gastroenterology 60:1–15

Combs GF, Scott ML (1974) Antioxidant effects of selenium and vitamin E function in the chick. J Nutr 104:1297–1303

Compston JE, Creamer B (1977) Plasma levels and intestinal absorption of 25-hydroxyvitamin D in patients with small bowel resection. Gut 18:171–175

Compston JE, Merrett AL, Ledger JE, Creamer B (1982) Faecal tritium excretion after intravenous administration of ^{3}H-25-hydroxyvitamin D_3 in control subjects and in patients with malabsorption. Gut 23:310–315

Courtenay Evans RJ, Howard AN, Hyams DE (1973) An effective treatment of hypercholesterolaemia using a combination of Secholex and clofibrate. Angiology 24:22–28
Crain FD, Lotspeich FJ, Krause RF (1967) Biosynthesis of retinoic acid by intestinal enzymes of the rat. J Lipid Res 8:249–254
Curtis AC, Ballmer RS (1939) The prevention of carotene absorption by liquid petrolatum. J Am Med Assoc 113:1785–1788
Curtis AC, Kline EM (1939) Influence of liquid petrolatum on blood content of carotene in human beings. Arch Intern Med 63:54–63
Danielsson A, Lorentzon R, Larsson SE (1982) Intestinal absorption and 25-hydroxylation of vitamin D in patients with primary biliary cirrhosis. Scand J Gastroenterol 17:349–355
David JSK, Ganguly J (1967) Further studies on the mechanism of absorption of vitamin A and cholesterol. Indian J Biochem Biophys 4:14–17
Davies M, Mawer EB, Krawitt EL (1980) Comparative absorption of vitamin D_3 and 25-hydroxyvitamin D_3 in intestinal disease. Gut 21:287–292
Davies T, Kelleher J, Smith CL, Walker BE, Lasowsky MS (1972) Effect of therapeutic measures which alter fat absorption on the absorption of alpha-tocopherol in the rat. J Lab Clin Med 79:824–831
De Haas GH, Postema NM, Nieuwenhuizen W, Van Deenen LLM (1968) Purification and properties of phospholipase A from porcine pancreas. Biochim Biophys Acta 159:103–117
Dobbins WO, Herrero BA, Mansbach CM (1968) Morphologic alterations associated with neomycin-induced malabsorption. Am J Med Sci 255:63–77
Doisy EA (1971) Vitamin K in human nutrition. Symp proc assoc of vitamin chemists, Chicago
Doisy EA, Matschiner JT (1970) Biochemistry of vitamin K. In: Morton RA (ed) Fat-soluble vitamins. Pergamon, Oxford
Drummond JC, Bell ME, Palmer ET (1935) Observations on the absorption of carotene and vitamin A. Br Med J i:1208–1210
Du Bois JJ, Holt PR, Kuron GW, Hashim SA, Van Itallie TB (1964) Effect of Tween 80 on cholestyramine-induced malabsorption. Proc Soc Exp Biol Med 117:226–229
Dueland S, Pedersen JI, Helgerud P, Drevon CA (1982) Transport of vitamin D_3 from rat intestine. J Biol Chem 257:146–150
Dunagin PE, Meadows EH, Olson JA (1965) Retinoyl beta-glucuronic acid: a major metabolite of vitamin A in rat bile. Science 148:86–87
Dutta SK, Costa BS, Russell RM, Connor TB (1979) Fat soluble vitamin deficiency in treated patients with pancreatic insufficiency. Gastroenterology 76:1126
Eden E, Sellers KC (1949) The absorption of vitamin A in ruminants and rats. Biochem J 44:264–267
El-Gorab M, Underwood BA (1973) Solubilization of β-carotene and retinol into aqueous solutions of mixed micelles. Biochim Biophys Acta 306:58–66
El-Gorab MI, Underwood BA, Loerch JD (1975) The roles of bile salts in the uptake of β-carotene and retinol by rat everted gut sacs. Biochim Biophys Acta 401:265–277
Elliott MC, Isaacs B, Ivy AC (1940) Production of "prothrombin deficiency" and response to vitamins A, D, and K. Proc Soc Exp Biol Med 43:240–245
Erlanson C, Borgström B (1968) The identity of vitamin A esterase activity of rat pancreatic juice. Biochim Biophys Acta 141:629–631
Fallat RW, Glueck CJ, Lutmer R, Mattson FH (1976) Short-term study of sucrose polyester a non-absorbable fat-like material as a dietary agent for lowering plasma cholesterol. Am J Clin Nutr 29:1204–1215
Faloon WW, Paes IC, Woolfolk D, Nankin H, Wallace K, Haro EN (1966) Effect of neomycin and kanamycin upon intestinal absorption. Ann NY Acad Sci 132:879–887
Fidge NH, Goodman DS (1968) The enzymatic reduction of retinal to retinol in rat intestine. J Biol Chem 243:4372–4379
Fidge NH, Shiratori T, Ganguly J, Goodman DS (1968) Pathways of absorption of retinal and retinoic acid in the rat. J Lipid Res 9:103–109

Forbes GB (1944) Chylothorax in infancy; observations on absorption of vitamins A and D and on intravenous replacement of aspirated chyle. J Pediatr 25:191–200

Forsgren L (1969) Studies on the intestinal absorption of labelled fat-soluble vitamins (A, D, E, and K) via the thoracic duct lymph in the absence of bile in man. Acta Chir Scand [Suppl] 399

Fraser DR, Kodicek E (1968) Investigations on vitamin D esters synthesised in rats. Biochem J 106:485–496

Fredrikzon B, Hernell O, Bläckberg L, Olivecrona T (1978) Bile salt-stimulated lipase in human milk: evidence of activity in vivo and of a role in the digestion of milk retinol esters. Pediatr Res 12:1048–1052

French JM, Gaddie R, Smith N (1956) Diarrhoea due to phenolphthalein. Lancet 1:551–553

Frick PG, Riedler G, Brogli H (1967) Dose response and minimal daily requirement for vitamin K in man. J Appl Physiol 23:387–389

Gagnon M, Dawson AM (1968) The effect of bile on vitamin A absorption in the rat. Proc Soc Exp Biol Med 127:99–102

Gallo-Torres H (1970 a) Obligatory role of bile for the intestinal absorption of vitamin E. Lipids 5:379–384

Gallo-Torres HE (1970 b) Intestinal absorption and lymphatic transport of DL-3,4-$^3H_2$-α-tocopheryl nicotinate in the rat. Int J Vitam Nutr Res 40:505–514

Gallo-Torres HE, Weber F, Wiss O (1971) The effect of different dietary lipids on the lymphatic appearance of vitamin E. Int J Vitam Nutr Res 41:504–515

Gallo-Torres HE, Ludorf J, Brin M (1978) The effect of medium-chain triglycerides on the bioavailability of vitamin E. Int J Vitam Nutr Res 48:240–249

Ganguly J (1969) Absorption of vitamin A. Am J Clin Nutr 22:923–933

Gascon-Barre M (1982) Biliary excretion of (^{3}H)-25-hydroxyvitamin D_3 in the vitamin D-depleted rat. Am J Physiol 242:G522–G532

Glueck CJ, Ford S, Scheel D, Steiner P (1972) Colestipol and cholestyramine resin. Comparative effects in familial type II hyperlipoproteinemia. J Am Med Assoc 222:676–681

Glueck CJ, Tsang RC, Fallat RW, Scheel BA (1974) Plasma vitamin A and E levels in children with familial type II hyperlipoproteinaemia during therapy with diet and cholestyramine resin. Pediatrics 54:51–55

Goodman DS, Huang HS (1965) Biosynthesis of vitamin A with rat intestinal enzymes. Science 149:879–880

Goodman DS, Blomstrand R, Werner B, Huang HS, Shiratori T (1966) The intestinal absorption and metabolism of vitamin A and β-carotene in man. J Clin Invest 45:1615–1623

Goodman DS, Huang HS, Kanai M, Shiratori T (1967) The enzymatic conversion of all-trans β-carotene into retinal. J Biol Chem 242:3543–3554

Greaves JD, Schmidt CLA (1933) The role played by bile in the absorption of vitamin D in the rat. J Biol Chem 102:101–112

Gross L, Brotman M (1970) Hypoprothrombinemia and hemorrhage associated with cholestyramine therapy. Ann Intern Med 72:95–96

Gustafson A, Lanner A (1974) Treatment of hyperlipoproteinaemia type II A with a new ion exchange resin Secholex. Eur J Clin Pharmacol 7:65–69

Haddad JG, Birge SJ (1975) Widespread specific binding of 25-hydroxycholecalciferol in rat tissues. J Biol Chem 250:299–303

Hamosh M, Klaeveman HL, Wolf RO, Scow R (1975) Pharyngeal lipase and digestion of dietary triglyceride in man. J Clin Invest 55:908–913

Harkins RW, Hagerman LM, Sarett HP (1965) Absorption of dietary fats by the rat in cholestyramine-induced steatorrhea. J Nutr 87:85–92

Hasegawa J, Tomono Y, Fujita T, Sugiyama K, Hamamura K (1981) The effect of food on the absorption of α-tocopheryl nicotinate in beagle dogs and human volunteers. Int Z Klin Pharmakol Ther Toxicol 19:216–219

Hashim SA, Van Itallie TB (1965) Cholestyramine resin therapy for hypercholesterolaemia. J Am Med Assoc 192:289–293

Hashim SA, Bergen SS, Van Itallie TB (1961) Experimental steatorrhea induced in man by bile acid sequestrant. Proc Soc Exp Biol Med 106:173–175

Heaton KW, Heaton ST, Barry RE (1971) An in vivo comparison of two bile salt binding agents, cholestyramine and lignin. Scand J Gastroenterol 6:281–286

Heaton KW, Lever JV, Barnard D (1972) Osteomalacia associated with cholestyramine therapy for postileectomy diarrhea. Gastroenterology 62:642–646

Hernell O, Olivecrona T (1974) Human milk lipases. II Bile salt-stimulated lipase. Biochim Biophys Acta 369:234–244

Heymann W (1937) Metabolism and mode of action of vitamin D. IV. Importance of bile in the absorption and excretion of vitamin D. J Biol Chem 122:249–256

Hoffman WS, Dyniewicz HA (1945) The effect of alumina gel upon the absorption of vitamin A from the intestinal tract. Gastroenterology 5:512–522

Hollander D (1973) Vitamin K_1 absorption by everted intestinal sacs of the rat. Am J Physiol 225:360–364

Hollander D (1976) Mechanism and site of small intestinal uptake of vitamin D_3 in pharmacological concentrations. Am J Clin Nutr 29:970–975

Hollander D (1980) Retinol lymphatic and portal transport: influence of pH, bile and fatty acids. Am J Physiol 239:G210–G214

Hollander D, Morgan D (1979) Aging: its influence on vitamin A intestinal absorption in vivo by the rat. Exp Gerontol 14:301–305

Hollander D, Muralidhara KS (1977) Vitamin A_1 intestinal absorption in vivo: influence of luminal factors on transport. Am J Physiol 232:E471–E477

Hollander D, Rim E (1976) Vitamin K_2 absorption by rat everted small intestinal sacs. Am J Physiol 231:415–419

Hollander D, Rim E (1978) Effect of luminal constituents on vitamin K_1 absorption into thoracic duct lymph. Am J Physiol 234:E54–E59

Hollander D, Ruble PE (1978) β-carotene intestinal absorption bile acid, pH, and flow rate effects on transport. Am J Physiol 235:E686–E691

Hollander D, Truscott TC (1974a) Mechanism and site of vitamin K_3 small intestinal transport. Am J Physiol 226:1516–1522

Hollander D, Truscott TC (1974b) Colonic absorption of vitamin K_3. J Lab Clin Med 83:648–656

Hollander D, Rosenstreich SJ, Volwiler W (1971) Role of the duodenum in vitamin D_3 absorption in man. Am J Dig Dis 16:145–149

Hollander D, Rim E, Muralidhara KS (1975) Mechanism and site of small intestinal absorption of α-tocopherol in the rat. Gastroenterology 68:1492–1499

Hollander D, Muralidhara KS, Rim E (1976) Colonic absorption of bacterially synthesized vitamin K_2 in the rat. Am J Physiol 230:251–255

Hollander D, Rim E, Muralidhara KS (1977a) Vitamin K_1 intestinal absorption in vivo: influence of luminal contents on transport. Am J Physiol 232:E69–E74

Hollander D, Rim E, Ruble PE (1977b) Vitamin K_2 colonic and ileal in vivo absorption: bile, fatty acids and pH effects on transport. Am J Physiol 233:E124–E129

Hollander D, Muralidhara KS, Zimmerman A (1978a) Vitamin D_3 intestinal absorption in vivo: influence of fatty acids, bile salts and perfusate pH on absorption. Gut 19:267–272

Hollander D, Wang HP, Chu CYT Badawi MA (1978b) Preliminary characterization of a small intestinal binding component for retinol and fatty acids in the rat. Life Sci 23:1011–1018

Hollander D, Rim E, Morgan D (1979) Intestinal absorption of 25-hydroxyvitamin D_3 in unanaesthetised rat. Am J Physiol 236:E441–E445

Holt PR, Dominguez AA (1981) Intestinal absorption of triglyceride and vitamin D_3 in aged and young rats. Dig Dis Sci 26:1109–1115

Howard AN, Courtenay Evans RJ (1974) Secholex®, clofibrate and taurine in hyperlipidaemia. Atherosclerosis 20:105–116

Howard AN, Hyans DE (1971) Combined use of clofibrate and cholestyramine or DEAE-Sephadex in hypercholesterolaemia. Br Med J 3:25–27

Huang HS, Goodman DS (1965) Vitamin A and carotenoids. I. Intestinal absorption and metabolism of ^{14}C-labelled vitamin A alcohol and β-carotene in the rat. J Biol Chem 240:2839–2844

Jacques LB, Millar GJ, Spinks JWT (1954) The metabolism of the K-vitamins. Schweiz Med Wochenschr 84:792–796

Javert CJ, Macri C (1941) Prothrombin concentration and mineral oil. Am J Obstet Gynecol 42:409–414

Johns WH, Bates TR (1970) Quantification of the binding tendencies of cholestyramine. II. Mechanism of interaction with bile salt and fatty acid salt anions. J Pharm Sci 59:329–333

Johnson P, Pover WFR (1962) Intestinal absorption of alpha-tocopherol. Life Sci 1:115–117

Johnston JM (1976) Triglyceride biosynthesis in the intestinal mucosa. In: Rommel K, Goebell H (eds) Lipid absorption: Biochemical and clinical aspects. MTP Press, Lancaster, pp 85–94

Jones CM, Culver PJ, Drummey GD, Ryan AE (1948) Modification of fat absorption in the digestive tract by the use of an emulsifying agent. Ann Intern Med 29:1–10

Juel-Jensen BE (1959) Sensitivity to phenindione. Report of a case of severe diarrhoea. Br Med J 2:173–174

Kasper H, Rabast U, Fassl H, Fehle F (1979) The effect of dietary fiber on the postprandial serum vitamin A concentration in man. Am J Clin Nutr 32:1847–1849

Katayama K, Fujita T (1972) Studies on lymphatic absorption of 1′,2′-(^{3}H)-coenzyme Q_{10} in rats. Chem Pharm Bull (Tokyo) 20:2585–2592

King RFGJ, Howdle PD, Kelleher J, Losowsky MS (1979) Synthetic detergents in bile-salt-deficient steatorrhoea. Clin Sci Mol Med 56:273–281

Klatskin G, Molander DW (1952) The absorption and excretion of tocopherol in Laennec's cirrhosis. J Clin Invest 31:159–170

Ko H, Royer ME (1974) In vitro binding of drugs to colestipol hydrochloride. J Pharm Sci 63:1914–1920

Konishi T, Baba S, Sone H (1973) Whole-body autoradiographic study of vitamin K distribution in rat. Chem Pharm Bull (Tokyo) 21:220–224

Kramer P (1967) The effect of antimotility and antidiarrheal drugs on the ileal excreta of human ileostomized subjects. Gastroenterology 52:1102

Kumar R, Nagubandi S, Mattox VR, Londowski JM (1980a) Enterohepatic physiology of 1,25-dihydroxyvitamin D_3. J Clin Invest 65:277–284

Kumar R, Nagubandi S, Londowski JM (1980b) The enterohepatic physiology of 24,25-dihydroxyvitamin D_3. J Lab Clin Med 96:278–284

Lawrence CW, Crain FD, Lotspeich FJ, Krause RF (1966) Absorption, transport and storage of retinyl-15-^{14}C palmitate-9,10-^{3}H in the rat. J Lipid Res 7:226–229

Lawson DEM, Wilson PW, Kodicek E (1969) Metabolism of vitamin D. A new cholecalciferol metabolite involving loss of hydrogen at C-1 in chick intestinal nuclei. Biochem J 115:269–277

Levine RA (1967) Effect of dietary gluten upon neomycin-induced malabsorption. Gastroenterology 52:685–690

Levine RA (1968) Steatorrhoea induced by para-aminosalicylic acid. Ann Intern Med 68:1265–1270

Levy E, Goldstein R, Freier S, Shafrir E (1981) Characterization of gastric lipolytic activity. Biochim Biophys Acta 664:316–326

Light RF, Alscher RP, Frey CN (1944) Vitamin A toxicity and hypoprothrombinaemia. Science 100:225–226

Lombardo D, Guy O (1980) Studies on the substrate specificity of a carboxyl ester hydrolase from human pancreatic juice. II. Action on cholesterol esters and lipid-soluble vitamin esters. Biochim Biophys Acta 611:147–155

Lombardo D, Deprez P, Guy O (1980) Esterification of cholesterol and lipid-soluble vitamins by human pancreatic carboxyl ester hydrolase. Biochimie 427–432

Longnecker JB, Basu SG (1965) Effect of cholestyramine on absorption of amino acids and vitamin A in man. Fed Proc 24:375

Loran MR, Althausen TL (1969) Transport of vitamin A in vitro across normal isolated rat intestine and intestine subjected to "partial" resection. Am J Physiol 197:1333–1336

Loran MR, Althausen TL, Spicer FW, Goldstein WI (1961) Transport of vitamin A across human intestine in vitro. J Lab Clin Med 58:622–626

Losito R, Owen CAS, Flock EV (1967) Metabolism of (^{14}C) menadione. Biochemistry 6:62–68

MacMahon MT, Neale G (1970) The absorption of α-tocopherol in control subjects and in patients with intestinal malabsorption. Clin Sci 38:197–210

MacMahon MT, Thompson GR (1970) Comparison of the absorption of a polar lipid, oleic acid and a nonpolar lipid, alpha-tocopherol from mixed micellar solutions and emulsions. Eur J Clin Invest 1:161–166

MacMahon MT, Neale G, Thompson GR (1971) Lymphatic and portal venous transport of alpha-tocopherol and cholesterol. Eur J Clin Invest 1:288–294

McDonald GB, Weidman M (1978) Portal versus lymphatic transport of absorbed long-chain fatty acids; the effect of saturation and chain length. Gastroenterology 74:1065

Mahadevan S, Seshadri Sastry P, Ganguly J (1963) Studies on metabolism of vitamin A. 4. Studies on the mode of absorption of vitamin A by rat intestine in vitro. Biochem J 88:534–539

Mahle AE, Patton MH (1947) Carotene and vitamin A metabolism in man: their excretion and plasma level as influenced by orally administered mineral oil and a hydrophilic mucilloid. Gastroenterology 9:44–53

Maislos M, Silver J, Fainaru M (1981) Intestinal absorption of vitamin D sterols: differential absorption into lymph and portal blood in the rat. Gastroenterology 80:1528–1534

Marks JS, Gleeson MH (1975) Steatorrhoea complicating therapy with mefenamic acid. Br Med J 4:442

Martius C (1967) Chemistry and function of vitamin K. In: Seegers WH (ed) Blood clotting enzymology. Academic, New York, pp 551–575

Mathias PM, Harries JT, Peters TJ, Muller DPR (1981) Studies on the in vivo absorption of micellar solutions of tocopherol and tocopheryl acetate in the rat: demonstration and partial characterization of a mucosal esterase localized to the endoplasmic reticulum of the enterocyte. J Lipid Res 22:829–837

Matschiner JT, Doisy EA (1962) Role of vitamin A in induction of vitamin K deficiency in the rat. Proc Soc Exp Biol Med 109:139–142

Matschiner JT, Hsia SL, Doisy EA (1967) Effect of indigestible oils on vitamin K deficiency in the rat. J Nutr 91:299–302

Mattson FH, Nolen GA (1972) Absorbability by rats of compounds containing from one to eight ester groups. J Nutr 102:1171–1176

Mattson FH, Volpenhein RA (1972a) Hydrolysis of fully esterified alcohols containing from one to eight hydroxyl groups by the lipolytic enzymes of rat pancreatic juice. J Lipid Res 13:325–328

Mattson FH, Volpenhein RA (1972b) Rate and extent of absorption of the fatty acids of fully esterified glycerol, erythritol, xylitol and sucrose as measured in thoracic duct cannulated rats. J Nutr 102:1177–1180

Mattson FH, Jandecek RJ, Webb MR (1976) The effect of a non-absorbable lipid, sucrose polyester, on the absorption of dietary cholesterol by the rat. J Nutr 106:747–752

Mattson FH, Hollenbach EJ, Kuehlthau CM (1979 The effect of a non-absorbable fat, sucrose polyester, on the metabolism of vitamin A by the rat. J Nutr 109:1688–1693

Mellors A, Barnes MMcC (1966) The distribution and metabolism of α-tocopherol in the rat. Br J Nutr 20:69–77

Mezick JA, Tompkins RK, Cornwell DG (1968) Absorption and intestinal lymphatic transport of ^{14}C-menadione. Life Sci 7:153–158

Miller NE, Clifton-Bligh P, Nestel PJ, Whyte HM (1973) Controlled clinical trial of a new bile acid sequestering resin, colestipol, in the treatment of hypercholesterolaemia. Med J Aust 1:1223–1227

Morgan JW (1941) The harmful effects of mineral oil (liquid petrolatum) purgatives. J Am Med Assoc 117:1335–1336

Morgan RGH, Barrowman J, Filipek-Wender H, Borgström B (1968) The lipolytic enzymes of rat pancreatic juice. Biochim Biophys Acta 167:355–366

Muller DPR, Harries JT, Lloyd JK (1974) The relative importance of the factors involved in the absorption of vitamin E in children. Gut 15:966–971

Muller DPR, Manning JA, Mathias PM, Harries JT (1976) Studies on the intestinal hydrolysis of tocopheryl esters. Int J Vitam Nutr Res 46:207–210

Muralidhara KS, Hollander D (1977) Intestinal absorption of α-tocopherol in the unanaesthetized rat. The influence of luminal constituents on the absorptive process. J Lab Clin Med 90:85–91

Nakamura T, Aoyama Y, Fujita T, Katsui G (1975) Studies on tocopherol derivatives: V. Intestinal absorption of several DL-3-4-$^3H_2$-α-tocopheryl esters in the rat. Lipids 10:627–633

Nechama H, Hoff D, Harell A, Edelstein S (1977) The intestinal absorption of vitamin D and its metabolites. J Mol Med 2:413–422

Nir I, Bruckental I, Ascarelli I, Bondi A (1967) Effect of dietary protein level on in vivo and in vitro vitamin A esterase activity in the chick. Br J Nutr 21:565–581

Ockner RK, Manning JA (1974) Fatty acid-binding protein in small intestine. Identification, isolation, and evidence for its role in cellular fatty acid transport. J Clin Invest 54:326–338

Olson JA (1961) The conversion of radioactive β-carotene into vitamin A by the rat intestine in vivo. J Biol Chem 236:349–356

Onisko BB, Esvelt RP, Schnoes HK, DeLuca HF (1980) Metabolites of 1α,25-dihydroxyvitamin D_3 in rat bile. Biochemistry 19:4124–4130

Paes IC, Searl P, Rubert MW, Faloon WW (1967) Intestinal lactase deficiency and saccharide malabsorption during oral neomycin administration. Gastroenterology 53:49–58

Parkinson TM (1967) Hypolipidemic effects of orally administered dextran and cellulose anion exchangers in cockerels and dogs. J Lipid Res 8:24–29

Parkinson TM, Schneider JC, Phillips WA (1973) Effects of colestipol hydrochloride (U-26, 597 A) on serum and fecal lipids in dogs. Atherosclerosis 17:167–179

Patton JS, Carey MC (1979) Watching fat digestion. The formation of visible product phases by pancreatic lipase is described. Science 204:145–148

Peake IR, Windmueller HG, Bieri JG (1972) A comparison of the intestinal absorption, lymph and plasma transport, and tissue uptake of α- and γ-tocopherols in the rat. Biochim Biophys Acta 260:679–688

Pearson CK, Barnes MMcC (1970) Absorption of tocopherols by small intestinal loops of the rat in vivo. Int J Vitam Nutr Res 40:19–22

Pearson CK, Legge AM (1972) Uptake of vitamin E by rat small-intestinal slices. Biochem J 129:16P–17P

Pihl O, Iber FL, Linscheer WG (1970) The enhancement of vitamin D_3 absorption in man by medium and long chain fatty acids. Clin Res 18:462

Ponchon G, Kennan AL, DeLuca HF (1969) Activation of vitamin D by the liver. J Clin Invest 48:2032–2037

Popper H, Volk BW (1944) Absorption of vitamin A in the rat. Arch Pathol Lab Med 38:71–75

Powell RC, Nunes WT, Harding RS, Vacca JB (1962) The influence of nonabsorbable antibiotics on serum lipids and the excretion of neutral sterols and bile acids. Am J Clin Nutr 11:156–168

Quick AJ, Stefanini M (1948) Experimentally induced changes in the prothrombin level of the blood. J Biol Chem 175:945–952

Race TF, Paes IC, Faloon WW (1970) Intestinal malabsortion induced by oral colchicine. Comparison with neomycin and cathartic agents. Am J Med Sci 259:32–41

Rautureau M, Rambaud JC (1981) Aqueous solubilisation of vitamin D_3 in normal man. Gut 22:393–397

Rao GA, Sorrels MF, Reiser R (1970) Biosynthesis of triglycerides from triose phosphates by microsomes of intestinal mucosa. Lipids 5:762–764

Ritland S, Fausa O, Gjone E, Blomhoff JP, Skrede S, Lanner A (1975) Effect of treatment with a bile-sequestering agent (Secholex®) on intestinal absorption, duodenal bile acids and plasma lipids. Scand J Gastroenterol 10:791–800

Robinson MJ, Kelley KL, Lehman EG (1964) Effect of cholestyramine, a bile acid binding polymer on vitamin K absorption in dogs. Proc Soc Exp Biol Med 115:112–115

Roe DA (1968) Essential hyperlipemia with xanthomatosis. Arch Dermatol 97:436–445

Saunders DR, Dawson AM (1963) The absorption of oleic acid in the bile fistula rat. Gut 4:254–260

Schachter D, Finkelstein JD, Kowarski S (1963) Pathways of transport and metabolism of C^{14}-vitamin D_2 in the rat. J Clin Invest 42:974–975

Schachter D, Finkelstein JD, Kowarski S (1964) Metabolism of vitamin D. I. Preparation of radioactive vitamin D and its intestinal absorption in the rat. J Clin Invest 43:787–796

Schade RWB, Van't Laar A, Majoor CLH, Jansen AP (1976) A comparative study of the effects of cholestyramine and neomycin in the treatment of type II hyperlipoproteinaemia. Acta Med Scand 199:175–180

Schmandke VH, Proll J (1964) Die α-tocopherol Ausscheidung in Gallen und Pankreassaft. Int Z Vitam Ernährungsforsch [Beih] 34:312–316

Schmandke H, Sima C, Maune R (1969) Die Resorption von alpha-Tokopherol beim Menschen. Int Z Vitamin Ernährungsforsch [Beih] 38:296–298

Schwartz KB, Goldstein PD, Witztum JL, Schonfeld G (1980) Fat-soluble vitamin concentrations in hypercholesterolemic children treated with colestipol. Paediatrics 65:243–250

Sedaghat A, Samuel P, Crouse JR, Ahrens EH (1975) Effects of neomycin on absorption, synthesis and/or flux of cholesterol in man. J Clin Invest 55:12–21

Shearer MJ, Barkhan P, Webster GR (1970) Absorption and excretion of an oral dose of tritiated vitamin K_1 in man. Br J Haematol 18:297–308

Shearer MJ, Mallinson CN, Webster GR, Barkhan P (1972) Clearance from plasma and excretion in urine, faeces and bile of an intravenous dose of a tritiated vitamin K_1 in man. Br J Haematol 22:579–588

Sinclair L (1967) Richets from liquid paraffin. Lancet i:792

Sitrin M, Bolt M, Rosenberg IH (1978) Characterization and quantitative analysis of the biliary excretion products of vitamin D and 25-OH-vitamin D (25-OH-D). Clin Res 26:285A

Sitrin MD, Pollack KL, Rosenberg IH (1981) Intestinal absorption of 1,25-$(OH)_2$ vitamin D_3 (1,25-D_3) in the rat. Gastroenterology 80:1288

Sitrin MD, Pollack KL, Bolt MJG, Rosenberg IH (1982) Comparison of vitamin D and 25-hydroxyvitamin D absorption in the rat. Am J Physiol 242:G326–G332

Smith JE, Milch PO, Muto Y, Goodman DS (1973) The plasma transport and metabolism of retinoic acid in the rat. Biochem J 132:821–827

Takahashi YI, Underwood BA (1974) Effect of long and medium chain length lipids upon aqueous solubility of α-tocopherol. Lipids 9:855–859

Taylor NB, Weld CB, Sykes JF (1935) The relation of bile to the absorption of vitamin D. Br J Exp Pathol 16:302–309

Thompson GR, Lewis B, Booth CC (1966) Absorption of vitamin D_3-^3H in control subjects and patients with intestinal malabsorption. J Clin Invest 45:94–102

Thompson GR, Ockner RK, Isselbacher KJ (1969) Effect of mixed micellar lipid on the absorption of cholesterol and vitamin D_3 into lymph. J Clin Invest 48:87–95

Thompson GR, MacMahon M, Claes P (1970) Precipitation by neomycin compounds of fatty acid and cholesterol from mixed micellar solutions. Eur J Clin Invest 1:40–47

Thompson GR, Barrowman J, Gutierrez L, Dowling RH (1971) Action of neomycin on the intraluminal phase of lipid absorption. J Clin Invest 50:319–323

Thompson SY, Braude R, Coates ME, Cowie AT, Ganguly J, Kon SK (1950) Further studies of the conversion of β-carotene to vitamin A in the intestine. Br J Nutr 4:398–421

Thompson WG, Thompson GR (1969) Effect of cholestyramine on the absorption of vitamin D_3 and calcium. Gut 10:717–722

Udall JA (1965) Human sources and absorption of vitamin K in relation to anticoagulation stability. J Am Med Assoc 194:127–129

Vahouny GV, Treadwell CR (1964) Absolute requirement for free sterol for absorption by rat intestinal mucosa. Proc Soc Exp Biol Med 116:496–498
Vaziri ND, Hollander D, Hung EK, Vo M, Dadufalza L (1983) Impaired intestinal absorption of vitamin D_3 in azotemic rats. Am J Clin Nutr 37:403–406
Vesell ES (1972) Individual variation in drug response. In: Orlandi F, Jezequel AM (eds) Liver and drugs. Academic, New York, pp 1–40
Visintine RE, Michaels GD, Fukayama G, Conklin J, Kinsell LW (1961) Xanthomatous biliary cirrhosis treated with cholestyramine. Lancet 2:341–343
Wagner VH, Wyler F, Rindi G, Bernhard K (1960) Resorption und Umwandlung von ^{14}C-β-Carotin bei der Ratte. Helv Physiol Pharmacol Acta 18:438–445
West RJ, Lloyd JK (1975) The effect of cholestyramine on intestinal absorption. Gut 16:93–98
Whiteside CH, Harkins RW, Fluckiger HB, Sarett HP (1965) Utilization of fat-soluble vitamins by rats and chicks fed cholestyramine a bile acid sequestrant. Am J Clin Nutr 16:309–314
Whyte M, Goodman DS, Karmen A (1965) Fatty acid esterification and chylomicron formation during fat absorption in the rat. 3. Positional relations in triglycerides and lecithin. J Lipid Res 6:233–240
Wiesner RH, Kumar R, Seeman E, Go VLW (1980) Enterohepatic physiology of 1,25-dihydroxyvitamin D_3 metabolites in normal man. J Lab Clin Med 96:1094–1100
Wilson FA, Sallee VL, Dietschy JM (1971) Unstirred water layers in intestine: rate determinant of fatty acid absorption from micellar solutions. Science 174:1031–1033
Wostmann BS, Knight PL (1965) Antagonism between vitamins A and K in the germ free rat. J Nutr 87:155–160
Woytkiw L, Esselbaugh NC (1951) Vitamin A and carotene absorption in the guinea pig. J Nutr 43:451–458
Yeh SD, Shils MF (1966) Effect of tetracycline on intestinal absorption of various nutrients by the rat. Proc Soc Exp Biol Med 123:367–370
Zile MH, Schnoes HK, DeLuca HF (1980) Characterization of retinoyl β-glucuronide as a minor metabolite of retinoic acid in bile. Proc Natl Acad Sci USA 77:3230–3233

Subject Index

Handbook of Experimental Pharmacology

Continuation of "Handbuch der experimentellen Pharmakologie"

Springer-Verlag
Berlin
Heidelberg
New York
Tokyo

Volume 25
Bradykinin, Kallidin and Kallikrein

Volume 26
Vergleichende Pharmakologie von Überträgersubstanzen in tiersystematischer Darstellung

Volume 27
Anticoagulantinen

Volume 28: Part 1
Concepts in Biochemical Pharmacology I

Part 3
Concepts in Biochemical Pharmacology III

Volume 29
Oral wirksame Antidiabetika

Volume 30
Modern Inhalation Anesthetics

Volume 32: Part 2
Insulin II

Volume 34
Secretin, Cholecystokinin Pancreozymin and Gastrin

Volume 35: Part 1
Androgene I

Part 2
Androgens II and Antiandrogens/Androgene II und Antiandrogene

Volume 36
Uranium - Plutonium - Transplutonic Elements

Volume 37
Angiotensin

Volume 38: Part 1
Antineoplastic and Immunosuppressive Agents I

Part 2
Antineoplastic and Immunosuppressive Agents II

Volume 39
Antihypertensive Agents

Volume 40
Organic Nitrates

Volume 41
Hypolipidemic Agents

Volume 42
Neuromuscular Junction

Volume 43
Anabolic-Androgenic Steroids

Volume 44
Heme and Hemoproteins

Volume 45: Part 1
Drug Addiction I

Part 2
Drug Addiction II

Volume 46
Fibrinolytics and Antifibronolytics

Volume 47
Kinetics of Drug Action

Volume 48
Arthropod Venoms

Volume 49
Ergot Alkaloids and Related Compounds

Volume 50: Part 1
Inflammation

Part 2
Anti-Inflammatory Drugs

Volume 51
Uric Acid

Handbook of Experimental Pharmacology

Continuation of "Handbuch der experimentellen Pharmakologie"

Springer-Verlag
Berlin
Heidelberg
New York
Tokyo

Volume 52
Snake Venoms

Volume 53
Pharmacology of Ganglionic Transmission

Volume 54: Part 1
Adrenergic Activators and Inhibitors I

Part 2
Adrenergic Activators and Inhibitors II

Volume 55
Psychotropic Agents

Part 1
Antipsychotics and Antidepressants

Part 2
Anxiolytics, Gerontopsychopharmacological Agents and Psychomotor Stimulants

Part 3
Alcohol and Psychotomimetics, Psychotropic Effects of Central Acting Drugs

Volume 56, Part 1+2
Cardiac Glycosides

Volume 57
Tissue Growth Factors

Volume 58
Cyclic Nucleotides

Part 1: **Biochemistry**

Part 2: **Physiology and Pharmacology**

Volume 59
Mediators and Drugs in Gastrointestinal Motility

Part 1: **Morphological Basis and Neurophysiological Control**

Part 2: **Endogenous and Exogenous Agents**

Volume 60
Pyretics and Antipyretics

Volume 61
Chemotherapy of Viral Infections

Volume 62
Aminoglycoside Antibiotics

Volume 63
Allergic Reactions to Drugs

Volume 64
Inhibition of Folate Metabolism in Chemotherapy

Volume 65
Teratogenesis and Reproductive Toxicology

Volume 66
Part 1: **Glucagon I**
Part 2: **Glucagon II**

Volume 67
Part 1
Antibiotics Containing the Beta-Lactam Structure I

Part 2
Antibiotics Containing the Beta-Lactam Structure II

Volume 68, Part 1+2
Antimalarial Drugs

Volume 69
Pharmacology of the Eye

Volume 71
Interferons and Their Applications

GPSR Compliance

The European Union's (EU) General Product Safety Regulation (GPSR) is a set of rules that requires consumer products to be safe and our obligations to ensure this.

If you have any concerns about our products, you can contact us on ProductSafety@springernature.com

In case Publisher is established outside the EU, the EU authorized representative is:

Springer Nature Customer Service Center GmbH
Europaplatz 3
69115 Heidelberg, Germany

Batch number: 10761697

Printed by Printforce, the Netherlands